THE GLAUCOMAS

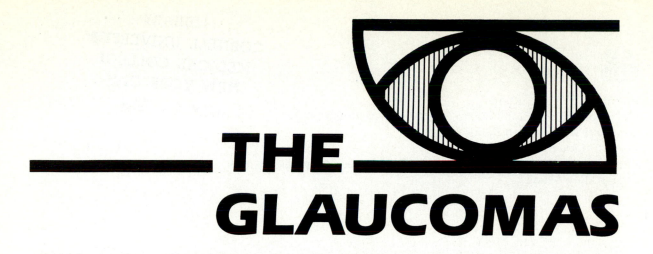

THE GLAUCOMAS

edited by

Robert Ritch, M.D.

Professor of Clinical Ophthalmology, The New York Medical College,
Valhalla, New York; Chief, Glaucoma Service, the New York Eye and Ear
Infirmary, New York, New York

M. Bruce Shields, M.D.

Professor of Ophthalmology; Director, Glaucoma Service, Duke University
Eye Center, Durham, North Carolina

Theodore Krupin, M.D.

Professor of Ophthalmology; Chief, Glaucoma Service, Scheie Eye Institute,
University of Pennsylvania School of Medicine, Philadelphia, Pennsylvania

with 1220 illustrations, including 36 illustrations in 4 color plates

THE C.V. MOSBY COMPANY

St. Louis · Baltimore · Philadelphia · Toronto   1989

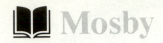 **Mosby**

Editor: Eugenia A. Klein
Developmental Editors: Elaine Steinborn, Kathryn H. Falk
Assistant Editor: Ellen Baker Geisel
Project Manager: Teri Merchant
Production Editors: Mary Stueck, Gail A. Brower, Betty Hazelwood
Design: Rey Umali

The C.V. Mosby Company
11830 Westline Industrial Drive, St. Louis, Missouri 63146

Library of Congress Cataloging-in-Publication Data

The Glaucomas/edited by Robert Ritch, M. Bruce Shields,
  Theodore Krupin.
    p.   cm.
  Includes bibliographies and index.
  ISBN 0-8016-4116-0
  1. Glaucoma. I. Ritch, Robert. II. Shields, M. Bruce.
III. Krupin, Theodore.
  [DNLM: 1. Glaucoma—diagnosis. 2. Glaucoma—
  therapy.   WN 290 5509]
RE871.G577 1989
617.7'41—dc19
DNLM/DLC

GW/MV/MV 9 8 7 6 5 4 3 2 1

CONTRIBUTORS

P. Juhani Airaksinen, M.D.
Professor and Chairman, Department of Ophthalmology, University of Oulu, Oulu, Finland

Stephen P. Bartels, Ph.D.
Assistant Professor of Ophthalmology, Harvard Medical School; Boston, Massachusetts; Associate Scientist, Department of Ophthalmology, Ophthalmic Pharmacology Unit, Eye Research Institute of Retina Foundation

A. Robert Bellows, M.D.
Assistant Clinical Professor of Ophthalmology, Harvard Medical School, Boston, Massachusetts

John E. Bourgeois, M.D.
Assistant Clinical Professor, Duke University Eye Center, Durham; Charlotte Eye, Ear, Nose, and Throat Associates, Charlotte, North Carolina

Michael E. Breton, Ph.D.
Assistant Research Professor of Ophthalmology, Scheie Eye Institute, University of Pennsylvania School of Medicine, Philadelphia, Pennsylvania

Richard F. Brubaker, M.D.
Professor and Chairman, Department of Ophthalmology, Mayo Clinic, Rochester, Minnesota

David G. Campbell, M.D.
Professor of Ophthalmology, Dartmouth Medical School, Hanover, New Hampshire

Louis B. Cantor, M.D.
Assistant Professor of Ophthalmology, Indiana University; Director, Glaucoma Service, Regenstrief Eye Clinic, Indianapolis, Indiana

Joseph Caprioli, M.D.
Associate Professor of Ophthalmology; Director of Glaucoma Service, Yale University School of Medicine, New Haven, Connecticut

Michael Cobo, M.D.
Associate Professor of Ophthalmology, Duke University, Durham, North Carolina

Marshall N. Cyrlin, M.D.
Assistant Clinical Professor of Ophthalmology, Michigan State University, East Lansing, Michigan

Christopher J. Dickens, M.D.
Associate Professor of Ophthalmology, University of California, San Francisco; Glaucoma Research Consultant, The Foundation for Glaucoma Research, San Francisco, California

Stephen M. Drance, M.D.
Professor and Chairman, Department of Ophthalmology, The University of British Columbia, Vancouver, British Columbia

Bruce A. Drum, Ph.D.
Assistant Professor of Ophthalmology, The Johns Hopkins University School of Medicine, Baltimore, Maryland

David L. Epstein, M.D.
Associate Professor of Ophthalmology, Howe Laboratory of Ophthalmology, Harvard Medical School; Massachusetts Eye and Ear Infirmary, Boston, Massachusetts

Marianne E. Feitl, M.D.
Instructor of Ophthalmology, Scheie Eye Institute, University of Pennsylvania School of Medicine, Philadelphia, Pennsylvania

Ronald L. Fellman, M.D.
Assistant Clinical Professor of Ophthalmology, University of Texas Southwestern Medical School, Dallas, Texas

Kathy Felts, B.A.
Research Associate, Department of Ophthalmology, University of Louisville School of Medicine, Louisville, Kentucky

Robert Folberg, M.D.
Director, Eye Pathology Laboratory; Associate Professor, Department of Ophthalmology, University of Iowa Hospitals and Clinics, Iowa City, Iowa

Thomas F. Freddo, M.D.
Fellow, Department of Ophthalmology,
University of Portland, Portland, Oregon

Beth R. Friedland
Clinical Assistant Professor of Ophthalmology,
University of North Carolina, Chapel Hill;
Survey of the Eye, Research Triangle Park, North
Carolina

Bruce J. Goldstick, M.D.
Fellow in Glaucoma, Department of
Ophthalmology, University of California, San
Diego, La Jolla, California

William R. Green, M.D.
Professor of Ophthalmology, Associate Professor
of Pathology, The Johns Hopkins University
School of Medicine, Baltimore, Maryland

Raymond Harrison, M.D.
Director, Glaucoma Service, Manhattan Eye, Ear,
and Throat Hospital, New York, New York

William M. Hart, Jr., M.D., Ph.D.
Associate Professor of Ophthalmology,
Washington University School of Medicine, St.
Louis, Missouri

Sohan Singh Hayreh, M.D., Ph.D.
Professor of Ophthalmology, University of Iowa,
Iowa City, Iowa

M. Rosario Hernandez, D.D.S.
Assistant Scientist, Department of
Ophthalmology, Ophthalmic Pharmacology Unit,
Eye Research Institute of Retina Foundation;
Instructor of Ophthalmology, Harvard Medical
School, Boston, Massachusetts

Jonathan Herschler, M.D.
Director, Glaucoma Service, Oregon Lions Sight
and Hearing Institute, Portland, Oregon

Helen Mintz Hittner, M.D.
Clinical Professor of Ophthalmology and
Pediatrics, Baylor College of Medicine, Houston,
Texas

H. Dunbar Hoskins, Jr., M.D.
Clinical Professor of Ophthalmology, University
of California, San Francisco, California

Shyun Jeng, M.D.
Research Fellow in Glaucoma, Department of
Ophthalmology, University of California, San
Diego, La Jolla, California

Tim Johnson, M.D.
Fellow, Department of Ophthalmology,
Washington University School of Medicine, St.
Louis, Missouri

Murray A. Johnstone, M.D.
Consultant in Glaucoma, Department of
Ophthalmology, University of Washington,
Seattle, Washington

Michael A. Kass, M.D.
Professor of Ophthalmology, Washington
University School of Medicine, St. Louis,
Missouri

L. Jay Katz, M.D.
Assistant Professor of Ophthalmology, Thomas
Jefferson University; Associate Surgeon, Wills
Eye Hospital, Philadelphia, Pennsylvania

Paul L. Kaufman, M.D.
Professor of Ophthalmology; Director, Glaucoma
Services, University of Wisconsin, Madison,
Wisconsin

Deen G. King, M.D.
Assistant Professor of Ophthalmology, University
of South Florida, Tampa, Florida

Joseph H. Krug, Jr., M.D.
Instructor of Ophthalmology, Harvard Medical
School; Ophthalmic Consultants of Boston, The
Glaucoma Consultation Service of the
Massachusetts Eye and Ear Infirmary, Boston,
Massachusetts

Theodore Krupin, M.D.
Professor of Ophthalmology; Chief, Glaucoma
Service, Scheie Eye Institute, University of
Pennsylvania School of Medicine, Philadelphia,
Pennsylvania

Yasuaki Kuwayama, M.D.
Assistant Professor of Ophthalmology, Osaka
University Medical School, Osaka, Japan

William E. Layden, M.D.
Professor and Chairman, Department of
Ophthalmology, University of South Florida,
Tampa, Florida

Julie S. Lee, M.D.
Lecturer, Department of Ophthalmology,
University of Louisville School of Medicine,
Louisville, Kentucky

Jeffrey M. Liebmann, M.D.
Clinical Instructor of Ophthalmology, the
New York Eye and Ear Infirmary, New York,
New York

Ronald F. Lowe, M.D.
Emeritus Ophthalmic Surgeon, The Royal
Victorian Eye and Ear Hospital, Melbourne,
Australia

Maurice H. Luntz, M.D.
Clinical Professor, Department of
Ophthalmology, Mount Sinai School of Medicine,
New York, New York

Elke Lütjen-Drecoll, M.D.
Professor and Chairperson, Department of
Anatomy, University of Erlangen/Nürnberg,
Erlangen, West Germany

John R. Lynn, M.D.
Professor of Ophthalmology, University of Texas
Southwestern Medical School, Dallas, Texas

Martin A. Mainster, M.D., Ph.D.
Professor of Ophthalmology, University of
Kansas Medical Center, Kansas City, Kansas

Robert M. Mandelkorn, M.D.
Clinical Assistant Instructor of Ophthalmology,
University of Pittsburgh, Pittsburgh,
Pennsylvania

Thomas H. Maren, M.D.
Graduate Research Professor of Pharmacology
and Therapeutics, University of Florida College
of Medicine, The J. Hillis Miller Health Center,
Gainesville, Florida

A. Edward Maumenee, M.D.
Emeritus Professor, Department of
Ophthalmology, The Johns Hopkins University
School of Medicine, Baltimore, Maryland

John A. McDermott, M.D.
Attending Physician, Glaucoma Service,
Department of Ophthalmology, the New York
Eye and Ear Infirmary, New York, New York

Thomas W. Mittag, Ph.D.
Professor of Ophthalmology and Pharmacology,
Mount Sinai School of Medicine, New York,
New York

Jose Morales, M.D.
Assistant Professor of Ophthalmology; Director,
Glaucoma Service, Departments of
Ophthalmology and Visual Science, Texas Tech
University Health Sciences Center School of
Medicine, Lubbock, Texas

John C. Morrison, M.D.
Assistant Professor of Ophthalmology, Oregon
Health Services, University of Portland, Portland,
Oregon

George F. Nardin, M.D.
Instructor of Ophthalmology, Kentucky Lions
Eye Research Institute, University of Louisville
School of Medicine, Louisville, Kentucky

Arthur H. Neufeld, Ph.D.
Senior Scientist and Head, Department of
Ophthalmology, Ophthalmic Pharmacology Unit,
Eye Institute of Retina Foundation; Professor of
Ophthalmology, Harvard Medical School,
Boston, Massachusetts

Randall J. Olson, M.D.
Professor and Chairman, Department of
Ophthalmology, University of Utah School of
Medicine, Salt Lake City, Utah

Paul Palmberg, M.D., Ph.D.
Associate Professor of Ophthalmology,
University of Miami School of Medicine;
Associate Professor, Bascom Palmer Eye
Institute, Miami, Florida

Richard Kenneth Parrish II, M.D.
Assistant Professor of Ophthalmology, Bascom
Palmer Eye Institute, University of Miami School
of Medicine, Miami, Florida

Jonathan E. Pederson, M.D.
Frank E. Burd Professor of Ophthalmology,
University of Minnesota, Minneapolis, Minnesota

Morris M. Podolsky, M.D.
Assistant Clinical Professor of Ophthalmology,
Mount Sinai School of Medicine, New York,
New York

Andrew M. Prince, M.D.
Clinical Instructor of Ophthalmology, New York
University Medical Center; Director, Glaucoma
Service, Catholic Medical Center of Brooklyn and
Queens, New York, New York

Ronald L. Radius, M.D.
Professor of Ophthalmology, Medical College of
Wisconsin, Milwaukee, Wisconsin

Alexander Reyes, M.D.
Glaucoma Fellow, the New York Eye and Ear
Infirmary, New York, New York

Thomas M. Richardson, M.D.
Assistant Clinical Professor of Ophthalmology,
Harvard Medical School; Assistant Surgeon,
Howe Laboratory of Ophthalmology,
Massachusetts Eye and Ear Infirmary, Boston,
Massachusetts

Claudia U. Richter, M.D.
Clinical Assistant in Ophthalmology, Harvard
University, Massachusetts Eye and Ear Infirmary,
Boston, Massachusetts

Robert Ritch, M.D.
Professor of Clinical Ophthalmology, The New
York Medical College, Valhalla, New York; Chief,
Glaucoma Service, the New York Eye and Ear
Infirmary, New York, New York

Johannes W. Rohen, M.D.
Professor and Chairman, Anatomisches Institut,
Universitat Erlangen/Nürnberg, Erlangen, West
Germany

Edwin M. Schottenstein, M.D.
Clinical Instructor of Ophthalmology, the New
York University Medical Center; Adjunct
Surgeon, the New York Eye and Ear Infirmary,
New York, New York

Jeffrey Schultz, M.D.
Assistant Professor of Ophthalmology; Director,
Glaucoma Service, Albert Einstein College of
Medicine/Montefiore Medical Center, Bronx,
New York

Carol L. Shields, M.D.
Clinical Fellow, Ocular Oncology Service, Wills
Eye Hospital, Jefferson Medical College, Thomas
Jefferson University, Philadelphia, Pennsylvania

Jerry A. Shields, M.D.
Director of Oncology Service, Department of
Ophthalmology, Wills Eye Hospital; Professor of
Ophthalmology, Thomas Jefferson University,
Philadelphia, Pennsylvania

M. Bruce Shields, M.D.
Professor of Ophthalmology; Director, Glaucoma
Service, Duke University Eye Center, Durham,
North Carolina

Richard J. Simmons, M.D.
Associate Clinical Professor of Ophthalmology,
Harvard Medical School, Boston, Massachusetts

Patricia Smith, M.D.
Assistant Professor of Ophthalmology and
Pathology, University of Virginia, Charlottesville,
Virginia

Ira S. Solomon, M.D.
Attending Ophthalmologist, Glaucoma Service,
the New York Eye and Ear Infirmary, New York,
New York

George L. Spaeth, M.D.
Professor of Ophthalmology, Thomas Jefferson
University; Director, William and Anne Goldberg
Glaucoma Service and Research Laboratories,
and Attending Surgeon, Wills Eye Hospital,
Philadelphia, Pennsylvania

Scott M. Spector, M.D.
Attending Ophthalmologist, Glaucoma Service,
the New York Eye and Ear Infirmary, New York,
New York

Richard J. Starita, M.D.
Assistant Clinical Professor of Ophthalmology,
University of Texas Southwestern Medical
School, Dallas, Texas

Walter J. Stark, M.D.
Professor of Ophthalmology, The Wilmer
Ophthalmological Institute, The Johns Hopkins
University School of Medicine, Baltimore,
Maryland

Richard A. Stone, M.D.
Associate Professor of Ophthalmology,
University of Pennsylvania School of Medicine,
Scheie Eye Institute, Philadelphia, Pennsylvania

John V. Thomas, M.D.
Clinical Assistant in Ophthalmology,
Massachusetts Eye and Ear Infirmary, Boston,
Massachusetts

Brenda J. Tripathi, Ph.D.
Research Associate Professor of Ophthalmology
and Visual Science, The University of Chicago,
Chicago, Illinois

Ramesh C. Tripathi, M.D., Ph.D.
Professor of Ophthalmology, The University of
Chicago, Chicago, Illinois

Anja Tuulonen, M.D.
Assistant Professor of Ophthalmology, University
of Oulu, Oulu, Finland

E. Michael Van Buskirk, M.D.
Professor and Vice Chairman, Department of
Ophthalmology, Oregon Health Sciences,
University of Portland, Portland, Oregon

Martin Wand, M.D.
Assistant Clinical Professor of Ophthalmology,
University of Connecticut Medical School,
Farmington, Connecticut

Peter G. Watson, M.D.
Head, Department of Ophthalmology,
Addenbrookes Hospital, University of
Cambridge, Cambridge, England

Martin Wax, M.D.
Assistant Professor of Ophthalmology and
Pharmacology, University of Pennsylvania School
of Medicine, Philadelphia, Pennsylvania

Robert N. Weinreb, M.D.
Professor and Vice Chairman, Department of
Ophthalmology, University of California, San
Diego, La Jolla, California

Jayne S. Weiss, M.D.
Corneal and External Disease of Ophthalmology,
University of Massachusetts Medical Center,
North Worcester, Massachusetts

Elliot B. Werner, M.D.
Associate Professor of Ophthalmology,
Hahnemann University, Philadelphia,
Pennsylvania

Moustafa K. Yaqub, M.D.
Glaucoma Fellow, New England Glaucoma
Research Foundation, Inc., Boston,
Massachusetts

Alan H. Zalta, M.D.
Assistant Professor of Ophthalmology; Chief,
Glaucoma Service, University of Cincinnati
College of Medicine, Cincinnati, Ohio

Ran C. Zeimer, Ph.D.
Research Associate Professor of Ophthalmology,
University of Illinois, Chicago, Illinois

Thom J. Zimmerman, M.D., Ph.D.
Professor and Chairman, Department of
Ophthalmology, University of Louisville School
of Medicine; Kentucky Lions Eye Research
Institute, Louisville, Kentucky

PREFACE

Glaucoma has come of age. Not long ago, the glaucomas were considered to consist of essentially primary open-angle, angle-closure, and congenital types. Now we recognize the addition of a multitude of secondary glaucomas. Improvements in diagnostic techniques, advances in scientific technology, and the intellectual thrust of biochemistry, cell biology, and molecular genetics have brought us to the beginning of a new era in the elucidation of these groups of mystifying disorders.

In 1951 a textbook devoted exclusively to glaucoma, entitled *The Glaucomas*, was published by H. Saul Sugar. A second edition appeared in 1957. This excellent text comprehensively covered the knowledge and understanding of the diagnosis and management of the glaucomas at that time.

As we now offer a new textbook with the same title, we are mindful of the contributions made by earlier pioneers in the field, whose work formed the foundation of our current achievements. At the same time, a comparison of the size and content of these present volumes to those of the textbooks of the 1950s reminds us of the immense strides that have been made in the intervening generation.

Consider the discipline of glaucoma of the 1950s. The diagnosis was still based largely on indentation tonometry, poorly standardized campimetry and arc perimetry, and evaluation of the optic nerve head with a direct ophthalmoscope. Morton Grant was just beginning to apply modern tonography to questions that would revolutionize our understanding of the mechanisms of the glaucomas as well as the actions of antiglaucoma drugs. Hans Goldmann was just introducing modern applanation tonometry and standardized bowl perimetry. It would be another two decades before the application of computer technology, leading to automated perimetry and image analysis of the optic nerve head.

Concomitant with the advances in understanding of mechanisms of the glaucomas and the development of diagnostic techniques during the past three decades has been the improvement of our ability to treat this broad group of disorders. Medical therapy for glaucoma in the early 1950s was limited to topical miotics and epinephrine. The carbonic anhydrase inhibitors were introduced through the work of Bernard Becker and Thomas Maren. It would be another quarter century before the introduction of the beta-blockers.

Glaucoma filtering surgery of the 1950s had not changed significantly from the time of its introduction at the turn of the century. Advances in microsurgery, guarded filtration techniques, improved setons, and pharmacologic modulation of wound healing were still in the future. The laser had not yet been invented; by the 1980s it would become the most commonly used tool for glaucoma surgery.

In pace with other disciplines, we can expect ever more rapid advances in our understanding and treatment of the glaucomas. Many diseases that have been regarded as single entities, such as diabetes or Marfan's syndrome, are now being recognized as groups of phenotypically similar disorders with multiple etiologies based on genetically determined defects in enzymes or structural proteins or both. We can expect that the same will hold true for what we now consider as primary open-angle glaucoma. We can expect to see further elucidation of the biochemistry of the trabecular meshwork, the role of cell surface molecules in aqueous outflow, and the nature of neural and endocrine control mechanisms regulating aqueous turnover. As more and more subtypes of the glaucomas are differentiated, a clearer understanding of the molecular or genetic defect in each of these can be expected to lead to more specific forms of treatment at a more basic level.

When one considers the rapid advances and the increasing number of specialized areas of scientific research being brought to bear on the field of glaucoma, it is not surprising that a large number of experts were needed to document comprehensively the knowledge that exists today. It is this goal that we hope to have accomplished in *The Glaucomas*.

Such an undertaking would never have been possible without the help of the many contributors to this text. To each of them, and to all who assisted in the preparation of their manuscripts, we offer our most sincere thanks. We also gratefully acknowledge the expert assistance of Ms. Eugenia Klein, Elaine Steinborn, and the excellent staff at The C.V. Mosby Co.

A special thanks to all who have served as our mentors through the years, including our residents and fellows, who continue to challenge us with provocative questions and who force us continually to seek new and better answers. It is our hope that these volumes will be an accurate record of the contributions of the past and present, so that all physicians may profit from this knowledge to further our common goal of preventing blindness from glaucoma.

Robert Ritch
M. Bruce Shields
Theodore Krupin

CONTENTS

Volume 1

PART ONE   Anatomy and Pathophysiology

1   Embryology of the anterior segment of the human eye, 3
Brenda J. Tripathi
Ramesh C. Tripathi

2   Morphology of aqueous outflow pathways in normal and
glaucomatous eyes, 41
Elke Lütjen-Drecoll
Johannes W. Rohen

3   Anatomy, microcirculation, and ultrastructure of the ciliary body, 75
John C. Morrison
E. Michael Van Buskirk
Thomas E. Freddo

4   Anatomy and pathophysiology of the retina and optic nerve, 89
Ronald L. Radius

5   Blood supply of the anterior optic nerve, 133
Sohan Singh Hayreh

6   The extracellular matrix of the trabecular meshwork and the
optic nerve head, 163
M. Rosario Hernandez
Arthur H. Neufeld

7   Functional testing in glaucoma: visual psychophysics and
electrophysiology, 179
Michael E. Breton
Bruce A. Drum

8   Aqueous humor formation: fluid production by a sodium pump, 199
Stephen P. Bartels

9   Pressure-dependent outflow, 219
Paul L. Kaufman

10   Uveoscleral outflow, 241
Jonathan E. Pederson

11 Episcleral venous pressure, 249
Ran C. Zeimer

12 The nervous system and intraocular pressure, 257
Richard A. Stone
Yasuaki Kuwayama

13 Ocular hypotony, 281
Jonathan E. Pederson

PART TWO Determination of Functional Status in Glaucoma

14 Tonography, 293
John A. McDermott

15 Intraocular pressure, 301
Edwin M. Schottenstein

16 Circadian variations in intraocular pressure, 319
Ran C. Zeimer

17 Measurement of aqueous flow by fluorophotometry, 337
Richard E. Brubaker

18 Goniscopy, 345
Paul Palmberg

19 Exploring the normal visual field, 361
John R. Lynn
Ronald L. Fellman
Richard J. Starita

20 Glaucomatous visual field defects, 393
Stephen M. Drance

21 Automated perimetry, 403
Marshall N. Cyrlin

22 Clinical evaluation of the optic disc and retinal nerve fiber layer, 467
P. Juhani Airaksinen
Anja Tuulonen
Elliot B. Werner

23 Quantitative measurements of the optic nerve head, 495
Joseph Caprioli

PART THREE   Pharmacology

24 Ocular cholinergic agents, 515
George F. Nardin
Thom J. Zimmerman
Alan H. Zalta
Kathy Felts

25 Adrenergic and dopaminergic drugs in glaucoma, 523
Thomas W. Mittag

26 Carbonic anhydrase inhibitors, 539
Beth R. Friedland
Thomas H. Maren

27 Hyperosmotic agents, 551
Marianne E. Feitl
Theodore Krupin

28 Alternative and future medical therapy of glaucoma, 557
Martin B. Wax

PART FOUR   Laser Surgery

29 Clinical laser physics, 567
Martin A. Mainster

30 Laser iridectomy and iridoplasty, 581
Robert Ritch
Jeffrey M. Liebmann
Ira S. Solomon

31 Laser treatment in open-angle glaucoma, 605
Bruce J. Goldstick
Robert N. Weinreb

32 Additional uses of laser therapy in glaucoma, 621
Jeffrey Schultz

PART FIVE   Glaucoma Surgery

33 Wound healing in glaucoma surgery, 633
Richard Kenneth Parrish II
Robert Folberg

34 Conventional surgical iridectomy, 645
Jose Morales
Robert Ritch

35 Filtration surgery, 653
L. Jay Katz
George L. Spaeth

36 Surgical management of coexisting cataract and glaucoma, 697
M. Bruce Shields

37 Surgery for congenital glaucoma, 707
Maurice H. Luntz
Raymond Harrison

38 Cyclodestructive surgery, 729
A. Robert Bellows
Joseph H. Krug, Jr.

39 Setons in glaucoma surgery, 741
Theodore Krupin
Scott M. Spector

Volume 2
PART SIX   Classifications and Mechanisms

40 Classifications and mechanisms of the glaucomas, 751
M. Bruce Shields
Robert Ritch
Theodore Krupin

PART SEVEN   The Primary Glaucomas

Section I   Congenital Glaucoma

41 Epidemiology and pathophysiology of congenital glaucoma, 761
Christopher J. Dickens
H. Dunbar Hoskins, Jr.

42 Diagnosis and treatment of congenital glaucoma, 773
Christopher J. Dickens
H. Dunbar Hoskins, Jr.

Section II   Open-angle Glaucoma

43 The epidemiology of primary open-angle glaucoma and ocular hypertension, 789
William M. Hart, Jr.

44 Low-tension glaucoma, 797
Elliott B. Werner

45 Primary open-angle glaucoma: a therapeutic overview, 813
Murray J. Johnstone

Section III Angle-closure Glaucoma

46 Angle-closure glaucoma: mechanisms and epidemiology, 825
Ronald F. Lowe
Robert Ritch

47 Angle-closure glaucoma: clinical types, 839
Ronald F. Lowe
Robert Ritch

48 Therapeutic overview of angle-closure glaucoma, 855
Robert Ritch
Ronald F. Lowe
Alexander Reyes

PART EIGHT The Secondary Glaucomas

Section I Glaucomas Associated with Developmental Disorders

49 Aniridia, 869
Helen Mintz Hittner

50 Axenfeld-Rieger syndrome, 885
M. Bruce Shields

51 Peters' anomaly, 897
Edwin M. Schottenstein

52 Glaucoma in the phakomatoses, 905
Jayne S. Weiss
Robert Ritch

53 Glaucoma associated with congenital disorders, 931
Louis B. Cantor

Section II Glaucomas Associated with Ocular Disease

54 Glaucomas associated with primary disorders of the corneal endothelium, 963
M. Bruce Shields
John E. Bourgeois

55 Pigmentary glaucoma, 981
Thomas M. Richardson

56 Exfoliation syndrome, 997
William E. Layden

57 Lens-induced open-angle glaucoma, 1017
Claudia U. Richter
David L. Epstein

58 Glaucoma secondary to lens intumescence and dislocation, 1027
Robert Ritch

59 Glaucoma associated with retinal disorders, 1047
Andrew M. Prince

60 Neovascular glaucoma, 1063
Martin Wand

61 Glaucomas associated with intraocular trauma, 1111
Jerry A. Shields
Carol L. Shields
M. Bruce Shields

Section III   Glaucomas Associated with Systemic Disease and Drugs

62 Glaucoma secondary to elevated episcleral venous pressure, 1127
Robert N. Weinreb
Shyun Jeng
Bruce J. Goldstick

63 Systemic diseases associated with elevated intraocular pressure and secondary glaucoma, 1141
Richard A. Stone

64 Corticosteroid-induced glaucoma, 1161
Tim Johnson
Michael A. Kass

65 Effects of nonsteroidal drugs on glaucoma, 1169
Robert M. Mandelkorn
Thom J. Zimmerman

Section IV   Glaucomas Associated with Inflammation and Trauma

66 Glaucoma secondary to keratitis, episcleritis, and scleritis, 1187
Peter G. Watson

67 Glaucoma associated with uveitis, 1205
Theodore Krupin
Marianne E. Feitl

68 Trauma and elevated intraocular pressure, 1225
Jonathan Herschler
Michael Cobo

69 Ghost cell glaucoma, 1239
David G. Campbell
M. Bruce Shields
Jeffrey M. Liebmann

Section V   Glaucomas Associated with Ocular Surgery

70 Malignant glaucoma, 1251
Richard J. Simmons
John V. Thomas
Moustafa K. Yaqub

71 Secondary glaucoma in aphakia, 1265
Morris M. Podolsky
Robert Ritch

72 Glaucoma and intraocular lens implantation, 1285
Deen G. King
William E. Layden

73 Epithelial, fibrous, and endothelial proliferation, 1299
Patricia Smith
Walter J. Stark
A. Edward Maumenee
William R. Green

74 Glaucoma associated with penetrating keratoplasty, 1337
Randall J. Olson

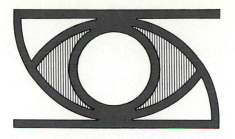

PART ONE

ANATOMY AND PATHOPHYSIOLOGY

1

Embryology of the Anterior Segment of the Human Eye

2

Morphology of Aqueous Outflow Pathways in Normal and Glaucomatous Eyes

3

Anatomy, Microcirculation, and Ultrastructure of the Ciliary Body

4

Anatomy and Pathophysiology of the Retina and Optic Nerve

5

Blood Supply of the Anterior Optic Nerve

6

*The Extracellular Matrix of the Trabecular Matrix
and the Optic Nerve Head*

7

*Functional Testing in Glaucoma: Visual Psychophysics and
Electrophysiology*

8

Aqueous Humor Formation: Fluid Production by a Sodium Pump

9

Pressure-dependent Outflow

10

Uveoscleral Outflow

11

Episcleral Venous Pressure

12

The Nervous System and Intraocular Pressure

13

Ocular Hypotony

Chapter 1

Embryology of the Anterior Segment of the Human Eye

Brenda J. Tripathi
Ramesh C. Tripathi

The anterior segment of the eye contains the approximately ellipsoidal cavity of the anterior chamber, which is bounded anteriorly by the inner surface of the cornea (endothelial lining), peripherally by the inner surface of the trabecular meshwork, and posteriorly by the anterior surface of the iris and the pupillary portion of the anterior surface of the lens. The apex of the anterior chamber angle terminates in the anterior face of the ciliary body, the so-called ciliary band seen gonioscopically; here the root of the iris and the inner surface of the trabecular meshwork approximate. The anterior chamber communicates posteriorly with the posterior chamber through the pupillary aperture, and anteriorly with the intercommunicating spaces of the trabecular meshwork, which constitutes the major outflow pathway for the aqueous humor (Fig. 1-1). Therefore, the structures of the anterior segment of the eye, which include the conjunctiva, cornea, limbus, anterior sclera, episclera, Tenon's capsule, anterior ciliary body, and iris-lens diaphragm, attain special significance in the pathogenesis of both primary and secondary glaucomas.

It is difficult to determine the precise time at which the anterior segment develops in the fetal human embryo, since various structures that constitute this segment appear at different stages of embryogenesis (Table 1-1). Embryologically, the human eye is derived from both ectoderm (surface and neural ectoderm including neural crest) and paraxial mesoderm. As is discussed below, many structures that were originally believed to have

been derived from mesoderm are now considered to be of neural crest origin (see the box on p. 5, *left*). This change in concept is particularly relevant to structures of the anterior segment, and even more so to the development of the outflow pathways of the aqueous humor and hence to the pathogenesis of glaucomatous disorders of the eye.

CHANGING CONCEPT OF THE EMBRYOLOGY OF THE ANTERIOR SEGMENT

The classical germ-layer theory of development of the human body perpetuated the idea that particular types of tissues could be matched with specific embryonic origins. Thus, it was originally believed that there were three layers in the developing embryo: the ectoderm, which gave rise to surface epithelia and to the nervous system; the endoderm, which formed the gut; and the mesoderm, which gave rise to all other structures that were not derived from either the ectoderm or endoderm. In accordance with this notion, early studies on the development of the eye* depicted the epithelium of the cornea, the retina, and the neural components of the uveal tract as being derived from ectoderm, and the remainder of the ocular structures as developing from mesoderm. Although it still may be true that the nonectodermal portions of the eye stem from mesenchymal cells (i.e., a dispersed population of undifferentiated

---

*References 25, 56-58, 82, 91, 107.

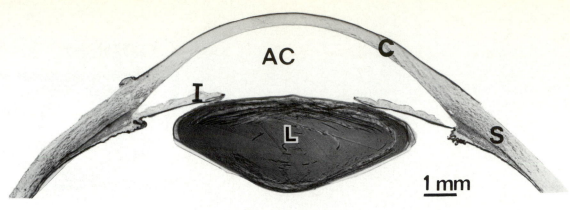

Fig. 1-1 Anterior segment of human eye in meridional section. Pupillary aperture is partly dilated. *C*, Cornea; *AC*, anterior chamber; *I*, iris; *L*, lens; *S*, sclera. (Original magnification ×9.) (From Tripathi, RC, and Tripathi, BJ: Functional anatomy of the anterior chamber of the angle. In Davson, HJ, editor: The eye, vol 1A, New York, 1984, Academic Press)

Table 1-1 Stages in development of anterior segment of the human eye

Age	Crown to rump length (mm)	Structure
EMBRYO (DAYS)		
24-25	3-4	Optic vesicle
		Conjunctival epithelium and stroma commence to develop
26-27	4.0-4.5	Lens placode
33	8-10	Lens vesicle separation
		Proliferation of skin ectoderm to form future upper lid
33-40	11-18	First mesenchymal ingrowth (corneal endothelium)
43	19	Second mesenchymal ingrowth (iris)
47-52	22-24	Third mesenchymal ingrowth (corneal stroma)
		Undifferentiated cells in angular region
		Anterior chamber: slitlike opening
56	31-34	Cornea consists of double layer of epithelial and endothelial cells, 5-8 rows of stromal cells, and few collagen fibrils
		Upper and lower lids visible; limbal conjunctiva is well demarcated
FETUS (WEEKS)		
10	43-48	Scleral stroma develops anteriorly
12-15	63-84	Lid margins fuse together
		Single layer endothelial cells cover central cornea
		Chamber angle defined by anterior iris surface meeting with corneal endothelium
		Angular region shows demarcation into corneoscleral region and ciliary-iris region
		Mesenchymal cells of future trabecular meshwork form a loose reticular network
		Schlemm's canal present as plexus of venous canaliculi
		Collector channels, aqueous veins, veins of deep and intrascleral plexuses
16-18	112-140	Corneal endothelium develops zonulae occludens
		Onset of aqueous humor production
		Differentiation of iris sphincter muscle and ciliary muscles
		Iris root consists of primitive stroma, vascular channels, pigmented and nonpigmented ciliary epithelium
		Development of scleral spur begins
		Mesenchymal cells of trabecular meshwork secrete collagen and elastic tissue
		Juxtacanalicular region differentiates
		Vacuolar configurations present in endothelial lining of Schlemm's canal
21-23	175-195	Angle recess at level with Schlemm's canal
		Trabecular meshwork consists of outer corneoscleral portion and inner uveal portion
		Corneoscleral meshwork organized as trabecular beams, and intertrabecular and intratrabecular spaces formed
28-30	220-260	Longitudinal fibers of ciliary muscle distinct and insert into scleral spur
		Uveal meshwork shows wide intercellular spaces
32-35	240-350	Circular fibers of ciliary muscle distinct
35-39	350-550	Angle recess reaches level of scleral spur

The times and length of the developing fetus are approximate.

CONTRIBUTIONS OF NEURAL CREST–DERIVED MESENCHYME AND OF MESODERMAL MESENCHYME TO OCULAR STRUCTURE IN HUMANS

A. Neural crest cell derivatives
  1. Sclera (except caudal region)
  2. Cornea
    a. Endothelium
    b. Keratocytes
  3. Uveal tract
    a. Fibroblasts of choroid
    b. Ciliary body muscles
    c. Stromal cells of iris
    d. Melanocytes
  4. Iridocorneal angle
    a. Trabecular meshwork endothelium
  5. Vascular system
    a. Pericytes, possibly
B. Mesodermal cell derivatives
  1. Caudal region of sclera
  2. Vascular endothelium, including lining of Schlemm's canal
  3. Extraocular muscles

CONTRIBUTIONS OF NEURAL CREST CELLS TO NONOCULAR TISSUES IN HUMANS

A. Cephalic structures
  1. Cartilages (except epiglottis)
  2. Bones
    a. Craniofacial and cervical skeleton
    b. Ossicles (malleus, incus, stapes) of middle ear
    c. Styloid process
    d. Hyoid bone
  3. Ligaments
    a. Stylohyoid ligament
    b. Anterior ligament of malleus
    c. Sphenomandibular ligament
  4. Leptomeninges (pia and arachnoid mater)
  5. Dental papillae (odontoblasts)
B. Noncephalic structures
  1. Nervous system
    a. Schwann cells
    b. Peripheral sensory and autonomic nerves
    c. Spinal ganglia
    d. Ganglia of cranial nerves V, VII, IX, and X
    e. Paraganglional cells (chromaffin and nonchromaffin)
  2. Skin
    a. Dermis
    b. Melanophores
  3. Neuroendocrine system
    a. Amine precursor uptake and decarboxylation (APUD) system
    b. C cells of thyroid
    c. Principal cells of parathyroid, possibly
    d. Neuroendocrine cells of digestive, urogenital, and bronchopulmonary tracts, possibly

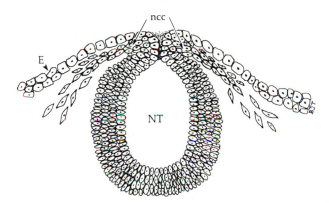

Fig. 1-2 Embryonic derivation of neural crest cells *(ncc).* These cells originate from neuroectoderm located at crest of neural folds at about the time folds fuse to form neural tube *(NT). E,* Surface ectoderm.

embryonic cells that are stellate-shaped and loosely arranged), it is now apparent that these cells differ in their embryonic origins. The importance of this realization lies in the fact that a number of congenital anomalies and other pathologic entities, especially disorders of the anterior segment, can be explained and more thoroughly understood if the classification incorporates consideration of the embryonic lineage of the cells involved.[8,46]

Recent experimental studies, most using the developing chick as the animal model, have shown that a major portion, if not all, of the ocular mes-

enchyme is derived from neural crest cells.* Neural crest cells may be defined as those neuroectodermal cells that proliferate from the crest of the neural folds at about the time the folds fuse to form the neural tube (Fig. 1-2). The neural crest cells that remain attached to the neural tube eventually differentiate into the cerebral and spinal ganglia and the roots of the dorsal nerves. However, many of the neural crest cells migrate away from the neural tube and form secondary mesenchyme, which differentiates into various body structures (see the box above).

The crest cells migrate into an extracellular matrix, devoid of cells, which is secreted by the surface epithelium and by the neural crest cells themselves and is rich in hyaluronic acid.[14,30,73] Because of hydration of the hyaluronic acid molecules, a space is formed into which the crest cells move. The extracellular matrix also contains type I collagen and the cell-associated glycoprotein fibronectin.[51] Fi-

---

*References 41, 50, 53, 54, 66-68.

bronectin is produced by all of the structures (ectoderm, somites, neural tube, and notochord) that surround the migrating crest cells, but the neural crest cells themselves do not synthesize detectable amounts of this glycoprotein.[50,51] In the early embryo, fibronectin is concentrated in the basement membrane of the tissues that serve as the limiting boundaries for crest cell migration.[94] In most embryos, the basal lamina of the neural tube also contains type IV collagen and laminin.[109]

The extracellular matrix through which the crest cells move has a complex chemical composition, and the role of each of the molecules that influence the migration of the cells is not known. Similarly, it has not been established whether the pattern of crest cell migration can be related to the differences in composition or structural organization of the extracellular matrix in the various tissues.[50,51] However, it is known that, once movement is initiated, the crest cells disperse from zones of high cell density to zones of lower density, and that they progress into the available cell-free space.[51]

From experimental studies of radioactively labeled embryonic cells and of chick-quail chimeras, the migratory pathways of the neural crest cells have been determined in the avian embryo.[40,41,50-54,111] However, it has been also realized that the interaction that takes place between the neural crest cells and the mesoderm is crucial to the normal growth of the eye and to the differentiation of all ocular and periocular tissues.[68]

In the developing chick embryo, the initial optic primordium (the optic vesicle) is apposed on its ventral and caudal surfaces by the most rostral extension of the paraxial mesoderm. Scanning electron microscopy has shown that a series of regions of slight condensation, called somitomeres, form in this cranial mesoderm.[64] Between adjacent somitomeres, the mesodermal mesenchymal cells are packed together less densely, and this formation may play an important role in the morphogenesis of the neural crest cells. In the avian embryo, the first neural crest cells develop in the region of the anterior mesencephalon; this is soon followed by similar formations in the regions of the diencephalon, posterior mesencephalon, and metacephalon. Most of the neural crest cells surrounding the optic vesicle have migrated rostrally from the mesencephalic region, but some originate in the region of the diencephalon.[66,68]

In mammals, however, the development of the cephalic neural crest cells differs considerably from that in the avian embryo. Although the neural crest cells appear first in the mesencephalic region, they develop before the apposition of the neural folds and before closure of the neural tube occurs. Presumably, this sequence of events takes place because, in mammals, closure of the neural tube begins at the cranial cervical region and proceeds both cranially and caudally.[68]

Although the later migratory pathways of the neural crest cells are established for the avian embryo, they are not well understood in mammals. In birds, the neural crest–mesoderm interface is known precisely, but in mammals it has not been possible to define the origin of the periocular mesenchymal cells that are located in the region corresponding to the avian interface. At the time when the neural crest cells form, the cranial population of mesodermal cells is larger in mammals than it is in birds, and this suggests that some of the ocular and periocular structures that are of crest origin in the chick would be formed by mesoderm in mammals.[68]

DEVELOPMENTAL ANATOMY

Optic Vesicle and Anterior Segment

The earliest development of the optic vesicle in humans appears as paired outpouchings, one on each side of the developing neural tube in the region that ultimately will form the diencephalon, or forebrain.[25,58,69,70] At the time of closure of the anterior neural tube (day 24; 3 mm embryo), the vesicles protrude from the primordial central nervous system and extend toward the surface ectoderm. By day 25, the vesicles have become pouch-shaped and, except in a small central region, are now surrounded by mesenchymal cells. As the optic vesicles extend farther toward the surface ectoderm, the superior and inferior walls of the neural tube constrict, so that each optic vesicle is connected to the wall of the forebrain by the so-called optic stalk (Fig. 1-3).

Induction of the lens is first seen as a thickening of the surface ectodermal cells (the lens placode) at about 27 days of gestation (4.0 to 4.5 mm). At this stage, the lens placode and its basal lamina are separated from the optic vesicle by a narrow space that contains fine filamentous material.[86] The interaction of the extracellular elements is thought to induce a gradual invagination of the lens placode and leads to formation of the lens vesicle, which initially remains attached to the surface ectoderm by the lens stalk. The formation of the lens vesicle is marked on the surface of the embryo as a depression referred to as a lens pit or pore (Fig. 1-3).

At the same time, the optic vesicle is devel-

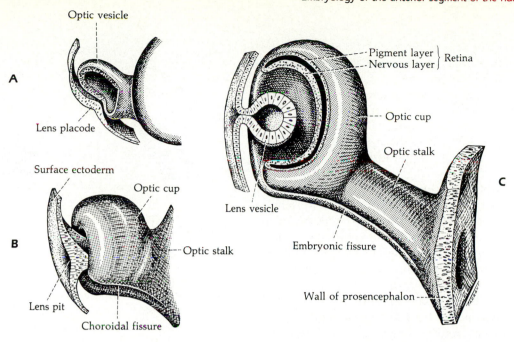

Fig. 1-3 Development of human optic cup. Lens is sectioned and optic cup in **A** and **C** has been partly cut away for clarity. **A,** 4.5 mm embryo. **B,** 5.5 mm embryo. **C,** 7.5 mm embryo. (From Tripathi, RC, and Tripathi, BJ: Functional anatomy of the anterior chamber angle. In Davson, HJ, editor: The eye, vol 1A, New York, 1984, Academic Press)

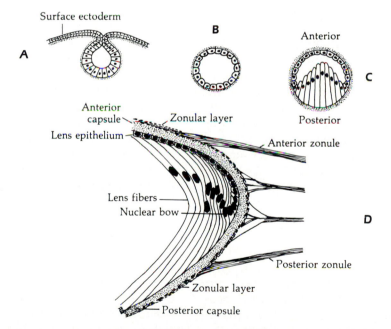

Fig. 1-4 Stages in development of lens and its capsule. **A,** Formation of lens vesicle from invagination of surface ectoderm together with its basal lamina in an embryo corresponding to 7 mm stage. **B,** Separation of lens vesicle from surface ectoderm and its surrounding basal lamina, which thickens with age and begins to form lens capsule at about 8 mm stage. **C,** Obliteration of lens vesicle by elongation of posterior cells of vesicle at about 13 mm stage. **D,** Equatorial region of fully formed lens. With formation of zonules, capsule is augmented by zonular layer. Attachment of zonules to anterior, posterior, and equatorial regions of lens becomes apparent at about 16 mm embryo stage. Note change in polarity of cells from anterior to posterior regions of lens. (From Tripathi, RC, and Tripathi, BJ: Anatomy of the human eye, orbit, and adnexa. In Davson, H, editor: The eye, vol 1A, New York, 1984, Academic Press)

oping into the optic cup. By 28 days (7.6 to 7.8 mm embryo), differential growth and movement of the cells of the optic vesicle cause the temporal and lower walls of the vesicle to move inward against the upper and posterior walls. The two laterally growing edges of the cup eventually meet and fuse. This process also involves the optic stalk and results in the formation of the embryonic or optic fissure (Fig. 1-3).

Further differentiation of the lens depends on the influence exerted by the optic cup. The lens vesicle separates from the surface ectoderm because of displacement as the vesicle sinks into the orifice of the optic cup. A zone of extreme attenuation and necrosis develops where the lens is joined to the surface ectoderm, and, by about 33 days gestation (8 to 10 mm), the separation is complete. Initially, the lens vesicle consists of a single layer of cells covered by a tenuous basal lamina (Fig. 1-4). As the vesicle closes, the posterior cells reduce their rate of DNA synthesis, but elongate markedly.[123] This process eventually obliterates the cavity of the lens vesicle by 45 days (20 mm). It is the optic (neural) cup that induces the transformation of lens cells into primary lens fibers.[70]

Cornea

The cornea begins to develop as soon as the lens vesicle separates from the surface ectoderm, at 33 days gestation. At this stage, the ectoderm consists of two layers of epithelial cells that rest on a thin basal lamina. Neural crest–derived mesenchymal cells grow from the margins of the rim of the optic cup into the developing eye, beneath the basal lamina of the epithelium. These cells participate in the first of three successive waves of ingrowth and are destined to form the corneal endothelium (Fig. 1-5). In the 17 to 18 mm embryo (about 40 days), the cornea consists of a superficial squamous cell layer and a basal cuboidal epithelial cell layer and of a double row of flattened cells posteriorly. At about the 19 mm stage, another wave of mesenchymal cells migrates from the rim of the optic cup in two directions. The lower (posterior) axial extension grows into the space between the lens epithelium and the corneal endothelium. These cells are destined to form the primary pupillary membrane, at 21 to 26 mm. The slitlike space left between these ingrowing cells and the developing corneal endothelium will result in the formation of the anterior chamber. At the 22 to 24 mm stage (approximately 7 weeks), the anterior (upper) extension of mesenchymal cells migrates between the epithelium and endothelium and will contrib-

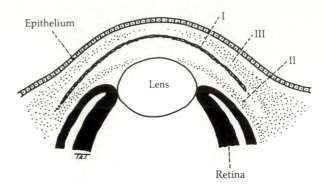

Fig. 1-5 Three successive waves of ingrowth of neural crest cells associated with differentiation of anterior chamber. *I*, First wave forms corneal endothelium; *II*, second wave forms iris and pupillary membrane, and, *III*, third wave forms keratocytes. (Modified from Tripathi, RC, and Tripathi, BJ: Functional anatomy of the anterior chamber of the angle. In Davson, HJ, editor: The eye, vol 1A, New York, 1984, Academic Press)

ute to the development of the corneal stroma. Initially, the central region of the stroma is acellular.

The ontogeny of the cornea has been studied in detail in the avian eye by Hay et al.[33,34] Once the lens is formed, the surface ectoderm is induced to form the primary stroma. The basal layer of epithelial cells secretes collagen fibrils and glycosaminoglycans that fill the space between the lens and the corneal epithelium.[24,33] At this stage, only macrophages, which engulf debris that remains after detachment of the lens vesicle, are present in the stroma. The primordial corneal endothelial cells that originate from the mesenchyme surrounding the optic vesicle use both the posterior surface of the primitive stroma and the fibronectin-containing basal lamina of the anterior lens cells as substrate for their migration.[10] At the time when the second wave of mesenchymal cells is about to invade the primitive cornea, the extracellular matrix of the stroma swells, apparently as a result of the hydration of hyaluronic acid, which seems to make space available for cell migration.[93] The superficial region of the stroma remains acellular, however, and forms Bowman's zone. It is remarkable that this zone maintains a unique feltlike arrangement of collagen fibrils that, if destroyed, are not regenerated. What contribution, if any, is made by the primitive epithelium to the development of Bowman's zone is unknown. It is also not known why the thickness of this region varies considerably among different species.[99] The stromal fibroblasts or keratocytes actively secrete the type I collagen fibrils and the matrix that will constitute the mature corneal stroma.[95]

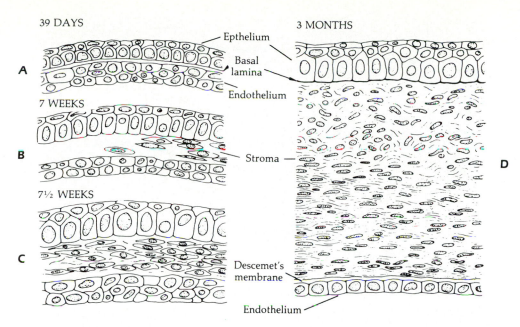

Fig. 1-6 Development of cornea in central region. **A,** At 39 days, two-layered epithelium rests on basal lamina and is separated from endothelium (two to three layers) by narrow acellular space. **B,** At 7 weeks, mesenchymal cells from periphery migrate into space between epithelium and endothelium. **C,** Mesenchymal cells (future keratocytes) are arranged in four to five incomplete layers by 7½ weeks, and a few collagen fibrils are present among cells. **D,** By 3 months, epithelium has two to three layers of cells, and stroma has about 25 to 30 layers of keratocytes that are more regularly arranged in posterior half. There is a thin, uneven Descemet's membrane between the most posterior keratocytes and now the monolayer of endothelium. (From Ozanics, V, and Jakobiec, FA: Prenatal development of the eye and its adnexa. In Biomedical foundations of ophthalmology, vol 1, Duane, TD, and Jaeger, EA, editors: Philadelphia, 1982, Harper & Row)

Initially, the secondary stroma is rich in fibronectin; but, as the corneal mesenchyme begins to condense, the fibronectin disappears.[51] At this time, the stroma attains its maximum width (approximately double the normal postembryonic width), but this soon decreases because of dehydration and compression of the connective tissue.[33] However, as pointed out by Hay,[34] there are certain fundamental differences between the development of the cornea in birds and that in mammals. The primary corneal stroma is not as well organized in mammals as it is in birds, and, in the former, it is composed of fine filaments, amorphous material, and only a few collagen fibrils. In the primate eye, furthermore, the primary (ectoderm) phase is deemphasized, the secondary (fibroblast) phase begins sooner than it does in birds, and the secondary stroma is not laid down on a well-organized primary stroma.

In the human embryo at 8 weeks (30 mm), the stroma consists centrally of five to eight rows of cells.[70] The most posterior layers of the stroma are confluent at the periphery with the condensed mesenchymal tissue of the future sclera, which is gradually spreading backward to enclose the eye. Soon afterward (35 mm), the cornea consists of two layers of epithelial cells (the middle wing cells do not develop until about the fourth or fifth month), a stroma with 15 layers of cells, and an endothelium that is still arranged as a double layer of cells (Fig. 1-6). By the third month, the endothelium in the central region has become a single layer of flattened cells that rest on an interrupted basal lamina, the beginnings of Descemet's membrane.[120,121] The cell apices of the endothelium are joined by zonulae occludentes by the middle of the fourth month of development, which corresponds to the onset of aqueous humor production.[122] By the sixth month of gestation, Descemet's membrane is clearly demarcated and the stroma consists of a primitive extracellular matrix and numerous active keratocytes (Fig. 1-7). The epithelium, however, is still only two to three cell layers thick.

At the 22 to 24 mm stage, the anterior chamber angle is undifferentiated and is occupied by loosely arranged mesenchymal cells, and the anterior chamber itself is a slitlike opening. The angle does not begin to differentiate until the canal of

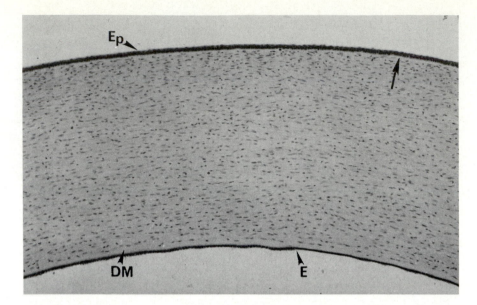

Fig. 1-7 Light micrograph of central cornea in a 6-month fetus. Epithelium *(Ep)* consists of two to three cell layers. Stroma contains numerous keratocytes, and there is an indistinct Bowman's zone *(arrow)*. Descemet's membrane *(DM)* is clearly demarcated. *E, Endothelium.* (Original magnification ×120.)

Schlemm appears, at about the fourth month. Approximately at this time, the iris proper begins to develop from the anterior rim of the optic cup (neuroepithelial layers), from mesoderm (vascular supply), and from neural crest–derived mesenchymal cells (anterior fibrocytic and melanocytic layers).

Angle of the Anterior Chamber, Ciliary Body, and Iris

Several hypotheses have been advanced in the attempt to explain the formation of the angle of the anterior chamber. Originally, it was thought that both the anterior chamber and the angle develop as a result of atrophy of the mesenchymal cells and that the tissue that remains adjacent to Schlemm's canal differentiates into the trabecular meshwork.* Another hypothesis suggested that the angle develops by a process of cleavage of the mesenchymal cells similar to that suggested for the formation of the anterior chamber. The cleavage was thought to result from an unequal rate of growth of the tissues of the anterior segment because the cornea grows more rapidly than do other structures.[3,17,60] The latter theory has been opposed, however, on the grounds that artifacts readily occur in the delicate embryologic tissues when these are prepared for histologic examination.[44,116,117] Other investigators

have been unable to confirm the theory of atrophy and reabsorption. A third hypothesis, which is based on electron microscopic studies, suggests that the angle of the anterior chamber is formed by a process of rarefaction and reorganization of the mesenchymal cells.[87] Although the precise mechanism of development of the angle is not established, it is apparent that the angle recess shows a progressive deepening that commences at about the third month of gestation (Fig. 1-8) and probably continues for a considerable time after birth (up to the age of 4 years).[102]

Several changes accompany the early remodeling of the anterior chamber angle. At 3 months in utero, the corneal endothelium extends to the angle recess. The posterior aspect of the angle is formed by loose mesenchymal tissue, by mesodermal cells that are developing into the vascular channels of the pupillary membrane, and by the pigment epithelium of the forward-growing optic cup. By the fifteenth fetal week, the chamber angle is well defined because the surface of the anterior iris and the primitive corneal endothelium meet (Fig. 1-9). Just anterior to this junction, there is a nest of mesenchymal cells that are destined to develop into the trabecular meshwork (described below). At this stage, the corneal endothelium that lines the chamber angle may be composed of several cell layers, but the cells flatten toward the iris root.[74] The anlage of the iris stroma is continuous

---

*References 5, 7, 9, 11, 56-58.

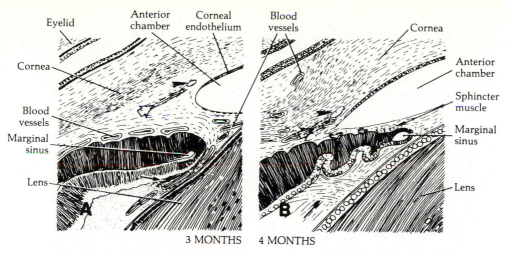

Eyelid — Anterior chamber — Corneal endothelium — Blood vessels — Cornea

Cornea — Anterior chamber — Sphincter muscle — Marginal sinus — Lens

Blood vessels — Marginal sinus — Lens

A **B**

3 MONTHS   4 MONTHS

Fig. 1-8 Progressive deepening of anterior chamber angle and its relation to neighboring tissues. **A,** At 3 months, corneal endothelium extends nearly to angle recess. There is an incipient Schlemm's canal *(arrowhead)* and a more posterior scleral spur condensation *(hollow arrow)* to its left. Pigment epithelium of forward-growing ectodermal optic cup is indented by blood vessels. **B,** At 4 months, angle recess has deepened and corneal endothelium has receded somewhat. There is a small aggregate of differentiating sphincter muscle fibers near tip of optic cup. Arrowhead points to Schlemm's canal. Condensed tissue just posterior to Schlemm's canal is developing scleral spur *(hollow arrow).* Angle recess is occupied by loose connective tissue separated by many spaces. Iris has grown, and only its ciliary portion is shown. Dilator muscle of iris has reached its root, which is still thick. (From Ozanics, V, and Jakobiec, FA: Prenatal development of the eye and its adnexa. In Biomedical foundations of ophthalmology, vol 1, Duane, TD, and Jaeger, EA, editors: Philadelphia, 1982, Harper & Row)

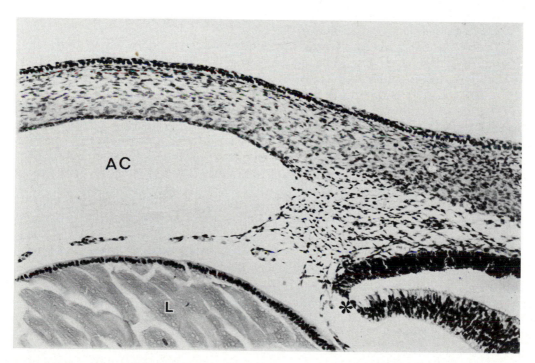

Fig. 1-9 Light micrograph of an eye of an 11-week fetus in meridional section. At this stage, angular region is ill defined and occupied by loosely arranged, spindle-shaped cells. Canal of Schlemm is unrecognizable, and ciliary muscles and ciliary processes are not yet formed; latter are derived from neural ectodermal fold *(asterisk).* Corneal endothelium appears continuous with cellular covering of primitive iris. *AC,* Anterior chamber; *L,* lens. (Original magnification ×230.) (From Tripathi, RC, and Tripathi, BJ: Functional anatomy of the anterior chamber angle. Duane, TD, and Jaeger, EA, editors: Biomedical foundations of ophthalmology, vol 1, Philadelphia, 1987, Harper & Row)

with the pupillary membrane and with the tunica vasculosa lentis, which ensheathes the developing lens. By the fourth month, the differentiating sphincter muscle fibers are seen aggregating at the tip of the optic cup. The cells in the apex of the angle are now beginning to differentiate into the fibers of the ciliary muscle. At this stage, the corneal endothelial cells still reach the apex of the anterior chamber angle and are contiguous with the cells on the surface of the iris stroma. At the end of the fourth month and the beginning of the fifth month, the iris root develops and consists of a primitive stroma, vascular channels, and the pigmented and nonpigmented ciliary epithelium. By the fifth month, the anterior chamber angle has become rounded and is lined by an unbroken but attenuated layer of corneal endothelial cells.[87] Even up to the sixth month, these flattened cells line the angle recess and join the cells of the developing anterior face of the iris root.[74]

As development proceeds, the peripheral margin or recess of the anterior chamber angle appears to move posteriorly. The so-called movement of tissues relative to one another is now being explained as resulting from a differential growth rate of the various tissue elements.[4] This process results in repositioning of the tissues so that the ciliary body (muscle and processes), which initially overlapped the developing trabecular meshwork, comes to lie posteriorly to the meshwork. Several authors believe that the exposure of the trabecular meshwork to the anterior chamber depends on the retraction of the corneal endothelium,[31,74,87,106] which lines the angle recess until about 7 months. Studies of the developing iridocorneal angle in human and monkey eyes by scanning electron microscopy have revealed the presence of a continuous layer of polyhedral cells (identified as corneal endothelium) up to a late stage in the final trimester of gestation. At this time, this cell layer develops fenestrations that expose the underlying well-developed trabecular meshwork.[31,106] Monkey eyes often have an operculum, which is a peripheral extension of the corneal endothelium and Descemet's membrane, and this structure partly covers the inner aspect of the anterior trabecular meshwork even in the adult eye.[99] Other investigators support the hypothesis that the trabecular meshwork does not have a distinct endothelial covering,[4,119] but that the exposed surface consists of multilayered mesenchymal cells that have not yet formed trabecular beams and intertrabecular spaces. This controversy has important clinical implications, especially with regard to the possible

mechanisms for the pathogenesis of congenital glaucoma.

Gradually, as the angle recess deepens and as the trabecular beams differentiate, the open spaces of the meshwork come into direct communication with the anterior chamber. This development can be correlated with the increase in the facility of aqueous outflow (0.09 μl/min/mm Hg before 7 months to 0.3 μl/min/mm Hg at 8 months).[49,72] By 7 months, the deepest part of the angle has receded to the level of Schlemm's canal, but at the time of birth, the apex of the angle is located beyond the canal and is at the level of the scleral spur.[44] The angle at birth differs from that in adulthood by having more uveal meshwork anterior to the ciliary muscle and in front of the scleral spur. Also, in the adult, the angle is open to the anterior face of the ciliary body.

Limbus

For descriptive purposes, the limbus can be divided into (1) the inner limbus (Schlemm's canal, trabecular meshwork, scleral spur, and Schwalbe's line), (2) the mid limbus (intrascleral collector channels and vascular plexus), and (3) the outer limbus (episcleral and conjunctival plexus) (Fig. 1-10).

Inner limbus

Schlemm's canal.   By the end of the third month of gestation, the future Schlemm's canal is present as a small plexus of venous canaliculi.* At first, these channels function as blood vessels, and, in fact, they are derived from mesodermal mesenchyme (Fig. 1-11). During the fourth month, other mesenchymal cells surround the canal of Schlemm and are enmeshed in a basal lamina–like material and in foci of collagen fibrils. This arrangement is destined to form the juxtacanalicular region, which remains, toward the anterior chamber, as a zone of loosely organized connective tissue.[102] The endothelial cells lining the canal of Schlemm are joined by tight junctions. Characteristic vacuolar configurations are apparent at about the beginning of the fifth month (Fig. 1-12), which is about the time of differentiation of the ciliary processes and of the onset of the circulation of aqueous humor.[99,118] Similar vacuoles have been recognized at about day 84 of gestation in the monkey *Macaca mulatta*, which has a gestation period of 160 to 162 days.[87] With the formation of macrovacuoles and the onset of aqueous circulation, the canal of Schlemm now functions as an aqueous sinus rather

---

*References 6, 9, 58, 82, 88, 118.

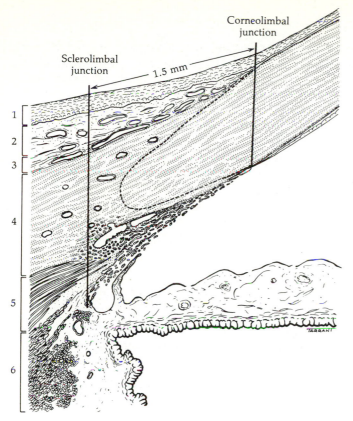

Sclerolimbal
junction

Corneolimbal
junction

1.5 mm

1
2
3
4
5
6

Fig. 1-10   Limbus, showing various structures from superficial to deep regions. *1,* Conjunctiva; *2,* conjunctival stroma; *3,* Tenon's capsule and episclera; *4,* limbal or corneoscleral stroma containing intrascleral plexus of veins and collector channels from Schlemm's canal; *5,* meridional portion of ciliary muscle; *6,* radial and circular portions of ciliary muscle. Pathologist's limbus is about a 1.5 mm wide zone extending posteriorly from line joining peripheral termination of Bowman's zone of cornea and of Descemet's membrane. Histologist's limbus *(dotted line)* is represented by a cone-shaped termination of corneal lamellae into sclera. (From Tripathi, RC, and Tripathi, BJ: Anatomy of the human eye, orbit, and adnexa. In Davson, H, editor: The eye, vol 1A, New York, 1987, Academic Press)

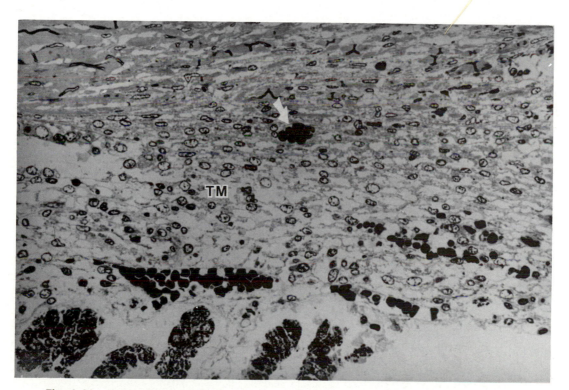

Fig. 1-11   Angular region of 18-week fetus in meridional section. Canal of Schlemm is present and filled with blood *(arrow).* Because of early appearance of fibrous component of trabeculae, trabecular meshwork region *(TM)* is more organized than 11-week fetus shown in Fig. 1-8. Trabecular spaces are apparent, although scleral spur and meridional fibers of ciliary muscle are barely recognizable. Ciliary processes *(below)* are partly differentiated. (Original magnification ×640.) (From Tripathi, RC, and Tripathi, BJ: Functional anatomy of the anterior chamber angle. In Duane, TD, and Jaeger, EA, editors: Biomedical foundations of ophthalmology, vol 1, Philadelphia, 1987, Harper & Row)

than a vascular channel.[102,118] During the subsequent months the endothelial cells lining the canal flatten and become thinner, and more vacuoles are formed. The vacuolar configurations (Fig. 1-13) are considered to be stages in a cyclic sequence of events that leads to the formation of transcellular channels, which allow the outflow of aqueous humor across the endothelial barrier of Schlemm's canal.[99,102] This unique biologic system has also been shown by us to be operative for the bulk outflow of the cerebrospinal fluid via arachnoid villi into the dural sinuses.[100,103]

At 6 months of gestation, Schlemm's canal and the scleral spur are still located posterior to the deepest part of the angle (Fig. 1-14). Although the positions of these two structures remain unchanged relative to each other, at approximately 7 months the apex of the angle has receded to the level of Schlemm's canal.[44] With the growth of the surrounding structures, Schlemm's canal ultimately comes to lie at the apex of the angle of the anterior chamber and is limited posteriorly by the scleral roll.[102]

Based on their structural studies of developing monkey and human eyes, Smelser and Ozanics[87] put forward the hypothesis that Schlemm's canal,

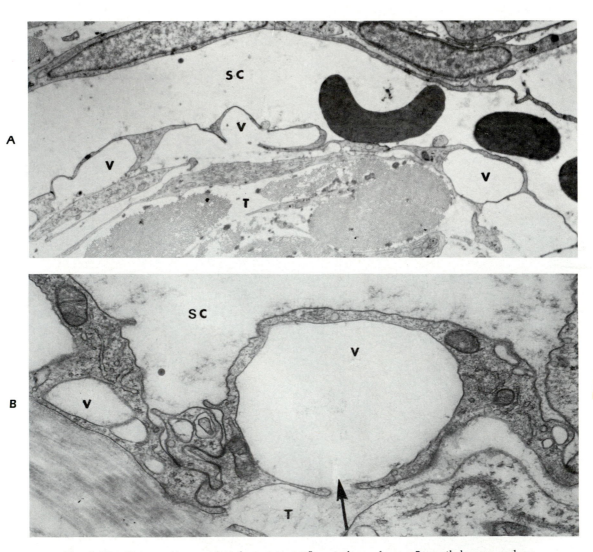

Fig. 1-12 Electron micrographs of aqueous outflow pathway from a 5-month human embryo. Unique giant vacuolar configurations *(V)* are present in endothelial cells that line inner wall of Schlemm's canal *(SC)*. Arrow in **B** denotes opening of vacuole on its basal aspect. *T,* part of the meshwork adjacent to Schlemm's canal. (**A,** Original magnification ×6000; **B,** original magnification ×18,200.) (From Wulle, K.G.: Adv Ophthalmol 26:269, 1972. Reproduced with permission from Tripathi, RC: Comparative aspects of the aqueous outflow pathway. In Davson, H, and Graham, LT, editors: The eye, vol 5A. New York, 1974, Academic Press)

which eventually becomes a ring-shaped structure around the entire circumference of the limbus, could have several points of origin. In some sections that passed through the angular region, no trace of the primitive Schlemm's canal is discernible at early stages of development. They suggest that the blind ends of the future collector channels grow through the scleral tissue and anastomose with one another to form the circumferential canal between the scleral tissue and the trabecular meshwork. Our own studies have shown that during the evolution of the vertebrate eye, the "angular aqueous plexus,"[99] which is analogous to Schlemm's canal in the primate eye, is not a circumferential structure. The plexus is present in a localized ventral segment in many fishes, and in the dorsal and ventral segments of the angle in amphibians; it is a circumferential plexus of chan-

nels only in reptiles and birds, and more so in higher primates.[99] Thus, it is possible that, during the ontogeny of Schlemm's canal, there is some repetition of its phylogeny.

Trabecular meshwork. The primitive trabecular meshwork is present initially as an approximately triangular or wedge-shaped structure formed by undifferentiated mesenchymal cells (see Fig. 1-9). Anteriorly, the apex of this structure lies between the endothelium and the deeper stroma of the cornea. Posteriorly, there is no clear distinction between the mesenchymal tissue that will differentiate into the ciliary muscle and that which will become the trabecular meshwork proper.[44] As discussed above, the corneal endothelium originally covers most, if not all, of the anterior face of the trabecular meshwork, thus delineating its border from the anterior chamber.

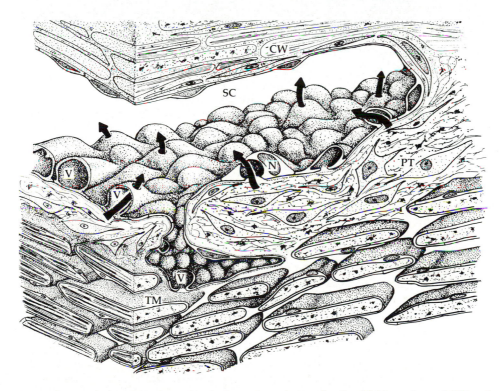

Fig. 1-13 Composite three-dimensional schematic rendering of walls of Schlemm's canal *(SC)* and adjacent trabecular meshwork *(TM)* in fully developed eye. Spindle-shaped cells lining trabecular wall of Schlemm's canal are characterized by luminal bulges corresponding to unique macrovacuolar configurations *(V)* accommodated by cells and nuclei *(N)*. Macrovacuolar configurations are formed by surface invaginations on basal aspect of individual cells and gradually enlarge to open eventually on apical aspect of cell surface, thus forming transcellular channels *(arrows)* for bulk flow of aqueous humor down a pressure gradient. Endothelial lining of trabecular wall is supported by variable zone of cell-rich pericanalicular tissue *(PT)* that borders organized superimposed trabecular sheets with intertrabecular and intratrabecular spaces that allow bulk flow of aqueous humor from anterior chamber to the canal of Schlemm. Compact corneoscleral wall *(CW)* of Schlemm's canal is formed by lamellar arrangement of collagen and elastic tissue. (From Tripathi, RC, and Tripathi, BJ: Anatomy of the human eye, orbit, and adnexa. In Davson, H, editor: The eye, vol 1A, New York, 1984, Academic Press)

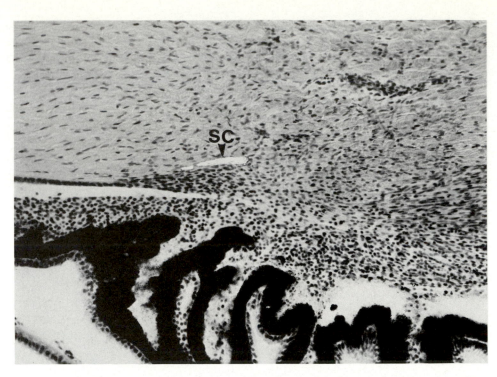

Fig. 1-14 Angular region of 6-month fetus. At this stage, trabecular meshwork is easily recognizable. Canal of Schlemm *(SC)* is functioning as an aqueous sinus. Meridional ciliary muscle fibers and scleral spur are defined, and radial and circular fibers are also recognizable. Ciliary processes are well formed. (Original magnification ×260.) (From Tripathi, RC, and Tripathi, BJ: Functional anatomy of the anterior chamber of the angle. In Duane, TD, and Jaeger, EA, editors: Biomedical foundations of ophthalmology, vol 1, Philadelphia, 1987, Harper & Row)

By the fifteenth week of gestation, a demarcation is thought to be discernible between the corneoscleral region and the ciliary-iris region based on the shape of the nuclei of the cells in these two regions, the former being spindle-shaped and the latter more round.[74] There is pronounced mitotic activity in both regions. The mesenchymal cells destined to form the trabecular meshwork are loosely attached without junctional specializations and form a reticular network (Fig. 1-15). Electron microscopy reveals that their cytoplasm contains distinct lysosomes, conspicuous ribosomes, and dilated cisternae of endoplasmic reticulum.[74] Small patches of collagen fibrils are recognizable between the mesenchymal cells; abundant unmyelinated nerve fibers can also be seen. Several small capillaries are present along the interface between the corneoscleral and ciliary-iris tissues.

Between the fourth and eighth months, the mesenchymal cells of the trabecular meshwork elongate and continue to secrete collagen fibrils and elastic elements. The next major change occurs between the twenty-second and the twenty-fourth week. It corresponds to the further development

of the scleral spur, which first appeared during the fourth month (see below). At this time, the ciliary muscle is discernible. Also, the primitive trabecular meshwork can now be divided into the corneoscleral portion, which is oriented longitudinally, and the inner uveal portion, which has a netlike arrangement. The trabecular beams of the deep corneoscleral meshwork are already organized as a core of collagen fibrils and elastic tissue, surrounded by endothelial cells with their tenuous basement membrane, the future cortical zone. The endothelial cells are interconnected through their numerous cytoplasmic processes (see Fig. 1-15). As the mesenchymal cells align themselves along the framework of the extracellular matrix, the intercellular spaces enlarge and interconnect to form intertrabecular and intratrabecular spaces. In contrast, the uveal meshwork, especially the posterior layer, still consists of randomly oriented mesenchymal cells with patches of collagen fibrils scattered in the extracellular compartment. The uveal portion of the meshwork is organized more loosely than is the deeper scleral meshwork. The shape and orientation of the individual trabecular beams

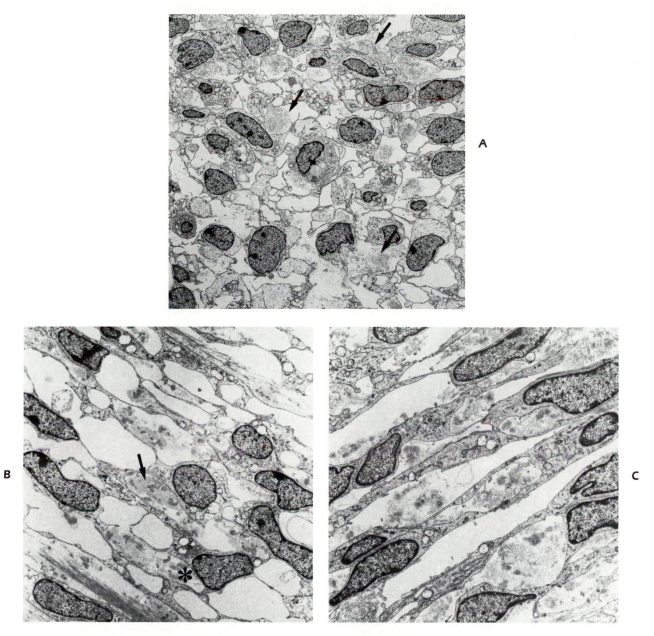

Fig. 1-15 **A,** Electron micrograph showing developmental stage of cellular elements of trabecular meshwork at fifteenth fetal week. Mesenchymal cells form angular tissue, and patches of collagen fibrils *(arrow)* are present among loosely connected cells. (Original magnification ×1666.) **B,** Electron micrograph showing development of corneoscleral trabeculae at twenty-second to twenty-fourth fetal week. Trabeculae are now oriented longitudinally, and trabecular cells have numerous cytoplasmic processes. In intercellular spaces, patches of collagen fibrils *(arrow)* and elastic tissue (asterisk) are seen. (Original magnification ×2500.) **C,** Electron micrograph of corneoscleral meshwork at twenty-eighth to thirtieth fetal week. Trabecular beams consist of a core of collagen fibrils and elastic tissue covered by cells that rest on a tenuous basement membrane. Cortical zone of beams has not yet formed. (Original magnification ×2500.) (From Reme, C, and d'Epinay, SL: Periods of development of the normal human chamber angle, Doc Ophthalmol 51:241, 1981.)

probably depend on mechanical influences such as the direction of the pull exerted on them.[99] Thus, the corneoscleral and deep uveal trabeculae are oriented circumferentially as flattened, perforated sheets, whereas the inner uveal trabeculae have a predominantly meridional position of their long axes, with a rounded, cordlike profile arranged in a netlike fashion so as to form a more resilient system.[99]

By the twenty-eighth to thirtieth week of fetal development, the longitudinal fibers of the ciliary muscle are distinct, and Schlemm's canal, which developed from a longitudinal vessel in the corneoscleral region, increases considerably in size. The trabecular beams of the corneoscleral meshwork are now elongated, and the endothelial cells covering each beam are connected by tight junctions and show only slender cytoplasmic processes (see Fig. 1-15). The uveal meshwork now shows wide intercellular spaces, some of which have become confluent. The scleral spur (see below) has become well developed, and, by the eighth month, both the circular and the meridional fibers of the ciliary muscle are also prominent. The trabecular beams continue to mature, and by the ninth month, the uveal trabeculae are well formed (Fig. 1-16).

With the development of the iris, iridotrabecular meshwork processes (corresponding to vestiges of the pectinate ligament in lower mammals) develop as a bridge between the iris root and the uveal meshwork during the formation of the angle recess.[28,36,44,99] Morphologically, the base of the process is similar to the iris stroma, but, as they taper and branch toward their anterior attachment with the uveal trabeculae, they become similar to the inner uveal cords (Fig. 1-17). Usually, iris processes are seen in no more than 35% of normal eyes. The size, shape, and number of iris processes vary widely among individuals, but usually no more than 100 such structures are present in normal eyes, and they tend to have a predilection for the nasal aspect of the eye. The processes can be seen gonioscopically in infants by about 1 year of age, in whom they appear as semitransparent bands that are wide at the base and join the uveal meshwork. Abnormalities in the configuration of the iris processess occur in various congenital disorders.

Scleral spur. The scleral spur, which is unique to higher primates, develops as a fibrous, wedge-shaped protrusion from the inner aspect of the anterior sclera and is oriented circumferentially (Fig. 1-18). Originally, the meridional fibers of the ciliary muscle are continuous with the trabecular meshwork, an arrangement that remains in the adult eyes of lower mammals. However, in primates, especially in humans, the scleral spur intervenes between these two tissues.[99] In humans, the scleral

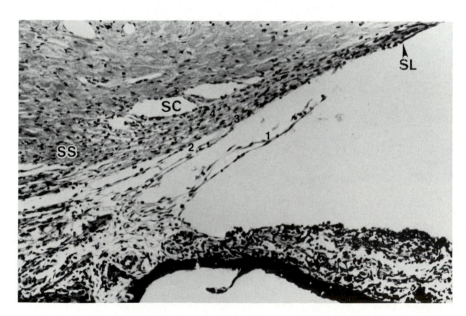

Fig. 1-16 Meridional section of angle of anterior chamber in 9-week-old infant. Angle recess is bridged by fine iris processes *(1)* that extend from root of iris and join uveal meshwork just anterior to midpoint. Inner uveal trabeculae *(2)* are well formed. Outer uveal trabeculae *(3)* pass just beneath scleral spur *(SS)*. *SL*, Schwalbe's line; *4*, corneoscleral trabeculae; *SC*, Schlemm's canal. (Original magnification ×180.)

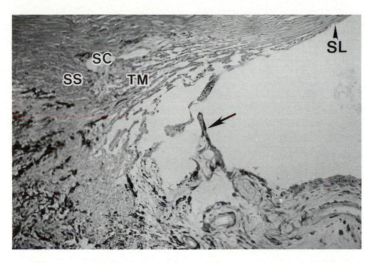

Fig. 1-17 Meridional section of anterior chamber angle in a juvenile. Iris processes *(arrow)* are well formed with a base consisting of iris tissue. Anteriorly, pigmented processes assume morphology of uveal trabeculae and join inner uveal meshwork by tapering and merging with it. *TM,* Trabecular meshwork; *SC,* Schlemm's canal; *SS,* scleral spur; *SL,* Schwalbe's line. (Original magnification ×170.)

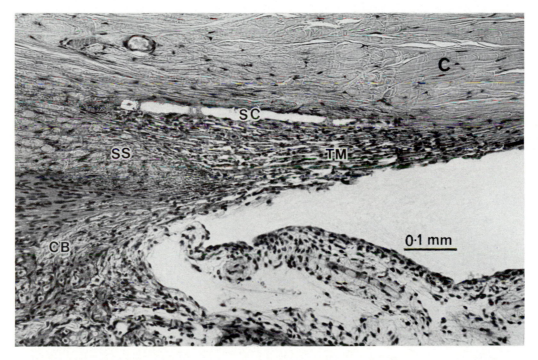

Fig. 1-18 Light micrograph of scleral spur *(SS)* in meridional section of human eye. Scleral roll forms posterior boundary of Schlemm's canal *(SC)* while sloping anteromedial border of spur provides attachment for corneoscleral trabecular sheets *(TM).* Meridional muscle fibers of ciliary body *(CB)* are inserted into posterior edge of spur. *C,* Peripheral cornea. (Original magnification ×240.) (From Tripathi, RC, and Tripathi, BJ: Functional anatomy of the anterior chamber angle. In Duane, TD, and Jaeger, EA, editors: Biomedical foundations of ophthalmology, vol 1, Philadelphia, 1987, Harper & Row)

spur is first evident during the fourth gestational month.[27] Its appearance corresponds to the retraction of the developing ciliary muscle fibers. The anterior ends of the longitudinal ciliary muscle fibers insert into the scleral spur, although this arrangement is not well established until about 7½ months. The outer portion of the trabecular meshwork, including a part of the uveal meshwork, bridges the scleral spur and the cornea, and hence it is referred to as corneoscleral meshwork. The collagen and elastic tissue of the scleral spur become oriented in a circular direction corresponding to that of the beams that constitute the corneoscleral trabeculae, and their collagen and elastic tissue components are continuous.[99] The meridional ciliary muscle fibers do not pass through the substance of the scleral spur.[36,102]

Schwalbe's line. The line of Schwalbe, which clinically marks the end of Descemet's membrane, forms the apex of the most anterior portion of the trabecular meshwork (Fig. 1-19). It is a prominent structure in only about 4% to 20% of human eyes, and its embryogenesis remains uncertain. It consists of 64 nm periodicity collagen fibrils intermixed with elastic fibers, both of which are oriented circumferentially. Clumps of "curly" collagen are encountered in aging eyes. The line of Schwalbe is considered to originate either as an unabsorbed remnant or as an excess of extracellular material that is produced by mesenchymal cells.[99]

Mid limbus

The mid limbus is a region where the collagenous frameworks of the cornea and sclera merge imperceptibly (Fig. 1-20). The mid limbal stroma is traversed by the veins of the deep and intrascleral plexuses, by a few small arteriolar channels, and by myelinated and unmyelinated nerves (mostly branches of the ciliary nerves) that pass through the trabecular meshwork to the cornea. Compar-

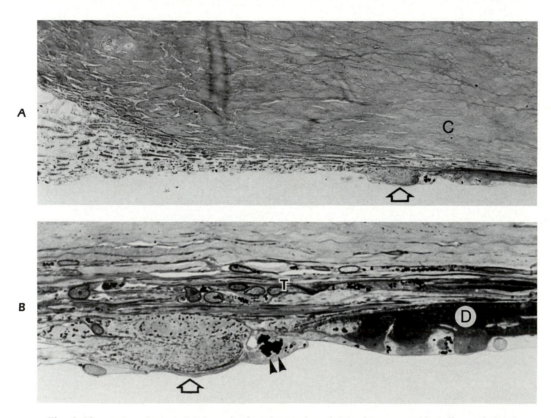

Fig. 1-19 **A,** Anterior termination of trabecular meshwork into deep corneal lamellae and anterior ring of Schwalbe *(arrow)* as seen in light micrograph of meridional section of human eye. (Original magnification ×220.) **B,** Higher magnification of ring of Schwalbe *(SR);* dotlike structures represent transversely cut elastic fibers. Descemet's membrane *(DM)* shows nodular profiles of Hassall-Henle bodies. Note termination of trabecular sheets *(T)* into deep corneal lamellae and transition of corneal endothelium into trabecular endothelium. Transitional endothelium *(arrow)* contains trapped pigment granules. (Original magnification ×895.) (From Tripathi, RC, and Tripathi, BJ: Functional anatomy of the anterior chamber angle. In Duane, TD, and Jaeger, EA, editors: Biomedical foundations of ophthalmology, vol 1, Philadelphia, 1987, Harper & Row)

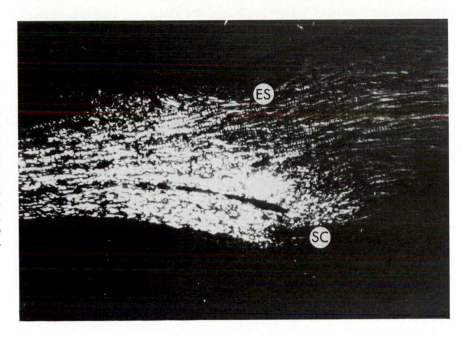

Fig. 1-20 Section of corneoscleral limbus viewed by polarized light. Note gradual transition of corneal collagen lamellae *(right)* into more birefringent scleral lamellae *(left)* and difficulty in demarcating transitional zone by a single line. *ES,* External scleral sulcus; *SC,* Schlemm's canal. (Original magnification ×60.) (From Tripathi, RC, and Tripathi, BJ: Anatomy of the human eye, orbit, and adnexa. In Davson, H, editor: The eye, vol 1A, New York, 1984, Academic Press)

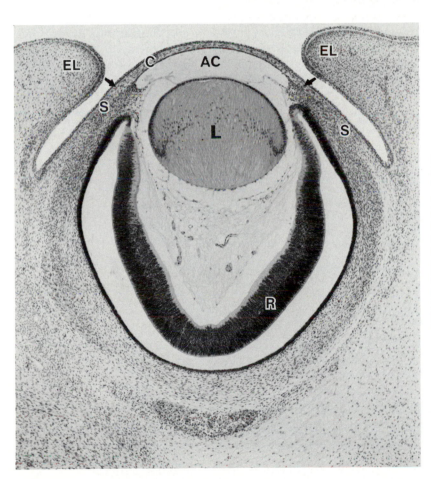

Fig. 1-21 Section through eye of a 30 mm human embryo showing an early stage in development of sclera. Sclera *(S)* is formed by condensation of mesenchymal tissue, which initially occurs anteriorly at limbus *(arrows)* and gradually proceeds posteriorly. *C,* Cornea; *AC,* anterior chamber; *L,* lens; *R,* neural retina (separated artifactually from the retinal pigment epithelium); *EL,* embryonic eyelids before fusion. (Original magnification ×84.) (From Tripathi, RC, and Tripathi, BJ: Functional anatomy of the anterior chamber angle. In Davson, HJ, editor: The eye, vol 1A, New York, 1984, Academic Press)

atively few detailed studies have documented the embryogenesis of this region or that of the outer limbus.

The sclera of the eye forms first at the limbus (Fig. 1-21) and gradually extends posteriorly.[70,71] Initially, it appears as a condensation of mesenchymal tissue, and the active fibroblast-like cells synthesize slender collagen fibrils and foci of elastic tissue. The mesenchymal tissue of the sclera is derived, for the most part, from neural crest cells. However, it is apparent that the caudal region of the sclera is derived from paraxial mesoderm because, at the time of neural crest cell formation, the caudomedial surface of the optic cup is already apposed by mesodermal cells. This apposition is maintained through the period of crest migration and of the development of the cranial and pontine flexures.[68] Studies of rhesus monkey fetuses reveal that development of the scleral stroma occurs at about 45 days' gestation, which is equivalent to 10 weeks in the human embryo.[71] At this stage, the corneal stroma is also being synthesized actively because of the activity of the keratocytes. In the early phase of development of the scleral stroma, its collagen fibrils are smaller in diameter than are those in the corneal stroma. However, the diameter of the collagen fibrils in the sclera increases rapidly; by the fifth month, the fibrils may be 100 nm or more.[81] In contrast, it has been shown that keratocytes form collagen at a faster rate than do the scleral fibroblasts; also, there are differences in the rate and amounts of noncollagenous proteins that they synthesize.[35] Therefore, it is apparent that, even though the keratocytes and scleral fibroblasts are derived from a common mesenchymal stock, these cells behave differently when they are established in their respective final positions.

The collector channels, aqueous veins, and veins of the deep and intrascleral plexuses first arise at about 12 weeks' gestation.[70] These vessels become differentiated from primitive mesoderm, but the factors that govern their arrangement into the fully formed, intricate plexuses are not known.

Outer limbus

The outer or anterior limbus consists of the conjunctival epithelium, the conjunctival stroma—which contains the episcleral and subconjunctival vascular plexuses, Tenon's capsule, and the loose fibrous tissue of the episclera (see Fig. 1-10).

The conjunctival epithelium and its stroma begin to develop soon after the optic vesicle is formed (at 4 weeks). They are derived from the surface ectoderm (epithelium) and mesenchyme (stroma), with mesodermal tissue contributing to the vascular plexuses. By the time the neural crest–derived mesenchymal cells have circumscribed the future cornea and iris region, the limbal vascular plexus is already established in the cell population.[10,68] The conjunctival epithelium is continuous with the cor-

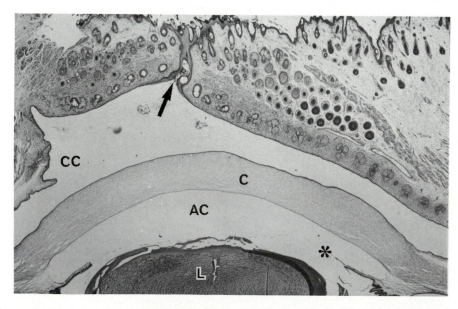

Fig. 1-22 Meridional section of fetal eye at fifth month of gestation. Eyelids are still fused *(arrow)*, and conjunctival cul-de-sac *(CC)* is well defined. Angle and anterior chamber *(AC)* are well formed, although the latter is still shallow. Pupillary membrane is still persistent *(asterisk)*. C, Cornea; L, lens. (Original magnification ×24.)

neal epithelium and with the surface ectoderm from which the eyelids will develop. Proliferation of the skin ectoderm in the region of the future upper lid begins at the outer canthus at 4 to 5 weeks (8 to 12 mm stage). By the 30 mm stage (end of the second month), both lids are visible, and the limbal conjunctiva is fairly well demarcated (Fig. 1-21). The lid folds continue to grow, so that the lid margins contact each other during the early part of the third month of gestation and remain fused until the fifth or sixth month (Fig. 1-22). During this period, the definitive development of the outer limbus occurs. It is believed that mesoderm of the second visceral arch migrates to the eye and forms the orbicularis palpebrae muscles of the lids[70]; however, there has been no detailed investigation of the origin of the mesenchyme that contributes to the outer limbus.

EMBRYOLOGIC BASIS FOR CONGENITAL AND DEVELOPMENTAL ANOMALIES (THE ANGULAR NEUROCRISTOPATHIES)

During ontogeny, the numerous dynamic interactions that take place between the mesenchymal cells and the ectodermal cells and within the individual cell populations are crucial to the normal development of the eye and to the differentiation of the ocular and periocular tissues. If the normal interactions are disrupted, congenital and developmental anomalies occur. Diseases and malformations of cells derived from the neural crest have been grouped together under the term *neurocristopathies*.[13] It has been recognized that neural crest–derived mesenchymal cells make a major contribution to the tissues of the anterior segment. Therefore, one would expect that a group of ocular diseases exists that involve the cornea, iris, and trabecular meshwork, either singly or in combination and often in association with glaucoma, and that are frequently accompanied by abnormalities of nonocular tissues that are also derived from neural crest cells (e.g., craniofacial and dental malformations, middle ear deafness, malformations of the base of the skull, and malformations of the shoulder girdle and upper spine).[45,46] Our discussion will be confined to those events in embryonic and fetal development that may help explain the pathogenesis of the disorders that are manifested early in life as glaucomatous disease of the eye.

In considering the glaucomas that develop congenitally or in early life, it is obviously important to have a clear understanding about the embryonic origins of the tissues of the aqueous outflow pathway, namely, the trabecular meshwork and Schlemm's canal. It is generally accepted that the endothelial lining of Schlemm's canal is derived from mesoderm, but the origin of the trabecular endothelial cells is not as well established. Based on the quail-chick transplant experiments mentioned earlier, it has generally been assumed that the trabecular cells in man are also derived from neural crest cells. However, in describing their experiments, Johnston et al.[41] did not report specifically on the ectomesenchymal identity of the trabecular endothelium, although Kupfer and Kupfer[46] cite Johnston, through a personal communication, as having found that, in birds, neural crest cells form the trabecular meshwork. Despite the fact that the aqueous outflow pathway and anterior chamber angle show significant differences between birds and man with respect to organization and morphology,[99] there is growing evidence that the trabecular endothelial cells in humans originate from the embryonic neural crest cells. During early development, the meshwork is in close proximity to the cornea, the ciliary body, and the iris, all of which have contributions from neural crest cells. The trabecular meshwork is involved in developmental anomalies that affect other neural crest–derived tissues of the anterior segment, and this suggests that these structures have a common embryonic ancestry.

A useful marker for cells of neural crest origin is the glycolytic enzyme neuron-specific enolase (NSE), the gamma-gamma form of which is believed to be specific for neuroectodermal cells.[77] Immunohistochemical techniques with anti-NSE antibodies have made it possible to map out derivatives of the neural crest not only in the human eye, but also in other body tissues. Thus, in normal tissues, neuronal cells of the autonomic ganglia, spinal cord, brainstem, cerebellum, cerebrum, and retina, as well as the neuroendocrine cells of the amine precursor uptake and decarboxylation (APUD) system (thyroid parafollicular cells, adrenal medullary chromaffin cells, and cells of the islets of Langerhans), stain positively with this technique.[12,39,80,112]

Recently, we have found that the corneal endothelium and the keratocytes in the posterior region of normal human corneas (Fig. 1-23) exhibit intensely positive staining with anti-NSE antibodies.[1,97] This immunohistochemical demonstration of NSE in the human corneal endothelium favors its neuroectodermal rather than mesodermal origin. However, the pattern of staining of the keratocytes has several implications. In contrast to the keratocytes in avian eyes, all keratocytes in the human cornea may not be derived from neural crest cells. Since the keratocytes in the posterior

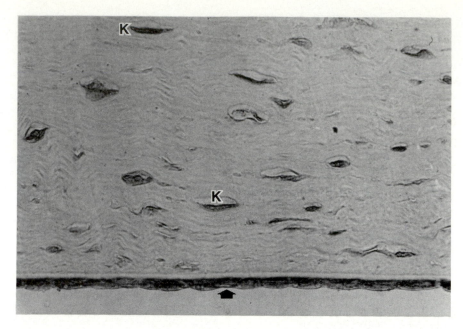

Fig. 1-23 Photomicrograph of section of formalin-fixed, paraffin-embedded human eye stained with affinity-purified antibodies against neuron-specific enolase according to peroxidase-antiperoxidase technique. Cytoplasm of corneal endothelial cells (arrow) stains intensely, as do keratocytes (K) in posterior aspect of stroma. (Original magnification x 1120.)

portion of the cornea stain more intensely for NSE than do the cells of the anterior stroma, we must consider the possibility that the proximity of the cells in the posterior region to the corneal endothelium may have a positive-inductive effect. Alternatively, it may be that all keratocytes are derived from neuroectoderm and that the cells in the anterior stroma lose the NSE during development. Another possibility is that there are two subpopulations of keratocytes that have mixed embryonic origins.[96]

By using the NSE staining technique, we have also examined the structures of the aqueous outflow pathway and found that the endothelial lining of Schlemm's canal does not stain positively. However, the endothelial cells do stain positively with antibodies against factor VIII–related antigen, which is a reliable marker for normal and neoplastic vascular endothelial cells.[1,79] These findings favor the mesodermal origin of Schlemm's canal. We have observed that the endothelial cells of the anterior portion of the trabecular meshwork at its termination into the peripheral cornea and of the inner uveal meshwork show a more intense staining reaction than do the cells of the posterior region of the trabecular meshwork (Fig. 1-24). By using an indirect immunofluorescence technique, Stone et al.[90] have shown localized NSE staining of isolated cells that is confined to the anterior portion of the

trabecular meshwork in rhesus monkey eyes. They attributed this finding to the presence of neuroregulatory cells in the meshwork. The differences in the results that were obtained could be explained by the fact that a peroxidase-antiperoxidase technique is more sensitive than the indirect immunofluorescence method and by the possibility that species variations exist. The finding that the endothelial cells of the posterior region of the trabecular meshwork in human eyes stain irregularly with anti-NSE antibodies indicates that either these cells have lost the ability to express NSE or they are not derived from neural crest cells. Alternatively, it is possible that the trabecular meshwork in humans is derived from a mixed population of cells in embryonic life. Other ocular structures—for example, the uveal tract and the sclera—are known to arise from neural crest cells and from other embryonic cell types. A definitive answer to the question of the origin of the trabecular endothelial cells, therefore, must await further studies.

Several ocular diseases involve one or more tissues of neural crest origin and are associated with chamber angle anomalies that are manifested in glaucoma and commonly accompanied by systemic abnormalities that also involve tissues of neural crest origin. These diseases include Axenfeld-Rieger syndrome, Peters' anomaly, iridocorneal endothelial (ICE) syndrome, posterior polymorphous

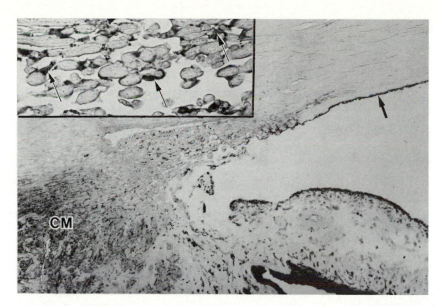

Fig. 1-24 Photomicrograph of section of formalin-fixed, paraffin-embedded human eye stained with affinity-purified antibodies against neuron-specific enolase according to peroxidase-antiperoxidase technique. Corneal endothelium *(arrow)* and anterior termination of trabecular meshwork show intense staining. Positive staining is also seen in ciliary muscle *(CM)* and iris. (Original magnification ×120.) *Inset:* Higher magnification of trabecular meshwork shows intense staining of cytoplasm of endothelial cells *(arrows).* (Original magnification ×470.)

dystrophy (PPMD), Sturge-Weber syndrome and other phakomatoses, and congenital glaucoma. All these disorders are believed to provide possible clinical evidence either of abnormalities in the migration of neural crest cells or of terminal interference with cellular interactions.[45]

Although Axenfeld-Rieger syndrome is characterized by a prominent, anteriorly displaced line of Schwalbe with attachment of tissue strands of peripheral iris, several reports have documented structural alterations in the trabecular meshwork and Schlemm's canal.[2,84,85,115] The trabecular beams are thickened, largely because of the increased size of the cortical zone, and the meshwork is compact (Fig. 1-25). Often the connective tissue of the trabeculae is fused because of an incomplete endothelial covering, or because thin endothelial cells cover two or more adjacent lamellae. Overall, there is a progressive narrowing of the free spaces in the trabecular meshwork from its inner to its outer aspect, so that, eventually, most of the trabecular spaces are obliterated. These changes may be accompanied by insertion of the peripheral iris stroma and ciliary body into the posterior third of the trabecular meshwork. A normal Schlemm's canal is usually absent and is represented only by one or more small endothelium-lined spaces at the periphery of the meshwork. Shields has postulated that the changes in the anterior segment of the eyes

in patients with Axenfeld-Rieger syndrome result from an arrest in the development of the tissue derived from neural crest cells that occurs late in gestation.[84,85] Primordial endothelial tissues are retained on the anterior iris and across the anterior chamber angle, and the arrested development of the angle structures is characterized by incomplete maturation of the trabecular meshwork and Schlemm's canal, and by the high insertion of the iris. A unique angle abnormality may be seen in which there is a complete lack of separation between the corneosclera and iris, together with a rudimentary development of the trabecular meshwork, scleral spur, ciliary muscle, and ciliary processes (Fig. 1-26). Because this entity also has a prominent Schwalbe's line, it could be regarded as a variant of Axenfeld-Rieger syndrome.

Peters' anomaly is characterized by a spectrum of changes in the anterior segment structures. These changes include defects in the posterior stroma, Descemet's membrane, and endothelium, with or without extension of iris tissue strands from the iris collarette to the edge of the corneal leukoma; they may also include a central keratolenticular stalk and cataract.[42,105,108] The corneal abnormalities are believed to result from incomplete migration of the neural crest–derived mesenchymal cells during early embryogenesis. Glaucoma commonly occurs and involves 50% to 70% of

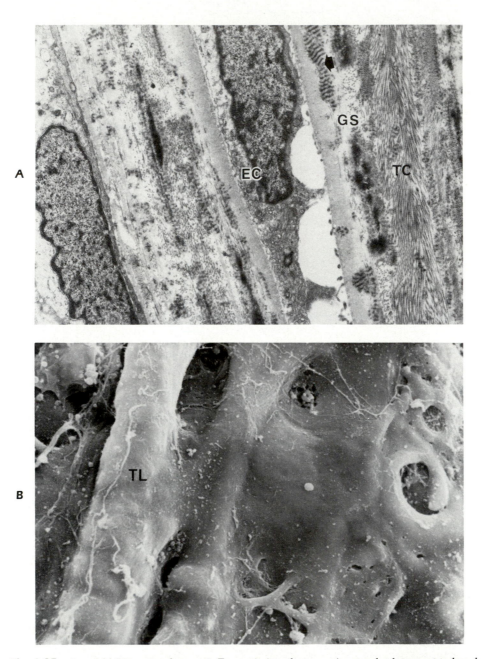

Fig. 1-25 Axenfeld-Rieger syndrome. **A,** Transmission electron micrograph of compact trabecular lamellae composed of cores of typical collagen with 64 nm periodicity *(TC)*, surrounded by ground substance *(GS)* that contains islands of broad-banded collagen with 128 nm periodicity *(arrow)*. Intervening endothelial cell *(EC)* fills most of the intertrabecular space with partial separation from one trabecular beam. (Original magnification ×15,150.) **B,** Scanning electron micrograph of innermost trabecular lamellae *(TL)* in midportion of meshwork covered by cellular layer that obliterates much of intertrabecular spaces. (Original magnification ×3400.)

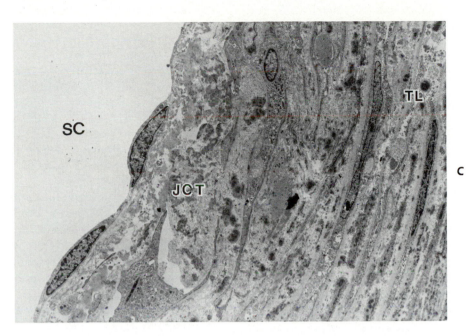

Fig. 1-25, cont'd   C, Transmission electron micrograph of outermost portion of trabecular mesh-work showing compact trabecular lamellae *(TL)*, amorphous material within zone of juxtacanalicular tissue *(JCT)*, and a portion of a rudimentary Schlemm's canal *(SC)*. (Original magnification ×5500.) (From Shields, MB: Axenfeld-Rieger syndrome: a theory of mechanism and distinctions from the iridocorneal endothelial syndrome, Trans Am Ophthalmol Soc 81:736, 1983)

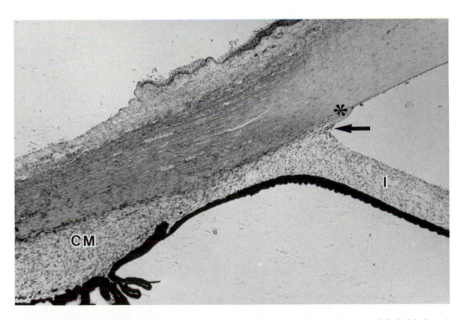

Fig. 1-26   Meridional section of the angular region of an eye from a 5-year-old child showing a unique angle abnormality. There is lack of separation between corneosclera and iris *(I)*. Line of Schwalbe is prominent *(asterisk)* and is attached to iris by prominent processes *(arrow)*. Ciliary muscle *(CM)* and ciliary processes are not well defined. Scleral spur and trabecular meshwork are rudimentary. (Original magnification ×72.)

cases.[2] Only a few studies have been reported on the structure of the trabecular meshwork and Schlemm's canal in patients with Peters' anomaly. In one patient who had total peripheral anterior synechiae, Schlemm's canal and the trabecular meshwork could not be identified.[78] Kupfer et al.[48] studied the trabeculectomy specimen from the eye of a 2-year-old child with Peters' anomaly and reported that the trabecular beams showed thickening, with the presence of "curly" collagen (Fig. 1-27). The endothelial cells contained an abnormal amount of phagocytosed pigment granules. Again, the authors suggested that the structural alterations could have resulted from a failure of differentiation of neural crest–derived cells that were destined to form the trabecular and corneal endothelia.[46,48]

The ICE syndrome is another disorder in which a spectrum of changes may be seen in the structures of the anterior segment. Because histopathologic studies have revealed proliferation of the corneal endothelium, with an abnormal basement membrane over the surface of the trabecular meshwork, extending across the apex of the anterior chamber angle and onto the anterior surface of the iris, it is generally believed that the glaucoma in ICE syndrome is a secondary phenomenon.[18,26,75,76] However, it has also been noted that the cellularity of the trabecular meshwork increases (Fig. 1-28),

which suggests that abnormalities in the trabecular endothelial cells exist independent of the other changes in the anterior segment.[26] In support of this hypothesis, there is a significantly decreased outflow facility, but no elevation of intraocular pressure, in the contralateral eye of patients with ICE syndrome.[47] Although further studies are necessary before a primary defect in the trabecular endothelium is confirmed, the cascade of alterations in patients with the ICE syndrome could be explained by a common defect in the neural crest cells that are destined to form structures of the anterior segment.[47]

Posterior polymorphous dystrophy also causes abnormalities that involve the cornea, anterior chamber angle, and the iris, and a spectrum of changes may be seen. Two forms of glaucoma have been identified in patients with PPMD. In one form, extension of the abnormal corneal endothelium and Descemet's membrane across the chamber angle and onto the anterior surface of the iris, peripheral anterior synechiae, and robust iris processes that extend to the prominent line of Schwalbe can be identified both clinically (Fig. 1-29) and histopathologically.[19,20,29,75,101] Although it may be assumed that, as in the ICE syndrome, the glaucoma is secondary because of the peripheral anterior synechiae, it is also possible that some primary defect exists in the trabecular meshwork.

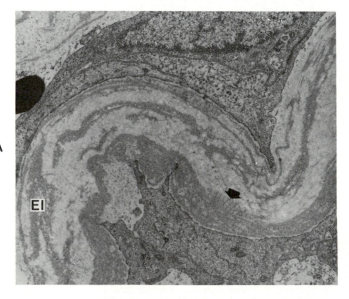
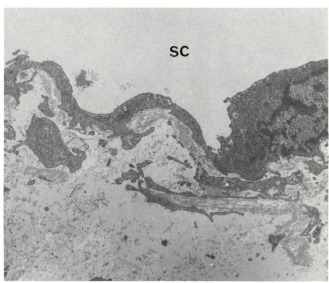

Fig. 1-27 Peters' anomaly. **A,** Trabecular meshwork showing fine structure of endothelial cells and wide-banded collagen fibers *(arrow)*. *EI,* Normal elastic tissue. (Original magnification ×30,000.) **B,** Electron micrograph of endothelial lining of Schlemm's canal *(SC)* and adjacent juxtacanalicular tissue. (Original magnification ×20,000.) (From Kupfer, C, Kuwabara, T, and Stark, WJ: The histopathology of Peters' anomaly, Am J Ophthalmol 80:653, 1975. Published with permission from The American Journal of Ophthalmology. Copyright by The Ophthalmic Publishing Company)

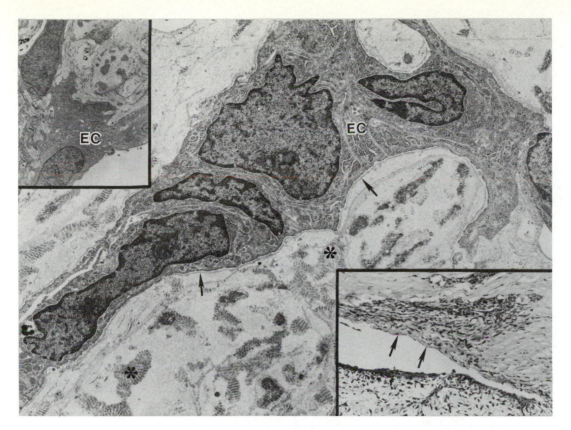

Fig. 1-28 Iridocorneal endothelial syndrome. Inset on right shows increased cellularity of trabecular meshwork with flat layer of endothelial cells that have laid down a thin cuticular membrane *(arrows)*. (Original magnification ×160.) Inset on left shows endothelial cell *(EC)* on surface of meshwork and extending into trabecular spaces. (Original magnification ×3600.) Main figure shows several endothelial cells *(EC)* filling spaces between trabecular beams. Latter typically contain patches of banded structures or "curly" collagen *(asterisk)*. Endothelial cells contain abundant rough-surfaced endoplasmic reticulum and have a thin basement membrane *(arrows)*. (Original magnification ×10,800.) (From Eagle, RCJ, Font, RL, and Yanoff, M: Proliferative endotheliopathy with iris abnormalities: the iridocorneal endothelial syndrome, Arch Ophthalmol 97:2104, 1979. Copyright 1974, American Medical Association)

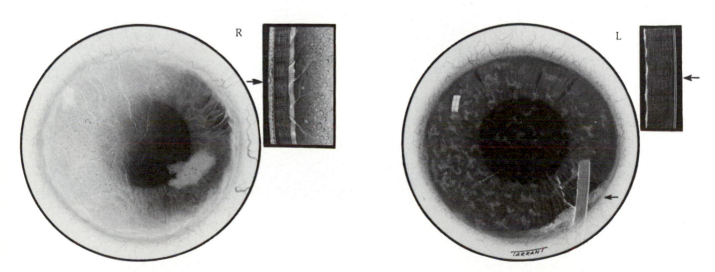

Fig. 1-29 Posterior polymorphous dystrophy. Artist's impression shows polymorphous pattern of opacities in corneal and angle abnormality. In right eye, there was a prominent line of Schwalbe and presence of goniosynechiae in a few places. Gonioscopy of left eye revealed a band of peripheral anterior synechiae between 4 and 6 o'clock, and robust iris processes, many of which extended to prominent Schwalbe's line, in remainder of angle. (From Tripathi, RC, Casey, TA, and Wise, G: Hereditary posterior polymorphous dystrophy: an ultrastructural and clinical report, Trans Ophthalmol Soc UK 94:211, 1974)

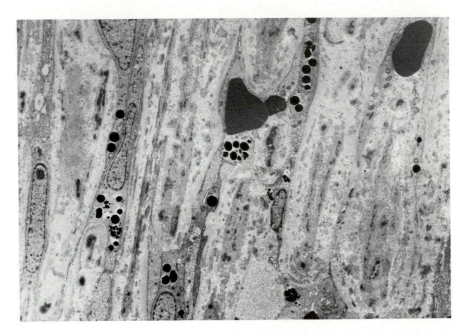

Fig. 1-30 Transmission electron micrograph of trabecular meshwork from a patient with posterior polymorphous dystrophy and associated open-angle glaucoma. Note compressed trabecular beams with almost total obliteration of trabecular spaces; many endothelial cells contain pigment granules. (Original magnification ×6000.) (From Bourgeois, J, Shields, MB, and Thresher, R: Open-angle glaucoma associated with posterior polymorphous dystrophy: a clinicopathologic study, Ophthalmology 42:420, 1984)

Fig. 1-31 Gonioscopic appearance of anterior chamber angle in a case of Sturge-Weber syndrome. Iris processes *(arrow)* adhere to trabecular meshwork similar to other types of congenital glaucoma. (From Cibis, GW, Tripathi, RC, and Tripathi, BJ: Glaucoma in Sturge-Weber syndrome, Ophthalmology 91: 1061, 1984)

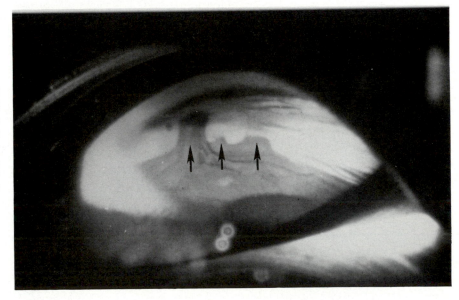

In the other form of glaucoma accompanying PPMD, the angle of the anterior chamber is not compromised by the corneal endothelium.[15] The insertion of the iris into the posterior portion of the trabecular meshwork is high. The intertrabecular spaces are compressed and obliterated. Curly collagen is present in the trabeculae, and many of the endothelial cells contain phagocytosed pigment granules (Fig. 1-30). It has been suggested that the configuration of the chamber angle structures results from a developmental anomaly,[15] and Kupfer[47] has characterized PPMD as part of the broad spectrum of diseases that involve abnormalities of tissue derived from neural crest cells.

Glaucoma occurs in about one third of the patients with Sturge-Weber syndrome, but its incidence is unknown for neurofibromatosis. Numerous theories have been put forward to account for the raised intraocular pressure in these conditions.[21,104,110] At least in some cases, the glaucoma may result secondarily—for example, from a neurofibroma that occludes the anterior chamber angle or from neovascularization. However, several investigators have reported primary defects in the structures of the aqueous outflow pathway in patients with neurofibromatosis. These abnormalities include malformation or absence of Schlemm's canal, persistence of embryonal tissue in the trabecular meshwork, and incomplete "cleavage" of the iridocorneal angle.* Neurofibromatosis is primarily a neuroectodermal dyplasia, and thus abnormalities in the neural crest cells that give rise to the structures of the anterior segment could explain the pathogenesis of the associated glaucoma in those patients who have no secondary obstruction to aqueous outflow.

Gonioscopically, patients with Sturge-Weber syndrome may show prominent iris processes adherent to the trabecular meshwork (Fig. 1-31), which indicates that there is a primary congenital defect in the development of the angle. A recent study of trabeculectomy specimens from patients with Sturge-Weber syndrome revealed not only a compact trabecular meshwork with hyalinization of the trabeculae, but also the presence of amorphous material in the intertrabecular spaces of the deeper uveal and corneoscleral regions.[21] Individual trabecular beams were thickened and had a prominent cortical zone that contained "curly" collagen (Fig. 1-32). Many trabecular endothelial cells showed degenerative changes. The juxtacanalicular region showed an excess of extracellular elements (granuloamorphous material, basal lamina material, banded and nonbanded structures), and degenerative changes were noted in the cellular component. The endothelial lining of Schlemm's canal was attenuated and had few vacuolar configurations.[21] These alterations in patients with Sturge-Weber syndrome are similar to those that occur in old age and in primary open-angle glaucoma, and they appear to represent a premature aging of the trabecular meshwork/Schlemm's canal system. It is also apparent that the defect in the aqueous outflow pathway can arise early in the development of the anterior chamber, because many of these patients have glaucoma and even buphthalmos soon after birth.

Whereas the glaucoma in many of the disorders already considered commonly develops during adulthood, congenital glaucoma is often present at birth, and infantile or juvenile glaucoma usually manifests itself within the first decade of life. It is, therefore, possible to rationalize the latter two disorders as arising during the development of the aqueous outflow pathway. Yet, considerable controversy exists concerning the pathogenesis of the congenital and juvenile glaucomas. One theory states that an impermeable membrane covers the inner aspect of the trabecular meshwork and occludes the intertrabecular spaces of the innermost uveal sheet.[11,83,116,117] This so-called Barkan's membrane is thought to be the corneal endothelial covering that is said to be present during the development of the angle of the anterior chamber and that, instead of receding and perforating during the final weeks of gestation, persists in eyes that develop glaucoma (Figs. 1-33 and 1-34). However, this theory has been refuted on the basis of histopathologic studies in which no evidence for such a membrane was found.*

Ultrastructural studies of the trabecular meshwork/Schlemm's canal system from patients with congenital glaucoma have shown thickened trabecular beams with excessive formation of basement membrane material and collagenous tissue[4,16,37,59,98] (Fig. 1-35). The thickening of the inner uveal cords is believed to prevent the posterior migration of the ciliary body and iris that normally occurs during the last weeks of gestation, thus causing incomplete differentiation of the angle.[4,37,89] The consequent traction, therefore, compacts the already thickened trabeculae and results

---

*References 22, 38, 43, 55, 65, 113, 114.

*References 4, 23, 32, 60-63, 98.

Text continued on p. 35.

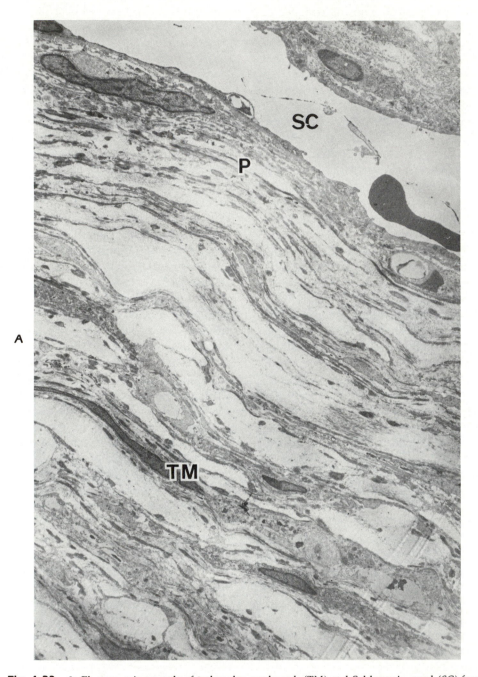

Fig. 1-32 A, Electron micrograph of trabecular meshwork *(TM)* and Schlemm's canal *(SC)* from a case of Sturge-Weber syndrome. Note compactness of meshwork, hyalinization of beams, and degenerate appearance of trabecular endothelial cells. *P,* Pericanalicular region. (Original magnification ×6340.)

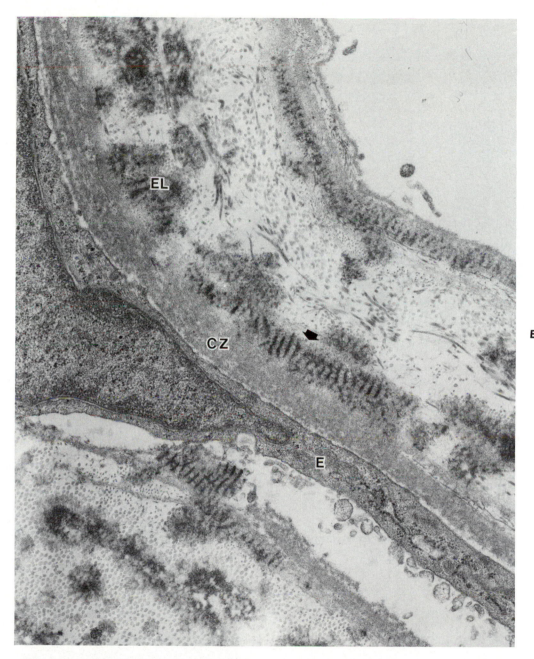

Fig. 1-32, cont'd   B, Electron micrograph of uveal trabeculae showing degenerative changes in endothelial covering *(E)* and thickened cortical zone *(CZ)* with accumulation of basement membrane material and long-spacing collagen *(arrow)*. Elastic tissue *(EL)* is also associated with long-spacing collagen. (Original magnification ×39,000.) (From Cibis, GW, Tripathi, RC, and Tripathi, BJ: Glaucoma in Sturge-Weber syndrome, Ophthalmology 91:1061, 1984)

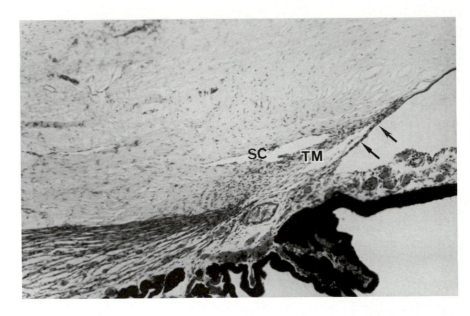

Fig. 1-33 Meridional section of angle of anterior chamber in infant with congenital glaucoma. Note that cellular membrane ("Barkan's membrane," *arrows*) is covering inner aspect of trabecular meshwork *(TM)* and is continuous with corneal endothelium. *SC,* Schlemm's canal. (Original magnification ×110.)

Fig. 1-34 Scanning electron micrograph of angle structures in a patient with infantile glaucoma. Trabecular meshwork *(TM)* is represented by compacted tissue, and the most superficial sheet *(arrow)* is imperforate. Specimen retrieved from paraffin block. (Original magnification ×95.) (From Anderson, DR: The development of the trabecular meshwork and its abnormality in primary infantile glaucoma, Trans Am Ophthalmol Soc 79:458, 1981)

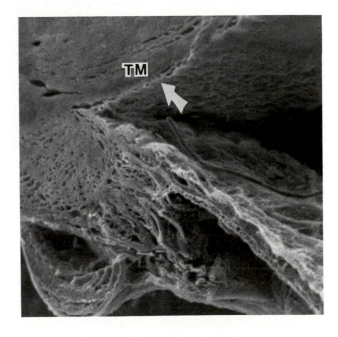

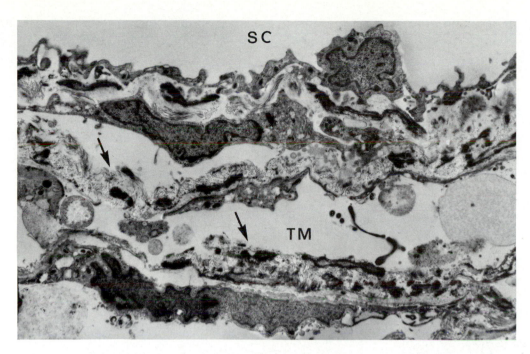

Fig. 1-35 Survey electron micrograph of trabecular wall of Schlemm's canal *(SC)* and adjacent trabecular meshwork *(TM)* in congenital glaucoma. Note attenuated endothelial lining of Schlemm's canal devoid of macrovacuolar configurations and disorganized trabecular meshwork together with a loss of trabecular endothelium in places *(arrow)*. (Original magnification ×7500.) (From Tripathi, RC: Aqueous outflow pathway in normal and glaucomatous eyes, Br J Ophthalmol 56:157, 1972)

in obstruction to outflow of the aqueous humor.[4] In another series of patients with congenital glaucoma that became evident within 6 months after birth, the ciliary body was displaced anteriorly so that it covered the inner aspect of the trabecular meshwork almost completely.[92] In these cases, the trabecular beams were not differentiated, and the meshwork consisted of endothelial cells embedded in a poorly organized extracellular matrix. Thus, it would appear that the posterior migration of the ciliary body and iris in embryonic life is necessary for the continued normal differentiation of the trabecular meshwork. It is also apparent that more than one type of alteration during development can produce clinically evident congenital glaucoma.

Several investigators have also noted that, in cases of congenital glaucoma, vacuolar configurations in the endothelial lining of Schlemm's canal are conspicuously absent, and that there is an excess of extracellular collagenous and amorphous materials in the juxtacanalicular region[4,92,98] (Fig. 1-35). Whether the lack of vacuoles in Schlemm's canal is a primary defect or occurs secondarily as a result of reduced aqueous flow, or is even a fixation artifact, must await further investigation.

In summary, there are certain similarities in the morphologic features of the trabecular meshwork/Schlemm's canal system in most of the disorders discussed briefly here. A disorder usually manifests itself as thickening of the trabecular beams caused by increased amounts of extracellular components (collagen, elastin, "curly" collagen, and basement membrane material), a consequent reduction of the intertrabecular spaces, and an attenuation of the endothelium. These findings have often been described as nondifferentiation of the trabecular meshwork or as persistence of embryonic characteristics. An embryonic angle is characterized by the anterior insertion of the iris, anteriorly displaced ciliary processes, a rudimentary scleral spur, insertion of meridional ciliary muscle fibers directly into the trabecular meshwork, and undifferentiated trabecular beams (Fig. 1-36). However, the similarity between the congenital abnormalities that occur in the trabecular meshwork/Schlemm's canal system and the normal age-related changes that occur in this region in senile eyes suggests that it would be better to regard many of the developmental anomalies as accelerated or premature aging of the endothelial cells.

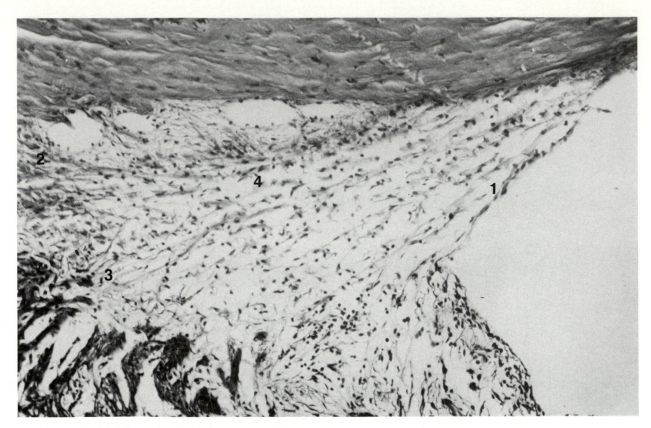

Fig. 1-36 Meridional section of angle of anterior chamber showing an embryonic configuration. The characteristic features include: *(1)* anterior insertion of iris; *(2)* rudimentary scleral spur; *(3)* insertion of ciliary muscle directly into the trabecular meshwork; *(4)* undifferentiated trabecular meshwork. (Original magnification ×190.)

Because the extracellular components are a product of the activity of these cells, the disease process is essentially one of the trabecular endothelium, which, in normal human eyes, is now presumed to be derived from neural crest cells. The trabecular endothelial cells not only produce the matrix macromolecules, but also control the manner in which these molecules are polymerized in the extracellular compartments. The cells form stable interactions with the molecules of the extracellular matrix. These molecules then dictate to the cell on questions of cellular shaping and spacing, cell metabolism, and other functions. The abnormal extracellular elements that are produced by the defective trabecular cells further impair normal cell function, with the result that there is increased resistance to aqueous outflow. This sequence of events can be characterized as a defective cell–extracellular matrix interaction.

It is also apparent that the endothelial cells lining the aqueous outflow pathway can respond in only a limited number of ways to adverse conditions, whether these conditions arise from abnormalities in the migration of the neural crest cells or in their terminal induction. What seems to be different among the various disorders is the age at which they produce clinical glaucoma, that is, in fetal life (congenital glaucoma), or at an early age (infantile or juvenile glaucoma), or at variable times during life (in association with other anomalies of the anterior segment such as PPMD, ICE syndrome, Axenfeld-Rieger syndrome, or Peters' anomaly). Perhaps primary open-angle glaucoma should be added to this spectrum of disorders, as an example of pathologic manifestation in older individuals.

An interesting finding is that, in several disorders, Schlemm's canal also shows abnormalities. Since its endothelial lining is considered to be mesodermal in origin, it could be postulated in explanation of the observed abnormalities that, during embryogenesis, there is a defective interaction between the endothelial cells of Schlemm's canal and those neural crest cells that are destined to form the trabecular meshwork. However, relatively little is known at present about the factors that induce the embryonic neural crest cells to differentiate into the structures of the anterior segment in the normal eye, and even less is understood about the causes of abnormalities that result in ocular neurocristopathies.

In this review, we have summarized the current knowledge, together with our personal observations, about the development of the structures of the anterior segment. Evidence is mounting that the neural crest makes a predominant contribution to the embryonic derivation of these structures, and this realization may help provide a better explanation for the pathogenesis of glaucomatous disorders of the eye, which has thus far remained an enigma. In view of the changing concept of the embryonic origin of the cells lining the trabecular beams and the posterior surface of the cornea, it is necessary to consider whether the traditional nomenclature of "endothelium" is indeed justified.[1,97]

REFERENCES

1. Adamis, P, et al: Neuronal-specific enolase in human corneal endothelium and posterior keratocytes, Exp Eye Res 41:665, 1985
2. Alkemade, PPH: Dysgenesis mesodermalis of the iris and the cornea, Assen, Netherlands, 1969, Van Gorcum
3. Allen, L, Burian, HM, and Braley, AE: A new concept of the development of the anterior chamber angle, Arch Ophthalmol 53:783, 1955
4. Anderson, DR: The development of the trabecular meshwork and its abnormality in primary infantile glaucoma, Trans Am Ophthalmol Soc 79:458, 1981
5. Bach, L, and Seefelder, R: Atlas zur Entwicklungsgeschichte des menschlichen Augen, Leipzig and Berlin, 1911-1914, Engelmann
6. Badtke, G: Zu Sondermanns These von der Entwicklung des Schlemmschen Kanals und der Ciliarfortsätze, Graefes Arch Klin Exp Ophthalmol 145:321, 1943
7. Badtke, G: Die normale Entwicklung des menschlichen Auges. In Velhagen der Augenarzt, vol, 1, Stuttgart, 1958, Thieme
8. Bahn, CF, et al: Classifications of corneal endothelium disorders based on neural crest origin, Ophthalmology 91:558, 1984
9. Barber, AN: Embryology of the human eye, St Louis, 1955, The CV Mosby Co
10. Bard, JBL, Hay, ED, and Meller, SM: Formation of the endothelium of the avian cornea: a study of cell movement in vivo, Dev Biol 42:334, 1975
11. Barkan, O: Pathogenesis of congenital glaucoma, gonioscopic and anatomic observations of the angle of the anterior chamber in the normal eye and in congenital glaucoma, Am J Ophthalmol 40:1, 1955
12. Bishop, AE, et al: Neuron specific enolase: a common marker for the endocrine cells and innervation of the gut and pancreas, Gastroenterology 83:902, 1982
13. Bolande, RP: The neurocristopathies: a unifying concept of disease arising in neural crest maldevelopment, Hum Pathol 5:409, 1974
14. Bolender, DL, Seliger, WG, and Markwald, RR: A histochemical analysis of polyanionic compounds found in the extracellular matrix encountered by migrating cephalic neural crest cells, Anat Rec 196:401, 1980
15. Bourgeois, J, Shields, MB, and Thresher, R: Open-angle glaucoma associated with posterior polymorphous dystrophy, Ophthalmology 91:420, 1984
16. Broughton, WL, Fine, BS, and Zimmerman, LE: Congenital glaucoma associated with a chromosomal defect: a histologic study, Arch Ophthalmol 99:481, 1981
17. Burian, H, Braley, AE, and Allen, L: A new concept of the development of the angle of the anterior chamber of the human eye, Arch Ophthalmol 55:439, 1956
18. Campbell, DG, Shields, MB, and Smith, TR: The corneal endothelium and the spectrum of essential iris atrophy, Am J Ophthalmol 86:317, 1978
19. Cibis, GW, Krachmer, JH, Phelps, CD, and Weingeist, TA: Iridocorneal adhesions in posterior polymorphous dystrophy, Trans Am Acad Ophthalmol Otolaryngol 81:770, 1976
20. Cibis, GW, Krachmer, JH, Phelps, CD, et al: The clinical spectrum of posterior polymorphous dystrophy, Arch Ophthalmol 95:1529, 1977
21. Cibis, GW, Tripathi, RC, and Tripathi, BJ: Glaucoma in Sturge-Weber syndrome, Ophthalmology 91:1061, 1984
22. Collins, ET, and Batten, RD: Neurofibroma of the eyeball and its appendages, Trans Ophthalmol Soc UK 25:248, 1905
23. DeLuise, VP, and Anderson, DR: Primary infantile glaucoma (congenital glaucoma), Surv Ophthalmol 28:1, 1983
24. Dodson, JW, and Hay, ED: Secretion of collagenous stroma by isolated epithelium in vitro, Exp Eye Res 65:215, 1971
25. Duke-Elder, S: System of ophthalmology, vol III, St Louis, 1964, The CV Mosby Co
26. Eagle, RCJ, Font, RL, and Yanoff, M: Proliferative endotheliopathy with iris abnormalities: the iridocorneal endothelial syndrome, Arch Ophthalmol 97:2104, 1979
27. Fischer, F: Entwicklungsgeschichtliche und anatomische Studieren über den Skeralsporn im menschlichen Auge, Albrecht von Graefes Arch Klin Exp Ophthalmol 131:318, 1933
28. Fritz, W: Über die Membrana Descemet's und das Ligamentum pectinatum iridis bei den Saugtieren

und Menschen, Sbr Akad Wissensch math-naturw Kl Wein 115:485, 1906

29. Grayson, M: The nature of hereditary deep polymorphous dystrophy in the cornea: its association with iris and anterior chamber dysgenesis, Trans Am Ophthalmol Soc 72:516, 1974

30. Greenberg, IH, and Pratt, RM: Glycosaminoglycan and glycoprotein synthesis by cranial neural crest cells in vitro, Cell Differ 6:119, 1977

31. Hansson, H-A, and Jerndal, T: Scanning electron microscopic studies on the development of the iridocorneal angle in the human eye, Invest Ophthalmol 10:252, 1971

32. Hansson, HA: Development of the angle of the anterior chamber and aetiology of congenital glaucoma, Br J Ophthalmol 56:298, 1972

33. Hay, ED, and Revel, JP: Fine structure of the developing avian cornea. In Wolsky, A, and Chen, PS, editors: Monographs in developmental biology; vol, 1, Basel 1969, S Karger

34. Hay, ED: Development of the vertebrate cornea, Int Rev Cytol 63:263, 1980

35. Herrmann, H: Tissue interaction and differentiation in the corneal and scleral stroma. In Smelser, GK, editor: Structure of the eye, New York, 1961, Academic Press

36. Hogan, MJ, Alvarado, JA, and Wedell, J: Histology of the human eye, Philadelphia, 1971, W B Saunders

37. Hoskins, HD, Hetherington, J, Jr, Shaffer, RN, and Welling, AM: Developmental glaucomas: diagnosis and classification. In Cairns, JE, editor: Symposium on glaucoma, St Louis, 1981, The CV Mosby Co

38. Hoyt, CM, and Billson, F: Buphthalmos in neurofibromatosis: is it an expression of giantism? J Ped Ophthalmol 14:228, 1977

39. Jiang, GJ, et al: Neuron specific enolase in the Merkel cells of mammalian skin: the use of specific antibody as a simple and reliable histological marker, Am J Pathol 104:63, 1981

40. Johnston, MC: A radioautographic study of the migration and fate of cranial neural crest cells in the chick embryo, Anat Rec 156:143, 1966

41. Johnston, MC, et al: Origins of avian ocular and periocular tissues, Exp Eye Res 29:27, 1979

42. Kenyon, KR: Mesenchymal dysgenesis in Peters' anomaly, sclerocornea and congenital endothelial dystrophy, Exp Eye Res 21:125, 1975

43. Knight, MS: A critical survey of neoplasms of the choroid, Am J Ophthalmol 8:791, 1925

44. Kupfer, C: A note on the development of the anterior chamber angle, Invest Ophthalmol 8:69, 1969

45. Kupfer, C, Datilies, MB, and Kaiser-Kupfer, M: Development of the anterior chamber of the eye: embryology and clinical implications. In Lütjen-Drecoll, E, editor: Basic aspects of glaucoma research, Stuttgart, 1982, Schattauer

46. Kupfer, C, and Kaiser-Kupfer, MI: New hypothesis of developmental anomalies of the anterior chamber associated with glaucoma, Trans Ophthalmol Soc UK 98:213, 1978

47. Kupfer, C, Kaiser-Kupfer, MI, Datilies, M, and McCain, L: The contralateral eye in the iridocorneal endothelial (ICE) syndrome, Ophthalmology 90: 1343, 1983

48. Kupfer, C, Kuwabara, T, and Stark, W: The histopathology of Peters' anomaly, Am J Ophthalmol 80:653, 1975

49. Kupfer, C, and Ross, K: The development of outflow facility in the human eye, Invest Ophthalmol 10:513, 1971

50. Le Douarin, N: Migration and differentiation of neural crest cells., In: Moscona, AA, and Monroy, A, editors: Current topics in developmental biology, vol, 16: Hunt, RK, editor: Neural development, part, II, New York, 1980, Academic Press

51. Le Douarin, NM: The neural crest, Cambridge, 1982, University Press

52. Le Douarin, NM: Characteristiques ultrastructurales du noyau intephasique chez la caille et chez le poulet et utilisation de cellules de caille comme 'marquers biologiques' en embryologie experimentale, Ann Embryol Morphol 4:125, 1971

53. Le Lievre, CS: Participation of neural crest–derived cells in the genesis of the skull in birds, J Embryol Exp Morphol 47:17, 1978

54. Le Lievre, C, and Le Douarin, N: Mesenchymal derivatives in the neural crest: analysis of chimeric quail and chick embryos, J Embryol Exp Morphol 34:125, 1975

55. Lieb, WA, Wirth, WA, and Geeraets, WJ: Hydrophthalmos and neurofibromatosis, Confin Neurol 19:239, 1958

56. Mann, I: The development of the human eye, Cambridge, 1928, University Press

57. Mann, I: The development of the human eye, New York, 1950, Grune & Stratton

58. Mann, I: The development of the human eye, Cambridge, England, 1964, Cambridge University Press

59. Maul, E, Strozzi, L, Munoz, C, and Reyes, C: The outflow pathway in congenital glaucoma, Am J Ophthalmol 89:667, 1980

60. Maumenee, AE: The pathogenesis of congenital glaucoma: a new theory, Trans Am Ophthalmol Soc 56:507, 1958

61. Maumenee, AE: The pathogenesis of congenital glaucoma: a new theory, Am J Ophthalmol 47:827, 1959

62. Maumenee, AE: Further observations on the pathogenesis of congenital glaucoma, Trans Am Ophthalmol Soc 60:140, 1962

63. Maumenee, AE: Further observations on the pathogenesis of congenital glaucoma, Am J Ophthalmol 55:1163, 1963

64. Meier, S: Development of the chick embryo mesoblast: morphogenesis of the prechordal plate and cranial segments, Dev Biol 83:49, 1981

65. Michelson-Rabinowitsch, C: Beitrag zur Kenntnis des Hydrophthalmus congenitus, Arch Augenheilkd 55:245, 1906

66. Noden, DM: An analysis of the migratory behavior of avian cephalic neural crest cells, Dev Biol 42:106, 1975

67. Noden, DM: The control of avian cephalic neural crest cytodifferentiation. I. Skeletal and connective tissue, Dev Biol 67:296, 1978

68. Noden, DM: Periocular mesenchyme: neural crest and mesodermal interactions. In Jakobiec, FA, editor: Ocular anatomy, embryology, and teratology, Hagerstown, Md, 1982, Harper & Row

69. O'Rahilly, R: The prenatal development of the human eye, Exp Eye Res 21:93, 1975

70. Ozanics, V, and Jakobiec, FA: Prenatal development of the eye and its adnexa. In Jakobiec, FA, editor: Ocular anatomy, embryology, and teratology, Hagerstown, Md, 1982, Harper & Row

71. Ozanics, V, Rayborn, M, and Sagun, D: Some aspects of corneal and scleral differentiation in the primate, Exp Eye Res 22:305, 1976

72. Pandolfi, M, and Astedt, B: Outflow resistance in the fetal eye, Acta Ophthal Kbh 49:344, 1971

73. Pratt, RM, Larsen, MA, and Johnston, MC: Migration of cranial neural crest cells in a cell-free hyaluronate rich matrix, Dev Biol 44:298, 1975

74. Reme, C, and D'Épinay, SL: Periods of development of the normal human chamber angle, Doc Ophthalmol 51:241, 1981

75. Rodrigues, MM, et al: Glaucoma due to endothelialization of the anterior chamber angle: a comparison of posterior polymorphous dystrophy of the cornea and Chandler's syndrome, Arch Ophthalmol 98:688, 1980

76. Rodrigues, MM, Streeten, BW, and Spaeth, GL: Chandler's syndrome as a variant of essential iris atrophy: a clinicopathological study, Arch Ophthalmol 96:643, 1978

77. Royds, JA, Parson, MA, Taylor, CB, and Timperley, WR: Enolase isoenzyme distribution in the human brain and its tumors, J Pathol 137:37, 1982

78. Scheie, HG, and Yanoff, M: Peters' anomaly and total posterior coloboma of retinal pigment epithelium and choroid, Arch Ophthalmol 87:525, 1972

79. Schmechel, DE, and Marangos, PJ: Neuron-specific enolase (NSE): specific cellular and functional marker for neurons and neuroendocrine cells., In: Barker, JL, and McKelvy, JF, editors: Current methods in cellular neurobiology, New York, 1983, John Wiley & Sons

80. Schmechel, DE, et al: Brain enolases as specific markers of neuronal and glial cells, Science 199:313, 1978

81. Schwarz, W: Electronen mikroscpische Untersuchungen uber die Differenzierung der Cornea- und Sklera-Fibrillen des Menschen, Z Zellforsch 38:78, 1953

82. Seefelder, R: Die Entwicklung des menschlichen Auges., In: Schieck-Brückner Kurzes Handbuch der Ophthalmolgie vol, I, Berlin, 1930, Springer

83. Shaffer, RN: Pathogenesis of congenital glaucoma: gonioscopic and microscopic anatomy, Trans Am Acad Ophthalmol Otolaryngol 59:297, 1955

84. Shields, MB: Axenfeld-Rieger syndrome: a theory of mechanism and distinctions from the iridocorneal endothelial syndrome, Trans Am Ophthalmol Soc 81:736, 1983

85. Shields, MB, Buckley, E, Klintworth, G, and Thresher, R: Axenfeld-Rieger syndrome: a spectrum of developmental disorders, Surv Ophthalmol 29:387, 1985

86. Silver, PHS, and Wakely, J: The initial stage in the development of the lens capsule in chick and mouse embryo, Exp Eye Res 19:73, 1974

87. Smelser, GK, and Ozanics, V: The development of the trabecular meshwork in primate eyes, Am J Ophthalmol 71:366, 1971

88. Sondermann, R: Über Entstehung Morphologie und Funktion des Schlemmschen-Kanals, Acta Ophthalmol 11:280, 1933

89. Speakman, JS, and Leeson, TS: Pathological findings in a case of primary congenital glaucoma compared with normal infant eyes, Br J Ophthalmol 48:196, 1964

90. Stone, RA, Kuwayama, Y, Laties, AM, and Marangos, PJ: Neuron specific enolase containing cells in the rhesus monkey trabecular meshwork, Invest Ophthalmol Vis Sci 25:1332, 1984

91. Streeter, GL: Developmental horizons in human embryos, Contrib Embryol 34:165, 1951

92. Tawara, A, and Inomata, H: Developmental immaturity of the trabecular meshwork in congenital glaucoma, Am J Ophthalmol 92:508, 1981

93. Toole, BP, and Trelstad, RL: Hyaluronate production and removal during corneal development in the chick, Dev Biol 26:28, 1971

94. Tosney, KW: The early migration of neural crest cells in the trunk region of the avian eye: an electron microscope study, Dev Biol 62:317, 1978

95. Trelstad, RL, and Coulombre, AJ: Morphogenesis of the collagenous stroma in the chick cornea, J Cell Biol 50:840, 1971

96. Tripathi, BJ, and Tripathi, RC: Expressivity of neuronal specific enolase by keratocytes, Invest Ophthalmol Vis Sci 28 (suppl):29, 1987

97. Tripathi, BJ, et al: Origin of corneal endothelium and keratocytes in human eyes, Invest Ophthalmol Vis Sci 26 (Suppl):174, 1985

98. Tripathi, RC: Aqueous outflow pathway in normal and glaucomatous eyes, Br J Ophthalmol 56:157, 1972

99. Tripathi, RC: Comparative physiology and anatomy of the aqueous outflow pathway. In Davson, H, and Graham, LT, editors: The eye, vol, 5, New York, 1974, Academic Press

100. Tripathi, RC: The functional morphology of the outflow systems of ocular and cerebrospinal fluids, Exp Eye Res 25 (suppl):65, 1977

101. Tripathi, RC, Casey, TA, and Wise, G: Hereditary posterior polymorphous dystrophy: an ultrastructural and clinical report, Trans Ophthalmol Soc UK 94:211, 1974

102. Tripathi, RC, and Tripathi, BJ: Functional anatomy of the anterior chamber of the angle. In Duane, TD, and Jaeger, EA, editors: Biomedical foundations of ophthalmology, vol., 1, Hagerstown, Md, 1982, Harper & Row

103. Tripathi, RC, and Tripathi, BJ: Bulk flow of the humors of the eye and brain through vacuolar transendothelial channels, Prog Appl Microcir 9:118, 1985

104. Tripathi, RC, Tripathi, BJ, and Cibis, GW: Sturge-Weber syndrome. In Gold, DH, and Weingeist, TA, editors: The eye in systemic disease, Philadelphia, 1987, Lippincott

105. Tripathi, RC, Tripathi, BJ, and Gaster, RN: Clinicopathologic study of Peters' anomaly., In: Trevor-Roper, P, editor: The cornea in health and disease, The Royal Society of Medicine Int Congr Symp Series No, 40 London, 1981, Academic Press

106. Van Buskirk, EM: Clinical implications of iridocorneal angle development, Ophthalmology 88:361, 1981

107. Von Kölliker, RA: Entwicklungsgeschichte d. Menschen und der höheren Tiere, Leipzig, 1861, W Engelmann

108. Waring, GO, Rodriques, MM, and Laibson, PR: Anterior chamber cleavage syndrome: a stepladder classification, Surv Ophthalmol 20:3, 1975

109. Wartiovaara, J, Leivo, I, and Vaheri, A: Matrix glycoproteins in early mouse development and in differentiation of teratocarcinoma cells. In Subtelny, S, and Wessells, NK, editors: The cell surface: mediator of developmental processes, New York, 1980, Academic Press

110. Weiss, JS, and Ritch, R: Glaucoma in the phakomatoses. In Ritch, R, and Shields, MB, editors: The secondary glaucomas, St. Louis, 1982, The CV Mosby Co

111. Weston, JA: A radioautographic study of the migration and localization of trunk neural crest cells in the chick, Dev Biol 6:279, 1963

112. Wharton, J, et al: Neuron-specific enolase as an immunocytochemical marker for the diffuse neuroendocrine system in human fetal lung, J Histochem Cytochem 29:1359, 1981

113. Wheeler, JM: Plexiform neurofibromatosis involving the choroid, ciliary body and other structures. Am J Ophthalmol 20:368, 1937

114. Wiener, A: A case of neurofibromatosis with buphthalmus, Arch Ophthalmol 54:481, 1925

115. Wolter, JR, Sandall, GS, and Fralick, FB: Mesodermal dygenesis of anterior eye with a partially separated posterior embryotoxon, J Pediatr Ophthalmol 4:41, 1967

116. Worst, JGF: The pathogenesis of congenital glaucoma, Springfield, Il, 1966, Charles C Thomas

117. Worst, JGF: Congenital glaucoma: remarks on the aspect of chamber angle, ontogenic and pathogenic background, and mode of action of goniotomy, Invest Ophthalmol 7:127, 1968

118. Wulle, KG: Electron microscopic observations of the development of Schlemm's canal in the human eye, Trans Am Acad Ophthalmol Otolaryngol 72:765, 1968

119. Wulle, KG: The development of the productive and draining system of the aqueous humor in the human eye, Adv Ophthalmol 26:296, 1972

120. Wulle, KG: Electron microscopy of the fetal development of the corneal endothelium and Descemet's membrane of the human eye, Invest Ophthalmol 11:897, 1972

121. Wulle, KG, and Lerche, W: Electron microscopic observations of the early development of the human corneal endothelium and Descemet's membrane, Ophthalmologica 157:451, 1969

122. Wulle, KG, Ruprecht, KW, and Windrath, LC: Electron microscopy of the development of the cell junctions in the embryonic and fetal human corneal endothelium, Invest Ophthalmol 13:923, 1974

123. Yamada, T: Morphological and biochemical aspects of cytodifferentiation: differentiation of lens cells. In Hagen, E, Wechsler, W, Zilliken, P, and Gardner, AF, editors: Experimental biology and medicine, I, Basel 1967, Karger

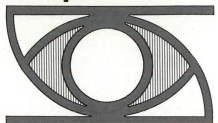

Chapter 2

Morphology of Aqueous Outflow Pathways in Normal and Glaucomatous Eyes

Johannes W. Rohen
Elke Lütjen-Drecoll

MORPHOLOGY OF THE NORMAL AQUEOUS OUTFLOW PATHWAYS

In the primate eye, aqueous humor is produced by the ciliary body. The ciliary epithelium plays an important role—energy-dependent, active-transport processes being the primary mechanism for aqueous humor production. The "primary aqueous humor" enters the posterior chamber, where its composition may be altered by reabsorption by either the iris or ciliary body or by the addition of metabolites and other compounds from the surrounding tissues, such as the lens. This "secondary aqueous humor" passes from the posterior chamber through the pupil into the anterior chamber. From the region of the anterior chamber angle aqueous humor can leave the eye by two routes. The first (direct) outflow pathway is through the trabecular meshwork into Schlemm's canal, the collector channels of Schlemm's canal, and then into the intrascleral and episcleral venus plexuses (see Chapter 8). The second (indirect) outflow pathway originates with passage of aqueous humor through the ciliary body. The aqueous humor flows along the interstitial spaces of the ciliary muscle and choroid or the suprachoroidal space through the sclera (transsclerally) or together with the vascular channels of the sclera into the connective tissue of the orbit. From there it probably drains via veins into the general circulation. This indirect fluid stream, which is called uveoscleral flow,[10,11,176] is independent of intraocular pressure and may be analogous to the drainage of lymphatic fluid in other organs of the body (see Chapter 8). In the monkey, the uveoscleral flow amounts to 0.8 μl/min.[12] In the human eye it accounts for less than 20% of the total drainage of aqueous humor.[13]

Aqueous humor may also leave the anterior chamber via iris vessels or iris stroma. In human and monkey eyes, the anterior leaf of the iris, particularly the endothelial lining, is incomplete. It contains variable-sized pores or crypts,[122,124,126,152] which allow aqueous humor to penetrate freely into the iris stroma and reach the vessel wall, which shows a number of structural peculiarities. The perivascular sheath of the iris vessels contains a high concentration of sulfated glycosaminoglycans and hyaluronidase-resistant substances such as keratan sulfate and heparan sulfate proteoglycans, the amount of which increases with age.[155] In rhesus monkeys it has been shown that horseradish peroxidase and anionic ferritin, perfused into the anterior chamber, can permeate into the stroma of the iris and iris vessels by transcellular vesicular transport.[107,108] Iridial vessels are, however, bidirectionally impermeable to cationic ferritin, that is, from the bloodstream to the stroma or from the anterior chamber toward the vessel lumen. There seems to be a unidirectional transport mechanism across the endothelium of iridial vessels responsible for the selective movements of anionic organic substances from aqueous humor or iris tissue into the bloodstream. Thus, iris vessels seem to behave in a way similar to that of vessels of the retina or brain.

Organization of the Trabecular Meshwork in Normal Eyes

Only higher primates and humans have developed a "trabecular" meshwork in the true sense of the word, consisting of lamellated sheets bordering on an organized vessel wall (Schlemm's canal). Lower monkeys (Prosimiae) and other mammals have a "reticular" meshwork, which covers a broader area of the sclera. Schlemm's canal is not seen, but instead many small vessel loops bend into the meshwork.[123,130] In these species, the chamber angle is filled with radial, interlacing strands of the so-called pectinate ligament, which includes the system of Fontana's spaces.[124,125,130]

In the course of primate evolution the pectinate ligament gradually becomes reduced (remnants can still be found in human eyes), and the ciliary body is "unified," a result of the greater differen-

tiation of the ciliary muscle. Also, the mechanisms for accommodation and Schlemm's canal both develop.[130] The morphologic and functional division of the human trabecular meshwork into three or four different portions is probably the result of that evolutionary process.

Anterior trabecular meshwork

The trabecular meshwork can be divided into two parts (Fig. 2-1). The most anterior portion lies adjacent to that portion of the limbus just posterior to Schwalbe's line. It has no contact with Schlemm's canal and is therefore termed the nonfiltering part of the trabecular meshwork. This part consists of three to five trabecular beams covered by small trabecular cells that often lie closely together, forming elongated bands or rows. They are in contact with the keratocytes of the posterior lamellae of the cornea. In experimental studies in monkeys, it has been hypothesized that the trabecular cells of the nonfiltering meshwork are regenerated by the keratocytes of the cornea.[71-73] If entire specimens of the chamber angle tissues are kept under tissue-culture conditions, these cells become enlarged and seem to proliferate. In the eyes of various monkey species, elongated bands or strands of cells are often seen in this region. These are termed opercular cells because, together with broad trabecular beams, they form a cover (oper-

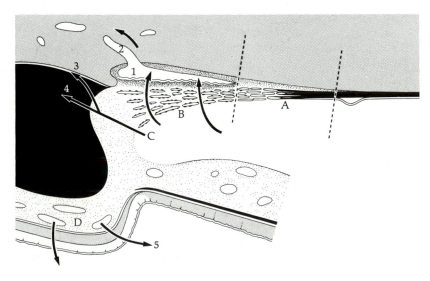

Fig. 2-1 Schematic drawing of human iridocorneal angle tissues (sagittal section). *A*, Area of nonfiltering trabecular meshwork. *B*, Filtration portion of trabecular meshwork; arrows indicate aqueous humor flow through meshwork into Schlemm's canal *(1)* and from canal into a collector channel *(2)*. *C*, Uveoscleral route of aqueous humor outflow; arrows indicate flow across root of iris *(3)* into ciliary body and suprachoridal space *(4)*. *D*, Aqueous humor flow from ciliary processes *(5)* into posterior chamber.

culum) over the anterior portion of the filtering meshwork.[37,38,85,138] Raviola[106] described a similar structure in the rhesus monkey. The opercular cells, termed by Raviola "Schwalbe's line cells," contain a high concentration of lamellar bodies, thought to be deposits of phospholipids. In recent immunohistochemical studies, enolase-containing cells were discovered in this region of the rhesus monkey eye.[168] These were considered to be neurosecretory.

Some authors believe that the cell population of the nonfiltering trabecular meshwork is derived from corneal endothelium. However, morphologically and histochemically, both cell systems differ significantly from each other; for example, the corneal endothelial cells contain a great amount of the enzyme carbonic anhydrase, whereas the trabecular cells do not. Positive staining of the corneal endothelium for carbonic anhydrase (Hansson histochemical stain) in the human eye stops at Schwalbe's line, whereas in the cynomolgus monkey, the staining extends posteriorly as far as the operculum.[75,76] Furthermore, in experimental and tissue-culture studies, cell degeneration or cell loss is often seen in corneal endothelial cells, whereas the cells of the nonfiltering and outer portions of the trabecular meshwork appear relatively stable. Although there is some evidence that the trabecular cells are different in structure and origin from the corneal endothelium, no final conclusion can as yet be drawn.

In the nonfiltering region, Descemet's membrane tapers off continuously toward its posterior end, splitting into several lamellae that are continuous with the basement-membrane-like sheets of the trabecular beams. This relationship between Descemet's membrane and the subendothelial membranes of the trabecular beams became evident with immunofluorescent studies using antibodies against laminin and collagen type IV.[69] With laminin-staining immunofluorescent techniques, it often seems that the subendothelial membrane can be divided into two parts. There is a very small intensely fluorescent line underneath the trabecular endothelial lining, whereas the adjacent broader band appears less intense. The small line may be the basal lamina of the trabecular cells, whereas the broader band may correspond to what the authors of earlier literature called "glass membranes."

In the transitional zone toward the cornea there are a number of peculiar morphologic structures.[137,179] Based on scanning electron micrographic studies, Svedbergh and Bill described four different zones in the adult human eye.[171] Zone I includes most of the cornea, and zone IV comprises the transitional area at the border of the trabecular meshwork. In the second zone, which measures about 500 to 1000 μm in width, the corneal endothelial cells possess a single, centrally located cilium 2 to 7 μm long. In the third zone (50 to 150 μm wide) the cells appear more irregular and without cilia. Here, the so-called Hassall-Henle's warts are often present. These warts consist of irregularly arranged collagen fibers forming clusters or knots that protrude into the anterior chamber. Among the collagenous fiber bundle homogeneous material and, as a rule, large amounts of long-spacing, curly or lattice collagen can be found.

The functional significance of the cilia of the posterior corneal endothelial cells is not clear. Using a replica technique, Wolf described a viscous layer covering the endothelial lining that he thought to contain glycoproteins and hyaluronic acid.[180] He assumed that this film is moved posteriorly toward the filtering portion of the trabecular meshwork by a coordinated movement of cilia. However, these assumptions remain hypothetical.

The transitional zone also contains holes, grooves, or small channels usually filled with cells or cytoplasmic processes. Whether these channels serve as fluid transport pathways or only as spaces for accessory cells needed for regeneration or repair is not known.

Filtering trabecular meshwork

The filtering portion of the trabecular meshwork covers the inner wall of Schlemm's canal. It consists of three morphologically distinct, and most probably functionally different portions (from outward to inward): (1) the cribriform layer, (2) the corneoscleral meshwork, and (3) the uveal meshwork (Fig. 2-2; see also Plate I, Fig. 1). At the inner surface of the uveal meshwork, remnants of the pectinate ligament in the form of radial, interlacing strands (iris processes) connecting the iris root with the trabecular meshwork or the cornea are often seen.

The *cribriform layer* (juxtacanalicular tissue; endothelial meshwork; pore tissue) comprises the outermost part of the trabecular meshwork adjacent to the inner wall endothelium of Schlemm's canal. It contains a network of fine fibrils, elastic-like fibers, and a number of elongated, fibroblast-like cells arranged in layers (Fig. 2-3). The cells are embedded within a homogeneous or fine fibrillar, extracellular material that in electron micrographs

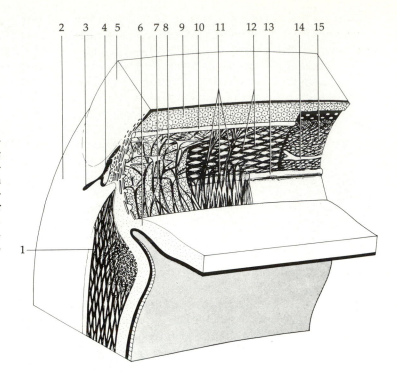

Fig. 2-2 Architecture of trabecular meshwork. Ciliary muscle *(1);* sclera *(2);* collector channel *(3);* Schlemm's canal *(4);* cornea *(5);* iris root *(6);* iris processes *(7);* uveal meshwork *(8);* corneal endothelium *(9);* Schwalbe's line *(10);* anterior ciliary muscle tendons *(11);* corneoscleral meshwork *(12);* scleral spur *(13);* Sondermann's channel *(14);* cribriform layer *(15).* (After Rohen, JW, and Unger, HM: Mainz, NR., 3, Wiesbaden, 1959, Steiner Verlag.) See also Plate I, Fig. 1.

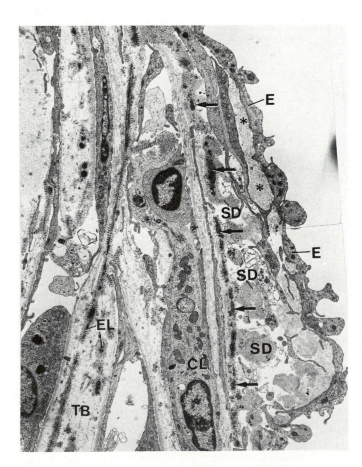

Fig. 2-3 Electron micrograph of cribriform layer. (Sagittal section, 50-year-old human, ×6000.) Subendothelial elastic-like fiber network of cribriform layer *(arrows);* subendothelial amorphous material *(asterisks);* endothelium of Schlemm's canal *(E);* elastic-like fibers *(EL);* cribriform layer cells *(CL);* trabecular beam *(TB);* sheath-derived plaques surrounding connecting fibrils *(SD).*

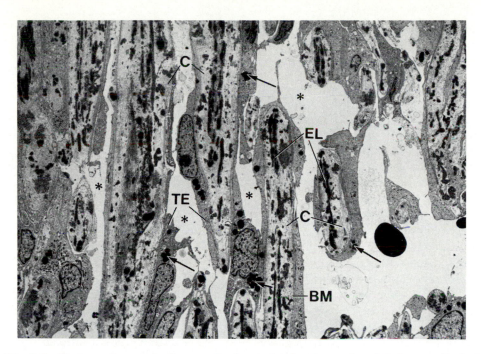

Fig. 2-4 Electron micrograph of corneoscleral part of trabecular meshwork in human. (Sagittal section, ×2310.) Pigment granules *(arrows)*; intertrabecular spaces *(asterisks)*; basement membrane *(BM)*; collageneous fibers *(C)*; elastic-like fibers *(EL)*; trabecular cells *(TE)*.

can appear as "empty spaces."[67] These "spaces" may represent preferential aqueous pathways through the cribriform layer toward the inner wall endothelium.

The *corneoscleral meshwork* extends from the scleral spur toward the cornea, filling the scleral sulcus. It comprises the main portion of the trabecular meshwork and consists of flat, interlacing beams or plates (Fig. 2-4). Each lamella contains a central core, consisting of ground-substance, collagenous, and elastic-like fibers. Normally, the lamellae are completely covered by a single layered endothelial lining that is supported by a basement membrane, called "glass membrane" in the earlier literature.

The *uveal meshwork* continues posteriorly with the ciliary body and iris root; anteriorly it tapers and is anchored at the inner layers of the corneal stroma or corneoscleral meshwork. The uveal meshwork consists of irregularly arranged strands or sheets, running mostly radially. These strands are connected with each other, forming a broad network with oval or round pores and openings 10 to 20 μm in diameter (Fig. 2-5). The strands are covered by endothelial cells that rest on a relatively thick basement membrane. The core of the uveal strands consists mostly of collagenous fibers, among which elastic-like fibers are distributed. The

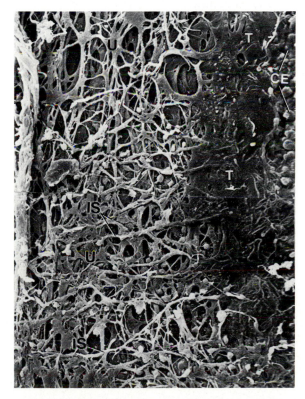

Fig. 2-5 Scanning electron micrograph of uveal meshwork and nonfiltering part of meshwork. (Internal aspect, ×1640.) Corneal endothelium *(CE)*; iris processes *(IS)*; transitional zone *(T)*; uveal meshwork *(U)*.

fiber system is arranged less regularly than the latticelike pattern of the corneoscleral portion.

Cell system of the trabecular meshwork

Trabecular cells produce glycosaminoglycans, extracellular glycoproteins, and fibrillar material.* They also are highly phagocytic,[149,151] removing particles, cellular debris, or protein molecules from the circulating aqueous humor (see Plate I, Fig. 5). Thus, the trabecular meshwork is capable of "cleaning" the aqueous humor and thereby preventing obstruction of the intertrabecular and cribriform pathways. The meshwork cells are capable of incorporating not only particles but also red blood cells, pigment granules of various sizes, and bacteria or microspheres.† Phagocytized material is enclosed in membrane-limited vacuoles that fuse with lysosomes forming phagolysosomes, which are stored within the cells. Macrophages or trabecular cells may lose contact with the trabecular beams and pass through the endothelium of Schlemm's canal, thus entering the circulatory system.[27,151] Normally, macrophages are also found within the trabecular meshwork, seeming to move freely through the intertrabecular spaces and inner wall endothelium.[35,151,161,179] They may enter the meshwork either via Schlemm's canal or from the iris and ciliary body.

Under tissue culture conditions, the trabecular cells are capable of synthesizing hyaluronic acid and glycosaminoglycans (GAGs), probably in the form of proteoglycans.‡ They also produce extracellular glycoproteins, such as fibronectin and laminin, which have been shown to play a role in cellular attachment and cell-matrix interaction.[100,101,180] Fibronectin has been recently demonstrated in human aqueous drainage channels, particularly in the inner and outer wall of Schlemm's canal. Interestingly, fibronectin staining is more abundant in the cribriform layer of Schlemm's canal than in the adjacent trabecular meshwork.[22]

In organ cultures derived from normal autopsy eyes, intense labeling of cribriform cells with ^{14}C-glucosamine was found, indicating that these cells in particular might be capable of synthesizing hyaluronic acid or GAGs.[146,148] After 2 to 4 days in culture the cribriform cells develop an elaborate system of rough-surfaced endoplasmic reticulum, many Golgi vesicles, and an increased number of mitochondria, indicating that they are highly metabolically active. In contrast, the uveal meshwork cells often degenerate or swell after in vitro cultivation.[141,147,148]

These and other observations lead to the assumption that the trabecular meshwork normally contains three basic cells:

1. The trabecular cells, which cover the beams of the corneoscleral meshwork or the strands and plates of the uveal meshwork in an epithelial-like manner, always resting on a basal lamina. They may be predominantly involved in the self-cleaning processes of the trabecular meshwork by phagocytosis, fibrillogenesis, and tissue repair.

2. The cribriform cells, which are distributed at random within the extracellular matrix of the cribriform layer beneath the endothelial lining of Schlemm's canal. They do not rest on a basement membrane, but the outermost cells contact the canal endothelium through mushroomlike cytoplasmic processes. They may be responsible for the production of the extracellular substances and fibrillar structures of the cribriform layer and their outflow channels. The cribriform cells might derive from perivascular cells such as pericytes or adventitial cells of Rouget and therefore enter the eye with the blood vessels. On the other hand, the trabecular cells are derived from neural crest cells, as are all other cells of the uvea and corneosclera except the cells of the vessel wall and the nerves.

3. The endothelial lining of Schlemm's canal, which clearly derives from mesodermal tissue.[61] These cells produce the underlying basement membrane material, but most probably not the plaque material deposited within the cribriform layer.[139,150] The inner wall endothelium is capable of developing pores, vacuoles, and transcellular microchannels through which aqueous fluid and particles and even erythrocytes can pass.[51,64,174]

Connection between the trabecular meshwork and the ciliary muscle system

The human ciliary muscle consists of smooth muscle fibers that form bundles surrounded by a sheath of fibroblasts.[52,121,126,178] These bundles are connected with each other so that a syncytium-like network is formed with a predominantly longitudinal orientation of fiber bundles in the outer part and more circular orientation in the inner part of

---

*References 22, 32, 70, 100, 101, 127, 134, 141, 181.
†References 27, 35, 64, 103, 161, 163, 165.
‡References 98-100, 101, 141, 145-147, 156-158.

the system.[119,120,126] The sheaths may enable the muscle bundles to glide between them, resulting in a gradual rearrangement of the entire network during muscle contraction. The longitudinal muscle fiber bundles taper off anteriorly, forming three different types of tendons, which penetrate into either the scleral spur or the trabecular meshwork[126,130,134,137,149] (Fig. 2-6). The type A tendons affix the outermost fiber bundles of the longitudinal portion to the sclera or scleral spur. The type B tendons consist of wide, flat strands of mainly collagenous material and pass through the entire trabecular meshwork without a major connection with the trabecular lamellae. They are anchored within the posterior corneal stroma layers. The type C tendons form brushlike terminations of elastic-like fibers that bend into the fiber system of the outermost corneoscleral meshwork and cribriform layer, thereby changing their course by about 90 degrees. A number of these tendons are connected with a delicate network of elastic-like fibers located within the cribriform layer, termed "cribriform plexus"[134] (Fig. 2-7). Bundles of fine fibrils derive from this plexus and run radially toward the endothelial lining of Schlemm's canal and are there-

fore termed "connecting fibrils"[134] (Fig. 2-8, A). According to recent histochemical studies, the connecting fibrils most probably represent oxytalan fibers.

The fibroblasts of the anterior ciliary muscle sheaths are continuous with the cells covering the trabecular lamellae. The muscle fiber tips become elongated, thereby forming fingerlike protrusions or indentations that develop many adhesion plaques at their cell membranes. Outside these membrane thickenings, elastic-like fibers originate, forming the type C tendons. These are surrounded by the same sheath material, also characteristic of the elastic-like fiber system of the trabecular lamellae (Fig. 2-8, B). Posteriorly, the intertrabecular spaces are continuous with the interstitial spaces of the longitudinal portion of the ciliary muscle system.

This elaborate connection between the longitudinal ciliary muscle bundles and the cribriform layer of the trabecular meshwork may well explain the functional relationship between the two. In monkeys as well as in humans, outflow resistance is significantly reduced after pilocarpine-induced ciliary muscle contraction.[6,7] After disinsertion of

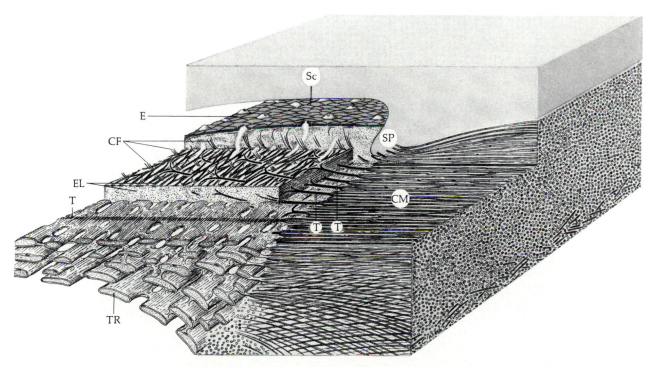

Fig. 2-6 Anterior ciliary muscle tendons *(T)* and their connections with trabecular meshwork. Connecting fibrils *(CF)*; ciliary muscle *(CM)*; endothelium of Schlemm's canal *(E)*; elastic-like fibers *(EL)*; Schlemm's canal *(Sc)*; scleral spur *(SP)*; ciliary muscle tendons *(T)*; trabecular meshwork (corneoscleral part) *(TR)*. (After Rohen, JW: Ophthalmology 90:758, 1983. Published courtesy of Ophthalmology)

the anterior ciliary muscle tendons, miotics lose much of their resistance-reducing effect.[55,74]

Analysis of sagittal sections shows that miotics cause the diameter of the entire trabecular meshwork to increase and the scleral spur to move posteriorly, causing a marked spreading of the trabecular meshwork lamellae.* Spreading alone, how-

ever, cannot explain the increase in outflow facility following administration of miotics, because the intertrabecular spaces and holes of the uveal and corneoscleral meshwork are too large to contribute significantly to changes in outflow resistance.

Experimental and theoretical studies suggest that the main part of outflow resistance is located not within the pores and microchannels of the canal endothelium itself[14] nor within the uveal and

---

*References 36, 37, 126, 130, 137, 149.

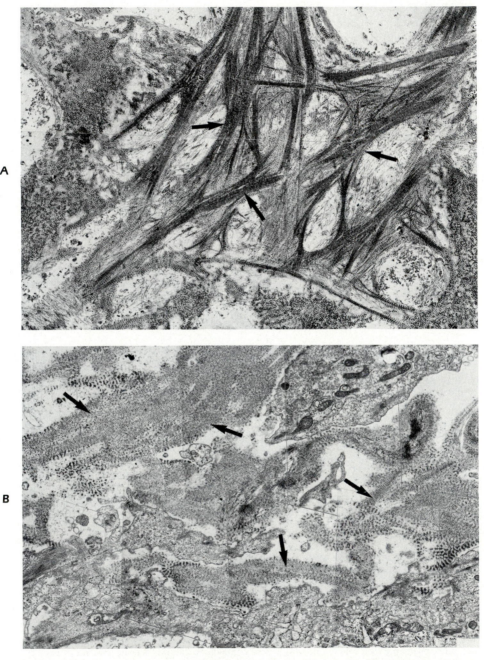

Fig. 2-7 Tangential sections through inner wall of Schlemm's canal at level of cribriform plexus (i.e., subendothelial elastic-like fiber network [arrows] in normal, **A,** and glaucomatous, **B,** eye). (Electron micrographs; **A,** ×6600, **B,** ×10,000.)

corneoscleral portion of the trabecular meshwork, but most probably within the cribriform layer.[67,88] Perfusion experiments with particles of various sizes or with tracers show preferential pathways for aqueous flow, located mainly within the cribriform region.[48-51] In stumptail macaques, there is a significant positive correlation between outflow facility and the area of "empty spaces" of the cribriform layer that are in close contact with the inner wall endothelium.[67] These electron microscopically "empty spaces" probably indicate the presence of actual filtering pathways for aqueous flow. These cribriform aqueous pathways are not thoroughly connected with each other, so that the inner wall is divided into a number of compartments sepa-

rated from each other by cribriform cells and extracellular material. If the number of these small pathways increases, the actual filtering area would increase significantly and lower the outflow resistance proportionally.

It is reasonable to assume that the delicate fiber system of the cribriform layer—the cribriform fiber plexus that is connected with the type C ciliary muscle tendons—could modify the diameter of the cribriform layer and thereby the number of the cribriform aqueous pathways. Inward pulling of the "cribriform fiber plexus" by the ciliary muscle tendons would increase the diameter of the cribriform layer, opening up the cribriform aqueous pathways, particularly in the anterior portion of the

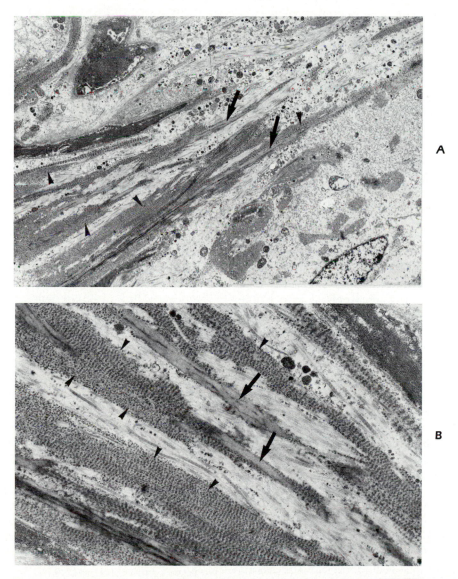

Fig. 2-8 Anterior ciliary muscle tendons consisting of elastic fibers *(arrows)* embedded in periodically banded sheath material *(arrowheads)*. (Electron micrographs; **A,** ×16,000, **B,** ×44,160.)

meshwork, which is often collapsed, and increase the area of filtration, thereby leading to a reduction in outflow resistance. In fact, Grierson et al.[36,40] found a significant increase in the frequency of giant vacuoles of the inner wall endothelium after topical administration of pilocarpine in the human eye, indicating that the filtering area and the number of cribriform pathways in immediate contact with the endothelium of Schlemm's canal had also increased.[39,64] The construction of the subendothelial fiber system also provides for the possibility of a stronger contraction of the ciliary muscle to widen the lumen of Schlemm's canal by an inward movement of its endothelial lining. Such changes might also affect outflow resistance and flow under certain conditions.[87-89]

After filtering operations such as trabeculectomy in monkeys, an increase in homogeneous material in the cribriform layer has been observed. This could be caused by an underperfusion of the nonoperated part of the trabecular meshwork.[68,141]

Collector Channels and Schlemm's Canal

Schlemm's canal represents a more or less complete circular channel embedded within the scleral sulcus, more comparable to a lymphatic vessel than to a vein or capillary. In sagittal sections, the diameter of the canal varies from 350 to 500 μm.[44,77,143] The canal is not uniform in shape and size, but frequently splits into branches separated by septa or tissue bridges. Anteriorly, the lumen is most often collapsed, whereas posteriorly it is wider and occasionally shows extensions into the trabecular meshwork, which Theobald[173] called "internal collector channels of Sondermann." The endothelial lining of Sondermann's channels is continuous with that of Schlemm's canal. It reveals no openings into the intertrabecular spaces, and these channels are simply diverticula of the canal. Their functional significance may be to increase the filtering area in a region where the diameter of the meshwork is maximal.

Schlemm's canal is covered with a single layered *endothelial lining*, the structure of which differs in the outer and inner wall. The endothelial cells of the inner wall normally show an elongated, spindlelike form with an average length of 160 μm (area about 408 μm²), whereas the outer wall cells are shorter and larger (area about 792 μm²).[78] Therefore, the number of cells is greater at the inner wall than at the outer wall. The inner wall cells are firmly connected with each other by maculae adhaerentes and zonulae occludentes and occasional gap junctions.[109]

Many of these cells contain giant vacuoles of various sizes[45] that are not found in the outer wall endothelium or the endothelial cells covering the septa or bridges of the canal. The intracellular giant vacuoles communicate both with the subendothelial layer and with the lumen of the canal by way of small pores or openings.* In humans, the diameter of the pores on the canal side varies between 0.5 and 1.5 μm, and on the meshwork side between 0.12 and 0.38 μm.[56] The number of pores on the meshwork side is greater than on the opposite side.

The existence of the giant vacuoles in vivo was questioned by Shabo et al.,[162,164] who considered them postmortem artifacts. They are not seen when the trabecular meshwork is fixed by perfusion from the canal side via episcleral veins. After perfusion of the anterior chamber with horseradish peroxidase in the monkey eye, the tracer passes through the vacuoles into the lumen of the canal[86] but not through the intercellular spaces. The frequency and size of the giant vacuoles are proportional to the pressure in the anterior chamber,† increasing with a rise in intraocular pressure or decreasing if the pressure is reduced.[28-30,96] Thus, giant vacuoles are preexisting structures forming transcellular microchannels by which aqueous humor can pass into Schlemm's canal.

The intercellular gaps or clefts, which are closed off by an elaborate system of tight junctions, seem to be insignificant for normal bulk flow.[109] These paracellular routes may, however, allow the penetration of macrophages or other cells into the lumen of the canal. It has been suggested that the inner wall may function as a one-way valve, preventing reflux of blood cells or proteins from the canal into the meshwork and anterior chamber.[26] After an abrupt paracentesis or sudden decrease of intraocular pressure, however, the inner wall endothelium can rupture and plasma proteins or (in experimental situations) tracer particles can enter the anterior chamber.[8,105,172] A moderate paracentesis leads only to a reduction in the number of giant vacuoles.[97] Small ruptures of the canal endothelium can be occluded by blood-borne thrombocytes.

The *outer wall* endothelium is supported by a complete basement membrane. However, the inner wall endothelium has hardly any basement membrane, because of regression during embryonic development.[178,182] Furthermore, the canal is

---

*References 45, 46, 51, 64, 164, 174.
†References 28-31, 34, 53, 64, 170.

surrounded by collagenous fiber bundles and by a network of elastic-like fibers embedded in a homogeneous ground substance rich in glycosaminoglycan-containing proteins. The elastic fiber network resembles that of the inner wall and is similarly connected with the endothelial lining of the canal by fine connecting fibrils. Recently deposits of plaque material were also found within the outer wall of Schlemm's canal that had the same appearance as that of the cribriform layer.[72] This plaque material develops from the sheaths of the elastic-like fibers and their connecting fibrils, particularly underneath the outer wall endothelium in the same manner observed in the inner wall region.

The outer wall normally contains three to six layers of fibroblast-like cells that, in organ culture, show a great tendency to proliferate. While proliferating, the cells increase considerably in size and develop an elaborate endoplasmic reticulum, many mitochondria, and ribosomes.[141,142,145,146] Cellular reactions of this kind were also seen in the cribriform layer. The biologic reactions of the inner and outer wall, which probably have the same origin, may therefore be of the same nature.

From the outer wall of Schlemm's canal, 25 to 35 *collector channels* emerge, which are connected to the vascular system of the limbal region.[5,143,144] The number and form vary around the circumference of the eye (Fig. 2-9). As a rule they are more numerous nasally than temporally.[5,58,59,173] Two different types of collector channels can be distinguished: (1) Direct channels (in humans normally only four to six) that run directly toward the episcleral venous plexus without anastomosing with the intrascleral vessels. They may also represent the so-called aqueous veins, observed in vivo.[3,24,58,59] (2) Indirect collector channels, which are smaller and more numerous and join the intrascleral capillary network only a short distance from the canal.

The openings of the collector channels in the outer wall of Schlemm's canal often show toruslike or liplike thickenings that might direct the flow from the lumen into these outlets. Flat, silver-impregnated specimens of the inner and outer wall show a very regular pattern of silver lines[78] that may mimic the directions of aqueous flow toward the collector channel openings. The entrance to the

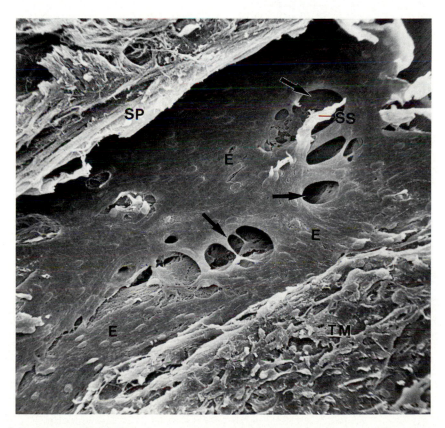

Fig. 2-9   Outer wall of Schlemm's canal in 60-year-old normal eye. Entrance to collector channels *(arrows)*; outer wall endothelium *(E)*; scleral spur *(SP)*; septum of Schlemm's canal *(SS)*; trabecular meshwork *(TM)*. (Scanning electron micrograph; ×4200.)

collector channels at the outer wall seems to correspond to preferential pathways in the inner wall of the canal.[177] Connective tissue bridges and septa of Schlemm's canal are often tortuous or oblique. They may facilitate the outflow current and ensure that the entrances of the collector channels remain open.

Structural Changes of the Outflow System with Increasing Age

In the aging eye, the trabecular beams thicken as a result of thickening of the subendothelial basement membranes or changes of the extracellular material within the central core.[138,139] The lattice collagen shows a regular banding with a periodicity of 100 to 120 nm (Fig. 2-10, *A*). Normal collagen fibers can enter the lattice collagen clusters, which then appear as small fibers among the dark bands, crossing them at right angles. After digestion with collagenase and testicular hyaluronidase, parts of the small collagen fibers are dissolved, while the dark, electron-dense bands remain unchanged.[69,70] With increasing age, protein-bound methionine is oxidized to methionine sulfoxide, which is probably incorporated into the clusters of lattice collagen.[47]

A regular banding with a smaller periodicity (40 to 50 nm) is found within the basement membranes. This occurs most often in the uveal and

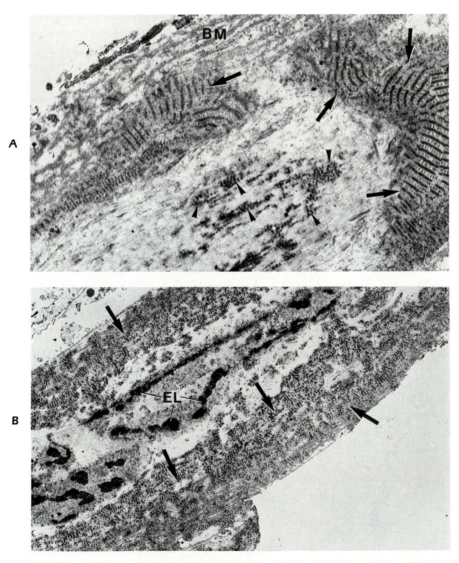

Fig. 2-10 Cross sections of trabecular beams with clusters of long-spacing or "lattice" collagen *(arrows).* **A,** Trabeculectomy specimen, pseudoexfoliation glaucoma. Note long-spacing lamellation of basement membrane *(BM)* and the deposits of atypical collagen *(arrowheads).* **B,** Trabeculectomy specimen, primary open-angle glaucoma. Note enormous thickening of basement membranes and their shagreenlike structure *(arrows). (EL),* Elastic-like fibers within central core. (**A,** ×44,160; **B,** ×9200.)

inner corneoscleral lamellae, and within the sheaths of the elastic-like fibers (Fig. 2-10,*B*). The sheaths of the elastic-like fibers consist of delicate, fine fibrils embedded in a homogeneous matrix that is less electron dense than the core. In contrast to the core, which remains unchanged with age, the sheath increases markedly in diameter, incorporating clusters of cross-banded material that shows periodicities of 40 to 50 nm or 100 to 120 nm[69,70] (Fig. 2-11). The core itself consists of electron-dense material intermingled with strands of an electron-transparent material. After digestion with pancreatic elastase, the electron-transparent strands are dissolved, indicating that only this small portion of the core consists of elastin. The sheaths can partly be digested by collagenases and chondroitinases; therefore they contain sulfated glycosaminoglycans, probably in the form of proteoglycans.[69,70] Here again, the clusters of banded structures (e.g., lattice collagen) remain almost unchanged.

With increasing age, there is a continuous loss of cells within the corneoscleral and uveal portion of the trabecular meshwork.[1,2,42] Denuded areas of trabecular lamellae show an increased amount of lattice collagen.[66,71] The decrease in cell number is slightly greater in the central part of the trabecular meshwork than in the anterior and posterior portions.

In the cribriform layer there also seems to be a continuous cell loss with increasing age. The main change is the development of extracellular material, which appears as irregular clusters, bands, or "plaques" (see Plate I, Fig. 3). Initially, three different types of plaques were distinguished.[150] Type I plaques are of relatively low electron density and are localized immediately beneath the inner wall endothelium. We assume that they derive from remnants of the basement membrane material that normally disappears in the course of postnatal development.[182,183] Type III plaques, which are highly electron dense, are crosssections of the elastic-like fibers. Type II plaques are the most important structures in this region. They often are immediately adjacent to the elastic-like fibers but can also appear as isolated plaquelike deposits in the neighborhood of the cribriform fiber plexus. They often contain cross-banded fibers with a periodicity of 45 to 50 nm or more.[128-130,132,133] Serial tangential sections oriented parallel to the inner wall endothelium reveal that the type II plaques are not plaques in the true sense of the word but extensions or thickenings of the sheaths of the elastic-like fibers. They often lose contact with these fibers and form broad interlacing plates or sheets within the cribriform layer.[134] This type of extracellular material has therefore been called sheath-derived plaque material (SD-plaques).[130,132]

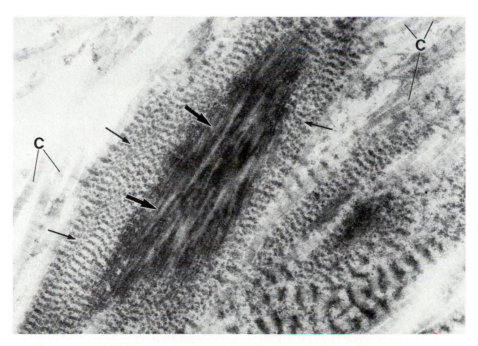

Fig. 2-11 Elastic-like fibers of trabecular meshwork after incubation with alcian-blue. *(Thick arrows)* Central core; *(small, long arrows)* sheath material with regular banding; *(C)*, collageneous fibers. (Electron micrograph; ×80,000.)

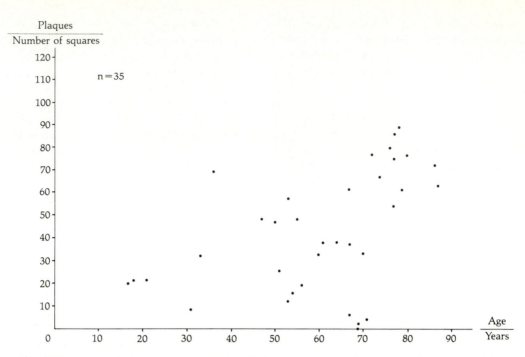

Fig. 2-12 Scatter diagram showing relationship between inner wall plaques and age in normal autopsy eyes. (After Lütjen-Drecoll, E, et al: Exp Eye Res 42:443, 1986)

This material also develops around the connecting fibrils, so that these fibrils are often completely masked (see Fig. 2-7, *B*). If, however, enzyme digestion methods are used, the plaque material can generally be dissolved so that the connecting fibrils become visible again.[70]

Within the cribriform layer, deposits of SD-plaque material continuously increase with age.[64,79,80,134,139] (Fig. 2-12). They contain hyaluronidase-digestible material, various kinds of chondroitin sulfates, and some dermatan sulfate proteoglycans.[70] Extracellular material of this kind also occurs within the outer wall of Schlemm's canal and between the anterior ciliary muscle bundle tips.[41] The amount of plaques increases with age. There is a positive correlation between the amount of the inner and outer wall plaques.[79,80] It might, therefore, be possible that the outer and inner wall of Schlemm's canal react in the same way.

With increasing age, the number of vacuoles and pores in the inner wall endothelium seems to become reduced.[33,42,84] The area covered by amorphous plaque material beneath the inner wall endothelium decreases with age, whereas the area of SD-plaques increases.[64,83] The reason for this increase in SD-plaque material is unclear. Surprisingly, there is no concomitant increase of intraocular pressure, probably because of a simultaneous reduction in the rate of aqueous formation with increasing age.[9,65]

In contrast, the collageneous fibers of the trabecular meshwork seem to be very stable. The diameter of the collageneous fibers in the sclera thickens with age. However, the diameter of the collageneous fibers of the cribriform and outer corneoscleral meshwork does not change with age. It remains constantly small (5 to 30 nm), as do the corneal fibers. The collageneous fibers of the uveal meshwork and innermost corneoscleral lamellae thicken slightly.[69,140] Aqueous humor is said to be capable of dissolving or distorting connective tissue. We have often observed that trabecular beams denuded from the protecting trabecular cells are partly dissolved, showing clusters of atypical collagen, swelling, and lamellation of basement membranes and development of great amounts of lattice (curly) collagen. Cell loss, therefore, could well be a reason for the so-called age-related changes in the structure of the extracellular material of the trabecular meshwork.

MORPHOLOGIC CHANGES OF THE OUTFLOW PATHWAYS IN DIFFERENT KINDS OF GLAUCOMA

Primary Open-angle Glaucoma (POAG)

There is much debate over the site of the increased outflow resistance in primary open-angle glaucoma.* Some authors believe that the major

---

*References 93, 94, 160, 164, 174, 175.

part of outflow resistance is located beyond Schlemm's canal, namely in the collector channels and aqueous veins.[4,60,62] However, calculations based on Poiseuille's law for laminar flow of fluid do not support this view.[91,92] Tripathi[174,175] postulated the cause to be a decrease in vacuolization of the inner wall endothelium of Schlemm's canal in glaucomatous eyes. Fink et al.,[21] however, did not find any difference in number and size of giant vacuoles, pores, or intercellular spaces between normal and glaucomatous eyes.[54]

Nesterov has developed the concept of "canalicular blockade" in the pathogenesis of primary open-angle glaucoma.[90,91] He feels that the main part of the outflow resistance is localized neither in the outer nor in the inner wall of Schlemm's canal but directly in its lumen.[92] In his opinion, a collapse of the canal is the essential change underlying structural changes in such places as the trabecular meshwork and outflow channels.

On the other hand, based on calculations of the circumferential flow along the canal within the excised human eye, Moses et al.[87,88] has suggested that the primary defect in primary open-angle glaucoma is the increased resistance of the inner wall of Schlemm's canal with the collapse of parts of the canal and the plugging of collector channels as a secondary effect.

Using scanning electron microscopy, Chaudry et al.[16] described in 10 trabeculectomy specimens from primary open-angle glaucoma "coating material of unknown nature" that covered the uveal part of the trabecular meshwork and was not seen in normal autopsy eyes. This material was thought to be responsible for the reduction of outflow facility in these cases. These observations could not be confirmed.[82,102] It has been argued that during surgery, plasma protein may enter the trabecular meshwork through the inner wall of Schlemm's canal and cause such changes.[23,82] In fact, protein leakage from Schlemm's canal could be induced experimentally in monkeys by paracentesis.[105]

Alvarado et al.[1] found a greater loss of trabecular cells in the inner than in the outer part of the meshwork in primary open-angle glaucoma. They assumed that the pathologic changes in primary open-angle glaucoma start in the innermost region rather than around Schlemm's canal.

Most of our knowledge about the morphologic changes of the trabecular meshwork in primary open-angle glaucoma is based on transmission or scanning electron microscopy of trabeculectomy specimens representing mostly the later stages of the disease. The initial changes in the tissue are, therefore, rarely observed.

Rohen and Witmer[150] first described clusters of extracellular material deposited within the cribriform layer of the trabecular meshwork as well as immediately underneath the endothelial lining of Schlemm's canal, which were termed "plaques."[128,130,132,134] These findings were confirmed later by Segawa,[159,160] Rodrigues et al.,[118] McMenamin and Lee,[83] Lee et al.,[64] and other investigators. As described above, most of this plaque material is derived from the sheath of the elastic-like fiber net underneath the endothelial lining of Schlemm's canal, so that the term sheath-derived plaque material (SD-plaques) was used[70,132,134] (Fig. 2-13).

In sagittal sections, broad strands of SD-material are occasionally seen running toward the endothelial lining of Schlemm's canal at an angle of 90 degrees, originating from the cribriform fiber plexus (see Fig. 2-3). These strands are considered to be "hyalinized" connecting fibrils embedded in or enveloped by sheath-derived plaque material.

The diameter of the core of the elastic-like fibers located within the cribriform or corneoscleral meshwork does not change significantly with age or in primary open-angle glaucoma.[69] On the contrary, the amount of SD-plaque material varies both in different age groups and in cases of primary open-angle glaucoma.

In normal autopsy eyes a significant correlation was seen between age and the area of SD-plaque material (see Fig. 2-12). However, in trabeculectomy specimens derived from cases of primary open-angle glaucoma no such correlation was observed (Fig. 2-14), but the total amount of SD-plaque material was found to be significantly greater in glaucomatous than in normal eyes.[79] This shows that primary open-angle glaucoma can not be considered simply as an age-dependent phenomenon.

Cytochemical study of trabeculectomy specimens reveals a number of additional fine fibrils adhering to the elastic-like fiber net and to the connecting fibrils.[70,134] These fibrils are embedded in proteoglycans and appear to be part of the elastic-like fiber sheath. The nature of these fine fibrils, which are not seen in normal eyes, is not known. One could speculate that they provide a base for the deposition of additional plaque material, which then forms the interlacing plates of extracellular material beneath the inner wall endothelium. These plates could block part of the filtering area of the inner wall of Schlemm's canal and be responsible for increased outflow resistance in glaucoma (Fig. 2-15; see also Plate I, Fig. 3).

Plaque material has also been found within the

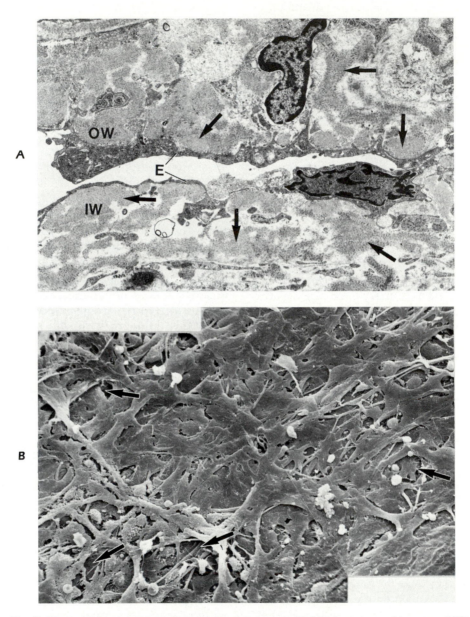

Fig. 2-13 **A,** Electron micrographs of inner and outer wall of Schlemm's canal in cases of POAG. Sheath-derived plaque material *(arrows);* endothelium of Schlemm's canal *(E);* inner wall *(IW);* outer wall *(OW).* (Sagittal section, trabeculectomy specimen; ×17,280.) **B,** Scanning electron micrograph of uveal meshwork in case of POAG. Note that openings of uveal meshwork are partly closed by hyalinized trabecular beams, partly still open *(arrows).* (Flat preparation, internal aspect; ×500.)

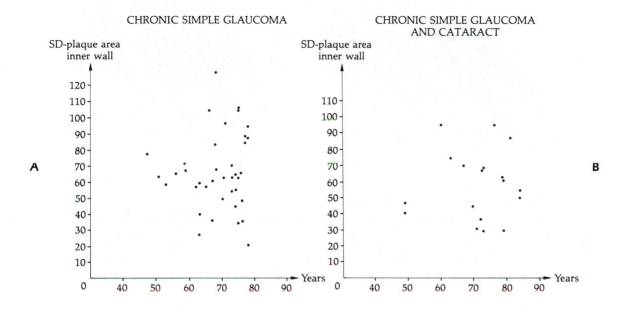

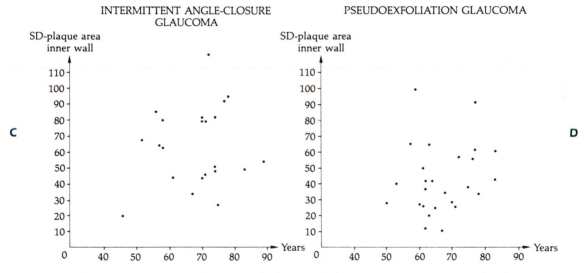

Fig. 2-14   Scatter diagrams showing relationship between inner-wall plaques and age in chronic simple glaucoma without, **A,** and with, **B,** cataract, in intermittent angle-closure glaucoma, **C,** and in pseudoexfoliation syndrome, **D.** (After Lütjen-Drecoll, E, et al: Exp Eye Res 42:443, 1986)

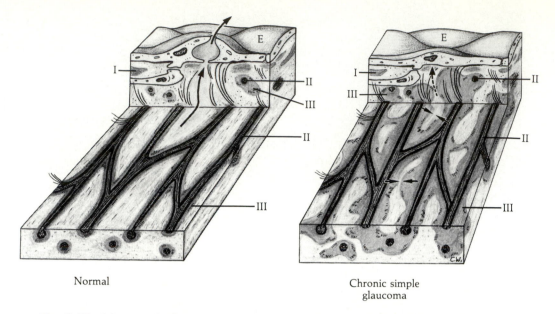

Normal

Chronic simple
glaucoma

Fig. 2-15 Schematic diagram illustrating development of SD-plaques *(III)* from sheaths of sub-endothelial elastic-like fiber network *(II)* in normal and glaucomatous eyes. Type I plaques *(I)* are probably remnants of basement membrane material. Endothelium of Schlemm's canal *(E)*. (From Rohen, JW: Ophthalmology 90:758, 1983. With permission of the American Academy of Ophthalmology) See also Plate I, Fig 3.

outer wall of Schlemm's canal (see Figs. 2-13 and Fig. 2-16). The amount is greater in glaucomatous than in age-matched normal eyes, but this increase is less than in the inner wall. No correlation between the outer and inner wall plaques was found in primary open-angle glaucoma. Since the amount of plaque material in glaucoma both in the inner and outer wall is greater than in normal elderly eyes, other factors must exist that lead to excessive plaque formation. The nature of such factors and the functional interrelationship between outer wall plaques and collector channels remain speculative. If plaque formation around the openings of collector channels becomes excessive, a narrowing or even a closing-off of these openings could occur, which then might also influence outflow mechanisms.

We also studied whether plaque formation occurs at places other than around Schlemm's canal. Characteristic plaque material was found only within the interstitial spaces between the anterior tips of the ciliary muscle fibers (Fig. 2-17). In this region, elastic-like fibers are also present. As these fibers also come in contact with aqueous humor by uveoscleral flow, it is possible that the additional extracellular material found in glaucomatous eyes accumulates in the sheath of these fibers.

In the iris, which normally does not contain elastic fibers, no plaque material was observed. However, morphologic changes of the extracellular material surrounding the vessel walls were seen in cases of primary open-angle glaucoma.[95] In contrast to age-matched nonglaucomatous eyes, the diameter of the collagen fibers remained relatively constant. At the same time, the composition and amount of the surrounding proteoglycans had changed. In glaucomatous eyes, a greater amount of keratan sulfate proteoglycans was found within the sheaths of the iris vessels.[155] It is not known whether the same substances that lead to the structural changes of the iris vessels also lead to plaque formation around Schlemm's canal and within the anterior ciliary muscle tips. On the other hand, it could also be possible that certain factors influence the cells located in these regions and that the changes seen in the extracellular material are secondary to the cellular changes.

In cases of primary open-angle glaucoma so-called *matrix vesicles* were found within the cribriform layer, indicating cellular degeneration[131] (Fig. 2-18). Matrix vesicles have been found in the vessel wall in various diseases (e.g., renal hypertension, arteriosclerosis).[113] In trabeculectomy specimens in primary open-angle glaucoma, both lysosomal and nonlysosomal matrix vesicles are found, usually located within the cribriform and juxtacanalicular layer. The nonlysosomal vesicles are usually greater in size and probably represent membrane-limited cytoplasmic remnants of trabecular or cribriform cells. Since lysosomal matrix vesicles still

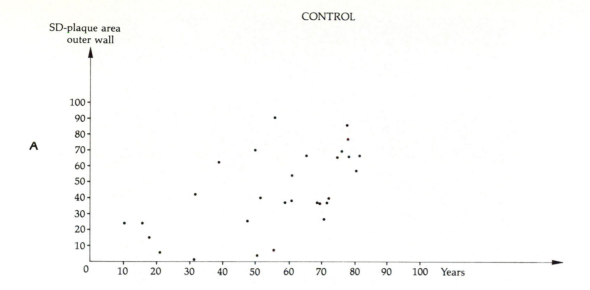

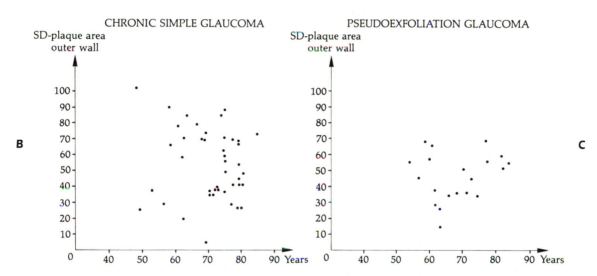

Fig. 2-16   Scatter diagrams showing relationship between out-wall plaques and age in normal eyes, **A,** in chronic simple glaucoma, **B,** and in pseudoexfoliation glaucoma, **C.** (After Lütjen-Drecoll, E, et al: Exp Eye Res 42:443, 1986)

contain a number of highly active enzymes, these vesicles can be considered "explosive bags" that might seriously injure the extracellular material of this region. The great amounts of atypical collagen, lattice (curly) collagen, and sheath-derived plaque material with periodic bandings found within the cribriform layer might be the result of such enzymatic interactions.[131]

A loss of trabecular cells has been described recently by Alvarado et al. in trabeculectomy specimens from primary open-angle glaucoma and in normal eyes.[1] These investigators state that loss of cells occurs in a gradient-like manner, with the inner tissues of the trabecular meshwork affected

most and the outermost tissues affected least. The decline in cellularity was found to be similar to but greater than what has been observed in advanced age. In the nonglaucomatous and glaucomatous meshwork the cellularity curves were parallel to each other from birth. They felt there could be a congenital basis for primary open-angle glaucoma in that the presumptive glaucoma patient is born with a decreased number of cells. The rate of cell loss with age would be the same, but later in life a "critical" depletion of the trabecular cell population might develop, resulting in a fusion of the innermost trabecular sheets and partial loss of patent aqueous channels.[1,20] Grierson et al.[42] found a

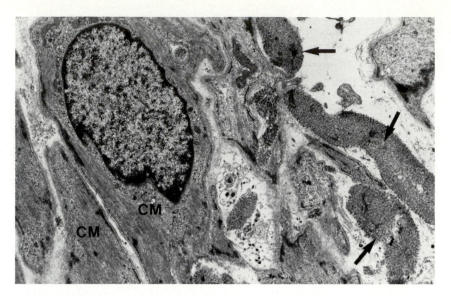

Fig. 2-17 Anterior ciliary muscle tips in a case of primary open-angle glaucoma. Note SD-plaques *(arrows)* deposited within interstitial spaces. Ciliary muscle fibers *(CM)*. (Electron micrograph; ×12,500.)

linear age-related increase in the frequency of fusions between trabecular beams.

In trabeculectomy specimens from primary open-angle glaucoma we often find an extreme "hyalinization" of the corneoscleral or uveal trabecular beams. Usually, there are a number of areas where the endothelial lining is lacking and where the subendothelial basement membranes can come in direct contact with the aqueous humor. At such sites the amount of lattice collagen appears greatly increased. The basement membranes are often enormously thickened, showing a great amount of lattice collagen inclusions. Sometimes, the basement membranes reveal a "shagreenlike" pattern with a regular banding of 40 to 50 nm (see Fig. 2-10, *B*). In some places, the basement membranes show a lamellation without inclusions of regular periodicity. Denuded trabecular beams can fuse with each other, so that the intertrabecular spaces appear obliterated in these areas. The uveal meshwork cells increase in size and spread out with elongated cytoplasmic processes that try to cover the denuded areas. These cells often appear electron dense and contain a large nucleus, many dark mitochondria, and a great amount of free ribosomes. It should be noted that the thickening of basement membranes usually begins at the internal surface of the trabecular beams and not at the canal side. Enlargement of the trabecular cells and thickening and fusion of the lamellae can result in a complete obstruction of the uveal and corneoscleral

aqueous pathways, a process that can be demonstrated best in scanning electron micrographs of flat preparations[16,102] (see Fig. 2-18). Based on our own scanning electron microscopic studies, we assume that these events appear mainly in more advanced stages of primary open-angle glaucoma and that in most cases of glaucoma the primary increase in outflow resistance lies in the cribriform layer of the meshwork.

Low-tension Glaucoma

We recently examined trabeculectomy specimens from five cases of low-tension glaucoma by electron microscopy.[135] In all cases, repeated measurements did not reveal an intraocular pressure above 20 or 21 mm Hg. The average pressure range was between 12 and 18 mm Hg. In all cases the trabecular beams appeared somewhat thickened. There were clusters of lattice (curly) collagen deposited predominantly within the elastic-like fiber sheaths. The basement membranes contained less of this material than found in primary open-angle glaucoma (Fig. 2-19).

The most surprising finding was the large amount of SD-plaque material, deposited beneath the endothelial lining of Schlemm's canal and within the cribriform layer (Fig. 2-20). The inner wall appeared thickened and somewhat distorted by these unevenly distributed clusters of plaques. In addition, masses of a fine fibrillar or amorphous material were seen immediately beneath the canal

Text continued on p. 64.

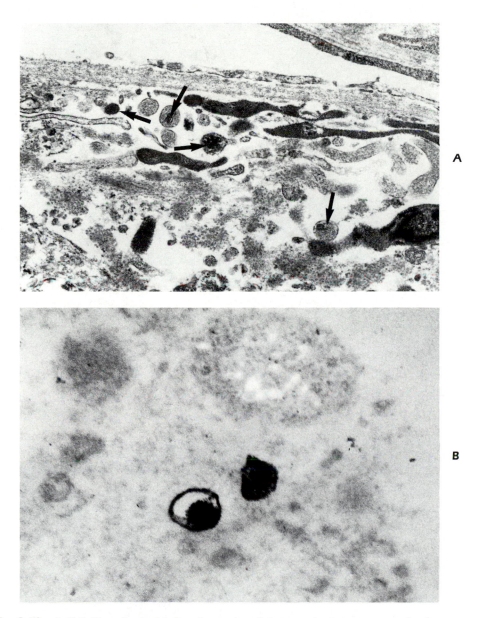

Fig. 2-18 **A,** Cribriform layer of trabecular meshwork in case of primary open-angle glaucoma showing various types of matrix vesicles *(arrows).* **B,** Two matrix vesicles showing positive reaction for acid phosphatase. (**A,** ×64,000; **B,** ×66,000.)

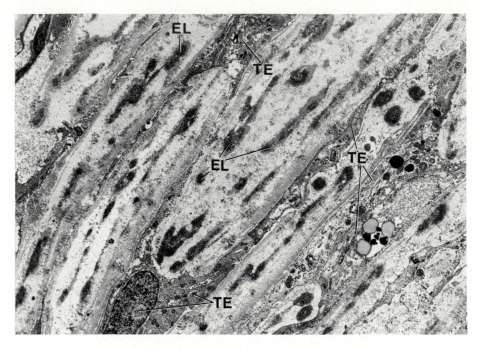

Fig. 2-19 Electron micrograph of corneoscleral part of trabecular meshwork in case of low-tension glaucoma. Elastic-like fibers within trabecular beams *(EL)*; trabecular cells *(TE)*. (Trabeculectomy specimen; ×6500.)

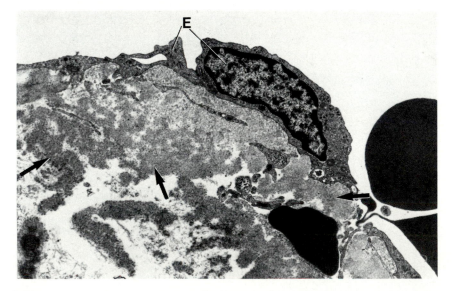

Fig. 2-20 Electron micrograph of inner wall of Schlemm's canal. Note numerous deposits of SD-plaques *(arrows)*. Endothelium of Schlemm's canal *(E)*. (Trabeculectomy specimen; ×19,200.)

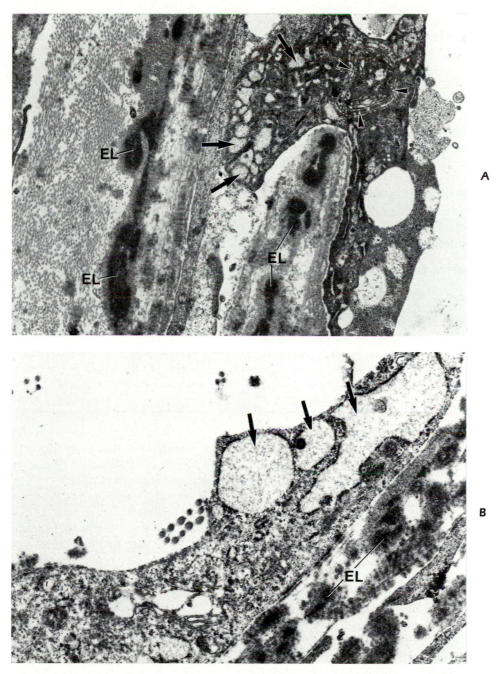

Fig. 2-21 Electron micrographs of trabecular cells in a case of low-tension glaucoma. Note great number of enlarged cisterns *(arrows)* and Golgi complex *(arrowheads)*. Elastic-like fibers *(EL)*. (Trabeculectomy specimen; **A,** ×26,880; **B,** ×42,560.)

endothelium in three of five cases. This substance could be fibrin or fibrinlike material, but might also be just protein that had reached the inner wall during surgery. Almost no empty spaces could be seen beneath the inner wall endothelium.

The morphology of the trabecular cells was also surprising. They appeared highly activated throughout the entire meshwork (Fig. 2-21). Between the trabecular lamellae, elongated and often enlarged trabecular cells were found that contained a well-developed endoplasmic reticulum with many cisternae, Golgi complexes, and mitochondria. The cisternae often appeared enlarged to form large membrane-limited vesicles that usually contained a granular or fibrillar material. Lipid inclusions were also occasionally seen.[135] These observations indicate that in low-tension glaucoma the trabecular cells are stimulated by some unknown factors to produce extracellular material, which appears to accumulate within the cribriform layer.

Pseudoexfoliative Glaucoma

In cases of pseudoexfoliative glaucoma the anterior surface of the lens, the ciliary processes and zonular apparatus, the posterior surface of the peripheral cornea, the iris, and the trabecular meshwork become partially covered by flakelike material. This material consists of randomly arranged fine fibrils without obvious periodicity embedded in a homogeneous matrix.[15,43,114-116,153] These fibrils, measuring 0.8 to 1 μm in length and 20 to 80 nm in diameter, appear to be composed of subunits of 8 to 10 nm.[17,43] Some authors have characterized the material as a basement-membrane-derived material,[25,63,169] whereas others considered it to be an amyloid-like structure.[18,117]

In a recent quantitative analysis we determined the amount of plaque material in 26 cases of pseudoexfoliative glaucoma. In both the inner and outer wall of Schlemm's canal the amount of this material was not greater than in normal eyes of the same age group.[79,81] On the other hand, usually a great amount of pseudoexfoliative material was found deposited beneath the inner wall endothelium as well as within the cribriform layer (Fig. 2-22, A). In a number of specimens, nearly all pathways through the cribriform region were filled with pseudoexfoliative material.

Deposits of pseudoexfoliative material were predominantly seen within the inner wall of Schlemm's canal and between the ciliary muscle tips, but seldom within the outer wall of Schlemm's canal. The distribution of the material indicates that it might penetrate the trabecular meshwork or the ciliary body by aqueous flow rather than be produced locally by trabecular cells or fibroblasts.[81]

The obstruction of the outflow pathways of the trabecular meshwork by pseudoexfoliative material might occur at the inner wall of Schlemm's canal or within the corneoscleral meshwork itself. In some cases we found areas of denuded trabecular lamellae where clusters of pseudoexfoliative fibrils were in direct contact with the basement membranes or the intratrabecular fiber network (Fig. 2-22, B). Similar observations have been made by Ringvold et al.,[116] Harnisch,[43] and Richardson and Epstein.[111,154] The aqueous pathways in such areas might be closed off if adhesions between contiguous trabecular beams develop on the basis of pseudoexfoliative material functioning as a kind of glue. If in previously normotensive eyes large amounts of pseudoexfoliative fibrils accumulate between the trabecular lamellae or within the inner wall of Schlemm's canal, aqueous outflow resistance might become elevated, resulting in the development of glaucoma. The origin of the pseudoexfoliative material is unknown.

Pigmentary Glaucoma

Pigment granules derived from the pigmented epithelium of the iris or of the ciliary body are commonly seen in the trabecular meshwork of older individuals (particularly those with diabetes) without elevation of intraocular pressure. Pigmentation of the trabecular meshwork is often more conspicuous inferiorly than superiorly.[167] The pigment granules are distributed between the trabecular beams, adhering to the trabecular or cribriform cells or within the cytoplasm of the trabecular cells after phagocytosis.[166]

It is not known whether pigmentary glaucoma is caused by pigmentary obstruction (mechanically) or by damage to the trabecular cells. In electron micrographs of trabeculectomy specimens, most of the trabecular cells are filled with pigment granules of various sizes, probably by phagocytosis.

Richardson et al.[112] assumed that plugging of the intertrabecular spaces by pigment granules, together with fragmentation and adhesion of trabecular beams, would cause decreased outflow facility. However, in our specimens an accumulation of free pigment granules beneath the inner wall of Schlemm's canal or clusters of granules deposited within the cribriform pathways were not seen (Fig. 2-23). The structure of the meshwork, particularly the trabecular beams and the cribriform layer, ap-

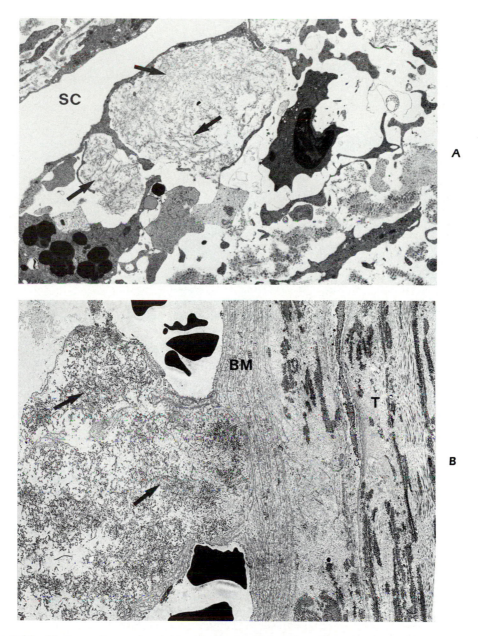

Fig. 2-22 Electron micrographs of trabecular meshwork in a case of pseudoexfoliation glaucoma. **A,** Cribriform layer with clusters of pseudoexfoliation fibrils *(arrows).* Schlemm's canal *(SC).* **B,** Trabecular beam. Pseudoexfoliation material *(arrows)* adhering to basement membrane *(BM).* Trabecular lamellae *(T).* (Trabeculectomy specimen; **A,** ×16,560; **B,** ×30,000.)

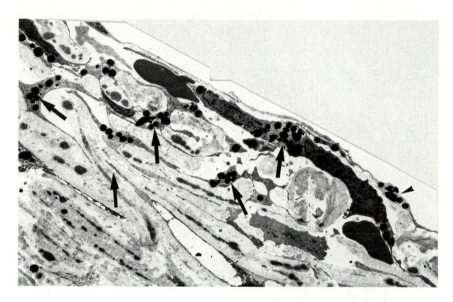

Fig. 2-23 Electron micrograph of inner wall of Schlemm's canal in a case of pigmentary glaucoma. Pigment granules are present within cells of cribriform layer *(arrows)* and within endothelium of Schlemm's canal *(arrowhead).* (Trabeculectomy specimen; ×4800.)

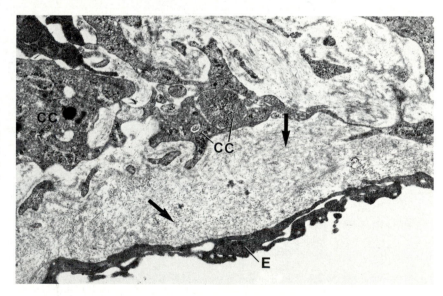

Fig. 2-24 Electron micrograph of trabecular meshwork in a case of corticosteroid-induced glaucoma. Note deposits of fine fibrillar material *(arrows)* underneath inner wall endothelium *(E).* Cribriform layer cells *(CC).* (Trabeculectomy specimen, ×44,160.)

peared relatively normal. Hyalinization of the trabecular sheets, thickening of their basement membranes, and development of lattice (long-spacing) collagen were in the normal range. Blockage of aqueous pathways through the meshwork by pigment granules might not be the sole cause of pigmentary glaucoma. The increase of outflow resistance might also be the result of changes in the biologic activity of trabecular meshwork cells.

A recent study showed that outflow facility decreases immediately after homologous pigment infusion into the anterior chamber of cynomolgus monkeys, but returns to normal after 1 week.[19] The infused pigment granules were immediately phagocytosed by polymorphonuclear leukocytes and later also by trabecular endothelial cells. In long-term experiments (42 and 105 days after pigment infusion) no changes in cellularity of the trabecular meshwork were found, despite an actual decrease in trabecular pigmentation. Seemingly, either there is replacement of the trabecular cells that had migrated from the trabecular beams, or the pigment is removed from the meshwork not by trabecular cells but by some other type of phagocytic cell, perhaps wandering macrophages.[19] The particles were neither toxic nor antigenic. Even repeated infusion of pigment granules did not cause the structural abnormalities in the meshwork, as have been described in human eyes with pigmentary glaucoma.[112] The results suggest that pigment accumulation by itself would not cause profound structural abnormalities leading to glaucoma.

Corticosteroid-induced Glaucoma

There are only a few studies on the morphologic changes of the trabecular meshwork in corticosteroid-induced glaucoma.[136] In a human eye enucleated for a melanoma, Kayes and Becker[57] did not find any changes in the trabecular meshwork after 8 weeks of topical administration of dexamethasone; the number and form of giant vacuoles and the appearance of the trabecular cells particularly appeared to be normal.

Electron microscopic analysis of trabeculectomy specimens in two cases of corticosteroid-induced glaucoma revealed a marked densification of the cribriform layer.[136] Masses of amorphous and fibrillar material deposited within the intertrabecular spaces and cribriform pathways completely blocked the outflow channels.

We have recently studied trabeculectomy specimens of two additional cases of corticosteroid-induced glaucoma. In both cases, the inner wall of

Schlemm's canal contained masses of fine fibrillar material embedded in a homogeneous matrix (Fig. 2-24). No free cribriform aqueous pathways were seen in these specimens. Many of the trabecular cells appeared greatly enlarged and contained vesicles filled with granular material. There were also signs of cell degeneration. Some cells contained lipid droplets of various sizes; other appeared swollen and filled with vesicles, fibrils, and large, electron-dense mitochondria.

Secondary Glaucoma in Combination with Mucopolysaccharidoses

Mucopolysaccharidoses are congenital disorders caused by the absence of enzymes needed for the degradation of certain glycosaminoglycans within the cells. Morphologically, all types of these diseases are characterized by the presence of mesenchyme-derived cells such as fibroblasts, chondrocytes, and keratocytes, which contain a great number of vacuoles filled with nondegraded glycosaminoglycan proteins. In a case of mucopolysaccharidosis type I Pfaundler-Hurler, vacuolated cells were found within the corneal epithelium and the conjunctiva.[104,110]

Recently we examined trabeculectomy specimens of cases of mucopolysaccharidoses (type I Pfaundler-Hurler and type II Hunter), in which secondary glaucoma had developed (unpublished data). In both cases, the trabecular endothelial cells contained a great number of vacuoles, varying in size and location (Fig. 2-25, *A*). The vacuoles apparently developed from the Golgi complex, from which they spread into the cytoplasm up to the most peripheral cytoplasmic processes. The vacuoles often contained an electron-dense core of fibrillar or homogeneous material; otherwise the vacuoles appeared empty, probably because their contents had been dissolved during the embedding procedures. In some areas the basement membranes of the trabecular beams were thickened, but otherwise the trabecular meshwork appeared normal.

In one case we obtained the entire eyeball, enabling us to study the ciliary body. The ciliary epithelium showed an enormous degree of vacuolization, whereas the ciliary muscle, the blood vessels of the uvea, and the iris appeared relatively normal. The basal membrane infoldings were reduced in size and number, as was the case with mitochondria. The nonpigmented endothelial cells and to a lesser degree the pigmented cells were also completely filled with membrane-limited vac-

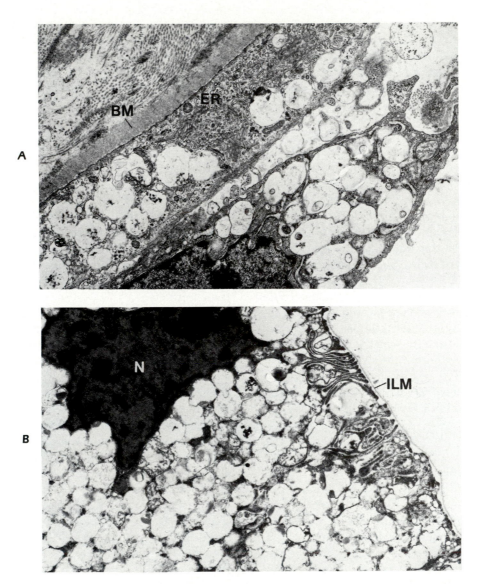

Fig. 2-25 Trabecular meshwork, **A,** and ciliary epithelium, **B,** in cases of mucopolysaccharidosis with glaucoma. **A,** Cross section of trabecular beam. Note enormous vacuolization of trabecular cells. Basement membrane *(BM);* smooth endoplasmic reticulum *(ER).* **B,** Nonpigmented ciliary epithelium with numerous cytoplasmic vacuoles. Internal limiting membrane *(ILM);* nucleus *(N).* (**A,** ×30,000; **B,** ×24,000.)

uoles (Fig. 2-25 *B*). This indicated that the ciliary epithelium was also involved in the production of proteoglycans.

The mechanism for this type of secondary glaucoma possibly results from the swollen and vacuolated trabecular cells, causing obstruction of the outflow pathways. It is also possible that metabolic disturbances of trabecular cells could lead to changes in the outflow mechanisms.

REFERENCES

1. Alvarado, J, Murphy, C, and Juster, R: Trabecular meshwork cellularity in POAG and non-glaucomatous normals, Ophthalmology 91:564, 1984
2. Alvarado, J, Murphy, C, Polansky, J, and Juster, R: Age-related changes in trabecular meshwork cellularity, Invest Ophthalmol Vis Sci 21:714, 1981
3. Ascher, KW: Aqueous veins: preliminary note, Am J Ophthalmol 25:31, 1942
4. Ascher, KW: The aqueous veins, Springfield, Ill, 1961, Charles C Thomas
5. Ashton, N: Anatomical study of Schlemm's canal and aqueous veins by means of neoprene casts, I. Aqueous veins, Br J Ophthalmol 35:291, 1951
6. Barany, EH: The mode of action of miotics on outflow resistance: a study of pilocarpine in the vervet monkey *(Cercopithecus ethiops)*, Trans Ophthalmol Soc UK 86:539, 1967
7. Barany, EH: The immediate effect on outflow resistance of intravenous pilocarpine in the vervet monkey *(Cercopithecus ethiops)*, Invest Ophthalmol 6:373, 1967
8. Bartels, SP, Pederson, JE, Gaasterland, DE, and Armaly, MF: Sites of breakdown of the blood-aqueous barrier after paracentesis of the rhesus monkey eye, Invest Ophthalmol Vis Sci 18:1050, 1979
9. Becker, B: The decline in aqueous secretion and outflow facility with age, Am J Ophthalmol 97:1667, 1979
10. Bill, A: The aqueous humor drainage mechanism in the cynomolgus monkey *(Macaca irus)* with evidence for unconventional routes, Invest Ophthalmol 4:911, 1965
11. Bill, A: Conventional and uveo-scleral drainage of aqueous humour in the cynomolgus monkey *(Macaca irus)* at normal and high intraocular pressures, Exp Eye Res 5:45, 1966
12. Bill, A: Aqueous humor dynamics in monkeys *(Macaca irus* and *Cercopithecus aethiops)*, Exp Eye Res 11:195, 1971
13. Bill, A, and Phillips, C: Uveoscleral drainage of aqueous humour in human eyes, Exp Eye Res 12:275, 1971
14. Bill, A, and Svedbergh, B: Scanning electron microscopic studies of the trabecular meshwork and the canal of Schlemm: an attempt to localize the main resistance to outflow of aqueous humor in man, Acta Ophthalmol 50:295, 1972
15. Blackstad, TW, Sunde, OW, and Traetteberg, J: On the ultrastructure of the deposits of Bussaca in eyes with glaucoma simplex and so-called senile exfoliation of the anterior lens capsule, Acta Ophthalmol 38:587, 1960
16. Chaudry, HA, et al: Scanning electron microscopy of trabeculectomy specimens in open-angle glaucoma, Am J Ophthalmol 88:78, 1979
17. Davanger, M: On the molecular composition and physico-chemical properties of the pseudoexfoliation material, Acta Ophthalmol 55:621, 1972
18. Davanger, M: The pseudo-exfoliation syndrome: a scanning electron-microscopic study. II. The posterior chamber region, Acta Ophthalmol 53:821, 1975
19. Epstein, DL, et al: Experimental obstruction to aqueous outflow by pigment particles in living monkeys, Invest Ophthalmol Vis Sci 27:387, 1986
20. Fine, BS, Yanoff, M, and Stone, RA: A clinicopathologic study of four cases of POAG compared to normal eyes, Am J Ophthalmol 91:88, 1981
21. Fink, A, Felix, MD, and Fletcher, RC: The electron microscopy of Schlemm's canal and adjacent structures in patients with glaucoma, Trans Am Ophthalmol Soc 70:82, 1972
22. Floyd, BB, Cleveland, PH, and Worthen, DM: Fibronectin in human trabecular drainage channels, Invest Ophthalmol Vis Sci 26:797, 1985
23. Gieser, DK, et al: Amorphous coating in open-angle glaucoma, Am J Ophthalmol 92:130, 1981
24. Goldmann, H: The drainage of the aqueous in man, Ophthalmologica 3:146, 1946
25. Ghosh, M, and Speakman, JS: The iris in senile exfoliation of the lens, Can J Ophthalmol 9:289, 1984
26. Grierson, I: Alterations in the outflow system in chronic simple glaucoma, Res Clin Forums 7:205, 1985
27. Grierson, I, and Lee, WR: Erythrocyte phagocytosis in the human trabecular meshwork, Br J Ophthalmol 57:400, 1973
28. Grierson, I, and Lee, WR: Changes in the monkey outflow apparatus at graded levels of intraocular pressure, Exp Eye Res 19:21, 1974
29. Grierson, I, and Lee, WR: The fine structure of the trabecular meshwork at graded levels of intraocular pressure. I. Pressure effects within the near-physiological range (8-30 mm Hg), Exp Eye Res 20:505, 1975
30. Grierson, I, and Lee, WR: The fine structure of the trabecular meshwork at graded levels of intraocular pressure. II. Pressure outside the physiological range (0 and 50 mm Hg), Exp Eye Res 20:523, 1975
31. Grierson, I, and Lee, WR: Pressure-induced changes in the ultrastructure of the endothelium lining of Schlemm's canal, Am J Ophthalmol 80:863, 1975
32. Grierson, I, and Lee, WR: Acid mucopolysaccharides in the outflow apparatus, Exp Eye Res 21:417, 1975

33. Grierson, I, and Lee, WR: Light microscopic quantitation of the endothelial vacuoles in Schlemm's canal, Am J Ophthalmol 84:234, 1977

34. Grierson, I, and Lee, WR: Pressure effects on flow channels in the lining endothelium of Schlemm's canal, Acta Ophthalmol 56:935, 1978

35. Grierson, I, and Lee, WR: Further observations on the process of haemophagocytosis in the human outflow system, v Graefe's Arch Klin Exp Ophthalmol 208:49, 1978

36. Grierson, I, Lee, WR, and Abraham, S: The effects of pilocarpine on the morphology of the human outflow apparatus, Br J Ophthalmol 62:302, 1978

37. Grierson, I, Lee, WR, and Abraham, S: The effects of topical pilocarpine on the morphology of the outflow apparatus of the baboon (Papio cynocephalus), Invest Ophthalmol Vis Sci 18:346, 1979

38. Grierson, I, Lee, WR, and Abraham, S: A light microscopic study of the effects of testicular hyaluronidase on the outflow system of the baboon (Papio cynocephalus), Invest Ophthalmol Vis Sci 18:356, 1979

39. Grierson, I, Lee, WR, and McMenamin, P: The morphological basis of drug action on the outflow system of the eye, Res Clin Forums 3:1, 1981

40. Grierson, I, Lee, WR, Moseley, H, and Abraham, S: The trabecular wall of Schlemm's canal: a study of the effects of pilocarpine by scanning electron microscopy, Br J Ophthalmol 63:9, 1979

41. Grierson, I, Howes, RC, Wang, Q: Age-related changes in the canal of Schlemm, Exp Eye Res 39:505, 1984

42. Grierson, I, Wang, Q, McMenamin, PG, and Lee, WR: The effects of age and antiglaucoma drugs on the meshwork cell population, Res Clin Forums 4:69, 1982

43. Harnisch, JP: Exfoliation material in different sections of the eye, v Graefe's Arch Klin Ophthalmol 203:181, 1977

44. Hogan, MJ, Alvarado, JA, and Weddell, JW: Histology of the human eye, Philadelphia, 1971, WB Saunders

45. Holmberg, A: The fine structure of the inner wall of Schlemm's canal, Arch Ophthalmol 62:935, 1003, 1959

46. Holmberg, A: Schlemm's canal and the trabecular meshwork: an electron microscopic study of the normal structure in man and monkey (Cercopithecus ethiops), Doc Ophthalmol 19:339, 1965

47. Horstmann, HJ, Rohen, JW, and Sames, K: Age-related changes in the composition of proteins in the trabecular meshwork of the human eye, Mech Ageing Dev 21:121, 1983

48. Huggert, A: An experiment in determining the pore-size distribution curve to the filtration angle of the eye. Part I, Acta Ophthalmol 35:12, 1957

49. Huggert, A: An experiment in determining the pore-size distribution curve to the filtration angle of the eye. Part II, Acta Ophthalmol 35:104, 1957

50. Huggert, A, Holmberg, A, and Esklund, A: Further studies concerning pore size in the filtration angle of the eye, Acta Ophthalmol Scand 33:429, 1955

51. Inomata, H, Bill, A, and Smelser, GK: Aqueous humor pathways through the trabecular meshwork and into Schlemm's canal in the cynomolgus monkey (Macaca irus): an electron microscopic study, Am J Ophthalmol 73:760, 1972

52. Ishikawa, T: Fine structure of the human ciliary muscle, Invest Ophthalmol 1:587, 1962

53. Johnstone, MA, and Grant, WM: Pressure-dependent changes in structure of the aqueous outflow system of human and monkey eye, Am J Ophthalmol 75:365, 1973

54. Karaganov, IL, Nesterov, AP, Batmanov, YrE, and Brikman, VG: Electronmicroscopic studies of the inner wall of Schlemm's canal in early open-angle glaucoma, Vest Oftalmol 2:5, 1979

55. Kaufman, PL, and Barany, EH: Residual pilocarpine effects on outflow facility after ciliary muscle disinsertion in the cynomolgus monkey, Invest Ophthalmol 15:558, 1976

56. Kayes, J: Pore structure of the inner wall of Schlemm's canal, Invest Ophthalmol 6:381, 1967

57. Kayes, J, and Becker, B: The human trabecular meshwork in corticosteroid-induced glaucoma, Trans Am Ophthalmol Soc 67:9, 1969

58. Kleinert, H: Der sichtbare Abfluß des Kamerwassers in den epibulbären Venen, v Graefe's Arch Klin Exp Ophthalmol 152:278, 1951

59. Kleinert, H: Die Vitalfärbung des Kammerwassers und seiner epibulbären Abflußwege nach Fluoreszeininjektion in die Vorderkammer, Klin Monatsbl Augenheilkd 122:665, 1953

60. Krasnov, MM: Antiglaucomatous operations on the outer and the inner walls of Schlemm's canal, Trans 3rd Congress of Ophthalmologists of the USSR 202, Volgograd Medicina 1966

61. Kupfer, C, Datiles, M, and Kaiser-Kupfer, M: Development of the anterior chamber of the eye: embryology and clinical implications. In Lütjen-Drecoll, E, editor: Basic aspects of glaucoma research, Stuttgart 1982, Schattauer Verlag

62. Larina, IN: On intrascleral outflow channels in glaucoma, Vest Oftalmol 2:18, 1967

63. Layden, WE, and Shaffer, RN: Exfoliation syndrome, Am J Ophthalmol 78:835, 1974

64. Lee, WR, Grierson, I, and McMenamin, PG: The morphological response of the primate outflow system to changes in pressure and flow. In Lütjen-Drecoll, E, editor: Basic aspects of glaucoma research, Stuttgart, 1982, Schattauer Verlag

65. Linnèr, E, and Strömberg, U: The course of untreated ocular hypertension, Acta Ophthalmol 42:835, 1964

66. Lütjen-Drecoll, E: Electron microscopic studies on reactive changes of the trabecular meshwork in human eyes after microsurgery, v Graefe's Arch Klin Exp Ophthalmol 183:267, 1972

67. Lütjen-Drecoll, E: Structural factors influencing outflow facility and its changeability under drugs: a study in *Macaca arctoides,* Invest Ophthalmol 12:280, 1973

68. Lütjen-Drecoll, E, and Bárány, EH: Functional and electron microscopic changes in the trabecular meshwork remaining after trabeculectomy in cynomolgus monkeys, Invest Ophthalmol 13:511, 1974

69. Lütjen-Drecoll, E, Dietl, T, Futa, R, and Rohen, JW: Age changes of the trabecular meshwork: a preliminary morphometric study. In Hollyfield, JG, editor: The structure of the eye, Holland, 1982, Elsevier Verlag

70. Lütjen-Drecoll, E, Futa, R, and Rohen, JW: Ultrahistochemical studies on tangential sections of the trabecular meshwork in normal and glaucomatous eyes, Invest Ophthalmol Vis Sci 21:563, 1981

71. Lütjen-Drecoll, E, and Kaufman, PL: Echothiophate-induced structural alterations in the anterior chamber angle of the cynomolgus monkey, Invest Ophthalmol Vis Sci 18:918, 1979

72. Lütjen-Drecoll, E, and Kaufman, PL: Biomechanics of echothiophate-induced anatomic changes in monkey aqueous outflow system, v Graefe's Arch Klin Exp Ophthalmol 224:564, 1986

73. Lütjen-Drecoll, E, and Kaufman, PL: Long-term timolol and epinephrine in monkeys. II. Morphological alterations in trabecular meshwork and ciliary muscle, Trans Ophthalmol Soc UK 105:196, 1986

74. Lütjen-Drecoll, E, Kaufman, PL, and Bárány, EH: Light and electron microscopy of the anterior chamber angle structures following surgical disinsertion of the ciliary muscle in the cynomolgus monkey, Invest Ophthalmol Vis Sci 16:218, 1977

75. Lütjen-Drecoll, E, and Lönnerholm, G: Carbonic anhydrase distribution in the rabbit eye by light and electron microscopy, Invest Ophthalmol Vis Sci 21:782, 1981

76. Lütjen-Drecoll, E, Lönnerholm, G, and Eichhorn, M: Carbonic anhydrase distribution in the human and monkey eye by light and electron microscopy, v Graefe's Arch Klin Exp Ophthalmol 220:285, 1983

77. Lütjen-Drecoll, E, and Rohen, JW: Histometrische Untersuchungen über die Kammerwinkelregion des menschlichen Auges bei verschiedenen Altersstufen und Glaukomformen, v. Graefe's Arch Klin Exp Ophthalmol 176:1, 1968

78. Lütjen-Drecoll, E, and Rohen, JW: Über die endotheliale Auskleidung des Schlemm'schen Kanals im Silberimprägnationsbild, v Graefe's Arch Klin Exp Ophthalmol 180:249, 1970

79. Lütjen-Drecoll, E, Shimizu, T, Rohrbach, M, and Rohen, JW: Quantitative analysis of "plaque material" in the inner and outer wall of Schlemm's canal in normal and glaucomatous eyes, Exp Eye Res 42:443, 1986

80. Lütjen-Drecoll, E, Shimizu, T, Rohrbach, M, and Rohen, JW: Quantitative analysis of "plaque material" between ciliary muscle tips in normal and glaucomatous eyes, Exp Eye Res 42:457, 1986

81. Lütjen-Drecoll, E, and Tamm, E: Differences in the amount of "plaque-material" in the outflow system of eyes with chronic simple and exfoliation glaucoma. In Krieglstein, GK, editor: Glaucoma update III, Berlin, 1987, Springer-Verlag

82. Maglio, M, McMahon, C, Hoskins, D, and Alvarado, J: Potential artifacts in scanning electron microscopy of the trabecular meshwork in glaucoma, Am J Ophthalmol 90:645, 1980

83. McMenamin, PG, and Lee, WR: Age-related changes in extracellular materials in the inner wall of Schlemm's canal, v Graefes Arch Klin Exp Ophthalmol 212:159, 1980

84. McMenamin, PG: Functional and morphological studies of the primate outflow apparatus, PhD thesis, University of Glasgow, 1981

85. McMenamin, PG, and Lee, WR: The normal anatomy of the pig-tailed macaque *(Macaca nemestrina)* outflow apparatus with particular reference to the presence of smooth muscle, v Graefe's Arch Klin Exp Ophthalmol 219:225, 1982

86. McRae, D, and Sears, ML: Peroxidase passage through the outflow channels of human and rhesus eyes, Exp Eye Res 10:15, 1970

87. Moses, RA: Circumferential flow in the canal of Schlemm: theoretical considerations, Am J Ophthalmol 88:585, 1979

88. Moses, RA, Grodzki, WJ,, Jr, Etheridge, EL, and Wilson, CD: Schlemm's canal: the effect of intraocular pressure, Invest Ophthalmol Vis Sci 20:61, 1981

89. Moses, RA, and Pickard, WF: Blood reflux in Schlemm's canal, Arch Ophthalmol 97:1307, 1979

90. Nesterov, AP: Diaphragms of the eye and their role in pathogenesis of primary glaucoma, Kazan Md J 6:38, 1968

91. Nesterov, AP: Role of blockade of Schlemm's canal in pathogenesis of primary open-angle glaucoma, Am J Ophthalmol 70:691, 1970

92. Nesterov, AP: Pathological physiology of primary open-angle glaucoma, the aqueous circulation. In Cairns, JE, editor: Glaucoma vol, I, London, 1986, Grune & Stratton

93. Nesterov, AP, and Batmanov, YrE: Study on morphology and function of the drainage area of the eye of man, Acta Ophthalmol 50:337, 1972

94. Nesterov, AP, and Batmanov, YE: Trabecular wall of Schlemm's canal in the early stage of primary open-angle glaucoma, Am J Ophthalmol 78:639, 1974

95. Okamura, R, and Lütjen-Drecoll, E: Elektronenmikroskopische Untersuchungen über die strukturellen Veränderungen der menschlichen Iris beim Glaukom, Graefes Arch 186:271, 1973

96. Okisaka, S: The effect of prostaglandin E₁ on the ciliary epithelium and the drainage angle of cynomolgus monkeys: a light and electron microscopic study, Exp Eye Res 22:141, 1976

97. Okisaka, S: Effects of paracentesis on the blood-aqueous barrier: a light and electron microscopic study on cynomolgus monkey, Invest Ophthalmol Vis Sci 15:824, 1976

98. Polansky, J, Gospodarowicz, D, Weinreb, R, and Alvarado, J: Human trabecular meshwork cell culture and glycosaminoglycan synthesis, Invest Ophthalmol Vis Sci 17(Suppl):207, 1978

99. Polansky, JR, Mood, IS, Maglio, MT, and Alvarado, JA: Trabecular meshwork cell culture in glaucoma research: evaluation of biological activity and structural properties of human trabecular cells in vitro, Ophthalmology 91:580, 1984

100. Polansky, J, Weinreb, R, Baxter, J, and Alvarado, J: Human trabecular cells. I. Establishment in tissue culture and growth characteristics, Invest Ophthalmol Vis Sci 18:1043, 1979

101. Polansky, JR, Weinreb, R, and Alvarado, JA: Studies on human trabecular cells propagated in vitro, Vision Res 21:155, 1981

102. Quigley, HA, and Addicks, EM: Scanning electron microscopy of trabeculectomy specimens from eyes with open-angle glaucoma, Am J Ophthalmol 90:854, 1980

103. Quigley, HA, and Addicks, EM: Chronic experimental glaucoma in primates. I. Production of elevated intraocular pressure by anterior chamber injection of autologous ghost red blood cells, Invest Ophthalmol Vis Sci 19:126, 1980

104. Quigley, HA, and Goldberg, MF: Scheie syndrome and macular corneal dystrophy, Arch Ophthalmol 85:553, 1971

105. Raviola, G: Effects of paracentesis on the blood-aqueous barrier: an electron microscope study on *Macaca mulatta* using horseradish peroxidase as a tracer, Invest Ophthalmol Vis Sci 13:828, 1974

106. Raviola, G: Schwalbe's line cells: a new cell type in the trabecular meshwork of *Macaca mulatta*, Invest Ophthalmol Vis Sci 22:45, 1982

107. Raviola, G, and Butler, JM: Unidirectional transport mechanism of horseradish peroxidase in the vessels of the iris, Invest Ophthalmol Vis Sci 25:827, 1984

108. Raviola, G, and Butler, JM: Asymmetric distribution of charged domains on the two fronts of the endothelium of iris blood vessels, Invest Ophthalmol Vis Sci 26:597, 1985

109. Raviola, G, and Raviola, E: Paracellular route of aqueous outflow in the trabecular meshwork and canal of Schlemm. A freeze-fracture study of the endothelial junctions in the sclerocorneal angle of the macaque monkey eye, Invest Ophthalmol Vis Sci 21:52, 1981

110. Reim, H, Rohen, JW, and Dittrich, JK: Klinische, histologische und e.m. Augenbefunde bei einem Säugling mit Mukopolysacharidose Typ Pfaundler-Hurler, Klin Monatsbl Augenheilkd 159:444, 1971

111. Richardson, TM, and Epstein, DL: Exfoliation glaucoma: a quantitative perfusion and ultrastructural study, Ophthalmology 88:968, 1981

112. Richardson, TM, Hutchinson, BT, and Grant, M: The outflow tract in pigmentary glaucoma, Arch Ophthalmol 95:1015, 1977

113. Riede, UN, and Staubesand, J: A unifying concept for the role of matrix vesicles and lysosomes in the formal pathogenesis of diseases of connective tissue and blood vessels, Beitr Pathol 160:3, 1977

114. Ringvold, A: Electron microscopy of the wall of iris vessels in eyes with and without exfoliation syndrome (pseudoexfoliation of the lens capsule), Virchows Arch (Path Anat) 348:328, 1969

115. Ringvold, A: Ultrastructure of exfoliation material, Virchows Arch (Path Anat) 350:95, 1970

116. Ringvold, A, and Vegge, T: Electron microscopy of the trabecular meshwork in eyes with exfoliation syndrome (pseudoexfoliation of the lens capsule), Virch Arch (Path Anat) 353:110, 1971

117. Ringvold, A: Pseudoexfoliation material: an amyloid-like substance, Exp Eye Res 17:289, 1973

118. Rodrigues, MM, Spaeth, GL, and Sivalingam, E: Histopathology of 150 trabeculectomy specimens in glaucoma, Trans Ophthalmol Soc UK 96:245, 1976

119. Rohen, JW: Der Ziliarkörper als funktionelles System, Gegenbaurs Morphologisches Jahrbuch 92:415, 1952

120. Rohen, JW: Kammerwinkelstudien (Zur funktionellen Struktur des Ziliarkörpers einiger Versuchstiere und des Menschen), v. Graefes Arch Klin Exp Ophthalmol 158:310, 1957

121. Rohen, JW: Anatomie des Auges. In Velhagen, K, editor: Der Augenarzt, Leipzig, 1969, Thieme Verlag

122. Rohen, JW: Comparative and experimental studies on the iris of primates, Am J Ophthalmol 52:384, 1961

123. Rohen, JW: The histologic structure of the chamber angle in primates, Am J Ophthalmol 52:529, 1961

124. Rohen, JW: Sehorgan. In Hofer, H, Schultz, AH, and Starck, D: Primatologia: handbook of primatology, vol II/1, Basel, 1962, Karger Verlag

125. Rohen, JW: Über das Ligamentum pectinatum der Primaten, Z Zellforschung 58:403, 1962

126. Rohen, JW: Das Auge und seine Hilfsorgane. In Möllendorff, W, and Bargmann, W, editors: Haut und Sinnesorgane: Handbuch der mikroskopischen Anatomie des Menschen vol III/4, Berlin, 1964, Springer Verlag

127. Rohen, JW: Über die reaktiven Veränderungen des Trabeculum corneosclerale im Primatenauge nach Einwirkung von Hyaluronidase, Z Zellforschung, 65:627, 1965

128. Rohen, JW: Feinstrukturelle Veränderungen im Trabekelwerk des menschlichen Auges bei verschiedenen Glaukomformen, Klin Monatsbl Augenheilkd 163:401, 1973

129. Rohen, JW: Chamber angle, functional anatomy physiology and pathology. In Heilmann, K, and Richardson, KT, editors: Glaucoma, Stuttgart, 1978, Thieme Verlag

130. Rohen, JW: The evolution of the primate eye in relation to the problem of glaucoma. In Lütjen-Drecoll, E, editor: Basic aspects of glaucoma research, Stuttgart, 1982, Schattauer Verlag

131. Rohen, JW: Presence of matrix vesicles in trabecular meshwork of glaucomatous eyes, v. Graefe's Arch Klin Exp Ophthalmol 218:171, 1982

132. Rohen, JW: Why is intraocular pressure elevated in chronic simple glaucoma? Anatomical considerations, Ophthalmology 90:758, 1983

133. Rohen, JW: Anatomy of the aqueous outflow channels. In Cairns, JE, editor: Glaucoma, vol I, London, 1986, Grune & Stratton

134. Rohen, JW, Futa, R, and Lütjen-Drecoll, E: The fine structure of the cribriform meshwork in normal and glaucomatous eyes as seen in tangential sections, Invest Ophthalmol Vis Sci 21:574, 1981

135. Rohen, JW, and Hoffmann, F: Electron microscopy of the trabecular meshwork in cases of low-tension glaucoma (submitted for publication)

136. Rohen, JW, Linnèr, E, and Witmer, R: Electron microscopic studies on the trabecular meshwork in two cases of cortisone glaucoma, Exp Eye Res 17:19, 1973

137. Rohen, JW, Lütjen, E, and Barany, EH: The reaction between the ciliary muscle and the trabecular meshwork and its importance for the effect of miotics on aqueous outflow resistance: A study in two contrasting monkey species, *Macaca irus* and *Cercopithecus aethiops*, v Graefe's Arch Klin Exp Ophthalmol 172:23, 1967

138. Rohen, JW, and Lütjen-Drecoll, E: Über die Altersveränderungen des Trabekelwerkes im menschlichen Auge, v Graefe's Arch Klin Exp Ophthalmol 175:285, 1968

139. Rohen, JW, and Lütjen-Drecoll, E: Age changes of the trabecular meshwork in human and monkey eyes. In Bredt, H, and Rohen, JW, editors: Ageing and development vol, I, Stuttgart, 1971, Schattauer Verlag

140. Rohen, JW, and Lütjen-Drecoll, E: Ageing and nonageing processes within the connective tissues of the anterior segment of the eye. In Müller, WEG, and Rohen, JW, editors: Biochemical and morphological aspects of ageing, Wiesbaden, 1981, Steiner Verlag

141. Rohen, JW, and Lütjen-Drecoll, E: Biology of the trabecular meshwork. In Lütjen-Drecoll, E, editor: Basic aspects of glaucoma research, Stuttgart, 1982, Schattauer Verlag

142. Rohen, JW, Lütjen-Drecoll, E, and Ogilvie, A: Histoautoradiographic and electron microscopic studies on short-term explant cultures of the glaucomatous trabecular meshwork, v Graefe's Arch Klin Exp Ophthalmol 223:1, 1985

143. Rohen, JW, and Rentsch, FJ: Über den Bau des Schlemm'schen Kanals und seiner Abflußwege beim Menschen, v Graefe's Arch Klin Exp Ophthalmol 176:309, 1968

144. Rohen, JW, and Rentsch, FJ: Elektronenmikroskopische Untersuchungen über den Bau der Außenwand des Schlemm'schen Kanals unter besonderer Berücksichtigung der Abflußkanäle und Altersveränderungen, v Graefe's Arch Klin Exp Ophthalmol 177:1, 1969

145. Rohen, JW, and Schachtschabel, DO: Morphologic and biochemical studies of the human trabecular meshwork in tissue culture, Invest Ophthalmol Vis Sci (Suppl):207, 1978

146. Rohen, JW, Schachtschabel, DO, and Berghoff, K: Histoautoradiographic and biochemical studies on human and monkey trabecular meshwork and ciliary body in short-term explant culture, v Graefe's Arch Clin Exp Ophthalmol 221:199, 1984

147. Rohen, JW, Schachtschabel, DO, Figge, H, and Bigalke, B: Die Struktur der Kammerwasserabflußwege und ihre Veränderungen beim Glaukom: in vivo und in vitro Untersuchungen. In Leydecker, W, editor: Glaukom Symposium Würzburg 1974, Stuttgart, 1976, F Enke Verlag

148. Rohen, JW, Schachtschabel, DO, and Wehrmann, R: Structural changes of human and monkey trabecular meshwork following in vitro cultivation, v Graefe's Arch Klin Exp Ophthalmol 218:225, 1982

149. Rohen, JW, and Unger, HH: Zur Morphologie und Pathologie der Kammerbucht des Auges, Abhandlung der Akademie der Wissenschaften und der Literatur, Mainz, Nr., 3, Wiesbaden, 1959, Steiner Verlag

150. Rohen, JW, and Witmer, R: Electron microscopic studies on the trabecular meshwork in glaucoma simplex, v Graefe's Arch Klin Exp Ophthalmol 183:251, 1972

151. Rohen, JW, and van der Zypen, E: The phagocytic activity of the trabecular meshwork endothelium: an electron microscopic study of the vervet *(Cercopithecus aethiops)*, v Graefe's Arch Klin Exp Ophthalmol 175:143, 1968

152. Rohen, JW, and Voth, D: Zur Irisstruktur der Primaten, Ophthalmologica 140:27, 1960

153. Roth, AM: Trabecular meshwork in glaucoma associated with the exfoliation syndrome: a scanning electron microscopy study, Glaucoma 1:35, 1979

154. Roth, M, and Epstein, DL: Exfoliation syndrome, Am J Ophthalmol 89:477, 1980

155. Sames, K, and Rohen, JW: Histochemical studies of the glycosaminoglycans in the normal and glaucomatous iris of human eyes, v Graefe's Arch Klin Exp Ophthalmol 207:157, 1978

156. Schachtschabel, DO, Bigalke, B, and Rohen, JW: Production of glycosaminoglycans by cell cultures of the trabecular meshwork of the primate eye, Exp Eye Res 24:71, 1977

157. Schachtschabel, DO, Rohen, JW, Wever, J, and Sames, K: Synthesis and composition of glycosaminoglycans by cultured human trabecular meshwork cells, v Graefe's Arch Klin Exp Ophthalmol 218:113, 1982

158. Schachtschabel, DO, Wever, J, Rohen, JW, and Bigalke, B: Changes in glycosaminoglycans synthesis during in vitro ageing of cultured WI-38 cells and trabecular meshwork cells of the primate eye. In Müller, WEG, and Rohen, JW, editors: Biochemical and morphological aspects of ageing, Abhandlung der Mainzer Akademie der Wissenschaften und der Literatur, Wiesbaden, 1981, Franz Steiner Verlag

159. Segawa, K: Ultrastructural changes of the trabecular tissue in primary open angle glaucoma, Jpn J Ophthalmol 19:317, 1975

160. Segawa, K: Electron microscopic changes of the trabecular tissue in primary open angle glaucoma, Ann Ophthalmol 11:49, 1979

161. Shabo, AL, and Maxwell, DS: Observations on the fate of blood in the anterior chamber: a light and electron microscopic study of the monkey trabecular meshwork, Am J Ophthalmol 73:25, 1972

162. Shabo, AL, and Maxwell, DS: The blood-aqueous barrier to tracer protein: a light and electron microscopic study of the primate ciliary process, Microvasc Res 4:142, 1972

163. Shabo, AL, and Maxwell, DS: The structure of the trabecular meshwork of the primate eye: a light and electron microscopic study with peroxidase, Microvasc Res 4:384, 1972

164. Shabo, AL, Reese, TS, and Gaasterland, D: Postmortem formation of giant endothelial vacuoles in Schlemm's canal of monkey, Am J Ophthalmol 76:896, 1973

165. Sherwood, M, and Richardson, TM: Kinetics of the phagocytic process in the trabecular meshwork of cats and monkeys, Invest Ophthalmol Vis Sci 20(suppl):65, 1981

166. Shimizu, T, Hara, K, and Futa, R: Fine structure of trabecular meshwork and iris in pigmentary glaucoma, v Graefe's Arch Klin Exp Ophthalmol 215:171, 1981

167. Spencer, WH: Pathological physiology of the secondary glaucomas. In Cairns, JE, editor: Glaucoma vol, I, London, 1986, Grune & Stratton Ltd

168. Stone, RA, Kuwayama, Y, Laties, AM, and Marangos, PJ: Neuron-specific enolase-containing cells in the rhesus monkey trabecular meshwork, Invest Ophthalmol Vis Sci 25:1332, 1984

169. Sugar, HS, Harding, C, and Barsky, D: The exfoliation syndrome, Ann Ophthalmol 8:1165, 1976

170. Svedbergh, B: Aspects of the aqueous humour drainage: functional ultrastructure of Schlemm's canal, the trabecular meshwork and the corneal endothelium at different intraocular pressures, Acta Univ Uppsl 256:1, 1976

171. Svedbergh, B, and Bill, A: Scanning electron microscopic studies of the corneal endothelium in man and monkeys, Acta Ophthalmol 50:321, 1972

172. Svedbergh, B, Lütjen-Drecoll, E, Ober, M, and Kaufman, PL: Cytochalasin B induced structural changes in the anterior ocular segment of the cynomolgus monkey, Invest Ophthalmol 17:718, 1978

173. Theobald, GD: Schlemm's canal: its anastomosis and anatomic relations, Trans Am Ophthalmol Soc 32:574, 1934

174. Tripathi, RC: Mechanism of the aqueous outflow across the trabecular wall of Schlemm's canal, Exp Eye Res 11:116, 1971

175. Tripathi, RC: Pathologic anatomy of the outflow pathways of aqueous humor in chronic simple glaucoma, Exp Eye Res 25(suppl):403, 1977

176. Tripathi, RC: Uveoscleral drainage of aqueous humour, Exp Eye Res 25(suppl):305, 1977

177. Ujiie, K, and Bill, A: The drainage routes for aqueous humor in monkeys as revealed by scanning electron microscopy of corrosion casts, Scan Electron Microsc II:849, 1984

178. van der Zypen, E: Licht- und elektronen-mikroskopische Untersuchungen über den Bau und die Innervation des Ziliarmuskels bei Mensch und Affe (Cercopithecus aethiops), v Graefe's Arch Klin Exp Ophthalmol 174:143, 1967

179. Vegge, T: The fine structure of the trabeculum cribriforme and the inner wall of Schlemm's canal in the normal human eye, Z Zellforsch 77:267, 1967

180. Wolf, J: Inner surface of regions in the anterior chamber taking part in the regulation of the intraocular tension, including the demonstration of the covering viscous substance, Docum Ophthalmol 25:113, 1968

181. Worthen, DM, and Cleveland, PH: Fibronectin production in cultured human trabecular meshwork cells, Invest Ophthalmol Vis Sci 23:265, 1982

182. Wulle, KG: Electron microscopic observations of the development of Schlemm's canal in the human eye, Trans Am Acad Ophthalmol Otolaryngol 72:765, 1968

183. Wulle, KG: The development of the productive and draining system of the aqueous humor in the human eye, Adv Ophthalmol 26:269, 1972

Chapter 3

Anatomy, Microcirculation, and Ultrastructure of the Ciliary Body

John C. Morrison
E. Michael Van Buskirk
Thomas F. Freddo

CILIARY BODY ANATOMY

The ciliary body and iris form the anterior uveal tract of the eye. Lying posterior to the iris as a ring of highly vascular tissue, the ciliary body comprises the ciliary muscle and ciliary processes. Both structures possess unique morphologic features that are essential to their highly specialized functions of accommodation, outflow facility regulation, and aqueous humor formation.

Viewed in cross-sectional profile, the ciliary muscle forms a triangle with its apex pointing posteriorly, ending at the ora serrata (Fig. 3-1). Its outermost longitudinal fibers insert as tendinous bands into the corneoscleral trabecular meshwork and scleral spur, whereas the middle radial and inner circular fibers form the base of the triangle. The longitudinal muscle fibers are only loosely adherent to the adjacent sclera via sparse collagen fibers, producing the potential, supraciliary space that can pathologically fill with blood and serous fluid. Ciliary muscle contraction decreases the resistance to outflow of aqueous humor, apparently through mechanical tension on the trabecular meshwork.

Lying internal to the ciliary muscle, the ciliary processes form the pars plicata, which, along with the more posterior pars plana, constitute the lateral wall of the posterior chamber (Fig. 3-2). Approximately 70 radially arrayed major ciliary processes project into the posterior chamber. Their anterior borders arise from the iris root, sweeping behind the iris to form the ciliary sulcus (Fig. 3-3). These major processes measure approximately 2 mm long, 0.5 mm wide, and 1 mm high and possess an irregular, knobby surface. Smaller, minor ciliary processes commonly lie between the major processes and do not project as far into the posterior chamber.

The pars plana extends from the posterior border of the ciliary processes to the ora serrata and is covered by a double layer of pigmented and nonpigmented epithelium. Although most ciliary zonules originate from between the inner, nonpigmented epithelial cells of the pars plana and their basement membrane,[19,24] some arise from between the ciliary processes. The zonules sweep anteriorly, fuse variably with the anterior vitreous and pars plicata basement membrane, and straddle the equator of the lens, inserting into its capsule. Thus on contraction, the ciliary muscle will shift anteriorly and reduce tension on the ciliary zonules, allowing the elastic increase in lens curvature that produces accommodation.

A light microscopic cross section of a major ciliary process demonstrates its three major components (Fig. 3-4): an inner capillary core, a surrounding loose stroma, and a double-layered epithelium continuous with that of the pars plana.

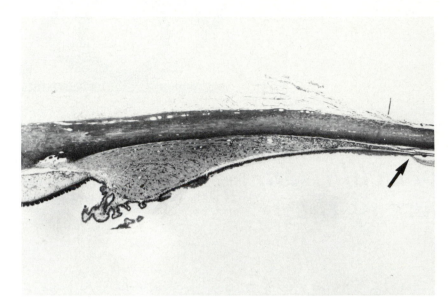

Fig. 3-1 Cross-sectional profile of primate ciliary body. Heavy pigmentation of triangular ciliary muscle outlines its longitudinal, radial, circular fibers. *Arrow* indicates ora serrata. (×15.)

Fig. 3-2 Scanning electron micrograph of lateral wall of posterior chamber with lens and zonules removed. Major, minor ciliary processes blend posteriorly with pars plana *(PP)*, which ends beneath vitreous base *(V)*. (×42.)

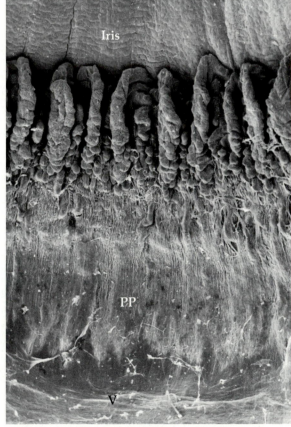

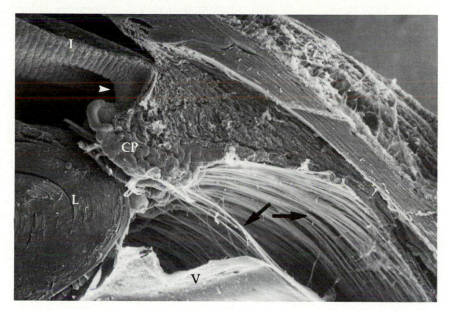

Fig. 3-3 Scanning electron micrograph of human ciliary body cut in cross-section demonstrates its relationship to iris *(I)*, zonules *(arrows)*, condensed anterior vitreous body *(V)*. Note ciliary sulcus *(arrowhead)* between iris, major ciliary processes *(CP)*. Shrinkage during processing has artifactually brought lens *(L)* into contact with ciliary processes. (×56.)

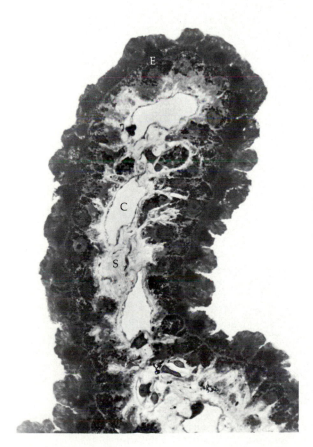

Fig. 3-4 Cross section of primate ciliary process illustrates capillary core *(C)*, stroma *(S)*, and double-layered pigmented and nonpigmented epithelium *(E)*. (×350.)

These components each possess unique morphologic features that reveal their roles in aqueous humor formation, a two-stage process that begins with passive ultrafiltration of plasma from the capillaries into the stroma followed by active secretion by the ciliary epithelium into the posterior chamber.

CILIARY BODY MICROVASCULATURE

Ciliary process vascular perfusion directly affects capillary hydrostatic pressure and ultrafiltration and indirectly influences active secretion by controlling delivery of oxygen and nutrients to the ciliary epithelium. The microvasculature responsible for ciliary body perfusion is a complex, three-dimensional system. Because of this complexity, the microvascular anatomy of the ciliary body is most easily understood by viewing carefully dissected methacrylate casts of its blood vessels with the scanning electron microscope after digestion of the surrounding tissues.[18]

The ciliary body receives blood from two sources: the anterior ciliary arteries and the long posterior ciliary arteries. Branches from both of these arteries anastomose freely with each other to produce a complex, redundant system characterized by numerous collateral channels that ensure consistent anterior segment perfusion even after partial interruption of its arterial supply, such as following strabismus and retinal detachment surgery.[16]

Derived from the ophthalmic artery, two anterior ciliary arteries approach the limbus from the insertions of each rectus muscle (with the exception of the lateral rectus, which contributes only one). Within the episclera, these arteries commonly branch and then interconnect, often forming a nearly complete anastomotic vascular ring, which occasionally can be observed clinically with biomicroscopy.

At the limbus several branches from each anterior ciliary artery turn inward, perforating the

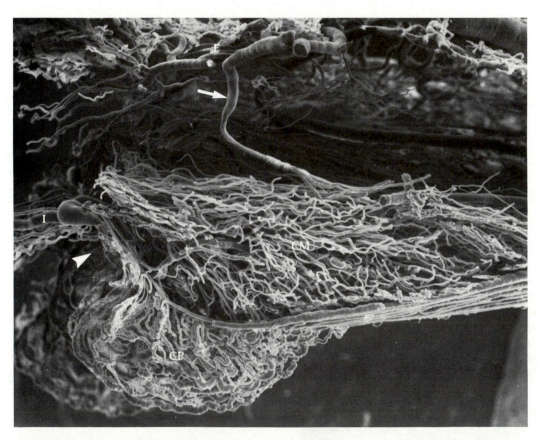

Fig. 3-5 Scanning electron micrograph of primate ciliary body methacrylate luminal casting. Profile view shows perforating branch (*arrow*) of anterior ciliary artery arising from episcleral microvasculature (*E*), traversing space once occupied by limbal sclera to enter ciliary muscle capillary bed (*CM*). Iris (*I*), ciliary processes (*CP*), outline ciliary sulcus (*arrowhead*). (×95.)

limbal sclera to enter the ciliary muscle capillary bed (Fig. 3-5). These branches arborize within the ciliary muscle and interconnect with each other and with branches from the nasal and temporal long posterior ciliary arteries.[16] These interconnections form a second anastomotic vascular ring, the intramuscular circle, which represents the major source of collateral blood flow to the ciliary body between the anterior and long posterior ciliary arterial systems (Fig. 3-6).

Numerous branches from the intramuscular circle supply capillaries to the ciliary muscle, which are densely packed and oriented parallel to the muscle fibers. Venous blood from the ciliary muscle drains primarily inward and posteriorly, into the choroidal veins.

Other branches from the intramuscular circle pass anteriorly to the root of the iris, where they bend and branch at right angles to form the major arterial circle, which lies tangential to the limbus. Because it consists of multiple vessels that often do not anastomose, the major arterial circle is often discontinuous and may be only a minor contributor to anterior segment collateral blood flow (Fig. 3-7).

The major arterial circle provides arterioles that supply both the iris and the ciliary processes. Iris arterioles arise either directly as separate branches from the major arterial circle or as the terminations of individual vessels comprising the major arterial circle.

Two types of arterioles, anterior and posterior, emanate from the major arterial circle to supply the ciliary processes.[17] Anterior arterioles arise in tufts,

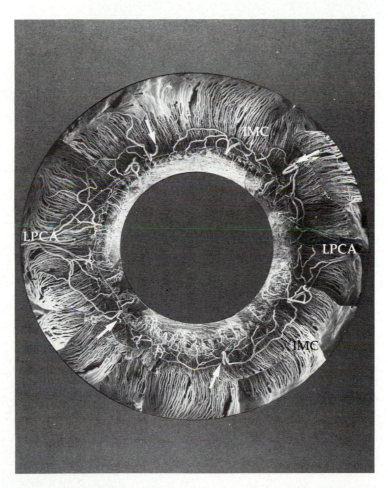

Fig. 3-6 Anterior view montage of primate ciliary body casting with episcleral, ciliary muscle capillary beds removed. Long posterior (*LPCA*), perforating anterior ciliary arteries *(arrows)* interconnect within ciliary bed to form nearly complete anastomotic vascular ring, intramuscular circle *(IMC)* (× 10.) (Modified from Morrison, JC, and Van Buskirk, EM: Ophthalmology 90:711, 1983.)

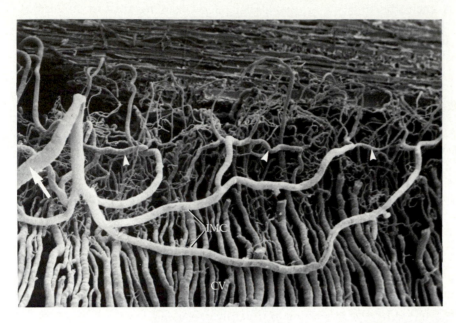

Fig. 3-7 Perforating anterior ciliary artery *(arrow)* supplies portion of intramuscular circle *(IMC)*, from which several branches pass to iris root to form circumferentially oriented but discontinuous major arterial circle *(arrowheads)*. Choroidal veins *(CV)*. (×65.) (Modified from: Morrison, JC, and Van Buskirk, EM: Ophthalmology 90:710, 1983)

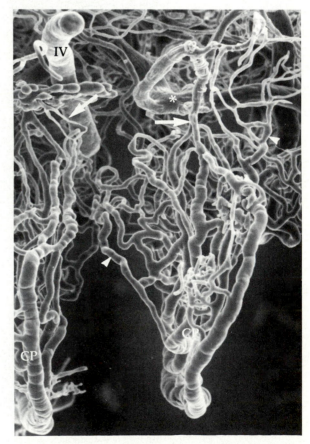

Fig. 3-8 Anterior view of two ciliary processes, looking into ciliary sulcus. Constricted-appearing anterior arterioles *(arrows)* arise from major arterial circle *(asterisk)* to supply dilated, veinlike capillaries of ciliary processes *(CP)*. *Arrowheads* indicate interprocess vascular connections; *IV* denotes severed iris vein. (×245.)

showing localized focal constrictions as they span the ciliary sulcus (Fig. 3-8). As they enter the processes, these arterioles rapidly dilate into irregular, large, veinlike capillaries that initially are directed anteriorly toward the ciliary process tip. These capillaries then turn and pass posteriorly within the internal margin of the process to empty into the choroidal veins (Fig. 3-9).

Whereas many anterior arterioles enter the ciliary processes directly, others branch to either side to enter the anterior regions of contiguous ciliary processes, forming interprocess vascular connections (see Fig. 3-8). In addition to providing vascular communication between ciliary processes, these interprocess connections commonly empty directly into the choroidal veins via veins lying along the base of the ciliary processes, providing a shunt that bypasses the ciliary processes entirely (see Fig. 3-9).

Arterioles that arise more posteriorly from the major arterial circle are generally less numerous and less constricted than the anterior arterioles (see Fig. 3-9). They enter the basal regions of the ciliary processes, providing irregular capillaries that serve the base and posterior regions of the ciliary processes. These capillaries also travel in a posterior direction, concentric to those from the anterior arterioles. Thus capillaries derived from anterior arterioles serve the ciliary process margins and those arising more posteriorly are situated within the base of the process.

Interprocess connections also arise from the posterior arterioles. These supply the minor ciliary processes on either side and the basal regions of neighboring major processes. Minor ciliary process capillaries resemble those of the major processes, being irregularly dilated and traveling posteriorly to drain into the choroidal veins.

The complex anatomy of the ciliary body microvasculature provides many potential avenues by which blood flow can be altered within this highly vascular organ (Fig. 3-10).[17] Constriction of anterior ciliary process arterioles would conceivably reduce perfusion of anterior and marginal capillaries and shunt blood to the minor ciliary processes and bases of major processes. Selective activation of other vascular sphincters could also shunt blood between major ciliary processes through interprocess connections. Finally, vascular pathways exist that would allow shunting of blood directly into the choroidal veins, bypassing the ciliary processes altogether.

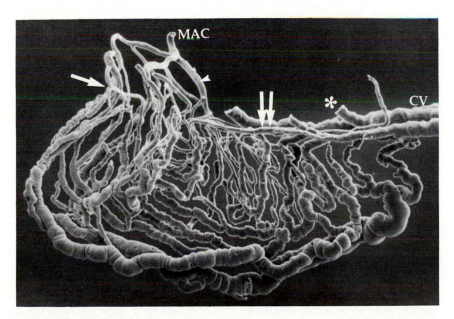

Fig. 3-9 Profile of individual major ciliary process casting indicates anterior (*arrow*), posterior (*arrowhead*) ciliary process arterioles arising from major arterial circle (*MAC*). Irregularly dilated capillaries from anterior arterioles pass posteriorly within ciliary process margin to empty into choroidal veins (*CV*). Capillaries supplied by posterior arterioles occupy base of process. *Double arrow* indicates choroidal vein extending along process base to drain interprocess connection. Severed branches (*asterisk*) represent drainage route of ciliary muscle capillaries (removed) into choroidal veins. (×145.)

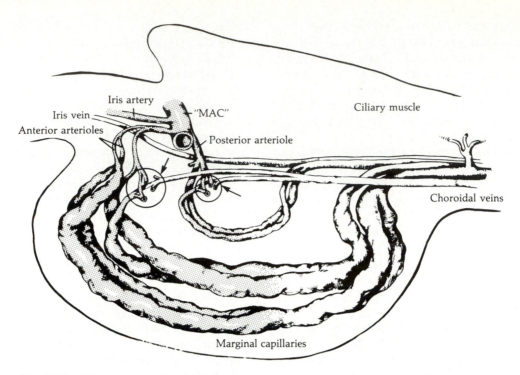

Fig. 3-10 Schematic representation of primate ciliary process microvasculature, illustrating anterior, posterior arteriolar supplies from major arterial circle *(MAC)*. Interprocess connections are circled, *arrows* indicate their relationship to choroidal veins providing possible shunt around ciliary process.

PHYSIOLOGY OF CILIARY BODY MICROCIRCULATION

Various physiologic, neurologic, and pharmacologic stimuli can alter ciliary body vascular resistance. Quantitative measurements using intravascularly injected radiolabeled microspheres have demonstrated that experimental increases in intraocular pressure do not change ciliary blood flow in either monkeys or cats, suggesting an autoregulatory decrease in vascular tone.[1,2] Similarly increasing systemic blood pressure in cats does not change ciliary body perfusion, probably because of a reflex increase in vascular resistance that may protect against the effects of elevated intravascular pressure.[7] Therefore vascular autoregulation exists within the ciliary body to protect and maintain its perfusion under varying physiologic conditions. Varying the tone of precapillary sphincters noted in castings of anterior ciliary process arterioles could contribute to this autoregulatory response.

Both adrenergic and cholinergic nerve endings have been identified histochemically in association with blood vessels of the ciliary processes and ciliary muscle in monkeys, man, and other animal species.[9,10,14] Radiolabeled microsphere studies indicate that unilateral stimulation of the sympathetic chain decreases blood flow in all parts of the ciliary body in monkeys,[4] rabbits,[6,7] and cats.[3] This response is decreased by pretreatment with nonspecific alpha-antagonists but is unaltered by propranolol, a nonspecific beta-antagonist. In addition, both alpha-1 and alpha-2 adrenergic drugs mimic this sympathetically induced decrease in ciliary body perfusion.[8,15] In contrast, the beta-stimulator isoproterenol has no measurable effect on anterior uveal blood flow.[15] It appears that adrenergic neural stimulation induces anterior uveal vasoconstriction, and that this is mediated primarily by alpha-adrenergic receptors.

The influence of parasympathetic nerves on ciliary blood flow is more complex. In monkeys, oculomotor nerve stimulation decreases iris blood flow but increases it in the ciliary processes.[23] In addition, the topical miotics pilocarpine and neostigmine increase ciliary body blood flow, an effect most evident in the ciliary processes.[5] These differing regional effects of cholinergic receptor stimulation indicate that ciliary body blood flow is not simply a passive response to a perfusion pressure dictated by the anterior and long posterior ciliary

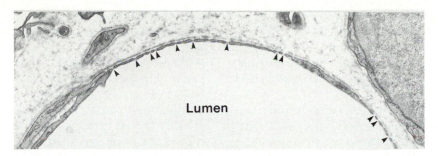

Fig. 3-11 Numerous fenestrations *(arrowheads)* are present along circumference of capillary in ciliary body stroma. (×22,000.)

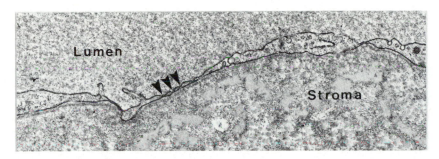

Fig. 3-12 Granular HRP reaction product leaks through fenestrations *(arrowheads)* of fenestrated capillary into surrounding ciliary body stroma. (×26,000.)

arteries. Instead, the individual microvascular beds of the iris, ciliary muscle, and ciliary processes appear capable of regulating their blood flow independently of each other. This is likely accomplished through the vessels of each of these components, which appear to possess distinctive structural characteristics, as well as unique pharmacologic and neurologic sensitivities.

ULTRASTRUCTURE OF THE CILIARY MICROVASCULATURE

Two different types of capillaries exist within the ciliary body. The ciliary muscle possesses continuous capillaries that are impermeable to intravenously injected tracers such as horseradish peroxidase (HRP) and play no known role in the process of aqueous humor production. The capillaries of the ciliary body stroma and those of individual ciliary processes, however, are fenestrated.[13] Such capillaries are lined by endothelial cells in which numerous circular pores appear in a variety of distributional patterns. For example, the fenestrations in endothelial cells of the choriocapillaris are confined to the side of the lumen that faces Bruch's membrane. The capillaries of the ciliary body stroma, however, are fenestrated around their entire circumference (Fig. 3-11).

Ciliary process capillaries do not constitute a significant barrier to the passage of macromolecules. Intravenously injected HRP rapidly escapes through the fenestrations of these capillaries and into the loose stromal matrix, finally reaching the ciliary epithelium (Fig. 3-12).[22]

ULTRASTRUCTURE OF THE CILIARY EPITHELIUM

The barrier that prevents macromolecules from reaching the posterior chamber resides within the ciliary epithelium, which consists of two layers of cells, the outer pigmented and the inner nonpigmented. Despite being bilayered, the ciliary epithelium is not compound but consists of two simple epithelia joined apex to apex with the basal lamina of the pigmented layer resting on the ciliary body stroma and that of the nonpigmented layer lining the posterior chamber (Fig. 3-13). This unusual arrangement results from invagination of the optic vesicle to form the optic cup during embryonic development.

The nonpigmented ciliary epithelium is continuous anteriorly with the pigmented epithelium of the iris and posteriorly with the neurosensory retina at the ora serrata. The pigmented epithelium continues anteriorly as the anterior myoepithelium of the iris and posteriorly as the retinal pigmented epithelium.

The cells of the pigmented ciliary epithelium are cuboidal, measuring 10 to 12 μm in height. Their basal surfaces are convoluted and rest on a basal lamina of variable thickness. Pigmented epithelial cells contain numerous melanosomes and a modest complement of mitochondria, rough endoplasmic reticulum, and Golgi complexes (see Fig. 3-13).

The nonpigmented ciliary epithelial cells of the

pars plicata are also cuboidal and possess a markedly infolded basal surface lying on a thin basal lamina that does not enter the myriad infoldings (see Fig. 3-3). These cells lack melanin and, compared with the cells of the pigmented epithelium, have more and larger mitochondria and rough endoplasmic reticulum, indicating a greater metabolic capacity. All of these features are amplified in the cells of the nonpigmented layer that lie in the anterior pars plicata, suggesting that this region makes a greater contribution overall to the production of aqueous humor.[12] These are also regions that casting studies suggest are perfused by capillaries that arise from the focally constricted, anterior ciliary process arterioles.[17]

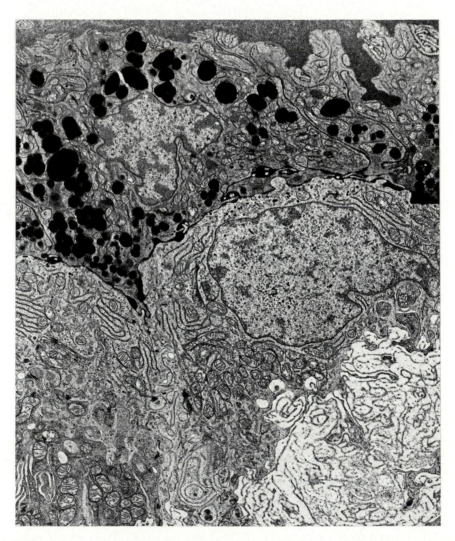

Fig. 3-13 Pigmented ciliary epithelium (above) with numerous black melanosomes, small mitochondria is easily distinguished from nonpigmented ciliary epithelium with larger, more numerous mitochondria. Note swirls of basal lamina from nonpigmented layer that line posterior chamber. (×12,500.)

Intercellular Epithelial Junctions

Both the pigmented and nonpigmented epithelial cells are interconnected by specialized intercellular junctions that control the passage of water, ions, and macromolecules into the aqueous humor.[20,21] Desmosomes and gap junctions are ubiquitous findings within and between both layers of the ciliary epithelium. In thin sections, desmosomes appear to maintain adjacent cells approximately 17 nm apart. The resulting intercellular cleft is spanned by branching filaments and, on the cytoplasmic surfaces of the adjoining cells, a thin plaque of filaments provides a point of insertion for bundles of 9 to 10 nm tonofilaments (Fig. 3-14, A). In freeze-fracture replicas, desmosomes appear as circular areas containing a heterogeneous population of intramembranous particles (Fig. 3-14, B).

Desmosomes provide attachment sites for the cytoskeleton of neighboring cells, a function likely shared by another type of intercellular junction called the *punctum adherens*. Within the nonpigmented ciliary epithelium, desmosomes also maintain the narrow width of the intercellular cleft that is necessary to concentrate solutes, an essential regulating step in maintaining the composition of aqueous humor.

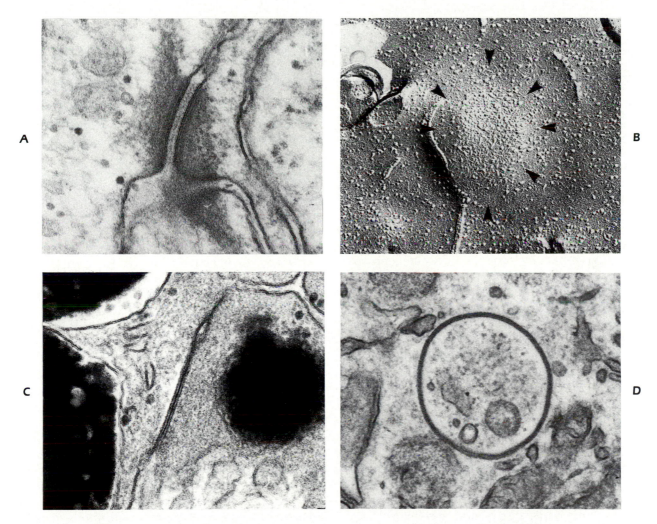

Fig. 3-14 **A,** Transmission electron micrograph of typical desmosome showing branching filaments extending across intercellular cleft. **B,** Freeze-fracture electron micrograph showing clustering of heterogeneous particles (*encircled by arrowheads*) that characterize a desmosome. **C,** Transmission electron micrograph of typical gap junction joining lateral surfaces of two pigmented ciliary epithelial cells. **D,** Transmission electron micrograph of invaginated gap junction seen here as complete circle. Cytoplasm confined within circle, cytoplasm outside circle belong to separate cells. (**A,** ×71,000; **B,** ×69,000; **C,** ×78,000; **D,** ×48,000.)

Continued.

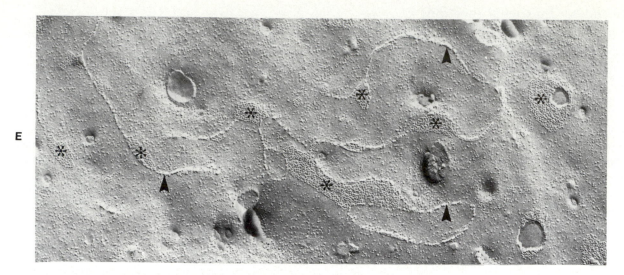

Fig. 3-14, cont'd **E,** Freeze-fracture replica of ciliary epithelium shows numerous gap junctions *(asterisks)* joining apical surfaces of two epithelial layers. In this location gap junctions are accompanied by discontinuous tight junctional strands *(arrowheads)*. **(E,** ×45,000.)

In thin sections, gap junctions usually appear straight or curved, with the junctional membranes of the adjoining cells invariably parallel and separated by a 2 to 4 nm space (Fig. 3-14, *C*). Variants called *invaginated gap junctions* are also seen in which the cytoplasm of one cell protrudes into the domain of its neighbor. Here the membranes of the two cells are joined by a gap junction over the entire vesicular protrusion (Fig. 3-14, *D*).

In freeze-fracture replicas, gap junctions appear as aggregates of intramembranous particles on the inner leaflet of the cell membrane and are complemented by similar arrays of pits on the outer leaflet (Fig. 3-14, *E*). When located between the apices of the pigmented and nonpigmented epithelial layers, gap junctions are commonly associated with discontinuous tight junctional strands (Fig. 3-14, *E*).

The particles seen in the freeze-fracture replicas of gap junctions represent proteins that bridge the "gap" to meet similar proteins from the apposing cell membrane. The resulting "connexons" are calcium-dependent and, when open, provide a 1.5 nm channel between the interiors of the two cells, allowing interchange of ions and small molecules such as amino acids, sugars, and nucleotides. Gap junctions thus mediate electrotonic and metabolic coupling of ciliary epithelial cells, permitting the two layers to operate as a functional syncytium in the coordinated production of aqueous humor. Indeed, the hypotonous stages of experimental anterior uveitis have been associated with a profound depletion of gap junctions from the inflamed ciliary epithelium.[11]

The Blood-Aqueous Barrier of the Ciliary Body

The blood-aqueous barrier function of the ciliary body lies within the nonpigmented ciliary epithelium.[20] Near their apical surfaces, nonpigmented ciliary epithelial cells are joined by zonulae occludens, or tight junctions, which form part of an apicolateral junctional complex, which also includes a zonula adherens and often a gap junction.

In thin sections, zonulae occludens appear as one or more areas of direct contact between intramembranous proteins of the adjacent plasma membranes, thus occluding the intercellular cleft (Fig. 3-15, *inset*). HRP leaked from the fenestrated capillaries of the ciliary body stroma freely permeates the intercellular spaces between adjacent pigmented epithelial cells and between the apices of the pigmented and nonpigmented layers. However, the zonula occludens of the nonpigmented epithelium prevent the tracer from reaching the posterior chamber (Fig. 3-15).

Freeze-fracture replicas demonstrate that zonulae occludens are a system of continuous branching and anastomosing strands that extend around the entire circumference of each cell (Fig. 3-16). The complexity of the junctional pattern varies, and junctional complexity and barrier permeability are known to be inversely related. The tight junctions located between the nonpigmented epithelial cells

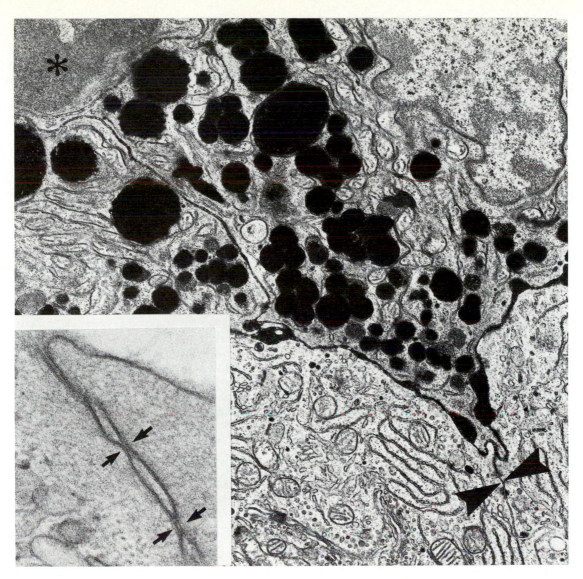

Fig. 3-15 Granular HRP reaction product in ciliary body stroma *(asterisk)* blackens intercellular clefts between adjacent pigmented ciliary epithelial cells, between apical surfaces of pigmented, nonpigmented layers. Further diffusion of HRP toward posterior chamber is blocked by tight junction at apicolateral surface of nonpigmented layer. No HRP reaction product is therefore seen in intercellular cleft between adjacent nonpigmented ciliary epithelial cells *(large arrowheads).* (×19,000.) *Inset,* Transmission electron micrograph shows point of fusion between membranes of adjacent nonpigmented ciliary epithelial cells *(arrows),* which are characteristic of zonulae occludens. (×131,000.)

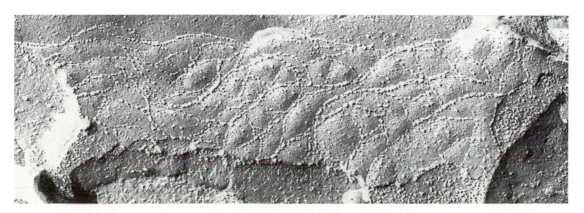

Fig. 3-16 Freeze-fracture replica of nonpigmented ciliary epithelium demonstrates branching, anastomosing strands of zonula occludens (×57,500).

represent a selective barrier that still allows diffusion of water and small molecules into the posterior chamber. In this manner, tight junctions help maintain the osmotic and electrical gradients across the ciliary epithelium that are required for the final, active step in aqueous humor production.

Tight junctions also prevent apical and basal nonpigmented epithelial cell receptors from floating to the opposite cell surface in the fluid mosaic of the cell membrane. This maintains the polarity of the ciliary epithelium.

REFERENCES

1. Alm, A, and Bill, A: The oxygen supply to the retina. II. Effects of high intraocular pressure and of increased arterial carbon dioxide tension on uveal and retinal blood flow in cats, Acta Physiol Scand 84:306, 1972

2. Alm, A: Ocular and optic nerve blood flow at normal and increased intraocular pressures in monkeys (Macaca irus): a study with radioactively labeled microspheres including flow determination in brain and some other tissues, Exp Eye Res 15:15, 1973

3. Alm, A: The effect of stimulation of the cervical sympathetic chain on retinal oxygen tension and on uveal, retinal and cerebral flow in cats, Acta Physiol Scand 88:84, 1973

4. Alm, A: The effect of sympathetic stimulation on blood flow through the uvea, retina and optic nerve in monkeys (Macaca irus), Exp Eye Res 25:19, 1977

5. Alm, A, Bill, A, and Young, FA: The effects of pilocarpine and neostigmine on the blood flow through the anterior uvea in monkeys: a study with radioactively labeled microspheres, Exp Eye Res 15:31, 1973

6. Beausang-Linder, M: Effects of sympathetic stimulation on cerebral and ocular blood flow: modification by hypertension, hypercapnia, acetazolamide, PGI-2, and papaverine, Acta Physiol Scand 114:217, 1982

7. Beausang-Linder, M: Sympathetic effects on cerebral and ocular blood flow in rabbits pretreated with indomethacin, Acta Physiol Scand 114:211, 1982

8. Bill, A, and Heilmann, K: Ocular effects of clonidine in cats and monkeys, Exp Eye Res 21:481, 1975

9. Ehinger, B: Adrenergic nerves to the eye and to related structures in man and in the cynomolgus monkey (Macaca irus), Invest Ophthalmol 5:42, 1966

10. Ehinger, B: Connections between adrenergic nerves and other tissue components in the eye, Acta Physiol Scand 67:57, 1966

11. Freddo, T: Intercellular junctions of the ciliary epithelium in anterior uveitis, Invest Ophthalmol Vis Sci 28:320, 1987

12. Hara, K, Lütjen-Drecoll, E, Prestle, H, and Rohen, JW: Structural differences between regions of the ciliary body in primates, Invest Ophthalmol Vis Sci 16:912, 1977

13. Holmberg, A: The ultrastructure of the capillaries in the ciliary body, Arch Ophthalmol 62:949, 1959

14. Laties, AM, and Jacobowitz, D: A comparative study of the autonomic innervation of the eye in the monkey, cat and rabbit, Anat Rec 156:383, 1966

15. Morgan, TR, Green, K, and Bowman, K: Effects of adrenergic agonists upon regional ocular blood flow in normal and ganglionectomized rabbits, Exp Eye Res 32:691, 1981

16. Morrison, JC, and Van Buskirk, EM: Anterior collateral circulation in the primate eye, Ophthalmology 90:707, 1983

17. Morrison, JC, and Van Buskirk, EM: Ciliary process microvasculature of the primate eye, Am J Ophthalmol 97:372, 1984

18. Morrison, JC, and Van Buskirk, EM: Sequential microdissection and scanning electron microscopy of ciliary microvascular castings, Scan Electron Microsc II:857, 1984

19. Raviola, G: The fine structure of the ciliary zonule and ciliary epithelium: with special regard to the organization and insertion of the zonular fibrils, Invest Ophthalmol Vis Sci 10:851, 1971

20. Raviola, G: The structural basis of the blood-ocular barriers, Exp Eye Res 25(suppl.):27, 1977

21. Raviola, G, and Raviola, E: Intercellular junctions in the ciliary epithelium, Invest Ophthalmol Vis Sci 17:958, 1978

22. Smith, RS, and Rudt, BA: Ultrastructural studies of the blood-aqueous barrier. II. The barrier to horseradish peroxidase in primates, Am J Ophthalmol 76:937, 1973

23. Stjernschantz, J, and Bill, A: Effect of intracranial stimulation of the oculomotor nerve on ocular blood flow in the monkey, cat and rabbit, Invest Ophthalmol Vis Sci 18:99, 1979

24. Streeten, BW: Zonular apparatus. In Duane, TD, Jaeger, EA, editors: Biomedical foundations of ophthalmology, Philadelphia, 1982, Harper & Row Publishers, Inc

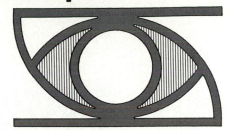

Chapter 4

Ronald L. Radius

Anatomy and Pathophysiology of the Retina and Optic Nerve

THE RETINA

Ganglion Cell Layer

Ganglion cells

Each optic nerve contains approximately 1.2 million axons. The ganglion cells of origin are located in the innermost nuclear layer of the retina (the ganglion cell layer).[124] Surrounding the fovea, the ganglion cell layer is from four to six cells thick[201] (Fig. 4-1). Within the fovea and the immediately adjacent retina, corresponding roughly to an area equivalent to that of the avascular zone, there are no ganglion cells. In the posterior pole, within the region circumscribed by the major retinal vessels, this layer is, on the average, two cells in thickness. In the more peripheral retina, it thins to a single cell layer.

The dendritic field of individual ganglion cells synapses within the inner plexiform layer with processes from bipolar and amacrine cells, the cell bodies of which lie within the inner nuclear layer of the retina.[22,39] There are several ganglion cell types, which are characterized by size and variation in their dendritic pattern[23,122] (Fig. 4-2). The smallest of the ganglion cells, "midget" cells, are approximately 10 μm in diameter. These cells have a more limited dendritic field and predominate in the posterior pole of the eye. Other ganglion cells range in size from 10 to 30 μm and vary considerably with respect to the extent of their dendritic

tree and synaptic pattern within the strata of the inner molecular layer.

Electrophysiology

In general, a given ganglion cell responds to a change in retinal illumination rather than to the absolute level of the light stimulus.[35,111] The ganglion cell response to retinal illumination is characterized by a change in the baseline rate of propagated action potentials. This firing rate is determined by a complex summation of the various inhibitory and excitatory impulses impinging on the ganglion cell body through its multiple synapses with amacrine and bipolar cells within the inner plexiform layer. Ganglion cells respond to changes in retinal illumination only if the stimulus involves their own receptive field.[63]

The receptive field, generally circular in shape, corresponds to a geographic region of the retina surrounding a ganglion cell, within which photostimulation of the receptor rods and cones increases or decreases the firing rate of the associated ganglion cell. Because the 1.2 million ganglion cells convey impulses from the several hundred million rods and cones, hundreds of individual receptor elements subserve each retinal ganglion cell. In the posterior pole, receptor fields are small and the ratio of receptors to ganglion cells is low. In the more peripheral retina, the receptor fields are

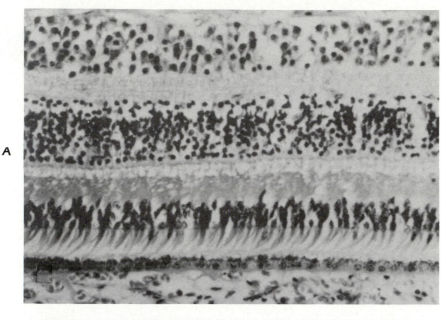

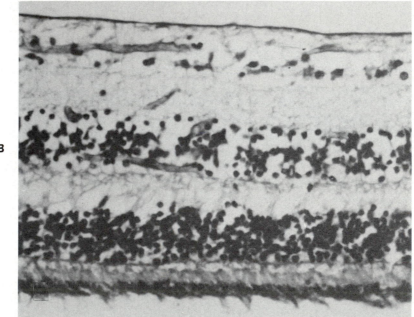

Fig. 4-1 Light photomicrographs of retina. **A,** Ganglion cell layer, the innermost nucleated layer within the retina, is from four to six cells thick within macular region. **B,** In retinal periphery, this same layer is from one to two cells thick. (Courtesy of WR Green. From Miller, NR: Walsh and Hoyt's neuro-ophthalmology, Baltimore, 1982, Williams & Wilkins)

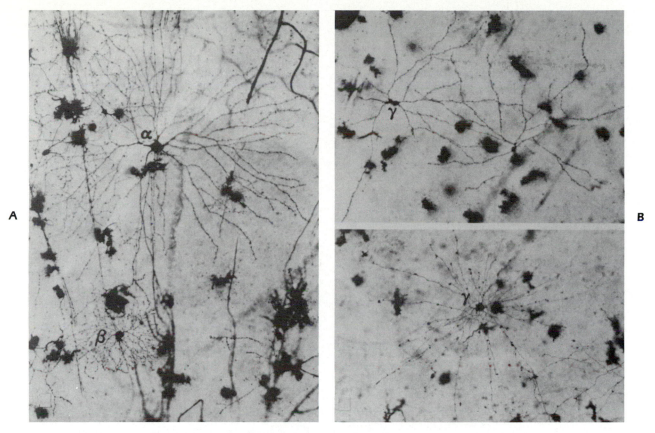

Fig. 4-2 Dendritic pattern of the retinal ganglion cell can be demonstrated by Golgi staining preparations. Retinal ganglion cells differ in size and extent of these dendritic patterns. Largest cell (**A,** ×160) is the alpha cell seen in upper left. Somewhat smaller beta cell is to lower left, and smallest cell, gamma cell, is pictured at upper right (×160) and at lower right (**B,** ×320) (From Boycott, BB, and Wassle, HJ Physiol [Lond] 240:397, 1974)

larger, and many more receptors affect the depolarization of a single ganglion cell.[80-82,111]

Receptor fields also overlap each other, particularly in the retinal periphery. Stimulation of individual receptors may influence the firing rate of several ganglion cells. Finally, although the center of a given receptor field is fixed according to the location of the individual ganglion cell, its diameter may vary over time, depending on the intensity, size, and frequency of the stimulus involved.[63,80,81,88]

The receptor field is generally organized into a center and surround opponent response to retinal illumination.[88,111] In a center-on ganglion cell, an increase in illumination of the central region of the receptor field increases the firing rate of the ganglion cell. In a center-off ganglion cell, a decrease in illumination of the center produces an increase in the ganglion cell firing. A change in illumination of the surround region within a single receptor field

produces exactly the opposite effect on the associated ganglion cell to that in the center.

Patterned after the description of retinal physiology characteristic of the cat eye, the primate retina has ganglion cells with X- and Y-type responses to retinal stimulation.* If the ganglion cell receptor field is alternately illuminated by a stimulus of the proper orientation and frequency, the X-type cell responds with a sustained change in firing rate. Y-type ganglion cells, on the other hand, respond to a change in retinal illumination with an abrupt but transient change in the baseline firing rate. These transient Y-type cells are also characterized by a center-surround receptor field. The transient response ganglion cells generally show shorter latency periods than the X-type cells. Finally, a third class of ganglion cells (W cells) do not demonstrate a center-surround receptor field and have the slow-

---

*References 29, 30, 35, 44, 82-84, 111.

est latency of conduction of the three ganglion cell populations.[188]

Neuroglia and blood flow

The neuroglia in the ganglion cell layer consist of processes of Müller cells, cell bodies of which are located within the inner nuclear layer. Retinal astrocyte processes envelop retinal capillaries and associated pericytes, isolating the ganglion cells from retinal blood flow.[212] Capillary endothelial cells are characterized by tight junctions between cells.[20,55,72,120,180] Blood flow to this retinal layer is ultimately derived from the retinal circulation.[6,12,64,65,94]

The Nerve Fiber Layer

Neuroglia

Throughout the central nervous system, the neuroglia provide a structural framework for support of the neural elements. This same pattern is evident within the optic nerve and retinal layers.

A single axon from each ganglion cell enters the overlying nerve fiber layer (Fig. 4-3). Within the retinal nerve fiber layer, axons are grouped into fiber bundles (Fig. 4-4 and 4-5). Individual fiber bundles are defined by incomplete channels formed by elongated sheetlike processes of Müller cell origin[152] (Fig. 4-6). The foot-plates of these same processes coalesce at the retinal surface to form a dense glial layer, the internal limiting membrane of the retina[72,111] (Fig. 4-7).

Within the fiber bundles, astrocyte processes envelop individual axons[114,212] (Fig. 4-8). Although this insulation by glial fibers is incomplete, with many instances of direct axon-axon contact, there is no evidence of any physiologic or electrochemical exchange between axons of the nerve fiber layer. This complex of astrocyte and Müller cell channels, established early in embryogenesis, may play some role in the development and orientation of axons as they grow from the ganglion cells toward the optic papillae.[181,182,187]

Blood flow

Blood flow to the nerve fiber layer is derived from the central retinal artery and is drained by the central retinal vein. The artery enters the optic nerve approximately 1 cm posterior to the globe as a branch of the ophthalmic artery.* Within the nerve and at the nerve head, the central retinal artery gives off small branches, which anastomose

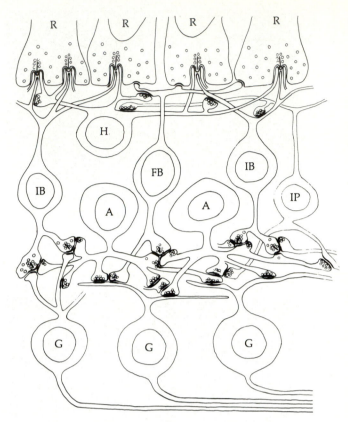

Fig. 4-3 Schematic representation of nucleated retinal layers including receptors *(R)* in outer nuclear layer, amacrine cell *(A)*, bipolar cells *(IB* and *FB)*, horizontal cell *(H)*, and interplexiform cell *(IP)*, all contained within inner nuclear layer and ganglion cell *(G)* within ganglion cell layer. A single axon from each retinal ganglion cell leaves this innermost nuclear layer and enters retinal nerve fiber layer, traveling in grouped fiber bundles to exit eye at optic nerve head. (Courtesy JE Dowling. From Miller, NR: Walsh and Hoyt's neuro-ophthalmology, Baltimore, 1982, Williams & Wilkins)

with the microcirculation of the more posterior portions of the nerve head derived primarily from the posterior ciliary circulation.* Although individual anatomy may vary, there is generally a single branching at or above the lamina cribrosa into a superior and inferior vessel and a second bifurcation within the nerve head into temporal and nasal branches. A single vessel goes to each of the four retinal quadrants. The superior and inferior temporal branches arch around the area centralis including the macula and fovea.

At the nerve head, the central retinal vessel is a true artery, complete with muscular coat. Within the retina, however, the muscular coat is lost and the vessels are actually arterioles. The retinal ar-

---

*References 6, 12, 49, 50, 64, 65, 68, 94.

*References 6, 12, 64, 65, 67, 68, 94, 174.

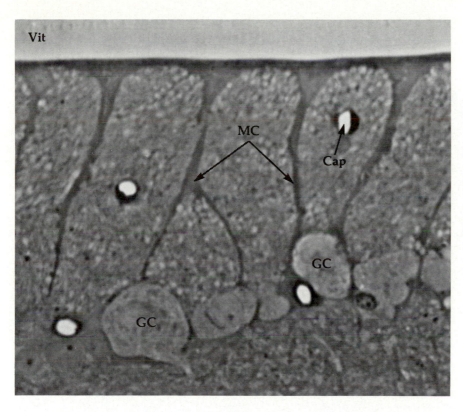

Fig. 4-4 Retinal nerve fiber layer cut in cross section reveals dense glial processes of Müller cell origin (*MC*) grouping axons into fiber bundles. *Vit*, Vitreous; *Cap*, capillary; *GC*, ganglion cell. (From Radius, RL, and Anderson, DR: Arch Ophthalmol 97:948, 1979. Copyright 1979, American Medical Association)

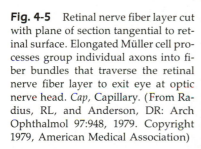

Fig. 4-5 Retinal nerve fiber layer cut with plane of section tangential to retinal surface. Elongated Müller cell processes group individual axons into fiber bundles that traverse the retinal nerve fiber layer to exit eye at optic nerve head. *Cap*, Capillary. (From Radius, RL, and Anderson, DR: Arch Ophthalmol 97:948, 1979. Copyright 1979, American Medical Association)

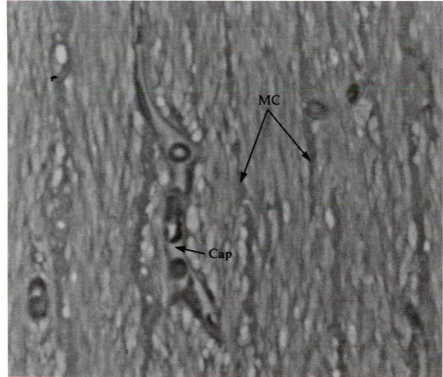

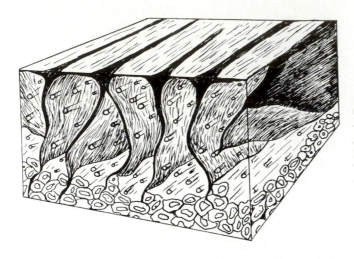

Fig. 4-6 Schematic representation of retinal nerve fiber layer depicting three-dimensional anatomy of nerve fiber layer axons grouped into individual fiber bundles by elongated sheetlike processes of Müeller cell origin. (From Radius, RL, and Anderson, DR: Arch Ophthalmol 97:948, 1979. Copyright 1979, American Medical Association)

Fig. 4-7 Low-power electron photomicrograph demonstrating internal limiting membrane (ILM) of retina comprising basement membrane formed by processes of Müller cell (MP) origin. N, Astrocyte nucleus. (Courtesy HA Quigley. From Miller, NR: Walsh and Hoyt's clinical neuro-ophthalmology, Baltimore, 1982, Williams & Wilkins)

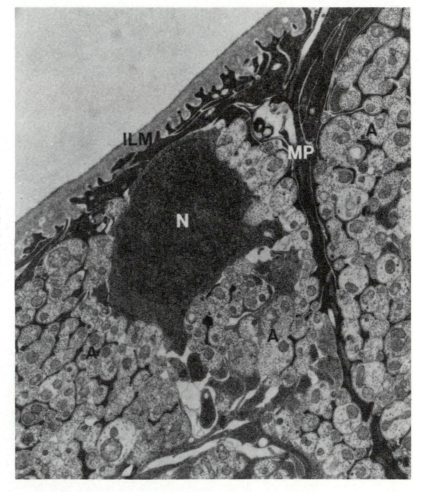

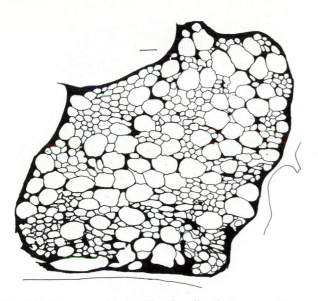

Fig. 4-8 Diagram of nerve fiber bundle of rhesus monkey, traced from montage of electron micrographs enlarged 30,000×. Glial tissue of both astrocyte and Müller cells is solid black. Of 508 fibers in this bundle, 188 had no glial contact and 52 contacted glia along 10% or less of their circumference. (Calibration 1 μm). (From Ogden, TE: Invest Ophthalmol Vis Sci 17:499, 1978.)

terioles progressively diminish in caliber, ultimately to the size of capillaries.[175] This capillary bed supplies the four inner layers of the retina, including the retinal nerve fiber layer, the ganglion cell layer, the inner molecular layer, and part of the inner nuclear layer. The microcirculation within these tissue layers, as well as the larger arterioles, are confined to the glial tissue framework and segregated by glial cell processes from direct contact with neuronal elements.

The capillaries, along with associated pericytes, are characterized by tight junctions.[55,180] Within the retina, this vasculature is an end-artery system, in which focal occlusion results in regional tissue infarction. The retinal circulation, however, exhibits a high degree of autoregulation.[2,3,53,142,184] Despite increasing intraocular pressure, retinal blood flow is maintained at a constant level until the intraocular pressure approaches the level of systolic blood pressure, at which point retinal blood flow decreases. When the intraocular pressure exceeds the systolic blood pressure, the vessel lumen collapses and ischemic infarction of the retina occurs. Irreversible morphologic changes in the retina can be seen after 2 hours of vascular occlusion.[87,155,157,162,168]

The retinal capillary bed is drained by small veins that converge into four major veins within the retina, a superior and inferior vein at the nerve head and a single central retinal vein within the nerve tissue. These veins roughly parallel the course of the retinal arterioles. The central retinal vein ultimately drains into the superior and inferior ophthalmic veins and the cavernous sinus.[6]

Topographic anatomy

Axon bundles within the nerve fiber layer generally follow a direct course from their ganglion cells of origin toward the optic nerve head.[103,115,116,151] Axons from regionally grouped ganglion cells are confined to adjacent fiber bundles. Although there may be some exchange of axons between adjacent fiber bundles, lateral dissemination of individual fibers within the retinal nerve fiber layer is not extensive (Fig. 4-9).

The pattern of fiber bundles can be recognized as bright striations in the retinal reflex by clinical ophthalmoscopy* (Fig. 4-10). This pattern is most obvious where the nerve fiber layer is thickest, such as within the papillomacular bundle temporal to the disc and in the superior and inferior arcuate bundles paralleling the major temporal branches of the central retinal artery.[143] Axons from the nasal retina pass directly into the nasal margin of the nerve. Axons from the temporal retina have a somewhat more complicated course.[73,75,78,111,151]

Fiber bundles from ganglion cells located between the nerve head and fovea travel within the papillomacular bundle to enter the temporal margin of the nerve head[173] (Fig. 4-11). Axons from ganglion cells located temporal to the fovea are divided into a superior and inferior arcade by the horizontal raphe extending from the macula into the temporal periphery of the retina.[202] Although this division is not anatomically exact, in general, ganglion cells above and below the raphe send the axons into the superior and inferior nerve fiber bundles, respectively. Fiber bundles arching around the macular region are joined by axons from more proximally located ganglion cells. The path roughly parallels that of the major retinal vessels. At the nerve head, these axon bundles enter the inferior and superior poles of the disc.

The vertical stratification of axons within the nerve fiber layer is not as well defined as the horizontal distribution in the human eye.[103,115,116,151] In the owl and rhesus monkeys, axons from peripheral retinal ganglion cells lie in the deeper layers of the nerve fiber layer.[103,116,151] As the fiber bundles pass toward the nerve head, axons from more prox-

---

*References 1, 77, 129, 151, 152, 161.

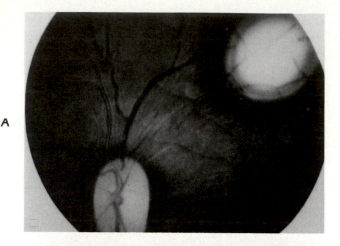

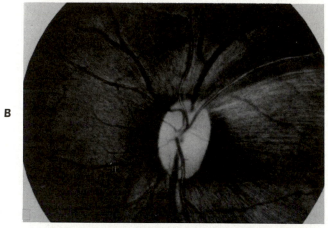

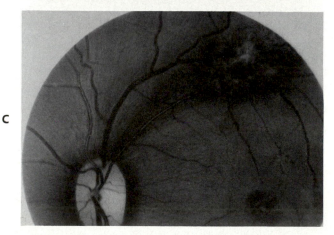

Fig. 4-9 Nerve fiber bundle defect photographed **A**, 3, **B**, 7, and **C**, 30 days after full-thickness retinal photocoagulation in monkey eye. Retinal nerve fiber layer striations of uninvolved retina border region of axon atrophy. Margins of arcuate defect are well defined, with little or no lateral spread of damaged axons. In histologic specimens, damaged axons within nerve fiber layer are confined to region of arcuate fiber bundle loss with little or no lateral extension into normal adjacent retina, *right*. (From Radius, RL, and Anderson, DR: Arch Ophthalmol 97:948, 1979)

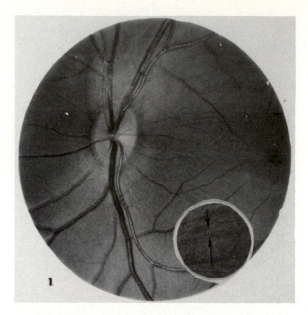

Fig. 4-10 Fundus photograph of normal monkey eye demonstrates striated pattern of nerve fiber bundles. In thicker regions of retinal nerve fiber layer within papillomacular bundle and arcuate regions paralleling major retinal vessels, this pattern is particularly well defined. Bright striated pattern of fiber bundle is offset by darker elongated processes of Müller cell origin. (From Radius, RL, and Anderson, DR: Arch Ophthalmol 97:948, 1979)

imally located cells penetrate overlying layers and lie in the more superficial strata of the nerve fiber layer. At the nerve head, axons from ganglion cells nearest the optic disc lie at the center of the nerve and axons from cells in the retinal periphery lie at the margins (Fig. 4-12). In the macaque monkey, the anatomy is exactly the opposite.[115] The anatomy of the human optic nerve posterior to the globe is most consistent with that of the owl and rhesus monkeys.[75,111,164,211]

Axonal transport

Axonal transport involves the intracytoplasmic transfer of materials.[8,11,34,178,210] In the neuron, the length of the axon in comparison to the size of the cell body makes this transcytoplasmic movement much more dramatic and more easily demonstrated.[205-207] Movement along the axon segment is bidirectional, orthograde transport being from the cell body to the axon terminal and retrograde transport being from the synapse back to the ganglion cell body (Fig. 4-13).

The predominant component of orthograde transport consists of membrane-bound protein synthesized in the rough endoplasmic reticulum of the cell body and transported within membrane-

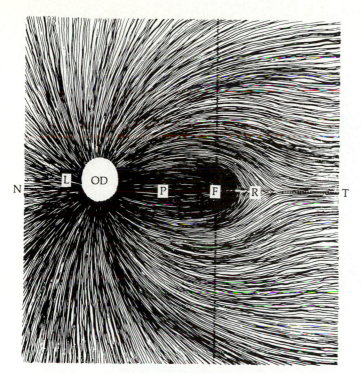

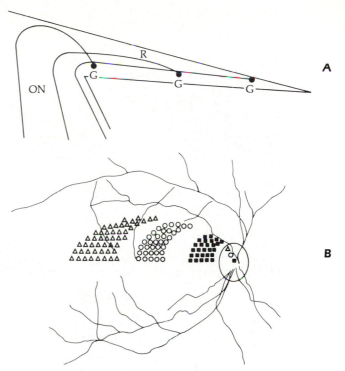

Fig. 4-11 Drawing of retinal nerve fiber layer depicts course of axon bundles. Axons from nasal *(N)* retina travel directly toward nerve head to enter along nasal margin of disc *(OD)*. Axons within papillomacular bundle *(P)* follow relatively direct course to enter temporal margin of disc. Fibers from temporal *(T)* retina arch around area centralis and fovea *(F)* to enter superior and inferior poles of optic nerve head. Horizontal raphe beginning just temporal to fovea and extending into temporal periphery separates superior and inferior bundles that originate from ganglion cells in temporal retina. (Courtesy JA Alvarado. From Hogan, MJ, Alvarado, JA, and Weddell, JE: Histology of the human eye: an atlas and textbook, Philadelphia, 1971, WB Saunders Co)

Fig. 4-12 **A,** Diagrammatic representation of vertical stratification of axons within retinal nerve fiber layer of rhesus monkey. Axons from peripheral ganglion cells *(G)* assume deeper position within nerve fiber layer as subsequent axons from ganglion cells closer to optic nerve, head are added to more superficial layers. **B,** Within optic nerve head itself, fibers from more peripheral retina assume more circumferential position *(triangles)*. Fibers from peripapillary retina assume more axial position within nerve *(squares)*, and axons from more central locations *(circles)* assume intermediate position. (From Minckler, DS: Arch Ophthalmol 98:1630, 1980. Copyright 1980, American Medical Association)

bound vesicles.[8,11,111] Likewise, pinocytotic vesicles of extracellular material from the region of the synapse at the lateral geniculate body move retrograde toward the cell body at a slightly slower rate by way of retrograde transport mechanisms. Various materials, including neurohormones, transmitter substances, ingested toxins, and even viral particles, can be moved by this transport system in either an orthograde or retrograde direction.

Materials move from the ganglion cell to the synapse at the lateral geniculate body in about 5 hours at a rate of 200 to 400 mm/day. Vesicles containing transported material can be identified microscopically along the surface of microtubules extending the length of the neuron. Neurofilaments complete with actin-like protein are also evident within the neuroplasm. Indeed, transport may be accomplished through some mechanism similar to

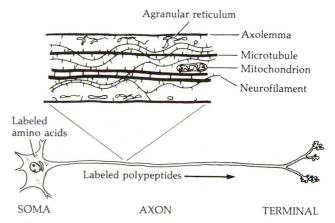

Fig. 4-13 Schematic drawing of composition of axoplasm as orthograde transport moves from cell body (SOMA) toward axon terminal. (Courtesy P Hoffman. From Miller, NR: Walsh and Hoyt's clinical neuro-ophthalmology, Baltimore, 1982, Williams & Wilkins)

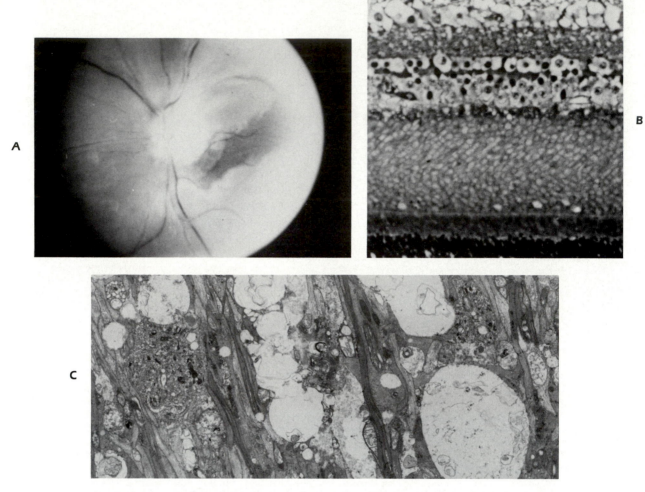

Fig. 4-14 **A,** Central retinal artery occlusion with preservation of some retinal tissue by cilioretinal artery. **B,** Gray discoloration of retina represents hydropic degeneration of inner layers similar to that seen in histologic specimens of animal eyes with experimental retinal artery occlusion. Dense white material superotemporal to nerve head lies along margin between perfused and ischemic tissue. **C,** Electron photomicrographs from similar regions with acute vascular occlusion demonstrate disruption of axonal cytoarchitecture with accumulation of swollen mitochondria, microvesicles, and dense membranous material. (From Radius, RL, and Anderson, DR: Br J Ophthalmol 65:767, 1981)

sliding of protein units seen in muscle fiber contraction.

Although the mechanisms of axonal transport are not well defined, metabolic energy using adenosine triphosphate (ATP) produced locally along the axon segment is required.[8,11,112,113] Focal anoxia will inhibit or block transport within the hypoxic segment, resulting in an accumulation of transported material upstream (orthograde) and downstream (retrograde) of the involved segment.[57,113,192,199] In an eye with a focal retinal arteriolar occlusion, transport interruption at the boundary between ischemic and normal nerve fiber layer can be recognized ophthalmoscopically as a dense white ring of intraretinal material concentric to the region of hypoxia[100-102,155,179] (Fig. 4-14).

Occlusion of the axon lumen by mechanical deformation, as well as such metabolic poisons as vincristine, will also inhibit or locally block normal transport mechanisms.* In an eye with elevated intraocular pressure, axonal transport interruption within the region of the posterior lamina cribrosa can be seen in both clinical disease and in experimental models of glaucoma† (Fig. 4-15). It is not clear whether this blockade results from focal isch-

---

*References 8, 11, 17, 18, 21, 40, 51, 205, 207.
†References 13, 52, 90, 104-106, 122, 127, 131, 135-137, 146, 158, 167, 183.

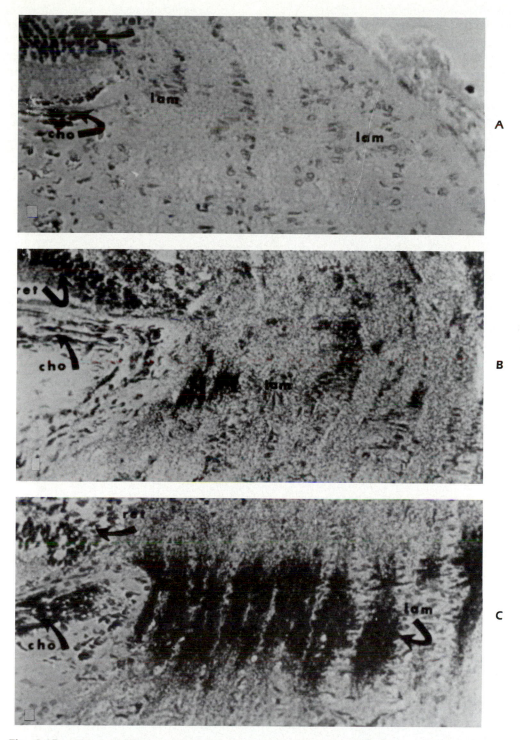

Fig. 4-15 Photomicrographs of optic nerve head radioautographs. Primate eyes were injected with tritiated leucine into vitreous cavity and examined 4 hours later. In normal eyes tagged leucine incorporated into protein can be recognized by exposed *(darkened)* emulsion grains throughout retinal tissue but concentrated within nucleated layers, **A.** In eyes with moderate, **B,** and maximal, **C,** pressure elevation during 4-hour test interval, accumulation of tritiated leucine is evident at level of the lamina cribrosa *(lam).* The accumulated material represents protein transported along ganglion cell axon through optic nerve to site of obstruction of axonal transport within lamina. *ret,* Retina; *cho,* choroid. (From Radius, RL, and Anderson, DR: Invest Ophthalmol Vis Sci 19:244, 1980)

emia within the axon segment, occlusion of the axon lumen by mechanical deformation within the nerve head, a combination of both phenomena, or other tissue changes.* It is also uncertain what role interruption in axonal transport plays in the development of pressure-induced axon damage. Nevertheless, complete blockade of retrograde transport mechanisms for more than 2 weeks may be expected to result in an end organ (lateral geniculate body) denervation atrophy of the axon and ganglion cell body.[7,126,136,150]

Microscopically, axons with focal regions of transport interruption show accumulation of materials moving up to but not through the blocked segment* (Fig. 4-16). This material moves toward the point of blockade via normal transport mech-

*References 11, 13, 52, 105, 136, 148, 149, 183.

*References 52, 90, 106, 131, 155, 156, 167, 215.

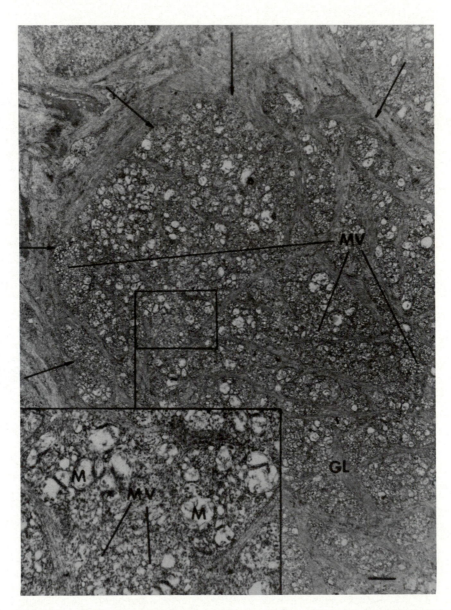

Fig. 4-16 Electron photomicrograph of primate eye with fast axonal transport interruption produced after 4 hours of elevated intraocular pressure. Accumulation of mitochondria *(M)*, microvesicles *(MV)*, dense granules, and other material occurs within axon lumen in these eyes with transport interruption at level of lamina cribrosa. (From Radius, RL, and Anderson, DR: Arch Ophthalmol 99:650, 1981. Copyright 1981, American Medical Association)

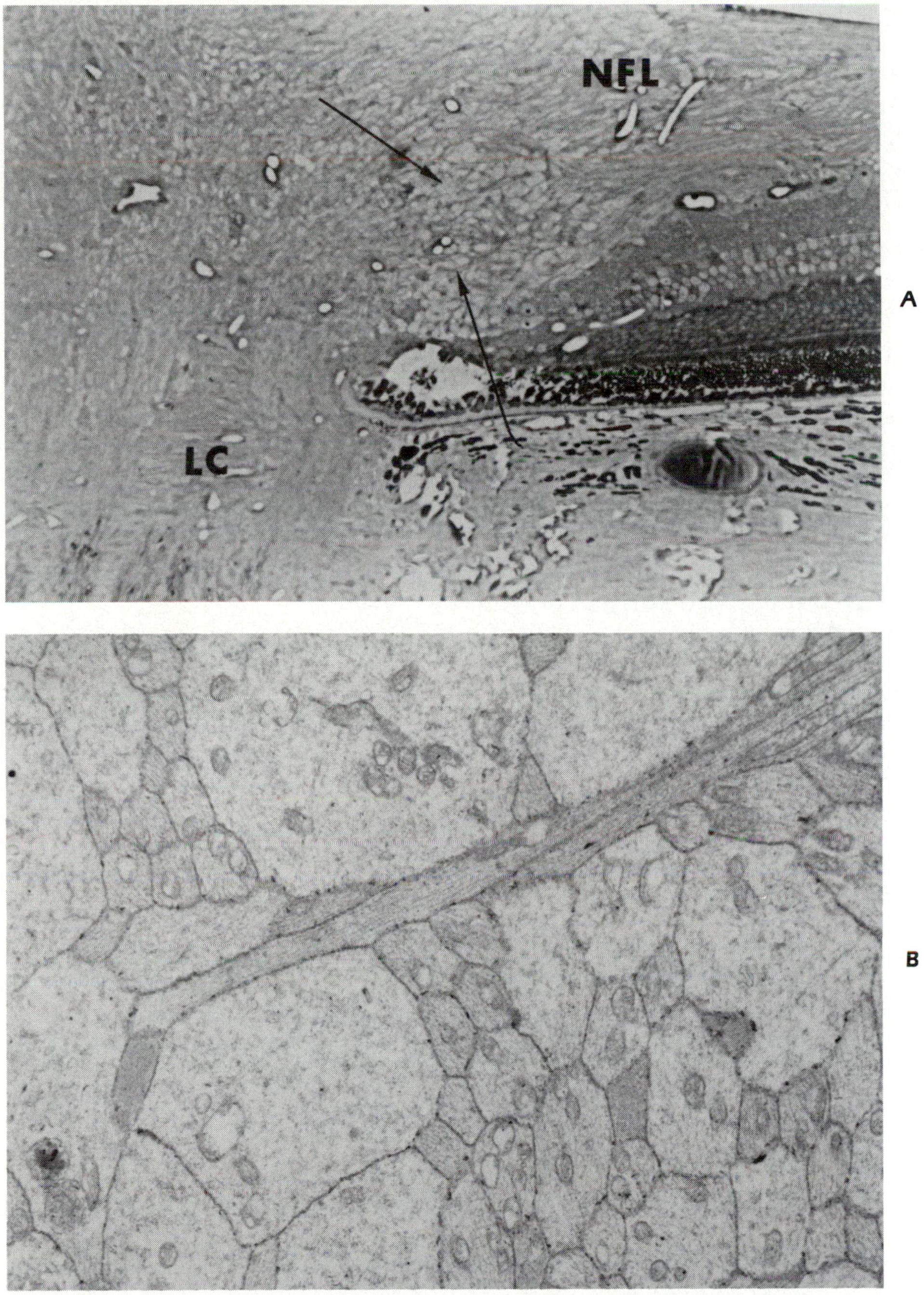

Fig. 4-17   Optic nerve head of primate eye with experimental disc edema associated with ocular hypotony. **A,** Anterior to lamina cribosa *(LC)* within nerve fiber layer *(NFL)* axon cylinders are dilated *(arrows),* and there is lateral displacement of disc tissue. **B,** Electron photomicrograph from same region demonstrates individual axons swollen by accumulation of axoplasm in these eyes with impaired slow axoplasmic flow. (**A** From Radius, RL, and Anderson, DR: Invest Ophthalmol Vis Sci 19:158, 1980; **B** from Radius, RL, and Anderson, DR: Br J Ophthalmol 65:767, 1981)

anisms in uninvolved axon segments. Microvesicles containing membrane-bound protein are among the more conspicuous of the accumulated materials. Mitochondria, which normally move in a to-and-fro motion at a comparable rate to that of the transported material, also accumulate at the point of blockage. Eventually the cytoplasm swells with disruption of the cytoarchitecture and ultimately with rupture of the cell membrane itself.[155,157] This cellular disintegration would seem to represent irreversible damage to the axon segment.

Axoplasmic flow

Slow axonal flow, a related phenomenon, can be described as bulk movement of soluble proteins synthesized within the cell body, moving along the axon segment at a slow rate of 1 to 3 mm/day.[70,71,113,206] This transport system may be thought of as a movement of the entire cytoplasmic column (including the cytoskeleton of microtubules and filaments) essentially replacing material catabolized downstream. Given the length of the axon (more than 5 cm) and the diameter of the axon (less than 5 μm), this movement cannot represent a force transmitted along the length of the axon by pressure generated at the cell body through material synthesis.

Slow axonal transport interruption can also be recognized clinically in eyes with papilledema or extreme hypotony. Swelling of the nerve head in these conditions reflects a slowdown or partial blockage of slow transport mechanisms at the nerve head.* Over several days, cytoplasmic material accumulates within the axons of the retinal nerve fiber layer, swelling the individual fibers and the nerve head tissue (Fig. 4-17). If the abnormality persists, the axonal cytoarchitecture may become disrupted. If the axon membrane ruptures, disintegration of the axon segment and the ganglion cell of origin will occur.

THE OPTIC NERVE HEAD

At the optic nerve head, axons of the retinal nerve fiber layer turn to exit the eye. Bundles of axons pass through some 200 to 300 irregular perforations in the sclera, forming the optic canal (Fig. 4-18).† The fiber bundles occupy the margins of the nerve head with the central retinal artery and vein slightly nasal of center within the nerve head tissue.

The orientation and dimensions of the canal show considerable variation in individual eyes,

---

*References 8, 9, 104, 109, 110, 154, 155, 193-197.
†References 4, 5, 15, 43, 128, 146, 159, 163.

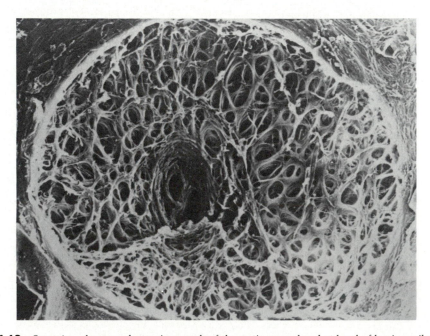

Fig. 4-18 Scanning electron photomicrograph of the optic nerve head at level of lamina cribrosa. Several hundred irregular perforations through sclera constitute scleral canal through which pass the 1.2 million optic nerve axons as they exit the eye. (From Miller, NR: Walsh and Hoyt's Clinical neuro-ophthalmology, Baltimore, 1982, Williams & Wilkins)

whereas the amount of neuronal tissue is relatively constant. The diameter of the optic nerve head is approximately 1.5 mm.[189] In eyes with a large optic canal, the central or physiologic depression, devoid of axons, will be larger[10,19,171,190] (Fig. 4-19). In eyes with a smaller optic canal, the cental cup will be smaller or even nonexistent. Since there is loss of axonal tissue with age, there may be a minor increase in the dimensions of the central cup with increasing age in the absence of optic nerve pathology.

The scleral canal is oriented nasal of the vertical as the nerve exits the eye. Axons from the nasal retina, therefore, make a more acute turn as they enter the nerve head than do axons from the fundus temporal to the nerve.[10,58,111] Viewed ophthalmoscopically, in those eyes in which the slant of the nerve is extreme, the nasal margin of the nerve head may appear undermined as the axons turn to leave the eye (Fig. 4-20). In the temporal nerve head, the neuroretinal tissue slopes gradually as the fibers pass from the retinal nerve fiber layer, across the nerve head and out the eye. The temporal margin of the central cup may be very difficult to define in these instances. In an eye in which the scleral canal is more vertically oriented, the nasal and temporal axons turn through more nearly equal angles as they leave the nerve fiber layer of the retina. The neuroretinal rim of tissue will be a concentric ring of pink tissue surrounding the central cup and retinal vessels.

The neurosensory retina deep to the nerve fiber layer, the retinal pigment epithelium, and the choroid, end at the nerve head. In many instances, however, all layers may not end at the very edge of the scleral canal. Frequently, a crescent, usually along the temporal margin of the nerve head, or even a ring of white sclera can be seen concentric to or surrounding the nerve head[4,10,41] (Fig. 4-21). If the retinal pigment epithelium ends short of the choroidal layer, the vascular pattern of this deeper layer can be seen concentric to the ring of bare sclera (Fig. 4-22). It is important clinically to recognize these variations and the precise margin of the scleral canal when describing the dimensions of the optic nerve head and central cup.

For the purpose of presentation, the optic nerve head may be conveniently divided into three vertical layers, which roughly parallel the layering of tissues adjacent to the nerve. The anterior optic nerve head is a continuation of the retinal nerve fiber layer into the nerve head. The lamina choroidalis is the region of the optic nerve head surrounded by the deeper retinal layers and the choroidal vasculature. The lamina scleralis marks the point of exit of the nerve through the sclera itself.

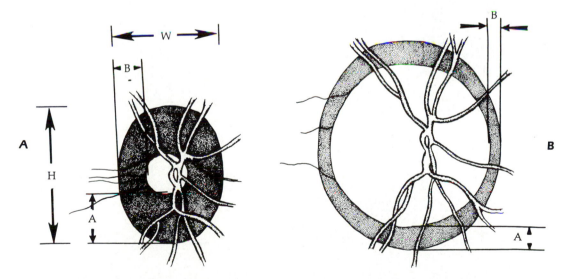

Fig. 4-19 A, Schematic drawing of normal optic nerve head. Height *(H)* of disc is somewhat greater than width *(W)*. Superior and inferior neural rim *(B)* is somewhat thicker than nasal and temporal rim. Thus, central cup is round. **B,** In eye with somewhat larger scleral canal the same amount of neural tissue (inferior and superior, *A,* nasal and temporal, *B*) will occupy the margins of the disc yielding a relatively large central physiologic cup. (From Anderson, DR: Thomas D. Duane's Clinical ophthalmology, Philadelphia, 1985, Harper & Row)

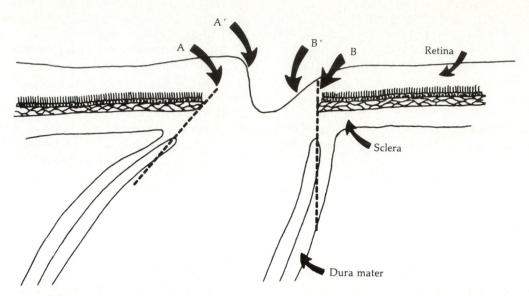

Fig. 4-20 Influence of tilt of scleral canal on slope of cup. Outward slope of canal *(A)* corresponds to steep often overhanging cup wall *(A')*. More perpendicular slope to the canal *(B)* corresponds to more gentle sloping wall to central optic cup *(B')*. (From Anderson, DR: Thomas C. Duane's Clinical ophthalmology, Philadelphia, 1985, Harper & Row)

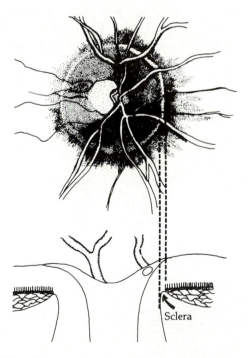

Fig. 4-21 Common anatomic variation in which concentric wedge or ring of sclera surrounds optic nerve head arises in instances in which a flange of sclera marks boundary of disc, separating choroid from nerve tissue. (From Anderson, DR: Thomas C. Duane's Clinical ophthalmology, Philadelphia, 1985, Harper & Row)

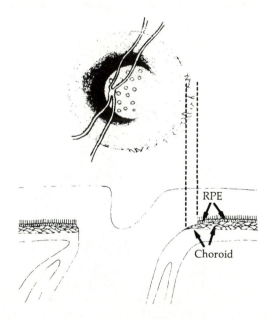

Fig. 4-22 In some instances, several retinal layers, including the choroid and retinal pigment epithelium *(RPE)*, are misaligned at optic disc. Clinically, this anatomy may be recognized as peripapillary crescent of choroidal vasculature uncovered by absence of overlying RPE. (From Anderson, DR: Thomas C. Duane's Clinical ophthalmology, Philadelphia, 1985, Harper & Row)

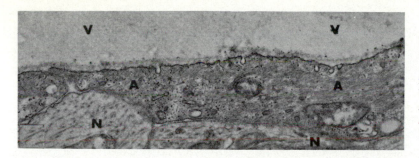

Fig. 4-23   Electron photomicrograph of anterior optic nerve head demonstrates thin strand of astrocyte cytoplasm *(A)* forming internal limiting membrane of Elschnig separating nerve fiber bundles *(N)* from vitreous *(V)* fibrils. (From Anderson, DR, Hoyt, WF, and Hogan, MJ: Trans Am Ophthalmol Soc 65: 275, 1967. Copyright 1967, American Medical Association)

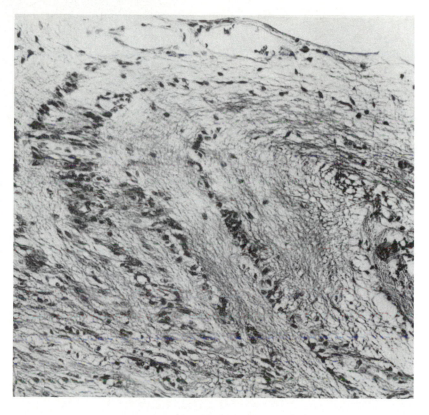

Fig. 4-24   Photomicrograph of anterior optic nerve head in primate eye demonstrates columns of glial cells and glial cell processes separating groups of axons into nerve fiber bundles. (From Anderson, DR, Hoyt, WF, and Hogan, MJ: Trans Am Ophthalmol Soc 65:275, 1967. Copyright 1967, American Medical Association)

Anterior Optic Nerve Head

Neuroglia

At the optic nerve head, the dense internal limiting membrane formed by the foot-plates of Müller cells is replaced by the much thinner limiting membrane of Elschnig[4,5,14,41,42] (Fig. 4-23). This membrane is formed by the fibrous astrocytes of the optic nerve head. It consists of cytoplasmic processes and a thin basement membrane covering the adventitia of the nerve head blood vessels and the bundles of axons as they turn to exit the eye.

Fiber bundle septae formed by elongated Müller cell processes within the retina are replaced by columns of astrocytes and glial processes (Fig. 4-24). At the nerve head, however, these septae are much less well defined and largely incomplete.

Glial processes intermix with axons within individual fiber bundles much as in the retinal nerve fiber layer.[213] The orientation of the glial processes roughly parallels that of the axons within the fiber bundles.

The astrocytes themselves are relatively pale cells with a thin rim of cytoplasm surrounding the nucleus. The cell bodies contain dense granules felt to represent lipofuscin, which are lysosomal in origin.[4,5,14,15] These inclusions are largely lipid in content and probably represent end products of normal cell metabolism. Their accumulation is frequently noted in cells that are usually long-lived and not normally replaced, such as the neuroglia of the central nervous system.

Gap junctions between processes of the glial

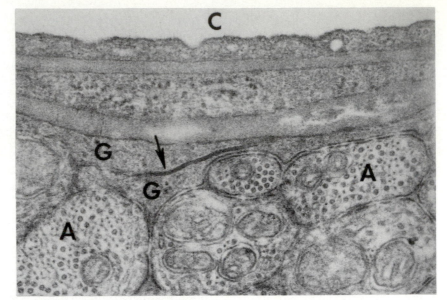

Fig. 4-25 Nerve head astrocytes (G) separate axons (A) from basement membrane of a capillary (C). Astrocyte processes in this region of nerve are joined by gap junctions (arrow). (From Quigley, HA: Invest Ophthalmol Vis Sci 16:582, 1977)

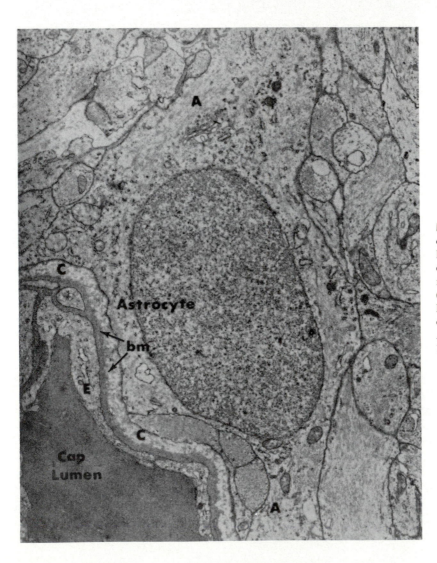

Fig. 4-26 Electron photomicrograph of capillary (Cap) within primate optic nerve head demonstrates basement membrane (bm) of endothelial cell and small amount of connective tissue (C) between adjacent astrocyte (A). Nerve tissue is isolated from capillary lumen by these two tissue layers. (From Anderson, DR, Hoyt, WF, and Hogan, MJ: Trans Am Ophthalmol Soc 65:275, 1967. Copyright 1967, American Medical Association)

cells allow electrical and biochemical coupling of individual cells[125] (Fig. 4-25). This functional syncytium of glial tissue provides a stable environment for the axons within the optic nerve.[54,121] In addition, glial cytoplasmic processes separate the blood vessels and associated adventitia from the neural elements. All nutrient and waste exchange between the axons and the microvasculature of the nerve head must pass through the astrocyte cytoplasm and basement membrane between the axons and the capillary lumen[4,5,14,15] (Fig. 4-26).

The glial processes may provide some degree of structural support for the axon bundles as they turn to enter the nerve head. The amount of glial tissue, however, is much reduced in this region in comparison to that of the retinal nerve fiber layer and more posterior portions of the optic nerve head itself. In instances of nerve injury, these nerve head astrocytes participate in the repair process, filling in spaces vacated by axon degeneration[7,133,134,153] The complex framework created by these cytoplasmic processes of glial tissue is established during the earliest stages of fetal development.[181,182,187] Axons pass through the syncytium as they grow from the ganglion cell layer toward the lateral geniculate body. The established anatomy within the glial network may program the orientation of this growth during embryogenesis of the optic nerve.

Blood vessels

The vasculature of the anterior optic nerve head consists of capillaries and the major retinal vessels (Fig. 4-27). The central retinal artery and vein are contained within their own adventitia and lie just nasal to the central optic cup. The capillaries vary in size from 7 to 20 μm in diameter[180] Characteristic of vessels within the central nervous system, the endothelial cells have tight junctions and associated pericytes.[198] The vasculature is confined to the glial support tissue, isolated from the axon columns.[4,5,14,15]

Blood supply to this portion of the nerve is derived from small branches of the central retinal artery.* There are anastomoses with the capillary bed of the deeper nerve head and the peripapillary retina (Fig. 4-28). In those eyes with cilioretinal vessels, usually involving the temporal nerve head, some blood flow may come directly from the posterior ciliary circulation.

Venous drainage of this capillary plexus is normally into the central retinal vein at the nerve head. In some pathologic conditions associated with obstruction of this normal egress, anastomoses with the peripapillary vessels and deeper choroidal vasculature may become dilated, shunting blood from the nerve head, through the choroid and ultimately out of the orbit via the superior and inferior orbital veins.[5]

Axons

At the level of the anterior optic nerve head, axons of the retinal nerve fiber layer comprise some 90% of the nerve head tissue volume.[107] The ultra-

---

*References 6, 12, 65, 68, 94, 174.

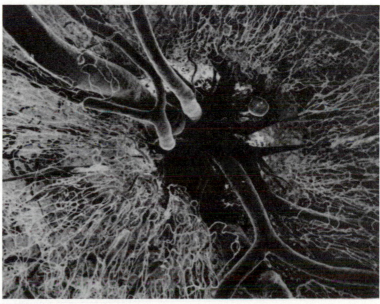

Fig. 4-27 Scanning electron photomicrograph showing intraocular vasculature of optic nerve head. (Courtesy HA Quigley. From Miller, NR: Walsh and Hoyt's Clinical neuro-ophthalmology, Baltimore, 1982, Williams & Wilkins)

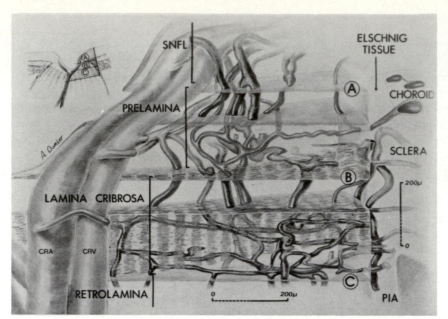

Fig. 4-28 Diagrammatic representation of optic nerve head vasculature demonstrates complex anastomoses between capillary beds of anterior optic nerve head, lamina choroidalis, lamina scleralis, and retroorbital optic nerve. *A*, superficial nerve fiber layer *(SNFL)* and prelaminar region. *B*, Prelaminar region and lamina cribrosa. *C*, Lamina cribrosa and retrolaminar optic nerve. Horizontal scale has been elongated and three contiguous regions expanded to facilitate illustration of anastomoses. *CRA*, Central retinal artery; *CRV*, central retinal vein. (From Lieberman, MF, Maumenee, AE, and Green, WR. Published with permission from the American Journal of Ophthalmology 82:405, 1976. Copyright by the Ophthalmic Publishing Co)

Fig. 4-29 Electron photomicrograph of anterior optic nerve head demonstrates astrocytes of anterior portion of lamina cribrosa. Plane of section cuts across longitudinal axis of astrocyte cell border and astrocyte processes. Little extracellular space is present between axon cylinders and processes of glial cell origin. (From Anderson, DR, Hoyt, WF, and Hogan, MJ: Trans Am Ophthalmol Soc 65:275, 1967. Copyright 1967, American Medical Association)

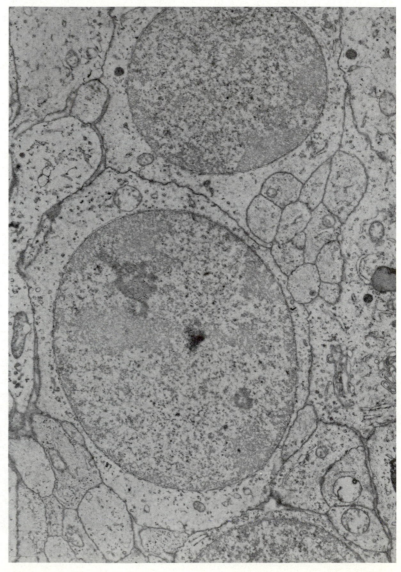

structure is unchanged from that of the axon segment within the retina, with the possible exception that the segment within the nerve head contains a greater concentration of mitochondria. There is little extracellular space in the normal nerve head (Fig. 4-29) (see Chapter 6).

The topographic grouping of regional axon bundles at the nerve head in the human eye has not been defined. Limited clinical information suggests that the axons from more peripheral retina assume a more circumferential position within the nerve head. Whatever the precise anatomy, grouping of axons into fiber bundles from adjacent retinal loci is probably preserved as the axons leave this most anterior layer of the nerve head.*

Lamina Choroidalis

The lamina choroidalis roughly parallels the level of the choroid and deeper layers of the retina adjacent to the disc[4,5,14,15] (Fig. 4-30). Anatomically it is characterized by increasing density and definition of interbundle glial columns with the percentage of nonneuronal tissue within the nerve head increasing from approximately 10% to nearly 50% more posteriorly.[4,5,14,15,107]

Neuroglia

This region of the nerve head is characterized by a glial lamina, with the relatively few connective

tissue elements confined primarily to the adventitia of the major retinal vessels.[4,5,15] Specialized astrocytes, arranged in columns, form glial tunnels containing the axon fiber bundles, now oriented perpendicular to the surface of the optic nerve head (Fig. 4-31).

These glial cells have a thin layer of cytoplasm surrounding the nucleus. Golgi apparatus, associated mitochondria, and sparse rough endoplasmic reticulum can be seen at the nuclear pole. Thin cytoplasmic arms extending from the main cell body, usually confined to the vertical cell columns, extend into the neuron bundles oriented perpendicular to the axon columns. The cytoplasm within these astrocyte processes demonstrates a dense cytoarchitecture of fibrillar material, presumably important to the structural role played by the glia in supporting the axonal columns within this region of the nerve head.[4,5,15]

Blood flow

The retinal artery and vein are centrally located within the lamina choroidalis. The only other vasculature within this region of the nerve are capillaries confined within the glial lamina. Collagen and connective tissue elements are largely absent within this microvasculature. Generally, the basement membrane of the enveloping astrocyte processes fuses directly with that of the capillary endothelium.[4,5,15]

This capillary bed shows extensive anastomoses with similar small vessels contained in the more

---

*References 73, 75, 77, 78, 103, 115, 116, 151, 152.

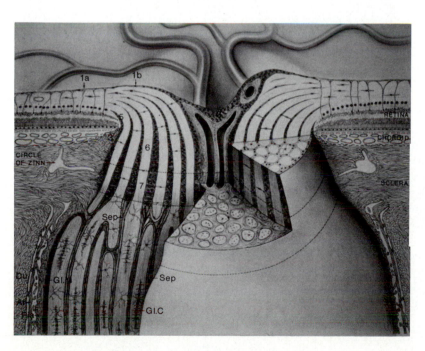

Fig. 4-30 Schematic drawing of optic nerve within and adjoining eyeball. *1a,* Inner limiting membrane of retina; *1b,* inner limiting membrane of Elschnig; *2,* central meniscus of Kuhnt; *3,* border tissue of Elschnig; *4,* border tissue of Jacoby; *5,* intermediary tissue of Kuhnt; *6,* anterior portion of lamina cribrosa; *7,* posterior portion of lamina cribrosa. (From Anderson, DR, and Hoyt, WF: Arch Ophthalmol 82:506, 1969. Copyright 1969, American Medical Association)

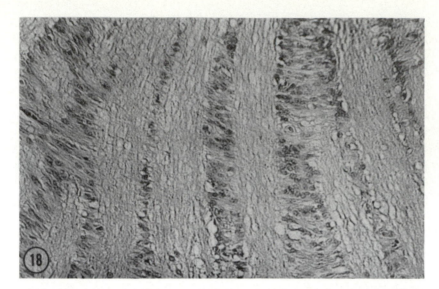

Fig. 4-31 Photomicrograph of primate optic nerve head in region of lamina choroidalis. Columns of astrocyte nuclei separate axons into fiber bundles. (From Anderson, DR, Hoyt, WF, and Hogan, MJ: Trans Am Ophthalmol Soc 65:275, 1967. Copyright 1967, American Medical Association)

Fig. 4-32 Schematic drawing of blood flow patterns in anterior optic nerve head, lamina cribrosa, and retroorbital optic nerve. Anastomotic channels exist between capillary beds of anterior optic nerve, lamina cribrosa, and retrolaminar optic nerve. Functional significance of these anastomoses in eyes with elevated intraocular pressure or reduced nerve head perfusion remains to be demonstrated. (From Lieberman, MF, Maumenee, AE, and Green, WR. Published with permission from the American Journal of Ophthalmology 82:405, 1976. Copyright by the Ophthalmic Publishing Co)

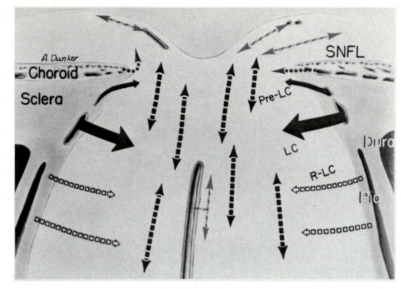

anterior nerve head and the lamina scleralis directly posterior to this region[12,94] (Fig. 4-32). Blood flow to this region is derived primarily from vessels branching off the posterior ciliary artery. These arterioles supply the capillaries within the lamina choroidalis. In addition, some vessels from the posterior ciliary circulation, passing through the adjacent choroidal tissue, contribute blood flow to this vascular plexus.[12,65,94]

Although the capillaries are characterized by tight junctions within the nerve itself, there is no barrier to diffusion between the adjacent choroid and optic nerve tissue.* Diffusion of material into the nerve from the choroid can be recognized in the late venous phase on fluorescein angiography[20,32,33,46,119] (Fig. 4-33). Venous drainage from the nerve tissue is primarily into the central retinal vein, although some blood may exit through the choroid.

Axons

The neuron segments within the lamina choroidalis are grouped into tight bundles by the surrounding columns of astrocytes. Adjacent axons come from ganglion cells located in spatially and probably functionally contiguous regions of the retina. Astrocyte processes from cell bodies located in glial columns contact portions of individual axons, much as in the retinal nerve fiber layer.

*References 11, 33, 48, 55, 56, 85, 120, 198.

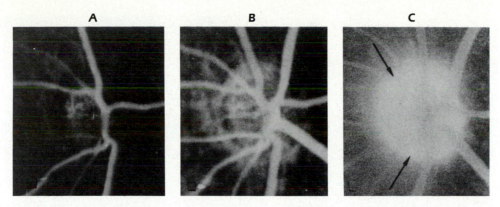

Fig. 4-33   A, Arterial, **B,** venous, and **C,** late (15 min) phases of fluorescein angiogram of normal monkey eye. Staining of peripheral optic nerve head tissue by fluorescein, **C,** depicts fluid flow through juxtapapillary tissue from choroidal vasculature. (From Radius, RL, and Anderson, DR: Invest Ophthalmol Vis Sci 19:244, 1980)

Lamina Scleralis

Neuroglia and connective tissue

The lamina scleralis is characterized by increasing numbers of fibroblasts and connective tissue elements with a gradual transition from the glial columns between axon bundles at the level of the lamina choroidalis to a region of dense connective tissue lamellae within the lamina scleralis[4,5,15] (see Fig. 4-30). Sheets of connective tissue with fibroblasts, collagen, ground substance, glycosaminoglycans, and basement membrane alternate with sheets of astrocytes oriented parallel to the outer eye wall and perpendicular to the axon bundles. Each tissue plane has 200 to 300 perforations (see Fig. 4-13). Lying roughly in register with those of adjacent tissue sheets, these form laminar tunnels encircling the fiber bundles. The sheets of connective tissue may be seen as a continuation of the adjacent sclera surrounding the optic foramen.

There is a gradual change in the astrocytes at deeper levels of the lamina corresponding to the increase in the density of connective tissue elements[4,5] (see Fig. 4-30). Anteriorly, within the lamina choroidalis, the only connective tissue between adjacent glial cells is a thin layer of basement membrane. The glial cells form a continuous layer separating the optic nerve bundles from the adjacent outer retinal layers and choroid. This border tissue of Kuhnt may be smooth, or, alternatively, irregular with interdigitations of glial tissue into the adjacent choroidal connective tissue.[4,5,15,89] Sheets of glial tissue also envelop the connective tissue adventitia surrounding the central retinal vessels.

With the transition into the lamina scleralis, fibroblasts and collagen are sandwiched between the astrocytes (Fig. 4-34). The astrocytes have multiple processes spreading in all directions between and around the axons of the fiber bundles, isolating individual axons from one another and from the connective tissue elements within the septae. The border tissue of Jacoby, consisting of vertical layers of connective tissue and astrocytes, surrounds the nerve and separates it from the adjacent sclera.[4,5,14,15,86] Sometimes a projection of sclera, the border tissue of Elschnig, extends more anteriorly, separating the optic nerve elements from the choroid.[4,5,42]

Blood vessels

All of the capillaries are contained within the glial connective tissue septae. Blood flow to this region is derived primarily from branches of the posterior ciliary artery penetrating either the adjacent sclera or choroid[6,12,65,94] (see Figs. 4-28 and 4-32). This capillary bed anastomoses extensively anteriorly and posteriorly with capillaries of adjacent portions of the optic nerve. Blood flow to the more posterior capillaries is derived primarily from branches of the pial vessels, which penetrate the retrobulbar optic nerve. Drainage is through the central retinal vein and pial vessels, which ultimately drain into the ophthalmic vein and cavernous sinus.

Axons

Within the lamina scleralis, axon bundles are confined in relatively rigid columns created by vertically oriented septae of astrocytes and connective tissue (see Fig. 4-34). These tissue tunnels, however, are incomplete or branching at multiple levels of the lamina, allowing some exchange of axons between adjacent bundles.

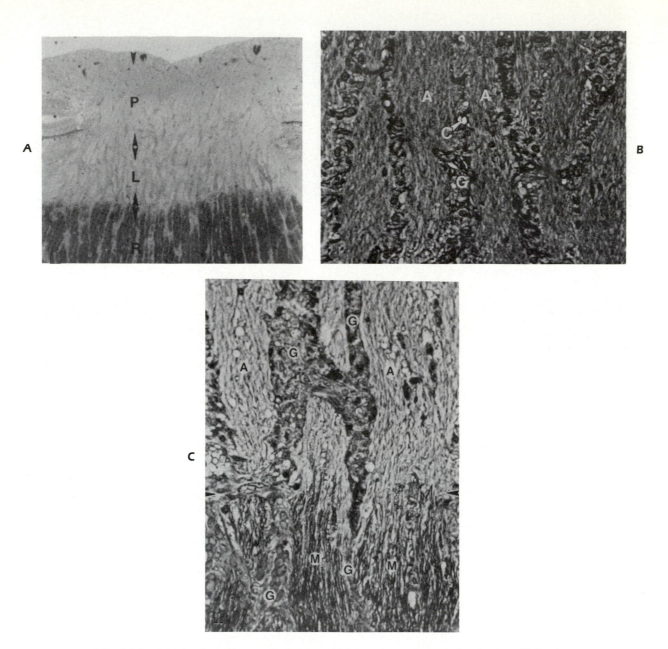

Fig. 4-34 **A,** Light photomicrograph showing architectural arrangement of prelaminar *(P)*, laminar *(L)*, and retrolaminar *(R)* portions of optic nerve. **B** and **C** show these regions in more detail. Moving posterior from retinal surface to level of myelinated axons *(M)* immediately behind globe, tissue columns of glial cells *(G)* separating axon bundles *(A)* contain increased amounts of connective tissue elements and become thicker. All microvasculature *(C)* within nerve head is confined to these tissue columns. (Courtesy of HA Quigley. From Miller, NR: Walsh and Hoyt's Neuro-ophthalmology, Baltimore, 1982, Williams & Wilkins)

Although the exact topography of axon bundles at this level is not defined in the human eye, in nonhuman primates, axons from adjacent areas of the retina are grouped tightly into one or a few adjacent fiber bundles at the level of the lamina scleralis (Fig. 4-35). Damage to the axon segments within a single bundle or group of bundles at this level could result in a focal loss of retinal ganglion cells. The primary lesion in pressure-induced axon damage may occur at this level, within the posterior lamina scleralis.*

Axons within this region of the lamina are similar to those throughout the course of the optic nerve,[4,5,117,118] abutting against adjacent axons or astrocyte processes. There is little if any extracellular space (see Fig. 4-29). Microtubules 200

---

*References 61, 62, 66, 98, 99, 105, 106, 108, 127, 128, 132, 135, 149.

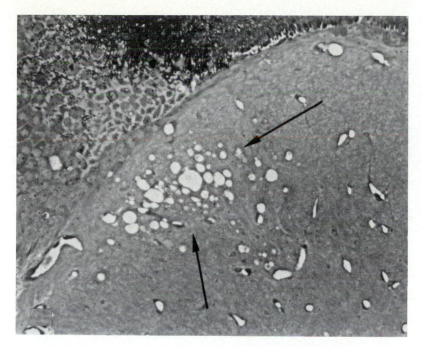

Fig. 4-35 Region of lamina cribrosa in monkey eye examined 3 days after xenon arc full-thickness destruction of retina immediately superior to macula within vascular arcade. Extent of retinal damage encompassed area of approximately 5 to 10 degrees. Burn destroyed all ganglion cells within region, as well as axons from peripheral ganglion cells traversing that area. Region of damaged axons, corresponding to Bjerrum's scotoma similar to that which might be seen in glaucoma (ignoring damage to peripheral axons within retina) is limited to a few fiber bundles at region of lamina cribrosa. (From Radius, RL, and Anderson, DR: Arch Ophthalmol 97:1154, 1979. Copyright 1979, American Medical Association)

Fig. 4-36 Histologic section showing four regions of optic nerve: *(1)* intraocular; *(2)* inraorbital; *(3)* intracanalicular; *(4)* intracranial; *(OC)* optic chiasm. (From Hogan, MJ, and Zimmerman, LE: Ophthalmic pathology. An atlas and textbook, Philadelphia, 1962, WB Saunders)

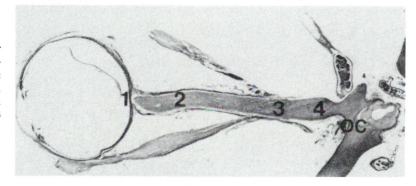

to 250 nm in diameter and neurofilaments 60 to 70 nm in diameter fill most of the cytoplasmic volume. There are scattered bits of smooth endoplasmic reticulum and mitochondria as well, but few if any other organelles are seen. The diameter of the axons varies from 0.2 to 5 μm with a mean of about 1.0 μm.*

EXTRAOCULAR OPTIC NERVE

Intraorbital Optic Nerve

Astroglia and connective tissue

The extraocular, intraorbital nerve is 2 to 3 cm long and extends from the posterior sclera to the optic foramen in the sphenoid bone[200] (Fig. 4-36).

The nerve is 3 to 4 mm in diameter and is surrounded by three vaginal sheaths, including the dense dura mater, which fuses with the sclera anteriorly and with the periosteum at the sphenoid bone. The nerve lies in a gentle S curve, longer than the orbital anteroposterior dimension, so that movement of the eye places no tension on the nerve tethered at the optic canal. The arachnoid and pia of the optic nerve are continuous with the meninges of the brain at the canal and fuse with the sclera at the eye. The subarachnoid space, continuous with that of the brain, ends as a blind pouch at the scleral wall.

Septae of pial origin enter the nerve substance forming incomplete columns the entire length of the nerve (Fig. 4-37). These columns of connective tissue divide the axons into fiber bundles much like

---

*References 16, 32, 79, 118, 124, 164, 176.

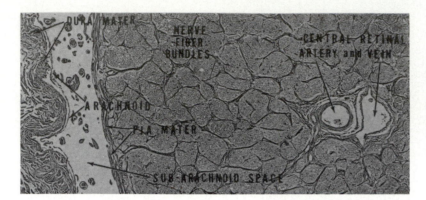

Fig. 4-37 Cross section of retroorbital optic nerve illustrating septae of pial origin that enter nerve substance separating axons into fiber bundles. (From Miller, NR: Walsh and Hoyt's Clinical neuroophthalmology, Baltimore, 1982, Williams & Wilkins)

Fig. 4-38 Capillary in anterior portion of lamina cribosa. Lumen is encircled by endothelial cells *(E)* with their basement membrane *(bm)*. Small amount of collagen accompanies capillary. Perivascular astrocyte cell sends processes around capillary separating mesodermal tissue from neurons. (From Anderson, DR, Hoyt, WF, and Hogan, MJ: Trans Am Ophthalmol Soc 65:235, 1967)

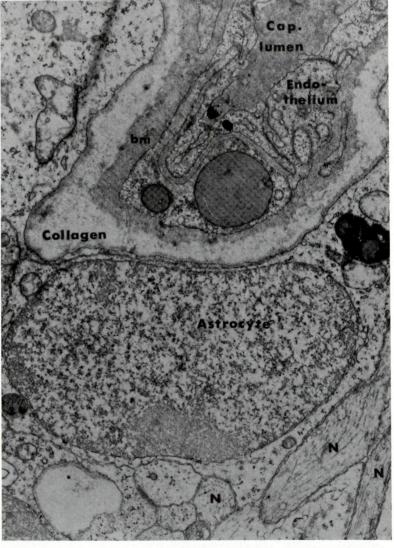

the glial septae more anteriorly in the nerve head and lamina cribrosa within the intraocular portion of the optic nerve.[4,5,14,15] Columns of glial cells including astrocytes and oligodendrocytes are located within the fiber bundles separate from the denser connective tissue septae. Astrocyte processes complete with basement membrane combine to form a continuous layer of glial tissue enveloping the connective tisssue septae and separating the tissue of mesodermal origin from the axon bundles and oligodendroglia (Fig. 4-38). A similar glial layer surrounds the adventitia of the central retinal artery and vein.

The astrocytes have relatively pale staining nuclei with few cytoplasmic organelles including rough endoplasmic reticulum, free ribosomes, glycogen, and Golgi apparatus concentrated primarily in or near the perikaryon of the cell. Filaments 6 to 7 nm in diameter predominate within the cytoplasm and microtubules are rare.

In contrast, the oligodendroglia have dense chromatin clumping within the nucleus, more cytoplasmic organelles, and increased numbers of microtubules. These cells give rise to the convoluted myelin sheath, which surrounds the individual axons, beginning at the posteriormost layers of the lamina cribrosa and extending to the optic nerve synapse within the lateral geniculate body[15,32,214] (Fig. 4-39).

Blood vessels

All blood supply to this segment of the optic nerve is derived from the pial vasculature arising in the meninges surrounding the nerve[12,94] (see Fig. 4-28). With the exception of the central retinal vessels, which exit the nerve approximately 1 to 2 cm behind the globe and a few isolated arterioles penetrating the nerve from the pia mater, all of the vasculature within the nerve consists of capillaries confined to the connective tissue septae.

The endothelium is complete, nonfenestrated, and characterized by tight junctions between adjacent cells.[4,5,14,15] The basement membrane of the endothelium fuses with that of associated pericytes and overlies a thin connective tissue core of the septae consisting of collagen fibrils and scattered fibroblasts. This layer, in turn, is separated from the glial tissue lining the septae by the basement membrane of the individual astrocytes. Throughout the extent of the optic nerve, there is no direct contact between the connective tissue elements of the septae and the axons or oligodendroglia of the fiber bundles.

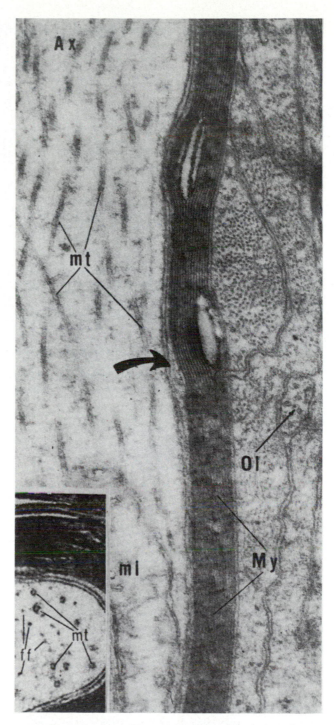

Fig. 4-39 Human optic nerve in longitudinal section at high magnification. Axoplasm *(Ax)* contains microtubules *(mt)* and mitochondria *(mi)*. Note small amount of oligodendrocyte cytoplasm *(arrow)* just within myelin sheath *(my)*. Oligodendrocyte process can be identified by presence of microtubules. Remainder of processes are of astrocyte origin and contain tonofilaments. Portion of human optic nerve axoplasm in cross section *(inset)*: note microtubules *(mt)* and neurofilaments *(ff)*. (From Anderson, DR, and Hoyt, WF: Arch Ophthalmol 82:452, 1969. Copyright 1969, American Medical Association)

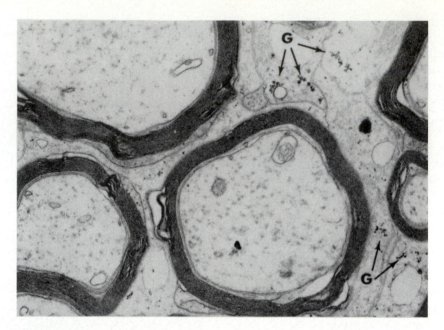

Fig. 4-40 Electron photomicrograph of intraorbital optic nerve cut in cross section. Cytoplasmic processes of glial cell origin fill most space between myelinated axons. Multiple wrappings of sheetlike processes of oligodendroglia around individual axon cylinders account for most of increased thickness of optic nerve at this level compared with that of intraocular nerve. (From Anderson, DR, Hoyt, WF, and Hogan, MJ: Trans Am Ophthalmol Soc 65:275, 1967. Copyright 1967, American Medical Association)

Axons

As axons exit the globe, they become enveloped by myelin sheaths characteristic of other myelinated tracts of the central nervous system.[5,14,15,32,214] The myelin sheaths enlarge the circumference of the optic nerve to between 3 and 4 mm as it exits the globe (Fig. 4-40). Elongated sheetlike processes of the oligodendroglia form multilaminated wrappings around individual axon cylinders. Though the membranes are unfused, there is little if any extracellular space interposed between the axon plasma membrane and glial membranes. A thin layer of glial cytoplasm can be seen within the multiple wrappings of the myelin sheath.

This segment of the optic nerve is characterized by saltatory conduction of neural response, with membrane depolarization occurring only at nodes of Ranvier where the myelin sheath becomes discontinuous.[11,111] At these junctions, individual layers of glial membrane within the sheath end in blind loops. Each loop contains an accumulation of cytoplasmic organelles including mitochondria and ribosomes, presumably important to maintenance of the nodal function. The axon cylinder is exposed to an adjacent astrocyte process filling the gap between myelin sheaths.

Occasionally, there is direct axon to axon contact within the nodal junction.

There is considerable axon exchange between fiber bundles confined within the incomplete connective tissue septae. A reorganization of fiber bundle topography occurs with axons from the macular region, both nasally and temporally to the fovea, assuming a more central position within the optic nerve rather than occupying the temporal sector as is characteristic of the more anterior nerve head and lamina cribrosa[73,75,78] (Fig. 4-41). The vertical organization is maintained with fibers from the superior retina lying in the superior nerve and axons from the inferior quadrants lying inferiorly. As the macular bundles assume a more axial position, the fibers from the more peripheral retina move temporarily around the circumference of the nerve cross section.

Posteriorly, the optic nerve enters the optic canal through the optic foramen. The canal itself is formed by a fusion of two roots of the lesser wing of the sphenoid bone and runs posteriorly and medially with the nerve, exiting the canal in the middle fossa at the dorsum sella to meet its fellow nerve at the optic chiasm[96] (Fig. 4-42). The canal tapers gradually in an anteroposterior direction and is vertically elongated.

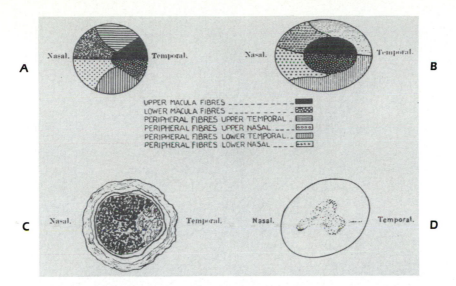

Fig. 4-41 Fiber arrangement in the optic nerve. **A,** Distal portion of optic nerve. **B,** Proximal portion of optic nerve. **C,** Degeneration of fibers in distal optic nerve after atrophy of papillomacular bundle. **D,** Fiber atrophy in proximal nerve following macular lesion. (From Duke-Elder, S: Textbook of ophthalmology, vol 1, St Louis, 1932, The CV Mosby Co)

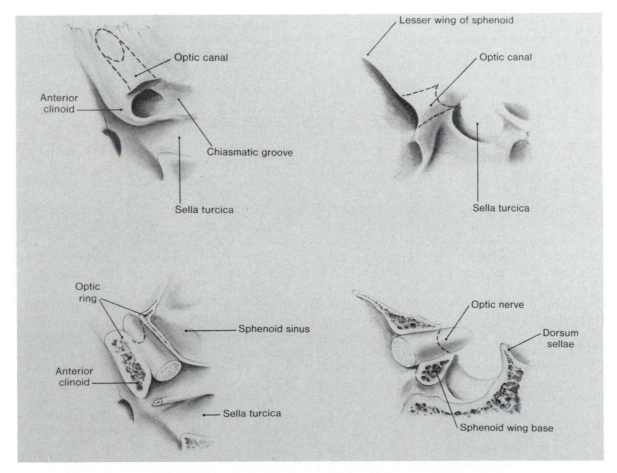

Fig. 4-42 Horizontal and lateral sketches of optic canal anatomy. Canal arises from base of lesser sphenoid wing. (From Maniscalco, JE, and Habal, MB: J Neurosurg 48:402, 1978)

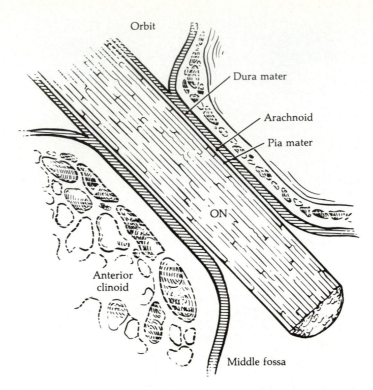

Fig. 4-43   Schematic drawing of optic nerve canal illustrating relationship of optic nerve to surrounding sphenoid bone. Dura is tightly adherent to bone within canal. Within orbit it divides into two sheaths, one of which continues as dura of optic nerve and other becomes periosteum of orbit. Intracranially, dura leaves optic nerve to become periosteum of sphenoid bone. (From Miller, NR: Walsh and Hoyt's Clinical neuro-ophthalmology, Baltimore, 1982, Williams & Wilkins)

The dura fuses with the periosteum of the optic canal and the nerve is enveloped by the arachnoid and pia mater[96,170] (Fig. 4-43). The nerve is relatively fixed in place, tethered by its attachments to the canal wall by the encircling meninges. The ophthalmic artery and branches of the carotid sympathetic plexus are also contained within the optic canal. The nerve is separated from the superior orbital fissure inferolaterally by the optic strut, a fusion between the lesser wing and the main body of the sphenoid bone.[31] Air cells of the sphenoid, ethmoid, and frontal sinuses surround the optic canal inferiorly, medially, and superiorly.[31,169]

Chiasm and Optic Tract

The intracranial optic nerve exits the optic canal moving upwards and medially, extending from 3 to 10 mm to the optic chiasm.[208] The chiasm, generally overlying the diaphragma sellae, is about 8 mm long, about 11 mm wide,[74,76,208] and approximately 4 mm thick. Approximately 20% of normal individuals have a more anteriorly (prefixed) or posteriorly (postfixed) located chiasm. Anatomic relationships with other structures within the mid-

dle fossa, including the carotid artery, oculomotor nerve, and pituitary gland, have been described in detail elsewhere* (Fig. 4-44).

The chiasm forms part of the anteroinferior wall of the third ventricle and is enveloped in meninges continuous with those of the optic nerve. Through this structure pass the more than 2 million axons from the two optic nerves.

There is a hemidecussation of fibers from the nasal retina of each eye, with approximately 43% of axons remaining uncrossed within the chiasm. Generally, the more peripheral fibers cross more anteriorly, with fibers from the inferior retina looping anteriorly into the substance of the contralateral optic nerve (von Willebrand's loop).[209] The more central fibers from the macular region cross more posteriorly within the chiasm. Simultaneously, there is a clockwise rotation within the right and a counterclockwise rotation within the left optic nerve such that the ventral retinal fibers assume a more medial position within the optic tract as it

---

*References 26-28, 36, 111, 170, 177.

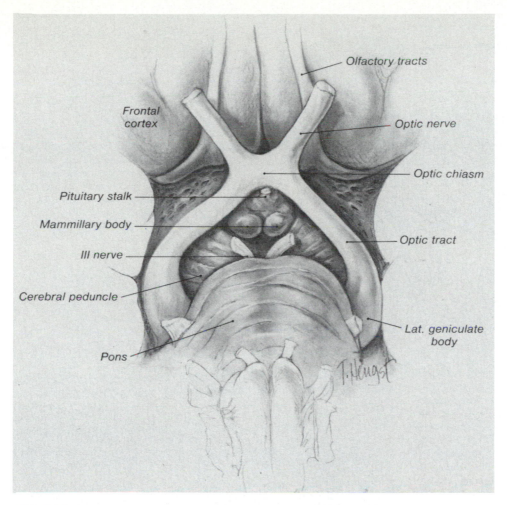

Fig. 4-44 Optic chiasm and optic tracts viewed from below. (From Ferner, H, editor: Atlas of topographical and applied human anatomy, vol 1, Philadelphia, 1963, WB Saunders Co)

exits the chiasm. Conversely, the axons from the superior retina assume a more medial position within the optic radiation.[74,76,123,172,173]

The optic tracts leave the chiasm and, passing laterally around the cerebral peduncles, synapse at the lateral geniculate body (see Fig. 4-44). Within the tract, fibers from anomalous retinal regions of contralateral eyes converge with macular fibers, assuming a dorsolateral position within the posterior tract. Fibers from the superior retina lie dorsomedially within the tract and axons from the inferior retina lie ventrolaterally.*

The optic tracts terminate at the lateral geniculate body, part of the inferior rostral thalamus.[69,91] The lateral geniculate body has a dorsal and ventral nucleus. Only the dorsal nucleus, however, com-

municates with the visual cortex through the optic radiation.[69,91] The dorsal nucleus consists of alternating layers of gray and white matter with six nucleated laminae numbered from 1 to 6 in a ventral to dorsal sequence. Axons from the contralateral eye project to layers 1, 4, and 6, and axons from the ipsilateral eye project to layers 2, 3, and 5. Layers 1 and 2 contain large (magnocellular) cell bodies, and layers 3 and 6 have relatively smaller (parvocellular) cells[91] (Fig. 4-45).

OPTIC NERVE IN GLAUCOMA

Pressure-induced changes in glaucomatous eyes occur throughout the optic nerve.* At the level of the retina, diffuse ganglion cell dropout leads to thinning or absence of this nuclear layer.[71,137,152] The

---

*References 24, 25, 95, 111, 172, 173.

*References 11, 108, 126, 127, 130, 137, 148, 167, 185, 186, 191, 215.

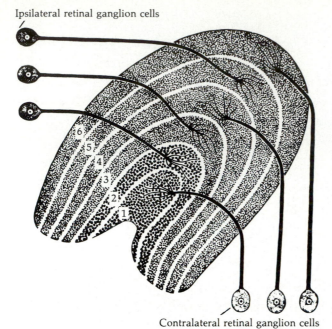

Ipsilateral retinal ganglion cells

Contralateral retinal ganglion cells

Fig. 4-45 Diagram of transverse section through lateral geniculate body. Layers are numbered from ventral to dorsal. *1* and *2* are the large areas. *3, 4, 5,* and *6* are the small layers. Contralateral fibers project onto layers *1, 4,* and *6.* Ipsilateral fibers project onto layers *2, 3,* and *5.* (From Glees, P: Verh Anat Ges 55:60, 1959)

Fig. 4-46 Cross section of retina through nerve fiber bundle defect in arcuate region of superotemporal vascular arcade. Within region of fiber bundle loss *(left)* there is thinning of nerve fiber layer *(NFL)* as seen in contrast to nerve fiber layer in more normal adjacent retina *(right).* GCL, Ganglion cell layer; *INL,* inner nuclear layer. (From Radius, RL, and Anderson, DR: Arch Ophthalmol 97:948, 1979)

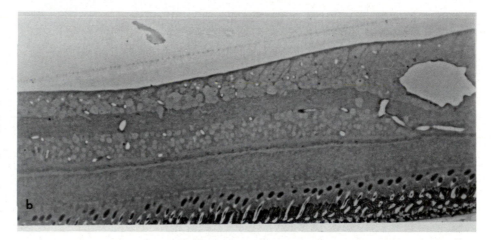

retinal nerve fiber layer is thinned by loss of axon cylinders (Fig. 4-46). Processes of glial cells fill much of the space vacated by axon loss. Nerve fiber bundle defects recognized clinically reflect moderate to advanced loss of neurons.[7,78,130,152] Remaining axons may show localized swelling without organelle accumulation.

The most profound changes occur at the optic nerve head. In moderately damaged eyes, axon loss is reflected by a general decrease in the tissue volume of the anterior optic nerve head. With severe damage, there is near total collapse of the anterior nerve structure[126,127,137,167] (Fig. 4-47). The lamina and remaining neurons are covered by a continuous sheet of astrocytes. The laminar sheets are collapsed and reduced in number. The lamina scleralis itself bows 0.5 to 1.0 mm posteriorly and undermines the adjacent choroid (Fig. 4-48). The size of the scleral opening itself is unchanged at the level of Bruch's membrane.[139,141] Capillaries are reduced in number, as are the sheets of astrocytes forming the glial columns of the anterior optic nerve head. There is, however, an increase in the overall surface area of the lamina. The total amount of glial tissue is reduced little, if at all. The increase in size of the physical cup at the nerve head is predominately a result of posterior bowing of the lamina scleralis and loss of axonal tissue.[126,137,140,167]

Diffuse axon loss occurs throughout the nerve,

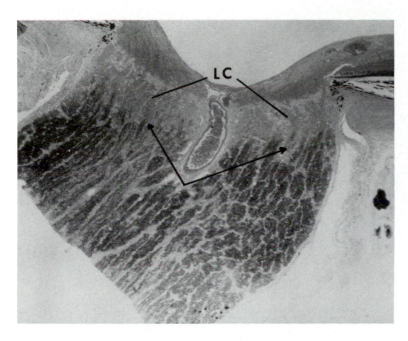

Fig. 4-47 Optic nerve head of primate eye with moderate glaucomatous optic neuropathy developing after several months of pressure elevation induced by trabecular photocoagulation. There is a reduction in volume of anterior optic nerve head with loss of axons and early bowing of posterior lamina cribrosa *(LC)*. Loss of myelin in the retroocular optic nerve is another sign of optic nerve damage in this eye with increased pressure *(arrows)*. (From Radius, RL, and Pederson, JE: Arch Ophthalmol 102:1693, 1984. Copyright 1984, American Medical Association)

Fig. 4-48 Optic nerve head from primate eye with extensive glaucomatous optic atrophy after months of pressure elevation induced by trabecular photocoagulation. There is almost total loss of axon cylinders. A few neurons *(AX)* can be identified by remaining myelin material seen in intraorbital portion of nerve behind globe. Lamina cribosa *(LC)* is bowed posteriorly, and there is undermining of scleral rim at optic nerve head *(arrows)*. Remaining sheets of glial and connective tissue *(GC)* are collapsed, and there is little if any tissue remaining of anterior optic nerve head. *N*, Nasal; *S*, superior; *T*, temporal. (From Radius, RL, and Pederson, JE: Arch Ophthalmol 102:1693, 1984. Copyright 1984, American Medical Association)

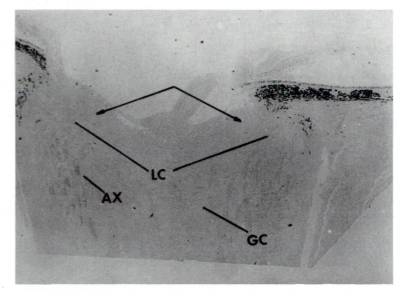

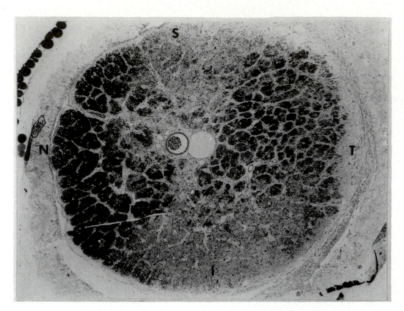

Fig. 4-49 Optic nerve cut in cross section taken from eye with moderate glaucomatous optic neuropathy. Although axon loss can be recognized throughout extent of nerve section, in this and many specimens, the superior (S) and inferior (I) poles are preferentially involved by neuron damage. N, Nasal; T, temporal. (From Radius, RL, and Pederson, JE: Arch Ophthalmol 102:1693, 1984. Copyright 1984, American Medical Association)

Fig. 4-50 Optic nerve head of primate eye with experimental glaucoma. Transport interruption (dark staining material, arrows) is frequently identified at level of lamina cribrosa in association with trabecular beams of connective tissue and glial cell elements as if increased pressure has damaged the axon segment by pressing it against lamellar plates of the lamina. (From Gaasterland, D, Tanishima, T, and Kuwabara, T: Invest Ophthalmol Vis Sci 17:838, 1978)

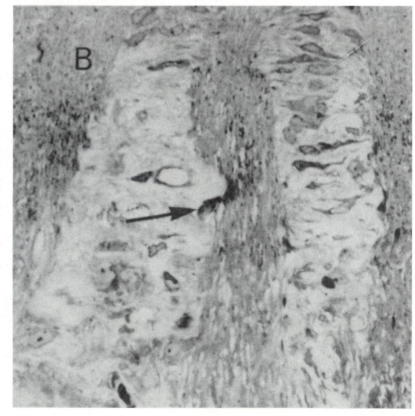

although frequently there is preferential involvement of specific nerve sectors (Fig. 4-49). Preferential loss most frequently involves the superior and inferior quadrants and least often involves the nasal sector. Remaining axons frequently demonstrate swellings and accumulation of organelles identical to that seen in experimental models of glaucoma in eyes with acute interruption of fast axonal transport mechanisms.[90,131,155,156] This transport blockage occurs at the level of the posterior lamina scleralis and at the edge of the scleral ring in more circumferentially placed axons. Astrocytes fill the spaces vacated by axon loss within the fiber bundle columns. The architecture of the laminar plates is distorted by the backward displacement of the lamina and undermining of the adjacent choroid.[43,92,93,139,167] Axons follow increasingly complex paths through the misaligned laminar pores. Transport interruption is seen frequently at bundle branchings in association with the connective tissue laminae[52] (Fig. 4-50). Occasionally, local ectasia, with loss of the lamina scleralis, can be identified, most frequently involving the inferior nerve sector.[163,166]

Posteriorly, there is a loss of axons and myelin.[126,127,137,167] Astrocytes fill the axon columns between the connective tissue septae. There is general thinning of the nerve diameter due to loss of the myelin sheaths. Frequently, active ascending (Wallerian) degeneration with disintegration of axon and myelin sheath can be seen along the length of the nerve.

The mechanism of pressure-induced axon damage remains poorly defined. Some inferences may be made by comparing the regional differences in the anatomy of the optic nerve at the lamina to the recognized pattern of preferential axon damage in eyes with elevated intraocular pressure.[148,149] For instance, the dimensions of the fiber bundle tunnels within the lamina and the density of the interbundle septae vary across the nerve section. In the nasal nerve, the laminar pores are smallest and the connective tissue and glial columns are thickest.* In the superior and inferior nerve quadrants, the interbundle septae are thinnest and the cross-section diameters of the fiber bundles are greatest (Fig. 4-51). The dimensions within the temporal nerve are intermediate. These regional differences in anatomy at the lamina may play some role in the specificity of optic nerve head damage in eyes with elevated intraocular pressure.

Regions of the lamina with relatively less in-

terbundle connective tissue and glial cell elements may provide less structural support of axon bundles in pressure-stressed eyes.* Regional collapse of the laminar structure may mechanically compress axon cylinders, causing segmental damage and ultimately ganglion cell loss.[43,52,140,163] Interruption of axonal transport caused by neuronal compression could damage the neuron at the lamina in eyes with elevated intraocular pressure.[17,18,59] In clinical and experimental models of glaucoma, transport interruption is seen within the posterior lamina scleralis,† frequently within axons adjacent to local projections of dense connective tissue and glial septa at branchings within fiber bundles (see Fig. 4-50). Direct compression of axon cylinders by the laminar plates may compromise normal neuron physiology. It has also been suggested that compression of axon cylinders may occur at the scleral rim as the fibers cross the margin of the disc. This region of the nerve head is most susceptible to mechanical distortion by acute pressure elevation.[92,93] The axons entering the temporal nerve may be most vulnerable to pressure-induced retrodisplacement of the lamina because of their relatively tangential course across the nerve head and scleral margin.

Alternatively, reduced blood flow within the nerve head of eyes with elevated intraocular pressure may play a role in axon damage.‡ Blood flow within the lamina cribrosa and optic nerve head is maintained within normal limits until extreme pressure levels are reached, usually in excess of diastolic pressures within the ophthalmic circulation.§ The autoregulatory capacity of the normal nerve seems to be somewhat less than that of the retinal circulation but exceeds that of the choroidal vasculature. The mechanism of autoregulation within the nerve head is unclear. Blood flow to this region is derived primarily from the posterior ciliary arteries, with lesser contributions from the central retinal artery and pial vasculature. It is unlikely that the posterior ciliary circulation would respond to tissue ischemia or reduced blood flow within the nerve head because 99% of the blood flow through the ciliary circulation is directed toward the choroidal circulation. It is possible that the capillary bed itself within the nerve head lamina may respond to local tissue conditions to regulate flow through the lamina.

Whatever the exact mechanism of blood flow

---

*References 128, 140, 146-149, 159, 160, 163.

*References 43, 98, 99, 128, 140, 146, 148, 149, 159, 160, 163.
†References 13, 43, 52, 105, 132, 145.
‡References 10, 11, 45, 47, 60-62, 65, 66.
§References 2, 3, 53, 184, 203, 204.

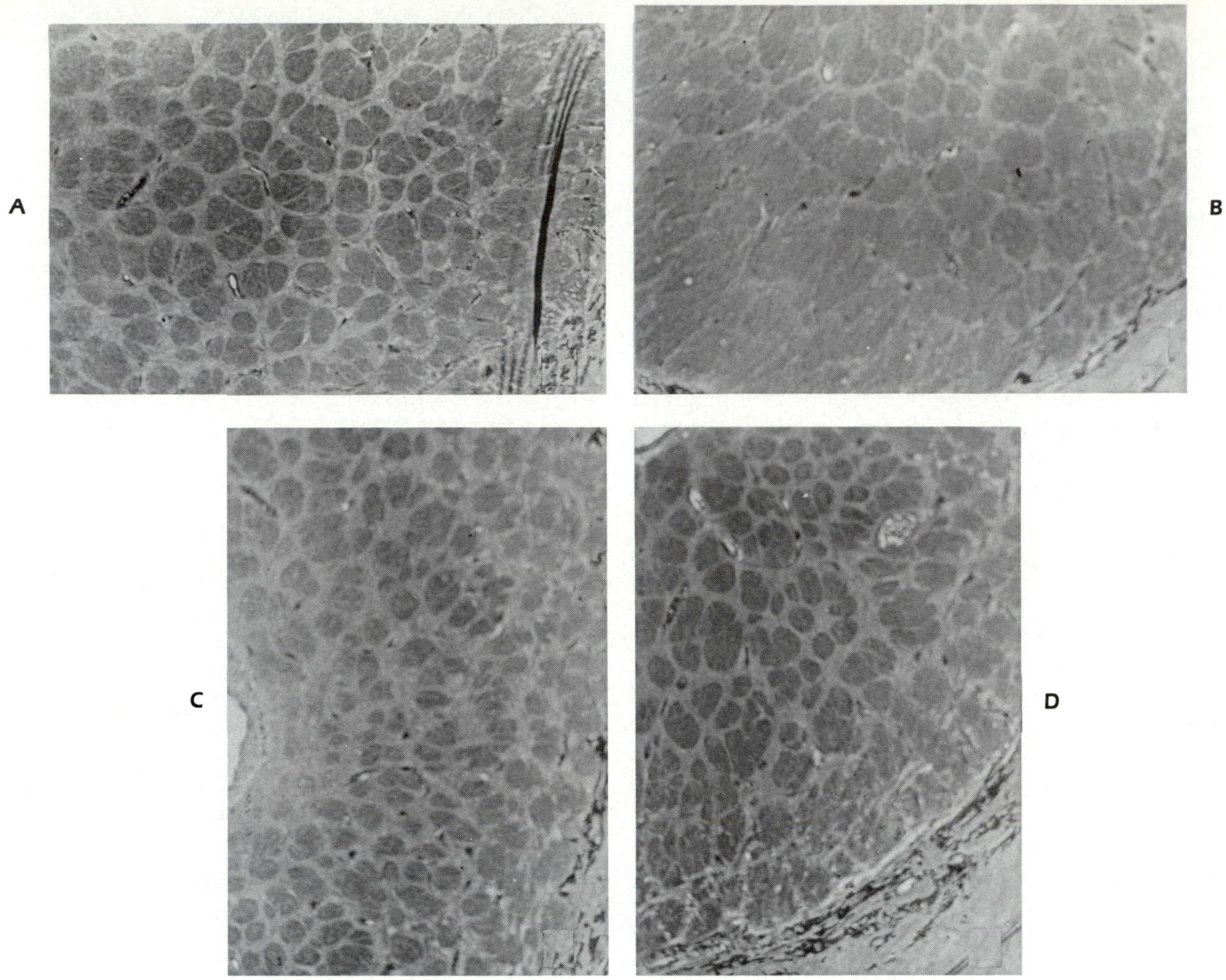

Fig. 4-51 Region of lamina scleralis cut in cross section in two monkey eyes. **A** and **C** are from the temporal and **B** and **D** are from the inferior nerve sectors. As in human specimens examined in much the same fashion, the cross-sectional area of laminar pores through which fiber bundles pass is largest and density of interbundle glial and connective tissue elements is less in those regions of the nerve (superior and inferior poles versus nasal and temporal sectors) preferentially vulnerable to a pressure insult. Collapse of laminar structure in these regions in response to elevated pressure may damage axon segments either through direct mechanical compression of the neuron, interruption of normal blood flow patterns within the microcirculation confined within the laminar tissue or other as yet unrecognized phenomena. (From Radius, RL: Arch Ophthalmol 99:478, 1981. Copyright 1981, American Medical Association)

regulation within the nerve head, it is unlikely that acute vascular collapse in eyes with elevated intraocular pressure is the cause of pressure-induced axon damage. Extreme pressure elevation in human eyes, frequently exceeding 60 mm Hg, can often be sustained without any demonstrable axon loss.[37,38,165] The effects of more moderate pressure elevation over longer periods of time on nerve head perfusion, however, are less well defined.[142]

It is possible that age- or disease-related abnormalities in autoregulation of blood flow at the nerve head are important to pressure-induced damage in glaucomatous eyes.[10,11,148,183,184] The vasculature within the lamina demonstrates extensive anastomoses with the microcirculation of the more anterior and posterior optic nerve.[7,12,94] The functional significance of these collateral channels, however, is uncertain. Like the retinal circulation, the capillary bed within the nerve head may represent an end-artery-type vasculature, with regional blood flow somewhat functionally isolated from adjacent capillary beds and dependent on feeding arterioles for adequate perfusion. It has been suggested that the vulnerability of the nerve head, and particularly the superior and inferior poles of the nerve head, to a pressure insult may reflect the anatomy of the posterior ciliary circulation.[65,67,144] The optic nerve papillae often lie within the watershed zone of choroidal perfusion by the lateral and medial posterior ciliary circulation. In eyes with compromised autoregulation within the nerve itself, elevated intraocular pressure may tax an already stressed tissue perfusion. The region functionally most distant from the blood supply would be most easily compromised and would show the greatest tissue effects as a result of the reduced tissue perfusion.

Alternatively, the anatomy within the microcirculation at the nerve head may define regional vulnerability to a pressure insult.[4,5,14,15] The distribution of capillaries across the nerve section at the lamina cribrosa is relatively uniform.[139] This pattern does not, in and of itself, explain the preferential damage of axons within the superior and inferior optic nerve head. On the other hand, the density of neurons within fiber bundles is greatest within these same regions.[128,146,159,163] The amount of blood flow available per unit volume of neuronal tissue within these more vulnerable sectors may be relatively compromised in eyes with increased intraocular pressure.[148,149] Moreover, all of the microcirculation within the nerve head at the lamina is confined to the same laminar plates. Mechanical compression of the interbundle septa and distortion of the laminar architecture in eyes with elevated intraocular pressure could compress or compromise regional blood flow with secondary neuronal ischemia as a mechanism of axon damage in eyes with elevated intraocular pressure. The combined features of the anatomy of the vasculature and of the lamina itself may define the preferential vulnerability of specific fiber bundles to the pressure insult.

Finally, differences in axon anatomy may help define individual fiber bundle susceptibility to a pressure insult. Psychophysical observations and examination of eyes with experimental glaucoma indicate that large diameter axons may be more vulnerable to pressure-induced optic atrophy.[97,138,148,149,167] Perhaps large diameter axons, with relatively reduced suface-to-volume ratios, may be more susceptible to local tissue ischemia than are small diameter axons with relatively large surface areas available for metabolic exchange. On the other hand, large diameter axons may be less able to withstand regional tissue distortion in eyes with increased intraocular pressure.

In the primate eye there are regional differences in the mean fiber dimensions of axons within the nerve head.[124,164,176] These differences, however, do not duplicate the pattern of preferential damage to fiber bundles in eyes with elevated pressure.[164,176] Axons from the nasal retina, on the average, are larger than the neurons from the temporal retina. The superior and inferior axons are intermediate in size. Likewise, axons at the margin of the disc are largest and axons located near the center of the nerve cross section are smallest. Axons in the intermediate regions are intermediate in size. There is a great deal of variation and range in axon dimensions in all regions of the nerve, but the mean axon diameters follow this pattern.[164] The distribution by size of fibers within regions of the nerve may be even more complex. The greatest fiber density and smallest axons are found in the inferotemporal nerve sector. The greatest proportion of large diameter axons are found in the superior disc. Although these regional variations in axon morphology may define, in part, fiber bundle vulnerability to a pressure insult, they do not, in and of themselves, explain the specificity of axon damage in the glaucomatous eye.

Notwithstanding these and other theories advanced to explain the pathogenesis or mechanism of pressure-induced axon damage in eyes with elevated intraocular pressure, the precise mechanism remains enigmatic. Perhaps a combination of factors in individual eyes accounts for the pattern of axon damage observed in the glaucomatous optic nerve.[148,149] Mechanically induced changes, either acute or chronic, within the lamina scleralis and at the scleral margin may compress axon cylinders and compromise blood flow to regional groups of fiber bundles.* Age-related changes in nerve head autoregulation may compound these anatomic changes.[11,183,184] As yet undefined pressure effects on nerve head astroglia may interfere with proper homeostasis around the axon cylinders, an important function of the glial tissue throughout the central nervous system, including the optic nerve.[148,149] Although different axon populations may be more or less vulnerable to these multiple insults, eventually compromise of normal axon physiology would occur, perhaps including a focal interruption in axonal transport mechanisms. In instances of irreversible damage to the involved axon segment, the end results would be ganglion cell loss and the visual deficits characteristic of the glaucomatous eye.

---

*References 92, 93, 128, 140, 146, 163, 166.

REFERENCES

1. Airaksinen, PJ, Niemenen, H, and Mustonen, E: Retinal nerve fiber layer photography with a wide angle fundus camera, Acta Ophthalmol (Copenh) 60:362, 1982
2. Alm, A, and Bill, A: The oxygen supply to the retina. II. Effects of high intraocular pressure and of increased arterial carbon dioxide on uveal and retinal blood flow in cats. A study with radioactively labelled microspheres including flow determinations in brain and other tissues, Acta Physiol Scand 84:306, 1972
3. Alm, A, and Bill, A: Ocular and optic nerve blood flow at normal and increased intraocular pressures in monkeys (Macaca irus): a study with radioactively labelled microspheres including flow determinations in brain and other tissues, Exp Eye Res 15:15, 1973
4. Anderson, DR: Ultrastructure of human and monkey lamina cribrosa and optic nerve head, Arch Ophthalmol 82:800, 1969
5. Anderson, DR: Ultrastructure of the optic nerve head, Arch Ophthalmol 83:63, 1970
6. Anderson, DR: Vascular supply to the optic nerve of primates, Am J Ophthalmol 70:341, 1970
7. Anderson, DR: Ascending and descending optic atrophy produced experimentally in squirrel monkeys, Am J Ophthalmol 76:693, 1973
8. Anderson, DR: Axonal transport in the retina and optic nerve. In Glaser, JS, editor: Neuro-ophthalmology; symposium of the University of Miami and the Bascom Palmer Eye Institute, vol, 9, St Louis, 1977, The CV Mosby Co
9. Anderson, DR: Papilledema and axonal transport. In Thompson, HS, et al, editors: Topics in neuro-ophthalmology, Baltimore, 1979, Williams & Wilkins
10. Anderson, DR: The optic nerve in glaucoma. In Duane, TD, and Jaeger, ER, editors: Clinical ophthalmology, Philadelphia, 1985, Harper & Row
11. Anderson, DR: The optic nerve. In Moses, RA, and Hart, W, editors: Adler's physiology of the eye, ed, 8, St Louis, 1985, The CV Mosby Co
12. Anderson, DR, and Braverman, S: Reevaluation of the optic disk vasculature, Am J Ophthalmol 82:165, 1976
13. Anderson, DR, and Hendrickson, A: Effect of intraocular pressure on rapid axoplasmic transport in monkey optic nerve. Invest Ophthalmol 13:771, 1974
14. Anderson, DR, Hoyt, WF, and Hogan, MJ: The fine structure of the astroglia in the human optic nerve and optic nerve head, Trans Am Ophthalmol Soc 65:275, 1967
15. Anderson, DR, and Hoyt, WF: Ultrastructure of the intraorbital portion of human and monkey optic nerve, Arch Ophthalmol 82:506, 1969
16. Arey, LB, and Schaible, AJ: The nerve fiber composition of the optic nerve, Anat Rec Suppl 58:3, 1934
17. Bárány, E: Experiments on axoplasmic flow. In Etienne, R, and Paterson, GD, editors: International Glaucoma Symposium (Albi, 1974), Marseille, 1975, Diffusion Generale de Librarie
18. Bárány, E: Ability of retrograde axoplasmic flow to overcome pressure gradients; preliminary communication, Doc Ophthalmol 16:215, 1978
19. Bengtsson, B: The variation and covariation of cup and disc diameters, Acta Ophthalmol (Copenh) 54:804, 1976
20. Ben-Sira, I, and Riva, CE: Fluorescein diffusion in the human optic disc, Invest Ophthalmol 14:205, 1975
21. Blumcke, S, Niedorf, HR, and Rode, J: Axoplasmic alterations in the proximal and distal stumps of transected nerves, Acta Neuropathol (Berl) 7:44, 1966
22. Boycott, BB, and Dowling, JE: Organization of the primate retina: light microscopy, Philos Trans R Soc Lond (Biol) 255:109, 1969
23. Boycott, BB, and Wassle, H: The morphologic types of ganglion cells of the domestic cat's retina, J Physiol (Lond) 240:397, 1974
24. Brouwer, B, and Zeeman, WPC: Experimental anatomical investigations concerning the projection of the retina on the primary optic centers in apes, J Neurol Psychopathol 6:1, 1925
25. Brouwer, B, and Zeeman, WPC: The projection of the retina in the primary optic neuron in monkeys, Brain 49:1, 1926
26. Bull, J: The normal variations in the position of the optic recess of the third ventricle, Acta Radiol [Diagn] (Stockh) 46:72, 1956
27. Burgland, RM, Ray, RS, and Torack, RM: Anatomical variations in the pituitary gland and adjacent structures in 225 human autopsy cases, J Neurosurg 28:93, 1968
28. Camp, JD: The normal and pathologic anatomy of the sella turcica as revealed by roentgenograms, Am J Roentgenol Radium Ther Nucl Med 12:143, 1924
29. Cleland, BG, Dubin, MW, and Levick, WR: Sustained and transient neurons in the cat retina and lateral geniculate nucleus, J Physiol (Lond) 217:473, 1971
30. Cleland, BG, Levick, WR, and Sanderson, KJ: Properties of sustained and transient ganglion cells in the cat retina, J Physiol (Lond) 228:649, 1973
31. Cares, HL, and Bakey, L: The clinical significance of the optic strut, J Neurosurg 34:355, 1971
32. Cohen, AI: Ultrastructural aspects of the human optic nerve, Invest Ophthalmol 6:294, 1967
33. Cohen, AI: Is there a potential defect in the blood-retinal barrier at the choroidal level of the optic nerve canal? Invest Ophthalmol 12:513, 1973
34. Dahlstroem, A: Axoplasmic transport (with particular respect to adrenergic neurons), Philos Trans R Soc Lond (Biol) 261:325, 1961

35. deMonasterio, FM: Properties of concentrically organized cells of the macaque retina, J Neurophysiol 41:1394, 1978

36. DiChiro, G: The width (third dimension) of the sella turcica, Am J Roentgenol Radium Ther Nucl Med 84:26, 1960

37. Douglas, GR, Drance, SM, and Schultzer, M: The visual field and nerve head in angle-closure glaucoma; a comparison of the effects of acute and chronic angle-closure glaucoma, Arch Ophthalmol 56:186, 1972

38. Douglas, GR, Drance, SM, and Schultzer, M: The visual field and nerve head following acute angle closure glaucoma, Can J Ophthalmol 9:404, 1974

39. Dowling, JE, and Boycott, BB: Organization of the primate retina: electron microscopy, Proc R Soc Lond (Biol) 166:80, 1966

40. Duce, IR, and Keen, P: Proceedings: a light and electron microscopic study of the accumulation of material in sectioned rat dorsal roots and the effect of demecolcine, Br J Pharmacol 55:265, 1975

41. Elschnig, A: Das Colobom am Sehnerveneintritte und der Conus nach unten, Graefes Arch Clin Exp Ophthalmol 51:391, 1900

42. Elschnig, A: Der normal Sehnerveneintritt des menschlichen Auges, Denkschriften der Mathematische-Naturwissenschaftische Classe der Kaiserlichen Akademie der Wissenschaften in Wein, 70:219, 1901

43. Emery, JK, Landis, D, and Paton, D: The lamina cribrosa in normal and glaucomatous eyes. Trans Am Acad Ophthalmol Otolaryngol 78:OP-290, 1974

44. Enroth-Cugell, C, and Robson, JG: The contrast sensitivity of retinal ganglion cells in the cat, J Physiol (Lond) 187:552, 1966

45. Ernest, JT: Pathogenesis of glaucomatous optic nerve disease, Trans Am Ophthalmol Soc 73:366, 1975

46. Ernest, JT, and Archer, D: Fluorescein angiography of the optic disk, Am J Ophthalmol 75:973, 1973

47. Ernest, JT, and Potts, AM: Pathophysiology of the distal portion of the topic nerve. I. Tissue pressure relationships, Am J Ophthalmol 66:373, 1968

48. Flage, T: Permeability properties of the tissues in the optic nerve head region in the rabbit and the monkey; an ultra-structural study, Acta Ophthalmol (Copenh) 55:652, 1977

49. François, J, and Neetens, A: Central retinal artery and central optic nerve artery, Br J Ophthalmol 47:21, 1963

50. François, J, and Neetens, A: Functional importance of the anterior optic nerve supply, Ophthalmologica 168:122, 1974

51. Friede, RL: Axon swellings produced in vivo in isolated segments of nerves, Acta Neuropathol (Berl) 3:229, 1964

52. Gaasterland, D, Tanishima, T, and Kuwabara, T: Axoplasmic flow during chronic experimental glaucoma. I. Light and electron microscopic studies of the monkey optic nerve head during development of glaucomatous cupping, Invest Ophthalmol Vis Sci 17:838, 1978

53. Geijer, C, and Bill, A: Effects of raised intraocular pressure on retinal, preliminar, laminar and retrolaminar optic nerve blood flow in monkeys, Invest Ophthalmol Vis Sci 18:1030, 1979

54. Gill, TH, Young, OM, and Tower, DB: The uptake of 36 Cl into astrocytes in tissue culture by potassium-dependent, saturable process, J Neurochem 23:1011, 1974

55. Grayson, MC, and Laties, AM: Ocular localization of sodium fluorescein; effects of administration in rabbit and monkey, Arch Ophthalmol 85:600, 1971

56. Grayson, M, Tsukahara, S, and Laties, AM: Tissue localization in rabbit and monkey eye of intravenously-administered fluorescein. In Shimizu, K, editor: Fluorescein angiography; proceedings of the International Symposium on Fluorescein Angiography, Tokyo, 1972, Toyko, 1974, Igaku Shoin Ltd

57. Grehn, F, and Prost, M: Function of retinal nerve fibers depends on perfusion pressure: neurophysiologic investigations during acute intraocular pressure elevation, Invest Ophthalmol Vis Sci 24:347, 1983

58. Guist, G: Coincident ophthalmoscopy and histology of the optic nerve, Vienna, 1934, Guist

59. Hahnenberger, RW: Effects of pressure on fast axoplasmic flow. An in vitro study in the vagus nerve of rabbits, Acta Physiol Scand 104:299, 1978

60. Harrington, DO: The Bjerrum scotoma, Am J Ophthalmol 59:646, 1969

61. Harrington, DO: Pathogenesis of the glaucomatous visual field defects: individual variations in pressure sensitivity. In Newell, FW, editor: Glaucoma: transactions of the fifth conference, Princeton, NJ, 1960, New York, 1961, Josiah Macy Jr Foundation

62. Harrington, DO: Differential diagnosis of the arcuate scotoma, Invest Ophthalmol 8:96, 1969

63. Hartline, HK: The response of single optic nerve fibers of the vertebrate eye to illumination of the retina, Am J Physiol 121:400, 1938

64. Hayreh, SS: The central artery of the retina: its role in the blood supply of the optic nerve, Br J Ophthalmol 45:651, 1963

65. Hayreh, SS: Blood supply of the optic nerve head and its role in optic atrophy, glaucoma, and oedema of the optic disc, Br J Ophthalmol 53:721, 1969

66. Hayreh, SS: Pathogenesis of visual field defects and the role of the ciliary circulation, Br J Ophthalmol 54:289, 1970

67. Hayreh, SS: Individual variation in blood supply of the optic nerve head, Doc Ophthalmol 3:217, 1985

68. Henkind, P, and Levitsky, M: Angioarchitecture of the optic nerve head, Am J Ophthalmol 68:979, 1969

69. Hines, MN: Recent contributions to localization of vision in the central nervous system (review), Arch Ophthalmol 28:913, 1942

70. Hoffman, PN, Clark, W, Carroll, PT, and Price, DL: Slow axonal transport of neurofilament proteins:

impairment by, B,B'-iminodipropionitrile administration, Science 202:633, 1978

71. Hoffman, PN, and Lasek, RJ: The slow component of axonal transport: identification of major structural polypeptides of the axon and their generality among mammalian neurons, J Cell Biol 66:351, 1975

72. Hogan, MJ, Alvarado, JA, and Weddell, JE: Histology of the human eye. An atlas and textbook, Philadelphia, 1971, WB Saunders Co

73. Hoyt, WF: Anatomic considerations of arcuate scotomas associated with lesions of the optic nerve and chiasm. Nauta axon degeneration study in the monkey, Bull Johns Hopkins Hospital 111:57, 1962

74. Hoyt, WF: Correlative functional anatomy of the optic chiasm, Clin Neurosurg 17:189, 1969

75. Hoyt, WF, and Luis, O: Visual fiber anatomy in the infrageniculate pathway of the primate; uncrossed and crossed retinal quadrant fiber projections studied with Nauta silver stain, Arch Ophthalmol 68:94, 1962

76. Hoyt, WF, and Luis, O: The primate chiasm, Arch Ophthalmol 70:69, 1963

77. Hoyt, WF, Schlicke, B, and Eckelhoff, RJ: Fundoscopic appearance of a nerve fiber bundle defect, Br J Ophthalmol 56:577, 1972

78. Hoyt, WF, and Tudor, RC: The course of peripapillary temporal retinal axons through the anterior optic nerve: a Nauta degeneration study in the primate, Arch Ophthalmol 69:503, 1963

79. Hughes, A, and Wassel, H: The cat optic nerve: fiber total count and diameter spectrum, J Comp Neurol 169:171, 1976

80. Ikeda, H, and Hill, RM: Can a peripheral ganglion cell respond differentially to images in and out of focus, Nature 229:557, 1971

81. Ikeda, H, and Wright, MJ: How large is the receptive field of a single retinal ganglion cell? J Physiol (Lond) 217:52, 1971

82. Ikeda, H, and Wright, MJ: Differential effects of refractive errors and receptive field organization of central and peripheral ganglion cells, Vision Res 12:1465, 1972

83. Ikeda, H, and Wright, MJ: Receptive field organization of "sustained" and "transient" retinal ganglion cells which subserve different functional roles, J Physiol (Lond) 222:769, 1972

84. Ikeda, H, and Wright, MJ: Is amblyopia due to inappropriate stimulation of the "sustained" pathway during development? Br J Ophthalmol 58:165, 1974

85. Isukahara, I, and Yamashita, H: An electron microscopic study on blood-optic nerve and fluid-optic nerve barrier, v Graefes Arch Clin Exp Ophthalmol 196:239, 1975

86. Jacoby, E: Uber den Neuroglia der Sehnerven, Klin Mbl Augenheilk 43:129, 1905

87. Kroll, AJ: Experimental central retinal artery occlusion, Arch Ophthalmol 79:453, 1968

88. Kuffler, SW: Discharge patterns and functional organization of mammalian retina, J Neurophysiol 16:37, 1953

89. Kuhnt, H: Zur Kenntnis des Sehnerven und der Netzhaut, v Graefes Arch Clin Exp Ophthalmol 25:179, 1879

90. Lampert, PW, Vogel, MH, and Zimmerman, LE: Pathology of the optic nerve in acute experimental glaucoma. Electron microscopic studies, Invest Ophthalmol 7:199, 1968

91. Les Gros Clark, WE, and Penman, GG: The projection of the retina in the lateral geniculate body, Proc R Soc Lond (Biol) 114:291, 1934

92. Levy, NS, Crapps, EE, and Bonney, RC: Displacement of the optic nerve head: response to acute intraocular pressure elevation in primate eyes, Arch Ophthalmol 99:2166, 1981

93. Levy, NS, and Crapps, EE: Displacement of the optic nerve in response to short term intraocular pressure elevation in human eyes, Arch Ophthalmol 102:782, 1984

94. Lieberman, MF, Maumenee, AE, and Green, WR: Histologic studies of the vasculature of the anterior optic nerve, Am J Ophthalmol 82:405, 1976

95. Mackenzie, I, Meighan, S, and Pollack, EN: On the projection of the retinal quadrants on the lateral geniculate bodies, and the relationship of the quadrants to the optic radiations, Trans Ophthalmol Soc UK 53:142, 1933

96. Maniscalco, JE, and Habel, MB: Microanatomy of the optic canal, J Neurosurg 48:402, 1978

97. Marx, JR, et al: Flash and pattern electro-retinogram in normal and laser induced glaucomatous primate eyes, Invest Ophthalmol Vis Sci 27:378, 1986

98. Maumenee, AE: The pathogenesis of visual field loss in glaucoma. In Brockhurst, RJ, Boruchoff, SA, Hutchinson, BT, and Lessell, S, editors: Controversy in ophthalmology, Philadelphia, 1977, WB Saunders Co

99. Maumenee, AE: Visual field loss in glaucoma. In Symposium on glaucoma, Transactions of the New Orleans Academy of Ophthalmology 1981, The CV Mosby Co

100. McLeod, D: Clinical signs of obstructed axoplasmic transport, Lancet 2:954, 1975

101. McLeod, D: Ophthalmoscopic signs of obstructed axoplasmic transport after ocular vascular occlusion, Br J Ophthalmol 60:551, 1976

102. McLeod, D: The role of axoplasmic transport in the pathogenesis of retinal cotton-wool spots, Br J Ophthalmol 61:177, 1977

103. Minckler, DS: The organization of nerve fiber bundles in the primate optic nerve head, Arch Ophthalmol 98:1630, 1980

104. Minckler, DS, and Bunt, AH: Axoplasmic transport in ocular hypotony and papilledema in the monkey, Arch Ophthalmol 95:1430, 1977

105. Minckler, DS, Bunt, AH, and Johanson, GW: Orthograde and retrograde axoplasmic transport during acute ocular hypertension in the monkey, Invest Ophthalmol Vis Sci 16:426, 1977

106. Minckler, DS, Bunt, AH, and Klock, IB: Radiologic and cytochemical ultrastructural studies of axoplasmic transport in the monkey optic nerve head, Invest Ophthalmol Vis Sci 17:33, 1978

107. Minckler, DS, McLean, IW, and Tso, MOM: Distribution of axonal and glial elements in the rhesus optic nerve head studied by electron microscopy, Am J Ophthalmol 82:179, 1976

108. Minckler, DS, and Spaeth, GL: Optic nerve damage in glaucoma, Surv Ophthalmol 26:128, 1981

109. Minckler, DS, and Tso, MOM: Experimental papilledema produced by cyclocryopexy, Am J Ophthalmol 82:577, 1976

110. Minckler, DS, Tso, MOM, and Zimmerman, LE: A light microscopic, autoradiographic study of axoplasmic transport in the optic nerve head ocular hypotony, increased intraocular pressure and papilledema, Am J Ophthalmol 82:741, 1976

111. Miller, NR: Walsh and Hoyt's clinical neuro-ophthalmology, Baltimore, 1982, Williams & Wilkins

112. Ochs, S: Local supply of energy to the fast axoplasmic transport mechanism, Proc Natl Acad Sci USA, 68:1279, 1971

113. Ochs, S: Systems of material transport in nerve fibers (axoplasmic transport) related to nerve function and trophic control, Ann NY Acad Sci 228:202, 1974

114. Ogden, TE: Nerve fiber layer astrocytes of the primate retina: morphology, distribution and density, Invest Ophthalmol Vis Sci 17:499, 1978

115. Ogden, TE: Nerve fiber layer of the macaque retina: retinotopic organization, Invest Ophthalmol Vis Sci 24:85, 1983

116. Ogden, TE: Nerve fiber layer of the owl monkey retina: retinotopic organization, Invest Ophthalmol Vis Sci 24:265, 1983

117. Ogden, TE: Nerve fiber layer of the primate retina: morphometric analysis, Invest Ophthalmol Vis Sci 25:19, 1984

118. Ogden, TE, and Miller, RF: Studies of the optic nerve of the rhesis monkey: nerve spectrum and physiology, Vision Res 6:485, 1966

119. Okinami, S, Ohkuma, M, and Tsukahara, I: Kuhnt intermediary tissue as a barrier between the optic nerve and retina, v Graefes Arch Clin Exp Ophthalmol 201:57, 1976

120. Olsson, Y, and Kristensson, K: Permeability of blood vessels and connective tissue sheaths in retina and optic nerve, Acta Neuropathol 26:147, 1973

121. Orkland, RK, Nicholls, JG, and Kuffler, SW: Effect of nerve impulses on the membrane potential of glial cells in the central nervous system of amphibia, J Neurophysiol 29:788, 1966

122. Polyak, S: The vertebrate visual system, Chicago, 1957, University of Chicago Press

123. Polyak, SL, Projection of the retina upon the cerebral cortex. In Rhoton, AL, Harris, FS, and Renn, WH: Neuro-ophthalmology, St. Louis, 1977, The CV Mosby Co

124. Potts, AM, et al: Morphology of the primate optic nerve, Invest Ophthalmol 11:980, 1972

125. Quigley, HA: Gap junctions between optic nerve head astrocytes, Invest Ophthalmol Vis Sci 16:582, 1977

126. Quigley, HA, and Addicks, EM: Chronic experimental glaucoma in primates. II. Effect of extended intraocular pressure elevation on optic nerve head and axonal transport, Invest Ophthalmol Vis Sci 19:137, 1980

127. Quigley, HA, Addicks, EM, Green, WR, and Maumenee, AE: Optic nerve damage in human glaucoma. II. The site of injury and susceptibility to damage, Arch Ophthalmol 99:635, 1981

128. Quigley, HA, and Addicks, EM: Regional differences in the structure of the lamina cribrosa and their relation to glaucomatous optic nerve damage, Arch Ophthalmol 99:137, 1981

129. Quigley, HA, and Addicks, EM: Quantitative studies of nerve fiber layer defects in glaucoma, Arch Ophthalmol 100:807, 1982

130. Quigley, HA, Addicks, EM, and Green, WR: Optic nerve damage in human glaucoma. III. Quantitative correlation of nerve fiber loss and visual field defect in glaucoma, ischemic neuropathy, papilledema, and toxic neuropathy, Arch Ophthalmol 100:135, 1982

131. Quigley, HA, and Anderson, DR: The dynamics and location of axonal transport blockade by acute intraocular pressure elevation in primate optic nerve, Invest Ophthalmol 15:606, 1976

132. Quigley, HA, and Anderson, DR: Distribution of axonal transport blockade by acute intraocular pressure elevation in the primate optic nerve head, Invest Ophthalmol Vis Sci 16:640, 1977

133. Quigley, HA, and Anderson, DR: Descending optic nerve degeneration in primates, Invest Ophthalmol Vis Sci 16:814, 1977

134. Quigley, HA, and Anderson, DR: The histologic basis of optic disc pallor in experimental optic atrophy, Am J Ophthalmol 83:709, 1977

135. Quigley, HA, Flower, RW, Addicks, EM, and McLeod, DS: The mechanism of optic nerve damage in acute experimental intraocular pressure elevation, Invest Ophthalmol Vis Sci 19:505, 1980

136. Quigley, HA, Guy, J, and Anderson, DR: Blockade of rapid axonal transport, Arch Ophthalmol 97:525, 1979

137. Quigley, HA, and Green, WR: The histology of human glaucoma cupping and optic nerve damage: clinicopathologic correlation in 21 eyes, Ophthalmology, 86:1803, 1979

138. Quigley, HA, and Hendrickson, A: Chronic experimental glaucoma in primates: blood flow study with iodoantipyrine and pattern selective ganglion

cell loss. Invest Ophthalmol Vis Sci 25(ARVO suppl):225, 1984

139. Quigley, HA, Hohman, RM, and Addicks, EM: Quantitative study of optic nerve head capillaries in experimental optic disk pallor, Am J Ophthalmol 93:689, 1982

140. Quigley, HA, Hohman, RM, Addicks, EM: Morphologic changes in the lamina cribrosa correlated with neural loss in open-angle glaucoma, Am J Ophthalmol 95:673, 1983

141. Quigley, HA, Hohman, RM, and Addicks, EM: Blood vessels of the glaucomatous disc in experimental primate and human eyes, Invest Ophthalmol Vis Sci 25:918, 1984

142. Quigley, HA, Hohman, RM, Sanchez, R, and Addicks, EM: Optic nerve head blood flow in chronic experimental glaucoma, Arch Ophthalmol 103:956, 1986

143. Radius, RL: Thickness of the retinal nerve fiber layer in primate eyes, Arch Ophthalmol 98:1625, 1980

144. Radius, RL: Optic nerve fast axonal transport abnormalities in primates: occurrence after short posterior ciliary artery occlusion, Arch Ophthalmol 98:2018, 1980

145. Radius, RL: Distribution of pressure-induced fast axonal transport abnormalities in primate optic nerve—an autoradiographic study, Arch Ophthalmol 99:1253, 1981

146. Radius, RL: Regional specificity in anatomy at the lamina cribrosa, Arch Ophthalmol 99:478, 1981

147. Radius, RL: Pressure-induced fast axonal transport abnormalities and the anatomy at the lamina cribrosa in primate eyes, Invest Ophthalmol Vis Sci 24:343, 1983

148. Radius, RL: The optic nerve head in experimental glaucomatous optic neuropathy, Presented 2nd Annual Snow-Light Glaucoma Symposium, Niigata, Japan, 1985

149. Radius, RL: Optic nerve head anatomy, Surv Ophthalmol (In press)

150. Radius, RL, and Anderson, DR: Retinal ganglion cell degeneration in experimental optic atrophy, Am J Ophthalmol 86:673, 1978

151. Radius, RL, and Anderson, DR: The course of axons through the retina and optic nerve head, Arch Ophthalmol 97:1154, 1979

152. Radius, RL, and Anderson, DR: The histology of retinal nerve fiber bundles and bundle defects, Arch Ophthalmol 97:948, 1979

153. Radius, RL, and Anderson, DR: The mechanism of disc pallor in experimental optic atrophy; a fluorescein angiographic study, Arch Ophthalmol 97:532, 1979

154. Radius, RL, and Anderson, DR: Fast axonal transport in early experimental disc edema, Invest Ophthalmol Vis Sci 19:158, 1980

155. Radius, RL, and Anderson, DR: Morphology of axonal transport abnormalities in primate eyes, Br J Ophthalmol 65:767, 1981

156. Radius, RL, and Anderson, DR: Rapid axonal transport in primate optic nerve. Distribution of pressure-induced interruption, Arch Ophthalmol 99:650, 1981

157. Radius, RL, and Anderson, DR: Reversibility of optic nerve damage in primate eyes subjected to intraocular pressure above systolic blood pressure, Br J Ophthalmol 65:111, 1981

158. Radius, RL, and Bade, B: Pressure-induced optic nerve axonal transport abnormalities in cat eyes, Arch Ophthalmol 99:2163, 1981

159. Radius, RL, and Bade, B: The anatomy of the lamina cribrosa in normal cat eyes, Arch Ophthalmol 100:1658, 1982

160. Radius, RL, and Bade, B: Axonal transport interruption and anatomy at the lamina cribrosa, Arch Ophthalmol 100:1661, 1982

161. Radius, RL, and DeBruin, J: Anatomy of the retinal nerve fiber layer, Invest Ophthalmol Vis Sci 21:745, 1981

162. Radius, RL, and Finklestein, D: Central retinal artery occlusion (reversible) in sickle trait with glaucoma, Br J Ophthalmol 60:428, 1976

163. Radius, RL, and Gonzales, M: Anatomy at the lamina cribrosa in human eyes, Arch Ophthalmol 99:2159, 1981

164. Radius, RL, and Klewin, KM: Axon morphology at the lamina cribrosa in monkey eyes, Jpn J Ophthalmol 30:203, 1986

165. Radius, RL, and Maumenee, AE: Visual field changes following acute elevation of intraocular pressure, Trans Am Acad Ophthalmol Otolaryngol 83:OP-61, 1977

166. Radius, RL, Maumenee, AE, and Green, WR: Pit-like changes of the optic nerve head in open-angle glaucoma, Br J Ophthalmol 62:389, 1978

167. Radius, RL, and Pederson, JE: Laser-induced primate glaucoma. II. Histology, Arch Ophthalmol 102:1693, 1984

168. Reinecke, RD, Kuwabara, T, Cogan, DG, and Weiss, OR: Retinal vascular patterns, V. Experimental ischemia of the cat eye, Arch Ophthalmol 67:470, 1962

169. Renn, WH, and Rhoton, AL: Microsurgical anatomy of the sellar region, J Neurosurg 43:288, 1975

170. Rhoton, AL, Harris, FS, and Renn, WH: Microsurgical anatomy of the sellar region and cavernous sinus. In Smith, JL, editor: Neuro-ophthalmology, St. Louis, 1977, The CV Mosby Co

171. Robin, AL, et al: An analysis of visual acuity, visual fields and disc cupping in childhood glaucoma, Am J Ophthalmol 88:847, 1979

172. Ronne, H: Der anatomische Projektion der Macula im Corpus geniculatum externa, Z Gesell Neurol Pschiat 22:469, 1914

173. Ronne, H: Uber doppleseitige Hemianopsie mit erhaltener Macula, Klin Monatsbl Augenheilk 53:470, 1914

174. Risco, JM, Grimson, BS, and Johnson, PT: Angioarchitecture of the ciliary artery circulation of the posterior pole, Arch Ophthalmol 99:864, 1981

175. Salzmann, M: The anatomy and histology of the human eyeball in the normal state. Its development and senescence. Chicago, 1912, University of Chicago Press

176. Sanchez, RM, Dunkelberger, GR, and Quigley, HA: The number and diameter distribution of axons in the monkey optic nerve, Invest Ophthalmol Vis Sci 27:1342, 1986

177. Schaeffer, JP: Some points in the regional anatomy in the optic pathway, with special reference to tumors of the hypophysis cerebri; and resulting ocular changes, Anat Rec 28:243, 1924

178. Schwartz, JH: Axonal transport: components, mechanisms and specificity, Annu Rev Neurosci, 2:457, 1979

179. Shakib, M, and Ashton, N: Ultrastructural changes in focal retinal ischemia, Br J Ophthalmol 50:325, 1966

180. Shakib, M, and Cunha-Vaz, JG: Studies of the permeability of the blood-retinal barrier. IV. Junctional complexes of the retinal vessels and their role in the permeability of the blood-retinal barrier, Exp Eye Res 5:229, 1966

181. Silver, J, and Robb, RM: Studies on the development of the eye cup and optic nerve in normal mice and in mutants with congenital optic nerve aplasia, Dev Biol 68:175, 1978

182. Silver, J, and Sidman, RL: A mechanism for the guidance and topographic patterning of retinal ganglion cell axons, J Comp Neurol 189:101, 1980

183. Sossi, N, and Anderson, DR: Blockage of axonal transport in optic nerve induced by elevation of intraocular pressure; effects of arterial hypertension induced by angiotensin I. Arch Ophthalmol 101:94, 1983

184. Sossi, N, and Anderson, DR: Effect of elevated intraocular pressure on blood flow; occurrence in cat optic nerve head studied with iodoantipyrine I 125. Arch Ophthalmol 101:98, 1983

185. Spaeth, GL: Morphologic damage of the optic nerve. In Heilman, K, and Richardson, KT, editors: Glaucoma: concepts of disease; pathogenesis, diagnosis, therapy, Philadelphia, 1978, WB Saunders Co

186. Spaeth, GL: Appearance of the optic disc in glaucoma: a pathologic classification. Transactions of the New Orleans Academy of Ophthalmology: Symposium on glaucoma, St Louis, 1981, The CV Mosby Co

187. Suburo, A, Carri, N, and Adler, R: The environment of axonal migration in the developing chick retina: a scanning electron microscopic (SEM) study, J Comp Neurol 184:519, 1979

188. Stone, J, and Hoffman, KP: Very slow conducting ganglion cells in the cat's retina: a major new functional type? Brain Res 43:610, 1972

189. Straatsma, BR, Foos, RY, and Spencer, LM: The retina—topography and clinical correlation. In Transactions of the New Orleans Academy of Ophthalmology, 1969, The CV Mosby Co

190. Teal, PK, Morin, JD, and McCulloch, C: Assessment of the normal disc, Trans Am Ophthalmol Soc 70:164, 1972

191. Thompson, AH: Physiological and glaucomatous cups, Trans Ophthalmol Soc UK 40:334, 1920

192. Trump, BF, Mergner, WJ, Won Kahng, M, and Saladino, AJ: Studies on the subcellular pathophysiology of ischemia, Circulation 53(suppl, 1):1, 1976

193. Tso, MOM: Axoplasmic transport in papilledema and glaucoma, Trans Am Acad Ophthalmol Otolaryngol 83:OP-771, 1977

194. Tso, MOM: Pathology and pathogenesis of papilledema. In Thompson, HS, Daroff, R, Frisen, L, et al, editors: Topics in neuro-ophthalmology, Baltimore, 1979, Williams & Wilkins

195. Tso, MOM, and Fine, BS: Electron microscopic study of human papilledema, Am J Ophthalmol 82:424, 1976.

196. Tso, MOM, and Hayreh, SS: Optic disc edema in raised intracranial pressure. III. A pathologic study of experimental papilledema, Arch Ophthalmol 95:1448, 1977

197. Tso, MOM, and Hayreh, SS: Optic disc edema in raised intracranial pressure. IV. Axoplasmic transport in experimental papilledema, Arch Ophthalmol 95:1458, 1977

198. Tso, MOM, Shih, CY, McLean, IW: Is there a blood-brain barrier of the optic nerve head? Arch Ophthalmol 93:815, 1975

199. Tucek, S, Hanslikova, V, and Stranikoca, D: Effect of ischemia on axonal transport of acetyltransferase and acetylcholine-esterase and on ultrastructural changes of isolated segments of rabbit nerves in situ. J Neurol Sci 36:237, 1978

200. Unsold, R, deGroot, J, and Newton, TH: Images of the optic nerve. Anatomic-CT correlation, Am J Roentgenol 135:767, 1980

201. Van Buren, JM: The retinal ganglion cell layer, Springfield, IL, 1963, Charles C Thomas Publisher

202. Vrabec, F: The temporal raphe of the human retina, Am J Ophthalmol 62:926, 1966

203. Weinstein, JM, Duckrow, DB, Beard, B, and Brennan, RW: Regional optic nerve blood flow and its autoregulation, Invest Ophthalmol Vis Sci 24:1559, 1982

204. Weinstein, JM, Funsch, D, Page, RB, and Brennan, RW: Optic nerve blood flow and its regulation, Invest Ophthalmol Vis Sci 23:640, 1982

205. Weiss, PA: Neuronal dynamics and neuroplasmic ("axonal") flow, Symp Int Soc Cell Biol 8:3, 1969

206. Weiss, PA: Neuronal dynamics and axonal flow. V. The semisolid state of the moving axonal column, Proc Nat Acad Sci USA 69:620, 1972

207. Weiss, PA, and Hiscoe, HB: Experiments on the mechanism of nerve growth, J Exp Zool 107:315, 1948

208. Whitnall, SE: An anatomy of the human orbit and accessory organs of vision, ed, 2, London, 1932, Oxford University Press

209. Willebrand, HL: Schema des Verlaufs der Sehnervenfasern durch das Chiasm, Z Augenheilk 59:135, 1926

210. Wilson, DL, and Stone, GC: Axoplasmic transport of proteins, Annu Rev Biophys Bioeng 8:27, 1979

211. Wolff, E, and Penman, GG: The position occupied by the peripheral retinal fibers in the nerve fiber layer and at the nerve head, Trans Ophthalmol Soc UK 70:35, 1950

212. Wolter, JR: The cells of Remak and the astroglia of the normal human retina, Arch Ophthalmol 53:832, 1955

213. Wolter, JR: The human optic papilla: a demonstration of new anatomic and pathologic findings, Am J Ophthalmol 44:48, 1957

214. Yamamoto, T: Electron microscopic observation of the human optic nerve, Jpn J Ophthalmol 10:40, 1966

215. Zimmerman, LE, deVenecia, G, and Hamasaki, DI: Pathology of the optic nerve in experimental acute glaucoma, Invest Ophthalmol 6:109, 1967

Chapter 5

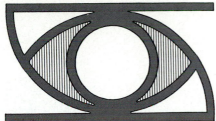

Blood Supply of the Anterior Optic Nerve

Sohan Singh Hayreh

The anterior portion of the optic nerve is affected in glaucoma and allied disorders. There is evidence that vascular disturbance in this part of the optic nerve may be the major cause of the optic disc changes and visual field defects in glaucoma.[45] Hence for a proper understanding of the optic nerve changes in glaucoma, it is essential to understand the complex nature of the blood supply and in vivo blood flow in the anterior optic nerve. Over the last 3 decades the advent of fluorescein fundus angiography and other in vivo techniques has resulted in a tremendous amount of new information on the subject, particularly in vivo blood flow.

BLOOD SUPPLY OF THE ANTERIOR OPTIC NERVE

Fig. 5-1 shows a schematic representation of the blood supply of the anterior optic nerve,[38,41,44] which can be divided into the optic nerve head and the retrolaminar part (see also Plate I, Fig. 2). The optic nerve head from back to front consists of the lamina cribrosa, prelaminar region, and surface nerve fiber layer.[37,39,41,44] The details of the blood supply of the various parts follow.

Lamina Cribrosa Region

The lamina cribrosa region is almost entirely supplied by centripetal branches from the short posterior ciliary arteries, and in a few cases, by the so-called arterial circle of Zinn and Haller. A typical circle of Zinn and Haller is an uncommon finding in humans and, when seen, it is usually an incomplete circle. Unfortunately, because of ignorance of this fact, undeserved importance is commonly given to this circle in the blood supply of the optic nerve head. The central retinal artery gives off no branches in this region,* although claims of a capillary branch from this artery to the lamina cribrosa have been made.[62,78] The blood vessels, 10 to 20 μm in diameter, lie in the fibrous septa and form a dense capillary plexus that makes the lamina cribrosa a highly vascular structure.[61]

Prelaminar Region

Although there is general agreement that centripetal branches arising from the peripapillary choroidal arteries (not the choriocapillaris[4,42]) are the main source of blood supply to the prelaminar region,† conflicting opinions have been voiced occasionally.[6,23,62] The interpretations of these conflicting investigators, however, are open to criticism, as discussed elsewhere. The prelaminar region may also receive some contribution from the vessels in the region of the lamina cribrosa. When a cilioretinal artery is present (in 32% to 40% of human eyes),[56,70] it gives branches to its respective segment of the prelaminar region.[25,70,80] Occasionally (4% to 5%) the cilioretinal artery may be small

---

*References 9, 13, 27, 28, 31, 34, 61, 63, 65, 69, 72, 77.
†References 3-5, 7, 22, 24, 25, 29, 30, 37, 38, 52, 54, 55, 67, 68, 74, 75, 80.

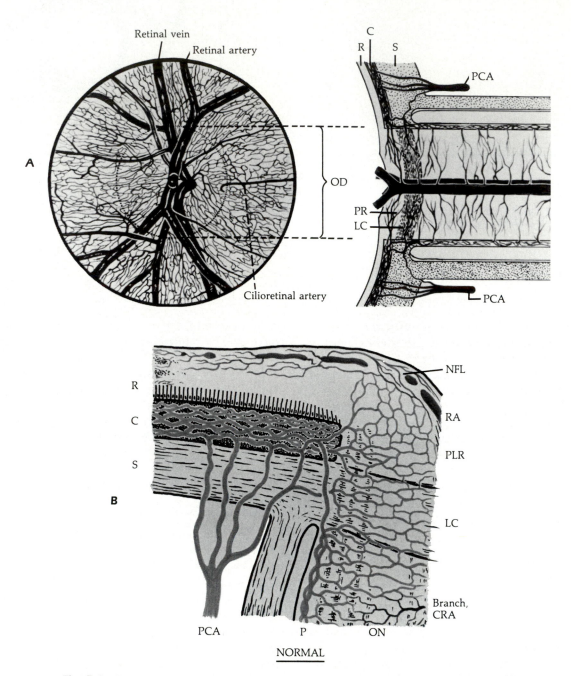

NORMAL

Fig. 5-1 Schematic representations of blood supply of anterior part of optic nerve. **A** also shows, on left side, ophthalmoscopic view of optic disc, adjacent retina. Choroid *(C)*; central retinal artery *(CRA)*; lamina cribrosa *(LC)*; surface nerve fiber layer of disc *(NFL)*; optic disc *(OD)*; optic nerve *(ON)*; pia *(P)*; posterior ciliary artery *(PCA)*; prelaminar region *(PLR/PR)*; retina *(R)*; retinal arteriole *(RA)*; sclera *(S)*. (**A,** From Hayreh, SS: Arch Ophthalmol 95:1565, 1977, and **B,** From Hayreh, SS. In Heilmann, M, and Richardson, KT: Glaucoma: conceptions of a disease, Stuttgart, 1978, Georg Thieme Publishers) See also Plate I, Fig. 2.

and terminate in the prelaminar region instead of going all the way to the retina. Such an artery has been called a "ciliopapillary arteriole"[25,70,80] and may supply one fourth to one third of the prelaminar region in the temporal part of the optic disc.[25] Fluorescein fundus angiographic studies strongly suggest that the temporal part of the prelaminar region is much more vascular than the rest of the region and receives the maximum contribution from the adjacent peripapillary choroid.[37] Fluorescein angiographic studies have clearly demonstrated the segmental nature of the blood supply in this region.*

Surface Layer of Nerve Fibers

The surface layer of nerve fibers on the optic nerve head is mainly supplied by branches from the retinal arterioles. These branches most commonly arise from the main retinal arterioles in the peripapillary region† and less often from capillaries on the surface of the optic disc, which are continuous with the retinal peripapillary capillaries. Branches from the prelaminar region also commonly supply this region (particularly in the temporal sector), as well as the ciliopapillary arterioles in some eyes.

Retrolaminar Region

The retrolaminar region has *peripheral centripetal* and *axial centrifugal* vascular systems.

Peripheral centripetal vascular system

The peripheral centripetal vascular system is seen in all nerves and is formed by pial branches derived from multiple sources. Usually the major contribution is from the multiple recurrent branches from the peripapillary choroid, as well as the arterial circle of Zinn and Haller (when present) or its substitute.‡ Other sources of these pial branches may be the central retinal artery§ and other branches of the ophthalmic artery.[35,36] The branches from the pial vessels enter the optic nerve along the septa in the nerve to supply the optic nerve.

Axial centrifugal vascular system

The axial centrifugal vascular system is formed by branches from the intraneural part of the central

retinal artery.* These may be present in 75% of the nerves—not necessarily in the retrolaminar region in all of them.[34,36,69] Hence in a significant proportion of eyes, the retrolaminar region has no axial vascular system and the entire blood supply is from the peripheral vascular system. Thus the major source of blood supply to the retrolaminar optic nerve is usually the peripapillary choroid.

In conclusion, the posterior ciliary arteries (PCAs), via the peripapillary choroid or the short posterior ciliary arteries, are the main source of blood supply to the anterior part of the optic nerve.

INDIVIDUAL VARIATIONS OF ANTERIOR OPTIC NERVE BLOOD SUPPLY

For a proper understanding of the role of the blood supply of the anterior part of the optic nerve in glaucoma and various ischemic disorders, it is essential to appreciate the marked individual variations in the blood supply. A detailed discussion of the subject is available elsewhere.[51] The various factors that produce this interindividual variation include the following.

Variations of Blood Flow in the Optic Nerve Head

Blood flow in the various intraocular vascular beds, including the optic nerve head, depends on the following four parameters:
1. Intraocular pressure
2. Mean arterial blood pressure (that is, diastolic blood pressure plus one third of the difference between the systolic and diastolic blood pressures)
3. Peripheral vascular resistance
4. Presence or absence of blood flow autoregulation

The blood flow in the optic nerve head can be calculated by dividing perfusion pressure by peripheral vascular resistance, where perfusion pressure equals the mean blood pressure minus intraocular pressure. Thus blood flow in the optic nerve head can be reduced under the following conditions:
1. An increase in intraocular pressure
2. A fall in the mean blood pressure
3. An increase in peripheral vascular resistance, for example, in various cardiovascular disorders (arterial hypertension, arteriosclerosis, atherosclerosis) and hematologic disorders

---

*References 25, 38, 42, 43, 67, 70, 80.
†References 5, 25, 37, 42, 52, 55.
‡References 5, 8, 34, 36, 60, 69.
§References 9, 13, 32, 34, 69, 72, 77, 79.

---

*References 9, 13, 32, 34, 36, 60, 63, 69, 72, 79.

4. An impaired autoregulation

All of these factors can operate individually or in various combinations to reduce the blood flow.

It is important to note that, of the four parameters on which the blood flow depends, we have no means of measuring the mean blood pressure in the capillaries of the optic nerve head, the peripheral vascular resistance, or the autoregulation in those vessels. We can measure only intraocular pressure. Systemic blood pressure is not a true reflection of the blood pressure in the intraocular vessels in every eye. For example, in patients with arterial hypertension, an increase in peripheral vascular resistance raises the systemic blood pressure but lowers the blood pressure in the capillaries. Our lack of information on three of the four parameters influencing the blood flow in the optic nerve head introduces unknown factors that are not constant, but vary from eye to eye and also change from time to time in the same individual. For example, during sleep there can be a marked fall in the mean blood pressure. There may also be a transient rise in the intraocular pressure at one time of the day and not at other times as part of the diurnal variation in the intraocular pressure.

Autoregulation of blood flow in the optic nerve head

The object of autoregulation in a tissue is to keep its blood flow relatively constant during changes in its perfusion pressure. Autoregulation of blood flow has been demonstrated in many organs of the body, including the brain,[73] retina,* and optic nerve head.[21,33,71,76] Although earlier studies denied the presence of autoregulation in the vessels of the optic nerve head,[2] some recent studies have demonstrated its presence.[21,33,71,76] This discrepancy is the result of the technical problems involved in dealing with the small amount of tissue in the optic nerve head. Regardless of which findings are correct, an important factor to consider is that it is not at all clear what controls this autoregulation.[49] Autoregulation is considered a feature of the arterioles and small arteries, but the exact size limit of the participating vessels is not known.[73] Even if autoregulation is present in the optic nerve head, there is evidence that it does not always effectively protect the tissue. For example, the blood vessels in the central nervous system have an efficient autoregulation, but transient ischemic attacks are not unusual. When the perfusion pressure falls below a critical level, autoregulation fails. Similarly, in anterior ischemic optic neuropathy, where there is a segmental acute ischemia of the optic nerve head, evidence indicates that the acute ischemia is primarily the result of a transient collapse of the circulation resulting from a fall of perfusion pressure, usually during sleep.[48] This would suggest that, if autoregulation does exist in the optic nerve head, it does not protect the optic nerve head during such a fall of perfusion pressure in its vessels. Studies suggest that whenever optic nerve head perfusion pressure falls below a critical level, the autoregulation decompensates.[15,33,71] The possibility that the efficiency of autoregulation diminishes with age has been suggested,[71] as well as the possibility that the autoregulation may fluctuate from time to time.

Variations of Anatomic Pattern of the Blood Supply of the Anterior Part of the Optic Nerve

Blood supply to the anterior part of the optic nerve shows a marked individual variation, so that each optic nerve has a unique pattern. The peripapillary choroid, circle of Zinn and Haller (when present), short posterior ciliary arteries, central retinal artery, and pial branches from other orbital arteries contribute to this blood supply. Some of the differences of the vascular anatomy reported in the literature can be explained on this basis, and there is no true "standard" vascular pattern. In my studies of the anatomic distribution of the central retinal artery and blood supply of the optic nerve in 100 human specimens, no 2 specimens, not even the 2 eyes of the same person, had an identical pattern.[34,69]

Variations of Posterior Ciliary Artery Circulation

As concluded above, the posterior ciliary arteries (PCAs), via the peripapillary choroid or the short PCAs, are the main source of blood supply to the anterior part of the optic nerve. In view of this, variations in the pattern of PCA circulation should influence the blood supply pattern markedly. Multiple variations in the pattern of PCA circulation include variations in the number of the PCAs, variations in the area of supply by each PCA, and differences in blood pressure in various PCAs, as well as short PCAs.

Variations in the number of the PCAs

An eye may be supplied by one (3%), two (48%), three (39%), four (8%), or five (2%) PCAs arising from the ophthalmic artery.[35,38] Thus in 90%

---

*References 1, 2, 14, 20, 64, 66.

of cases there are usually 2 to 3 PCAs. I have designated the PCAs "medial," "lateral," and "superior" according to their distribution in the choroid. An eye may have one (70%) or two (30%) medial PCAs, none (3%), one (75%), two (20%), or three (3%) lateral PCAs, and an additional one (2%) or two (7%) superior PCAs. These variations in the number of PCAs and their location influence the blood supply of the anterior part of the optic nerve.

Variations in the area of supply by each PCA

When there are two PCAs (for example, lateral and medial) there is a wide variation in the area supplied by the two arteries, and their supply in the posterior part of the fundus (including the optic nerve head) varies accordingly.[43,46-48,50] Figs. 5-2 and 5-3, respectively, show medial and lateral PCAs supplying medial and lateral halves of the optic nerve head. Figs. 5-4 and 5-5 show the medial PCA supplying the entire optic disc except for a tiny temporal part (containing some of the maculopapillar nerve fibers), which is supplied by the lateral PCA. Fig. 5-6 shows almost the entire disc supplied by the medial PCA with the lateral PCA supply just touching the superotemporal margin of the disc. In Figs. 5-7 to 5-9 the entire optic disc is supplied by the medial PCA without any contribution from the lateral PCA. Thus when there are two PCAs (lateral and medial PCAs), the border between the distribution of the two PCAs may be situated anywhere between the fovea and the nasal peripapillary choroid (Fig. 5-10). When there are three PCAs, the area of the optic nerve head supplied by each may again vary markedly (Fig. 5-11).

Watershed zone.   Experimental and clinical studies have demonstrated that the various PCAs do not anastomose with one another, nor do they anastomose with the anterior ciliary arteries; they act as end-arteries.[43,50] The border between the territories of distribution of any two end-arteries is called the *watershed zone.* The location of the watershed zone between the various PCAs depends on the area of supply by each PCA, in which there is a marked individual variation. Figs. 5-12 to 5-21 illustrate the presence and location of the watershed zone in eyes with two PCAs. The watershed zone may be located anywhere between the fovea and the nasal peripapillary choroid (see Fig. 5-10). Fig. 5-22 illustrates schematically five such locations. Shimizu et al.[68] found the watershed zone between the medial and lateral PCAs to be situated between the optic disc and fovea in 20% of cases studied, and passing through the tem-

Text continued on p. 147.

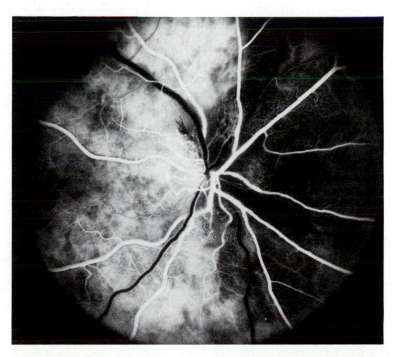

Fig. 5-2   Fluorescein fundus angiogram of right eye of 75-year-old man with anterior ischemic optic neuropathy (negative temporal artery biopsy for arteritis), showing normal filling of area supplied by lateral PCA but no filling of area supplied by medial PCA. (From Hayreh, SS: Doc Ophthalmol 59:217, 1985)

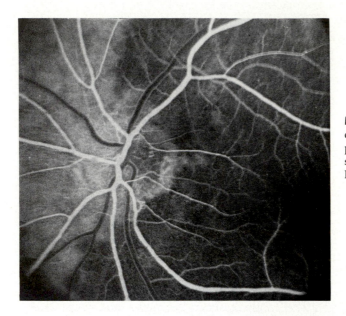

Fig. 5-3 Fluorescein fundus angiogram of left eye of 78-year-old man with anterior ischemic optic neuropathy (negative temporal artery biopsy for arteritis), showing normal filling of area supplied by medial PCA but no filling of area supplied by lateral PCA. (From Hayreh, SS: Br J Ophthalmol 58:955, 1974)

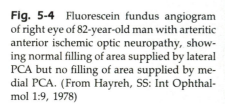

Fig. 5-4 Fluorescein fundus angiogram of right eye of 82-year-old man with arteritic anterior ischemic optic neuropathy, showing normal filling of area supplied by lateral PCA but no filling of area supplied by medial PCA. (From Hayreh, SS: Int Ophthalmol 1:9, 1978)

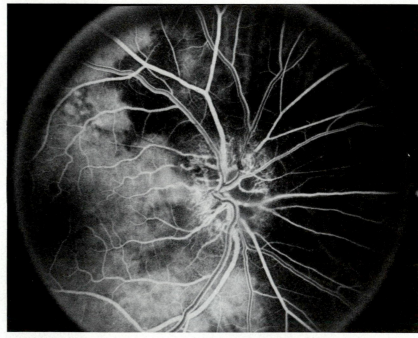

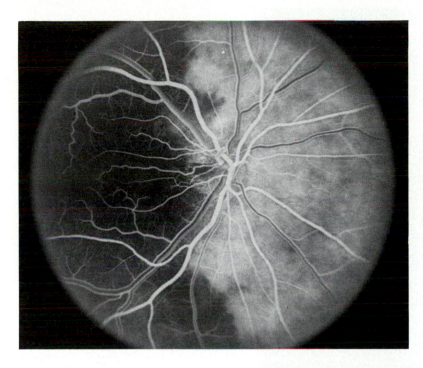

Fig. 5-5 Fluorescein fundus angiogram of right eye of 70-year-old man with anterior ischemic optic neuropathy (negative temporal artery biopsy for arteritis), showing normal filling of area supplied by medial PCA but no filling of area supplied by lateral PCA. (From Hayreh, SS: Doc Ophthalmol 59:217, 1985)

Fig. 5-6 Fluorescein fundus angiogram of right eye of 67-year-old woman with arteritic anterior ischemic optic neuropathy, showing normal filling of area supplied by lateral PCA but no filling of area supplied by medial PCA. (From Hayreh, SS: Doc Ophthalmol 59:217, 1985)

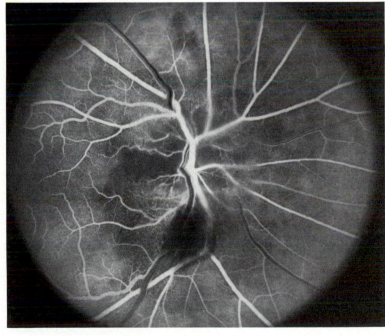

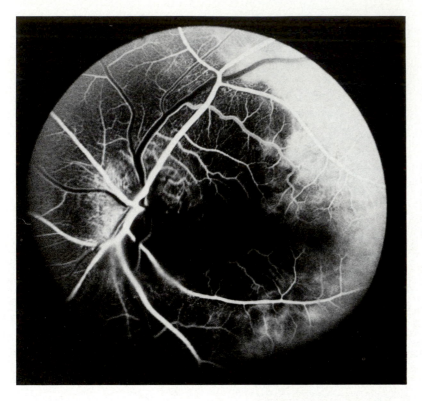

Fig. 5-7 Fluorescein fundus angiogram of left eye of 63-year-old woman with arteritic anterior ischemic optic neuropathy, showing normal filling of area supplied by lateral PCA, but no filling of area supplied by medial PCA. (From Hayreh, SS: Int Ophthalmol 1:9, 1978)

Fig. 5-8 Fluorescein fundus angiogram of left eye of 78-year-old woman with arteritic anterior ischemic optic neuropathy, partial central retinal artery occlusion, showing normal filling of area supplied by lateral PCA but much delayed filling of area supplied by medial PCA and of central retinal artery (because of almost complete occlusion of common trunk of central retinal artery, medial PCA at its origin from ophthalmic artery[34,35]). (From Hayreh, SS: Doc Ophthalmol 59:217, 1985)

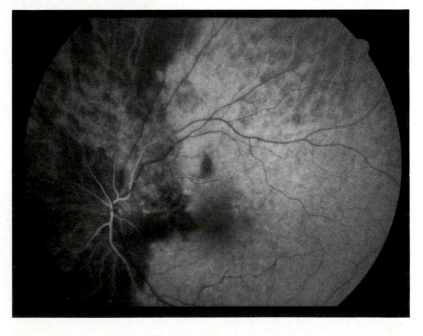

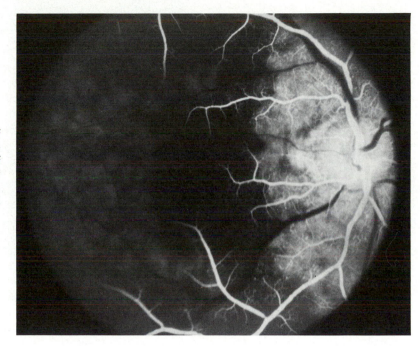

Fig. 5-9 Fluorescein fundus angiogram of right eye of 61-year-old man with internal carotid artery occlusion, showing good filling of area supplied by medial PCA, extremely early patchy filling of area supplied by lateral PCA. (From Hayreh, SS et al: Arch Ophthalmol 100:1585, 1982)

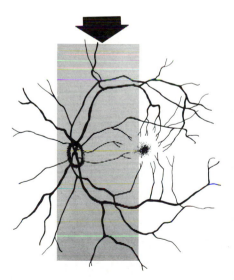

Fig. 5-10 Shaded area *(arrow)* shows broad area of choroid between fovea, nasal peripapillary choroid. Watershed zone between medial, lateral PCAs may be situated *anywhere* within this area. (From Hayreh, SS: Doc Ophthalmol 59:217, 1985)

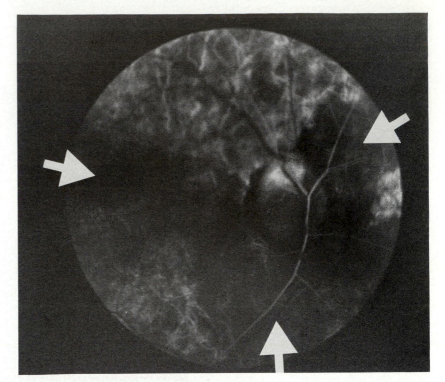

Fig. 5-11 Fluorescein fundus angiogram of normal human right eye, showing Y-shaped watershed zone *(arrows)* between superior, lateral, medial PCAs. (From Hayreh, SS: Br J Ophthalmol 58:955, 1974)

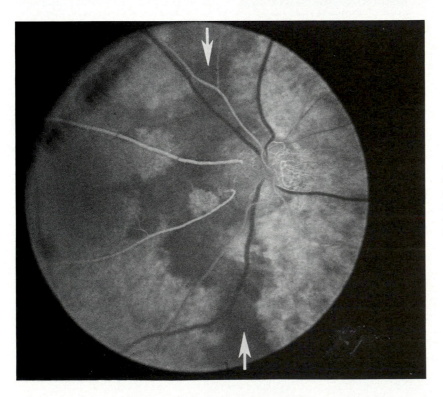

Fig. 5-12 Fluorescein fundus angiogram of right eye of 66-year-old man with old central retinal artery occlusion, showing nonfilling of watershed zone *(arrows)* between lateral, medial PCAs. (From Hayreh, SS: Br J Ophthalmol 59:631, 1975)

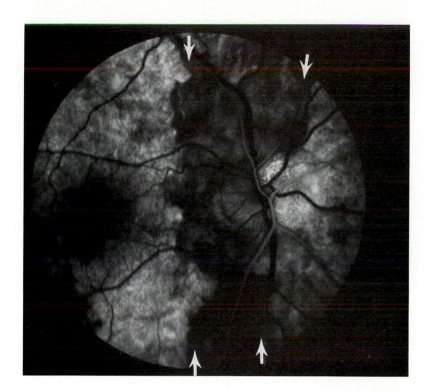

Fig. 5-13 Fluorescein fundus angiogram of right eye of 14-year-old girl with pseudopapilledema, showing delayed filling of watershed zone *(arrows)* between lateral, medial PCAs. (From Hayreh, SS: Doc Ophthalmol 59:217, 1985)

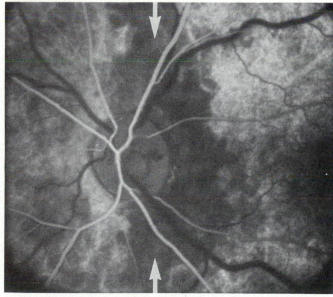

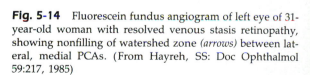

Fig. 5-14 Fluorescein fundus angiogram of left eye of 31-year-old woman with resolved venous stasis retinopathy, showing nonfilling of watershed zone *(arrows)* between lateral, medial PCAs. (From Hayreh, SS: Doc Ophthalmol 59:217, 1985)

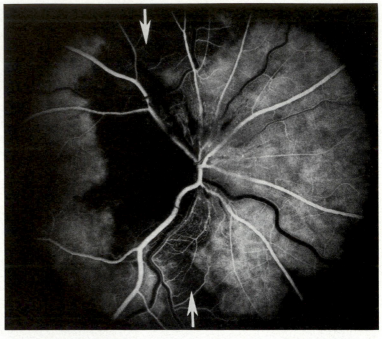

Fig. 5-15 Fluorescein fundus angiogram of right eye of 60-year-old man with nonarteritic anterior ischemic optic neuropathy, showing nonfilling of watershed zone *(arrows)* between lateral, medial PCAs. (From Hayreh, SS: Doc Ophthalmol 59:217, 1985)

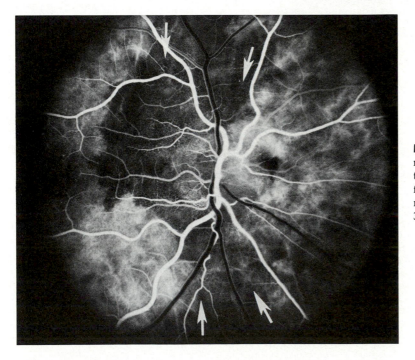

Fig. 5-16 Fluorescein fundus angiogram of right eye of 52-year-old man with nonarteritic anterior ischemic optic neuropathy, showing nonfilling of watershed zone *(arrows)* between lateral, medial PCAs. (From Hayreh, SS: Arch Neurol 38:675, 1981)

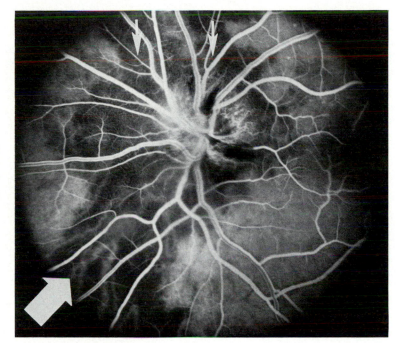

Fig. 5-17 Fluorescein fundus angiogram of left eye of 74-year-old man with arteritic anterior ischemic optic neuropathy, showing nonfilling of watershed zone *(arrows)* between lateral, medial PCAs. (From Hayreh, SS: Doc Ophthalmol 59:217, 1985)

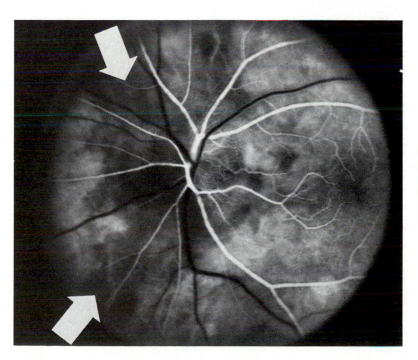

Fig. 5-18 Fluorescein fundus angiogram of left eye of 45-year-old woman with nonarteritic anterior ischemic optic neuropathy, showing nonfilling of watershed zone *(arrows)* between lateral, medial PCAs. (From Hayreh, SS: Doc Ophthalmol 59:217, 1985)

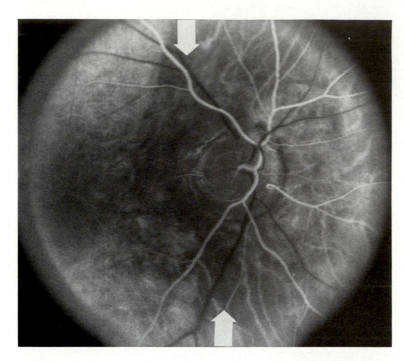

Fig. 5-19 Fluorescein fundus angiogram of right eye of 67-year-old man with low-tension glaucoma, shows filling of area supplied by lateral PCA; poor, early filling of area supplied by medial PCA and almost no filling of watershed zone *(arrows)*, optic disc. (From Hayreh, SS: Doc Ophthalmol 59:217, 1985)

Fig. 5-20 Fluorescein fundus angiogram of right eye of 68-year-old man with low-tension glaucoma, shows poor, patchy filling of watershed zone *(arrows)*, optic disc, peripapillary choroid. (From Hayreh, SS: Doc Ophthalmol 59:217, 1985)

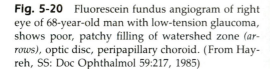

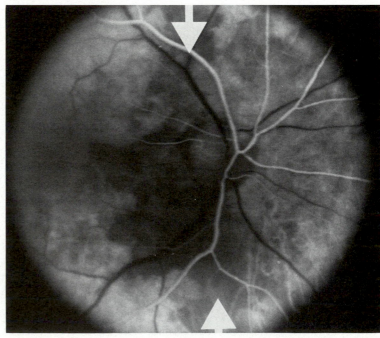

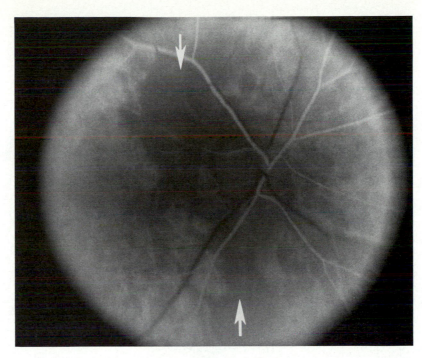

Fig. 5-21 Fluorescein fundus angiogram of right eye of 83-year-old woman with low-tension glaucoma, shows nonfilling of watershed zone *(arrows)*, optic disc. (From Hayreh, SS: Doc Ophthalmol 59:217, 1985)

poral half of the optic disc and temporal peripapillary choroid in 27% of the cases. In the remainder, they could not define a distinct watershed zone.

In normal eyes it is often difficult to outline the watershed zone between the PCAs on routine fluorescein fundus angiography because of the extremely fast filling of the choroidal vascular bed. In view of this technical limitation, we have no information as to the relative incidence in the general population of the various positions of the watershed zone between the various PCAs. In our studies on eyes with anterior ischemic optic neuropathy, because of a fall in perfusion pressure in the distribution of the PCAs, the watershed zone is seen comparatively more commonly than in normal eyes. In our studies on primary open-angle glaucoma, low-tension glaucoma, and ocular hypertension, we found the main locations of the watershed zones as shown in Fig. 5-23, so that in 60% of the cases it passed through the temporal part of the optic disc and adjacent peripapillary choroid, in 16% it passed through the entire disc (see Fig. 5-17), and in 10% it passed through the nasal part of the disc and adjacent nasal peripapillary choroid (see Fig. 5-18). Figs. 5-11, and 5-24 to 5-26 show the location and pattern of the watershed zone when there are three PCAs.

IMPORTANCE OF LOCATION OF THE WATERSHED ZONE. The watershed zone, being an area of comparatively poor vascularity, is most vulnerable to a fall in perfusion pressure and ischemic disorders. There is ample proof of this from various organs having end-arterial supply and watershed zones (for example, the brain and kidney). In the choroid, in the event of a fall of the perfusion pressure in the PCAs, the watershed zone between the PCAs is vulnerable to nonperfusion or hypoperfusion (and ischemia). Thus when the watershed zone between the PCAs passes through one or the other part of the optic disc or the peripapillary choroid, that part of the disc is more vulnerable to ischemia, but when the watershed zone is situated away from the disc or the peripapillary choroid (see Figs. 5-7 to 5-9) the disc is in a comparatively safe zone. Figs. 5-15 to 5-18 and 5-24, from eyes with anterior ischemic optic neuropathy, and Figs. 5-19 to 5-21, 5-25 and 5-26, from eyes with low-tension glaucoma, primary open-angle glaucoma, and ocular hypertension respectively, illustrate the special susceptibility of the watershed zone to develop filling defects.

It is not essential that the entire vertical length of the watershed zone between the medial and lat-

Text continued on p. 152.

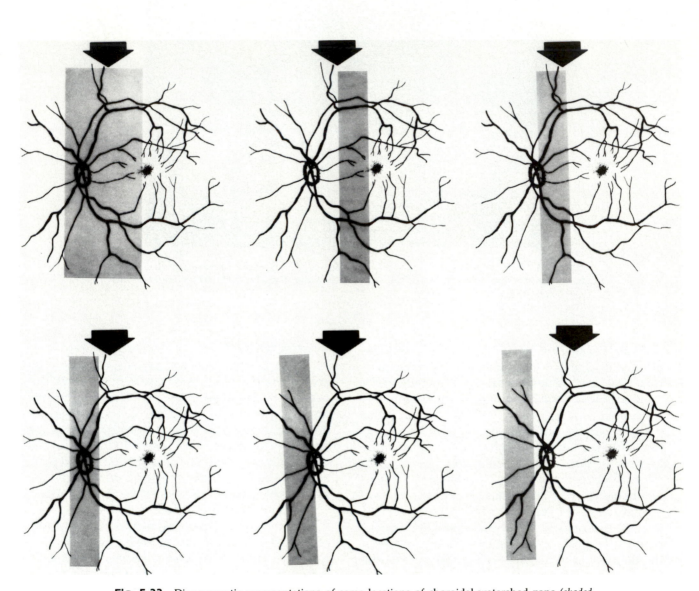

Fig. 5-22 Diagrammatic representations of some locations of choroidal watershed zone *(shaded band)* seen in humans. *(Top left diagram)* Same as shown in Fig. 5-10, showing area within which watershed zone may be located anywhere. Remaining five figures show five variations in location of watershed zone.

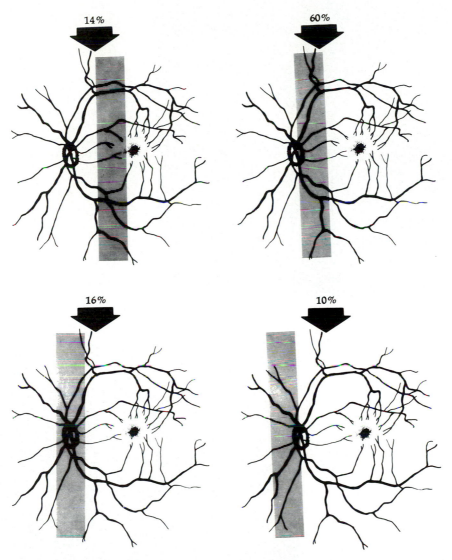

Fig. 5-23   Diagrammatic representations incidence of four locations of choroidal watershed zone seen in our studies on primary open-angle glaucoma, low-tension glaucoma, and ocular hypertension.

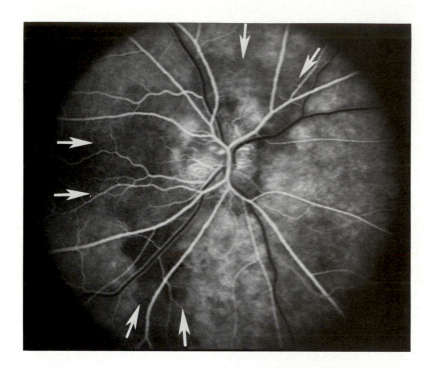

Fig. 5-24 Fluorescein fundus angiogram of right eye of 61-year-old man with nonarteritic anterior ischemic optic neuropathy, showing markedly delayed filling of Y-shaped watershed zone *(arrows)* between superior, medial, lateral PCAs. (From Hayreh, SS: Doc Ophthalmol 59:217, 1985)

Fig. 5-25 Fluorescein fundus angiogram of right eye of 25-year-old woman with primary open-angle glaucoma, total cupping of optic disc, and intraocular pressure of 31 mm Hg in eye, shows nonfilling of watershed zones *(arrows)*, peripapillary choroid. (From Hayreh, SS: Doc Ophthalmol 59:217, 1985)

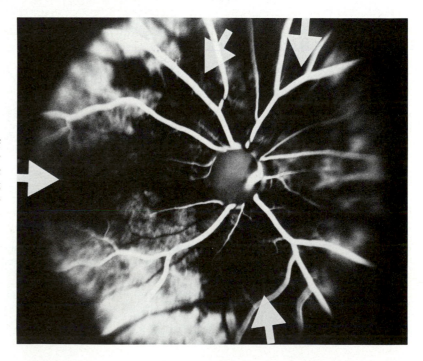

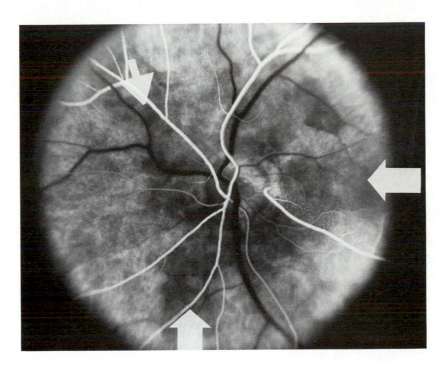

Fig. 5-26 Fluorescein fundus angiogram of left eye of 53-year-old man with ocular hypertension (intraocular pressure 25 mm Hg), shows poor, patchy filling of watershed zone, peripapillary choroid *(arrows)*. (From Hayreh, SS: Doc Ophthalmol 59:217, 1985)

Fig. 5-27 Fluorescein fundus angiogram of right eye of 72-year-old man with arteritic ischemic optic neuropathy, showing nonfilling of upper half of watershed zone *(arrows)*, peripapillary choroid, and upper half of optic disc. (From Hayreh, SS: Br J Ophthalmol 58:964, 1974)

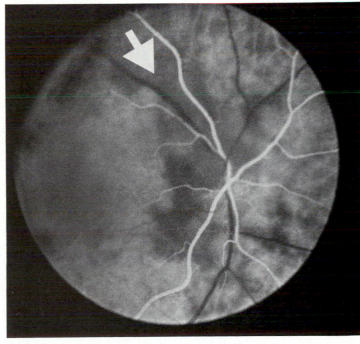

eral PCAs show pathologic filling defects; only the upper or lower half may have them. For example, Figs. 5-27 to 5-29 show a filling defect in the upper half of the watershed zone and adjacent disc, resulting in inferior visual field defects, and Figs. 5-30 and 5-31 show the filling defect in the lower half of the watershed zone and adjacent part of the disc, and superior visual field defect. The precise reason why only the upper or lower half of the watershed zone should show a filling defect remains obscure. Most probable in such eyes there are two medial or lateral PCAs so that only one of the PCAs' distribution has a poor perfusion pressure in its vascular bed (see below).

Thus the tremendous variation in the distribution by the various PCAs and in the location of the watershed zone in the choroid plays an important role in determining the site and extent of involvement of the anterior part of the optic nerve in acute and chronic ischemic disorders of the optic disc.

Peripapillary choroid. The fluorescein angiograms reproduced here also demonstrate that in the vast majority of eyes the peripapillary choroid is the main source of blood supply to the optic disc (in contradistinction to some claims that the peripapillary choroid plays little or no role). The peripapillary choroid not only plays an essential role in the blood supply of the anterior part of the optic nerve but also shows evidence of more susceptibility to obliteration or delayed filling (when the perfusion pressure in the PCA circulation falls appreciably) than the rest of the choroidal vascular bed. This has been documented in a large number of experimental studies of raised intraocular pressure in animals[19,37,53,57,74] (Fig. 5-32), and clinical studies of ocular hypertension, primary open-angle glaucoma, low-tension glaucoma, and anterior ischemic optic neuropathy* (see Figs. 5-19 to 5-21, 5-25 to 5-30, 5-33). The reasons for the special susceptibility of the peripapillary choroid to obliteration or delayed filling are still obscure.[37] The fact that the peripapillary choroid is usually a part of the choroidal watershed zone and as such shares in its properties may be partly responsible for this phenomenon.

Difference in blood pressure in various PCAs

It is always taken for granted that the mean blood pressure in all of the major arteries arising from the ophthalmic artery is the same (that is, in the central retinal artery, lateral PCA, and medial PCA). Our clinical and experimental observations have suggested that the mean blood pressure in these arteries may differ in health, as well as in disease. In the event of a fall of perfusion pressure, the vascular bed supplied by one artery may be affected earlier and more than others.

For example, the choroidal vascular bed filled uniformly at normal intraocular pressure in a normal healthy eye of a monkey (Fig. 5-34, *A*), but, when the intraocular pressure was elevated, the fluorescein angiogram (Fig. 5-34, *B*) showed no filling of the choroid in the territory of the medial PCA, while the choroid supplied by the lateral PCA filled (that is, the medial PCA had a lower mean blood pressure than the lateral PCA), and a few seconds later, (Fig. 5-34, *C*) showed early filling of the area supplied by the upper of the two medial PCAs. In an eye with low-tension glaucoma, the area of the choroid supplied by the inferior lateral PCA showed a delayed filling compared with the rest of the choroid (Fig. 5-31, *A*). In Fig. 5-9, from an eye with ocular ischemia resulting from internal carotid artery occlusion, the choroidal vascular bed supplied by the medial PCA is filled, while there is little filling in the area supplied by the lateral PCA, although after many minutes the latter did show filling.

In an eye with low-tension glaucoma (Fig. 5-35), the area supplied by one of the inferior medial short PCAs did not fill initially, although most of the rest of the choroid filled. This appreciable delayed filling of the choroid in the distribution of one or the other PCA or short PCA reflects a lower mean blood pressure in that artery compared with the fellow arteries. This may explain the greater tendency of one half (superior or inferior half) of the choroidal watershed zone to show nonfilling or delayed filling, as seen in Figs. 5-27 to 5-31.

In conclusion, when all of the variations and the various factors that influence the blood flow are considered, it can be seen that enormous individual variations in the blood supply of the anterior part of the optic nerve make the subject complex. These complexities of the optic nerve in health and disease must be appreciated to understand the role of vascular disturbances in various ischemic disorders of the optic nerve head, including glaucomatous damage. It is wrong to assume that the pattern of blood supply of the optic nerve is almost identical in all eyes, and that all ischemic lesions are explainable on one standard vascular pattern.

---

*References 10-12, 16-18, 26, 39, 40, 42, 58, 59.

Text continued on p. 158.

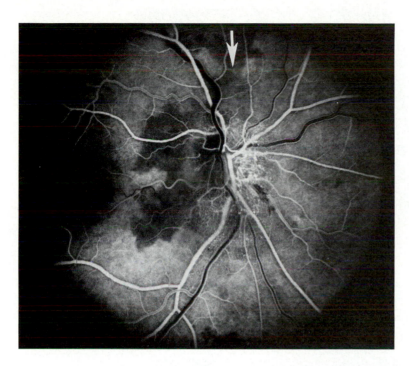

Fig. 5-28 Fluorescein fundus angiogram of right eye of 46-year-old man with nonarteritic anterior ischemic optic neuropathy, showing nonfilling of upper half of watershed zone *(arrow)*, peripapillary choroid, and temporal part of optic disc. (From Hayreh, SS: Doc Ophthalmol 59:217, 1985)

Fig. 5-29 Fluorescein fundus angiogram of right eye of 47-year-old diabetic man with nonarteritic anterior ischemic optic neuropathy, showing nonfilling of upper half of watershed zone *(arrow)*, peripapillary choroid, and temporal part of disc. (From Hayreh, SS: Doc Ophthalmol 59:217, 1985)

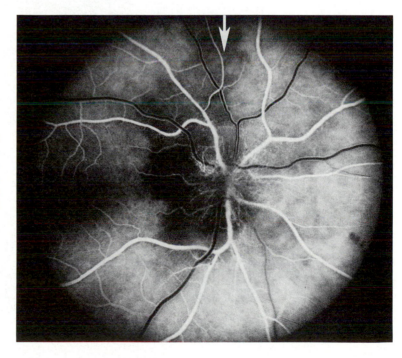

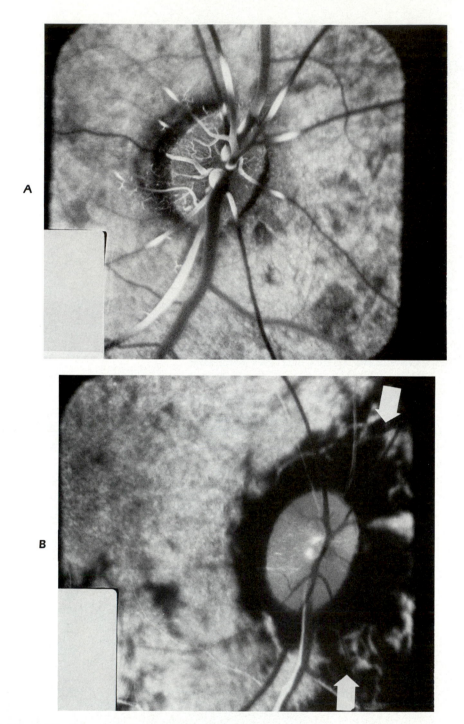

Fig. 5-30 Fluorescein fundus angiograms of right eye of healthy, normal cynomolgus monkey (after experimental central retinal artery occlusion). **A** shows normal filling of entire choroid at normal intraocular pressure, but **B,** at 70 mm Hg intraocular pressure, shows no filling of peripapillary choroid and sparse patchy filling of watershed zone *(arrows)*.

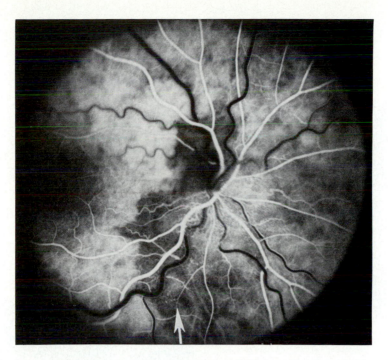

Fig. 5-31   Fluorescein fundus angiogram of right eye of 63-year-old man with internal carotid artery occlusion and nonarteritic anterior ischemic optic neuropathy, shows nonfilling of lower half of watershed zone *(arrow)*, superior peripapillary choroid, and superior temporal part of optic disc. (From Hayreh, SS: Doc Ophthalmol 59:217, 1985)

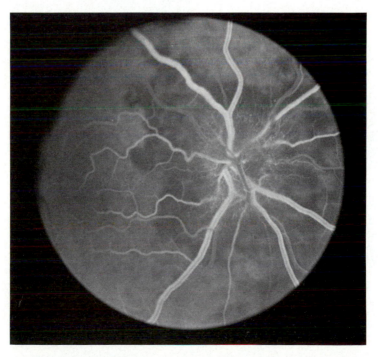

Fig. 5-32   Fluorescein fundus angiogram of right eye of 72-year-old woman with arteritic anterior ischemic optic neuropathy and no perception of light in that eye. Retinal venous phase of angiography shows no filling of optic disc and peripapillary choroid, with filling of rest of the choroid except inferior watershed zone. (From Hayreh, SS: Br J Ophthalmol 58:964, 1974)

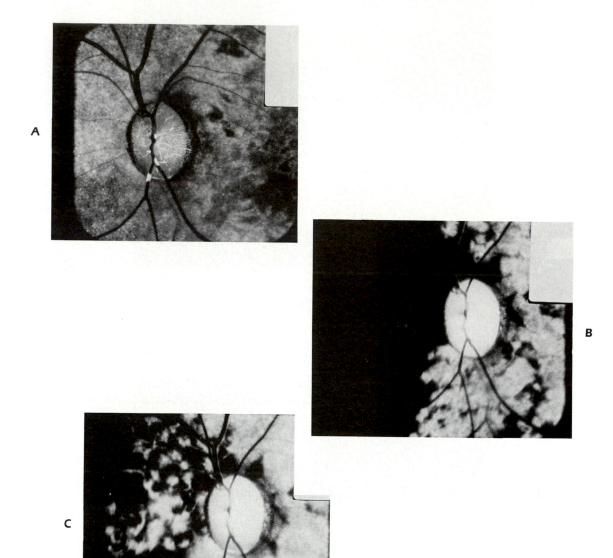

Fig. 5-33   Fluorescein fundus angiograms of left eye of normal, healthy cynomolgus monkey (after experimental central retinal artery occlusion), at **A,** normal, **B** and **C,** 70 mm Hg intraocular pressure, show normal choroidal filling in **A,** filling of area supplied only by lateral PCA in **B,** and of additional early filling of area supplied by upper of two medial PCAs a few seconds later in **C.**

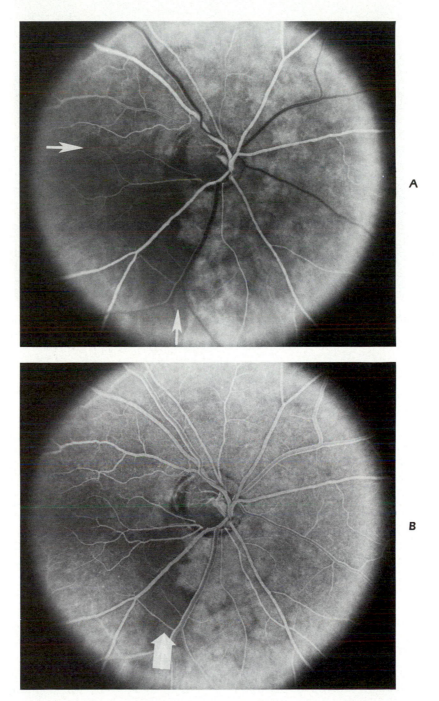

Fig. 5-34   Fluorescein fundus angiograms of right eye of 69-year-old woman with low-tension glaucoma. **A** shows filling defect (indicated by arrows) in inferior temporal quadrant of choroid, lower half of optic disc. **B** (5 seconds after **A**) shows nonfilling of lower half of watershed zone (*arrow*), peripapillary choroid, and lower half of optic disc. (From Hayreh, SS: Doc Ophthalmol 9:217, 1985)

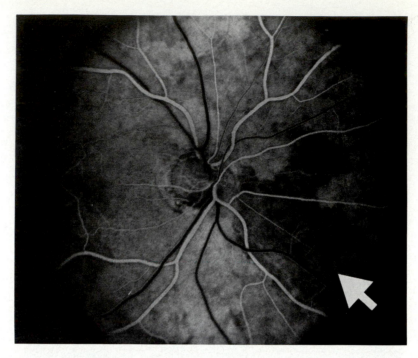

Fig. 5-35 Fluorescein fundus angiogram of right eye of 72-year-old woman with low-tension glaucoma, shows no filling in distribution of inferior medial short PCA *(arrow)*, lower part of optic disc. (From Hayreh, SS: Doc Ophthalmol 59:217, 1985)

Misconceptions about the Blood Supply of the Optic Nerve Head

Following are some of the misconceptions regarding the blood supply of the optic nerve head.

1. All eyes have a basically similar vascular pattern and blood flow. Individual variations in the blood supply of the anterior part of the optic nerve have been discussed in detail previously and elsewhere.[51] The blood supply and blood flow in different eyes are not identical, and there is no standard vascular pattern; there are enormous individual variations.

2. The peripapillary choroid does not supply the anterior part of the optic nerve. As discussed previously, the peripapillary choroid is the main source of blood supply to the optic nerve head and the retrolaminar region of the optic nerve. Occasional reports have alleged that the peripapillary choroid has no significant role.[62] These reports have argued that if the peripapillary choroid supplies the optic nerve head, then why, in eyes where ophthalmoscopy shows a white peripapillary ring, is there no optic atrophy? This question is based on the erroneous impression that a white peripapillary ring is indicative of complete atrophy of the choroidal vascular bed in that area and thus loss

of blood supply from the peripapillary choroid to the optic nerve head. Fluorescein fundus angiographic studies in eyes with a white peripapillary ring, however, show in that region normal, large peripapillary choroidal arteries, and fine branches arising from them and going to the prelaminar region.[37] The white peripapillary ring is an ophthalmoscopic artifact caused by reflection of incident light from the Bruch's membrane and complete masking of the underlying vascular bed; it does not represent sclera. Bruch's membrane is transparent to the transmitted fluorescent light from the underlying peripapillary choroidal vessels. In vivo fluorescein fundus angiographic studies on the choroidal vascular bed have demonstrated the segmental nature of the peripapillary choroid in experimental occlusion of the PCAs and their subdivision[43,50] by the segmental filling defects in the peripapillary choroid and by the occurrence of segmental anterior ischemic optic neuropathy in more than 90% to 95% of cases.

3. Capillary anastomoses in the anterior part of the optic nerve prevent ischemia of the optic nerve head. In the entire length of the optic nerve, the presence of a continuous capillary network—arranged in longitudinal and transverse chan-

nels—has been documented since 1903 in histologic studies by many authors.[31,60,77] This capillary network in the prelaminar region becomes continuous anteriorly with the adjacent retinal capillary network. Lieberman et al. in a histologic study,[62] emphasized the presence of so-called longitudinal vascular systems in the anterior part of the optic nerve (that is, the longitudinally arranged capillaries[31,60,70]). They stressed that these produce free anastomoses in this part of the optic nerve and that the blood supply in the optic nerve head is therefore not sectoral. They further suggested that the "longitudinal vascular system" is of great importance, implying that in the event of occlusion of one or more feeders to the system, the blood supply to the involved sector of the optic nerve head can be maintained by these anastomotic channels. They argued that this freely communicating capillary network (because of the presence of the longitudinal vascular system) protects the optic nerve head from developing ischemia. This view, however, is not supported by the available evidence about the in vivo circulation in health and disease.

In the event of an acute or subacute occlusion of an arteriole, the capillary anastomoses cannot protect the involved region from ischemic damage because they are incapable of rapidly establishing collateral circulation. In the retina, for example, fluorescein angiography and retinal digest preparations have shown that the retinal capillary network is one continuous vascular bed; yet occlusion of a precapillary arteriole is always associated with focal ischemia and development of a cotton-wool spot. Similarly, the presence of segmental anterior ischemic optic neuropathy is a well-established and common entity; in over 500 eyes with anterior ischemic optic neuropathy we have demonstrated on fluorescein angiography segmental filling defects in the optic disc and adjacent peripapillary choroid. Thus in conclusion, from the functional point of view, these anastomoses of capillaries within the anterior part of the optic nerve do not establish collateral circulation in the event of occlusion of their afferent arterioles. Although the nutritional exchange takes place at the level of the capillaries, it is really the afferent arterioles that are of great significance in any consideration of ischemic disorders of the optic nerve head, and intercapillary anastomoses in the optic nerve have no role at all to play in establishing collateral circulation to protect the optic nerve tissue from ischemic damage.

4. Morphologic studies on the optic nerve are useful in evaluation of the blood flow. Many authors have used these studies as the basis for theories about various disorders of the blood flow in the optic nerve head. In vivo fluorescein angiography has demonstrated that one cannot extrapolate in vivo blood flow and circulation from anatomic studies, particularly histologic and ultrastructural ones. Whereas such studies give useful information about the morphologic changes in the tissues of the optic nerve head, they are not much help in giving information about the disturbances in the blood flow in vivo in the optic nerve head. For example, it has been claimed that because many capillaries are seen on histopathologic examination of the optic nerve head in glaucomatous eyes with early and moderate glaucomatous loss of nerve fibers, no vascular disorder can be considered responsible for the optic nerve head changes in glaucoma. However, one must bear in mind two well-established facts: (1) capillaries are far more resistant to ischemic damage than the neural tissue, and (2) the presence of capillaries, as seen on histologic section, in no way proves that there is normal blood flow or that there is no ischemia. Fluorescein angiography has revolutionized our knowledge on the in vivo blood supply of the optic nerve head in health and disease and is useful for such evaluation, but it does have limitations, including inadequate resolution of the optic disc microvasculature, difficulty in outlining the prelaminar capillaries, inadequate knowledge of the optic disc fluorescence, significance of presence or absence of a filling defect on angiography, and unknown reliability of a single angiographic examination.

REFERENCES

1. Alm, A, and Bill, A: The oxygen supply to the retina. II. Effects of high intraocular pressure and of increased arterial carbon dioxide tension on uveal and retinal blood flow in cats; a study with radioactively labelled microspheres including flow determinations in brain and some other tissues, Acta Physiol Scand 84:306, 1972

2. Alm, A, and Bill, A: Ocular and optic nerve blood flow at normal and increased intraocular pressures in monkeys (Macaca irus); a study with radioactively labelled microspheres including flow determinations in brain and some other tissues, Exp Eye Res 15:15, 1973

3. Anderson, DR: Vascular supply to the optic nerve of primates, Am J Ophthalmol 70:341, 1970

4. Anderson, DR, and Braverman, S: Reevaluation of the optic disk vasculature, Am J Ophthalmol 82:165, 1976

5. Araki, M: Anatomical study of the vascularization of the optic nerve, Acta Soc Ophthalmol Jpn 79:101, 1975

6. Araki, M: The role of blood circulation of prelaminar capillaries in producing glaucomatous cupping, Acta Soc Ophthalmol Jpn 80:201, 1976

7. Araki, M, and Honmura, S: The collateral communications of the retinal circulation with the choroidal circulation at the optic nerve head, Acta Soc Ophthalmol Jpn 77:1557, 1973

8. Armaly, MF, and Araki, M: Optic nerve circulation and ocular pressure: contribution of central retinal artery and short posterior ciliary arteries and the effect on oxygen tension, Invest Ophthalmol 14:475, 1975

9. Beauvieux, J, and Ristitch, K: Les vaisseaux centraux du nerf optique, Arch Ophthalmol 41:352, 1924

10. Begg, IS, Drance, SM, and Goldmann, H: Fluorescein angiography in the evaluation of focal circulatory ischaemia of the optic nervehead in relation to the arcuate scotoma in glaucoma, Can J Ophthalmol 7:68, 1972

11. Best, M, Blumenthal, M, Galin, MA, and Toyofuku, H: Fluorescein angiography during induced ocular hypertension in glaucoma, Br J Ophthalmol 56:6, 1972

12. Best, M, and Toyofuku, H: Ocular hemodynamics during induced ocular hypertension in man, Am J Ophthalmol 74:932, 1972

13. Bignell, JL: Investigations into the blood supply of the optic nerve with special reference to the lamina cribrosa region, Trans Ophthalmol Soc Australia 12:105, 1952

14. Bill, A: Effects of acetazolamide and carotid occlusion on the ocular blood flow in unanesthetized rabbits, Invest Ophthalmol 13:954, 1974

15. Bill, A: Some aspects of the ocular circulation, Invest Ophthalmol Vis Sci 26:410, 1985

16. Blumenthal, M, Best, M, Galin, MA, and Toyofuku, H: Peripapillary choroidal circulation in glaucoma, Arch Ophthalmol 86:31, 1971

17. Blumenthal, M, Gitter, KA, Best, M, and Galin, MA: Fluorescein angiography during induced ocular hypertension in man, Am J Ophthalmol 69:39, 1970

18. Boyd, TAS, and Rosen, ES: A new method of clinical assessment of an intraocular pressure sensitive ischaemic mechanism in glaucoma, Can J Ophthalmol 5:12, 1970

19. De Freitas, F, and Morin, JD: The changes in the blood supply of the posterior pole of rabbits with ocular hypertension, Can J Ophthalmol 6:139, 1971

20. Dollery, CT, Hill, DW, and Hodge, JV: The response of normal retinal blood vessels to angiotensin and noradrenaline, J Physiol 165:500, 1963

21. Ernest, JT: Autoregulation of optic-disk oxygen tension, Invest Ophthalmol Vis Sci 13:101, 1974

22. Ernest, JT: Pathogenesis of glaucomatous optic nerve disease, Trans Am Ophthalmol Soc 73:366, 1975

23. Ernest, JT, and Archer, D: Fluorescein angiography of the optic disc, Am J Ophthalmol 75:973, 1973

24. Ernest, JT, and Potts, AM: Pathophysiology of the distal portion of the optic nerve. II. Vascular relationships, Am J Ophthalmol 66:380, 1968

25. Evans, P, et al: Fluorescein cineangiography of the optic nerve head, Trans Am Acad Ophthalmol Otolaryngol 77:OP260, 1973

26. Francois, J, and de Laey, JJ: Fluorescein angiography of the glaucomatous disc, Ophthalmologica 168:288, 1974

27. Francois, J, and Neetens, A: Vascularization of the optic pathway. I. Lamina cribrosa and optic nerve, Br J Ophthalmol 38:472, 1954

28. Francois, J, and Neetens, A: Vascularization of the optic pathway. III. Study of intra-orbital and intra-cranial optic nerve by serial sections. Br J Ophthalmol 40:45, 1956

29. Francois, J, and Neetens, A: The fine angio-architecture of the anterior optic nerve. In Cant, JS, editor: The optic nerve, Proc Second Mackenzie Symposium London, 1972, Kimpton

30. Francois, J, and Neetens, A: Comparative anatomy of the vascular supply of the eye in vertebrates. In Davson, H, and Graham, P, editors: The eye, vol., 5, London, 1975, Churchill Livingstone

31. Francois, J, Neetens, A, and Collette, JM: Vascular supply of the optic pathway. II, Further studies by microarteriography of the optic nerve. Br J Ophthalmol 39:220, 1955

32. Fryzkowski, A: Branches of the extravaginal, intravaginal and intraneural parts of the central retinal artery of man, Pol Med J 11:1305, 1972

33. Geijer, C, and Bill, A: Effects of raised intraocular pressure on retinal, prelaminar, laminar, and retrolaminar optic nerve blood flow in monkeys, Invest Ophthalmol 18:1030, 1979

34. Hayreh, SS: A study of the central artery of the retina in human beings, master's thesis, India, 1958, Punjab University

35. Hayreh, SS: The ophthalmic artery. III. Branches, Br J Ophthalmol 46:212, 1962

36. Hayreh, SS: The central artery of the retina—its role in the blood supply of the optic nerve, Br J Ophthalmol 47:651, 1963

37. Hayreh, SS: Blood supply of the optic nerve head and its role in optic atrophy, glaucoma and oedema of the optic disc, Br J Ophthalmol 53:721, 1969

38. Hayreh, SS: Pathogenesis of visual field defects—role of the ciliary circulation, Br J Ophthalmol 54:289, 1970

39. Hayreh, SS: Optic disc changes in glaucoma, Br J Ophthalmol 56:175, 1972

40. Hayreh, SS: Anterior ischaemic optic neuropathy. II. Fundus on ophthalmoscopy and fluorescein angiography, Br J Ophthalmol 58:964, 1974

41. Hayreh, SS: Anatomy and physiology of the optic nerve head, Trans Am Acad Ophthalmol Otolaryngol 78:OP-240, 1974

42. Hayreh, SS: Anterior ischemic optic neuropathy, New York, 1975, Springer

43. Hayreh, SS: Segmental nature of the choroidal vasculature, Br J Ophthalmol 59:631, 1975

44. Hayreh, SS: Structure and blood supply of the optic nerve. In Heilmann, K, and Richardson, KT, editors: Gluacoma—conceptions of a disease: pathogenesis, diagnosis, therapy, Stuttgart, 1978, Georg Thieme Publishers

45. Hayreh, SS: Pathogenesis of optic nerve damage and visual field defects. In Glaucoma—conceptions of a disease: pathogenesis, diagnosis, therapy, Stuttgart, 1978, Georg Thieme Publishers

46. Hayreh, SS: Ischemic optic neuropathy, Int Ophthalmol 1:9, 1978

47. Hayreh, SS: Acute choroidal ischaemia, Trans Ophthalmol Soc UK 100:400, 1980

48. Hayreh, SS: Anterior ischemic optic neuropathy, Arch Neurol 38:675, 1981

49. Hayreh, SS: Effects of elevated IOP on blood flow, Arch Ophthalmol 101:1948, 1983

50. Hayreh, SS: Physiological anatomy of the choroidal vascular bed, Int Ophthalmol 6:85, 1983

51. Hayreh, SS: Inter-individual variation in blood supply of the optic nerve head. Its importance in various ischemic disorders of the nerve head, and glaucoma, low-tension glaucoma and allied disorders, Doc Ophthalmol 59:217, 1985

52. Hayreh, SS, and Perkins, ES: Clinical and experimental studies on the circulation at the optic nerve head. In Cant, JS, editor: Proc Wm Mackenzie Centenary Symposium on the Ocular Circulation in Health and Disease, London, 1968, Kimpton

53. Hayreh, SS, Revie, IHS, and Edwards, J: Vasogenic origin of visual field defects and optic nerve changes in glaucoma, Br J Ophthalmol 54:461, 1970

54. Henkind, P, and Levitzky, M: Angioarchitecture of the optic nerve. I. The papilla, Am J Ophthalmol 68:979, 1969

55. Itoh, K: Fluorescein angiographic finding of normal optic disc, Acta Soc Ophthalmol Jpn 77:1543, 1973

56. Justice, J, and Lehmann, RP: Cilioretinal arteries: a study based on review of stereo fundus photographs and fluorescein angiographic findings, Arch Ophthalmol 94:1355, 1976

57. Kalvin, NH, Hamasaki, DI, and Gass, JDM: Experimental glaucoma in monkeys. I. Relationship between intraocular pressure and cupping of the optic disc and cavernous atrophy of the optic nerve, Arch Ophthalmol 76:82, 1966

58. Laatikainen, L: Fluorescein angiographic studies of the peripapillary and perilimbal regions in simple, capsular and low-tension glaucoma, Acta Ophthalmol Suppl 111, 1971

59. Laatikainen, L, and Mäntylä, P: Effects of a fall in the intraocular pressure level on the peripapillary fluorescein angiogram in chronic open-angle glaucoma, Acta Ophthalmol 52:625, 1974

60. Leber, T: Graefe-Saemisch Handbuch der gesamten Augenheilkunde, ed., 2, vol., 2, Leipzig, 1903, Engelmann

61. Levitzky, M, and Henkind, P: Angioarchitecture of the optic nerve. II. Lamina cribrosa, Am J Ophthalmol 68:986, 1969

62. Lieberman, MF, Maumenee, AE, and Green, WR: Histologic studies of the vasculature of the anterior optic nerve, Am J Ophthalmol 82:405, 1975

63. Magitot, A: Thèse de Paris, Paris, 1908, Vigot Frères

64. Porsaa, K: Experimental studies on the vasomotor innervation of the retinal arteries, Acta Ophthalmol Suppl 18, 1941

65. Redslob, E: La lame cribrée: sa morphologie, son développement, Ann Oculist (Paris) 189:749, 1956

66. Russell, RWR: Evidence for autoregulation in human retinal circulation, Lancet 2:1048, 1973

67. Schwartz, B, Rieser, JC, and Fishbein, SI: Fluorescein angiographic defects of the disc in glaucoma, Arch Ophthalmol 95:1961, 1977

68. Shimizu, K, Yokochi, K, and Okano, T: Fluorescein angiography of the choroid, Jpn J Ophthalmol 18:97, 1974

69. Singh, S, and Dass, R: The central artery of the retina. II. A study of its distribution and anastomoses, Br J Ophthalmol 44:280, 1960

70. Sodeno, Y: Cilioretinal artery and the microcirculation of the optic disc, Acta Soc Ophthalmol Jpn 78:561, 1974

71. Sossi, N, and Anderson, DR: Effect of elevated intraocular pressure on blood flow; occurrence in cat optic nerve head studied with iodoantipyrine I 125, Arch Ophthalmol 101:98, 1983

72. Steele, EJ, and Blunt, MJ: The blood supply of the optic nerve and chiasma in man, J Anat 90:486, 1956

73. Strandgaard, S: Autoregulation of cerebral circulation in hypertension, Acta Neurol Scand 57(suppl 66):1, 1978

74. Swietliczko, I, and David, NJ: Fluorescein angiography in experimental ocular hypertension, Am J Ophthalmol 70:351, 1970

75. Theodossiadis, GP: Über die Vaskularisation in der Regio praelaminaris der Papilla Optica, Klin Monatsbl Augenheilkd 158:646, 1971

76. Weinstein, JM, Duckrow, RB, Beard, D, and Brennan, RW: Regional optic nerve blood flow and its autoregulation, Invest Ophthalmol Vis Sci 24:1559, 1983

77. Wolff, E: Some aspects of the blood supply of the optic nerve, Trans Ophthalmol Soc UK 59:157, 1939

78. Wolff, E: The blood supply to the lamina cribrosa, Trans Ophthalmol Soc UK 60:69, 1940

79. Wybar, KC: Anastomoses between the retinal and ciliary arterial circulation, Br J Ophthalmol 40:65, 1956

80. Yokochi, K, Maruyama, H, and Sodeno, Y: Microcirculation of the disc and peripapillary choroid, Acta Soc Ophthalmol Jpn 77:1534, 1973

6

The Extracellular Matrix of the Trabecular Matrix and the Optic Nerve Head

7

Functional Testing in Glaucoma: Visual Psychophysics and Electrophysiology

8

Aqueous Humor Formation: Fluid Production by a Sodium Pump

9

Pressure-Dependent Outflow

10

Uveoscleral Outflow

11

Episcleral Venous Pressure

12

The Nervous System and Intraocular Pressure

13

Ocular Hypotony

Chapter 6

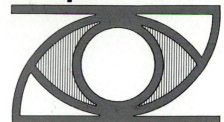

The Extracellular Matrix of the Trabecular Meshwork and the Optic Nerve Head

M. Rosario Hernandez
Arthur H. Neufeld

CHARACTERISTICS OF EXTRACELLULAR MATRIX

The extracellular matrix is the structural support that allows groups of cells to function as a tissue. The extracellular matrix is made up of specific macromolecules assembled in geometric relationships to provide strength, flexibility, elasticity, and surfaces to the tissues that they serve. Study of the extracellular matrix has become a major objective in many laboratories because changes in this structure are clearly related to changes in development, aging, disease, and various aspects of cellular behavior.

There is apparently a continuum between the molecules of the extracellular matrix, the cell membrane, and the interior of the cell. Thus, many cellular functions are dependent on and regulated by the extracellular matrix, which provides a scaffold for cell migration, attachment sites for cell adhesion, and instructions for cell differentiation, which are often expressed in the cell shape. Most important, the architecture of tissues and organs is dependent on extracellular matrix biosynthesis and degradation. Thus, the growth, shape, and maintenance of tissues and organs are completely dependent on remodeling of the extracellular matrix. Therefore, pathologic changes in a tissue or organ are also related to changes in regulation of the biosynthesis or degradation of extracellular matrix molecules.

The major components of the extracellular matrix are collagens, elastin, proteoglycans, and attachment factors. These are all large structural macromolecules that exist outside the cell with no apparent enzymatic activity. Producing these macromolecules throughout life, cells are in constant contact and interaction with their own extracellular matrix, as well as that produced by other neighboring cells. In some tissues, the turnover of extracellular matrix (i.e., synthesis and degradation) is slow, for example, bone, cartilage, tendons, and perhaps sclera. In other tissues, a more rapid turnover occurs, for example, in loose connective tissues. Nevertheless, the turnover of extracellular matrix components is regulated and is dependent on hormones, growth factors, or other trophic and environmental influences.

There are two major types of extracellular matrices: basement membranes and interstitial matrix. The basement membrane is a unique but universal type of extracellular matrix that separates the cell responsible for its synthesis from the underlying interstitial matrix, often a stroma. The basement membrane is deposited on one side of endothelial and epithelial cells, usually the basal surface, and around all sides of fat, muscle, and Schwann cells. The basement membrane, or basal lamina, is approximately 100 nm in thickness and is a continuous sheet of extracellular matrix composed of collagen, noncollagenous proteins and proteoglycans.

Functionally, the basement membrane provides attachment sites for a sheet of cells, a filtration barrier for the movement of molecules, and, because of its flexibility and elasticity, the interface between two different tissue types with different physical qualities.[10]

The interstitial matrix is characteristic of connective tissues and is synthesized by cells of the fibroblast family, such as osteoblasts, chondroblasts, and fibroblasts. Interstitial matrix surrounds cells of a similar type, separating them from each other, and has primary responsibility for the maintenance of the shape of an organ. The interstitial matrix consists of a complex skeleton of collagens, elastic fibers, proteoglycans, and glycoproteins, which provides strength and mechanical support to an organ or tissue, as well as providing the scaffold that supports the blood vessels and nerves that supply and regulate the functional cells of the tissue.[17]

MACROMOLECULES OF THE EXTRACELLULAR MATRIX

Collagen (see Plate I, Fig. 4)

Collagens are the most abundant fibrillar proteins in the body and the major components of the extracellular matrix. Collagens have a structural role in giving support and tensile strength to tissues. This heterogeneous class of macromolecules is made up of several genetically distinct types. Collagens from mammalian tissues have been characterized biochemically and have some common chemical and functional characteristics.[34,35] They are often classified according to their supramolecular organization as fibrous, nonfibrous, and filamentous.

Fibrous collagens are characteristic of the interstitial matrices. These macromolecules form striated fibrils with a characteristic axial repeat pattern of 67 nm. Fibrils may aggregate to form larger collagen fibers. This group of collagens is comprised of collagens type I, II and III; two other collagen types, V and K, are also included in this class but their supramolecular structures are not well characterized.[35] Type I collagen is the major collagen of skin, tendon, bone, sclera, and cornea; type II collagen is the major collagen of cartilage and vitreous humor; and type III is found in loose connective tissue, blood vessel walls, and placenta.

Nonfibrous collagens are not organized as fibrils but aggregate as loose networks of individual molecules bound together in a lattice structure to form sheets that may appear stacked. Collagen type IV, the major collagenous component of basement membranes, is the best studied collagen of

this group. Its supramolecular organization is optimally adapted to the highly elastic and mechanically stable, sheetlike structure of basement membranes.[30]

Filamentous collagens form the microfibrillar component present in many tissues. An example of this group is collagen type VI, present in the intima of the aorta.[23] Other filamentous collagens are types VII, VIII, IX, and X.[35] The functional significance of these recently characterized collagen types may be in connecting different forms of fibrous and nonfibrous collagens.

Although collagen has a structural role, in most tissues these molecules are continuously turned over in the extracellular matrix. Collagen biosynthesis, secretion, and degradation are complex processes that offer several potential sites for regulation. Disturbance of these normal processes, either through an acquired or inherited defect, may cause malfunction, resulting in a variety of pathologic changes. Furthermore, age-related changes in tissues and organs are associated with changes in the extracellular matrix. For example, excessive cross linking of collagen molecules may change the properties of collagen fibers, such as their flexibility or their interaction with other extracellular components, as well as interfere with their physiologic degradation.[3,43]

During the growth, maintenance, and aging of a tissue, the synthesis and degradation of collagens is strictly regulated physiologically by feedback mechanisms that can stimulate or inhibit collagen production or breakdown.[37] Hormones and humoral factors, such as growth factors, are therefore important in the regulation of collagen metabolism.[8]

Elastin (see Plate I, Fig. 4)

Elastin is a fibrillar protein present in the extracellular matrix of many tissues. This macromolecule, which is perhaps the least soluble protein in the body, lasts the lifetime of the organism. Elastin has a unique physiologic role in tissues as the biologic rubber that absorbs mechanical stress with perfect recoil. Tissues of the lung, vascular system, and certain specialized elastic ligaments are characterized by the presence of elastin.[12]

Elastin is organized in tissues as elastic fibers. The elastic fibers have two components: an insoluble amorphous material, which is elastin, and a microfibrillar component, a glycoprotein, which provides the matrix into which elastin is incorporated. This microfibrillar component presumably controls the shape and size of the elastic fiber. However, elastin can occur in a tissue alone, independent of an elastic fiber. Elastin usually co-distributes with collagen and the relative proportion of these macromolecules determines the physical strength of the tissue and its elasticity.[9,12]

Although elastin is the most stable macromolecule of the extracellular matrix, degradation of elastin can occur. During inflammation, invading inflammatory cells are capable of degrading elastin, which may have major pathologic consequences for the function of the tissue. Under normal conditions, elastin turnover is apparently minimal.[9]

In the eye, as in other organs, elastin is present in those tissues that are exposed to mechanical distortion caused by changes in pressure or movement. These tissues include the trabecular meshwork, lens zonules, and the lamina cribrosa.

Proteoglycans

Proteoglycans are complex macromolecules consisting of a core protein and one or more types of glycosaminoglycan chains, covalently bound to the core protein. Proteoglycans are the amorphous, gellike material of the extracellular matrix. Decades ago, this material was called "amorphous ground substance."

These macromolecules are negatively charged and have large amounts of water associated with them; therefore, they occupy an extended hydrodynamic volume relative to their molecular weights, and can compress under a load and expand again when the load is removed. This unique property of the proteoglycans is provided by the side chains of glycosaminoglycans.

Glycosaminoglycans, previously called "mucopolysaccharides," are long-chain polymers of repeating disaccharides that contain a hexosamine-type sugar and either a carboxylated or sulfated ester producing the linear array of negative charges. There are five major types of glycosaminoglycans: hyaluronic acid, heparan sulfate, dermatan sulfate, chondroitin sulfate, and keratan sulfate. Only hyaluronic acid exists alone as a glycosaminoglycan in tissues; all the others are attached to a protein core as part of a proteoglycan.[16]

Within the extracellular matrix, proteoglycans are dynamic molecules, and alterations in the amounts or types of proteoglycans can affect tissue function. These macromolecules can rapidly polymerize and depolymerize, thereby altering their hydrodynamic volume and affecting the physiology of the tissue.[7] In tissues, such as blood vessel walls and cartilage, that are exposed to transient changes in pressure, proteoglycans interact with collagens and elastic components to buffer these changes. Furthermore, proteoglycans and the as-sociated glycosaminoglycans are rapidly synthesized and degraded in the extracellular matrix. Because turnover of these elements is more rapid than the collagens, these molecules have the potential to play an important role in plasticity and remodeling of the extracellular matrix.[49]

Attachment Factors

The best-known macromolecules in this heterogeneous group of glycoproteins are fibronectin and laminin. Both of these molecules are important for normal attachment of cells to their substrate and for cell attachment following injury and repair of tissue. Laminin and fibronectin condition the surface of the damaged substrate, thus permitting cellular migration and adhesion.

Fibronectin occurs in two forms with similar molecular properties but different biologic activities. The cellular form is found in all interstitial matrices and some basement membranes; the plasma form is found in blood, amniotic fluid and cerebral spinal fluid. When found in extracellular matrices of tissues, fibronectin binds to the cell surface as well as to collagen fibrils and glycosaminoglycans, acting as a specific gluelike molecule between the components of the extracellular matrix and the cells. In addition to promoting cell migration, fibronectin also has a role in the control of growth and cellular differentiation. Interestingly, the behavior of malignant cells may be correlated inversely with fibronectin; the lack of surface fibronectin is generally associated with the tumorigenic potential of malignant cells.[24]

Laminin is one of the major, universal components of basement membranes. This glycoprotein promotes the attachment of epithelial or endothelial cells to collagen type IV, the other major component of basement membranes.[52] Laminin is not an attachment factor for fibroblasts or the other collagen types that are characteristic of interstitial matrices. Laminin may play a key role in the development and regeneration of the central nervous system. This attachment factor is synthesized after birth for the short period associated with the postnatal development of the central nervous system.[5] Furthermore, laminin supports the growth of neurites in tissue culture and increases in concentration in vivo after neural injury.[32]

Experimental Determinations

The macromolecules of the extracellular matrix can be determined quantitatively by biochemical techniques, while cytochemical techniques can be used to determine their anatomic distributions within tissues. For quantitation, extraction of tissues is followed by biochemical identification using amino acid analysis, electrophoretic mobility, or sensitivity to specific enzymes. Synthesis and degradation of the macromolecules of the extracellular matrix is studied by using radiolabeled precursors. Furthermore, the new techniques of molecular biology are providing the means to study genetic expression and regulation of the different components of the extracellular matrix. Biochemical determinations of the macromolecules of the extracellular matrix of ocular tissues have been limited by the size of the tissues. Some advances have been made using tissue culture to characterize the synthetic products of specific cells.

The development of immunocytochemical techniques has allowed the study of the distribution of the macromolecules of the extracellular matrix in different tissues. Using this technique, a specific antibody to the macromolecule is reacted with tissue sections or cells in tissue culture. Antibodies can distinguish between the different types of collagens, as well as the different types of attachment factors and other macromolecules present in the extracellular matrix. Current techniques have provided a wide variety of antibodies for use in these investigations.

Two kinds of antibodies are available for immunocytochemistry. In the past, conventional (polyclonal) antibodies were raised by injecting the antigen in an animal, and then affinity chromatography was used to purify the antibody. These conventional antibodies, although somewhat specific, usually have an affinity for a variety of antigenic sites along macromolecules and show cross-reactivity among species and similar molecules. More recently, monoclonal antibodies have been produced by mouse or rat lymphocyte-myeloma hybrids called hybridomas. These hybridomas produce one homogeneous antibody that has a high degree of specificity and, once fully characterized, is available indefinitely with no variation. To visualize the antibody associated with the antigenic site in the tissue section, a second antibody directed against the first antibody is tagged with a fluorescent or enzyme label and is reacted with the tissue sections or cells in tissue culture.

TRABECULAR MESHWORK

Description and Importance

The major route for the exit of aqueous humor from the eye is the outflow pathway. As the aqueous humor leaves the anterior chamber, the fluid passes through the trabecular meshwork and the juxtacanalicular tissue, across the inner wall of the canal of Schlemm and into the lumen of the canal. From the canal, the fluid passes through collector channels and mixes with blood in the episcleral veins. There is a reduction of hydrostatic pressure between the anterior chamber and the canal of Schlemm; therefore, a major component of the resistance to the flow of aqueous humor must be located somewhere between these two points. In primary open-angle glaucoma, the elevated intraocular pressure is due to decreased aqueous humor flow through the outflow pathway. The decreased aqueous humor outflow is due to an increased resistance, which apparently occurs somewhere in the corneoscleral areas of the trabecular meshwork or the juxtacanalicular tissue. Many investigations have therefore focused on the cells and the extracellular matrix of this area.

The trabecular meshwork functions as a self-cleaning filter, capable of allowing flow of aqueous humor while removing cellular debris and particulate matter. The trabecular meshwork also serves as a one-way valve for the flow of aqueous humor out of the eye, preventing backflow from the canal of Schlemm, which can occasionally contain blood, into the eye. The flow of aqueous humor may be influenced by the tension on the trabecular meshwork arising from the ciliary muscle, by the action of several drugs useful in the treatment of glaucoma, and the architecture of the tissue as governed by its macromolecular components.

The trabecular meshwork is a spongelike connective tissue made up of trabecular beams, which gradually thicken as the distance from the anterior chamber increases, thus narrowing the intratrabecular spaces through which aqueous humor flows. This circular meshwork, which fills the chamber angle, eventually becomes the juxtacanalicular tissue, rich in extracellular matrix and cells, but with no apparent space for aqueous humor flow. Thus, the properties of the extracellular matrices of these connective tissues may contribute significantly to the resistance to the outflow of aqueous humor normally, in glaucoma, and in response to drugs.

Trabecular Beams and Juxtacanalicular Tissue

The trabecular meshwork beams are covered by a layer of endothelial cells, which are not continuously joined together, and a subendothelial region, which corresponds to a discontinuous basement membrane. The core of the beam is an extracellular matrix consisting of fibrillar forms of collagen, elastic fibers, and amorphous substance. As the beams increase in thickness, the core becomes denser. The cells of the juxtacanalicular tissue are star-shaped cells embedded in an extracellular matrix made up of fibrillar collagen, elastic fibers, and ground substance. In this region, the presence of curly collagen, or long spacing collagen, is characteristic and increases with age. The juxtacanalicular tissue ends at the discontinuous basement membrane of the inner wall of the canal of Schlemm.[53]

The macromolecular components of the extracellular matrix of the trabecular meshwork are known.[38] The central core of the trabecular beams is formed by collagen type III (Fig. 6-1). Collagen type I is present in the center of the core but is less prominent. Elastin is also found in the central portion of the core of the trabecular beams (Fig. 6-2). Fibronectin, laminin, and collagen type IV are not present in the core of the trabecular meshwork beams.

In the subendothelial region, there is collagen types IV and V, laminin, fibronectin, and the glycosaminoglycan, heparan sulfate (Fig. 6-3).[11,22,38,42,44] These components are associated with basement membranes, except for collagen type V, which is an unusual finding in this region. Perhaps its presence in the subendothelial space is to link

Text continued on p. 171.

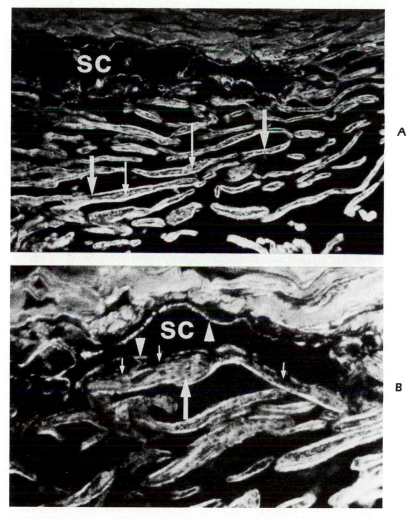

Fig. 6-1 Localization of collagen type III in trabecular meshwork and Schlemm's canal. **A,** Semithin section of meshwork and canal *(SC),* showing dual localization of type III stain, in both subendothelial *(thick arrows)* and core *(thin arrows)* regions of beams. Staining in outer wall of canal is also apparent. (× 240.) **B,** Subendothelial portion of both inner and outer walls of Schlemm's canal *(SC)* reacts positively for type III *(arrowheads).* Note stain in outer wall. There is also stain in juxtacanalicular meshwork *(large arrow)* but extensive regions remain unstained *(small arrows).* (× 600.) (From Murphy, CG, Andersen, JY, Newsome, DA, and Alvarado, JA. Published with permission from the American Journal of Ophthalmology 104:33, 1987. Copyright by the Ophthalmic Publishing Co)

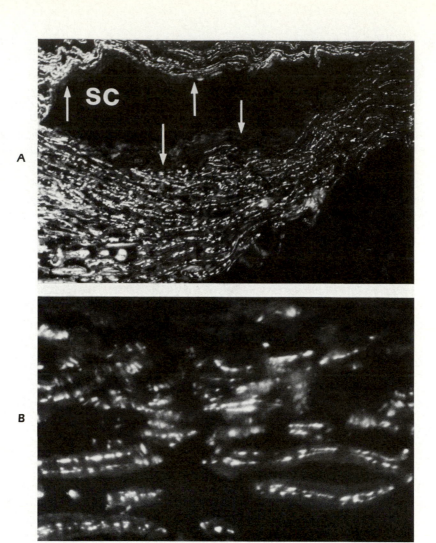

Fig. 6-2 Distribution of elastin in the trabecular meshwork. **A,** Unique punctate staining pattern for this protein is shown in meshwork and canal *(SC)*. Note that stain also extends into tissues beyond outer wall of canal. Both inner and outer walls, as well as juxtacanalicular tissue *(arrows)*, are devoid of stain for elastin and are barely visible (× 240). **B,** Higher magnification of trabecular meshwork beams. Stain appears as double row of dots within beam cores. Remainder of beams, including the subendothelial portion, does not stain (× 600.) (From Murphy, CG, Andersen, JY, Newsome, DA, and Alvarado JA. Published with permission from the American Journal of Ophthalmology 104:33, 1987. Copyright by the Ophthalmic Publishing Co)

Fig. 6-3 Membrane-associated proteins in trabecular meshwork. Outer meshwork and Schlemm's canal *(SC)* are above and inner meshwork and anterior chamber *(ac)* are below. **A** through **G,** 1 to 2 μm sections; **H,** 6 μm section. **A,** Type IV collagen surrounds trabecular beams and is found in subendothelial region of Schlemm's canal. (× 240.) **B,** Type IV collagen is sharply localized to subendothelial region of trabecular beams. Cores *(arrows)* are unstained. (× 600.) **C,** In trabecular meshwork, type V collagen also has subendothelial distribution. (× 260.) **D,** Subendothelial regions *(arrows)* of inner *(iw)* and outer *(ow)* walls of Schlemm's canal showing staining for type V collagen. (× 600.) **E,** Laminin is also found subendothelially, as seen in this section of anterior *(s,* Schwalbe's ring) end of trabecular meshwork. Cornea *(c)* is unstained. (× 240.) **F,** Midregion of inner meshwork of same specimen stained for laminin. Stain is absent from core regions of beams *(arrows)*. (× 600.) **G,** Fibronectin is localized beneath trabecular cells *(arrows)* and "cores" lack staining. (× 600.) **H,** Thick section (6 μm) of meshwork stained for heparan sulfate proteoglycan. Although resolution is not as high as in semithin sections (**A** through **G**), subendothelial localization is conspicuous in trabecular beams. (× 240.) (From Murphy, CG, Andersen, JY, Newsome, DA, and Alvarado, JA. Published with permission from the American Journal of Ophthalmology 104:33, 1987. Copyright by the Ophthalmic Publishing Co)

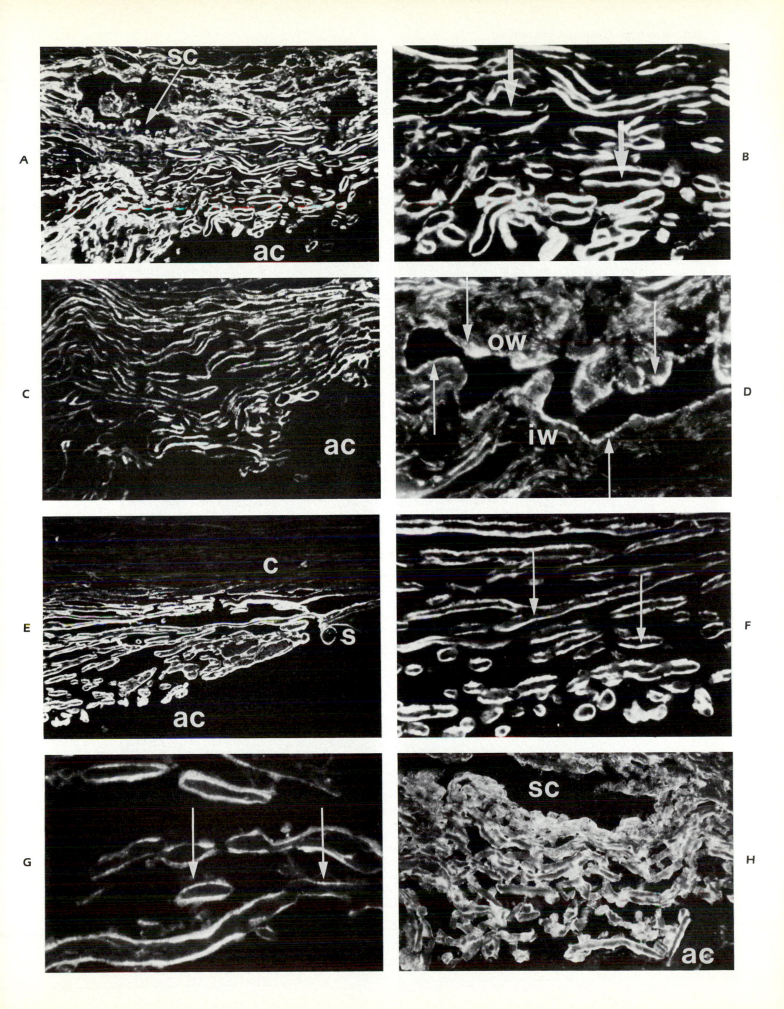

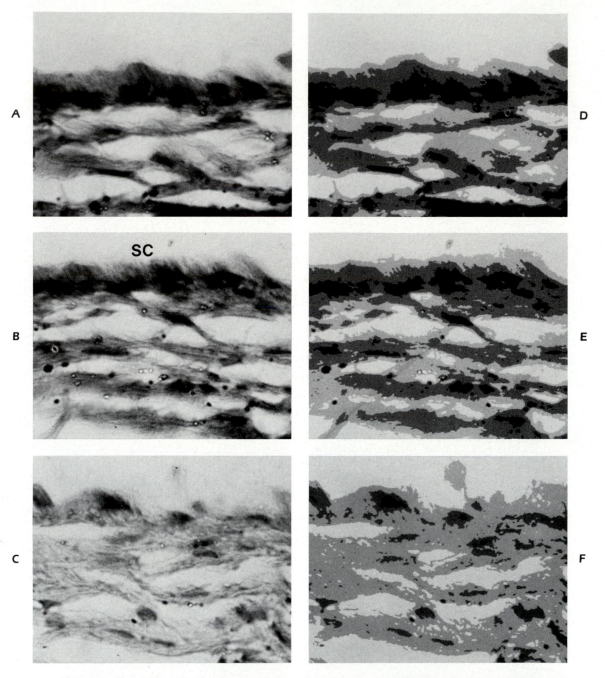

Fig. 6-4 Composite of light micrographs (**A** to **C**) and computer images (**D** to **F**) of the intensity of Alcian blue staining of buffer- or enzyme-treated 8 μm serial sections of the inner trabecular meshwork of a primate eye. **A,** Control sections incubated with buffer. **B,** Hyaluronic lyase (degrades only hyaluronic acid). **C,** Chondroitin ABC lyase (degrades the chondroitin sulfates at pH 8.6). Staining intensity is coded in percent transmission on a gray scale (e.g., 40, representative of a presence of staining) to 100, representative of the absence of staining). *SC,* Schlemm's canal. (× 1500.) (From Knepper, PA, and McLone, DG: Pediatr Neurosci 12:240, 1985)

basement membrane components and interstitial collagen in the beams.

Collagen type III (see Fig. 6-1), IV and V, laminin, heparan sulfate and fibronectin (see Fig. 6-3) are present in the subendothelial region of Schlemm's canal. In the rest of the juxtacanalicular tissue, only patchy staining for collagen type III has been described (see Fig. 6-1).[38] Ultrastructural observations indicate the presence of collagen fibrils, elastic-like material and "curly collagen."[33,53] In this region, there is an age-related appearance of an extracellular material, "plaques," that is made up of abnormal collagen with a particular periodicity and electron-dense granular material. Enzymatic digestion to identify the components of this material has not proven successful.[33] In glaucoma, there may be abnormally high amounts of this material.[45,46]

The extracellular spaces of the trabecular meshwork and the juxtacanalicular tissue contain a gel-like substance, which may play a large part in producing the resistance to the flow of aqueous humor. This material consists of a complex variety of proteoglycans of which the glycosaminoglycan side chains have been studied extensively.

The juxtacanalicular tissue contains the largest quantities of proteoglycans. The glycosaminoglycans represented in these molecules include dermatan sulfate, heparan sulfate, chondroitin sulfate, and keratan sulfate.[1,28] Hyaluronic acid is present throughout the tissue in significant amounts as a free glycosaminoglycan not bound to a protein core (Fig. 6-4). The glycosaminoglycans are also found within the trabecular beams, perhaps as the ground substance surrounding the collagen in the cores. In addition, there is a glycosaminoglycan lining on the surfaces of the trabecular endothelial cells that lines the trabecular spaces, providing an interface between aqueous humor and tissue.[6,28]

Human trabecular meshwork has been explanted in tissue culture. The cells grown from these explants, presumably the endothelial cells lining the trabecular beams, grow as a monolayer, have an epithelial morphology, and synthesize extracellular matrix macromolecules.* Trabecular meshwork cells in tissue culture synthesize the basement membrane components present in the subendothelial region of the trabecular meshwork in vivo: collagen type IV, laminin, and fibronectin.[22,39]

Human and monkey trabecular meshwork

cells have been used to study the synthesis of glycosaminoglycans in tissue culture.[15,31,39,56] These cells have been used to study the synthesis of glycosaminoglycans in tissue culture.[15,31,39,56] These cells synthesize hyaluronic acid, chondroitin sulfate, dermatan sulfate, heparan sulfate, and keratan sulfate, all of which have been demonstrated histochemically and biochemically in the human trabecular meshwork in vivo.[1,6,28] Trabecular meshing that they may be capable of regulating their extracellular environment in vivo.[55]

Functional Significance

The fibrillar forms of collagen that form the core of the trabecular beams are structural and have important mechanical implications for the function of the tissue. Collagen types I and III give the tissue tensile strength to maintain the shape and to withstand the fluctuations in intraocular pressure and the forces on the tissue due to accommodation. Elastin, the other major component of the core of the trabecular beams, may serve to return the trabecular meshwork to its original structure following accommodative changes.

Functionally, the macromolecules of the basement membrane attach the endothelial cells to the trabecular beams and, although the layer covering the beams is incomplete, may provide a permeability barrier. There is interaction between the cytoarchitecture through the intracellular filaments and the underlying extracellular matrix of the basement membrane. An extensive network of actin-like filaments is present in trabecular meshwork cells, and some drugs may act to alter the interaction between the cell and its basement membrane.

Because of their ability to bind water, the glycosaminoglycans lining the trabecular beams and in the juxtacanalicular tissue may be important in regulating the flow of aqueous humor through this tissue. Hyaluronic acid, present in the highest concentrations of all the glycosaminoglycans in the trabecular meshwork, has the greatest ability to bind water. The classic experiments using hyaluronidase have demonstrated that perfusion of an eye with this enzyme increases the outflow of aqueous humor.[4] Furthermore, the experimental use of hyaluronic acid during intraocular surgery increases intraocular pressure.[28] Knepper[28] suggests that hyaluronic acid acts as a gel filtration system in the outflow pathway and conceptually postulates that the tightness or looseness of the lattice of hyaluronic acid molecules may regulate the exclusion volume and the water-binding characteristics of the

---

*References 14, 15, 22, 31, 39, 47, 48, 54-56.

tissue, which will influence the flow of aqueous humor through this area.

In primary open-angle glaucoma and glucocorticoid-induced glaucoma, glycosaminoglycan-like deposits have been identified in the trabecular meshwork and the juxtacanalicular tissue.[13,33,45,46,50] There is also a material made up of unknown components on the surface of trabecular endothelial cells, as well as in the intertrabecular matrix in glaucomatous tissue.[33] Rohen[45] has identified plaque-like deposits that may contain glycosaminoglycans in the juxtacanalicular tissue in increased amounts in the trabecular meshwork from glaucomatous eyes.

Glucocorticoids elevate the intraocular pressure in susceptible individuals (see Chapter 64). The mechanism by which these hormones affect intraocular pressure is probably related to the regulatory function that glucocorticoids have on extracellular matrix synthesis and degradation. Dexamathasone produces a significant decrease in the synthesis of collagen in human trabecular meshwork in organ culture.[21] In human trabecular meshwork cells in tissue culture, dexamethasone increases the accumulation of hyaluronic acid.[15] The use of in vitro systems, such as cell and organ culture, may provide new information about the potential for pharmacologic manipulation of the extracellular matrix of the trabecular meshwork.

OPTIC NERVE HEAD

Description and Importance

The corneal and scleral tissue constitute most of the walls of the eye and form a strong, nondistensible shell for the contents of the eye.

The optic nerve head fills the scleral canal, which is an interruption in the shell of the globe. The optic nerve head is a weaker portion of the ocular wall that is adapted to provide several important functions. This tissue must supply mechanical and nutritional support to the optic nerve fibers while resisting the distension due to intraocular pressure changes and the distortion caused by ocular movements.

Three regions are described histologically in the optic nerve head. The retinal portion, where the nerve fiber layers converge to take a 90-degree turn to form the optic nerve, is referred to as the prelaminar area. This region consists of nonmyelinated nerve fiber bundles separated by columns of astroglia. Within the glial columns and completely surrounded by astroglia, capillaries are regularly found that have a continuous basement membrane. These capillaries are similar to retinal and central nervous system capillaries.

Posterior to the prelaminar area is the lamina cribrosa, which is divided into two parts. The choroidal lamina cribrosa is situated at the level of the choroid, and the scleral lamina cribrosa is posterior and situated at the level of the sclera. In the choroidal region of the lamina cribrosa, the nerve bundles are nonmyelinated and astrocytes send out processes that are perpendicular to the course of the nerve and provide support by forming tubelike channels for the bundles of nerve fibers. The posterior, scleral portion of the lamina cribrosa is composed of 10 plates of collagenous, connective tissue, which appear to be stretched across the scleral canal. Each plate is perforated by several hundred openings, which are aligned between plates to permit the exit of the bundles of nerve fibers. These connective tissue plates, called cribriform plates, are composed of a core of connective tissue, which include capillaries, and are lined by astrocytes. Much evidence has accumulated to indicate that this particular region of the optic nerve head is associated with degeneration of nerve fibers observed in glaucoma.

Posterior to the scleral portion of the lamina cribrosa is the retrolaminar region. Here, the nerve fibers become myelinated, resulting in an increased diameter of the optic nerve. The nerve bundles are separated by pial septae containing blood vessels and lined by astroglia. The pial septae are continuous with the tissue forming the cribriform plates but are parallel to the nerve bundles and organized longitudinally.

The work of Quigley[40,41] demonstrates that the cupping associated clinically with glaucoma results from the compression, stretching, and rearrangement of the connective tissues of the optic nerve head in response to elevated intraocular pressure. The cribiform plates appear to collapse together, much like a closing accordion, making the floor of the cup recede deeper. The lamina cribrosa is pushed outward and behind Bruch's membrane, producing a backward or outward bowing of the tissue in some cases. Thus, the increase in cup size results from the loss of nerve fibers and the rearrangement of the tissue is due to compression of the cribriform plates.

The Lamina Cribrosa

The cribriform plates of the lamina cribrosa are composed of a core of extracellular matrix made up of histologically identified collagen and elastic fibers and containing capillaries, surrounded by basement membranes, and the occasional fibroblastic appearing cell.[2] The cribriform plates are lined by astrocytes that extend processes into the nerve fiber bundles. The astrocytes are separated from the core of the cribriform plates by a continuous and well-defined basement membrane. At the sclera, the astrocytes are also separated from the interstitial matrix by a continuous basement membrane.[2]

Many investigations of the glaucomatous changes in this region of the optic nerve head have described the gross appearance of the connective tissue elements that remain after digestion of the neural elements. Using the scanning electron microscope, Quigley[40] has demonstrated that the stacks of cribriform plates retain the distortion characteristic of glaucoma. Therefore, the macromolecular components of the extracellular matrix of the cribriform plates may play an important role in the changes in the optic nerve head due to glaucoma.

Immunofluorescent staining for collagen types in the human lamina cribrosa has provided new insights into the structure of this tissue. The most conspicuous finding is that of collagen type IV in transverse patterns throughout the cribriform plates[18,20,25] (Fig. 6-5) and codistributing with laminin.[18] These lamellar structures oriented across the nerve bundles are presumably stacks of basement membranes. By comparison to the neighboring sclera, the cribriform plates are relatively sparse in the collagens of the interstitial matrix. Thus, the lamina cribrosa appears not to be an extension of the sclera but rather a specialized extracellular matrix of the central nervous system.

In the lamina cribrosa of young adults, the core of the cribriform plates contains substantial amounts of elastin in the form of long fibers[20] (Fig. 6-5). The presence of this macromolecule is consistent with the ultrastructural demonstration of elastic fibers in the core of the cribriform plates.[2] Collagen type III co-distributes with elastin, appearing as patches within the core (Fig. 6-6). The density of this fibrillar form of collagen may increase with age. Collagen type I is present as a minor component disposed transversely as fine fibrils in the core of the plates.[18] The presence of these specific forms of collagens is consistent with the ultrastructural demonstration of striated collagen fibrils in this tissue.[2] Within the core, the blood vessels are delimited by collagen type IV (Fig. 6-5) and laminin, consistent with the distribution of their basement membranes, and are also surrounded by collagen type III and fibronectin (see Fig. 6-5). Fibronectin does not appear elsewhere in the core of the cribriform plates in the human.[18]

Separating the core of the cribriform plates from the surrounding astrocytes is a well-defined, continuous layer of collagen type IV and laminin, which are apparently part of the basement membranes of the astrocytes and extend linearly into the core of the cribriform plates.[20]

Immunofluorescent staining has also revealed the relationships between lamellae of the cribriform plates. For example, linear patterns of collagen type IV and elastin are continuous between plates at different levels and connect different plates transversely within this tissue.[18,20]

The macromolecular organization of the insertion area of the lamina cribrosa in the sclera indicates that this is a specialized structure. Concentric, circumferential, tightly packed fibers of elastin surround the laminar and prelaminar region of the optic nerve head (Fig. 6-6).[20] Furthermore, the fibers of elastin of the cribriform plates, running perpendicularly to the nerve bundles, are continuous with and appear to arise from the concentric, circumferential fibers of the insertion. Fibers of elastin are found in the adjacent sclera, where they are short, sparse, do not show any special orientation, and are easily distinguished from those of the insertion region. The processes of the astrocytes of the lamina cribrosa extend through the bundles of elastin fibers and form an anchoring network in the insertion region (Fig. 6-6). The macromolecular components of the basement membranes of the astrocytes, collagen type IV and laminin, extend beyond the cell processes into the sclera (Fig. 6-6; see also Plate II, Fig. 1).[20]

Thus, the cribriform plates and the insertion of the lamina cribrosa have different macromolecular components, with different distributions than the neighboring sclera. Sclera is composed primarily of fibrillar forms of collagen type III.[27] Elastin is present randomly and in minor amounts throughout the sclera.[36] The presence of collagen type IV, laminin, and fibronectin has been described in the sclera surrounding the blood vessels. Collagen type IV and laminin are not present in the scleral stroma.[20,29]

The other regions of the optic nerve head have an extracellular matrix different from that of the lamina cribrosa.[18,20] In the prelaminar area, collagen type IV, laminin, fibronectin, and collagen type III are associated with the extracellular matrix of the blood vessel walls. In the optic nerve proper, the extracellular matrix of the pial septa is continuous and has similar characteristics as the pia mater. The basement membrane of the pial septa is continuous with the basement membrane of the cribriform plates. Thus, there is a transition in the orientation of the extracellular matrix support elements from

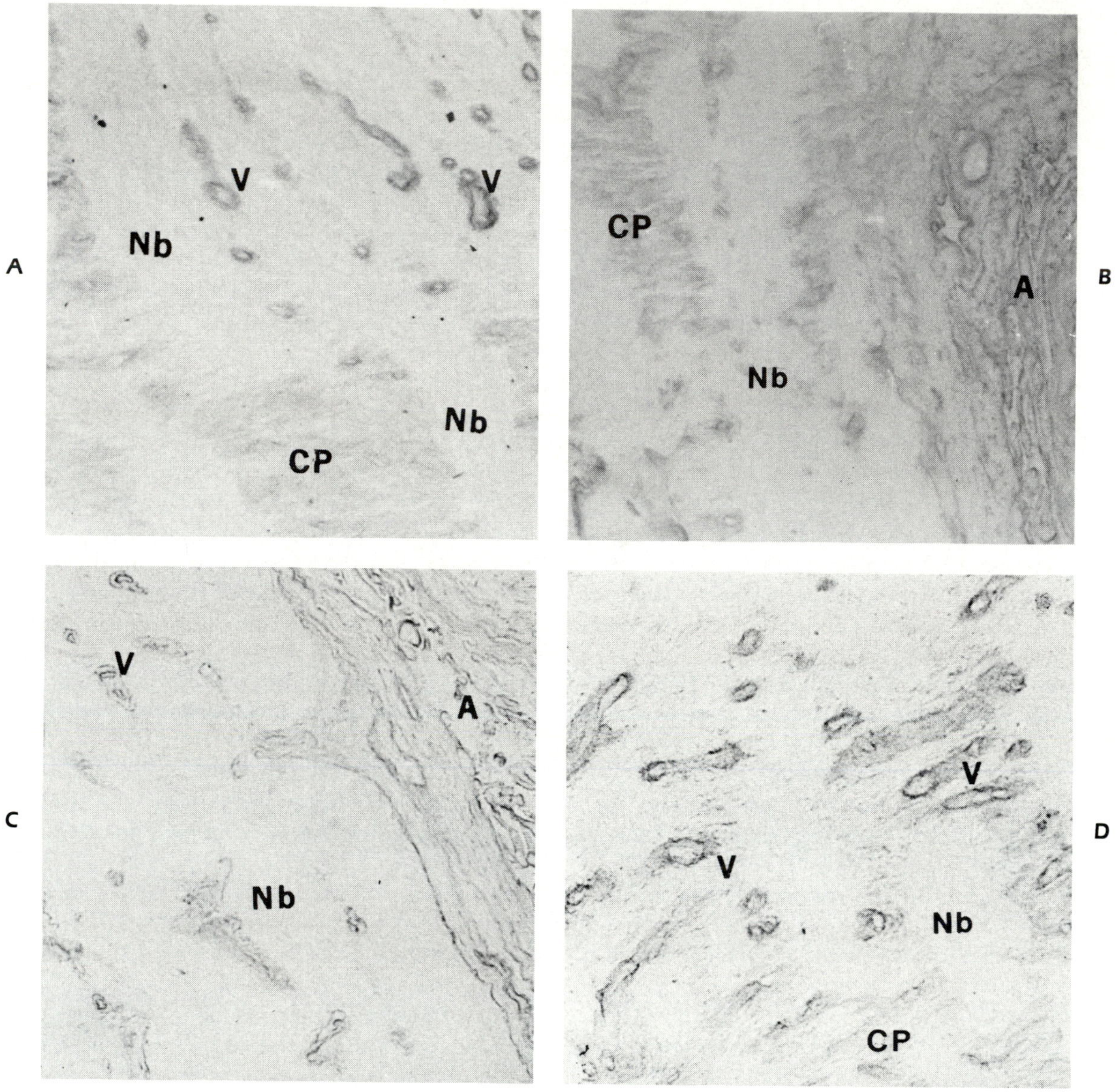

Fig. 6-5 Immunoperoxidase staining for human collagen type III and human fibronectin. **A,** Staining for collagen type III is positive in blood vessels (*V*), cribriform plates (*CP*) show faint, diffuse staining. Nerve bundles *(NB).* (× 100.) **B,** Positive staining is seen in arachnoid *(A).* (× 100.) **C,** Positive staining for human fibronectin in arachnoid and blood vessels. (× 100.) **D,** Positive staining for human fibronectin in blood vessels of lamina cribrosa; cribriform plates are not stained. (× 100.) (From Hernandez, MR, Xing, XXL, Igoe, F, and Neufeld, AH. Published with permission from the American Journal of Ophthalmology 104:567, 1987. Copyright by the Ophthalmic Publishing Co)

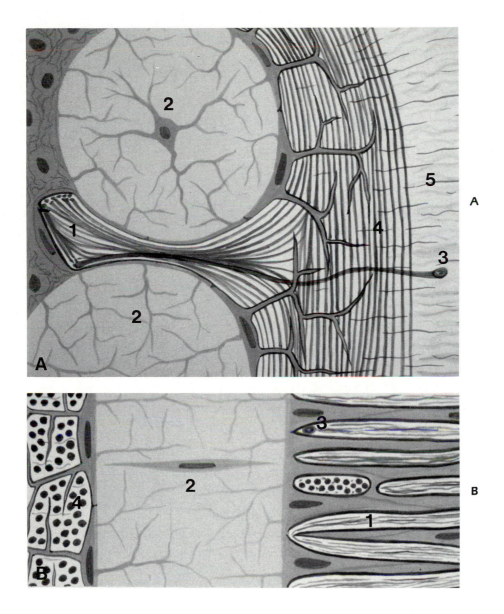

Fig. 6-6 Schematic drawing of lamina cribrosa showing different extracellular matrix components and their relationships with nerve bundles, astrocytes, and surrounding tissues. **A,** Cross section of lamina cribrosa. **B,** Longitudinal section. Cribriform plates *(1)*; nerve bundles *(2)*; blood vessels *(3)*; insertion region *(4)*; sclera *(5)*. (From Hernandez, MR, Xing, XXL, Igoe, F, and Neufeld, AH. Published with permission from the American Journal of Ophthalmology 104:567, 1987. Copyright by the Ophthalmic Publishing Co) See also Plate II, Fig. 1.

the transverse aspect of the lamina cribrosa to the longitudinal columns of the pial septa.

Several cell types contribute macromolecules to the extracellular matrix of the cribriform plates. As in other tissues and throughout the retina, the vascular endothelium and pericytes contribute the basement membrane macromolecules and surrounding collagens to the blood vessel walls. However, the extracellular matrix of the cribriform plates may receive contributions from a variety of cell types. The astrocytes, which form the lining throughout this region, presumably synthesize, at least in part, the basement membrane macromolecules, collagen type IV, and laminin, which coat the core of the cribriform plates. Cells that synthesize the macromolecules found in the core of the cribriform plates are less apparent. Few fibroblasts are present in this region, and fibroblasts do not grow in tissue culture when the lamina cribrosa is explanted. However, a "fibroblastoid" cell is grown in tissue culture from explants of human lamina cribrosa.[19] This cell is large, flat, broad and does not appear to be either a fibroblast or an astrocyte. In tissue culture, the lamina cribrosa cells synthesize collagen type IV, collagen type III, and elastin. The distribution of these cells in situ and their ability to synthesize the macromolecules in the core of the cribriform plates in vivo remains to be determined.

Functional Significance

The macromolecular components of the extracellular matrix of the lamina cribrosa provide this tissue with functional characteristics different from those of sclera. Although lacking the tensile strength of sclera, the lamina cribrosa is apparently a compliant tissue that may be resilient to acute, mechanical changes. The interconnected lamellar stacks of collagen type IV presumably form a loose macromolecular network with characteristics of the elastic and mechanically stable sheetlike organization of basement membranes. These sheetlike structures suspended transversely across the nerve fiber bundles may fulfill the elastic needs of the tissue to absorb stresses. The presence of elastin, a unique macromolecule that functions as a biologic rubber to absorb stress with perfect recoil, in combination with collagen type IV, may further adapt the tissue to resist the distension due to pressure changes in the eye or the distortion due to ocular movements and may provide the ability to recover the original structure.

The presence of collagens type I and III in the core of the cribriform plates undoubtedly provides some rigidity to this tissue. Increases in the amounts of these fibrillar forms of collagens with age may cause loss of compliance, elasticity, and flexibility of the lamina cribrosa. Age-related increases in the total collagen content of this tissue have been demonstrated by the histologic appearance of increased connective tissue in this region, as well as the biochemical determination of increased collagen-associated amino acids.[51]

In the insertion region, the formation of a network of collagen type IV extending beyond the elastin fibers into the sclera indicates a strong anchoring function for the extracellular matrix in this area. The concentric fibroelastic components of the insertion region represent a peripheral support of the nonmyelinated fiber bundles, an elastic sleeve that is tightly organized and holds the nerve bundles as they pass through this area. This fibroelastic ligament functions to attach firmly the lamina cribrosa to the surrounding connective tissue of the sclera via the network of collagen type IV extending beyond the elastin fiber and to return the tissue to its original shape upon the reestablishment of normal intraocular pressure via the continuity with the elastic fibers in the core of the cribriform plates.

The long-term glaucomatous process that causes a compressive realignment of the cribriform plates may be reflected in, or even caused by, the extracellular matrix. These changes occur in a relatively weak point in the wall of the eye, are age-related, and show individual variability. Therefore, the characteristics, relative composition, and spatial distribution of the macromolecules of the extracellular matrix in the lamina cribrosa may provide an explanation for the glaucomatous changes in this tissue.

Further knowledge of the types of macromolecular components and how they alter with age will help distinguish among several possibilities that can account for glaucomatous changes in the optic nerve head. For example, the relative amounts of extracellular matrix macromolecules may show a normal distribution of individual variability. Changes associated with elevated intraocular pressure may only occur in certain individuals at one end of this continuum, whereas most individuals would be unaffected. Individuals with low tension glaucoma may have an extracellular matrix unable to provide normal functions even at normal intraocular pressure. Alternatively, there may be age-related changes in the extracellular matrix of the lamina cribrosa associated with alterations in the amounts or distributions of the macromolecules or the actual, biochemical nature of the macromolecules. Depending on the rate at which these age-related changes occur and the relative level of intraocular pressure, certain individuals may be predisposed to or protected from the glaucomatous changes in this region. Finally, the lamina cribrosa may be a tissue with the ability to respond to stress. For example, in response to elevated intraocular pressure the lamina cribrosa cells may change their production of collagen amounts or types in some individuals; whereas in other individuals, this change in biosynthetic ability may not occur. Reactive responses could either encourage the damage or protect an individual from elevated intraocular pressure.

REFERENCES

1. Acott, TS, Wescott, M, Passo, MS, and Van Buskirk, EM: Trabecular meshwork glycosaminoglycans in human and cynomolgus monkey eye, Invest Ophthalmol Vis Sci 26:1320, 1985
2. Anderson, DR: Ultrastructure of human and monkey lamina cribrosa and optic nerve head, Arch Ophthalmol 82:800, 1969
3. Bailey, AJ: Structure, function and aging of the collagens of the eye, Eye 1:175, 1987
4. Barany, EH, and Scotchbrook, S: Influence of testicular hyaluronidase on the resistance to flow through the angle of the anterior chamber, Acta Physiol Scand 30:240, 1954
5. Carbonetto, S: The extracellular matrix of the nervous system, Trends Neurosci, October 1984, p 382
6. Collins, JA, Gum, GG, Palmberg, PF, and Knepper, PA: Microscale analysis of glycosaminoglaycans from single human trabecular meshwork, Invest Ophthalmol Vis Sci 27(suppl):162, 1986
7. Comper, WD, and Laurent, TC: Physiological function of connective tissue polysaccharides, Physiol Rev 58:255, 1978
8. Cutroneo, KR, Sterling Jr, KM, and Shull, S: Steroid hormone regulation of extracellular matrix proteins. In Mecham, R, editor: Regulation of matrix accumulation, Orlando, 1986, Academic Press, Inc
9. Davidson, JM, and Giro, MG: Control of elastin synthesis: molecular and cellular aspects. In Mecham, R, editor: Regulation of matrix accumulation, Orlando, 1986, Academic Press, Inc
10. Farquhar, MG: The glomerular basement membrane. A selective macromolecular filter. In Hay, ED, editor: Cell biology of extracellular matrix, ed 2, New York, 1983, Plenum Press
11. Floyd, BB, Cleveland, PH, and Worthen, DM: Fibronectin in human trabecular drainage channels, Invest Ophthalmol Vis Sci 26:797, 1985
12. Franzblau, C, and Faris, B: Elastin. In Hay, ED, editor: Cell biology of the extracellular matrix, New York, 1981, Plenum Press
13. Goossens, W, Higbee, RG, Palmberg, PF, and Knepper, PA: Histochemical identification of glycosaminoglycans in primary open angle glaucoma, Invest Ophthalmol Vis Sci 27(suppl):162, 1986
14. Grierson, I, Marshall, J, and Robins, E: Human trabecular meshwork in primary culture: a morphological and autoradiographic study, Exp Eye Res 37:349, 1983
15. Hajek, AS, Palmberg, P, Sossi, G, and Ocon, M: Dexamethasone-induced accumulation of glycosaminoglycans in human trabecular endothelial cultures is dependent on serum. Invest Ophthalmol Vis Sci 26(suppl):111, 1985
16. Hascall, VC, and Hascall, GK: Proteoglycans. In Hay, ED: Cell biology of the extracellular matrix, ed 2, New York, 1983, Plenum Press
17. Hay, ED, editor: Cell biology of extracellular matrix, ed 2, New York, 1983, Plenum Press
18. Hernandez, MR, Igoe, F, and Neufeld, AH: Extracellular matrix of the human optic nerve head, Am J Ophthalmol 102:139, 1986
19. Hernandez, MR, Igoe, F, and Neufeld, AH: Cell culture of the human lamina cribrosa, Invest Ophthalmol Vis Sci (In press)
20. Hernandez, MR, Xing, XXL, Igoe, F, and Neufeld, AH: Extracellular matrix of the human lamina cribrosa; a pressure-sensitive tissue, Am J Ophthalmol 104:567, 1987
21. Hernandez, MR, Weinstein, BI, Dunn, MW, Gordon, GG, et al: The effect of dexamethasone on the synthesis of collagen in normal human trabecular meshwork explants, Invest Ophthalmol Vis Sci 26:1784, 1985
22. Hernandez, MR, et al: Human trabecular meshwork cells in culture: morphology and extracellular matrix components, Invest Ophthalmol Vis Sci 28:1655, 1987
23. Hessle, H, and Engvall, E: Type VI collagen, J Biol Chem 259, 6:3955, 1984
24. Hynes, RO: Fibronectin and its relation to cellular structure and behavior. In Hay, ED, editor: Cell biology of the extracellular matrix, New York, 1981, Plenum Press
25. Jeng, S, Goldbaum, MH, Logemann, RB, and Weinreb, RN: Extracellular matrix of the optic nerve, Invest Ophthalmol Vis Sci 28(suppl):61, 1987
26. Kaufman, PL: The effects of drugs on the outflow of aqueous humor. In Drance, SM, and Neufeld, AH, editors: Glaucoma: applied pharmacology in medical treatment, Orlando, 1984, Grune & Stratton, Inc
27. Keeley, FW, Morin, JD, and Vesely, S: Characterization of collagen from normal human sclera, Exp Eye Res 39:533, 1984
28. Knepper, PA, and McLone, DG: Glycosaminoglycans and outflow pathways of the eye and brain, Pediatr Neurosci 12:240, 1985
29. Konomi, H, et al: Immunohistochemical localization of type I, III, and IV collagens in the sclera and choroid of bovine, rat, and normal and pathological human eyes, Biomedical Research 4:451, 1983

30. Kuhn, K, et al: The structure of type IV collagen in biology, chemistry and pathology of collagen, Ann NY Acad Sci 460:14, 1985

31. Kurosawa, A, et al: Cultured trabecular-meshwork cells: immunohistochemical and lectin-binding characteristics, Exp Eye Res 45:239, 1987

32. Liesi, P: Laminin and fibronectin in normal and malignant neuroectodermal cells, Med Biol 61:163, 1984

33. Lütjen-Drecoll, E, Futa, R, and Rohen, JW: Ultrahistochemical studies on tangential sections of the trabecular meshwork in normal and glaucomatous eyes, Invest Ophthalmol Vis Sci 21:563, 1981

34. Martin, GR, Timpl, R, Müller, PK, and Kühn, K: The genetic distinct collagens, Trends in Biochemistry 10:285, 1985

35. Miller, EJ: The structure of fibril-forming collagens, in biology, chemistry and pathology of collagen. Ann NY Acad Sci 460:1, 1985

36. Moses, RA, Grodzki, WJ Jr, Starcher, BC, and Gailione, MJ: Elastin content of the scleral spur, trabecular meshwork, and sclera, Invest Ophthalmol Vis Sci 17:817, 1978

37. Muller, PK, Nerlich, AG, Bohm, J, and Phan-Than, L: Feedback regulation of collagen synthesis. In Mecham, R, editor: Regulation of matrix accumulation, Orlando, 1986, Academic Press, Inc

38. Murphy, CG, Yun, AJ, Newsome, DA, and Alvarado, JA: Localization of extracellular proteins of the human trabecular meshwork by indirect immunofluorescence, Am J Ophthalmol 104:33, 1987

39. Polansky, JR, Wood, IS, Maglio, MT, and Alvarado, JA: Trabecular meshwork cell culture in glaucoma research: evaluation of biological activity and structural properties of human trabecular cells in vitro, Ophthalmology 91:580, 1984

40. Quigley, HA, et al: Morphological change in the lamina cribrosa correlated with neural loss in open-angle glaucoma, Am J Ophthalmol 95:673, 1983

41. Quigley, HA: Changes in the appearances of the optic disk, Surv Ophthalmol 30:111, 1985

42. Radda, TM, Aberer, W, and Klemen UM: Immunfluoreszenzuntersuchungen des menschlichen Trabekelwerkes, Klin Mbl Augenheilk 182:141, 1983

43. Robins, SP, and Bailey, AJ: Age-related changes in collagen, Biochem Biophys Res Commun 48:76, 1972

44. Rodrigues, MM, Katz, SI, Foidart, J-M, and Spaeth, GL: Collagen, factor VIII antigen, and immunoglobulins in the human aqueous drainage channels, Trans Am Acad Ophthalmol Otolaryngol 87:337, 1980

45. Rohen, JW: Why is intraocular pressure elevated in chronic simple glaucoma? Ophthalmology 90:758, 1983

46. Rohen, JW, Linner, E, and Witmer, R: Electron microscopic studies on the trabecular meshwork in two cases of corticosteroid-glaucoma, Exp Eye Res 17:19, 1973

47. Schachtschabel, DO, Rohen, JW, Wever, J, and Sames, K: Synthesis and composition of glycosaminoglycans by cultured human trabecular meshwork cells, v Graefes Arch Clin Exp Ophthalmol 218:113, 1982

48. Schachtschabel, DO, Wilke, K, and Wehrmann, R: In vitro cultures of human and monkey trabecular meshwork. In Lütjen-Drecoll, E, editor: Basic aspects of glaucoma research, Stuttgart/New York, 1982, FK Schattauer

49. Spooner, BS, and Thompson-Pletscher, HA: Matrix accumulation and the development of form: proteoglycans and branding morphogenesis. In Mecham, RP, editor: Regulation of matrix accumulation, Orlando, Fl, 1986, Academic Press

50. Stocker, S, et al: Collagene trabeculaire cornéoscleral: modifications ultrastructurales et immunotypage dans le glaucome chronique et cortisone, J Fr Ophthalmol 3:415, 1980

51. Tengroth, B, and Ammitzboll, T: Changes in the content and composition of collagen in the glaucomatous eye—basis for a new hypothesis for the genesis of chronic open angle glaucoma, Acta Ophthalmol (Copenh) 62:999, 1984

52. Timpl, R, et al: Laminin: a glycoprotein from basement membranes, J Biol Chem 254:9933, 1979

53. Tripathi, RC, and Tripathi, BJ: Functional anatomy of the anterior chamber angle. In Duane, TD, and Jaeger, EA, editors: Biomedical foundations of ophthalmology, Philadelphia, 1982, Harper & Row

54. Tripathi, RC, and Tripathi, BJ: Human trabecular endothelium, corneal endothelium, keratocytes, and scleral fibroblasts in primary cell culture: a comparative study of growth characteristics, morphology, and phagocytic activity by light and scanning electron microscopy, Exp Eye Res 35:611, 1982

55. Yue, BYJT, Elner, VM, Elner, SG, and Davis, HR: Lysosomal enzyme activities in cultured trabecular meshwork cells, Exp Eye Res 44:891, 1987

56. Yue, BYJT, and Elvart, JL: Biosynthesis of glycosaminoglycans by trabecular meshwork cells in vitro, Curr Eye Res 6:959, 1987

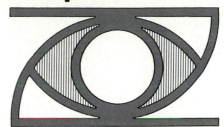

Chapter 7

Functional Testing in Glaucoma

Michael E. Breton
Bruce A. Drum

Visual psychophysics and electrophysiology

Visual psychophysics provides noninvasive measurement techniques designed to answer the question of how we see. Conclusions about visual function are based on data obtained by asking patients about their perception of controlled stimuli. Using the assumption of psychoneural congruency (the retina and brain are solely responsible for transforming light into vision), and by applying appropriate physiologic-psychophysical linking hypotheses,[18] we can draw conclusions about visual system function based on the psychophysical data.

Psychophysics treats vision as an input-output problem in which the visual system is the "black box." As a noninvasive technique, the objective of psychophysics is to describe the logic of the black box rather than to uncover its physiologic structure directly.[71] Typically, psychophysics makes use of mathematic models that, in combination with neurophysiologic knowledge, may be used to infer the functional status of retinal or optic nerve elements. Knowledge of the physiologic mechanisms that underlie psychophysical performance may also lead to more specific testing methods with increased diagnostic power. On the research level, psychophysics, single-cell electrophysiology, and neuro-

physiology often come together in a synergistic relationship.

From the point of view of functional testing, glaucoma is not a well-defined or well-documented disease. One psychophysical test, *perimetry*, has played a central role in defining the disease and in documenting its progression. Until recently, a virtual congruence between visual field loss and loss of optic nerve fibers (a true defining property of the disease) has been assumed. In the past decade, however, evidence from psychophysics, electrophysiology, and histology has shown convincingly that visual field loss is not generally, if ever, the first sign of optic nerve compromise.[85] Moreover, visual field loss, when present, may not be proportional to the loss of optic nerve fibers.[85] Nevertheless, perimetry remains the yardstick by which all other tests and physiologic findings are measured.

Progress in understanding the mechanisms that produce functional loss in glaucoma is being made on a broad front that includes psychophysics and electrophysiology. The current flood of new data can present apparent contradictions, the resolutions of which require a thorough knowledge of the basis of the testing techniques, as well as a sound understanding of neurophysiology.

This chapter presents a selective and critical review of studies in psychophysics and clinical electrophysiology as they relate to glaucoma. It also presents an integrated summary of recent research findings from relevant studies in psychophysics, neurophysiology, and single-cell electrophysiology. We hope that approach will enable the reader to better evaluate the continuing flow of new information in this exciting field. We believe that each of these test techniques, when used properly and within the limits of its basic assumptions, can provide valuable information on the current status and possibly the prognosis of glaucoma.

BASIC ELEMENTS OF THE VISUAL PROCESS

An understanding of the role of the basic visual elements is helpful in interpreting abnormal test results, as well as in devising new tests that may improve our ability to diagnose glaucomatous damage of the ganglion cell layer and optic nerve.

Variability in performance for psychophysical tests depends partly on variability in the sensitivity of the biologic detection elements and partly on the generation of biologic noise events in the visual detection system. The organization of the visual system appears to be designed to maximize performance for a variety of tasks under a wide range of adaption conditions.

Receptors

Four photopigments are present in the receptors of the eye. One, rhodopsin, accounts for about 95% of all the photopigment and is contained in rod receptors, which are organized to optimize perception at low-light levels. Because visual performance in the rod system is mediated by a single photopigment, discrimination on the basis of wavelength is not possible, and the rod system does not participate in color perception. The other three photopigments present in the normal eye are differentiated by their peak absorption efficiencies into three classes of cone receptors. The cone system is optimized for perception at moderate to high light intensities and, because of its three independent cone (trivariant) organization, can mediate wavelength discrimination, which is expressed behaviorally as color perception.

Absolute threshold detection experiments performed under conditions that optimize either rod- or cone-mediated perception have shown no difference in the ability of rod and cone photopigments to absorb photons. For rods, only one photon is required to be captured by one photopigment chromophore to initiate a visually significant event under completely dark adapted conditions. This rod requirement is maintained for an area of 5 to 7 rod outer segments within a time frame of about 50 milliseconds.[45] Similarly for cones, between 2 and 5 photon absorptions per receptor appear sufficient for stimulation.[14,108] However, under certain conditions, much larger differences have been recorded for overall rod system sensitivity compared with cone system sensitivity that can be accounted for on the basis of photopigment absorption. For example, dark adaptation thresholds recorded at retinal locations centered about 10 degrees in the periphery for a 5-degree target spot of white light show sensitivity differences of about 2.5 to 3.0 log units (a factor of 300 to 1000) between the cone and rod systems.[21]

Postreceptor Organization

Interpretation of test results depends partly on understanding postreceptor events. Photoreceptor responses are not simply transmitted to the centers of visual perception but are repeatedly transformed at successive stages along the visual pathway. For example, most of the enhanced sensitivity of the rod system compared with the cone system depends not on fundamental differences at the point of photon capture but on differences in transmission efficiency associated with the receptor[12,75] and on its postreceptoral organization, which pools information from thousands of receptors. Differences between rod and cone organization are greatest in the central foveal region where the cones have one-to-one connections as centers of midget ganglion cells, chromatically antagonistic receptive fields.[40,82] Thus organization of the rod system appears to be optimized to detect light signals at the lowest possible level and apparently to orient the cone-dominated fovea toward an area of interest. The cone system, by comparison, appears to be optimized in several ways to extract detailed feature information, such as edges, shapes, fine motion, texture, and color from an image at somewhat higher light levels.

Photoreceptors in a retinal pool form the receptive field of the ganglion cell to which they project and control. In addition to pooling or amplifying a weak signal, receptive fields for both rods and cones provide a spatial antagonistic arrangement optimized to accentuate or extract certain features from the stimulus. The classic receptive field described by Kuffler[64] for the cat and by Hubel and Wiesel[53] for the monkey, demonstrates a concentric arrangement of inhibitory elements surrounding an excitatory center. Nearly all primate receptive fields exhibit this antagonistic arrangement. Lateral communication is probably accomplished through amacrine and horizontal cell interneurons, but the mechanisms of interaction are not well understood.

Classification of ganglion cells based on temporal responses

In an important demonstration of functional differentiation, Gouras[40] identified two major classes of primate ganglion cells on the basis of their temporal response properties. A class of cells labeled *phasic* responds transiently to changes of stimulus intensity, whereas cells classified as *tonic* respond in a sustained fashion. Tonic and phasic ganglion cells are effectively segregated at the level of the lateral geniculate nucleus, where Kaplan and Shapley[59] found that tonic and phasic cells project, respectively, to the parvocellular and magnocellular layers.

Phasic ganglion cells appear to be responsible for high temporal frequency response at relatively low spatial frequencies. Nearly all phasic cells have both rod and cone input from rod and cone receptive fields of similar size.[33,42] These large cells make up about 10% of all ganglion cells in the peripheral retina and possibly less than 10% of the fovea. Based on anatomic evidence, phasic ganglion cells have correspondingly large, highly overlapping receptive fields,[79] with thick, fast-conducting axons. Most of the phasic cells summate linearly over their receptive field center, but about 20% to 30% of the largest phasic cells exhibit a nonlinear response, as evidenced by a flicker component at twice the stimulating frequency.[58] As expected for large receptive fields, spatial contrast sensitivity functions of phasic cells typically peak at low spatial frequencies of about 2 cycles/degree. The phasic cell reponse increases rapidly with contrast and approaches its maximum at a relatively low contrast of about 30%.[59]

Tonic ganglion cells are complementary to phasic cells in nearly every respect and are part of the midget system[82] in which most ganglion cells receive receptive field center input from only a single cone. Although a few tonic cells receive both rod and cone input, most receive only cone input.[112] The cells are small, with small receptive fields and slender, slowly conducting axons. Cells with short wavelength cone-center inputs have somewhat larger, faster-conducting axons than cells with only long and middle wavelength cone inputs.[26] Tonic cells include about 80% of all ganglion cells, and, unlike phasic cells, their foveal representation is amplified severalfold at the lateral

geniculate nucleus and cortical levels.[79] Their dendritic fields overlap by a factor of about two, although it is not clear how dendritic field size relates to functionally defined receptive field size for centers that have only single-cone input. Tonic ganglion cells respond less vigorously to luminance contrast than phasic cells and their response does not saturate quickly but continues to increase up to high luminance contrasts.[59]

Chromatic-achromatic classification of ganglion cells

The cone receptive fields vary in their ability to respond to light differing in spectral distribution. Primate microelectrode studies designed to reveal response characteristics of cone-driven single ganglion cells have identified cell types that respond differentially to different colors of light (chromatic cells), as well as cell types that are not able to differentiate on the basis of wavelength (achromatic cells).[27,40] These results have led to theories of parallel processing models for visual system function that separate chromatic from achromatic processing.[44,56] However, more recent data do not show complete separation of chromatic and achromatic function at the physiologic level. Thus virtually all cells that can be identified as tonic are chromatic under conditions of low temporal and spatial stimulation but respond as achromatic cells at high spatial and temporal frequencies. Phasic cells are achromatic independent of stimulus conditions.

The theoretical work of Ingling and colleagues[54,55] has provided important insights into the dual response charcteristics of tonic ganglion cells in both spatiotemporal and color vision. At low spatial and temporal frequencies, tonic cells function as color-opponent cells with spectral sensitivities that are differences between their center and surround cone inputs (Fig. 7-1). For example, a red (long wavelength) cone center and green (middle wavelength) cone surround would give rise to a $+R-G$ cell with the spectral sensitivity shown in Fig. 7-1. Cells with $-G+R$ are also found at the retinal level, as are color-opponent cells for yellow and blue ($+Y-B$ and $+B-Y$ cells).

At high spatial or temporal frequencies, however, these tonic chromatic cells are predicted to function as achromatic cells with spectral sensitivities equal to the sums of their center and surround inputs. Fig. 7-2 show the spectral response of a cell that is chromatically antagonistic at low rates (5 Hz) of temporal stimulation but that is completely additive at higher stimulation rates (30 Hz).[43,114,115] In other words, tonic cells should respond as achro-

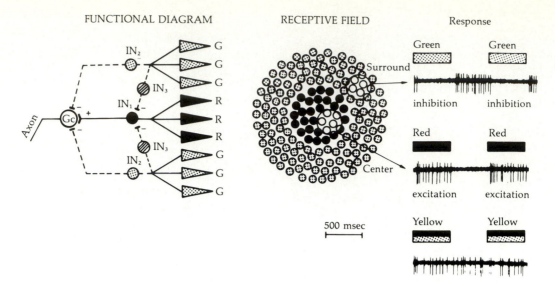

FUNCTIONAL DIAGRAM   RECEPTIVE FIELD   Response

Fig. 7-1 Simplified functional diagram showing receptive field structure, responses of color-opponent ganglion cell *(Gc)*. Red-sensitive cones in center act excitatorily (+), whereas green-sensitive cones in the surround act inhibitorily (−) by way of interneurons (IN_1 - IN_3). Yellow light, which stimulates both red- and green-sensitive cones, produces no modulated response to light, since center and surround contributions cancel each other. A stimulus covers entire receptive field with time course indicated by bar. (From Zrenner, E: Neurophysiological aspects of color vision in primates. Comparative studies on simian retinal ganglion cells and the human visual system. In Braitenberg, V, et al. In Braitenberg, V, editor: Studies of brain function, vol. 9, Berlin, 1983, Springer Verlag)

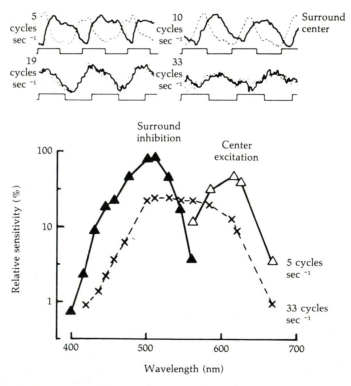

Fig. 7-2 Action spectrum of red/green color-opponent ganglion cell. Action spectrum is obtained for flicker threshold criterion at low (5 Hz, *triangles*) and at high (33 Hz, *crosses*) frequencies of stimulation in presence of white adapting light of 30,000 td. As reported by Gouras and Zrenner,[43,116] these cells lose color-opponency at higher flicker frequencies because of phaseshift between center and surround response as shown above. (From Zrenner, E: Neurophysiological aspects of colour vision mechanisms in the primate retina. In Mollon, JD, and Sharpe, LT: Colour vision physiology and psychophysics, New York, 1983, Academic Press)

matic cells to rapid flicker or to fine spatial detail, but they also respond to color-opponent cells to large, uniform, static targets.[117] These predicted transformations from chromatic to achromatic responses occur experimentally in single tonic cells.[27,43]

New test design

A detailed understanding of ganglion cell function is important in the design and interpretation of psychophysical and electrophysiologic tests for glaucomatous optic nerve damage. For example, the poor sensitivity of conventional perimetry to glaucomatous damage is not surprising when we consider that each point on the retina is normally covered by the receptive field centers of more than five ganglion cells, and that single ganglion cell responses can be measured for stimuli that are near psychophysical threshold. Diffuse ganglion cell loss should merely reduce redundancy (and thus increase variability) long before a measurable gap appears in the receptive field coverage. This argument suggests that tests designed to sample only a subset of ganglion cells (such as test of rod sensitivity or short wavelength cone sensitivity) should be more sensitive to diffuse loss because a smaller percentage of loss is needed to produce gaps in coverage. Tests can also be designed to test hypotheses about selective ganglion cell loss (for example, selective loss of cells with large axons, or selective loss of cells in short wavelength cone pathways), and to take advantage of any tendencies for selective loss that are confirmed. However, it is not always clear that "informed" test design will in fact lead to greater sensitivity.

Basis of Color Vision Testing

Mediation of color vision at the retinal level is accomplished in a two-stage process initiated by photon capture in the cones and transformed through the middle retinal layers into two opponently coded color signals at the level of the ganglion cells (Fig. 7-3). The three photoactive pigments present in the cone outer segment membranes mediate the capture of light photons. The electronic structure of the photopigment chromophore is transformed in shape when a photon of appropriate energy passes in close proximity and is "caught" or "captured." The transformed chromophore is released from its much larger opsin molecule, initiating a series of biochemical events that result in propagation of a signal along the cone outer segment membrane, through the cone inner segment, and into the network of interconnecting neurons of the middle retinal layers. The proba-

bility of a photon being caught by a cone photopigment depends on the energy of the photon (and thus its wavelength) compared with the optical energy needed to change the shape and to release the photopigment molecule from the opsin.

Once a photon is caught, all information concerning its wavelength is lost according to the principle of univariance.[74] The cone sensitivity functions illustrated in Fig. 7-3 are thus probability functions relating the photon's wavelength to the likelihood of initiating a visual event. From the point of photon capture in the cones, wavelength information is represented only in the relative ratios of photon hits in the three different cone classes and is apparently encoded by a transformation of the cone signals through the middle retinal layers. The mechanisms for this transformation are not completely understood, but the outcome at the ganglion cell level appears to correspond as a first approximation to some major attributes of perception.

The most important neural-perceptual correspondence is the apparent coding of the neural signal into opponent color pairs. At the level of perception, Hering[48] and others have described the opponent pairing of red with green and of yellow with blue. Members of a given pair cannot be perceived together in the same spatial area but can mix with either member of the opponent pair. Thus the appearance of red excludes the appearance of green in the same spatial extent at one time, but red may mix with yellow or blue. Color names reflect this exclusive pairing, since reddish greens and yellowish blues are not part of our color vocabulary.

The neural explanation for opponent color perception appears to depend on an antagonistic synapse scheme at the ganglion cell level. For example, inputs from long and middle wavelength cones synapse antagonistically on the same ganglion cell[40,41] producing the neural substrate for a red-green channel (see Fig. 7-1). Depending on the excitatory or inhibitory nature of the specific cone inputs, a given ganglion cell can either increase or decrease its firing rate from its resting level to signal a net imbalance in photon catches for the two types of cone.

Wavelength information in the form of the ratio of photon catches in the three cone classes is reflected in the relative firing rate of ganglion cells. However, a cell's firing rate cannot increase and decrease at the same time, which accounts for perceptual opponency to a first approximation. For example, a red (long wavelength) light will result in more photon catches in the long wavelength-

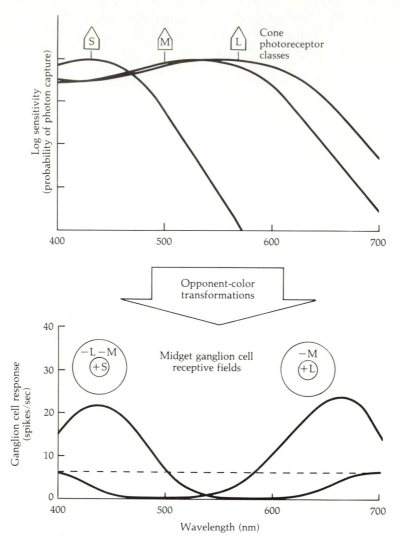

Fig. 7-3 Transformation of cone spectral sensitivities to opponent-color functions at ganglion cell level. Cone spectral sensitivities represent probability of capturing a photon of a given wavelength. Information concerning wavelength of a flux of photons is encoded at cone level only as a relative difference in cone firing rates. At a higher level, differences are represented as relative increases or decreases in ganglion cell firing rates, as shown by opponent functions at the bottom of the figure.

sensitive receptor and cause all red-green opponent cells to have unbalanced outputs in favor of red. At the same time, yellow-blue cells will be receiving net unbalanced inputs from both long and middle wavelengths (green) receptors, which pool their signals in opposition to the inputs from the short wavelangth (blue) cones. These yellow-blue ganglion cells will signal yellow. The relative strengths of the red and yellow signals are hypothesized to determine the perceived hue.

This simple picture of cone antagonism is complicated for the short wavelength cones, since short wavelength visible light produces a reddish sensation mixed with blue. The usual interpretation of this phenomenon is that some blue cones send

their signals to the R side of a proportion of R-G channels. Other new evidence indicates that middle wavelength cones may also contribute to the sensation of blue.[32]

The opponent explanation of color processing provides a way of interpreting the finding of disproportionate loss of yellow-blue color discrimination in glaucoma patients. Since color signals are separated into red-green and yellow-blue classes at the ganglion cell level, it follows that ganglion cell axons that form the optic nerve can also be separately identified. It is conceivable that glaucomatous optic nerve damage may differentially affect one or the other class of fibers. This might happen, for example, if yellow-blue fibers are more

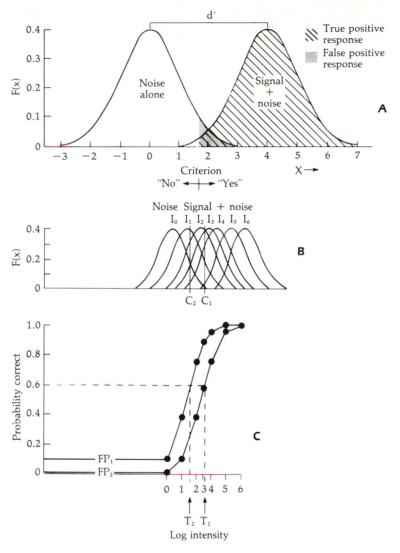

Fig. 7-4 Schematic of signal detection analysis of threshold behavior. **A,** Distance between the means of noise alone and signal-plus-noise distributions is labeled d', and is an index of how detectable (different) the signal-plus-noise distribution is. Area under curve of noise distribution to right of observer response criterion gives false positive rate, while area under signal-plus-noise distribution gives probability of true positive response. **B,** Different signal strengths (I_0 to I_6) produce different signal-plus-noise distributions, each characterized by a different d'. **C,** Setting response criterion allows prediction of response behavior in terms of probability of true positive (correct) response and in terms of false positive rate. Use of criterion C_1 yields right-hand response curve with low false positive rate (FP_1). Criterion C_2 yields greater sensitivity of response (curve moved to left) but higher error rate (FP_2). Actual threshold values (T_1, T_2) are determined by arbitrary assignment of desired probability of correct response, 60% in this case.

vulnerable to damage because they are larger in size than red-green fibers (but smaller than phasic cell fibers) or because they pass through the lamina cribrosa in disproportionate numbers within a zone particularly susceptible to mechanical disruption.[86,87,94] However, differential loss in blue sensitivity may also result from a loss of blue cone receptors or from a yellowing of the lens with increasing age. These processes would not be ex-

pected a priori to correlate with the glaucomatous process and therefore must be differentiated from optic nerve damage as a contributing cause of any observed yellow-blue color deficit.

PSYCHOPHYSICS

Concepts of Threshold Testing

All psychophysical tests used in the study of glaucoma are based on the concept of threshold testing. Intuitively, the concept of a visual threshold may be defined as that level of the critical variable of a visual task below which the subject fails to perform the task. For example, conventional visual field testing requires the detection of a spot of white light on a homogeneous white background. One can easily conceive of values for variables such as the intensity and spot size of a target light below which the spot will not be detected. However, on careful study, the apparent threshold value for a given observer is found to change from moment to moment. Instead of a single stable threshold value, a range of values is needed to define a transition zone from seeing to not seeing. Increasing values in this range are associated monotonically with increasing probabilities of detecting the spot of light (Fig. 7-4, *B*).

Threshold variation depends on the type of threshold task being presented (for example, the detection of light with or without a background, or discrimination between different patterns or colors) and on some behavioral characteristics of the observer.[92] For completely dark adapted detection of a small spot of light with no background (absolute threshold), variability in the threshold value may be accounted for by the unavoidable quantal fluctuations in the "constant intensity" light source.[45,101] However, most clinical tests are increment or discrimination threshold tasks at adaptation levels far above absolute threshold, where quantal fluctuations as a source of signal variation are insignificantly small, and the stimulus intensity is effectively constant.

Even when stimulus fluctuations are negligible, some "noise" or moment-to-moment biologic variation in the observer's visual system is always present. For example, the adaptation state and the sensitivity of the observer may drift, and spurious events may occur in the system that imitate the effect of true light stimulation. The task of the observer then is to detect a signal in the presence of background noise (noise distribution). The effect of stimulus presentation is to produce a new distribution of "events" in the system (signal-plus-noise) with a higher mean value than the mean value for the noise distribution alone. The success of the observer in detecting the signal depends on the separation between the noise and the signal-plus-noise distributions (Fig. 7-4, *A*). The separation between the means of the noise and the signal-plus-noise distributions is an important measure of signal detectability.

The ultimate response of the observer also depends on the "decision rule" that he adopts. For example, the observer may choose a certain (criterion) value along the dimension of interest (for example, brightness), above which he will always say the stimulus is present (answer "yes") and below which he will always conclude it is not present (answer "no"; see Fig. 7-4, *A*). The observer's basis for setting the criterion may be the desire to produce a limited percentage of false positive answers and may be manipulated at the will of the observer. Such decision rules, in conjunction with the characteristics of the noise and the signal-plus-noise distributions, finally determine the observer's response behavior.

A well-developed body of signal detection theory and experimentation supports this understanding of threshold performance.[34] From the physician's point of view, it is not as important to understand the mathematic details of signal detection theory as it is to appreciate the nature of threshold variation in diagnostic tests. For example, a naive patient may, for a number of reasons, set a criterion that is not stable throughout a test session, or one that varies between test sessions. The characteristics of the noise distribution may also vary, either in relation to the disease process (an outcome that might profitably be analyzed) or in response to other physiologic variables such as illness or lack of sleep.

Application of Threshold Techniques to Visual Field Testing

Visual field testing, or perimetry, is an adaptation of methods developed originally to investigate the nature of light detection at threshold. Clinical perimetric techniques differ from research paradigms primarily in the need to test many locations in the visual field. Although many perimetric methods have been tried, only two, kinetic and automated static perimetry, are used clinically. The kinetic method, as exemplified by the Goldmann perimeter, explores the limits of the visual field by measuring equal sensitivity contours, or isopters, using a moving, continuously illuminated test spot projected on a homogeneous white background. The spot is most often moved from an area of nonseeing to an area of seeing at some constant velocity. Although the Goldmann technique has provided the clinical standard for many years, major difficulties in obtaining quantitatively repeatable kinetic visual fields arise from variations in target speed, threshold criterion, and reaction time.

Computerized static perimetric methods have been developed recently in an attempt to improve the quantitative aspects of visual field testing. Static testing techniques are a direct adaptation of classical detection paradigms in that the patient is required to respond to a briefly flashed stimulus at many test locations in the visual field. As originated by Sloan[97] and developed by Aulhorn and Harms,[10] static perimetry consisted of manually measuring detection thresholds at regular intervals along one or more meridians in the visual field, usually without withholding knowledge of the test position from the subject. The advent of inexpensive microcomputers has allowed the development of automated static perimetry in which randomized stimulus sequences for many test locations in the visual field can be kept track of simulaneously. Inaccurate results caused by the patient attempting to fixate the ecentric target are minimized, since the next presentation position is unknown to the patient. However, thresholds tend to be higher and more variable when positional uncertainty is present compared with paradigms where the next presentation position is known.[9,23] In spite of positional uncertainty effects, automated static perimetry appears superior to manual kinetic methods in detecting early glaucomatous defects.[46,73,84]

A further problem with static perimetry is that, even with optimized automated protocols, the visual field cannot be examined in as much detail or as quickly as with kinetic methods. A new development by Drum[29] proposes a "hybrid" perimetry method that can produce detailed and accurate isopter maps with static stimuli. A constant-luminance flashing stimulus is moved in steps between flashes until the isopter boundary is found. The technique is faster than static perimetry and eliminates the reaction time errors inherent in kinetic perimetry. Preliminary studies indicate that variability is similar to static and kinetic thresholds.

Adaptation level effects

The effects of light and dark adaptation on glaucomatous visual defects have not been systematically investigated. The level of illumination in most current perimeters is dictated by compatibility or engineering considerations rather than by optimization studies. Threshold contrast (the ratio of test target luminance to background luminance) decreases with increasing adaptation level, suggesting that shallow scotomas might be more detectable on high-luminance backgrounds. On the other hand, Drum[30] has shown that scotopic thresholds are elevated substantially more than photopic thresholds in glaucoma, indicating that neural pathways receiving rod input may be selec-

tively damaged. However, the selective scotopic loss appears to be largely diffuse, in that localized scotomas appear to be of similar depth under photopic and scotopic conditions. It remains to be seen whether midphotopic or scotopic conditions will provide significant advantages over the mesopic and low-photopic conditions currently used in clinical perimetry.

Spatial and Temporal Vision in Glaucoma

Snellen acuity is the best known measure of visual spatial processing. The test letters are presented at the highest contrast possible as black figures on a white background, and the patient's performance depends on his ability to resolve the separation between elements in a letter. Thus visual acuity is a test only of high spatial frequency response at contrast levels far above threshold. In recent years methods of testing spatial vision have been borrowed from engineering concepts of system analysis that measure spatial processing at threshold contrast levels and at a full range of sinusoidal spatial frequencies.

Spatial contrast sensitivity

In tests of spatial contrast sensitivity, the patient is presented with alternating light and dark sinusoidal bars at different spatial frequencies and is then asked what is the minimum (threshold) contrast at which the bars can be seen at each frequency. As illustrated in Fig. 7-5, a contrast sensitivity test produces a modulation transfer function that, under an assumption of visual system linearity, can be used to infer performance for any arbitrary stimulus configuration. Fig. 7-5, *B* shows the relative modulation depth needed to see low-, medium-, and high-frequency stimuli at threshold.

Application of these techniques to glaucoma diagnostic testing demonstrates deficits in performance on a group basis. Based on the results of studies into the mechanisms of spatial contrast performance,[19,35] Arden and Jacobsen devised a clinically simple plate test and measured its usefulness in glaucoma patients.[4] The results showed a clear separation of hypertensive (glaucoma suspect) and normal scores from those of patients judged to be in various stages of glaucoma. Additional work with these plates[51,106] and with a CRT display[6,8,113] by Atkin et al. have shown that this type of test is capable of separating glaucomatous eyes from normal eyes. However, a high false positive rate is associated with this technique depending on scoring criteria.[99]

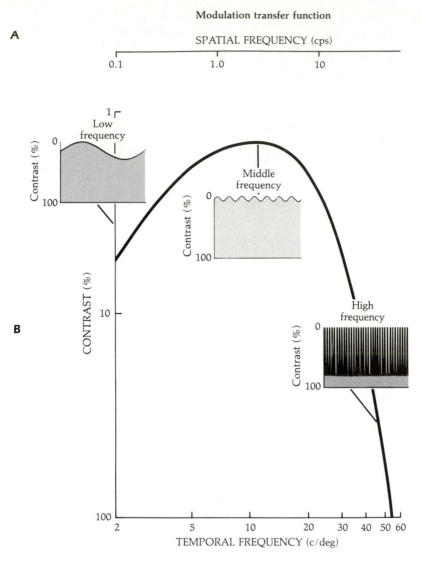

Fig. 7-5 Modulation transfer functions (MTF) for, **A,** spatial and, **B,** temporal paradigms. At each frequency, MTF gives contrast necessary for threshold detection of sine-wave grating (spatial paradigm) or pulse train (temporal paradigm). MTF is shown in schematic form for three frequencies in low, middle, and high ranges. The least "ripple" or smallest modulation is needed for detecting mid-frequency range spatial and temporal stimuli.

Other spatial discrimination tests

New testing techniques that rely on spatial discriminations other than detection of a spot of light on a homogeneous field have been introduced recently. These tests are based on the assumption that detection of a small spot of light is a perceptually simple task that potentially can be mediated by isolated ganglion cells, but that the perceptual ability to distinguish between differing spatial patterns requires a relatively intact matrix of receptive fields mediated by many neighboring ganglion cells at once.

Given their similar motivational basis, these techniques show considerable diversity in the method of stimulus presentation. Phelps et al.[80] have developed an acuity perimetry method in which the task is to resolve a grating produced on the retina with a laser interferometer. Regan et al.[88] have developed a set of letter acuity charts in which both contrast and letter size are varied parametrically. Taking an entirely different approach to low-contrast acuity, Frisen[39] has developed a visual field test in which the stimuli are low-contrast rings with the same space-average luminance as the uniform background field. In this test, ring diameter is varied until the ring is at detection threshold. Drum et al.[31] have developed a class of pattern discrimination tests in which the task is to detect a patch of nonrandom dots against a dynamic random dot surround. Although results from all of these new tests are encouraging, none has conclusively demonstrated greater sensitivity to early glaucomatous damage than conventional perimetry. Such a demonstration would, of course, require a prospective study of glaucoma suspects to determine whether early defects found only with the new test could predict glaucomatous damage measured by established parametric techniques.

Temporal contrast sensitivity

In a method similar to that used for spatial contrast sensitivity testing, modulation transfer functions can be generated for time-related (temporal) processing in the visual system by presenting a uniform target field modulated sinusoidally in time rather than as a function of spatial position.[25] Temporal discrimination testing demonstrates abnormalities in patients with glaucomatous damage. Tyler[105] measured modulation transfer functions for 5-degree diameter stimuli at the fovea and above the blind spot, and found significant midfrequency range defects both inside and outside conventional scotomas. Rossi et al.[91] reported that critical flicker fusion for small, threshold-level stimuli is reduced in glaucoma, but that the reduction is much smaller than would be measured using constant-luminance stimuli that ignore increment threshold defects. More recently, Stelmach et al.[100] have found losses of two-pulse temporal resolution, both in glaucoma suspects and in confirmed glaucoma patients.

In summary, both spatial and temporal contrast sensitivity testing yields significantly more complete and systematic data on the status of visual performance than conventional tests of visual acuity and critical flicker fusion. Both techniques show promise in detecting glaucomatous optic nerve damage at a stage earlier than is possible with conventional visual field methods. However, neither method has been evaluated in a longitudinal study that could firmly establish its false-positive as well as its false-negative rate in identifying those patients at greater risk of developing progressive visual loss.

Color Testing in Glaucoma

Color perception depends on differential photon absorptions in the three cone classes found in the normal retina. Disruption by a disease process of the cone receptors or the subsequent elements in the neural-visual chain may produce deficits in color vision, which may be measured clinically as abnormalities in color matching, spectral sensitivity, color arrangement (mediated by color appearance), and color discrimination. Studies of color vision deficits in glaucoma have employed variations of these and other techniques in a long history that dates from the end of the nineteenth century. Color vision defects have been consistently demonstrated using these foveally mediated testing methods in both glaucoma patients and suspects.

Testing methods

The Farnsworth-Munsell 100-hue test of color discrimination is the most used clinical method of assessing color vision in glaucoma. This test requires the patient to arrange in correct color order 85 desaturated (near white) color samples that are evenly distributed around the color circle. The color differences are small enough that normal observers generally make at least some mistakes. The test's clinical popularity derives primarily from its ease of use. It provides valid information on color discrimination ability that tends to correlate with other measures of color visual performance.

The D-15 test is another easily administered test, designed by Farnsworth, that is much used in clinical practice. The color differences are large compared with the 100-hue test and arrangement is based on a perceived color order in which dissimilar colors (reds and greens or blues and yellows) are not placed next to each other. The test is designed as a pass/fail screening test for congenital color defects and does not readily provide quantitative information suitable for clinical interpretation. It is also generally not as sensitive as the 100-hue test for clinical purposes. A derivative of the D-15, the Lanthony New Color Test incorporates more desaturated levels in an effort to gain sensitivity and is in limited use.[1]

Less commonly used for clinical purposes is the anomaloscope, in which two monochromatic primary colors are matched to a monochromatic test color. Although quantitative data interpretable in terms of receptor mechanisms may be obtained, a relatively expensive instrument and considerable examiner expertise are required.[65]

Classification of deficits

Deficits in color performance may be classed either as (1) congenital deficits, which are present at birth and are most often associated with otherwise normal visual function, or (2) acquired deficits, which are associated with either a disease process, a toxic process, aging of visual system elements, or any other environmentally induced or later-occurring genetic event.[81] Color test results may also be interpreted in terms of prereceptor or postreceptor neural loss. Prereceptor factors include the ocular media, especially the lens, and the yellowish macular pigment overlying the receptors in the macular region. Changes in the spectral filtering characteristic of these elements may affect color matching and discrimination, but basic trichromacy is not affected.

Receptoral loss, in contrast, may reduce the number of color dimensions. Total loss of one receptor class effectively reduces the normal trichromat to a dichromat, where only two, rather than three, primary colors are needed for color matching. Progressive disease almost never produces acquired, perfectly selective loss, either of receptors or of subsequent neural elements. Also, it is not possible from the clinical color test results to unequivocally specify the site of disease-related neural changes. Instead, the site of damage is commonly inferred from other supporting data on the disease state. Since glaucoma is a disease of the optic nerve, it is commonly presumed that color defects measured with these tests are associated with ganglion cell or optic nerve deterioration. This presumption may not always be well founded, since normal color deficits associated with the aging lens may mimic those produced by glaucoma.

Color deficits may show differentially greater disturbance along either the red-green or yellow-blue color axes, or the disturbance may be randomly distributed around the color circle. The classification of defects as either red-green or yellow-blue may be purely descriptive of the color regions where most errors are made, such as for the 100-hue or D-15 tests, or it may be tied to a physiologic interpretation of a defect that appeals to an opponent color's theoretical framework. The consensus of color vision studies is that differentially greater yellow-blue or tritan defects compared with red-green occur in a large percentage of glaucoma patients and in a somewhat smaller, but still greater than normal, percentage of glaucoma suspects. Francois and Verriest,[38] for example, reported in an early study using the 100-hue test that about 60% of 30 primary open-angle glaucoma patients showed differential yellow-blue defects compared with 3% (1 patient) who showed a red-green defect. Other studies report incidence rates for yellow-blue

defects in primary open-angle glaucoma using the 100-hue test that range from a low of 34%[66] to a high of 85%.[37]

Incidence of glaucoma-related color deficits

Factors that appear to effect the incidence rate of color deficits in glaucoma include the level of illumination during testing, the inclusion criteria used for defining a glaucoma patient or glaucoma suspect, and the normal limits used to decide if a patient shows a defect. The effect of illumination level on the absolute 100-hue error score is demonstrated in a study by Ourgaud et al.,[76] where illuminance level was set at 200 and 2200 lux for repeat tests on the same 14 primary open-angle glaucoma patients. The incidence rate for yellow-blue defects was 71% at 200 lux but declined to 9% at 2200 lux.

More recently, Breton et al.[15] reported a difference in intensity-response functions for primary open-angle glaucoma patients compared with normal. The intensity-response function was measured using the 100-hue test over a 3 log unit range of intensity from 1.6 to 1600 lux. An analysis of slope, range, and asymptote values for the function allowed identification of a color deficit in 83% of 24 primary open-angle glaucoma patients compared with a 58% incidence of color deficits based on a single score taken at 160 lux. The additional information provided by the intensity-response function may help in differentiating patients from normals on the basis of color performance. It may also increase the sensitivity of color testing in glaucoma, without loss of specificity.

Inclusion and exclusion criteria for defining patient categories also influence the reported color defect incidence rates. Lakowski and Drance[66] defined two ocular hypertensive categories on the basis of treatment status, and they defined three glaucoma categories according to severity of visual field defect. They reported a higher incidence of color defects for ocular hypertensives on treatment (50%) compared with those not on treatment (19%), and they reported increasing rates of yellow-blue errors (34% to 74%) for increasing severity of glaucomatous visual field defect. For this study, the treated ocular hypertensives showed a higher rate of color defects than the most mildly affected glaucoma group, suggesting some overlap in pathology not revealed by the extent of the glaucomatous visual field loss.

Demonstration that a visual functional deficit is associated with glaucoma is generally accomplished by statistically comparing glaucoma patients or glaucoma suspects with a normal age-matched control group. For example, Drance et al.[28] demonstrated a higher incidence of progression to glaucomatous visual fields for ocular hypertensives with elevated 100-hue scores. However, knowledge of the statistical correlation for the ocular hypertensive group was not of much help in predicting exactly which individuals would progress. Verification of a deficit for an individual patient is accomplished by comparing the individual score with the limits of normal for the appropriate age-matched group. Because of the relatively wide limits of the currently accepted normative data,[109,110] an individual score must be quite high to be judged abnormal. It is less difficult to demonstrate a statistical difference between two groups than to demonstrate a difference between an individual and a normal group mean.

In practice, color vision tests have not proved useful in diagnosing early stages of glaucomatous optic nerve damage. The level of color deficit required to demonstrate pathologic change usually cannot be recorded before other signs of optic nerve damage, such as progressive or asymmetric cupping and minimal visual field loss. Also adding to the uncertainty surrounding the use of color vision as an early indication of optic nerve damage is the failure to demonstrate foveally mediated color deficits in all cases of glaucoma where definitive visual field loss is present. This problem is shared with other tests, such as spatial and temporal contrast sensitivity. The assumption is that if foveally mediated color loss is a reliable sign of early damage, color deficits should be demonstrable whenever clear cut optic nerve damage is present as documented by visual field deficits.

In an effort to better understand the mechanisms leading both to color deficits and visual field loss, Breton and Krupin[17] looked at the correlation between color discrimination as measured by the 100-hue test and visual fields for both primary open-angle glaucoma patients and glaucoma suspects. No correlation between color discrimination and visual fields was found for suspects when age covariance was taken into account, as might be expected. However, the data also failed to demonstrate a significant correlation for glaucoma patients who showed definite visual field loss. This was true even though color deficits were clearly associated with visual field loss for the glaucoma group. These results suggest that other factors unrelated to the glaucomatous process may be contributing to the color deficit recorded for glaucoma patients.

Interpreting individual results

Depending on the instrument of color measurement, several factors contribute to "noise" variation in measurements on normals that in turn control the limits of a confidence interval used for deciding if an individual patient falls within a normal response range. These factors include (1) the effects of learning and other performance variables, (2) the degree to which lens density varies from the expected mean value for age, and (3) the variation in pupil size in the normal population compared with that of a glaucoma population undergoing treatment that might produce a fixed miotic pupil. In addition, it is possible for a mechanism such as loss of blue cones to contribute to a measured yellow-blue deficit, but also for this mechanism to not correlate with progressive optic nerve damage.

Particularly for the 100-hue test, learning effects may seriously interfere with attempts to record serial data on an individual. Breton et al.[16] reported a significant improvement in scores for about one third of their naive normal observers over the course of four retests. Without a pretest training procedure, it was impossible to record reliable serial intensity-response data in a substantial number of patients.

ELECTROPHYSIOLOGY

Electrophysiologic tests such as the electroretinogram (ERG) and visual evoked potential (VEP) provide information on the gross electrical functioning of certain physiologic structures. As with psychophysics, the techniques are minimally invasive (for example, contact lens and skin electrodes) but are objective in the sense that an instrument directly reads the "response" from the patient.

Electrophysiology is an attempt to gain objective information on the state of visual system functioning and thereby to bypass many of the most troublesome problems of psychophysical testing, such as an unstable response criterion, learning effects, and the need for competent behavioral response. The most reliable clinical electrophysiologic tool, the flash ERG has not provided useful information on optic nerve and ganglion cell function. Neither has the VEP been of much diagnostic use in glaucoma, even though it provides direct information on optic nerve function.

Electroretinogram

The ERG is the gross electrical response of the retina to a transient light stimulus, which, for clin-

Pattern ERG variability

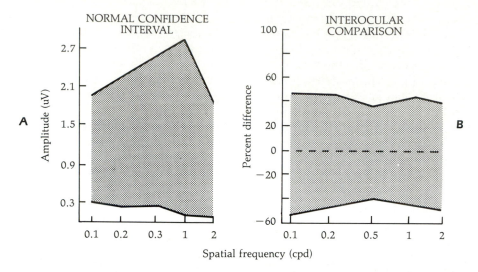

Fig. 7-6 Statistical variation in pattern electroretinogram (PERG) recordings. **A,** Variability in PERG recordings for normal eyes is such that 99% confidence interval as function of stimulus frequency extends close to zero. **B,** Interocular variability of PERG in normal subjects at 99% confidence level takes in response range of ±50%. (From Hess, et al: Invest Ophthalmol Vis Sci 26:1610, 1985)

ical testing, is usually a bright, brief pulse of light that uniformly illuminates the entire retina. The patient's eye is dark-adapted before the test to maximize the amplitude of the primarily rod response, which ranges from 300 to 600 μV in normal eyes. The ERG is clinically recorded with a corneal contact lens electrode connected to an amplifier and (usually) a computer system for displaying and saving the response waveform.

The ERG as obtained clinically from flashed stimuli has not been a useful test for glaucoma, since it reflects only the activity of radial retinal elements such as photoreceptors, bipolar, and Müller cells and not the activity of the ganglion cells and their axons that are affected in glaucoma. This origin of the flash ERG explains why the response amplitude is normal in patients with severe glaucomatous optic nerve damage.[2,47]

However, a recent technique using alternating checkerboard, bar or sine wave patterns has demonstrated a "pattern-evoked" ERG response that may reflect inner retinal activity.* In particular, Maffei and Fiorentini showed the pattern ERG to be absent in cats whose optic nerves had been severed, causing retrograde degeneration at the ganglion cell level.[68] Some evidence, which shows that the pattern ERG can be recorded in some cases of

severe optic nerve and retrograde ganglion cell disruption,[96,107] has challenged the hypothesis put forward by Maffei and Fiorentini that the ganglion cells are the origin of the pattern ERG.[68] Also, challenging this hypothesis in another way, Riemslag et al.[89,90,98,107] have argued that the so-called pattern ERG is merely a nonlinear component of the luminance response, having little to do with patterned stimuli per se. Partially reconciling these points of view are studies that have concluded the pattern ERG is a complex potential that depends on both luminance and pattern parameters.[11,31,61,93,116]

The origin of the pattern ERG is a matter of intense interest for glaucoma specialists, who are searching for a reliable clinical test of early glaucomatous optic nerve damage. Quigley et al. have shown that visual field tests,[85,87] which historically have been the definitive test of glaucomatous damage, do not show localized defects until more than half of the optic nerve axons have been destroyed. If the pattern ERG could reliably detect damage before field loss is recorded, it would be of great diagnostic value in glaucoma.

The amplitude of the pattern ERG is small (<10 μV) and variable, even in normal subjects.[50,60,104] Fig. 7-6, *A* shows that confidence limits for normal pattern ERG amplitudes extend nearly to zero, and Fig. 7-6, *B* shows that substantial amplitude differences between eyes are common in normal sub-

*References 5, 11, 24, 30, 36, 49, 61, 62, 69, 72, 111.

jects. Even though there is much evidence that pattern ERG amplitudes are significantly reduced in glaucoma,* it still is not clear that these reductions can be reliably detected in individual patients who may have (1) both eyes similarly affected but by unknown amounts, (2) preretinal opacities that have unknown effects on amplitudes, (3) large normal differences between left and right eye amplitudes,[50,60] or (4) normal pattern ERG amplitudes that are much larger or smaller than mean values.

Several investigators have reported that "far-field" pattern ERG response from a stimulated fellow eye can be recorded from the electrode placed on the unstimulated eye at almost the amplitude recorded for the stimulated fellow eye.[67,78,95] More recently, Arden et al. have confirmed that far-field artifacts are measurable with certain electrode configurations,[3] but at much lower amplitudes than are recorded for the stimulated eye. They note that all the studies reporting large artifacts used gold foil electrodes, which are quite sensitive to eyelid and eye movement artifacts that have been shown to mimic bioelectric potentials.[57]

In summary, the source of the pattern ERG response is not fully understood. There is abundant evidence that the pattern ERG is related at least partially to ganglion cell function, and that its amplitude is reduced by glaucomatous damage to the optic nerve. However, the pattern ERG, as it is measured with current techniques, is a small and variable potential that is difficult to record reliably, even in normal eyes. Major advances in recording and analysis techniques will be necessary for the pattern ERG to become clinically useful for early detection of glaucoma.

Visual Evoked Potential

The VEP is the gross electrical response of the cerebral cortex to visual stimulation. It is recorded clinically with scalp electrodes positioned over the primary occipital visual areas. The most potent stimulus is a centrally fixated, high-contrast reversing checkerboard, bar, or sine wave grating pattern displayed on a CRT screen that subtends about 10 to 15 degrees of visual angle. Although the visual angle is small, little is added to the response by increasing visual area. Studies of VEP amplitude as a function of stimulus area have shown that nearly all of the response comes from macular stimulation.[22] Unless foveal stimulation is explicitly avoided,[20] VEP abnormalities in glaucoma tend to reflect diffuse foveal damage more than the localized paracentral damage that is so often evident in early visual field defects.

The evidence available for VEP abnormalities in glaucoma is not impressive. Numerous studies have been done showing defects for patients with established glaucomatous visual field loss,* but these studies have not attempted to determine whether the VEP or the visual field showed the greater defect. As with the pattern ERG, advanced glaucomatous damage can produce a clearly abnormal VEP, but the abnormality usually is not pronounced enough to reliably detect early damage in individual patients. However, comparisons of VEPs in the two eyes of asymmetric glaucoma patients may be sensitive enough to be useful in assessing progression.[20,52] Interestingly, the delay in the VEP is correlated with glaucomatous visual field damage better than is the amplitude of the response.[7,20,102] The opposite is true of the pattern ERG.[52]

Mathematic models are used in clinical electrophysiology, as in psychophysics, in an attempt to understand the consequences of specific neurophysiologic loss. However, the output of any such model is limited by the elemental nature of the data and cannot be interpreted directly in visual functional terms. Therefore the results of an electrophysiologic test may tell us little about actual visual performance, although they may tell us much about the local electrical activity of specific neural and associated elements in the visual chain.

REFERENCES

1. Adams, AJ, Rodic, R, Husted, R, and Stamper, R: Spectral sensitivity and color discrimination changes in glaucoma and glaucoma suspect patients, Invest Ophthalmol Vis Sci 23:516, 1982
2. Alvis, DL: Electroretinographic changes in controlled chronic open-angle glaucoma, Am J Ophthalmol 61:121, 1966
3. Arden, GB, Hogg, CR, and Carter, RM: Uniocular recording of pattern ERG, Vision Res 26:281, 1986
4. Arden, GB, and Jacobsen, JJ: A simple grating test for contrast sensitivity: preliminary results indicate value in screening for glaucoma, Invest Ophthalmol 17:23, 1978
5. Arden, GB, Vaegen, and Hogg, CR: Clinical and experimental evidence that the pattern electroretinogram (PERG) is generated in more proximal retinal layers than the focal electroretinogram (FERG), Ann NY Acad Sci 388:580, 1982

6. Atkin, A, et al: Interocular comparison of contrast sensitivities in glaucoma patients and suspects, Br J Ophthalmol 64:858, 1980

7. Atkin, A, et al: Flicker threshold and pattern VEP latency in ocular hypertension and glaucoma, Invest Ophthalmol Vis Sci 24:1524, 1983

8. Atkin, A, et al: Abnormalities of central contrast sensitivity in glaucoma, Am J Ophthalmol 88:205, 1979

9. Aulhorn, E, and Durst, W: Comparative investigation of automatic and manual perimetry in different visual field defects, Doc Ophthalmol Proc Ser 14:17, 1977

10. Aulhorn, E, and Harms, H: Visual perimetry. In Jameson, D, Hurvich, L, editors: Handbook of sensory physiology, vol 8, no. 4, Visual Psychophysics, New York, 1972, Springer

11. Baker, CL, and Hess, RF: Linear and nonlinear components of human electroretinogram, J Neurophysiol 51:952, 1984

12. Baylor, DA, Nunn, BJ, and Schnapf, JL: the photocurrent noise and spectral sensitivities of the monkey *Macaca fasicularis*, J Physiol 357:575, 1984

13. Bobak, P, et al: Pattern electroretinograms and visual-evoked potentials in glaucoma and multiple sclerosis, Am J Ophthalmol 96:72, 1983

14. Bouman, MA, and Van de Velden, HA: The two quanta explanation of the dependence of the threshold values and visual acuity on the visual angle and the time of observation, J Opt Soc Am 37:908, 1947

15. Breton, ME, Fletcher, DE, and Krupin, T: Intensity response color test functions in glaucoma, Invest Ophthalmol Vis Sci 28(Suppl):62, 1987

16. Breton, ME, Fletcher, DE, and Krupin, T: The influence of serial practice on Farnsworth-Munsell 100-hue scores: the learning effect, Appl Opt (In press)

17. Breton, ME, and Krupin, T: Age and covariance between 100-hue color scores and quantitative perimetry in primary open-angle glaucoma, Arch Ophthalmol 105:642, 1987

18. Brindley, GS: Physiology of the retina and visual pathway, Baltimore, 1970, The Williams & Wilkins Co 19. Campbell, FW, and Robson, JG: Application of fourier analysis to the visability of gratings, J Physiol 197:551, 1968

20. Cappin, JM, and Nissim, S: Visual evoked responses in assessment of field defects in glaucoma, Arch Ophthalmol 93:9, 1975

21. Chapanis, A: The dark adaptation of the color anomalous measured with lights of different hues, J Gen Physiol 30:423, 1947

22. Chiappa, KH: Evoked potentials in clinical medicine, New York, 1983, Raven Press

23. Cohn, TE, and Lasley, DJ: Detectability of a luminance increment: effect of spatial uncertainty, J Opt Soc Am 64:1715, 1974

24. Dawson, WW, Maida, TM, and Rubin, ML: Human pattern-evoked retinal responses are altered by optic atrophy, Invest Ophthalmol Vis Sci 22:796, 1982

25. De Lange, H: Research into the dynamic nature of the human fovea-cortex systems with intermittent light. I. Attenuation characteristics with white colored light, J Opt Soc Am 48:777, 1958

26. De Monasterio, FM, Asymmetry of on- and off-pathways of blue-sensitive cones of the retina of macaques, Brain Res 166:39, 1979

27. De Valois, RL, and Pease, PL: Contours and contrast: responses of monkey lateral geniculate nucleus cells to luminance and color figures, Science 171:694, 1971

28. Drance, SM, Lakowski, R, Schuler, M, and Douglas, GR: Acquired color vision changes in glaucoma: use of 100-hue test and Pickford anomaloscope as predictors of glaucoma field change, Arch Ophthalmol 99:829, 1981

29. Drum, B: Hybrid perimetry: a blend of static and kinetic techniques, Appl Opt 26:1415, 1987

30. Drum, B, Armaly, MF, and Huppert, WE: Scotopic sensitivity loss in glaucoma, Arch Ophthalmol 104:712, 1986

31. Drum, B, et al: Pattern discrimination perimetry: a new concept in visual field testing, Doc Ophthalmol Proc Ser 49:433, 1987

32. Drum, B: Color naming of near-threshold monochromatic increments on white background. Topical Meeting Color Appearance, Technical Digest Series (Optical Society of America, Washington, DC), 15:50, 1987

33. D'Zmura M, and Lennie, P: Shared pathways for rod and cone vision, Vision Res 26:1273, 1986

34. Egan, JP: Signal detection theory, New York, 1975, Academic Press

35. Enroth-Cugel, C, and Robson, JG: The contrast sensitivity of retinal ganglion cells of the cat, J Physiol 187:517, 1966

36. Fiorentini, A, Maffei, L, Pirchio, M, Sinelli, D, et al: The ERG response to alternating gratings in patients with disease of the peripheral visual pathway, Invest Ophthalmol Vis Sci 21:490, 1981

37. Fishman, GA, Krill, AE, and Fishman, M: Acquired color defects in patients with open-angle glaucoma and ocular hypertension. In Verriest, G, editor: Modern problems in ophthalmology, ed 13, Basal, 1972, Karger

38. François, J, and Verriest, G: Les dychromatopsies acquises dans le glaucome primaire, Ann Oculist (Paris) 192:191, 1959

39. Frisén, L: A computer-graphics visual field screener using high-pass spatial frequency resolution targets and multiple feedback devices, Doc Ophthalmol Proc Ser 49: 441, 1987

40. Gouras, P: Identification of cone mechanisms in monkey ganglion cells, J Physiol 199:533, 1968

41. Gouras, P: Antidromic responses of orthodromically identified ganglion cells in monkey retina, J Physiol (London) 204:407, 1969

42. Gouras, P, and Link, K: Rod and cone interaction in dark-adapted monkey ganglion cells, J Physiol 184:499, 1966

43. Gouras, P, and Zrenner, E: Enhancement of luminance flicker by color-opponent mechanisms, Science 205:587, 1979

44. Guth, SL, and Lodge, HR: Heterochromatic additivity, foveal spectral sensitivity and a new color model, J Opt Soc Am 63:450, 1973

45. Hecht, S, Schlaer, S, and Pirenne, MF: Energy, quanta, and vision, J Gen Physiol 25:819, 1942

46. Heijl, A, and Drance, SM: Computerized profile perimetry in glaucoma, Arch Ophthalmol 98:2199, 1980

47. Henkes, HE: The electroretinogram in glaucoma, Ophthalmologica 121:44, 1951

48. Hering, E: Outlines of a theory of the light sense, Hurvich, LM, and Jameson, D, translators, Cambridge, MA, 1964, Harvard University Press

49. Hess, RF, and Baker, CL: Human pattern-evoked electroretinogram, J Neurophysiol 51:939, 1984

50. Hess, RF, et al: The pattern evoked electroretinogram: its variability in normals and its relationship to amblyopia, Invest Ophthalmol Vis Sci 26:1610, 1985

51. Hitchings, RA, Powell, DJ, Arden, GB, and Carter, RM: Contrast sensitivity gratings in glaucoma family screenings, Br J Ophthalmol 65:515, 1981

52. Howe, JW, and Mitchell, KW: Simultaneous recording of pattern electroretinogram and visual evoked cortical potential in a group of patients with chronic glaucoma, Doc Ophthalmol Proc Ser 40:101, 1984

53. Hubel, DH, and Wiesel, TN: Receptive fields of optic nerve fibers in the spider monkey, J Physiol 154:572, 1960.

54. Ingling, CR, Jr, and Drum, B: Retinal receptive fields: correlations between psychophysics and electrophysiology, Vision Res 13:1151, 1973

55. Ingling, CR, Jr, and Martinez, E: The spectral sensitivity of the R-G X-cell channel, Vision Res 25:33, 1985

56. Ingling, CR, and Tsou, BH: Orthogonal combination of the three visual channels, Vision Res 17:1075, 1977

57. Johnson, MA, and Massof, RM: The photomyoclonic reflex: an artifact of the clinical electroretinogram, Br J Ophthalmol 66:368, 1982

58. Kaplan, E, and Shapley, RM: X and Y cells in the lateral geniculate nucleus of macaque monkeys, J Physiol 330:125, 1982

59. Kaplan, E, and Shapley, RM: The primate retina contains two types of ganglion cells with high and low contrast sensitivity, Proc Natl Acad Sci USA 83:2755, 1986

60. Kirkham, TH, and Coupland, SG: Pattern ERGs and check size: absence of spatial frequency tuning, Curr Eye Res 2:511, 1983

61. Korth, M, and Rix, R: Effect of stimulus intensity and contrast on pattern ERG, Ophthalmic Res 16:60, 1984

62. Korth, M, Rix, R, and Sembritzki, O: Spatial contrast transfer functions of the pattern-evoked electroretinogram, Invest Ophthalmol Vis Sci 26:303, 1985

63. Krogh, E: VER in intraocular hypertension, Acta Ophthalmol 58:929, 1980

64. Kuffler, SN: Discharge patterns and function organization of mammalian retina, J Neurophysiol 16:37, 1953

65. Lakowski, R, Bryett, J, and Drance, SM: A study of colour in ocular hypertensives, Can J Ophthalmol 7:86, 1972

66. Lakowski, R, and Drance, SM: Acquired dyschromatopsias: the earliest functional losses in glaucoma, Doc Ophthalmol Proc Ser 19:159, 1979

67. Leguire, LE, and Rogers, GL: Pattern electroretinogram: use of non-corneal electrodes, Vision Res 25:867, 1985

68. Maffei, L, and Fiorentini, A: Electroretinographic responses to alternating gratings before and after section of the optic nerve, Science 211:953, 1981

69. Maffei, L, Fiorentini, A, Bisti, S, and Hollander, H: Pattern ERG in the monkey after section of the optic nerve, Exp Brain Res 59:423, 1985

70. Marx, MS, et al: Flash and pattern electroretinograms in normal and laser-induced glaucomatous primate eyes, Invest Ophthalmol Vis Sci 27:378, 1986

71. Massof, RM: Vision psychophysics and retinal cell biology. In Adler, R, editor: The retina part II, San Diego, 1986, Academic Press, Inc

72. May, JG, Ralston, JV, Reed, JL, and Van Dyk, HJL: Loss in pattern-elicited electroretinograms in optic nerve dysfunction, Am J Ophthalmol 93:418, 1982

73. Mills, RP, Hopp, RH, and Drance, SM: Comparison of quantitative testing in the Octopus, Humphrey, and Tubingen perimeters, Am J Ophthalmol 102:496, 1986

74. Naka, KI, and Rushton, WAH: S-potentials from colour units in the retina of fish (Cyprinidae), J Physiol 185:536, 1966

75. Nunn, BJ, Schnapf, and Baylor, DA: Spectral sensitivity of single cones in the retina of Macaca fascicularis, Nature 309:264, 1984

76. Ourgaud, AG, Vola, JL, Jayle, GE, and Baud, CE: A study on the influence of the illumination level and pupillary diameter on chromatic discrimination in glaucomatous patients. In Verriest, G, editor: Modern problems in ophthalmology II, Basel, 1972, Karger

77. Papst, N, Bopp, M, and Schnaudigel, OE: Pattern electroretinogram and visually evoked cortical potentials in glaucoma, v Graefes Arch Clin Exp Ophthalmol 222:29, 1984

78. Peachey, NS, Sokol, S, and Moskowitz, A: Recording the contralateral PERG: effect of different electrodes, Invest Ophthalmol Vis Sci 24:1514, 1983

79. Perry, VH, and Cowey, A: The ganglion cell and cone distributions in the monkey's retina: implications for central magnification factors, Vision Res 25:1745, 1985

80. Phelps, CD, Blondeau, P, and Carney, B: Acuity perimetry: a sensitive test for the detection of glaucomatous optic nerve damage, Doc Ophthalmol Proc Ser 42:359, 1984

81. Pokorny, J, Smith, VS, Verriest, G, and Pinckers, AJLG: Congenital and acquired color vision defects, New York, 1979, Grune & Stratton, Inc

82. Polyak, SL: The retina, Chicago, 1941, University of Chicago Press

83. Porciatti, V, and von Berger, GP: Pattern electroretinogram and visual evoked potential in optic nerve disease: early diagnosis and prognosis, Doc Ophthalmol Proc Ser 40:117, 1984

84. Portnoy, GL, and Krohn, MA: The limitations of kinetic perimetry in early scotoma detection, Ophthalmol 85:287, 1978

85. Quigley, HA, Addicks, EM, and Green, WR: Optic nerve damage in human glaucoma. III. Quantitative correlation of nerve fiber loss and visual field defect in glaucoma, ischemic neuropathy, papilledema and toxic neuropathy, Arch Ophthalmol 100:135, 1982

86. Quigley, HA, Dunkelberger, GR, and Sanchez, RM: Chronic experimental glaucoma causes selectively greater loss of larger optic nerve fibers, Invest Ophthalmol Vis Sci 27(suppl):42, 1986

87. Quigley, HA, et al: Morphologic changes in the lamina cribrosa correlated with neural loss in open-angle glaucoma, Am J Ophthalmol 95:673, 1983

88. Regan, D, and Neima, D: Low-contrast letter charts in early diabetic retinopathy, ocular hypertension, glaucoma, and Parkinson's disease, Br J Ophthalmol 68:885, 1984

89. Riemslag, FCC, and Heynen, HGM: Depth profile of pattern local electroretinograms in macaque, Doc Ophthalmol Proc Ser 40:143, 1984

90. Riemslag, FCC, Ringo, JL, Spekreijse, H, and Lunel, HFV: The luminance origin of the pattern electroretinogram in man, J Physiol 363:191, 1985

91. Rossi, P, Ciulo, G, and Calabria, G: Time resolution in glaucomatous visual field defects, Doc Ophthalmol Proc Ser 35:149, 1983

92. Sakitt, B: Counting every quantum, J Physiol 223:131, 1972

93. Schuurmans, RP, and Beringer, T: Luminance and contrast responses recorded in the man and cat, Doc Ophthalmol 59:187, 1985

94. Sanchez, RM, Dunkelberger, GR, and Quigley, HA: The number and diameter distribution of axons in the monkey optic nerve, Invest Ophthalmol Vis Sci 27:1342, 1986

95. Seiple, WH, and Siegel, IM: Recording the pattern electroretinogram: a cautionary note, Invest Ophthalmol Vis Sci 24:796, 1983

96. Sherman, J: Simultaneous pattern reversal electroretinograms and visual evoked potentials in diseases of the macula and optic nerve, Ann NY Acad Sci 388:214, 1982

97. Sloan, LL: Instruments and techniques for the clinical testing of light sense. III. An apparatus for studying regional differences in light senses, Arch Ophthalmol 22:223, 1939

98. Spekreijse, H, Estevez, O, and van der Tweel, LH: Luminance responses to pattern reversal, Doc Ophthalmol Proc Ser 10:205, 1973

99. Stamper, RL: Hsu-Winges, C, and Sopher, M: Arden contrast sensitivity testing in glaucoma, Arch Ophthalmol 100:947, 1982

100. Stelmach, LB, Drance, SM, and Di Lollo, V: Two-pulse temporal resolution in patients with glaucoma, suspected glaucoma, and in normal observers, Am J Ophthalmol 102:617, 1986

101. Teich, MC, et al: Multiplication noise in the human vision system at threshold. I. Quantum fluctuations and minimum detectable energy, J Opt Soc Am 72:419, 1982

102. Towle, VL, Moskowitz, A, Sokil, S, and Schwartz, B: The visual evoked potential in glaucoma and ocular hypertension: effects of check size, field size and stimulation rate, Invest Ophthalmol Vis Sci 24:175, 1983

103. Trick, GL: Retinal potentials in patients with primary open-angle glaucoma: physiological evidence for temporal frequency tuning deficits, Invest Ophthalmol Vis Sci 26:1750, 1985

104. Trick, GL, and Trick, LR: An evaluation of variation in pattern reversal retinal potential characteristics, Doc Ophthalmol Proc Ser 40:57, 1984

105. Tyler, CW: Specific deficits of flicker sensitivity in glaucoma and hypertension, Invest Ophthalmol Vis Sci 20:204, 1981

106. Vaegan, and Halliday, BL: A forced choice test improves clinical contrast sensitivity testing, Br J Ophthalmol 66:477, 1982

107. van den Berg, TJ, Riemslag, FC, deVos, GW, and Verguyn Lunel, HF: Pattern ERG and glaucomatous visual field defects, Doc Ophthalmol 61:335, 1986

108. van de Velden, HA: The number of quanta necessary for perception of light in the human eye, Ophthalmologica 111:321, 1946

109. Verriest, G: Further studies on acquired deficiency of color discrimination, J Opt Soc Am 53:185, 1963

110. Verriest, G, Laethem, J, and Uvijils, A: A new assessment of the normal range of the Farnsworth-Munsell 100-hue test scores, Am J Ophthalmol 93:635, 1982

111. Wanger, P, and Persson, HE: Pattern-reversal electroretinograms in unilateral glaucoma, Invest Ophthalmol Vis Sci 24:749, 1983

112. Wiesel, TN, and Hubel, DH: Spatial and chromatic interactions in the lateral geniculate body of the rhesus monkey, J Neurophysiol 29:1115, 1966

113. Wolkstein, M, Atkin, A, and Bodis-Wollner, I: Contrast sensitivity in retinal disease, Ophthalmol 87:1140, 1980

114. Zrenner, E: Neurophysiological aspects of color vision in primates. Comparative studies on simian retinal ganglion cells and the human visual system. Monograph. In Braitenberg, V, et al, editors: Studies of brain function, vol 9, Berlin, 1983, Springer Verlag

115. Zrenner, E: Neurophysiological aspects of colour vision mechanisms in the primate retina. In Mollon, JD, and Sharpe, LT, editors: Colour vision physiology and psychophysics, New York, 1983, Academic Press, Inc

116. Zrenner, E, Baker, CL, Hess, RF, and Olsen, BV: Current source density analysis of linear and nonlinear components of the primate electroretinogram, Invest Ophthalmol Vis Sci 27(Suppl):242, 1986

117. Zrenner, E, and Gouras, P: Retinal ganglion cells lose color opponency at high flicker rates, Invest Ophthalmol Vis Sci 17(suppl):130, 1978

Chapter 8

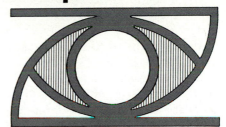

Aqueous Humor Formation

Stephen P. Bartels

Fluid production by a sodium pump

The biologic mechanisms responsible for the production of aqueous humor remain inadequately defined despite intensive scientific efforts that have been directed toward their elucidation. Our current understanding of aqueous humor production relates to improvements in analytic techniques and equipment rather than to any fundamental change in plausible hypotheses. Aqueous humor is produced primarily by a secretory process, although a small fraction may be produced by ultrafiltration. The focus of this chapter is on the role of secretion in aqueous humor formation and the ionic pump mechanisms that drive this process. Other aspects of the aqueous humor composition and biochemistry have been discussed in more comprehensive detail elsewhere.*

HISTORICAL PERSPECTIVE

It has long been debated whether aqueous humor is formed by ultrafiltration or by secretion. At the beginning of the twentieth century, Leber proposed that aqueous humor was a transudate of plasma.[35] In 1906, Henderson and Starling concluded that "the production of intra-ocular fluid is strictly proportional to the difference in pressure between the blood in the capillaries of the eyeball and the intraocular fluid."[43] In contrast, Seidel vigorously espoused the role of secretion in aqueous humor formation.[35] Because aqueous humor turnover proceeds at a very slow rate (1% to 2% min^{-1}), alternative hypotheses based on either ultrafiltrative (dialysis under pressure) or secretory mechanisms provided plausible explanations. However, a number of biochemical observations unequivocally supported secretion as the primary mechanism of aqueous humor production, including: (1) the effect of aqueous humor outflow on steady-state solute concentrations, (2) the rates of entry and turnover of radioactive tracers into the aqueous humor, (3) the higher concentration of ascorbate in the posterior rather than in the anterior chamber or the plasma, and (4) the low concentration of nonionized, freely diffusible urea in aqueous humor. These measurements indicated that active rather than passive forces were important in aqueous humor production.

In the late 1920s, Duke-Elder concluded that the hydrostatic pressures in the various vessels supplying and draining the ciliary body were compatible with ultrafiltration being the driving force behind aqueous humor formation.[29-31] He observed, however, that "in complicated physiological experiments the number of imperfectly con-

*References 10, 25, 26, 35, 73, 79.

199

trollable variables frequently leads to equivocal results."[32] Biochemical studies of horse and rabbit aqueous humor indicated that a correction had to be made for the unequal mass of solutes in plasma and aqueous humor when comparing the distribution of diffusible constituents. The deficit of sodium and excess of chloride supported the hypothesis that aqueous humor was in a Donnan equilibrium with plasma.[32] Plasma was found to have a greater osmotic pressure than aqueous humor ($\sim$20 mosm/L); the refraction and electrical conductivity of plasma did not change following equilibration with aqueous humor; and intraocular pressure responded predictably to changes in either the blood pressure or the osmotic pressure of either plasma or aqueous humor.[33,34] Duke-Elder concluded that the physical forces involved in the production of aqueous humor did not necessitate the intervention of any special secretory mechanism. Since the hydrostatic pressure in the vessels was comparatively greater than the intraocular pressure and because the osmotic pressure was greater in the capillary plasma than in the aqueous humor, the hypothesis that aqueous humor was a dialysate of plasma and that the two fluids were in a Donnan equilibrium was compatible with the physiologic data.

On the other hand, Duke-Elder also made the clinical observation that there was a low correlation between intraocular pressure and blood pressure, and consequently he provided a strong empiric foundation in favor of secretion having a role in aqueous humor formation. Friedenwald recognized that "if no through and through circulation of the aqueous exists [as distinguished from a closed thermal circulation or random diffusion], then obstructive theories of glaucoma are untenable."[38] Synechiae and adhesions in secondary glaucoma, iris bombé, and lens dislocation into the anterior chamber were suggested as examples of obstructions that caused ocular hypertension, and thereby supported his proposal that aqueous humor did indeed flow. He reasoned that, because aqueous humor was similar to a dialysate of plasma, aqueous flow would have to be small when compared with the diffusion of crystalloids into the ocular fluids. He went on to measure aqueous humor flow using the Smith-Leber-Niesnamoff method. Friedenwald cannulated the eyes of dogs and maintained normal intraocular pressure via an external reservoir. The calculated rate of aqueous flow was found to be 1 μl min^{-1} by blocking the outflow of aqueous humor via trabecular pathways with intracamerally injected serum. The movement of fluid out of the anterior chamber was measured by determining the displacement of an air bubble in a calibrated capillary tube situated between the eye and the reservoir.

Urea is a nonionic, metabolic end-product that, in solution, is freely diffusible across membranes. If aqueous humor is a true dialysate, equal concentrations of urea should be found in aqueous humor and in plasma. Adler found 25% less urea in aqueous humor than in blood, and concluded that aqueous humor is not a dialysate of plasma, and that "the membrane which separates the blood from the aqueous is not an inert semi-permeable membrane."[1]

Human studies finally resolved the question of whether aqueous humor was simply a dialysate of plasma. In 1938, Benham et al. found that the osmotic pressure of aqueous humor actually was greater than that of plasma.[6] They used cocaine to locally anesthetize patients' eyes before paracentesis and thereby eliminated artifacts caused by systemic anesthesia. Because the osmotic pressure of aqueous humor and plasma of glaucoma patients was not significantly different from normotensive controls, the obvious conclusion was "that pathologically raised tension in the eye is not a simple function of the osmotic balance between the aqueous humour and the blood."[6] Hodgson reported that the chloride concentration in human aqueous humor was much higher than could be expected if aqueous humor was in a Donnan equilibrium with plasma and that there were no significant differences in the aqueous humor/plasma ratios in normotensive patients compared with glaucomatous patients.[44] The authors concluded that variations in intraocular pressure could not be a simple function of chloride concentration:

> The conclusion to be drawn from this investigation is that the blood plasma and aqueous humour cannot be considered to be separated by inert membranes, which distribute ions in accordance with the requirements of a Gibbs-Donnan equilibrium. . . . The membranes in the eye, therefore, must possess the property of concentrating chloride in the aqueous humor. . . . It is possible that the high chloride of aqueous humour ensures the circulation of intraocular fluid and the maintenance of intra-ocular pressure.[44]

In the early 1930s Friedenwald investigated where and how aqueous humor could be secreted.[39] He found that fluid could pass easily from the ciliary capillaries to the posterior chamber, but that fluid did not pass in the reverse direction. This phenomenon was characterized as the *irreciprocal permeability to water* of the ciliary body. Thus, a boundary was identified where water could secrete if there was a local energy source that could generate a transbarrier potential energy difference. The presence of the necessary metabolic machinery was suggested by the behavior of dyes. Anionic, acidic dyes (e.g., eosin, bromphenol blue, rose bengal) penetrated the ciliary epithelium and accumulated in the stroma, although cationic, basic dyes (e.g., crystal violet, malachite green, night blue) accumulated in the epithelium.[40] This anomolous distribution pattern was interpreted as representing a vectoral transport mechanism dependent on oxidative metabolism, and the ciliary body's "veritable exuberance in pushing things around" made it the likely site of the secretory system for aqueous humor.[37] Results of reacting ciliary bodies with redox indicator dyes and grading the bleaching of the dyes indicated that an apparent redox potential difference of 230 mV existed between the ciliary epithelium (+100 mV) and stroma (−130 mV).[40] Friedenwald reasoned that, if this epithelial-stromal boundary could be reversibly oxidized, ionic transfer from the stroma to the epithelium could occur producing a fluid with excess sodium bicarbonate. While the staining patterns of these dyes do not appear directly related to aqueous humor transport, his view of "a dim but intriguing vista of integrative relations at the intercellular level" predicted an energy-dependent transport mechanism localized in the ciliary body and secreting a slightly hypertonic aqueous humor.[37]

In 1942 Kinsey et al. used deuterium oxide, heavy water, to measure the entry and exit rates of water in the eye. The half-life periods for measurements from blood-to-aqueous and from aqueous-to-blood ranged from 3 to 7 minutes and indicated that half of the water in aqueous humor is renewed every 2½ to 3 minutes.[57] The formation rate of aqueous humor would have to equal about 50 μl min^{-1} to account for these short half-life periods. Plasma water is constantly exchanging with extravascular water, and extravascular water continually exchanges with intracellular water. The rapid dispersion of deuterium oxide throughout the eye demonstrates clearly that the diffusion of water does not equal the slow net bulk flow of aqueous humor. In addition, Kinsey et al. performed investigations using radioisotopes of sodium, chloride, and phosphorus.[9] Following intraperitoneal injection, levels of radioactive sodium and chloride accumulated in the aqueous at a much slower rate (half-life period ~40 min) than did heavy water. By their calculations, an equivalent aqueous humor formation rate would be about 4 μl min^{-1}.[59]

Kinsey and Grant extended the observation that the chemical composition of the aqueous presented boundary conditions with which any quantitative characterization of flow would have to be compatible.[56] They proposed that, by determining the time course of a tracer substance in the blood and aqueous humor, mathematical models could be used to quantitate the blood-to-aqueous transfer rate and to infer whether the transfer occurred via an ultrafiltrative or secretory mechanism. They used their models to show that, when a substance was secreted into the aqueous humor and left the anterior chamber by bulk flow, its steady-state aqueous humor/plasma concentration ratio equaled the ratio of its coefficient of transfer from blood-to-aqueous to its coefficient of transfer out of the anterior chamber by flow.

$$\left(\frac{C_{aq}}{C_{pl}}\right)_{Steady\ State} = \frac{k_{in}}{k_{out}}$$

However, because neither the coefficient of transfer from blood-to-aqueous (k_{in}), nor the coefficient of transfer out of the anterior chamber by flow (k_{out}) can be directly derived from the steady-state aqueous humor/plasma concentration ratio, these steady-state ratios were not readily useful in determining the mechanisms involved in aqueous humor formation. But, following administration of a tracer substance, if the time course of the changing tracer concentrations in the blood and the aqueous humor could be determined, these data could be used "to infer by what process the transfer is taking place."[56]

Using this approach, Kinsey and Grant analyzed the aqueous humor/plasma ratio data for sodium, chloride, thiocyanate, lithium, bromide, and urea.[55,56,59] For each substance a number of aqueous humor/plasma ratios had been measured over the time course of the experiments. For a given ratio, a series of values for the blood-to-aqueous transfer coefficient could be calculated by using progressively increasing values for the transfer coefficient based on flow (Fig. 8-1). These values differed depending on whether the ultrafiltration model or the secretion model was used. Lines were plotted relating the flow coefficient to the corresponding blood-to-aqueous coefficent for each substance, and the point at which these lines intersected the line representing the coefficients at steady-state was identified. Thus, values were determined for the two transfer coefficients that characterized each substance during both dynamic and steady-state conditions. Two very different values were consistently predicted for the coefficient of transfer by flow: 0 μl min^{-1} with the ultrafiltration model and 4 μl min^{-1} with the secretion model. The ultrafiltration model predicted that, with any substantial outflow of aqueous humor, a substance would have to enter from the blood at a much greater rate than the data indicated if its steady-state ratio were to approach 1. The observed electrolyte concentrations that were close to 1 at steady-state (notably, sodium and chloride) could be attained despite significant outflow if they entered by a secretory process. These studies could not, however, be used to determine which ion was actually being secreted and which was the counterion.

Confirmation of the existence of a secretory mechanism and methods for quantitating the rate

of aqueous humor formation were sought during the late 1940s and throughout the 1950s. Davson et al. used a miniaturized system to dialyze plasma and aqueous humor.[27] Sodium and chloride consistently were found to move from the aqueous humor into the plasma. Because this excess could not be accounted for by either ultrafiltrative or outflow mechanisms, a secretory process by the ciliary epithelial cells was strongly indicated. Davson reported that inulin (MW ~5000), perfused into the anterior chamber under normal intraocular pressure, left the eye rapidly.[26] In case the cannulation had compromised the blood-aqueous barrier, an even higher concentration of inulin was perfused into the blood. The higher concentration of intravascular inulin would prevent diffusion out of the anterior chamber via iridial vessels. Because the inulin could not leave by diffusion and was not metabolized, it had to leave the eye by bulk flow. A clever method for measuring flow was developed by Bárány and Kinsey.[2] Following intravenous injection, paraaminohippuric acid, ^{131}I-Rayopake, and ^{131}I-Diodrast would enter the aqueous humor but would also be rapidly cleared by the kidney from the plasma. Two hours after injection, the concentration in the plasma was below that in the aqueous humor, and aqueous humor from one eye was removed. An hour later, aqueous humor from

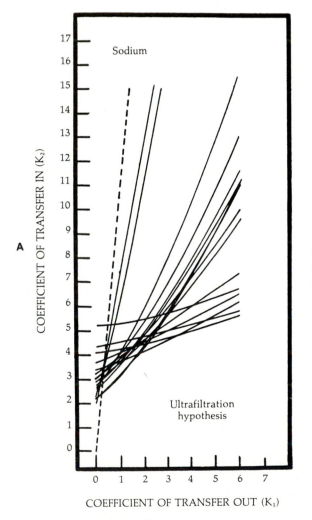

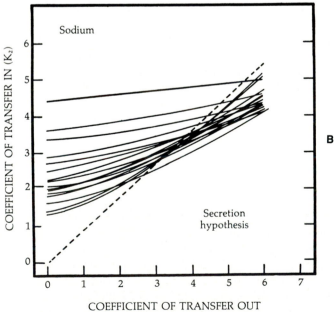

Fig. 8-1 Blood-to-aqueous transfer coefficient by flow for sodium. Different values obtained depend on whether **A,** ultrafiltration, or **B,** secretion model was used. (From Kinsey, VE: J Gen Physiol 26:131, 1942)

the opposite eye was removed. The difference in tracer concentration was used to determine a constant rate of disappearance from the anterior chamber, and this value was corrected for residual tracer in the plasma. The extreme limits for the rate of disappearance (k_{flow}) of these tracers were found to be 1.02% to 1.43% min⁻¹ irrespective of whether they entered by diffusion or secretion.[54] This translates to a flow rate of 2.75 μl min⁻¹, assuming an anterior chamber volume of 250 μl. The shortcomings of the individual methods notwithstanding, the cumulative data indicated that aqueous humor flowed at a slow but significant rate and, the data strongly supported the idea that a secretory mechanism functions in aqueous humor production.

Based on the high concentration of bicarbonate ions in rabbit anterior chamber aqueous humor, Kinsey proposed a system of aqueous humor production that emphasized a secretory mechanism for bicarbonate coupled to its counterion sodium.[50] At a relatively macroscopic level, the primary product of secretion by the ciliary processes was the

fluid behind the iris in the posterior chamber. By sampling this fluid, Kinsey found that an even higher concentration of bicarbonate and of ascorbate existed here than in the anterior chamber aqueous humor. However, the concentrations of both chloride and phosphate were lower in the posterior chamber than in the anterior chamber[51] Fig. 8-2). These results refuted the idea that iris vessels were impermeable to ions and suggested that aqueous humor was undergoing constant modification by diffusion across these vessels. Relative to the mechanism of secretion of aqueous humor, Kinsey postulated the existence of an energy-dependent bicarbonate-transport process that created hypertonicity in the posterior chamber.[51] The mathematical model of the data was improved to include exchange between the posterior chamber aqueous humor and the vitreous and lens.[52] A better approximation of time actually required for tracer entry could be made by allowing for the fact that the vitreous is not a well-stirred compartment, accounting for variable tracer plasma concentra-

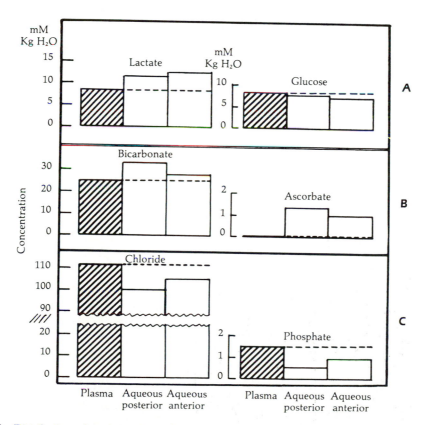

Fig. 8-2 Distribution of concentrations of various substances in plasma and aqueous humors of posterior and anterior chambers. Mode of entry into posterior chamber may account for distribution differences. These are **A**, diffusion, **B**, secretion, and **C**, diffusion with distribution altered by production (lactate) or utilization (glucose) by lens or other metabolizing tissue in anterior chamber. (From Kinsey, VE: Arch Ophthalmol 50:401, 1953)

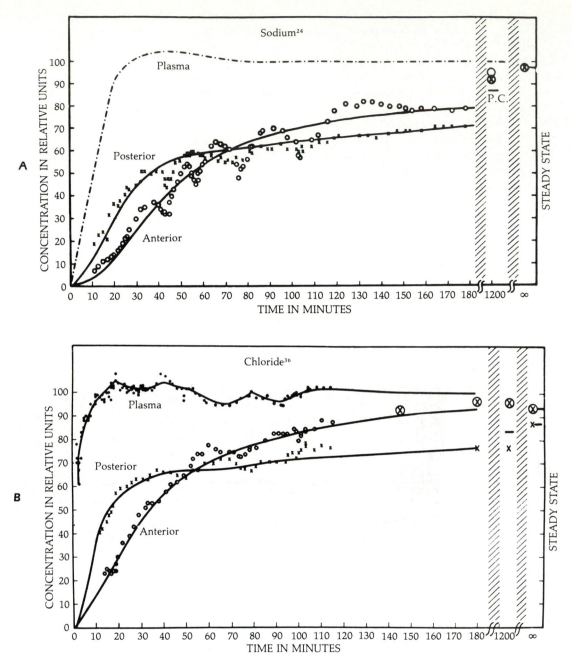

Fig. 8-3 **A,** Concentration of Na[24] in plasma and in posterior and anterior chambers of rabbit eye at various times after parenteral administration. **B,** Concentration of Cl[36] in plasma and in posterior and anterior chambers of rabbit eye at various times after parenteral administration. (Original data from Kinsey, VE: Doc Ophthalmol 13:7, 1959. From Kinsey, VE: Circulation 21:968, 1960)

tion, and by applying computer-aided data analysis.[58] The rates of accumulation of ^{24}Na, ^{36}Cl, and $H^{14}CO_3$ were used to determine transfer coefficients and to estimate the ionic composition of the posterior chamber fluid (Fig. 8-3). The high level of bicarbonate clearly indicated that it is an impor-

tant ion (Fig. 8-4). The aqueous humor/plasma distribution ratios in species other than rabbits did not consistently show a deficit of chloride or an excess of bicarbonate (Table 8-1).[25] This led Davson to deduce "that the essential factor in the production of aqueous humour may rather be the excess of so-

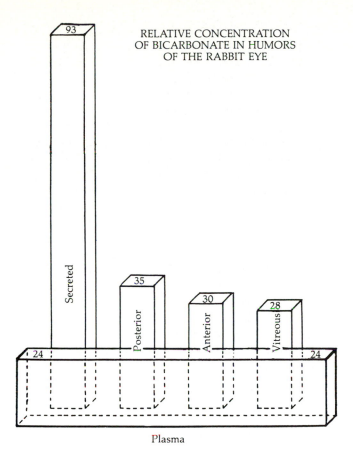

RELATIVE CONCENTRATION
OF BICARBONATE IN HUMORS
OF THE RABBIT EYE

Fig. 8-4   Relative intraocular concentrations of bicarbonate in rabbit eye. (From Kinsey, VE: Doc Ophthalmol 13:7, 1959)

Table 8-1   Distributions of chloride and bicarbonate between plasma and aqueous humor of various species

Species	Distribution-ratio (R_{Aq})	
	Cl^-	HCO_3^-
Horse	1·14	0·82
Ox	1·15	—
Sheep	1·16	0·83
Goat	1·09	0·67
Monkey	1·09	0·77
Man	1·13	0·93
Man	1·08	0·83
Galago	1·10	0·88
Dog	1·07	1·13
Cat	1·055	1·27
Rabbit	1·01	1·28
Guinea pig	0·935	1·35
Rat	1·025	1·15

From Cole, DF: Ocular fluids. In Davson, H, editor: The eye, ed 3, vol 1a, New York, 1984, Academic Press, Inc

dium."[26] In 1960, Kinsey concluded that "the probable hypertonicity of the fluid indicates that the mechanism involves a sodium pump and probably a diffusional transport of water as a result of osmotic forces."[53]

SODIUM/POTASSIUM - ADENOSINE TRIPHOSPHATASE (Na/K-ATPase) AND THE EYE

In 1957 Skou isolated from membrane fragments of crab peripheral nerve an ATPase whose activity depended on the relative concentrations of Na^+, K^+, Mg^{+2}, and Ca^{+2}.[85] In concentrations of K^+ equal to that found in the nerve, the activity of this Mg^{+2}-activated ATPase was highly dependent on the Na^+ concentration, and increased approximately linearly over a range of 10 to 100 mM. By analogy, an influx of sodium following depolarization of the nerve activated the enzyme. It was proposed that this ATPase, because of its affinities for Na^+ and K^+, could function as a regulatory enzyme controlling the intracellular concentration of these ions.[86] Today we believe that active transport involves one of three enzymes: Na/K-ATPase, H/K-ATPase, or Ca-ATPase. Generally, these are the only enzymes in the extramitochondrial membranes of animal cells that directly convert chemical work into osmotic work.[48,64,74] Fueled by metabolic energy, molecules are moved by these enzymes against a concentration gradient.

In animals, the net exchange across a plasma membrane of most other substances against their concentration gradient involves coupling their movement to the sodium electrochemical gradient. This gradient is generated by Na/K-ATPase, a large polypeptide chain (900 to 1200 residues) and cross-linked alpha-beta heterodimer. The alpha subunit (MW 120,000) is the catalytic subunit and is relatively hydrophobic. The beta subunit (MW 55,000) is a sialoglycoprotein. The enzyme spans the plasma membrane and has numerous membrane-associated regions that are distributed throughout the catalytic subunit. The most plausible hypothesis is that a cation channel is formed by the juxtaposition of the subunits. Neither rotational nor translational diffusion of NA/K-ATPase across the membrane is involved in the transmembrane active transport of Na^+ and K^+. Cations pass through the center of the enzyme. Catalysis is stimulated by covalent phosphorylation of an aspartic acid residue of the polypeptide. The source for phosphorylation is the gamma phosphate of ATP. In the presence of Na$^+$, the phosphorylated intermediate is formed; in the presence of K$^+$, the phosphorylated intermediate is hydrolyzed.

The native enzyme has two unique conformations, and these conformational changes are believed to be responsible for the movement of the respective cations from one side of the membrane to the other. The conformational differences are small structural changes in the geometry of the channel. Conformation E$_1$ provides access from the inside of the cell; conformation E$_2$ provides access from the outside. Transition from E$_1$-P to E$_2$-P requires Na$^+$ to be bound to the enzyme. The transition from E$_2$ to E$_1$ requires K$^+$ to be bound to the enzyme. During conformational changes, each cation remains in the compartment and then departs into the medium on the opposite side. Functionally, Na/K-ATPase creates electrochemical gradients for sodium.

BIOCHEMICAL LOCALIZATION OF Na/K-ATPase

Bonting et al. reported in 1961 that about 31% of the total ATPase activity in the human ciliary body was Na/K-ATPase.[13] This value was considered an underestimate because of the probability that contamination by the iris and the ciliary muscle would reduce the specific activity. Riley compared activity in ciliary epithelial cell suspensions, strips of epithelial cells, stroma, and homogenates with biochemically localized ATPase activity[75] (Table 8-2). Na/K-ATPase activity was 30 times greater in the ciliary epithelium than in the stroma. In cells fractionated on a Percoll gradient, both Na/K-ATPase and anion-stimulated ATPase activities were greater in nonpigmented ciliary epithelial cells compared with pigmented cells.[77] Upon subcellular fractionation, 90% of the anion-ATPase activity and 95% of the mitochondial marker, cytochrome oxidase, were found in the supernatant fraction; whereas, 80% of the Na/K-ATPase activity was found in the plasma-membrane fraction. In addition, the specific activity of the Na/K-ATPase in the plasma-membrane fraction of ciliary epithelial cells was 11 times greater than that in the supernatant fraction. These studies indicated that the ciliary epithelial cells had Na/K-ATPase in their plasma membrane and that the activity in nonpigmented ciliary epithelial cells was greater than that in pigmented ciliary epithelial cells.

To transport ions, Na/K-ATPase requires energy in the form of adenosine triphosphate (ATP). ATP can be made by either oxidative phosphorylation or glycolysis. Both pathways have been found to be more active in the nonpigmented ciliary epithelial cells than in the pigmented cells, and both oxygen consumption and glycolysis are inhibited by ouabain.[*] Thus, while sodium transport across the ciliary epithelium depends largely on energy generated by oxidative metabolism in mitochondria, Na/K-ATPase can also use glycolytic ATP as an energy source.

HISTOCHEMICAL LOCALIZATION OF Na/K-ATPase

Histochemical techniques have been used to determine the location of Na/K-ATPase in the ciliary body.[23,70,81,82,87] The localization of Na/K-ATPase in the basolateral regions of nonpigmented epithelial cells or in the numerous infoldings of their basal plasma membranes would strongly support the idea that the cellular mechanism mediating aqueous humor secretion is a standing-gradient osmotic flow system[28] (Fig. 8-5). Our current working hypothesis is that a hyperosmotic sodium gradient is produced and maintained in the intercellular spaces between adjacent nonpigmented ciliary ep-

*References 14, 15, 22, 63, 76, 78, 80

Table 8-2 ATPase of rabbit ciliary body in preparations made by different procedures

Preparation	Total activity (μmoles P$_i$ liberated/ mg N per hr)	Inhibition by ouabain (%)	Na–K-Dependent activity
(1) Beaded suspension	52	44	23
Beaded suspension after homogenization (tight)	42	18	7.6
"Processes"	—	56	—
(2) Whole homogenate (loose fitting pestle)	10	30	3.0
Stroma	8	6	0.5
Epithelial strip	29	63	18

From Riley, MV: Exp Eye Res 3:76, 1964

ithelial cells by the Na/K-ATPase active transport system. The excess sodium dilutes the water concentration in these spaces. Water flows down its concentration gradient from a higher concentration, intracellularly or intercellularly between pigmented and nonpigmented cells, to a lower concentration in the intercellular space, that is hyperosmotic as a result of the high concentration of sodium. Posterior chamber-to-stroma bulk flow of water is constrained by the tight junctions occluding the intercellular space around the nonpigmented cells at their apical ends. Net flow of aqueous humor is into the posterior chamber.

At the light microscopic level, ouabain-sensitive staining of the nonpigmented epithelium was observed in frozen sections incubated with ATP. However, whether the pigmented cells contained the enzyme was uncertain.[23] Using both fixed and frozen tissue, a dense, diffuse reaction product indicative of nucleoside phosphatase activity was found at the free surface and intercellular junctions of the nonpigmented cells.[70,81] The pigmented cells showed slight staining except at the nonpigmented-pigmented cell interface. At the electron microscopic level, staining resulting from hydro-

lysis of ATP occurred most prominently on the interdigitated cell membranes between adjacent nonpigmented epithelial cells and at the boundary between the nonpigmented and the pigmented epithelium[82] (Fig. 8-6). Intravitreal injection of 0.5 μg ouabain reduced staining of the ciliary epithelium.[81] Because this decrease in staining coincided with a reduction in intraocular pressure, the results suggested that the positive stain was indicative of transport enzyme activity. However, this nucleoside phosphatase activity could not be inhibited in vitro despite incubation with 10^{-2} to 10^{-8} M ouabain.[81] Tormey concluded, based on his evaluation of the histochemical methods for localizing Na/K-ATPase, that "there was no necessary relationship between histochemically demonstrated ATPase and transcellular transport."[87] He found that most of the stain was localized in the basal and lateral interdigitations of the nonpigmented epithelium (Fig. 8-7). However, he could not demonstrate ouabain or calcium inhibition, any difference in intensity of stain between sodium-containing and sodium-free incubation media, or a greater amount of staining in transporting ciliary epithelia as compared with nontransporting ocular epithelia (e.g.,

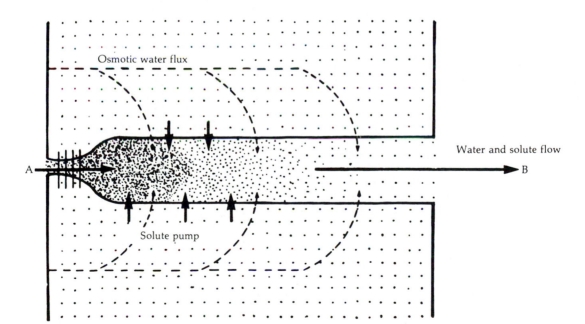

Fig. 8-5 Representation of standing gradient osmotic flow system consisting of a long, narrow channel, with restricted entry at left-hand end. *(A)*, Dot density indicates solute concentration. Solute is actively transported from cells into intercellular channel by a solute pump, making channel fluid hypertonic. As solute diffuses toward open end of channel at right-hand side. *(B)*, Osmotic differential allows water to enter across the walls. In steady state, a standing gradient is maintained as osmolarity decreases from the restricted to the open end as volume flows toward the open end. (From Cole, DF: Ocular fluids. In Davson, H, editor, The eye, ed 3, vol 1a, New York, 1984, Academic Press, Inc)

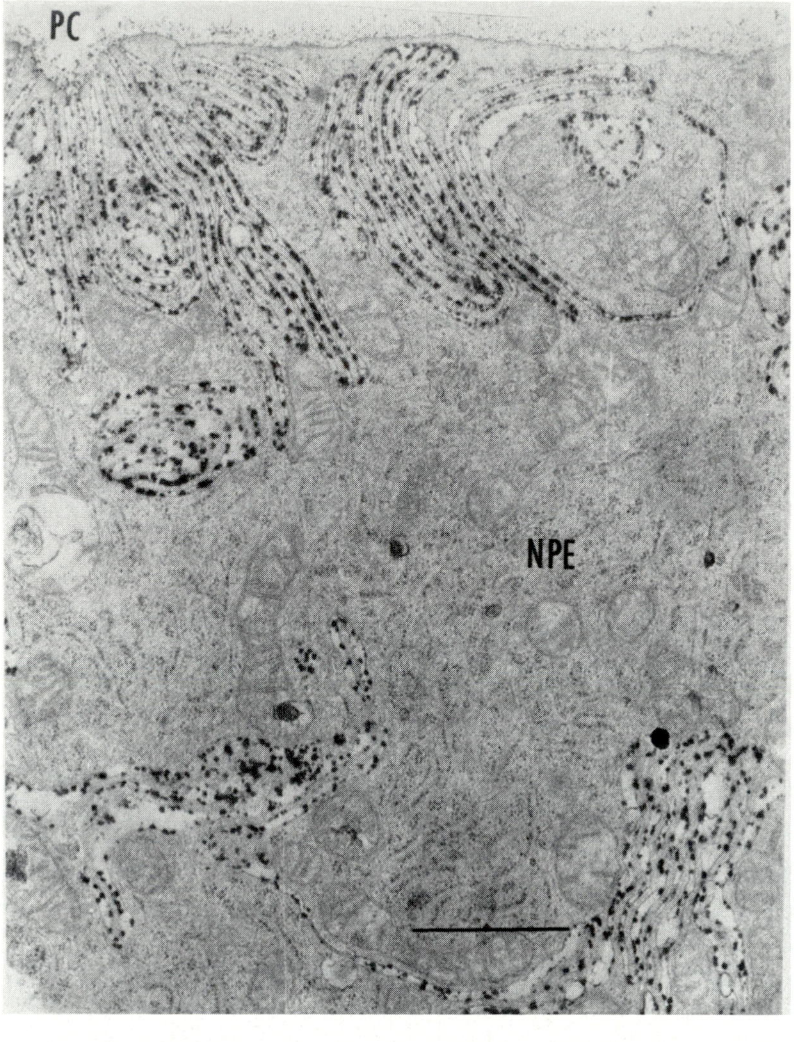

Fig. 8-6   Nucleoside phosphate activity in ciliary epithelium of albino rabbits. Frozen section incubated in Wachstein-Meisel medium at 37° C for 25 minutes with ATP substrate. Reaction product occurs equally on cell membranes near apical and lateral interdigitations. Sparse deposition observed along internal limiting membrane. *PC,* posterior chambers; *NPE,* nonpigmented epithelium. (2% glutaraldehyde fixation; ×27,900.) (From Shiose, Y et al.: Invest Ophthalmol 5:152, 1966)

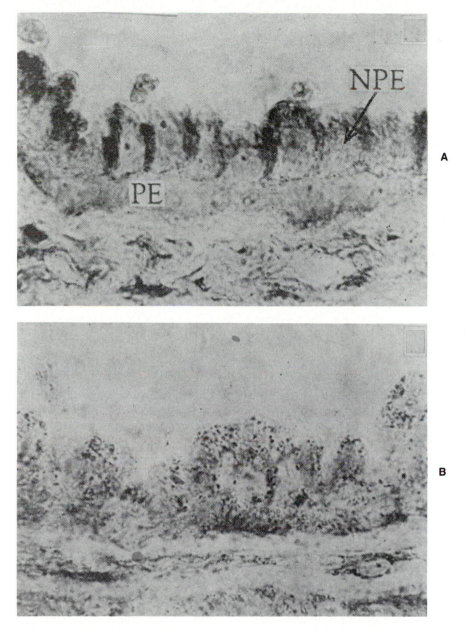

Fig. 8-7 Photomicrographs of ciliary epithelium of albino rabbit stained with Wachstein-Meisel ATPase medium ($\times$1100). **A,** Fixed 15 min with 3% glutaraldehyde shows membrane associated ATPase activity. Most of reaction product is found in *nonpigmented* epithelial layer *(NPE),* where it is localized adjacent to lateral cell borders and, to a lesser extent, near free cell surfaces. This distribution corresponds to distribution of plasma membrane interdigitations (infoldings) as seen by electron microscopy. Very small amounts of reaction product are also found in the basal portion of *pigmented* epithelium *(PE)* and between the two epithelial layers. **B,** Fixed 5 min with 2.5% hydroxyadipaldehyde, punctate reaction product corresponds to distribution of mitochondria through cytoplasm of both cell layers. Considerably weaker, diffuse staining is associated with interdigitations. (From Tormey, JM: Nature 210:820, 1966)

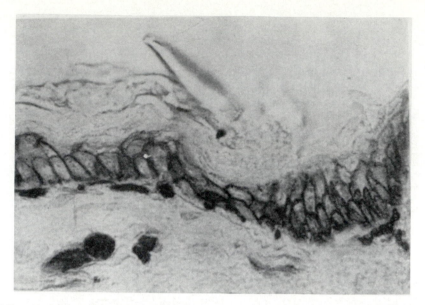

Fig. 8-8 Photomicrograph of albino rabbit eyelid epidermis, stained with Wachstein-Meisel ATPase medium. Cornified layers contain no reaction product. In the more basal layers, epidermal cell margins are outlined by an intense ATPase reaction. Localization demonstrated in this nontransporting epithelium resembles that found in frog skin ×530. (From Tormey, JM: Nature 210:820, 1966)

bulbar conjunctiva, palpebral conjunctiva, and palpebral epidermis)[87] (Fig. 8-8). Confirmation of the microscopic location of Na/K-ATPase in the ciliary epithelium will depend on whether the resolution of electron microscopic autoradiography will be adequate to locate radiolabeled markers such as ouabain. Immunohistochemical techniques may further refine our knowledge of the localization of the enzyme in the ciliary epithelium.

IN VIVO STUDIES

There is little doubt that Na/K-ATPase is integral to aqueous humor secretion. Turnover of ^{24}Na in the posterior and anterior chambers, aqueous humor flow, and intraocular pressure all decrease following systemic hypothermia by cold water immersion.[3,72] A temperature-related reduction in metabolic and enzymatic processes resulting in decreased sodium transport and aqueous humor secretion is suggested by these results. Cole measured the effects of two metabolic inhibitors, dinitrophenol and fluoracetamide, by blocking the drainage angle with silicone, collecting aqueous humor continuously through an anterior chamber cannula, and measuring the flow with a calibrated measuring capillary.[19] Both inhibitors caused about a 33% reduction of flow and influx of Na, Cl, and K. In other experiments involving insertion of a capillary electrode into the posterior chamber of rabbits, potential differences of 5 to 10 mV were found and the aqueous humor was positive relative to the plasma. Blood-aqueous potentials of similar magnitude and sign were found when the intraocular electrode was placed in the anterior chamber.[66] Cole calculated the active transport of sodium across the blood-aqueous barrier to be about 0.6 μEq min^{-1} based on its total flux (0.89 μEq min^{-1}) and determined the fraction of influx, when not inhibited by dinitrophenol (0.3 μEq min^{-1}).[20] Ouabain, administered via the lingual artery, decreased sodium influx, aqueous flow, potential difference, and short-circuit current (Table 8-3, Fig. 8-9).

Ouabain (65 μg kg^{-1}, IV) was found to specifically inhibit cat ciliary body Na/K-ATPase (41%), decrease intraocular pressure (19%) coincident with a drug-induced increase in systemic blood pressure, and reduce the rate of recovery of intraocular pressure (70%), following removal of aqueous humor.[83] The sensitivity of Na/K-ATPase to ouabain was species specific. In fact, the half-maximal inhibition concentration for rabbits was 3.6 times higher than for cats.[12] Ouabain in rabbits inhibited Na/K-ATPase following lingual artery or intravitreal administration.[4,11,20] Following intravitreal injection of 0.5 μg ouabain, intraocular pressure in rabbits remained reduced for days (7 mm Hg at 4 to 5 days after injection) without significant alteration of outflow facility.[4] This was compatible

Table 8-3 Effect of ouabain upon water and sodium influx and blood-aqueous potential difference

	Mean values ± SEM*	
	Before treatment	Change
Potential difference (mV)	6.10 ± 0.36	−4.40 ± 0.23
Inflow (μl min^{-1})	5.71 ± 0.50	−3.56 ± 0.54
Na influx (μEq min^{-1})	0.854 ± 0.08	−0.532 ± 0.09
Short-circuit current (μA)	435 ± 67	−350

From Cole, DF: Br J Ophthalmol 45:202, 1961
*SEM, Standard error of the mean.

with a 32% reduction in the rate of aqueous humor secretion. However, intravenous injection of 100 to 250 μg kg^{-1} ouabain (i.e., ~LD$_{50}$) had no effect on intraocular pressure. In cats, the inhibitory effect of intravenous ouabain on aqueous humor flow was found to be dose dependent over 18 to 67 μg kg^{-1}.[65] The 40% decrease in aqueous humor flow following intravenous ouabain (67 μg kg^{-1}) was correlated with decreased entry into the aqueous humor of 29% and 19%, respectively, for sodium and chloride.[41,69] In glaucoma patients, digoxin decreased intraocular pressure (14%) and calculated flow (33%) and reduced the rate of recovery of intraocular pressure (46%) following bulbar compression.[83] Unfortunately, however, even though the cardiac glycosides effectively reduce aqueous humor secretion and intraocular pressure, their side effects severely limit their clinical usefulness.[84]

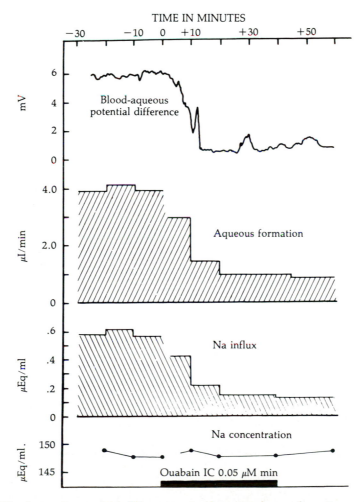

Fig. 8-9 Blood-aqueous potential difference, rate of aqueous humor formation, sodium influx, and plasma concentration during close arterial administration of ouabain. (From Cole, DF: Ocular fluids. In Davson, H, editor, The eye, ed 3, New York, 1984, Academic Press, Inc)

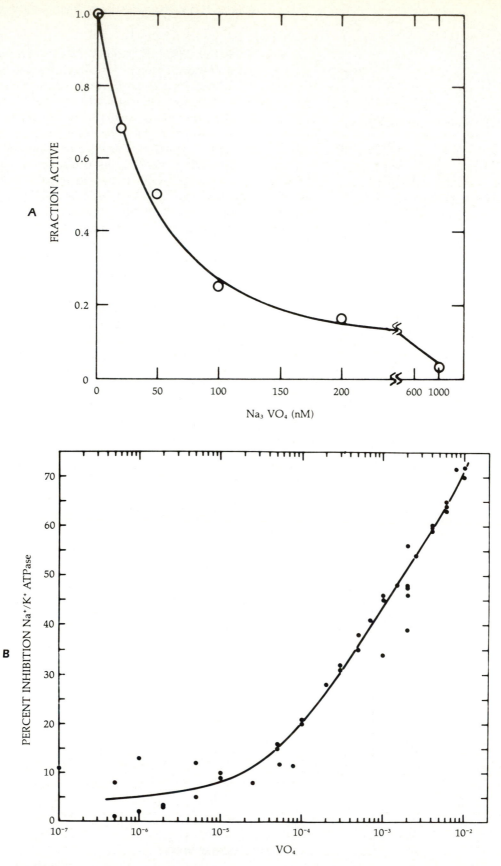

Fig. 8-10 **A,** Fraction of dog kidney Na/K-ATPase active at steady state as a function of Na_2VO_4 concentration. **B,** Inhibition by in vitro metavanadate of ATPase in deoxycholate extracted membrane fragments from normal rabbit iris and ciliary body. Total vanadate-sensitive ATPase (7.85 ± 0.23 μmol/mg protein/hr) was determined with 50 mM $NaVO_3$ and comprised about 40% of total ATPase activity. (**A** From Cantley, LC, et al.: J Biol Chem 252:7421, 1977; **B** from Mittag, TW, et al: Invest Ophthalmol Vis Sci 25:1335, 1984)

VANADATE

Vanadate is an inorganic anion that inhibits kidney Na/K-ATPase at low concentrations (K_i = 10 to 100 nM) and iris–ciliary body enzyme at higher concentrations (K_i = 50 to 100 μM)[16,62,68] (Fig. 8-10). Vanadate binds to the cytoplasmic portion of Na/K-ATPase where hydrolysis of ATP occurs and probably inhibits the phosphatase site of the enzyme. This mechanism is suggested because the high-affinity vanadate binding site is also the ATP binding site that stimulates Na/K-ATPase activity, and because competitive binding occurs between phosphate and vanadate.[17,49] Intraocular pressure decreased after 1% or 2% NaVO$_3$ or after 0.3%, 0.5%, 1%, or 2% Na$_3$VO$_4$.[61] Measured tonographically, facility of outflow did not change. The posterior chamber ascorbate concentration increased, indicating reduced aqueous humor flow.[5] Unfortunately the exciting possibility that topical vanadate can inhibit Na/K-ATPase in the ciliary processes is unlikely.

Na/K-ATPase activity was assayed in vitro by measuring intracellular uptake of radiolabeled rubidium (^{86}Rb), an element with chemical properties similar to potassium.[5] The iris–ciliary body accumulated ^{86}Rb against a concentration gradient. The rate of accumulation was time and temperature dependent and was inhibited by ouabain (IC_{50} = 1 μM). Vanadate also inhibited ^{86}Rb accumulation but required a much higher concentration (IC_{50} = 3 mM) (Table 8-4), probably because vanadate needs to penetrate the cell to inactivate Na/K-ATPase, whereas ouabain interacts with the enzyme at the extracellular surface. Following topical ocular administration, iris–ciliary body concentrations of vanadate in only the micromolar range were found, and no enzyme inhibition was detected using a membrane ATPase assay.[68] Although the membrane preparation procedures could have masked some inhibitory activity, the low tissue concentration of vanadate and relative insensitivity of iris–ciliary body Na/K-ATPase to vanadate suggested that its hypotensive effect was mediated by some other pathway.

IN VITRO STUDIES

Another method of examining transport mechanisms involved in secreting aqueous humor is to study the ciliary body tissue in vitro, isolated from cardiovascular, hormonal, and nervous regulatory pathways. Ciliary bodies can be removed surgically and placed in chambers designed to measure electrical characteristics, ion fluxes, and fluid flow. Most of these studies have been done in rabbits, although other mammals (ox, cat, monkey) have been studied.[18,21,46] Microelectrode studies have shown that the transmembrane electrical potential is negative relative to outside the cell, and that ciliary epithelial cells are electrically coupled.[7,24,42,67] Cardiac glycosides (strophanthidin and ouabain) produce only slow transmembrane depolarization of normal ciliary epithelial cells and partial inhibition of the volume regulatory response in swollen cells.[36,42,67] Transepithelial measurements indicate that the stroma-to-posterior chamber electrical potential is small and that the polarity depends on the composition of the incubation medium.[7,21,46,60,63]

Without exception, the experimental results of various in vitro methods support the hypothesis that the sodium pump is involved in ion transport by the ciliary epithelium and in the flow of aqueous humor into the posterior chamber. Swollen ciliary processes shrink by a mechanism that is sodium dependent and inhibited by ouabain.[8] The transepithelial potential difference depends on the presence of sodium.[21] The net influx of sodium ions persists in the short-circuited cat ciliary body and the coupled transport of chloride depends on the presence of sodium[45,47] (Fig. 8-11).

The short-circuit current (SCC), the current necessary to eliminate the electrical potential difference across the epithelium, is also sensitive to ouabain.[60,63,71] More recent observations have led to the evolution of a more comprehensive model of ionic transport across ciliary epithelium. Cole's model (1961) recognized the importance of the sodium pump[21] (Fig. 8-12, *A*). The model proposed by Krupin et al. in 1984 incorporates other important properties of the ciliary epithelium that affect ion transport[63] (Fig. 8-12, *B*). Based on the effect of ouabain on SCC, significant amounts of Na/K-ATPase are believed to be located not only on the

Table 8-4 *Inhibitors of ^{86}Rb accumulation by rabbit ciliary body (in vitro)*

Agent	Concentration (50% inhibition)
Ouabain	1×10^{-6}M
Vanadate	3×10^{-2}M
Prazosin	1×10^{-4}M
Phentolamine	7×10^{-4}M
Propranolol	3×10^{-4}M
Timolol	1×10^{-2}M
Cyanide	1×10^{-2}M
Iodoacetate	2×10^{-2}M
Dinitrophenol	2×10^{-3}M

From Becker, B: Invest Ophthalmol Vis Sci 19:1156, 1980

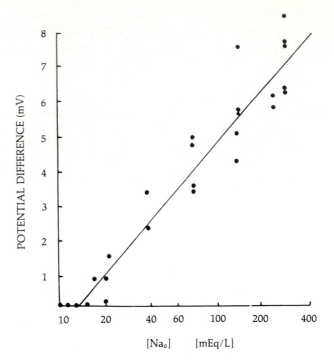

Fig. 8-11 Relationship between ciliary body potential difference (ordinate) and outside sodium concentration (Na_o). Abscissa scale is logarithmic, and regression line represents the equation:

$$E = 4.5 \log (Na_o) - 4.28$$

(From Cole, DF: Br J Ophthalmol 45:646, 1961)

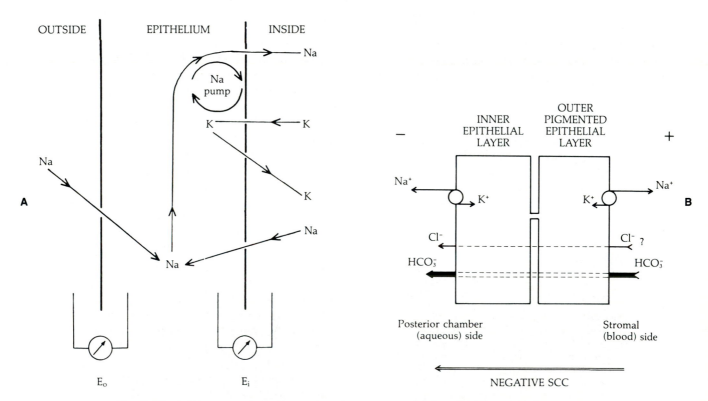

Fig. 8-12 **A,** Diagrammatic representation of cation permeabilities of blood-aqueous barrier at its outer (stromal) and inner (epithelial) surfaces. **B,** Proposed model of rabbit ciliary epithelial transport system. (**A** From Cole, DF: Br J Ophthalmol 45:641, 1961; **B** from Krupin, T, et al.: Exp Eye Res 38:115, 1984)

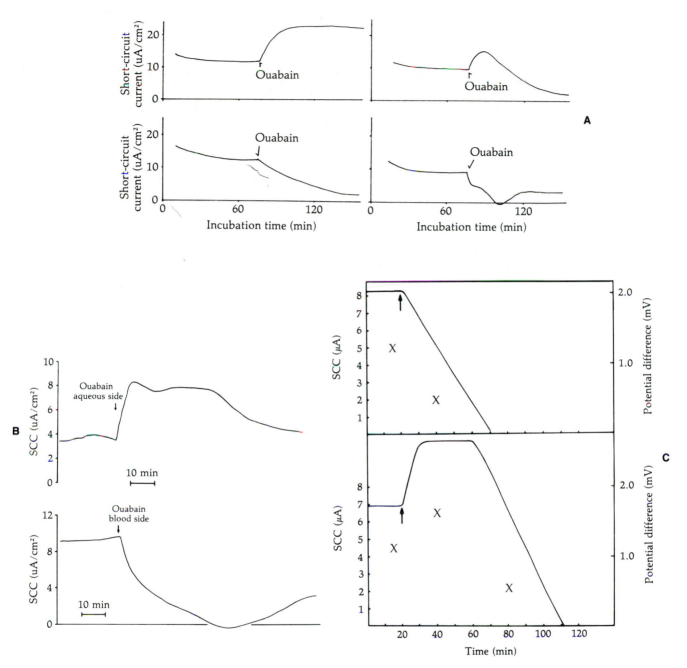

Fig. 8-13 **A,** Effects of ouabain (10^{-5} M) on short-circuit current (SCC) from aqueous side *(upper)* and from stromal side *(lower)*. **B,** Effect of ouabain (5×10^{-5} M) on SCC of isolated rabbit iris ciliary body. *(Upper)* Ouabain addition to aqueous side. *(Lower)* Ouabain addition to blood side. **C,** A typical effect of ouabain on rabbit iris ciliary body SCC when added to either ciliary body (blood) side *(upper)* or to ciliary process (aqueous) side *(lower)* of chamber. Measured potential difference is shown by *X*. (**A** From Kishida, K, et al: Jpn J Ophthalmol 25:407, 1981; **B** from Pepsin, SR, et al: Curr Eye Res 2:815, 1982; **C** from Krupin, T, et al: Exp Eye Res 38:115, 1984)

basolateral region of the nonpigmented epithelium, but also on the basolateral region of the pigmented epithelium. This conclusion is based on the observation that inhibition of SCC is especially pronounced when ouabain is delivered to the solution on the stromal side of the barrier but, when delivered to the solution on the posterior chamber side, the SCC transiently increases (Fig. 8-13). This difference in response suggests that there are two discrete populations of sodium pumps—one readily accessible from the stromal side, the other readily accessible from the posterior chamber side. Regardless of whether ouabain (0.1 mM) is added to the posterior chamber aqueous humor side or to the stromal side, the SCC across monkey ciliary epithelium is eliminated within 30 to 40 minutes[18] (Fig. 8-14).

Regarding the general question of aqueous humor formation, it has been consistently demonstrated with in vitro organ preparations that inhibition of Na/K-ATPase will completely inhibit electrogenic ionic transport. It would be ideal if these in vitro systems produced fluid at a rate similar to the aqueous humor formation rate in vivo. Then the more direct correlation between Na/K-ATPase and flow could be examined. Although this goal remains an objective of future research, there remains little doubt that aqueous humor is a fluid produced by a sodium transport mechanism in the ciliary epithelium. Consequently, any treatment regimen for glaucoma leading to reduced aqueous humor formation will probably involve a decrease in either the rate or efficiency of the sodium pump or in the total number of available pump sites.

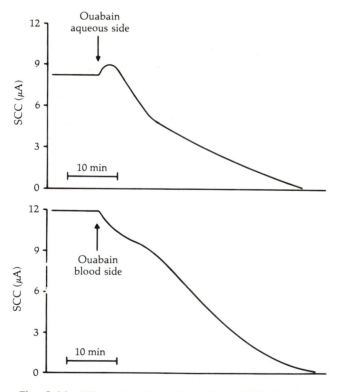

Fig. 8-14 Effects of ouabain (0.1 mM) on SCC of isolated monkey iris ciliary body. *Upper panel,* ouabain addition to aqueous side. *Lower panel,* ouabain addition to blood side. (From Chu, TC, et al.: Invest Ophthalmol Vis Sci 28:1644, 1987)

REFERENCES

1. Adler, FH: Is the aqueous humour a dialysate? Arch Ophthalmol 10:11, 1933
2. Bárány, E and Kinsey, VE: The rate of flow of aqueous humor. 1. The rate of disappearance of para-aminohippuric acid, radioactive Rayopake, and radioactive Diodrast from the aqueous humor of rabbits, Am J Ophthalmol 32:177, 1949
3. Becker, B: The effect of hypothermia on aqueous humor dynamics. 3. Turnover of ascorbate and sodium, Am J Ophthalmol 51:1032, 1961
4. Becker, B: Ouabain and aqueous humor dynamics in the rabbit eye, Invest Ophthalmol 2:325, 1963
5. Becker, B: Vanadate and aqueous humor dynamics, Invest Ophthalmol Vis Sci 19:1156, 1980
6. Benham GH, Duke-Elder WS, and Hodgson TH: The osmotic pressure of the aqueous humor in the normal and glaucomatous eye, J Physiol 92:355, 1938
7. Berggren, L: Intracellular potential measurements from the ciliary processes of the rabbit eye in vivo and in vitro, Acta Physiol Scand 48:461, 1960
8. Berggren, L: Effect of composition of medium and of metabolic inhibitors on secretion in vitro by the ciliary processes of the rabbit eye, Invest Ophthalmol 4:83, 1965
9. Besancon, RM: The encyclopedia of physics, New York, 1966, Reinhold Publishing Corp
10. Bill, A: Blood circulation and fluid dynamics in the eye, Physiol Rev 55:383, 1975
11. Bonting, SL and Becker, B: Studies on sodium-potassium-activated adenosine triphosphatase. 14. Inhibition of enzyme activity and aqueous humor flow in the rabbit eye after intravitreal injection of ouabain, Invest Ophthalmol 3:523, 1964
12. Bonting, SL, Caravaggio, LL, and Hawkins, HM: Studies on sodium-potassium-activated adenosine triphosphatase. 4. Correlation with cation transport sensitive to cardiac glycosides, Arch Biochem Biophys 98:413, 1962
13. Bonting, SL, Simon, KA, and Hawkins, NM: Studies on sodium-potassium-activated adenosine triphosphatase. 1. Quantitative distribution in several tissues of the cat, Arch Biochem Biophys 95:416, 1961

14. Braunagel, SC and Yorio, T: Aerobic and anaerobic metabolism of bovine ciliary process: effects of metabolic and transport inhibitors, J Ocular Pharmacol 3:141, 1987

15. Cameron, E and Cole, DF: Succinic dehydrogenase in the rabbit ciliary epithelium, Exp Eye Res 2:25, 1963

16. Cantley, LC, Cantley, LG, and Josephson, L: A characterization of vanadate interactions with the (Na,K)ATPase: mechanistic and regulatory implications, J Biol Chem 253:7361, 1978

17. Cantley, LC, et al.: Vanadate is a potent (Na,K)ATPase inhibitor found in ATP derived from muscle, J Biol Chem 252:7421, 1977

18. Chu, TC, Candia, OA, and Podos, SM: Electrical parameters of the isolated monkey ciliary epithelium and effects of pharmacological agents, Invest Ophthalmol Vis Sci 28:1644, 1987

19. Cole, DF: Effects of some metabolic inhibitors upon the formation of the aqueous humour in rabbits, Br J Ophthalmol 44:739, 1960

20. Cole, DF: Electrochemical changes associated with the formation of the aqueous humour, Br J Ophthalmol 45:202, 1961

21. Cole, DF: Electrical potential across the isolated ciliary body observed in vitro, Br J Ophthalmol 45:641, 1961

22. Cole, DF: Utilization of carbohydrate metabolites in rabbit ciliary epithelium, Exp Eye Res 2:284, 1963

23. Cole, DF: Location of ouabain-sensitive adenosine triphosphatase in ciliary epithelium, Exp Eye Res 3:72, 1964

24. Cole, DF: Aqueous humor formation, Doc Ophthalmol 21:116, 1966

25. Cole, DF: Ocular Fluids. In Davson, H editor: The eye, ed 3, vol 1a, New York, 1984, Academic Press Inc

26. Davson, H: Physiology of the ocular and cerebrospinal fluids, Boston, 1956, Little, Brown & Co

27. Davson, H, Duke-Elder, WS, and Maurice, DM: Changes in ionic distribution following dialysis of aqueous humour against plasma, J Physiol 109:32, 1949

28. Diamond, JR and Bossert, WH: Standing-gradient osmotic flow: a mechanism of coupling of water and solute transport in epithelia, J Gen Physiol 50:2061, 1968

29. Duke-Elder, WS: The venous pressure of the eye and its relation to the intraocular pressure, J Physiol 61:409, 1926

30. Duke-Elder, WS: The arterial pressure in the eye, J Physiol 62:1, 1926

31. Duke-Elder, WS: The ocular circulation: its normal pressure relationships and their physiological significance, Br J Ophthalmol 10:513, 1926

32. Duke-Elder, WS: The biochemistry of the aqueous humour, Biochem J 21:66, 1927

33. Duke-Elder, WS: The osmotic pressure of the aqueous humour and its physiological significance, J Physiol 62:315, 1927

34. Duke-Elder, WS: The pressure equilibrium of the eye, J Physiol 64:78, 1927

35. Duke-Elder, WS: The aqueous humour. In System of ophthalmology, vol 4, St Louis, 1968, The CV Mosby Co

36. Farahbakhsh, NA, and Fain, GL: Volume regulation of non-pigmented cells from ciliary epithelium, Invest Ophthalmol Vis Sci 28:934, 1987

37. Friedenwald, JS: The formation of the intraocular fluid, Am J Ophthalmol 32:8, 1949

38. Friedenwald, JS, and Pierce, HF: Circulation of aqueous. I. Rate of flow, Arch Ophthalmol 7:538, 1932

39. Friedenwald, JS, and Pierce, HF: Circulation of the aqueous. II. Mechanism of reabsorption of fluid, Arch Ophthalmol 8:9, 1932

40. Friedenwald, JS, and Stiehler, RD: Circulation of the aqueous. VII. A mechanism of secretion of the intraocular fluid, Arch Ophthalmol 20:761, 1938

41. Garg, LC, and Oppelt, WW: The effect of ouabain and acetazolamide on transport of sodium and chloride from plasma to aqueous humor, J Pharmacol Exp Ther 175:237, 1970

42. Green, K, Bountra, C, Georgiou, P, and House, CH: An electrophysiologic study of rabbit ciliary epithelium, Invest Ophthalmol Vis Sci 26:371, 1985

43. Henderson, EE, and Starling, EH: The factors which determine the production of intraocular fluid, Proc R Soc Lond [Biol] 77:294, 1906

44. Hodgson, TH: The chloride content of blood serum and aqueous humor, J Physiol 94:118, 1938

45. Holland, MG: Chloride ion transport in the isolated ciliary body. II. Ion substitution experiments, Invest Ophthalmol 9:30, 1970

46. Holland, MG, Mallerich, D, Bellestri, J, and Tischler, B: In vitro membrane potential of the cat ciliary body, Arch Ophthalmol 64:693, 1960

47. Holland, MG, and Stockwell, M: Sodium ion transport of ciliary body in vitro, Invest Ophthalmol 6:401, 1967

48. Jorgenson, PL: Structure, function, and regulation of Na,K-ATPase in the kidney, Kidney Int 29:10, 1986

49. Josephson, L, and Cantley, LC: Isolation of a potent (Na-K)ATPase inhibitor from striated muscle, Biochem 16:4572, 1977

50. Kinsey, VE: A unified concept of aqueous humor dynamics and the maintenance of intraocular pressure: an elaboration of the secretion-diffusion theory, Arch Ophthalmol 44:215, 1950

51. Kinsey, VE: Comparative chemistry of aqueous humor in posterior and anterior chambers of rabbit eye, Arch Ophthalmol 50:401, 1953

52. Kinsey, VE: Posterior and anterior chamber aqueous humor formation, Arch Ophthalmol 52:330, 1955

53. Kinsey, VE: Ion movement in the eye, Circulation 21:968, 1960

54. Kinsey, VE, and Bárány, E: The rate of flow of aqueous humor. 2. Derivation of rate of flow and its physiological significance, Am J Ophthalmol 32:189, 1949

55. Kinsey, VE, and Grant, WM: Further chemical studies on blood-aqueous humor dynamics, J Gen Physiol 26:119, 1942

56. Kinsey, VE, and Grant, WM: The mechanisms of aqueous humor formation inferred from chemical studies on blood-aqueous humor dynamics, J Gen Physiol 26:131, 1942

57. Kinsey, VE, Grant, WM, and Cogan, DG: Water movement and the eye, Arch Ophthalmol 27:242, 1942

58. Kinsey, VE, and Reddy, DVN: An estimate of the ionic composition of the fluid secreted into the posterior chamber, inferred from a study of aqueous humor dynamics, Doc Ophthalmol 13:7, 1959

59. Kinsey, VE, et al.: Sodium, chloride and phosphorus movement and the eye: determined by radioactive isotopes, Arch Ophthalmol 27:1126, 1942

60. Kishida, K, Sasabe, T, Manabe, R, and Otori, T: Electrical characteristics of the isolated rabbit ciliary body, Jpn J Ophthalmol 25:407, 1981

61. Krupin, T, Becker, B, and Podos, SM: Topical vanadate lowers intraocular pressure in rabbits, Invest Ophthalmol Vis Sci 19:1360, 1980

62. Krupin, T, Podos, SM, and Becker, B: Ocular effects of vanadate. In Krieglstein, GL and Leydhecker, W, editors: Glaucoma update II, Berlin, 1983, Springer-Verlag

63. Krupin, T, Reinach, PS, Candia, OA, and Podos, SM: Transepithelial electrical measurements on the isolated rabbit iris-ciliary body, Exp Eye Res 38:115, 1984

64. Kyte, J: Molecular considerations relevant of the mechanism of active transport, Nature 292:201, 1981

65. Macri, FJ, Dixon, R, and Rall, DP: Aqueous humor turnover rates in the cat, Invest Ophthalmol 5:386, 1966

66. Miller, JE: Alterations of the blood-aqueous potentials in the rabbit, Invest Ophthalmol 1:59, 1962

67. Miller, JE, and Constant, MA: The measurement of rabbit ciliary epithelial potentials in vitro, Am J Ophthalmol 50:855, 1960

68. Mittag, TW, et al.: Vanadate effects on ocular pressure, (Na^+,K^+)-ATPase and adenylate cyclase in rabbit eyes, Invest Ophthalmol Vis Sci 25:1335, 1984

69. Oppelt, WW, and White, ED: Effect of ouabain on aqueous humor formation rate in cats, Invest Ophthalmol 7:328, 1968

70. Palkama, A, and Uusitalo, R: The histochemical demonstration of sodium-potassium-activated adenosine triphosphatase activity in rabbit ciliary body, Ann Med Exp Biol Fenn 48:49, 1970

71. Pepsin, SR, and Candia, OA: Na^+ and Cl^- fluxes, and effects of pharmacological agents in the short-circuit current of the isolated rabbit iris-ciliary body, Cur Eye Res 2:815, 1982

72. Pollack, IP, Becker, B and Constant, MA: The effect of hypothermia on aqueous humor dynamics. 1. Intraocular pressure and outflow facility of the rabbit eye, Am J Ophthalmol 49:1126, 1960

73. Reddy, VN: Biochemistry of aqueous humor. In Lutjen-Drecoll, editor: Basic aspects of glaucoma research, Stuttgart, 1982, FK Schattauer Verlag

74. Repke, KR: A model of allosteric regulation of Na/K-transporting ATPase, Biochim Biophys Acta 864(2):195, 1986

75. Riley, MV: The sodium-potassium-stimulated adenosine triphosphatase of rabbit ciliary epithelium, Exp Eye Res 3:76, 1964

76. Riley, MV: The tricarboxylic acid cycle and glycolysis in relation to ion transport by the ciliary body, Biochem J 98:898, 1966

77. Riley, MV, and Kishida, K: ATPases of ciliary epithelium: cellular and subcellular distribution and probable role in secretion of aqueous humor, Exp Eye Res 42:559, 1986

78. Russmann, W: Levels of glycolytic enzymatic activity in the ciliary epithelium prepared from bovine eyes, Ophthalmic Res 2:205, 1971

79. Sears, ML: The aqueous. In Moses, RA, editor: Adler's physiology of the eye: clinical application, ed 7, St Louis, 1981, The CV Mosby Co

80. Shimizu, H, Riley, MV, and Cole, DF: The isolation of whole cells from the ciliary epithelium together with some observations on the metabolism of the two cell types, Exp Eye Res 6:141, 1967

81. Shiose, Y, and Sears, M: Localization and other aspects of the histochemistry of nucleoside phosphatases in the ciliary epithelium of albino rabbits, Invest Ophthalmol 4:64, 1965

82. Shiose, Y, and Sears, M: Fine structural localization of nucleoside phosphatase activity in the ciliary epithelium of albino rabbits, Invest Ophthalmol 5:152, 1966

83. Simon, KA, Bonting, SL, and Hawkins, NM: Studies on sodium-potassium-activated adenosine triphosphatase. 2. Formation of aqueous humor, Exp Eye Res 1:253, 1962

84. Simon, KA, and Bonting, SL: Possible usefulness of cardiac glycosides in treatment of glaucoma, Arch Ophthalmol 68:227, 1962

85. Skou, JC: Influence of some cations on an adenosine triphosphatase from peripheral nerves, Biochim Biophys Acta 23:394, 1957

86. Skou, JC: Further investigations on a Mg + Na-activated adenosine triphosphatase, possibly related to the active, linked transport of Na and K across nerve membrane, Biochim Biophys Acta 42:6, 1960

87. Tormey, JMcD: Significance of the histochemical demonstration of ATPase in epithelia noted for active transport, Nature 210:820, 1966

Chapter 9

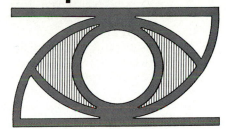

Pressure-dependent Outflow

Paul L. Kaufman

Aqueous humor enters the posterior chamber from the ciliary processes as a result of hydrostatic and osmotic gradients between the posterior chamber and the ciliary process vasculature and stroma,[19,53,180,221] and action ion transport across the ciliary epithelium.[147,174] The aqueous humor then flows around the lens and through the pupil into the anterior chamber, leaving the eye by passive bulk flow via the following pathways at the anterior chamber angle:

1. The trabecular or conventional route: through the trabecular meshwork, across the inner wall of Schlemm's canal, and then into collector channels, aqueous veins, and the general venous circulation
2. The posterior, unconventional, or uveoscleral route[53] (see Chapter 10): across the iris root and the anterior face of the ciliary muscle, through the connective tissue between muscle bundles, into the suprachoroidal space, and then out through the sclera

In various monkey species, the trabecular route accounts for 45% to 70% of the total drainage of aqueous humor, the uveoscleral pathway draining the remainder.[47] In the normal eye, the importance of the uveoscleral pathway has not been well quantitated. In the eyes of middle-aged or elderly people with posterior segment tumors, this pathway accounts for 5% to 20% of total aqueous humor drainage.[49] There is relatively little uveoscleral drainage of aqueous humor in cats[36] or rabbits.[37] Other potential routes of aqueous humor egress include reabsorption of nascent fluid by the ciliary processes themselves,[53] and flow posteriorly across the vitreoretinal interface. There is little net water movement across the iris vasculature.[52,55]

FLUID MECHANICS

The chamber angle tissues offer a certain normal resistance to fluid outflow. Intraocular pressure builds up, in response to the inflow of aqueous humor, to a level sufficient to drive fluid across that resistance at the same rate at which it is produced by the ciliary body; this is the steady-state intraocular pressure. In the glaucomatous eye, this resistance is unusually high, causing an elevated pressure. Although the proportionate distribution of this resistance within the chamber angle tissues is unsettled, the general consensus is that in the normal monkey eye and in the normal and glaucomatous human eye, most of the resistance lies across and within the trabecular meshwork,[17,106,107] perhaps in the cribriform region adjacent to the inner wall of Schlemm's canal.[50,53,125,165]

Understanding the factors governing normal and abnormal aqueous humor formation, aqueous humor outflow, intraocular pressure, and their interrelationships and manipulation is vital to understanding and treating glaucoma. Briefly, let

F	=	flow ($\mu l \times min^{-1}$)
F_{in}	=	total aqueous humor inflow
F_s	=	inflow from active secretion
F_f	=	inflow from ultrafiltration
F_{out}	=	total aqueous humor outflow
F_{trab}	=	outflow via trabecular pathway
F_u	=	outflow via uveoscleral pathway
P	=	pressure (mm Hg)
P_i	=	intraocular pressure

P_e = episcleral venous pressure
R = resistance to flow (mm Hg × min × $\mu1^{-1}$)
C = facility or conductance of flow ($\mu1 \times min^{-1} \times mm\ Hg^{-1}$) = 1/R
C_{tot} = total aqueous humor flow facility
C_{trab} = facility of outflow via trabecular pathway
C_u = facility of outflow via uveoscleral pathway
C_{ps} = facility of inflow

Then

F_{in} = F_s + F_f
F_{out} = F_{trab} + F_u
C_{tot} = C_{trab} + C_u + C_{ps}

At steady-state

F = F_{in} = F_{out}

The simplest hydraulic model, represented by the classic Goldmann equation, views aqueous humor flow as passive, non-energy-dependent, bulk fluid movement down a pressure gradient, with aqueous humor leaving the eye only via the trabecular route, where $\Delta P = P_i - P_e$, so that $F = C_{trab} (P_i - P_e)$. This relationship, although correct, is vastly oversimplified. Since there is no delimitation of the spaces between the trabecular beams and the spaces between the ciliary muscle bundles,[122] fluid can pass from the chamber angle into the tissue spaces within the ciliary muscle. These spaces in turn open into the suprachoroid, from which fluid can pass through the scleral substance or the perivascular/perineural scleral spaces into the episcleral tissues. Along this route, the fluid mixes with tissue fluid from the ciliary muscle, ciliary processes, and choroid. Thus, this flow pathway may be analogous to lymphatic drainage of tissue fluid in other organs (there are no ocular lymphatics) by providing an important means of ridding the eye of potentially toxic tissue metabolites.*

Flow from the anterior chamber across the trabecular meshwork into Schlemm's canal is pressure dependent, but drainage via the uveoscleral pathway is virtually independent of pressure at intraocular pressure levels greater than 7 to 10 mm Hg in the uninflamed eye.[38,42,53] Although the actual drainage rates ($\mu1 \times min^{-1}$) via the trabecular and uveoscleral routes in the monkey may be approximately equal, the measured facility of uveoscleral outflow (C_u, determined by measuring F_u at two

*References 33-35, 38, 40-42, 47, 49, 53, 55, 124.

different pressure levels) is only about 0.01 to 0.02 $\mu1 \times min^{-1} \times mm\ Hg^{-1}$.[38,241] Thus, uveoscleral facility constitutes at most only about 5% of total facility. The reasons for the relative pressure-independence of the uveoscleral pathway are not entirely clear but might be consequent to the complex nature of the pressure and resistance relationships between the various fluid compartments within the intraocular tissues along the route.[53]

The ultrafiltration component of aqueous humor formation is pressure-sensitive, decreasing with increasing intraocular pressure. This phenomenon is quantifiable and is termed *pseudofacility*, because a pressure-induced decrease in inflow will resemble an increase in outflow facility when tonography and constant pressure perfusion are used without special modification[39,61,157] to measure outflow facility.* Pseudofacility was initially thought to constitute as much as 15% to 35% of total facility as measured by tonography or perfusion in the human[95,97,157-159] and the monkey† eye respectively. However, direct measurements of aqueous humor formation in monkeys by isotope dilution at different intraocular pressures, incorporating techniques to circumvent various technical and physiologic artifacts, suggest that pseudofacility is considerably lower, averaging about 0.02 $\mu1 \times min^{-1} \times mm\ Hg^{-1}$ [48,55,133] and thus amounting to no more than 5% to 10% of total facility. This seems consistent with the predominant role of active secretion, which is rather unaffected by intraocular pressure within the near-physiologic range, as opposed to passive ultrafiltration in the entry of newly formed aqueous humor into the posterior chamber.[51,53,174,190,221] In situations in which the blood–aqueous humor barrier is disrupted, such as inflammation, ultrafiltration may become more pronounced and pseudofacility thus increases.[175] This blunts the tendency for intraocular pressure to increase under such conditions.

C_{trab} is not completely independent of intraocular pressure or episcleral venous pressure. In human[63] and monkey[27] eyes, C_{trab} declines by about 1% to 2% per mm Hg increase in pressure, and is perhaps related to compression of the trabecular meshwork or Schlemm's canal.[28,177-179,181,182] C_{trab} increases with increasing P_e, presumably by inflating Schlemm's canal and opening collapsed segments.[28] Intraocular pressure also increases with increasing P_e, but slightly less than mm Hg for mm Hg.[180]

*References 19, 22, 23, 39, 48, 180.
†References 26, 39, 42, 43, 62, 63.

Since, under normal steady-state conditions, C_{ps} and C_u are so low compared with C_{trab}, the intraocular pressure-dependence of C_{trab} is so small, and P_e varies but little, the hydraulics of aqueous humor dynamics may be reasonably approximated for clinical purposes by

$$F_{in} = F_{out} = C_{trab}(P_i - P_e) + F_u$$

Typical values for these parameters in the normal human eye are as follows:

$$F_{in} = F_{out} = 2.5 \ \mu1 \times min^{-1}$$
$$C_{trab} = 0.3 \ \mu1 \times min^{-1} \times mm \ Hg^{-1}$$
$$P_i = 16 \ mm \ Hg$$
$$P_e = 9 \ mm \ Hg$$
$$F_u = 0.4 \ \mu1 \times min^{-1}$$

so that

$$2.5 = 0.3 \ (16 - 9) + 0.4$$

FLUID MOVEMENT ACROSS THE INNER WALL OF SCHLEMM'S CANAL

Over the years, there has been considerable debate as to the route and mechanism by which aqueous humor passes from the trabecular to the luminal side of the endothelium of the inner wall of Schlemm's canal. At present, it seems reasonably certain that most of the fluid transfer occurs via a pressure-dependent system of transcellular channels,* rather than via intercellular pathways.[223] These transcellular channels begin as invaginations on the trabecular (basal) side of the inner wall endothelial cell. The invaginations enlarge progressively, concurrent with the thinning of the cytoplasm on the luminal (apical) aspect of the cell. Eventually, the *giant vacuole* thus formed opens to the canal lumen, forming a through-and-through channel, with a *pore* opening to both sides (albeit not necessarily simultaneously). This is a dynamic intraocular pressure-dependent process, but it is probably not energy dependent. Such transcellular channels and pores can also occur without the formation of giant vacuoles. An analogous process occurs in the arachnoid villi during drainage of the cerebrospinal fluid.[244] Micropinocytosis and paracellular pathways probably contribute very little to fluid movement across the inner wall. Particulate sieving probably does not occur to any meaningful degree during fluid passage across the inner wall endothelium, but occurs rather in the juxtacanalicular region of the meshwork, where the flow pathways narrow progressively as the inner wall is approached from the meshwork side.[125] This system

*References 109, 110, 112, 113, 125, 127, 173, 244.

may act as a one-way valve, permitting fluid and particulate matter to exit the anterior chamber into Schlemm's canal while preventing reflux. However, it probably provides no more than 10% to 25% of the overall resistance to aqueous humor outflow; the majority of the resistance resides in the juxtacanalicular region of the meshwork.[50]

The hydrodynamics of fluid movement through the entire conventional pathway obey all the laws of passive bulk flow. However, the synthetic, phagocytic, contractile, and other properties of the biologically active endothelial cells are undoubtedly crucial to the normal functioning of the system, and its response to hormones, autacoids, and drugs. The earlier concept of the trabecular meshwork/Schlemm's canal as an inert "black box" is clearly erroneous. Rather, we are dealing with a biologically active tissue that mediates and modulates a passive physical process.

INNERVATION OF THE AQUEOUS HUMOR OUTFLOW APPARATUS

The primate trabecular meshwork is very sparsely innervated. Although occasional fibers of a variety of nerve types have been identified (e.g., adrenergic, cholinergic, vasoactive intestinal polypeptide (VIP)–like, substance P–like, neuropeptide Y–like), they are mainly confined to the posterior uveal and posterior corneoscleral regions and are not currently known to play any role in outflow physiology.[188,211,227,229-232] As in some other tissues,[14,31,32,163] the beta-adrenergic receptors in the meshwork endothelium[126,196,197] are probably not innervated. Rather, they respond to ambient free catecholamines. The non-selective beta-adrenergic antagonist timolol does not itself alter outflow facility in humans,[264] but it does prevent the facility-increasing effect of exogenous epinephrine,[2,238] and so indicates that the meshwork is normally under little or no beta-adrenergic tone.

Different nerve types are also present in the ciliary muscle, but other than the adrenergic and cholinergic mechanisms associated with muscle contraction and relaxation, they have no currently known relationship to outflow physiology.[211,227,229-232,238] Indeed, many of the nerves identified in the ciliary muscle and posterior meshwork probably do not represent endings to those tissues, but rather are fibers on their way elsewhere.

More intriguing is the recent immunohistochemical localization of neuron-specific enolase to a discontinuous band of cell clusters in the anterior trabecular meshwork of the rhesus monkey. This might indicate a neuroendocrine or regulatory function for such cells.[228] Since so little is known about endogenous regulation of outflow facility, such findings clearly deserve further study.

TRABECULAR MESHWORK BIOCHEMISTRY

The biochemistry and metabolism of the trabecular meshwork have long been a mystery. Recent studies have begun to define enzymatic pathways and metabolic requirements of excised bovine meshwork,[5-7,217] and suggest the importance of trabecular cell membrane sulfhydryl groups in maintaining normal outflow resistance.[84,85,95,164] Chemical agents that react with sulfhydryl groups may increase or decrease outflow facility when perfused through the anterior chamber of calf or primate eyes. The differing effects of various agents may depend on the nature and specificity of the interaction and the presence of different populations of sulfhydryl groups. Inhibition of meshwork glycolytic metabolism and energy production cannot explain the functional effects, which may be the result of morphologic alterations in the meshwork and inner canal wall. Thus iodoacetamide and N-ethylmaleimide produce an increase in facility associated with enlargement of the subendothelial spaces within the cribriform region and disruption of the inner canal wall, while p-chloromercuribenzene sulfonate or p-chloromercuribenzene decreases facility associated with trabecular cell swelling.

UNDERPERFUSION OF THE MESHWORK

Underperfusion of the trabecular meshwork by aqueous humor can occur in the following experimental settings:

1. Following filtration surgery, aqueous humor flows preferentially through the surgical sclerostomy site, thereby bypassing the remaining meshwork[166]
2. Peripheral anterior synechiae[168] or opercular overgrowth[167] prevent aqueous humor from reaching the meshwork
3. Canal and meshwork shape changes shunt aqueous humor away from certain portions of the meshwork[172]

These situations all lead to a characteristic light and electron microscopic appearance of meshwork densification, activation of meshwork endothelial cells, and increased extracellular material within the cribriform region. Monkeys treated chronically with acetazolamide exhibit similar meshwork abnormalities (Lütjen-Drecoll, E, personal communication, 1985), suggesting that chronic reduction of the rate of aqueous humor formation, as during clinical glaucoma treatment, may not be as innoc-

uous as has been thought.[150] Alteration of the chemical composition of the aqueous humor may also be a factor, as has been shown for the decrease in outflow resistance occurring during experimental perfusion of the anterior chamber of monkeys.[86,100]

CHOLINERGIC MECHANISMS

In primates the iris root inserts into the ciliary muscle and the uveal meshwork just posterior to the scleral spur; the ciliary muscle inserts at the scleral spur and the posterior inner aspect of the trabecular meshwork.[122,207] The influence of these two contractile, cholinergically innervated structures on resistance to aqueous humor outflow has long been a source of speculation. Voluntary accommodation (human[8]), electrical stimulation of the third cranial nerve (cat[9-11] and monkey[243]), topical, intracameral, or systemically administered cholinergic agonists (monkey and human[21,180]), and in enucleated eyes (monkey and human) pushing the lens posteriorly with a plunger through a corneal fitting,[249] all decrease outflow resistance, whereas ganglionic blocking agents and cholinergic antagonists increase resistance.[21,25,101,115,214] Furthermore, the resistance-decreasing effect of intravenous pilocarpine in monkeys is virtually instantaneous, implying that the effect is mediated by an arterially perfused structure or structures.[24]

These findings collectively suggest that iris sphincter and ciliary muscle contraction physically alter meshwork configuration so as to decrease resistance, whereas muscle relaxation deforms it so as to increase resistance.[66,180] However, not all of the experimental evidence supports this strictly mechanical view of cholinergic and anticholinergic effects on meshwork function. Thus in monkeys intravenous atropine rapidly reverses some but not all of the pilocarpine-induced resistance decrease,[18,22] and topical pilocarpine causes a much greater resistance decrease per diopter of induced accommodation than does systemic pilocarpine (monkey[22]) or voluntary accommodation (human[222]). Such findings raise the possibility of a resistance-decreasing pharmacologic effect directly on the endothelium of the trabecular meshwork or Schlemm's canal.[18,22]

A means of distinguishing secondary mechanical effects of drugs from primary pharmacologic ones was achieved with the development of techniques in the living monkey eye for totally removing the iris at its root,[129] and for disinserting the anterior end of the ciliary muscle over its entire circumference and retrodisplacing it to a more posterior position on the inner scleral wall.[130] In these preparations, the ciliary muscle retains its normal morphology and its contractibility in response to pilocarpine, and the meshwork exhibits essentially its normal light and electron microscopic appearance.[167] Aniridia has no effect on intraocular pressure, resting outflow resistance, or resistance responses to intravenous (Table 9-1) or intracameral pilocarpine.[135] After total iris removal and ciliary muscle disinsertion, however, there is virtually no acute resistance response to either intravenous or intracameral pilocarpine (Fig. 9-1),[130] and no response to topical pilocarpine given at 6-hour intervals for 18 to 24 hours.[131]

It thus seems virtually certain that the acute resistance-decreasing action of pilocarpine, and presumably of other cholinomimetics, is mediated entirely by drug-induced ciliary muscle contraction, with no direct pharmacologic effect on the meshwork itself. This is consistent with the absence of cholinergic receptors, as measured by specific ³H-quinuclidinyl benzilate (^{3}H-QNB) binding,

Table 9-1 Effect of total iridectomy on outflow facility and its response to intravenous pilocarpine in 11 cynomolgus monkeys

Co	
I	0.37 ± 0.04
O	0.39 ± 0.05
I/O	0.96 ± 0.06
Cpp	
I	0.91 ± 0.18
O	1.07 ± 0.22
I/O	0.95 ± 0.12
Cpp/Co	
I	2.40 ± 0.24
O	2.55 ± 0.23
I/O	0.98 ± 0.10

Modified from Kaufman, PL: Invest Ophthalmol Vis Sci 18:870, 1979. With permission.

I = iridectomized eye; O = opposite eye. For each eye, Co = mean of three determinations of total outflow facility ($\mu l \times min^{-1} \times mm\ Hg^{-1}$) during the 20 minutes immediately preceding intravenous pilocarpine; Cpp = mean of two determinations of total outflow facility for the period 10 to 26 minutes after intravenous pilocarpine HCl (1.0 mg/kg). Atropine sulfate, 0.1 mg/kg, given intramuscularly before perfusion. Each value in the table is the mean ±S.E.M. for 11 eyes or pairs of eyes.

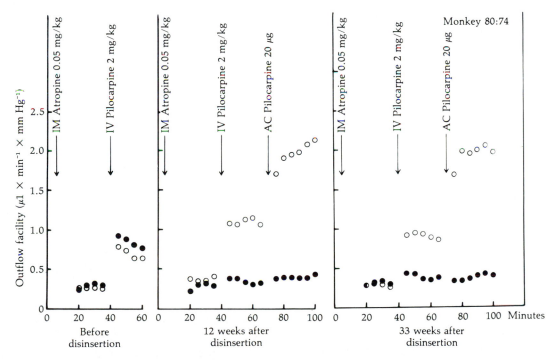

Fig. 9-1 Outflow facility and facility responses to intravenous (IV) and intracameral (AC) pilocarpine hydrochloride before and after unilateral ciliary muscle disinsertion in a typical bilaterally iridectomized cynomolgus monkey. Intramuscular atropine sulfate (IM atropine) was given before each perfusion to minimize systemic effects of intravenous pilocarpine. Note absence of facility increase following intravenous and intracameral pilocarpine in the iridectomized and disinserted eye *(solid circles)*, as opposed to the large facility increases in the opposite iridectomized-only eye *(open circles)*. (From Kaufman, PL, and Bárány, EH: Invest Ophthalmol 15:793, 1976)

in cultured meshwork endothelium (Polansky, JR, personal communication, 1985). The inability of atropine to reverse the pilocarpine-induced facility increases in normal eyes rapidly and completely, and could be the result of mechanical hysteresis of the meshwork. Ciliary muscle contraction forces a rapid structural change on the meshwork, but muscle relaxation cannot itself reverse this change; elasticity of the meshwork is involved, and its effects may be exerted slowly.[131] The variation in the relative magnitude of pilocarpine-induced accommodation and decrease in the resistance when the drug is administered by different routes might reflect differences in bioavailability of the drug to different regions of the muscle. No information is available regarding the possible existence of very slowly developing (weeks or longer) primary cholinomimetic effects on meshwork function, but there seems little reason to postulate such a phenomenon.

Light and electron microscopic studies of the trabecular meshwork and Schlemm's canal have demonstrated pilocarpine-induced alterations in the size and shape of the intertrabecular spaces and in various characteristics, including vacuolization, of the inner canal wall endothelium.* However, these alterations are considered to be secondary to pilocarpine-induced ciliary muscle contraction and augmented transtrabecular outflow.[111] We do not know what precise structural alterations in the meshwork or canal account for the ciliary muscle contraction-induced decrease in resistance to passive bulk fluid outflow. Possibilities include opening entirely new channels, decreasing the resistance of some or all existing channels, and alleviating collapse of Schlemm's canal.[28,165,177,182] There remains much to learn about the physics behind the physiology.

ADRENERGIC MECHANISMS

Topical and intracameral epinephrine increase outflow facility in rabbit and primate eyes.† Much work has been done attempting to define the time course, type of receptor (alpha, beta) and biochemical pathways (prostaglandins, cyclic adenosine 5' monophosphate [cAMP]) involved in these responses. However, the site and mechanism of the facility-increasing effect of adrenergic compounds remain unknown. These agents affect smooth muscle tone in the iris and ciliary body; they may alter intraocular, intrascleral, and extrascleral vascular

tone; and they may have direct effects on the endothelium lining the outflow pathways, all of which may alter outflow facility. These potential sites of action are not mutually exclusive, and indeed that multiplicity may account for much of the variability and confusion in the literature.

Iris and Ciliary Muscle

Anatomic relationships suggest that the tone of the iris dilator muscle could influence outflow facility.[26] Both smooth muscles of the iris are sympathetically innervated.[78,161] The iris dilator contracts strongly to alpha-adrenergic agonists.[247,248] The function of the sympathetic innervation of the iris sphincter muscle remains unclear. The role of the ciliary muscle in modulating outflow facility has been detailed above. The ciliary muscle is sympathetically innervated,[78,161] and there appears to be a weak beta-adrenergic relaxant response of at least some portions of the muscle.[69,181,242,247,248]

The intracameral epinephrine or norepinephrine dose–outflow facility response relationship and the maximum facility increase induced by each drug respectively are virtually identical in surgically untouched, aniridic, and ciliary muscle disinserted monkey eyes. Facility-increasing doses dilate the pupil in most surgically untouched monkey eyes. These findings indicate that neither the iris nor the ciliary muscle are involved in the responses.[136,137]

Ocular Vasculature

It has been proposed that the outflow facility–increasing action of adrenergic agonists is primarily related to their effects on intrascleral and extrascleral vasculature.[160] Intracameral infusion of the noncatecholamine vasoconstrictors ergotamine and angiotensin II, and the vasoactive agents histamine, serotonin, and bradykinin (which may have either vasoconstricting or vasodilating effects, depending on the particular vascular bed) decrease outflow facility in surgically untouched, aniridic, and ciliary muscle disinserted monkey eyes.[136-138] Although different vascular beds may react differently to any given vasoconstrictor or vasodilator, these results do not support the contention that the outflow facility–increasing effects of catecholamines such as epinephrine and norepinephrine are the result of their vascular actions.

Trabecular Meshwork

In surgically untouched, aniridic, and disinserted monkey eyes, which have widely varying baseline outflow facilities, epinephrine and nor-

---

*References 1, 13, 89, 91, 92, 117, 123, 180, 206, 246.
†References 15, 26, 29, 44, 46, 75, 153-156, 185, 200, 219, 220, 250.

epinephrine respectively increase outflow facility by a constant percentage of the initial (baseline) outflow facility. This suggests that the drugs exert their effects on whatever is responsible for the major part of the variation in baseline outflow facility. To attribute entirely to pseudofacility or facility of uveoscleral routes the constant percentage of increase in outflow facility observed in eyes with baseline outflow facilities varying over a fourfold to fivefold range would require that virtually all of the baseline outflow facility consist of pseudofacility or uveoscleral facility.[136,137] However, this is not the case.[26,38,133]

Could the sclera, including its vasculature, be the main site of action of the drugs? Since pilocarpine exerts its resistance-decreasing effect by way of ciliary muscle traction on the trabecular meshwork,[130] and since in the normal monkey eye pilocarpine markedly decreases and ganglionic blockade with hexamethonium markedly increases both outflow resistance and its interindividual variability,[21] most of the variability in baseline resistance must reside at sites other than the sclera.[136,137]

The preceding arguments leave only the trabecular meshwork and inner wall of Schlemm's canal as potential sites of action. Epinephrine and norepinephrine exert their action on whatever characteristic of the meshwork/canal that accounts for interindividual variability in starting facility. One possibility would be an increase in the hydraulic conductivity of a unit filtering area.[136,137]

Biochemical evidence also points to the meshwork as the target tissue. Trabecular cells in culture possess beta-adrenergic receptors, probably of the $beta_2$ subtype, as measured by radioligand binding and radioautography.[126,196] Isolated trabecular tissue[184] and trabecular cells in culture[197] produce cAMP when exposed to adrenergic agonists. Topically applied adrenergic agonists elevate aqueous humor cAMP levels; intracameral administration of cAMP or its analogues, but not the inactive metabolite adenosine 5'-monophosphate (AMP), lowers intraocular pressure and increases outflow facility.[141,143,183-186] The cAMP-induced facility increase is not additive to that induced by adrenergic agonists, and vice versa.[187] Thus, the adrenergic agonist–induced facility increase seems to be mediated through the adenylate cyclase–cAMP pathway. The ability of timolol (a mixed $beta_1$, $beta_2$-adrenergic antagonist)[2,238] but not betaxolol (a relatively selective $beta_1$-antagonist)[2] to inhibit the facility-increasing effect of epinephrine further points to a $beta_2$-adrenergic receptor–mediated effect.

All the available data from different species,

utilizing different drug administration and facility-measuring techniques, are remarkably consistent with respect to the surprisingly large epinephrine and norepinephrine levels required to produce consistent increases in outflow facility. It seems that effective anterior chamber concentrations are on the order of 3×10^{-4} M.* Of course, there is no way of knowing how closely anterior chamber levels reflect drug concentration at the physiologically active site, which might be relatively sequestered from the anterior chamber aqueous humor.

OUTFLOW RESISTANCE AND MESHWORK BIOLOGY

In the primate eye, approximately 75% of the resistance to aqueous humor outflow resides in the tissues between the anterior chamber and the lumen of Schlemm's canal.† A small percentage of the resistance, perhaps 10% to 25%, resides in the inner wall of Schlemm's canal.[50,233,234] However, most of the resistance is in the cribriform portion of the meshwork‡—the outermost part of the meshwork consisting of several layers of endothelial cells embedded in a ground substance composed of a wide variety of macromolecules, including hyaluronic acid, other glycosaminoglycans, collagen, fibronectin, and other glycoproteins.§ These macromolecules are presumably produced by meshwork endothelial cells‖ although, if this is the case, the mechanisms regulating their synthesis are totally unknown.[94]

In eyes with primary open-angle glaucoma, there appears to be deposition of an as yet only partially characterized electron-dense material in the cribriform region, although the influence of the confounding variables of age and prior medical therapy needs further assessment.[169-171, 209] Pigmentary and pseudoexfoliation glaucoma may be more certain examples of glaucoma caused by deposition of specific materials clogging or damaging the meshwork.

The endothelial cells of the meshwork have phagocytic capabilities.[74,108,208] It has been proposed that the meshwork is in effect a self-cleaning filter and that in most of the open-angle glaucomas, the self-cleaning (that is, phagocytic) function is deficient or at least inadequate to cope with the amount

---

*References 26, 44, 46, 116, 121, 136, 137, 140, 142, 156, 185, 189, 199, 218.
†References 50, 53, 79, 80, 107, 125, 165, 233.
‡References 50, 53, 79, 80, 107, 125, 165.
§References 73, 74, 90, 198, 205, 210, 212, 213, 262.
‖References 73, 74, 148, 195, 198, 221.

of material present.[54] Perfusion of the anterior chamber in normal primate eyes is associated with a progressive time-dependent decrease in outflow resistance.* This occurs even when pooled homologous aqueous humor or an artificial solution closely resembling it is used as the perfusate[99,100] and, albeit perhaps to a lesser degree, even when the ciliary muscle has been detached from the scleral spur.[145,146] Although the precise mechanism responsible for this phenomenon is not known, and ciliary muscle contraction may play some role,[45,46] washout of resistance-contributing extracellular material from the trabecular meshwork has been a leading hypothesis.[99,100]

Combining the clogged filter concept of glaucoma with the washout concept of perfusion-induced resistance decrease has inevitably led to interest in compounds that may disrupt the structure of the meshwork and canal inner wall so as to promote washout of normal and pathologic resistance-producing extracellular material. Such compounds may provide insight into cellular and extracellular mechanisms governing outflow resis-

tance in normal and glaucomatous states. Additionally, if normal or pathologic extracellular material requires many years to accumulate to the extent that intraocular pressure becomes elevated, perhaps a one-time washout would provide years of normalized outflow resistance and intraocular pressure.[55]

Cytochalasins

Monkey and human trabecular and Schlemm's canal inner wall endothelial cells contain cytoplasmic actin microfilaments and may therefore possess contractile properties.* Cytochalasins are fungal metabolites that interfere with the polymerization process by which globular cytoplasmic actin aggregates into actin microfilaments.[59,60,77,103] Anterior chamber infusion of microgram doses of cytochalasins B and D in cynomolgus and rhesus monkeys caused distension of the cribriform meshwork, separation of its cells, and ruptures of the inner canal wall endothelium, leading to washout of extracellular material (Fig. 9-2)[128,235] and up to a sixfold increase in conventional outflow facility

---

*References 18, 20, 45, 46, 86, 99, 100, 132, 136, 137.

*References 102, 107, 108, 112, 125, 203, 245.

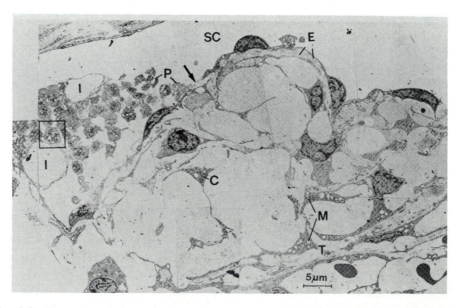

Fig. 9-2 Transmission electron microscopy of Schlemm's canal and cribriform meshwork approximately 30 minutes after intracameral infusion of 5 μg of cytochalasin B. Inner wall endothelium (SC) demonstrates ruptures (arrow) and abnormally large invaginations (I). Extracellular material (E) has been lost from some areas between inner wall endothelium and first subendothelial cell layer (and replaced by plasma [asterisk]) and is completely absent from most parts of the cribriform meshwork. Degranulated platelets (P); cells of cribriform meshwork (C); swollen mitochondria (M); first corneoscleral trabeculum (T). (From Svedbergh, B, Lütjen-Drecoll, E, Ober, M, and Kaufman, PL: Invest Ophthalmol Vis Sci 17:718, 1978)

(Fig. 9-3).[128,132,133,138,144] This is completely unrelated to ciliary muscle contraction, since the effect is similar whether or not the ciliary muscle has been surgically disinserted.[132,134] The in vivo dose-response relationships for different cytochalasin analogues confirm that the effect is indeed caused by actin filament disruption[139] rather than some other cytochalasin action.[194] In vitro studies with cultured human and monkey trabecular cells confirm the alteration of cell shape.[197]

Despite different mechanisms of action and primary attack points on the outflow apparatus, nearmaximal or supramaximal intracameral pilocarpine and cytochalasin B doses are not additive, and they actually cancel each other out in their facility-increasing effect.[144] The following are two possible explanations for this observation:

1. Both drugs ultimately attack the same high-resistance pathways with equal effectiveness, so that maximal resistance reduction

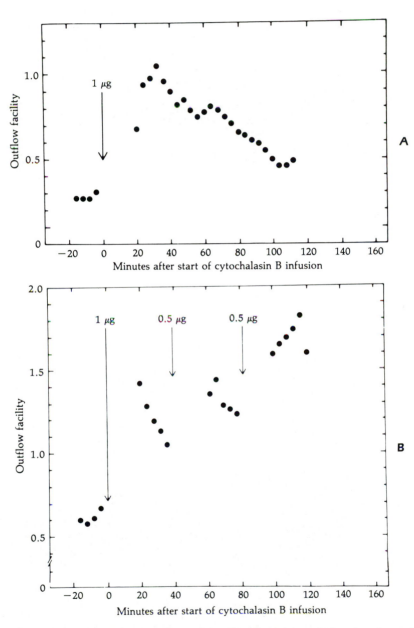

Fig. 9-3 Time course of cytochalasin B effects on outflow facility (μ1/min/mm Hg) in normal eyes of two monkeys (opposite eyes not shown). **A,** Single intracameral dose of 1 μg cytochalasin B, followed by uninterrrupted measurement of facility. **B,** Single dose of 1 μg and booster doses of 0.5 μg. (From Kaufman, PL, and Bárány, EH: Invest Ophthalmol Vis Sci 16:47, 1977)

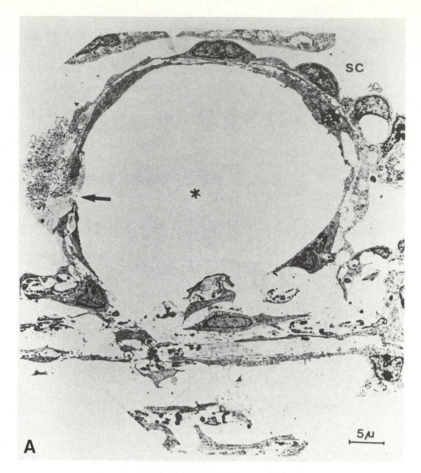

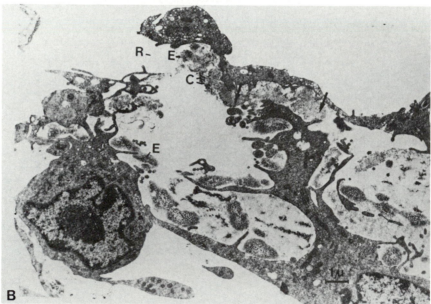

Fig. 9-4 **A,** Transmission electron microscopy of Schlemm's canal *(SC)* and trabecular meshwork after 40-minute perfusion, 6 mM Na$_2$ EDTA. Inner wall endothelium and first subendothelial cell layer are detached from underlying cribriform meshwork and balloon into Schlemm's canal lumen. Balloon *(asterisk)* shows large rupture *(arrow),* allowing swollen collagen fibers and cell debris to pass out. **B,** Schlemm's canal and cribriform meshwork after 80-minute perfusion, 4 mM Na$_2$ EDTA. Inner wall endothelium shows large rupture *(R).* Homogeneous material accumulation *(arrows),* curly collagen *(C),* elastic material *(E)* under intact part of inner wall endothelium. Note many small, intracellular empty vesicles. (From Bill, A, Lütjen-Drecoll, E, and Svedbergh, B: Invest Ophthalmol Vis Sci 19:492, 1980)

by the first drug precludes any effect of the second. Since pilocarpine and cytochalasin B both produce mechanical distortion of the meshwork and canal, albeit by different primary actions and attack points, it is conceivable that in both instances the same crucial areas are affected.

2. Each drug specifically attacks the resistance of an entirely separate flow pathway, but the resistances are parallel, so that markedly reducing the second resistance has little additional overall effect once the first has been reduced. The parallel resistance hypothesis has potential clinical implications for combined antiglaucoma therapy with *any* two drugs facilitating aqueous humor outflow. If no increase of facility or reduction of intraocular pressure occurs when the second drug is added, one may not necessarily conclude that this drug is ineffective in that particular patient. It may simply indicate that the effect of the second drug is masked by the effect of the first drug. If the patient subsequently becomes resistant to or intolerant of the first drug, the substitution of a second drug may be dramatically effective.[144]

Chelators

Perfusion of the monkey anterior chamber with calcium- and magnesium-free mock aqueous humor containing 4 to 6 mM disodiumethylenediamine-tetraacetate (EDTA) or with calcium-free mock aqueous humor containing 4 mM ethylene glycol *bis* (aminoethylether) tetraacetate (EGTA) also causes large increases in facility and ultrastructural changes (Fig. 9-4) similar to those induced by cytochalasins.[57] Because EDTA chelates both calcium and magnesium, whereas EGTA is much more specific for calcium,[204] calcium would appear to be the critical cation in maintaining the structural and functional integrity of the conventional outflow pathway.

With all four cytochalasins and chelators thus far studied, facility falls toward normal when they are removed from the anterior chamber.[57,132,139] Morphologic recovery, so far studied only for cytochalasin B, begins at least within hours and is largely complete within 1 week.[235] No long-term physiologic, biomicroscopic, or histologic effects are apparent at the dosages used.[132,140,167,235] The rapid reversibility of the drug's effect when the agent is removed is characteristic of the action of cytochalasin B in other cellular systems.[68,103,105]

Hyaluronidases and Proteases

Nearly three decades ago it was shown that intracameral infusion of hyaluronidase produced a marked increase in facility in the bovine eye, presumably because of washout of acid mucopolysaccharide–rich extracellular material in the chamber angle tissues.[16] Studies in primates gave much more variable results.[92,107,191,193] In the enucleated human eye perfused at room temperature, alpha-chymotrypsin had little effect on facility.[107] However, in vitro experiments have shown that effects of trypsin may be masked at low temperatures[202] and that a combination of trypsin and EDTA may have a marked effect in dissociating cultured cells not easily dissociated by either agent alone.[240] Perfusion of the anterior chamber of living monkeys with 50 units/ml of alpha-chymotrypsin gave a large facility increase, which persisted for several hours even after the enzyme was removed from the infusate.[56] The increase in facility induced by intracameral 0.5 mM Na_2 EDTA was augmented and prolonged by alpha-chymotrypsin.[56]

Although neither the subcellular events nor the exact pathophysiologic sequences responsible for the chamber angle alterations produced by these agents has yet been elucidated, it seems that agents that alter the cytoskeleton, cell junctions, contractile proteins, or extracellular material produce a "pharmacologic trabeculotomy" and "cleansing" of the meshwork. Much work remains before clinical trials of such agents can be considered, but the prospect is enormously exciting.

Cell-induced and Other Particulate-induced Facility Decreases

Normal erythrocytes are deformable and pass easily from the anterior chamber through the tortuous pathways of the trabecular meshwork and the inner wall of Schlemm's canal.[125] However, nondeformable erythrocytes such as sickled or clastic (ghost) cells may become trapped within and obstruct the meshwork, elevating outflow resistance and intraocular pressure.[64,65,104] Similarly, macrophages swollen with ingested lens proteins leaking from a hypermature cataract,[88] or breakdown products from intraocular erythrocytes,[87] or pigmented tumors (or the tumor cells themselves)[263] may produce meshwork obstruction. Pigment liberated from the iris spontaneously (pigment dispersion syndrome) or iatrogenically (following argon-laser iridotomy) may clog the meshwork, presumably without prior ingestion by wandering macrophages,[107,192,201] as may zonular fragments following iatrogenic enzymatic zonulo-

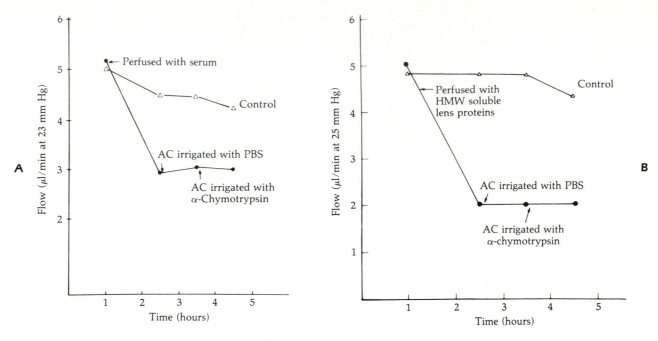

Fig. 9-5 A, Effect of specially isolated high-molecular-weight (HMW) soluble lens proteins from human cataracts (1 mg/ml; MW greater than 150 × 10⁶) on fluid outflow. Ten enucleated human eyes were perfused for 1 hour with HMW soluble lens proteins *(filled circles)*. Six controls were sham-treated with a protein-free solution *(open triangles)*. Attempts were made to reverse the effect by washing out the anterior chamber with alpha-chymotrypsin. **B,** Effect of normal human serum on fluid outflow. Serum was perfused into the experimental eyes for 30 minutes following a preliminary 1-hour aqueous perfusion and measurement of outflow *(arrow)*. Results are shown for 38 serum-treated eyes *(solid circles)* and 24 sham-treated controls *(open triangles)*. Attempts were made to reverse the effect by washing out the anterior chamber with alpha-chymotrypsin (7 eyes). Anterior chamber *(AC)*; phosphate-buffered salt solution *(PBS)*. (**A,** From Epstein, DL, Jedziniak, JA, and Grant, WM: Invest Ophthalmol Vis Sci 17:272, 1978; **B** from Epstein, DL, Hashimoto, JM, and Grant, WM: Am J Ophthalmol 86:101, 1978. Published with permission from The American Journal of Ophthalmology. Copyright by The Ophthalmic Publishing Company)

lysis[4,260] or lens capsular fragments following neodymium:yttrium-aluminum-garnet (Nd:YAG) laser posterior capsulotomy.[70]

Protein-induced and Other Macromolecule-induced Facility Decreases

Glaucoma secondary to hypermature cataract (phacolytic glaucoma) or uveitis has long been ascribed to trabecular obstruction. In the former entity, the presence of protein-laden macrophages lining the chamber angle seemed adequate to account for the increased outflow resistance.[88] The uveitis-related glaucomas comprise many different entities (see Chapter 67), and the etiology of the increased outflow resistance seems less clear. Postulated mechanisms include trabecular involvement by the primary inflammatory process, trabecular obstruction by inflammatory cells, or secondary alteration of trabecular cellular physiology by inflammatory mediators or byproducts released elsewhere in the eye.

Recently, it has been shown that small amounts of purified high–molecular-weight, soluble lens proteins[81,83] or serum itself,[81] when perfused through the anterior chamber of freshly enucleated human eyes, cause an acute and marked increase in outflow resistance (Fig. 9-5). Thus, it may be that specific proteins, protein subfragments, or other macromolecules are themselves capable of obstructing or altering the meshwork so as to increase outflow resistance, perhaps contributing to the elevated intraocular pressure in entities such as the phacolytic, uveitic, exfoliation,[76] and hemolytic[87] glaucomas.

CORTICOSTEROIDS

Topical or systemic glucocorticoids may induce elevation of intraocular pressure in susceptible individuals,[12,30,150,151,215] apparently as a result of decreased outflow facility (see Chapter 64). Although glucocorticoid receptors have been identified in the cells of the outflow pathways,[119,236,251] the biochemical and consequent physical processes causing the decrease in facility are poorly understood.

Recent preliminary evidence suggests that glucocorticoids may play a major role in the normal physiologic regulation of outflow facility and intraocular pressure, perhaps by modulation of macromolecular metabolism or prostaglandin-adrenergic interactions in the outflow system. The glucocorticoid effect on the physiology of the outflow pathways may be more rapid than previously believed—perhaps hours rather than weeks.[253] Dexamethasone alters complex carbohydrate, hyaluronic acid, protein, and collagen synthesis and distribution in the cells and tissues of the rabbit and human aqueous humor outflow systems.[118,120,148,197] Prostaglandins are produced by human trabecular endothelial cells in culture; dexamethasone inhibits trabecular cell prostaglandin synthesis by up to 90%.[252]

Cortisol metabolism in cultured trabecular cells differs in normal and open-angle glaucoma lines.

$$\underset{I}{Cortisol \rightarrow 5\alpha, 5\beta\text{-dihydrocortisol}} \underset{II}{\rightarrow 5\alpha, 5\beta\text{-tetrahydrocortisol}}$$

Reaction I is catalyzed by a Δ^4-reductase and reaction II by a 3-oxidoreductase. In normal cell lines, there is no accumulation of the active dihydrocortisol intermediates; all cortisol is rapidly metabolized to the inactive tetrahydrocortisols. In glaucomatous cell lines, Δ^4-reductase activity is increased by greater than 100-fold, whereas 3-oxidoreductase activity is decreased by greater than fourfold, leading to a significant accumulation of the dihydrocortisol intermediates.[224,255] 5β-dihydrocortisol potentiates cortisol- and dexamethasone-induced nuclear translocation of the cytoplasmic glucocorticoid receptor in rabbit iris-ciliary body,[254] and also potentiates the action of topically applied dexamethasone in raising intraocular pressure in young rabbits.[225]

Although these observations need to be confirmed and extended, they appear to herald a new phase not only in steroid-glaucoma research, but also in unraveling the mysteries of trabecular meshwork biology.

PROSTAGLANDINS

Prostaglandins (PG) are synthesized by human trabecular endothelial cells in culture, and therefore could conceivably play a role in the normal physiologic regulation of aqueous humor outflow.[252] However, the marked intraocular pressure–lowering effect of exogenously administered PGF$_{2\alpha}$ in monkeys[58,67,71,162,226] is not the result of al-

tered trabecular outflow facility (which changes only slightly or not at all),[71,145,162] but rather it is caused by increased uveoscleral drainage.[72] Given the extraordinarily small topical PGF$_{2\alpha}$ doses required to produce this effect (<1 μg),[3] it seems possible that PG produced by the trabecular endothelium could be carried with the aqueous humor through the uveoscleral routes, where it exerts its action. Thus, the meshwork itself might regulate uveoscleral outflow, with PG acting as the regulatory autacoid.

OUTFLOW BIOMECHANICS AND PHARMACOLOGIC RESPONSES

Pharmacologic Manipulation

Aqueous humor outflow via the conventional drainage pathway is a physical process that can be altered pharmacologically. Several classes of pharmacologic agents unequivocally alter aqueous humor outflow in the primate: cholinomimetics, catecholamines, cytochalasins, chelators, alpha-chymotrypsin, ergotamine,[136,137] and angiotensin[136,137] to name some. Some of these compounds (e.g., cytochalasins,[132,235] chelators[56,57] produce structural alterations in the chamber angle that would seem to account for their effects on outflow. Other agents may affect outflow secondarily, such as pilocarpine-induced ciliary muscle contraction.[24,130] However, in no instance is the complete sequence of physical events by which a drug alters aqueous humor outflow known. For instance, what characteristics of the meshwork and/or the canal are altered by ciliary muscle contraction so as to increase aqueous humor outflow? Narrowing or collapse of Schlemm's canal may decrease outflow facility.[28,177-179,181,182] Ciliary muscle tendons connect directly with the cribriform meshwork and inner canal wall in such a way that muscle contraction might spread the cribriform meshwork and widen the canal, whereas muscle relaxation might tend to collapse them.[209] Such studies begin to address the real issues but do not explain conclusively the physics behind the physiology. Even with agents such as cytochalasins, which have a presumably specific subcellular action (interference with actin filament formation)[59,60] and a clearly disruptive effect on the structural integrity of the outflow pathways,[132,235] the precise pathophysiologic sequence of events is unclear. In the case of the catecholamines, there is no knowledge whatsoever about the biophysical response.

Physical Manipulation

A nonpharmacologic approach to altering physical characteristics of the meshwork and/or canal has been the application of laser energy to the trabecular meshwork. Initial efforts were directed at puncturing holes in the meshwork and inner canal wall. Such holes resulted in increased outflow facility and decreased intraocular pressure, but patency was nearly always transient; the openings scarred over, and facility and intraocular pressure usually returned to their former levels.* It was shown that, in monkeys, intensive circumferential treatment of the meshwork with argon-laser energy produced sufficient scarring to significantly decrease facility and increase intraocular pressure on a long-term basis.[97]

Recently it has become clear that spacing about 100 small (50 μm), less intensive, continuous-wave argon laser burns evenly around the circumference of the meshwork of the glaucomatous human eye can result in a significant and longer-term increase in outflow facility and a decrease in intraocular pressure, apparently without actually producing a "hole" in the meshwork or inner canal wall.[216,257-259] Indeed, histologic studies demonstrate the expected scar formation at the lasered sites.[176,258] Although the presence of an undetected puncture leading from the anterior chamber into the canal lumen cannot be unequivocally excluded, an intriguing alternate hypothesis is that localized contracture of the laser-produced scars tightens and narrows the trabecular ring, and the distortion somehow promotes the egress of aqueous humor.[256,258,259] This may be somewhat analogous to the effect of ciliary muscle contraction, although in neither case can we say precisely how such distortion eases fluid passage. Still another possibility is that the laser energy produces a fundamental change in trabecular cell biology and/or meshwork extracellular material, leading to decreased resistance. The responses of the outflow apparatus to pharmacologic agents following argon laser trabeculoplasty have not been systematically studied, but knowledge of these responses may be extremely important from both clinical therapeutic and basic physiologic standpoints.

The basic biomechanics of aqueous humor outflow and their manipulation are vitally important areas, and have been too long neglected. Better understanding will be crucial in developing new pharmacologic approaches to improve aqueous humor outflow in glaucomatous states.

*References 114, 152, 237, 239, 257, 261.

REFERENCES

1. Allan, L, and Burian, HM: The valve action of the trabecular meshwork: studies with silicone models, Am J Ophthalmol 59:382, 1965
2. Allen, RC, and Epstein, DL: Additive effect of betaxolol and epinephrine in primary open angle glaucoma, Arch Ophthalmol 104:1178, 1986
3. Alm, A, and Villumsen, J: Intraocular pressure and ocular side effects after prostaglandin $F_{2\alpha}$ eye drops: a single dose-response study in humans, Proc Int Soc Eye Res 4:14, 1986
4. Anderson, DR: Experimental alpha chymotrypsin glaucoma studied by scanning electron microscopy, Am J Ophthalmol 71:470, 1971
5. Anderson, PJ, Wang, J, and Epstein, DL: Metabolism of calf trabecular (reticular) meshwork, Invest Ophthalmol Vis Sci 19:13, 1980
6. Anderson, PJ, Karageuzian, LN, Cheng, H-M, and Epstein, DL: Hexokinase of calf trabecular meshwork, Invest Ophthalmol Vis Sci 25:1258, 1984
7. Anderson, PJ, Karageuzian, LN, and Epstein, DL: Phosphofructokinase of calf trabecular meshwork, Invest Ophthalmol Vis Sci 25:1262, 1984
8. Armaly, MF, and Burian, HM: Changes in the tonogram during accommodation, Arch Ophthalmol 60:60, 1958
9. Armaly, MF: Studies on intraocular effects of the orbital parasympathetic pathway. I. Technique and effects on morphology, Arch Ophthalmol 61:14, 1959
10. Armaly, MF: Studies on intraocular effects of the orbital parasympathetics. II. Effects on intraocular pressure, Arch Ophthalmol 62:117, 1959
11. Armaly, MF: Studies on intraocular effects of the orbital parasympathetic pathway. III. Effect on steady state dynamics, Arch Ophthalmol 62:817, 1959
12. Armaly, MF: Steroids and glaucoma. In Transactions of the New Orleans Academy of Ophthalmology: Symposium on glaucoma, St Louis, 1967, The CV Mosby Co, p 74
13. Asayama, J: Zur Anatomie des Ligamentum Pectinatum, Albrecht von Graefes Arch Ophthalmol 53:113, 1902
14. Auerbach, GD: Beta-adrenergic receptors, cyclic AMP, and ion transport in the avian erythrocyte, Adv Cyclic Nucleotide Res 5:117, 1975
15. Ballintine, EJ, and Garner, LL: Improvement of the coefficient of outflow in glaucomatous eyes, Arch Ophthalmol 66:314, 1961
16. Bárány, EH, and Scotchbrook, S: Influence of testicular hyaluronidase on the resistance to flow through the angle of the anterior chamber, Acta Physiol Scand 30:240, 1954
17. Bárány, EH: Resistance to aqueous outflow. In Newell, FW, editor: Glaucoma, transactions of the first conference, New York, 1955, Josiah Macy Jr Foundation

18. Bárány, EH: The mode of action of pilocarpine on outflow resistance in the eye of a primate *(Cercopithecus ethiops)*, Invest Ophthalmol 1:712, 1962

19. Bárány, EH: A mathematical formulation of intraocular pressure as dependent on secretion, ultrafiltration, bulk outflow, and osmotic reabsorption of fluid, Invest Ophthalmol 2:584, 1963

20. Bárány, EH: Simultaneous measurement of changing intraocular pressure and outflow facility in the vervet monkey by constant pressure infusion, Invest Ophthalmol Vis Sci 3:135, 1964

21. Bárány, EH: Relative importance of autonomic nervous tone and structure as determinants of outflow resistance in normal monkey eyes *(Cercopithecus ethiops* and *Macaca irus)*, In Rohen, JW, editor: The structure of the eye, Second symposium, Stuttgart, 1965, Schattauer

22. Bárány, EH: The mode of action of miotics on outflow resistance: a study of pilocarpine in the vervet monkeys, *Cercopithecus ethiops,* Trans Ophthalmol Soc UK 86:539, 1966

23. Bárány, EH: Pseudofacility and uveo-scleral outflow routes: some nontechnical difficulties in the determination of outflow facility and rate of formation of aqueous humor, Glaucoma symposium, Tützing Castle, Basel, 1966, Karger

24. Bárány, EH: The immediate effect on outflow resistance of intravenous pilocarpine in the vervet monkey, *Cercopithecus ethiops,* Invest Ophthalmol 6:373, 1967

25. Bárány, EH, and Christensen, RE: Cycloplegia and outflow resistance, Arch Ophthalmol 77:757, 1967

26. Bárány, EH: Topical epinephrine effects on true outflow resistance and pseudofacility in vervet monkeys studied by a new anterior chamber perfusion technique, Invest Ophthalmol 7:88, 1968

27. Bárány, EH, Linner, E, Lütjen-Drecoll, E, and Rohen, JW: Structural and functional effects of trabeculectomy in cynomolgus monkeys. I. Light microscopy, V Graefes Arch Klin Exp Ophthalmol 184:1, 1972

28. Bárány, EH: The influence of extraocular venous pressure on outflow facility in *Cercopithecus ethiops* and *Macaca fascicularis,* Invest Ophthalmol Vis Sci 17:711, 1978

29. Becker, B, Pettit, TH, and Gay, AJ: Topical epinephrine therapy of open angle glaucoma, Arch Ophthalmol 66:219, 1961

30. Becker, B, and Hahn, K: Topical corticosteroids and heredity in primary open-angle glaucoma, Am J Ophthalmol 57:543, 1964

31. Bilezikian, JP: A beta-adrenergic receptor of the turkey erythrocyte. I. Binding of catecholamine and relationship to adenylate cyclase activity, J Biol Chem 248:5577, 1973

32. Bilezikian, JP: A beta-adrenergic receptor of the turkey erythrocyte. II. Characterization and solubilization of the receptor, J Biol Chem 248:5584, 1973

33. Bill, A: The aqueous humor drainage mechanism in the cynomolgus monkey *(Macaca irus)* with evidence for unconventional routes, Invest Ophthalmol 4:911, 1965

34. Bill, A: The protein exchange in the eye with aspects on conventional and uveoscleral bulk drainage of aqueous humor in primates. In Rohen, JW, editor: The structure of the eye, Second Symposium, Stuttgart, 1965, Schattauer-Verlag

35. Bill, A, and Hellsing, K: Production and drainage of aqueous humor in the cynomolgus monkey *(Macaca irus).* Invest Ophthalmol 4:920, 1965

36. Bill, A: Formation and drainage of aqueous humor in cats, Exp Eye Res 5:185, 1966

37. Bill, A: The routes for bulk drainage of aqueous humor in rabbits with and without cyclodialysis, Doc Ophthalmol 20:157, 1966

38. Bill, A: Conventional and uveo-scleral drainage of aqueous humor in the cynomolgus monkey *(Macaca irus)* at normal and high intraocular pressures, Exp Eye Res 5:45, 1966

39. Bill, A, and Bárány, EH: Gross facility, facility of conventional routes, and pseudofacility of aqueous humor outflow in the cynomolgus monkey: the reduction in aqueous humor formation rate caused by moderate increments in intraocular pressure, Arch Ophthalmol 75:665, 1966

40. Bill, A, and Wålinder, P-E: The effects of pilocarpine on the dynamics of aqueous humor in a primate *(Macaca irus)*, Invest Ophthalmol 5:170, 1966

41. Bill, A: Effects of atropine and pilocarpine on aqueous humor dynamics in cynomolgus monkeys *(Macaca irus)*, Exp Eye Res 6:120, 1967

42. Bill, A: Further studies on the influence of the intraocular pressure on aqueous humor dynamics in cynomolgus monkeys, Invest Ophthalmol 6:364, 1967

43. Bill, A: The effect of ocular hypertension caused by red cells on the rate of formation of aqueous humor, Invest Ophthalmol 7:162, 1968

44. Bill, A: Early effects of epinephrine on aqueous humor dynamics in vervet monkeys *(Cercopithecus ethiops)*, Exp Eye Res 8:35, 1969

45. Bill, A: Effects of atropine on aqueous humor dynamics in the vervet monkey *(Cercopithecus ethiops)*, Exp Eye Res 8:284, 1969

46. Bill, A: Effects of norepinephrine, isoproterenol, and sympathetic stimulation on aqueous humor dynamics in vervet monkeys, Exp Eye Res 10:31, 1970

47. Bill, A: Aqueous humor dynamics in monkeys *(Macaca irus* and *Cercopithecus ethiops)*, Exp Eye Res 11:195, 1971

48. Bill, A: Effects of long-standing stepwise increments in eye pressure on the rate of aqueous humor formation in a primate *(Cercopithecus ethiops)*, Exp Eye Res 12:184, 1971

49. Bill, A, and Phillips, CI: Uveoscleral drainage of aqueous humor in human eyes, Exp Eye Res 12:275, 1971

50. Bill, A, and Svedbergh, B: Scanning electron microscopic studies of the trabecular meshwork and the canal of Schlemm—an attempt to localize the main resistance to outflow of aqueous humor in man, Acta Ophthalmol 50:295, 1972

51. Bill, A: The role of ciliary blood flow and ultrafiltration in aqueous humor formation, Exp Eye Res 16:287, 1973

52. Bill, A: The role of the iris vessels in aqueous humor dynamics, Jpn J Ophthalmol 18:30, 1974

53. Bill, A: Blood circulation and fluid dynamics in the eye, Pharmacol Rev 55:383, 1975

54. Bill, A: The drainage of aqueous humor, Invest Ophthalmol 14:1, 1975

55. Bill, A: Basic physiology of the drainage of aqueous humor. In Bito, LZ, Davson, H, and Fenstermacher, JD, editors: The ocular and cerebrospinal fluids, Fogarty International Center Symposium, Exp Eye Res 25(Suppl):291, 1977

56. Bill, A: Effects of Na$_2$ EDTA and alpha-chymotrypsin on aqueous humor outflow conductance in monkey eyes, Ups J Med Sci 85:311, 1980

57. Bill, A, Lütjen-Drecoll, E, and Svedbergh, B: Effects of intracameral Na$_2$ EDTA and EGTA on aqueous outflow routes in the monkey eye, Invest Ophthalmol Vis Sci 19:492, 1980

58. Bito, LZ, Draga, A, Blanco, J, and Camras, CB: Long-term maintenance of reduced intraocular pressure by daily or twice daily topical application of prostaglandins to cat or rhesus monkey eyes, Invest Ophthalmol Vis Sci 24:312, 1983

59. Brenner, SL, and Korn, ED: Substoichiometric concentrations of cytochalasin D inhibit actin polymerization: additional evidence for an F-actin treadmill, J Biol Chem 254:9982, 1979

60. Brown, SS, and Spudich, JA: Mechanism of action of cytochalasin: evidence that it binds to actin filament ends, J Cell Biol 88:487, 1981

61. Brubaker, RF, and Kupfer, C: Determination of pseudofacility in the eye of the rhesus monkey, Arch Ophthalmol 75:693, 1966

62. Brubaker, RF: The measurement of pseudofacility and true facility by constant pressure perfusion in the normal rhesus monkey eye, Invest Ophthalmol 9:42, 1970

63. Brubaker, RF: The effect of intraocular pressure on conventional outflow resistance in the enucleated human eye, Invest Ophthalmol 14:286, 1975

64. Campbell, DG, Simmons, RJ, and Grant, WM: Ghost cells as a cause of glaucoma, Am J Ophthalmol 81:441, 1976

65. Campbell, DG, and Essingman, EM: Hemolytic ghost cell glaucoma, Arch Ophthalmol 97:2141, 1979

66. Camras, CB, and Bito, LZ: Reduction of intraocular pressure in normal and glaucomatous primate (Aotus trivirgatus) eyes by topically applied prostaglandin F$_{2\alpha}$, Curr Eye Res 1:205, 1981

67. Camras, CB, et al: Multiple dosing of prostaglandin F$_{2\alpha}$ or epinephrine on cynomolgus monkey eyes. I. Aqueous humor dynamics, Invest Ophthalmol Vis Sci 28:463, 1987

68. Carter, SB: Effects of cytochalasins on mammalian cells, Nature 213:261, 1967

69. Casey, WJ: Cervical sympathetic stimulation in monkeys and the effects on outflow facility and intraocular volume: a study of the East African vervet (Cercopithecus ethiops), Invest Ophthalmol 5:33, 1966

70. Channell, M, and Beckman, H: Intraocular pressure changes after Neodymium-YAG laser posterior capsulotomy, Arch Ophthalmol 102:1024, 1984

71. Crawford, K, Kaufman, PL, and True-Gabelt, B: Effects of topical PGF$_{2\alpha}$ on aqueous humor dynamics in cynomolgus monkeys, Curr Eye Res 6:1035, 1987

72. Crawford, K, and Kaufman, PL: Pilocarpine antagonizes PGF$_{2\alpha}$-induced ocular hypotension in monkeys: evidence for enhancement of uveoscleral outflow by PGF$_{2\alpha}$, Arch Ophthalmol 105:1112, 1987

73. Crean, EV, et al: Establishment of calf trabecular meshwork cell cultures, Exp Eye Res 43:503, 1986

74. Crean, EV, Tyson, SL, and Richardson, TM: Factors influencing glycosaminoglycan synthesis by calf trabecular meshwork cell cultures, Exp Eye Res 43:365, 1986

75. Criswick, VG, and Drance, SM: Comparative study of four different epinephrine salts on intraocular pressure, Arch Ophthalmol 75:768, 1966

76. Davanger, M: On the molecular composition and physicochemical properties of the pseudoexfoliation material, Acta Ophthalmol 55:621, 1977

77. Davies, P, and Allison, AC: Effects of cytochalasin B on endocytosis and exocytosis. In Tannenbaum, SW, editor: Cytochalasins, biochemical and cell biological aspects, Amsterdam, 1978, North Holland, p 143

78. Ehinger, B: Adrenergic nerves to the eye and to related structures in man in the cynomolgus monkey (Macaca irus), Invest Ophthalmol 5:42, 1966

79. Ellingsen, BA, and Grant, WM: Influence of intraocular pressure and trabeculotomy on aqueous outflow in enucleated monkey eyes, Invest Ophthalmol 10:705, 1971

80. Ellingsen, BA, and Grant, WM: Trabeculotomy and sinusotomy in enucleated human eyes, Invest Ophthalmol 11:21, 1972

81. Epstein, DL, Hashimoto, JM, and Grant, WM: Serum obstruction of aqueous outflow in enucleated eyes, Am J Ophthalmol 86:101, 1978

82. Epstein, DL, Jedziniak, JA, and Grant, WM: Obstruction of aqueous outflow by lens particles and heavy molecular weight soluble protein, Invest Opthalmol Vis Sci 17:272, 1978

83. Epstein, DL, Jedziniak, JA, and Grant, WM: Identification of heavy molecular weight soluble lens protein in aqueous humor in phakolytic glaucoma, Invest Ophthalmol Vis Sci 17:298, 1978

84. Epstein, DL, Hashimoto, JM, Anderson, PJ, and Grant, WM: Effect of iodoacetamide perfusion on outflow facility and metabolism of the trabecular meshwork, Invest Ophthalmol Vis Sci 20:625, 1981

85. Epstein, DL, Patterson, MM, Rivers, SC, and Anderson, PJ: N-ethylmaleimide increases the facility of aqueous outflow of excised monkey and calf eyes, Invest Ophthalmol Vis Sci 22:752, 1982

86. Erickson, KA, and Kaufman, PL: Comparative effects of three ocular perfusates on outflow facility in the cynomolgus monkey, Curr Eye Res 1:211, 1981

87. Fenton, RH, and Zimmerman, LE: Hemolytic glaucoma, Arch Ophthalmol 70:236, 1963

88. Flocks, M, Littwin, CS, and Zimmerman, LE: Phacolytic glaucoma: clinicopathologic study of 138 cases of glaucoma associated with hypermature cataract, Arch Ophthalmol 54:37, 1955

89. Flocks, M, and Zweng, HC: Studies on the mode of action of pilocarpine on aqueous outflow, Am J Ophthalmol 44:380, 1957

90. Floyd, BB, Cleveland, PH, and Worthen, DM: Fibronectin in human trabecular drainage channels, Invest Ophthalmol Vis Sci 26:797, 1985

91. Fortin, EP: Canel de Schlemm y ligamento pectineo, Arch Ophthalmol 4:454, 1925

92. Fortin, EP: Action du muscle ciliaire sur la circulation de l'oeil; insertion du muscle ciliaire sur la paroi du canal de Schlemm: signification physiologique et pathologique, CR Soc Biol 102:432, 1929

93. François, J, Rabaey, M, and Neetens, A: Perfusion studies on the outflow of aqueous humor in human eyes, Arch Ophthalmol 55:193, 1956

94. François, J: The importance of the mucopolysaccharides in intraocular pressure regulation, Invest Ophthalmol 14:173, 1975

95. Freddo, TF, Patterson, MM, Scott, DR, and Epstein, DL: Influence of mercurial sulfhydryl agents on aqueous outflow pathways in enucleated eyes, Invest Ophthalmol Vis Sci 25:278, 1984

96. Gaasterland, D, Kupfer, C, Ross, K, and Gabelnick, HL: Studies of aqueous humor dynamics in man. III. Measurements in young normal subjects using norepinephrine and isoproterenol, Invest Ophthalmol 12:267, 1973

97. Gaasterland, D, and Kupfer, C: Experimental glaucoma in the rhesus monkey, Invest Ophthalmol 13:455, 1974

98. Gaasterland, D, Kupfer, C, and Ross, K: Studies of aqueous humor dynamics in man: IV. Effects of pilocarpine upon measurements in young normal volunteers, Invest Ophthalmol 14:848, 1975

99. Gaasterland, D, Pederson, JE, and MacLellan, HM: Perfusate effects upon resistance to aqueous humor outflow in the rhesus monkey eye: a comparison of gluthathione-bicarbonate Ringer's solution to pooled aqueous humor as perfusate, Invest Ophthalmol Vis Sci 17:391, 1978

100. Gaasterland, DE, Pederson, JE, MacLellan, HM, and Reddy, VN: Rhesus monkey aqueous humor composition and a primate ocular perfusate, Invest Ophthalmol Vis Sci 18:1139, 1979

101. Galin, MA: Mydriasis provocative test, Arch Ophthalmol 66:353, 1961

102. Gipson, IK, and Anderson, RA: Actin filaments in cells of human trabecular meshwork and Schlemm's canal, Invest Ophthalmol Vis Sci 18:547, 1979

103. Godman, GC, and Miranda, AF: Cellular contractility and the visible effects of cytochalasin. In Tannenbaum, SW, editor: Cytochalasins, biochemical and cell biological aspects, Amsterdam, 1978, North Holland

104. Goldberg, MF: The diagnosis and treatment of sickled erythrocytes in human hyphemas, Trans Am Ophthalmol Soc 76:481, 1978

105. Goldman, RD, et al: Fibrillar systems in cell motility. In Porter, RW, and Fitzsimons, DW, editors: Locomotion of tissue cells, Ciba Foundation Symposium 14 (new series), Amsterdam, 1973, Associated Scientific

106. Goldmann, H: L'origine de l'hypertension oculaire dans le glaucome primitif, Ann Occul (Paris) 184:1086, 1951

107. Grant, WM: Experimental aqueous perfusion in enucleated human eyes, Arch Ophthalmol 69:783, 1963

108. Grierson, I, and Lee, WR: Erythrocyte phagocytosis in the human trabecular meshwork, Br J Ophthalmol 57:400, 1973

109. Grierson, I, and Lee, WR: Pressure-induced changes in the ultrastructure of the endothelium lining Schlemm's canal, Am J Ophthalmol 80:862, 1975

110. Grierson, I, and Lee, WR: The fine structure of the trabecular meshwork at graded levels of intraocular pressure. I. Pressure effects within the near-physiological range (8-30 mm Hg), Exp Eye Res 20:505, 1975

111. Grierson, I, Lee, WR, and Abraham, S: Effects of pilocarpine on the morphology of the human outflow apparatus, Br J Ophthalmol 62:302, 1978

112. Grierson, I, and Rahi, AHS: Microfilaments in the cells of human trabecular meshwork, Br J Ophthalmol 63:3, 1979

113. Grierson, I, and Johnson, NF: The post-mortem vacuoles of Schlemm's canal, v Graefes Arch Klin Exp Ophthalmol 215:249, 1981

114. Hager, H: Besondere mikrochirurgische Eingraffe. II. Erste Erfahrungen mit dem Argon Laser Gerat 800, Klin Monatsbl Augenheilkd 162:437, 1973

115. Harris, LS: Cycloplegic-induced intraocular pressure elevations, Arch Ophthalmol 79:242, 1968
116. Harris, LS, Galin, MA, and Lernor, R: The influence of low-dose l-epinephrine on aqueous outflow facility, Ann Ophthalmol 2:455, 1970
117. Heine, L: Die Anatomie des akkommodierten Auges—mikroskopische Fixierung des Akkommodationspaltes, v Graefes Klin Exp Ophthalmol 49:1, 1900
118. Hernandez, MR, et al: The effect of dexamethasone on the in vitro incorporation of precursors of extracellular matrix components in the outflow pathway region of the rabbit eye, Invest Ophthalmol Vis Sci 24:704, 1983
119. Hernandez, MR, et al: Glucocorticoid target cells in human outflow pathway: autopsy and surgical specimens, Invest Ophthalmol Vis Sci 24:1612, 1983
120. Hernandez, MR, et al: The effect of dexamethasone on the synthesis of collagen in normal human trabecular meshwork explants, Invest Ophthalmol Vis Sci 26:1784, 1985
121. Hoffmann, F: Effect of noradrenalin on intraocular pressure and outflow in cynomolgus monkeys, Exp Eye Res 7:369, 1968
122. Hogan, MJ, Alvarado, JA, and Weddell, JE: Histology of the human eye: an atlas and textbook, Philadelphia, 1971, WB Saunders Co
123. Holmberg, Å, and Bárány, EH: The effect of pilocarpine on the endothelium forming the inner wall of Schlemm's canal: an electron microscopic study in the monkey *Cercopithecus aethiops,* Invest Ophthalmol 5:53, 1966
124. Inomata, H, Bill, A, and Smelser, GK: Unconventional routes of aqueous humor outflow in cynomolgus monkey *(Macaca irus),* Am J Ophthalmol 73:893, 1972
125. Inomata, H, Bill, A, and Smelser, GK: Aqueous humor pathways through the trabecular meshwork and into Schlemm's canal in the cynomolgus monkey *(Macaca irus):* an electron microscopic study, Am J Ophthalmol 73:760, 1972
126. Jampel, HD, et al: β-adrenergic receptors in human trabecular meshwork, Invest Ophthalmol Vis Sci 28:772, 1987
127. Johnstone, MA, and Grant, WM: Pressure-dependent changes in structures of the aqueous outflow system of human and monkey eyes, Am J Ophthalmol 75:365, 1973
128. Johnstone, M, Tanner, D, Chau, B, and Kopecky, K: Concentration dependent morphologic effects of cytochalasin B in the aqueous outflow system, Invest Ophthalmol Vis Sci 19:835, 1980
129. Kaufman, PL, and Lütjen-Drecoll, E: Total iridectomy in the primate in vivo: surgical technique and postoperative anatomy, Invest Ophthalmol 14:766, 1975
130. Kaufman, PL, and Bárány, EH: Loss of acute pilocarpine effect on outflow facility following surgical disinsertion and retrodisplacement of the ciliary muscle from the scleral spur in the cynomolgus monkey, Invest Ophthalmol 15:793, 1976
131. Kaufman, PL, and Bárány, EH: Residual pilocarpine effects on outflow facility after ciliary muscle disinsertion in the cynomolgus monkey, Invest Ophthalmol 15:558, 1976
132. Kaufman, PL, and Bárány, EH: Cytochalasin B reversibly increases outflow facility in the eye of the cynomolgus monkey, Invest Ophthalmol Vis Sci 16:47, 1977
133. Kaufman, PL, Bill, A, and Bárány, EH: Formation and drainage of aqueous humor following total iris removal and ciliary muscle disinsertion in the cynomolgus monkey, Invest Ophthalmol Vis Sci 16:226, 1977
134. Kaufman, PL, Bill, A, and Bárány, EH: Effect of cytochalasin B on conventional drainage of aqueous humor in the cynomolgus monkey. In Bito, LZ, Davison, H, and Fenstermacher, JD, editors: The ocular and cerebrospinal fluids, Fogarty International Symposium, Exp Eye Res 25(Suppl):415, 1977
135. Kaufman, PL: Aqueous humor dynamics following total iridectomy in the cynomolgus monkey, Invest Ophthalmol Vis Sci 18:870, 1979
136. Kaufman, PL, and Bárány, EH: Adrenergic drug effects on aqueous outflow facility following ciliary muscle retrodisplacement in the cynomolgus monkey, Invest Ophthalmol Vis Sci 20:644, 1981
137. Kaufman, PL, and Rentzhog, L: Effect of total iridectomy on outflow facility responses to adrenergic drugs in cynomolgus monkeys, Exp Eye Res 33:65, 1981
138. Kaufman, PL, Bárány, EH, and Erickson, KA: Effect of serotonin, histamine, and bradykinin on outflow facility following ciliary muscle retrodisplacement in the cynomolgus monkey, Exp Eye Res 35:191, 1982
139. Kaufman, PL, and Erickson, KA: Cytochalasin B and D dose-outflow facility response relationships in the cynomolgus monkey, Invest Ophthalmol Vis Sci 23:646, 1982
140. Kaufman, PL: The effects of drugs on the outflow of aqueous humor. In Drance, SM, and Neufeld, AM, editors: Glaucoma: applied pharmacology in medical treatment, Orlando, 1984, Grune & Stratton
141. Kaufman, PL: Total iridectomy does not alter outflow facility responses to cyclic AMP in cynomolgus monkeys, Exp Eye Res 43:441, 1986
142. Kaufman, PL: Epinephrine, norepinephrine, and isoproterenol dose-outflow facility response relationships in cynomolgus monkeys with and without ciliary muscle retrodisplacement, Acta Ophthalmol 64:356, 1986

143. Kaufman, PL: cAMP and outflow facility in monkey eyes with intact and retrodisplaced ciliary muscle, Exp Eye Res 44:415, 1987

144. Kaufman, PL: Non-additivity of maximal pilocarpine and cytochalasin effects on outflow facility, Exp Eye Res 44:283, 1987

145. Kaufman, PL: Effects of intracamerally infused prostaglandins on outflow facility in cynomolgus monkey eyes with intact or retrodisplaced ciliary muscle, Exp Eye Res 43:819, 1986

146. Kaufman, PL, True-Gabelt, B, and Erickson-Lamy, KA: Time-dependence of perfusion outflow facility in the cynomolgus monkey, Curr Eye Res Submitted 1987

147. Kinsey, VE: Ion movement in ciliary processes. In Bittar, EE, editor: Membranes and ion transport, vol 3, New York, 1971, Wiley & Sons

148. Knepper, PA, Collins, JA, and Frederick, R: Effect of dexamethasone, progesterone, and testosterone on IOP and GAGs in the rabbit eye, Invest Ophthalmol Vis Sci 26:1093, 1985

149. Knepper, PA, Collins, JA, Weinstein, HG, and Breen, M: Aqueous outflow pathway complex carbohydrate synthesis in vitro, Invest Ophthalmol Vis Sci 24:1546, 1983

150. Kolker, AE, and Becker, B: Topical corticosteroids and glaucoma: current status. In Bellows, JG, editor: Contemporary ophthalmology, Baltimore, 1972, Williams & Wilkins

151. Kolker, AE, and Hetherington, J, Jr: Becker-Shaffer's diagnosis and therapy of the glaucomas, ed 5, St Louis, 1983, The CV Mosby Co

152. Krasnov, MM: Laser puncture of anterior chamber angle in glaucoma, Am J Ophthalmol 75:674, 1973

153. Krill, AE, Newell, FW, and Novak, KM: Early and long-term effects of levoepinephrine on ocular tension and outflow, Am J Ophthalmol 59:833, 1965

154. Kronfeld, PC: Dose-effect relationships as an aid to the evaluation of ocular hypotensive drugs, Invest Ophthalmol 3:258, 1964

155. Kronfeld, PC: The efficacy of combinations of ocular hypotensive drugs, Arch Ophthalmol 78:140, 1967

156. Kronfeld, PC: Early effect of single and repeated doses of l-epinephrine in man, Am J Ophthalmol 72:1058, 1971

157. Kupfer, C, and Sanderson, P: Determination of pseudofacility in the eye of man, Arch Ophthalmol 80:194, 1968

158. Kupfer, C, and Ross, K: Studies of aqueous dynamics in man. I. Measurements in young normal subjects, Invest Ophthalmol 10:518, 1971

159. Kupfer, C, Gaasterland, D, and Ross, K: Studies of aqueous humor dynamics in man. II. Measurements in young normal subjects using acetazolamide and l-epinephrine, Invest Ophthalmol 10:523, 1971

160. Langham, ME: The aqueous outflow system and its response to autonomic receptor agonists. In Bito, LZ, Davson, H, and Fenstermacher, JD, editors: The ocular and cerebrospinal fluids, Fogarty International Center Symposium, Exp Eye Res 25 (Suppl):311, 1977

161. Laties, AM, and Jacobowitz, D: A comparative study of the autonomic innervation of the eye in monkey, cat and rabbit, Anat Rec 156:383, 1966

162. Lee, P, Podos, SM, and Severin, C: Effect of prostaglandin $F_{2\alpha}$ on aqueous humor dynamics of rabbit, cat and monkey, Invest Ophthalmol Vis Sci 25:1087, 1984

163. Levitzki, A: The binding characteristics and number of beta-adrenergic receptors in the turkey erythrocyte, Proc Natl Acad Sci USA 71:2773, 1974

164. Lindenmayer, JM, Kahn, MG, Hertzmark, E, and Epstein, DL: Morphology and function of the aqueous outflow system in monkey eyes perfused with sulfhydryl reagents, Invest Ophthalmol Vis Sci 24:710, 1983

165. Lütjen-Drecoll, E: Structural factors influencing outflow facility and its changeability under drugs, Invest Ophthalmol 12:280, 1973

166. Lütjen-Drecoll, E, and Bárány, EH: Functional and electron microscopic changes in the trabecular meshwork remaining after trabeculectomy in cynomolgus monkeys, Invest Ophthalmol 13:511, 1974

167. Lütjen-Drecoll, E, Kaufman, PL, and Bárány, EH: Light and electron microscopy of the anterior chamber angle structures following surgical disinsertion of the ciliary muscle in the cynomolgus monkey, Invest Ophthalmol Vis Sci 16:218, 1977

168. Lütjen-Drecoll, E, and Kaufman, PL: Echothiophate-induced structural alterations in the anterior chamber angle of the cynomolgus monkey, Invest Ophthalmol Vis Sci 18:918, 1979

169. Lütjen-Drecoll, E, Futa, R, and Rohen, JW: Ultrahistochemical studies on tangential sections of the trabecular meshwork in normal and glaucomatous eyes, Invest Ophthalmol Vis Sci 21:563, 1981

170. Lütjen-Drecoll, E, Shimizu, T, Rohrbach, M, and Rohen, JW: Quantitative analysis of plaque material in the inner- and outer wall of Schlemm's canal in normal and glaucomatous eyes, Exp Eye Res 42:443, 1986

171. Lütjen-Drecoll, E, Shimizu, T, Rohrbach, M, and Rohen, JW: Quantitative analysis of plaque material between ciliary muscle tips in normal and glaucomatous eyes, Exp Eye Res 42:457, 1986

172. Lütjen-Drecoll, E, and Kaufman, PL: Biomechanics of echothiophate-induced anatomic changes in monkey aqueous outflow system, v Graefes Arch Clin Exp Ophthalmol 224:564, 1986

173. MacRae, D, and Sears, ML: Peroxidase passage through the outflow channels of human and rhesus eyes, Exp Eye Res 10:15, 1970

174. Maren, TH: HCO_3 formation in aqueous humor: mechanism and relation to the treatment of glaucoma, Invest Ophthalmol 13:179, 1974

175. Masuda, K, and Mishima, S: Effects of prostaglandins on inflow and outflow of aqueous humor in rabbits, Jpn J Ophthalmol 17:300, 1973

176. Melamed, S, Pei, J, and Epstein, DL: Argon laser trabeculoplasty in monkeys, Invest Ophthalmol Vis Sci 26(ARVO Suppl):158, 1986

177. Moses, RA: The effect of intraocular pressure on resistance to outflow, Surv Ophthalmol 22:88, 1977

178. Moses, RA: Circumferential flow in Schlemm's canal, Am J Ophthalmol 88:585, 1979

179. Moses, RA, Hoover, GS, and Oostwouder, PH: Blood reflux in Schlemm's canal, Arch Ophthalmol 97:1307, 1979

180. Moses, RA: Intraocular pressure. In Moses, RA, editor: Adler's physiology of the eye: clinical application, ed 7, St Louis, 1981, The CV Mosby Co

181. Moses, RA, Grodzki, WJ, Jr, Etheridge, EL, and Wilson, CD: Schlemm's canal: the effect of intraocular pressure, Invest Ophthalmol Vis Sci 20:61, 1981

182. Moses, RA, Etheridge, EL, and Grodzki, WJ, Jr: The effect of lens depression on the components of outflow resistance, Invest Ophthalmol Vis Sci 22:37, 1982

183. Neufeld, AH, Jampol, LM, and Sears, ML: Cyclic-AMP in the aqueous humor: the effects of adrenergic agents, Exp Eye Res 14:242, 1972

184. Neufeld, AH, and Sears, ML: Cyclic-AMP in ocular tissues of the rabbit, monkey and human, Invest Ophthalmol 13:475, 1974

185. Neufeld, AH, Dueker, DK, Vegge, T, and Sears, ML: Adenosine 3',5'-monophosphate increases the outflow of aqueous humor from the rabbit eye, Invest Ophthalmol 14:40, 1975

186. Neufeld, AH, and Sears, ML: Adenosine 3',5'-monophosphate analogue increases the outflow facility of the primate eye, Invest Ophthalmol 14:688, 1975

187. Neufeld, AH: Influences of cyclic nucleotides on outflow facility in the vervet monkey, Exp Eye Res 27:387, 1978

188. Nomura, T, and Smelser, GK: The identification of adrenergic and cholinergic nerve endings in the trabecular meshwork, Invest Ophthalmol 13:525, 1974

189. Obstbaum, SA, Kolker, AE, and Phelps, CD: Low-dose epinephrine: effect on intraocular pressure, Arch Ophthalmol 92:118, 1974

190. Pedersen, JE: Fluid permeability of monkey ciliary epithelium in vivo, Invest Ophthalmol Vis Sci 23:176, 1982

191. Pedler, WS: The relationship of hyaluronidase to aqueous outflow resistance, Trans Ophthalmol Soc UK 76:51, 1956

192. Petersen, HP: Can pigmentary deposits on the trabecular meshwork increase the resistance of the aqueous outflow? Acta Ophthalmol 47:743, 1969

193. Peterson, WS, and Jocson, VL: Hyaluronidase effects on aqueous outflow resistance: quantitative and localizing studies in the rhesus monkey eye, Am J Ophthalmol 77:573, 1974

194. Plagemann, PGW, Wohlheuter, RM, Graff, JC, and Marz, R: Inhibition of carrier-mediated and non-mediated permeation processes by cytochalasin B. In Tannenbaum, SW, editor: Cytochalasins, biochemical and cell biological aspects, Amsterdam, 1978, North Holland

195. Polansky, JR, Weinreb, RN, Baxter, JD, and Alvarado, J: Human trabecular cells. I. Establishment in tissue culture and growth characteristics, Invest Ophthalmol Vis Sci 18:1043, 1979

196. Polansky, JR, Weinreb, R, and Alvarado, JA: Studies on human trabecular cells propagated in vitro, Vision Res 21:155, 1981

197. Polansky, JR, et al: Cultured human trabecular cells: evaluation of hormonal and pharmacological responses in vitro. In Ticho, U, and David, R, editors: Recent advances in glaucoma, Amsterdam, 1984, Elsevier Science Publishers BV

198. Polansky, JR, Wood, IS, Maglio, MT, and Alvarado, JA: Trabecular meshwork cell culture in glaucoma research: evaluation of biological activity and structural properties of human trabecular cells in vitro, Ophthalmology 91:580, 1984

199. Pollack, IP, and Rossi, H: Norepinephrine in treatment of ocular hypertension and glaucoma, Arch Ophthalmol 93:173, 1975

200. Prijot, E: Contribution à l' étude de la tonometrie et de la tonographie en opthalmologie, Doc Ophthalmol 15:1, 1961

201. Quigley, HA: Long-term follow-up of laser iridotomy, Ophthalmology 88:218, 1981

202. Rees, D, Lloyd, CW, and Thom, D: Control of grip and stick in cell adhesion through lateral relationships of membrane glycoproteins, Nature 267:124, 1977

203. Ringvold, A: Actin filaments in trabecular endothelial cells in eyes of the vervet monkey (Cercopithecus ethiops), Acta Ophthalmol 56:217, 1978

204. Rodewald, R, Newmann, SB, and Karnovsky, MJ: Contraction of isolated brush borders from the intestinal epithelium, J Cell Biol 70:541, 1976

205. Rodrigues, MM, Katz, SI, Foidart, JM, and Spaeth, GL: Collagen, factor VIII antigen, and immunoglobulins in the human aqueous drainage channels, Trans Am Acad Ophthalmol 87:337, 1980

206. Rohen, JW: Handbuch der mikroskopischen Anatomie des Menschen, Berlin, 1964, Springer

207. Rohen, JW, Lütjen, E, and Bárány, EH: The relation between the ciliary muscle and the trabecular meshwork and its importance for the effect of miotics on aqueous outflow resistance, v Graefes Arch Klin Exp Ophthalmol 172:23, 1967

208. Rohen, JW, and Van der Zypen, E: The phagocytic activity of the trabecular meshwork endothelium: an electron microscopic study of the vervet (*Cercopithecus ethiops*), v Graefes Arch Klin Exp Ophthalmol 175:143, 1968

209. Rohen, JW, Futa, R, and Lütjen-Drecoll, E: The fine structure of the cribriform meshwork in normal and glaucomatous eyes as seen in tangential sections, Invest Ophthalmol Vis Sci 21:574, 1981

210. Rohen, JW, Schachtschabel, DO, and Wehrmann, R: Structural changes in human and monkey trabecular meshwork following in vitro cultivation, v Graefes Arch Klin Exp Ophthalmol 218:225, 1982

211. Ruskell, GL: Innervation of the anterior segment of the eye. In Lütjen-Drecoll, E, editor: Basic aspects of glaucoma research, Stuttgart, 1982, Schattauer Verlag

212. Schachtschabel, DO, Bigalke, B, and Rohen, JW: Production of glycosaminoglycans by cell cultures of the trabecular meshwork of the primate eye, Exp Eye Res 24:71, 1977

213. Schachtschabel, DO, Rohen, JW, Wever, J, and Sames, K: Synthesis and composition of glycosaminoglycans by cultured human trabecular meshwork cells, v Graefes Arch Klin Exp Ophthalmol 218:113, 1982

214. Schimek, R, and Lieberman, WJ: The influence of Cyclogyl and Neo-synephrine on tonographic studies of miotic control in open angle glaucoma, Am J Ophthalmol 51:781, 1961

215. Schwartz, B: The response of ocular pressure to corticosteroids. In Schwartz, B, editor: Corticosteroids and the eye, Int Ophthalmol Clin 6:929, 1966

216. Schwartz, AL, Whitten, ME, Bleiman, B, and Martin, D: Argon laser trabecular surgery in uncontrolled phakic open-angle glaucoma, Ophthalmology 88:203, 1981

217. Scott, DR, Karageuzian, LN, Anderson, PJ, and Epstein, DL: Glutathione peroxidase of calf trabecular meshwork, Invest Ophthalmol Vis Sci 25:599, 1984

218. Sears, ML, and Sherk, TE: The trabecular effect of noradrenalin in the rabbit eye, Invest Ophthalmol 3:157, 1964

219. Sears, ML: The mechanism of action of adrenergic drugs in glaucoma, Invest Ophthalmol 5:115, 1966

220. Sears, ML, and Neufeld, AH: Adrenergic modulation of the outflow of aqueous humor, Invest Ophthalmol 14:83, 1975

221. Sears, ML: The aqueous. In Moses, RA, editor: Adler's physiology of the eye: clinical application, ed 7, St Louis, 1981, The CV Mosby Co

222. Shaffer, RN: In Newell, FW, editor: Glaucoma, transactions of the 5th conference, New York, 1961, Josiah Macy Jr Foundation

223. Shabo, AL, Reese, TS, and Gaasterland, D: Postmortem formation of giant endothelial vacuoles in Schlemm's canal of the monkey, Am J Ophthalmol 76:896, 1973

224. Southren, AL, et al: Altered cortisol metabolism in cells cultured from trabecular meshwork obtained from patients with primary open-angle glaucoma, Invest Ophthalmol Vis Sci 24:1413, 1983

225. Southren, AL, et al: 5β-dihydrocortisol: possible mediator of the ocular hypertension in glaucoma, Invest Ophthalmol Vis Sci 26:393, 1985

226. Stern, FA, and Bito, LZ: Comparison of the hypotensive and other ocular effects of prostaglandins E_2 and $F_{2\alpha}$ on cat and rhesus monkey eyes, Invest Ophthalmol Vis Sci 22:588, 1982

227. Stone, RA, Laties, AM, and Brecha, NC: Substance P-like immunoreactive nerves in the anterior segment of the rabbit, cat and monkey eye, Neuroscience 7:2459, 1982

228. Stone, RA, Kuwayama, Y, Laties, AM, and Marangos, PJ: Neuron-specific enolase-containing cells in the rhesus monkey trabecular meshwork, Invest Ophthalmol Vis Sci 25:1332, 1984

229. Stone, RA, and Kuwayama, Y: Substance P-like immunoreactive nerves in the human eye, Arch Ophthalmol 103:1207, 1985

230. Stone, RA: Neuropeptide Y and the innervation of the human eye, Exp Eye Res 42:349, 1986

231. Stone, RA, Laties, AM, and Emson, PC: Neuropeptide Y and the ocular innervation of rat, guinea pig, cat and monkey, Neuroscience 17:1207, 1986

232. Stone, RA, Tervo, T, Tervo, K, and Tarkkanen, A: Vasoactive intestinal polypeptide-like immunoreactive nerves to the human eye, Acta Ophthalmol 64:12, 1986

233. Svedbergh, B: Aspects of the aqueous humor drainage: functional ultrastructure of Schlemm's canal, the trabecular meshwork and the corneal endothelium at different intraocular pressures, Acta Universitatis Upsaliensis 256:1, 1976

234. Svedbergh, B: Effects of intraocular pressure on the pores of the inner wall of Schlemm's canal: a scanning electron microscopic study. In Yamada, S, and Mishima, S, editors: The structure of the eye, Jpn J Ophthalmol 127, 1976

235. Svedbergh, B, Lütjen-Drecoll, E, Ober, M, and Kaufman, PL: Cytochalasin B-induced structural changes in the anterior ocular segment of the cynomolgus monkey, Invest Ophthalmol Vis Sci 17:718, 1978

236. Tchernitchin, A, et al: Glucocorticoid localization by radioautography in the rabbit eye following systemic administration of ³H-dexamethasone, Invest Ophthalmol Vis Sci 19:1231, 1980

237. Teichmann, I, Teichmann, KD, and Fechner, PU: Glaucoma operation with the argon laser, Eye Ear Nose Throat Monthly 55:58, 1976

238. Thomas, JV, and Epstein, DL: Timolol and epinephrine in primary open angle glaucoma: transient additive effect, Arch Ophthalmol 99:91, 1981

239. Ticho, U, and Zauberman, H: Argon laser application to the angle structures in the glaucomas, Arch Ophthalmol 94:61, 1976

240. Tokiwa, T, Hoshika, T, Shiraishi, M, and Sato, J: Mechanism of cell dissociation with trypsin and EDTA, Acta Med Okayama 33:1, 1979

241. Toris, CB, and Pederson, JE: Effect of intraocular pressure on uveoscleral outflow following cyclodialysis in the monkey eye, Invest Ophthalmol Vis Sci 26:1745, 1985

242. Törnqvist, G: Effect of cervical sympathetic stimulation on accommodation in monkeys: an example of a beta-adrenergic, inhibitory effect, Acta Physiol Scand 67:363, 1966

243. Törnqvist, G: Effect of oculomotor nerve stimulation on outflow facility and pupil diameter in a monkey (Cercopithecus ethiops), Invest Ophthalmol 9:220, 1970

244. Tripathi, RC: The functional morphology of the outflow systems of ocular and cerebrospinal fluids. In Bito, JZ, Davson, H, and Fenstermacher, JD, editors: The ocular and cerebrospinal fluids, Fogarty International Center Symposium, Exp Eye Res 25(Suppl):65, 1977

245. Tripathi, RC, and Tripathi, BJ: Contractile protein alteration in primary open angle glaucoma, Exp Eye Res 31:725, 1980

246. Uga, S: Electron microscopy of the ciliary muscle. II. On the fine structure of the anterior terminal portion of the ciliary muscle, Acta Soc Ophthalmol Jpn 72:1019, 1968

247. Van Alphen, GWHM, Robinette, SL, and Macri, FJ: Drug effects on ciliary muscle and choroid preparations in vitro, Arch Ophthalmol 68:81, 1962

248. Van Alphen, GWHM, Kern, R, and Robinette, S: Adrenergic receptors of the intraocular muscles: comparison to cat, rabbit and monkey, Arch Ophthalmol 74:253, 1965

249. Van Buskirk, EM, and Grant, WM: Lens depression and aqueous outflow in enucleated primate eyes, Am J Ophthalmol 76:632, 1973

250. Weekers, R, Prijot, E, and Gustin, J: Recent advances and future prospects in the medical treatment of ocular hypertension, Br J Ophthalmol 38:742, 1954

251. Weinreb, RN, et al: Detection of glucocorticoid receptors in cultured human trabecular cells, Invest Ophthalmol Vis Sci 21:403, 1981

252. Weinreb, RN, Mitchell, MD, Alvarado, JA, and Polansky, JR: Glucocortocoid regulation of eicosanoid biosynthesis in cultured human trabecular cells. In Ticho, U, David, R, editors: Recent advances in glaucoma, Amsterdam, 1984, Elsevier Science Publishers BV

253. Weinreb, RN, Polansky, JR, Kramer, SG, and Baxter, JD: Acute effects of dexamethasone on intraocular pressure in glaucoma, Invest Ophthalmol Vis Sci 26:170, 1985

254. Weinstein, BI, Gordon, G, and Southren, AL: Potentiation of glucocorticoid activity by 5β-dihydrocortisol: its role in glaucoma, Science 222:172, 1983

255. Weinstein, BI, Munnangi, P, Gordon, GG, and Southren, AL: Defects in cortisol-metabolizing enzymes in primary open-angle glaucoma, Invest Ophthalmol Vis Sci 26:890, 1985

256. Wickham, MG, and Worthen, DM: Argon laser trabeculotomy: long-term follow-up, Ophthalmology 86:495, 1979

257. Wilensky, JT, and Jampol, LM: Laser therapy for open-angle glaucoma, Ophthalmology 88:213, 1981

258. Wise, JB, and Witter, SL: Argon laser therapy for open-angle glaucoma: a pilot study, Arch Ophthalmol 97:319, 1979

259. Wise, JB: Long-term control of adult open-angle glaucoma by argon laser treatment, Ophthalmology 88:197, 1981

260. Worthen, DM: Scanning electron microscopy after alpha chymotrypsin perfusion in man, Am J Ophthalmol 73:637, 1972

261. Worthen, DM, and Wickham, MG: Argon laser trabeculotomy, Trans Am Acad Ophthalmol Otolaryngol 78:371, 1974

262. Worthen, DM, and Cleveland, TH: Fibronectin production in cultured human trabecular meshwork cells, Invest Ophthalmol Vis Sci 23:265, 1982

263. Yanoff, M: Glaucoma mechanisms in ocular malignant melanomas, Am J Ophthalmol 70:898, 1970

264. Zimmerman, TJ, Harbin, R, Pett, M, and Kaufman, HE: Timolol and facility of outflow, Invest Ophthalmol Vis Sci 16:623, 1977

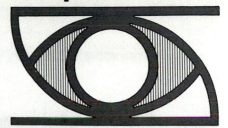

Chapter 10

Uveoscleral Outflow

Jonathan E. Pederson

Uveoscleral outflow may be defined as aqueous outflow through the intermuscular spaces of the ciliary muscle, into the supraciliary-suprachoroidal space, and out through the substance of the sclera or through the perivascular spaces of the emissarial channels.[22] The movement of tracers from the anterior chamber into the supraciliary-suprachoroidal space, which has been observed by numerous investigators, was dismissed originally as merely diffusion, phagocytosis, or an artifact.

In 1965, Bill reported that a substantial fraction of radioiodinated albumin perfused through the anterior chamber of the cynomolgus monkey could be recovered within the uveal tract and sclera.[6] In freshly killed cynomolgus monkeys, 25 minutes of anterior chamber perfusion with radioiodinated albumin resulted in high and nearly equal albumin concentrations in the anterior and posterior sclera. This observation argued against diffusion as a primary moving force for the tracer. In living cynomolgus monkeys, an anterior chamber perfusion of myoglobin, albumin, and gamma globulin was carried out for 90 minutes.[5] These three tracers left the anterior chamber at similar rates in spite of large differences in diffusion coefficients. It was thus concluded that these substances left the anterior chamber by bulk flow. Approximately one fourth of the albumin was recovered from the ocular tissues. This was interpreted as evidence for an unconventional route of bulk aqueous humor outflow, termed *uveoscleral outflow.* If there had been a combination of bulk outflow from the anterior chamber through the trabecular meshwork together with diffusion of the tracers into the uveal tissues and sclera, the tracers would have been expected to leave the anterior chamber at more dissimilar rates. Based on these preliminary findings suggesting bulk flow through a uveoscleral outflow pathway, numerous subsequent physiologic and anatomic studies have been performed.

ROUTE OF UVEOSCLERAL OUTFLOW

Anatomy

The anatomy of the uveoscleral outflow pathway has been carefully described by Bill et al.[19] To summarize, no epithelial barrier exists between the anterior chamber and the supraciliary space. For this reason alone, it may be inferred that the rate at which substances pass from the anterior chamber into the supraciliary space depends on the permeability of the ciliary muscle to them. The longitudinal fibers of the ciliary muscle extend posteriorly and disappear into the connective tissue between the choroid and sclera. The intermuscular spaces are filled with loose connective tissue and ground substance. The suprachoroidal space itself is composed of loose connective tissue and may be considered largely a potential space, since the normal volume of fluid in it is only approximately 10 μl.[36] In the hamster eye, separate anterior and posterior uveal compartments, separated by a "compact zone" have been described.[31] This compact zone contains tight-junctioned fibroblastic lamellae and separates the choriocapillaris and choroidal interstitium from the suprachoroidal space. It is not known whether such a functional structure exists in primates or humans. The sclera consists of tightly interwoven collagen bundles of fibroblasts.

Numerous perforations in the sclera exist for the passage of nerves and blood vessels, termed *emissarial channels*. Surrounding the nerves or vessels are loose connective tissue spaces. No true lymphatics exist within the eye, but it has been suggested that the loose connective tissue surrounding the nerves or vessels of the emissarial channel serves a lymphlike function.[33]

The existence of the uveoscleral outflow pathway can be readily demonstrated in the freshly enucleated monkey eye. Fluorescein-stained fluid perfused into the anterior chamber at a normal intraocular pressure will appear at the vortex vein exit site within about 10 or 15 minutes. Under this circumstance, fluorescein-stained fluid flows around the vortex vein, not within its lumen (Fig. 10-1).

Tracer Studies

A large number of diverse tracers have been employed in different species to delineate the uveoscleral outflow pathway. The use of different-

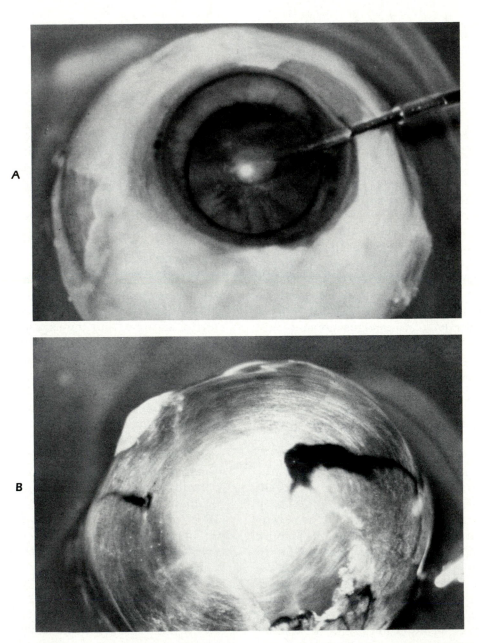

Fig. 10-1 **A,** Fluorescein-containing physiologic salt solution perfusion into anterior chamber of enucleated monkey eye at intraocular pressure of 15 mm Hg. **B,** Fluorescein-stained fluid flows out around vortex vein exit site.

sized tracers in various species has also been used to determine the relative "permeability" of the ciliary muscle. For the purpose of discussion, tracers will be divided into three categories based on size: (1) small tracers such as fluorescein, (2) medium-sized tracers such as proteins, and (3) large tracers such as latex spheres.

Fluorescein passes rapidly from the anterior chamber into the suprachoroidal space in cats, rabbits, and monkeys.[34] Fluorescein also penetrates blood vessels in the iris stroma and anterior ciliary body, leading to the designation uveovortex pathway.[30,40] In the rabbit, nitro blue tetrazolium dye passes into the ciliary cleft and into the perivascular aqueous channels of the ciliary body.[27]

Unlike the smaller tracers, species differences are noted with respect to medium-sized tracers such as fluorescein-labeled dextran. In the monkey eye, fluorescein isothiocyanate (FITC) dextran 70 rapidly penetrates the ciliary muscle and appears in the suprachoroidal space (Fig. 10-2).[42] Similar findings are noted in the hamster using horseradish peroxidase or ferritin.[31] In the rabbit, red dextran does not penetrate the eye posterior to the limbus.[10] However, subsequent studies with fluorescein-labeled dextrans and Thorotrast have revealed tracer within the suprachoroidal space.[23,45] Dye-labeled albumin can be seen in the iris and ciliary body of the rabbit eye but is not found in the suprachoroidal space.[34] In the dog, FITC dextran 40 can be seen in the suprachoroidal space.[29] Direct injection of red dextran into the suprachoroidal space penetrates the perivascular spaces of the sclera and to a lesser extent the sclera itself.[4]

Large tracers such as 0.1 μm latex spheres move from the anterior chamber to the suprachoroidal space near the optic nerve in only 20 minutes in the monkey eye.[19] 1 μm latex spheres reach the suprachoroidal region of the macula in 3 hours. From the suprachoroid, the latex spheres exit the sclera via the loose connective tissue around the long posterior ciliary arteries and nerves.[21] 1 to 3 μm vinyl particles also pass far into the suprachoroidal space in enucleated monkey eyes.[34] Vinyl particles do not penetrate beyond the ciliary muscle of the cat eye and only minimally infiltrate the ciliary body in the rabbit eye.[34] In the dog, 0.5 and 1.0 μm microspheres move into the suprachoroidal space, whereas 3 μm spheres do not.[24,39]

PHYSIOLOGY OF UVEOSCLERAL OUTFLOW

Methodology

In a typical experiment, the anterior chamber is perfused with a tracer for a suitable length of time. The anterior chamber is then flushed free of tracer and the eye is removed and dissected. The amount of tracer recovered in the tissues may then be expressed as equivalent volumes of aqueous, since the original anterior chamber concentration of tracer is known.[5] Radiolabeled tracers have

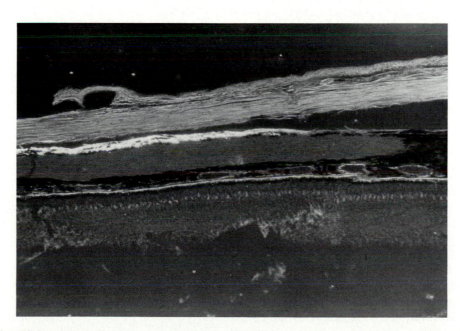

Fig. 10-2 Fluorescein-isothiocyanate dextran 70 perfusion in anterior chamber of monkey eye shows fluorescent material in suprachoroidal space after 30 minutes. (Reprinted from Toris, CB, and Pederson, JE: Invest Ophthalmol Vis Sci 26:1745, 1985)

proven suitable for this type of experiment, as well as covalently bound fluorescent tracers.[41]

It is important to recognize the assumptions underlying the determination of the rate of uveoscleral outflow. From the arguments outlined earlier, it is assumed that tracer moving into the uveal tract and sclera represents a bulk flow of fluid. Thus the tracer is merely a marker for fluid movement. Tritiated water cannot be used, since its high rate of diffusion makes interpretation of the data impossible. The choice of the proper-sized tracer is important, since smaller molecules may diffuse into the tissues, giving erroneous results. Furthermore, the duration of the experiment is important, since the tracer may actually be entirely lost from the eye if the perfusion is carried out too long, resulting in an underestimate of the actual flow.

Of these various assumptions, the most important question is the proportion of tracer that moves through the uveoscleral route as a result of being "swept along" by flow versus that portion caused by diffusion. This uncertainty is the most commonly held skepticism of uveoscleral outflow studies.

There is no clinical method to measure uveoscleral outflow. Fluorophotometry can measure anterior chamber aqueous humor flow, and conventional outflow can be calculated from outflow facility, intraocular pressure, and episcleral venous pressure. The difference between the fluorophotometry value and the conventional outflow value would theoretically yield the uveoscleral outflow value. However, the errors of each individual measurement are compounded, yielding uncertain results.

Diffusion Versus Flow

For flow to exist from the anterior chamber into the suprachoroidal space, a hydrostatic pressure differential must exist. In cats, the suprachoroidal pressure is 2 mm Hg lower than the anterior chamber pressure.[46] This experiment has not been repeated in other species. One method to differentiate between diffusion and flow would be to measure the rate of appearance of different-sized tracers in the suprachoroidal space. This has been performed in monkeys, using fluorescein, and FITC dextran 4, 40, 70, and 150.[43] The uveoscleral outflow rates for these different tracers are shown in Table 10-1 and are remarkably similar. This evidence argues against diffusion as a significant factor for tracer movement. Even stronger evidence was found in a unidirectional tracer flux experiment. The rate of movement of FITC dextran 70 from the anterior chamber into the suprachoroid

was determined in one series of experiments, and the rate of movement of the tracer from the suprachoroid into the anterior chamber was measured in a separate set of experiments following tracer injection into the suprachoroidal space (Fig. 10-3). The movement of the tracer was almost 200 times greater from the anterior chamber to suprachoroid than vice versa.[38] Were diffusion the predominant factor, these fluxes would be similar.

For smaller tracers, diffusion will undoubtedly occur. For example, in the monkey eye, 9% of anterior chamber fluorescein exits the eye via vortex vein blood.[36] Fluorescein may enter the uveal circulation by diffusion or possibly active transport into uveal vessels, as occurs in retinal vessels.[25] The amount of anterior chamber albumin recovered in the vortex vein blood is only 1% to 3%.[36] Similar findings are noted in rabbits where only 1% of albumin and 8% of inulin exits via the vortex veins.[3,34] The iris vessels themselves drain only a trivial amount of aqueous humor.[20] Once fluid has passed

Table 10-1 Uveoscleral outflow in monkey eyes with various tracer sizes[42,43]

Tracer	Uveoscleral outflow (μl/min)
Fluorescein	0.70
Fluorescein-isothiocyanate	
Dextran (molecular weight)	
4,000	0.78
40,000	0.79
70,000	0.70
150,000	0.70

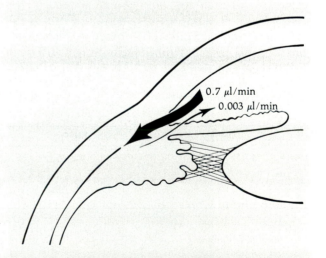

Fig. 10-3 Unidirectional fluxes of fluorescein isothiocyanate (FITC) dextran 70 from anterior chamber to suprachoroidal space and vice versa, expressed in equivalent volumes of aqueous humor. Results imply flow from anterior chamber to suprachoroid.

from the anterior chamber into the suprachoroidal space, it may possibly be osmotically absorbed by uveal vessels,[36] leave the sclera through emissarial channels, or flow through the sclera itself.

Rate of Uveoscleral Outflow

Species variation

The rate of uveoscleral outflow in various species is given in Table 10-2. In the monkey eye, rates between 0.2 and 1.0 µl/min at a normal intraocular pressure have been observed. In the human eye, two patients with malignant melanomas were found to have uveoscleral outflow rates of approximately 0.1 and 0.3 µl/min.[18] In cats, uveoscleral outflow is 0.36 µl/min[9] and in rabbits is 0.11 µl/min.[10] In the dog, 15% of aqueous outflow is via uveoscleral routes, corresponding to a rate of 0.5 µl/min.[1]

Intraocular pressure dependence

Three different studies on monkey eyes have indicated that uveoscleral outflow is largely pressure-independent. In one study, increasing the intraocular pressure from 12 to 22 mm Hg resulted in an increase of uveoscleral outflow from an original value of 0.44 to only 0.63 µl/min.[7] This change was statistically insignificant at the 0.01 confidence level. In a subsequent study on monkeys, the rate of uveoscleral outflow at an intraocular pressure of 8 mm Hg was 0.6 µl/min and was unchanged at an intraocular pressure of 4 mm Hg.[13] At an intraocular pressure of 35 mm Hg, uveoscleral outflow

Table 10-2 Species variation of uveoscleral outflow

Species	Uveoscleral outflow (µl/min)
Rabbit[10]	0.1
Cat[9]	0.4
Dog[1]	0.5
Vervet monkey[8,14,15,16]	0.2-0.6
Cynomolgus monkey*	0.3-1.0
Human[18]	0.2

*References 7, 10, 12, 13, 17, 40, 42, 43.

Table 10-3 Drug effects on uveoscleral outflow

Drug	Effect
Atropine[12,15]	↑↑↑
Pilocarpine[11]	↓↓↓↓
Norepinephrine[16]	—
Epinephrine[16]	↑↑
Isoproterenol[16]	↓
Prostaglandin (PGF$_{2\alpha}$)[34]	↑↑↑

rose to 0.75 µl/min. None of these values were significantly different from one another. However, at an intraocular pressure of 2 mm Hg, uveoscleral outflow was markedly reduced to 0.15 µl/min and at 1.5 mm Hg was 0.05 µl/min. Thus uveoscleral outflow is pressure-dependent at low intraocular pressures. These findings have been confirmed in more recent studies in which the facility of uveoscleral outflow was found to be about 0.01 µl/min/mm Hg.[42] When compared with the normal outflow facility of 0.3 µl/min/mm Hg,[28] uveoscleral outflow is virtually pressure-independent. However, cyclodialysis, which removes the barrier to tracer movement between the anterior chamber and the suprachoroidal space, results in a markedly pressure-dependent increase in uveoscleral outflow.[11,42] Presumably in that circumstance, fluid flow is governed by the difference between the intraocular pressure and the pressure on the external surface of the sclera.

The reason for the minimal variation in uveoscleral outflow at different intraocular pressures is not entirely clear. Presumably the driving force between the anterior chamber and the suprachoroid remains constant except at low intraocular pressures.

Since uveoscleral outflow is essentially pressure-independent and conventional outflow through the trabecular meshwork is highly pressure-dependent, expressing uveoscleral outflow as a percentage of total outflow can be misleading depending on the intraocular pressure. For example, with a high aqueous humor flow and an intraocular pressure of 20 mm Hg, the *percent* of uveoscleral outflow would be much lower than at an intraocular pressure closer to the episcleral venous pressure, at which conventional outflow would almost cease. Nevertheless, it is useful to use these percentages for species comparison. Thus it may be summarized that at normal intraocular pressure in the monkey, 30% to 65% of aqueous humor outflow is by uveoscleral routes, whereas in dogs it is 15%, in humans less than 10%, in cats 3%, and in rabbits 3%.

Pharmacologic alterations

Table 10-3 lists the effects of various drugs on the rate of uveoscleral outflow in the monkey eye. Alteration of the tone of the ciliary muscle has a profound effect on uveoscleral outflow. This would suggest that the ciliary body is the rate-limiting step in the pathway of uveoscleral outflow. Atropine causes a doubling of uveoscleral outflow[12,15] and pilocarpine causes a precipitous, more than tenfold drop in uveoscleral outflow.[11] Similar trends are also noted in human eyes.[18] The effect of adrenergic agents is less profound. Epinephrine causes an increase in uveoscleral outflow[14] whereas norepinephrine does not.[16] Isoproterenol also causes a slight increase in uveoscleral outflow.[16] Prostaglandin $F_{2\alpha}$ increases uveoscleral outflow.[35]

UVEOSCLERAL OUTFLOW IN OCULAR DISEASE

As a result of methodologic limitations, it is difficult to measure uveoscleral outflow in a clinical setting. Therefore direct measurements of uveoscleral outflow are confined to animal models of disease. Following cyclodialysis, a marked increase in uveoscleral outflow has been noted in both monkeys[41] and rabbits.[42] This is consistent with the hypothesis that the ciliary muscle is a rate-limiting step in uveoscleral outflow. Disinsertion of the ciliary muscle tendon from the sclera allows free communication between the anterior chamber and suprachoroid, leading to hypotony. The clinical aspects of this disorder are presented in Chapter 13. Disorders that result in enlargement of the intramuscular spaces of the ciliary muscle would be expected to increase uveoscleral outflow. Examples of these include iridocyclitis or ciliochoroidal detachment with edema of the ciliary muscle. In the monkey models of these disorders, uveoscleral outflow is enhanced in bovine serum albumin-induced ocular inflammation associated with reduced intraocular pressure.[43,44] In ciliochoroidal detachment in the monkey, aqueous flow is normal and the intraocular pressure is below the episcleral venous pressure, implying that uveoscleral outflow accommodates the aqueous humor produced.[37]

It has been suggested that reduced uveoscleral outflow may be partly responsible for the development of open-angle glaucoma in the human.[26] This hypothesis has not been tested and no recent data are available to confirm this. However, in one human eye with neovascular glaucoma, the uveoscleral outflow rate was found to be zero.[18] Furthermore, in the glaucomatous beagle, uveoscleral outflow accounted for only 3% of aqueous humor outflow compared with 15% in normal beagles.[2] These findings would strongly suggest that peripheral anterior synechiae, as in these two conditions, prevent egress of anterior chamber fluid into the suprachoroidal space.

REFERENCES

1. Barrie, KP, Gum, GG, Samuelson, DA, and Gelatt, KN: Quantitation of uveoscleral outflow in normotensive and glaucomatous beagles by ^{3}H-labeled dextran, Am J Vet Res 46:84, 1985

2. Barrie, KP, Glenwood, GG, Samuelson, DA, and Gelatt, KN: Morphologic studies of uveoscleral outflow in normotensive and glaucomatous beagles with fluorescein-labeled dextran, Am J Vet Res 46:89, 1985

3. Bill, A: The drainage of blood from the uvea and the elimination of aqueous humour in rabbits, Exp Eye Res 1:200, 1962

4. Bill, A: Movement of albumin and dextran through the sclera, Arch Ophthalmol 74:248, 1965

5. Bill, A: The aqueous humor drainage mechanism in the cynomolgus monkey *(Macaca irus)* with evidence for unconventional routes, Invest Ophthalmol 4:911, 1965

6. Bill, A, and Hellsing, K: Production and drainage of aqueous humor in the cynomolgus monkey *(Macaca irus)*, Invest Ophthalmol 4:920, 1965

7. Bill, A: Conventional and uveo-scleral drainage of aqueous humour in the cynomolgus monkey *(Macaca irus)* at normal and high intraocular pressures, Exp Eye Res 5:45, 1966

8. Bill, A: The routes for bulk drainage of aqueous humour in the vervet monkey *(Cercopithecus ethiops)*, Exp Eye Res 5:55, 1966

9. Bill, A: Formation and drainage of aqueous humour in cats, Exp Eye Res 5:185, 1966

10. Bill, A: The effects of pilocarpine on the dynamics of aqueous humor in a primate *(Macaca irus)*, Invest Ophthalmol 5:170, 1966

11. Bill, A: The routes for bulk drainage of aqueous humour in rabbits with and without cyclodialysis, Doc Ophthalmol 20:157, 1966

12. Bill, A: Effects of atropine and pilocarpine on aqueous humour dynamics in cynomolgus monkeys *(Macaca irus)*, Exp Eye Res 6:120, 1967

13. Bill, A: Further studies on the influence of the intraocular pressure on aqueous humor dynamics in cynomolgus monkeys, Invest Ophthalmol 6:364, 1967

14. Bill, A: Early effects of epinephrine on aqueous humor dynamics in vervet monkeys *(Cercopithecus ethiops)*, Exp Eye Res 8:35, 1969

15. Bill, A: Effects of atropine on aqueous humor dynamics in the vervet monkey *(Cercopithecus ethiops)*, Exp Eye Res 8:284, 1969

16. Bill, A: Effects of norepinephrine, isoproterenol and sympathetic stimulation on aqueous humour dynamics in vervet monkeys, Exp Eye Res 10:31, 1970

17. Bill, A: Aqueous humor dynamics in monkeys *(Macaca irus* and *Cercopithecus ethiops)*, Exp Eye Res 11:195, 1971

18. Bill, A: Uveoscleral drainage of aqueous humour in human eyes, Exp Eye Res 12:275, 1971

19. Bill, A, Inomata, H, and Smelser, GK: Unconventional routes of aqueous humor outflow in cynomolgus monkey *(Macaca irus)*, Am J Ophthalmol 73:893, 1972

20. Bill, A: The role of the iris vessels in aqueous humor dynamics, Jpn J Ophthalmol 18:30, 1974

21. Bill, A, and Inomata, H: Exit sites of uveoscleral flow of aqueous humor in cynomolgus monkey eyes, Exp Eye Res 25:113, 1977

22. Bill, A: Basic physiology of the drainage of aqueous humor, Exp Eye Res 25(suppl):291, 1977

23. Cole, DF, and Monro, PAG: The use of fluorescein-labeled dextrans in investigation of aqueous humour outflow in the rabbit, Exp Eye Res 23:571, 1976

24. Cruise, LJ, and McClure, R: Posterior pathway for aqueous humor drainage in the dog, Am J Vet Res 42:992, 1981

25. Cunha-Vaz, J, and Maurice, D: Fluorescein dynamics and the eye, Doc Ophthalmol 26:61, 1969

26. Fine, BS, Yanoff, M, and Stone, RA: A clinicopathologic study of four cases of primary open-angle glaucoma compared to normal eyes, Am J Ophthalmol 9:88, 1981

27. Fowlks, WL, and Havener, VR: Aqueous flow into the perivascular space of the rabbit ciliary body, Invest Ophthalmol 3:374, 1964

28. Gaasterland, DE, Pederson, JE, and MacLellan, HM: Perfusate effects upon resistance to aqueous humor outflow in the rhesus monkey eye, Invest Ophthalmol Vis Sci 17:391, 1978

29. Gelatt, KN, Gum, GG, Williams, LW, and Barrie, KP: Uveoscleral flow of aqueous humor in the normal dog, Am J Vet Res 40:845, 1979

30. Green, K, et al: The fate of anterior chamber tracers in the living rhesus monkey eye with evidence for uveo-vortex outflow, Trans Ophthalmol Soc UK 97:731, 1977

31. Kelly, DE, Hageman, GS, and McGregor, JA: Uveal compartmentalization in the hamster eye revealed by fine structural and tracer studies: implications for uveoscleral outflow, Invest Ophthalmol Vis Sci 24:1288, 1983

32. Kleinstein, RN, and Fatt, I: Pressure dependency of transcleral flow, Exp Eye Res 24:335, 1977

33. Last, RJ: Wolff's anatomy of the eye and orbit, ed 6, Philadelphia, 1968, WB Saunders Co

34. McMaster, PRB, and Macri, FJ: Secondary aqueous humor outflow pathways in the rabbit, cat, and monkey, Arch Ophthalmol 79:297, 1968

35. Nilsson, SFE, Stjernschantz, J, and Bill, A: $PGF_{2\alpha}$ increases uveoscleral outflow, Invest Ophthalmol Vis Sci 28(suppl):284, 1987

36. Pederson, JE, Gaasterland, DE, and MacLellan, HM: Uveoscleral aqueous outflow in the rhesus monkey: importance of uveal reabsorption, Invest Ophthalmol Vis Sci 16:1008, 1977

37. Pederson, JE, Gaasterland, DE, and MacLellan, HM: Experimental ciliochoroidal detachment: effect on intraocular pressure and aqueous flow, Arch Ophthalmol 97:536, 1979

38. Pederson, JE, and Toris, CJ: Uveoscleral outflow: diffusion or flow? Invest Ophthalmol Vis Sci 28:1022, 1987

39. Samuelson, DA, Gum, GG, Gelatt, KN, and Barrie, KP: Aqueous outflow in the beagle: unconventional outflow, using different-sized microspheres, Am J Vet Res 46:242, 1985

40. Sherman, SH, Green, K, and Laties, AM: The fate of anterior chamber fluorescein in the monkey eye. I. The anterior chamber outflow pathways, Exp Eye Res 27:159, 1978

41. Suguro, K, Toris, CB, and Pederson, JE: Uveoscleral outflow following cyclodialysis in the monkey eye using a fluorescent tracer, Invest Ophthalmol Vis Sci 26:810, 1985

42. Toris, CB, and Pederson, JE: Effect of intraocular pressure on uveoscleral outflow following cyclodialysis in the monkey eye, Invest Ophthalmol Vis Sci 26:1745, 1985

43. Toris, CB, Gregerson, DS, and Pederson, JE: Uveoscleral outflow using different-sized fluorescent tracers in normal and inflamed eyes, Exp Eye Res (In Press)

44. Toris, CB, and Pederson, JE: Aqueous humor dynamics in experimental iridocyclitis, Invest Ophthalmol Vis Sci 28:477, 1987

45. Tripathi, RC: Uveoscleral drainage of aqueous humour, Exp Eye Res 25(suppl):305, 1977

46. Van Alphen, GWHM: On emmetropia and ametropia, Ophthalmologica 142(suppl):47, 1961

Chapter 11

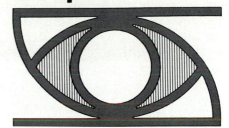

Episcleral Venous Pressure

Ran C. Zeimer

The measurement of the effect of increased episcleral venous pressure on intraocular pressure has helped clarify the processes governing aqueous humor dynamics. Episcleral venous pressure measurements have not been clinically valuable in primary open-angle glaucoma, and measured values are similar in open-angle glaucomatous, ocular hypertensive, and normal eyes. However, in several secondary glaucomas, an increase in episcleral venous pressure as a result of abnormal conditions in the extraocular circulation causes elevated intraocular pressure (see Chapter 62).

Ascher[1-3] first reported that clear aqueous humor flow could be observed in the episcleral veins of humans, confirming his histologic observations that Schlemm's canal was connected to episcleral veins. Ascher explained Lauber's earlier finding that blood in the anterior ciliary vein of dogs contained a lower erythrocyte concentration than systemic blood, on the basis of dilution with aqueous humor. Uribe-Troncoso[34] collected clear fluid from the perilimbal sclera of rabbit eyes immersed in oil in vivo, measured the rate of aqueous flow, and demonstrated patent connections between the anterior chamber and the episcleral veins. Seidel[26] injected India ink into the rabbit anterior chamber and observed its appearance in the episcleral veins.

Renewed interest in episcleral venous pressure measurement began after Ascher[1] emphasized the role of episcleral veins in aqueous humor dynamics. The pressure chamber method first used by Seidel[26] was improved and new methods devised. Goldmann[12] introduced a technique using a hard probe and a torsion balance; Stepanik[28] suggested an indirect method based on intraocular pressure dynamics after artificial reduction of pressure; and a noncontact method, using a jet of air, was introduced by Krakau et al.[14] Recently, the pressure chamber method was improved and made clinically practical by Zeimer et al.[37]

PHYSIOLOGY OF EPISCLERAL VENOUS PRESSURE

The physiology of episcleral venous pressure is directly related to aqueous humor dynamics.

The aqueous humor enters the posterior chamber of the eye, flows through the pupil into the anterior chamber, and returns to the bloodstream by two routes: (1) through the anterior surface of the ciliary body (the uveoscleral or unconventional outflow), and (2) through the trabecular meshwork into Schlemm's canal (conventional outflow). The uveoscleral outflow drains the aqueous humor at a steady rate that is unaffected by intraocular pressure or episcleral venous pressure. The trabecular outflow carries the greater portion of aqueous humor from the eye. The veins that drain Schlemm's canal carry aqueous humor through the sclera into the episcleral (recipient) veins. The aqueous may be observed in clear veins emerging from the limbus (aqueous veins) and in recipient laminated veins, in which aqueous humor flows within a column of blood before mixing with it. A pressure difference or gradient is necessary to force fluid through the aqueous veins. The higher pressure is the intraocular pressure (IOP), and the lower pressure is the episcleral venous pressure (EVP). The pressure gradient (IOP − EVP) drives the trabecular outflow, F_{trab}, which also depends on the trabecular resistance, R_{trab}. The relationship between these variables is given as follows:

(1) $$F_{trab} = (IOP - EVP) / R_{trab}$$

This equation indicates that the flow increases with the pressure gradient and decreases with the resistance. To obtain a constant flow, a rise in episcleral venous pressure must be accompanied by a rise in intraocular pressure. This relationship is complicated by the fact that R_{trab} is not strictly constant but seems to increase with the pressure gradient, probably as a result of some collapse of the outflow channels. Brubaker[7] has suggested a first approximation as presented in the following equation:

(2) $$R_{trab} = R_O + R_O Q (IOP - EVP)$$

where R_O is the trabecular resistance present when the intraocular pressure is equal to the episcleral venous pressure and Q is the fractional change in R_O brought about by a change in pressure gradient of 1 mm Hg, representing the increment in resistance resulting from obstruction of outflow channels caused by the rise in the pressure gradient.

We can summarize and write that:

(3) $$F_{trab} = (IOP - EVP) / (R_O + R_O Q (IOP - EVP))$$

expressing the fact that, in the presence of a constant flow, episcleral venous pressure may influence aqueous dynamics and intraocular pressure by two mechanisms. As an approximation, assuming that trabecular outflow in humans is approximately equal to the aqueous humor production (F_{in}), and R_{trab} is almost constant, one obtains Goldmann's equation:

(4) $$F_{in} = (IOP - EVP) / R_{trab}$$

The correlation between episcleral venous pressure and intraocular pressure in normotensive eyes and eyes with primary open-angle glaucoma and ocular hypertension is unclear. Talusan et al.[29] found a negative correlation in the above groups of eyes (about −0.4) between episcleral venous pressure and intraocular pressure. The best fit, which was obtained by a logarithmic function, predicted that an increase in pressure from 20 to 40 mm Hg would be accompanied by a drop in episcleral venous pressure from 8.5 to 6 mm Hg. This finding matched the observations of Talusan and Schwartz,[30] which indicated an episcleral venous pressure of 10.5 mm Hg in 40 normal eyes and 7.5 mm Hg in 50 eyes with ocular hypertension. This

finding also matched the observations of Kupfer,[15] who obtained means of 8.4 ± 0.3 and 7.7 ± 0.2 mm Hg in normal and ocular hypertensive eyes, respectively. The possible relationship between episcleral venous pressure and intraocular pressure was illustrated by the synchronicity between their circadian variations in normal and glaucomatous eyes.[5,18,33]

Contrary to these findings, Weigelin and Lohlein[35] reported a positive correlation (+0.59) between episcleral venous pressure and intraocular pressure in 172 subjects with intraocular pressures between 7 and 24 mm Hg. Podos et al.[23] observed that differences in episcleral venous pressure between the two eyes of the same patient did not appear to account for the difference in intraocular pressure. Also, little difference was found in episcleral venous pressure when normal eyes were compared with eyes with altered intraocular pressure, such as hypotony,[27] and before and after abrupt decreases in intraocular pressure in the same eye.[19]

MEASUREMENT OF EPISCLERAL VENOUS PRESSURE

Identification of Vessels

Gartner[11] stated that the layering of aqueous humor and blood often distinguishes aqueous veins. The tributaries of these veins carry clear aqueous humor and are not always seen as they exit the sclera beneath the conjunctiva and Tenon's capsule. Even on the conjunctival surface, aqueous veins lack the coloring that delineates blood vessels. However, when tributaries carrying aqueous humor and blood enter an aqueous vein, the red blood cells can be observed tumbling into the clear fluid, forming eddies, and flowing from the limbus. Episcleral veins can be differentiated from conjunctival veins by applying an applicator to the surface of the eye: episcleral veins remain fixed, whereas conjunctival veins move. Episcleral vessels are identified most easily between the 1 and 5 o'clock and the 7 and 11 o'clock positions, in a zone between the equator and the limbus.[3]

No difference in episcleral venous pressure is apparent in different meridians,[31] and only a small pressure gradient occurs along the recipient veins.[13,18,19] Linnér et al.[20] observed that the pressure in nonrecipient episcleral veins and conjunctival veins resembles the pressure in the recipient veins, thus justifying the use of conjunctival veins where nonrecipient episcleral veins are not readily accessible. In contrast, Krakau et al.[14] found the pressure in the recipient veins to be 3 to 4 mm Hg higher than in the conjunctival veins. They felt that this was not attributable to the fact that the episcleral veins are situated more deeply in the conjunctiva, since the lower pressure occurs in both superficial and deep conjunctival veins. The discrepancy between the findings by Krakau et al. and those of Linnér et al.[20] may be the result of different methods of measurement. Krakau et al. used an air jet to apply the measuring pressure, which may result in a different tissue pressure distribution from that acquired by placing a probe in contact with the eye over a restricted area.

Choice of Measurement End Point

All of the methods to calculate episcleral venous pressure use a measurable pressure (or force) applied externally to the vein until the wall deforms or collapses. It is assumed that the venous wall has little inherent rigidity, so that it begins to collapse as soon as the externally applied pressure exceeds the intraluminal pressure. The choice of the most accurate end point has been the subject of considerable discussion. Four possibilities have been considered: (1) when the earliest changes are detected, such as when the blood color becomes somewhat paler; (2) when the color is estimated to be 50% of its original value; (3) when the perfused width reaches half the original vessel width; and (4) when the flow is totally obstructed.

Measurements taken at the point of complete vessel collapse are expected to yield falsely elevated values, since the interruption of flow may increase the intravenous pressure. Mims and Holland[21] used a pressurized membrane to compare end points B and D. In ten measurements on six monkey eyes, they obtained a standard deviation of 0.85 and 1.71 mm Hg, respectively. A similar comparison on six rabbit eyes yielded standard deviations of 0.50 and 1.18 mm Hg, respectively.

Gaasterland and Pederson[10] compared measurements with a noninvasive pressurized membrane chamber and direct cannulation at the same venous site in seven eyes of four anesthetized rhesus monkeys and defined three end points: (1) slight indentation, (2) intermittent collapse, and (3) sustained collapse of the venous lumen corresponding to D above. The mean pressures in the measuring chamber corresponding to these end points were 9.9 ± 0.9, 23.5 ± 2.9, and 31.4 ± 4.0 mm Hg, respectively. After obtaining the noninvasive measurements, the pressure within the vein was determined by cannulation to be 11.3 ± 0.5 mm Hg. The first end point, which appears to be between end points A and B, was best correlated to and slightly underestimated the cannulated pressure, whereas the second and third end points

overestimated the episcleral venous pressure. They found an increase of 5 to 7 mm Hg between slight indentation and obliteration in normal young humans.

Brubaker[6] noted with the pressure chamber technique that end point D yielded results in close agreement with cannulation measurements. Conversely, measurements using the Goldmann force method deviated markedly at this end point. The error introduced by measuring at end point D tended to increase with the size of the vein.[17,36] This could be explained by the fact that some blood in an obstructed vessel is forced into collateral pathways. When the vessel is large, the collateral pathways may not accommodate the increased flow, which then causes a rise in pressure. In small vessels, where many anastomoses are present, only minimal change is expected.[17,22]

In conclusion, end point A appears to correspond to a pressure that underestimates episcleral venous pressure, whereas end point D overestimates it. The end points of choice thus becomes B (50% reduction in color)[6,21,22,36,37] and C (50% reduction in perfused vessel width).[14] Although these end points are not identified as easily as end point D, Zeimer et al.[37] have shown that practice and good visibility with stereoscopic vision and magnification should produce reproducible measurements.

Force Method

The force method of measurement (Fig. 11-1), described by Goldmann,[12] applies a variable force over a constant area of conjunctiva overlying an episcleral vein. Although commonly referred to as the *torsion balance method*, the technique is characterized by the force applied to a given area, which has been measured using a torsion balance[12] or a force-displacement transducer.[23]

The basis for the method is the assumption that a known force (F) applied over a known area (A) of conjunctiva elevates the tissue pressure in that area by an amount equal to $F \div A$. This assumption is correct if the force required to deform the tissue is negligible, the force is applied uniformly over the area of the probe, and the force is not applied over any other area. These conditions can be closely approximated when the vessel is near the surface and the applanation surface is small.

The size of the applanation surface has crucial limits. If the area is too small, transducer inaccuracies, vibrations, and surface tension will introduce large errors. Also, the tissue area affected by the probe will exceed the probe size. The use of too large a probe with a flat applanating tip on a

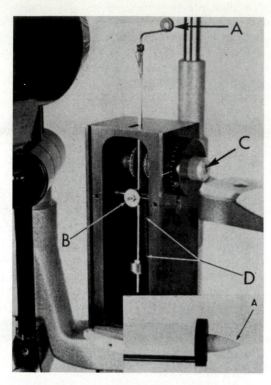

Fig. 11-1 Instrument based on force method for measurement of episcleral venous pressure is shown mounted on slit-lamp microscope. Hard probe *(A)*; torsion arm *(B)*; dial graduated in mm Hg *(C)*; and uniform weight chain *(D)*. Lateral view of tip *(A)* is shown below. (From Brubaker, RF: Arch Ophthalmol, 77:110, 1967. Copyright 1967, American Medical Association)

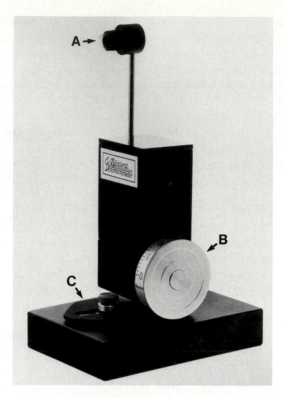

Fig. 11-2 Episcleral Venomanometer based on pressure chamber method. Membrane *(A)*; dial graduated in mm Hg *(B)*; and footplate for mounting on slit-lamp microscope *(C)*. (Courtesy Eyetech Ltd, Skokie, Illinois)

curved globe will lead to a nonuniform distribution of force, even when the instrument is perpendicular to the surface. Goldmann[12] used a probe diameter of 500 μm, whereas Brubaker[6] found that a tip diameter of 250 to 300 μm was satisfactory, since the force could be applied uniformly and the orientation of the plane of the conjunctiva was less critical. The reproducibility of the force method has been reported to be ±1.2 mm Hg.[23]

Pressure Chamber Method

Seidel[26] described the pressure chamber method in 1923. One side of the chamber is formed by a thin, transparent, elastic membrane placed against the eye. The other side is rigid and transparent, enabling the episcleral vein to be viewed. The pressure in the chamber is adjusted until the end point is reached. The pressure chamber method is also a partially occlusive method and is based on many of the assumptions of the force method to measure episcleral venous pressure. The episcleral venous pressure is assumed to be equal to the pressure recorded in the chamber at the end point. To achieve this equality, the pressures re-

quired to deform the conjunctiva, the interposed membrane, and the vessel wall must be negligible.

Ideally, the membrane should be not only transparent, thin, and elastic, but also nonrigid, tear resistant, airtight, nonirritating, easily obtainable, and rapidly fit to the instrument. Many materials have been recommended for the membrane: intestinal serosa,[26,35] latex film,[18,19] softened cellophane,[32] and pericardium of toads and frogs.[6,16] Phelps and Armaly[22] experimented with more than 25 different materials. They found that the least rigid, but most difficult to prepare, was toad pericardium and the most convenient was latex manufactured as a tonometer cover (Tonofilm). Although less transparent and stiffer than toad pericardium, the latex provided comparable results in paired measurements. Phelps and Armaly obtained a reproducibility better than ±1 mm Hg in 25 eyes, from ±1 to ±2 mm Hg in 27 eyes, and over ±2 mm Hg in only 4 eyes.

Zeimer et al.[37] developed an instrument that was easily operated by one observer, required no calibration, was compact, attached quickly to the slit-lamp, permitted stereopsis, and provided good

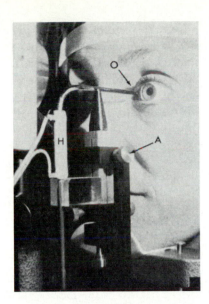

Fig. 11-3 Instrument based on air jet method for measurement of episcleral venous pressure is shown mounted on slit-lamp microscope. *Adjusting screw (A); heating wire (H); and mouthpiece (O).* (From Krakau, CET, Widakowich, J, and Wilke, K: Acta Ophthalmol, 51:185, 1973)

reproducibility. The Episcleral Venomanometer incorporates elements found separately in different devices (Fig. 11-2). A flexible transparent membrane is mounted on an air chamber, and the pressure is controlled through the rotation of a dial marked with gradations in millimeters of mercury. The latter moves a piston, which changes the volume of the air chamber and, thereby, its pressure. When the dial is on zero, the piston uncovers an opening in the chamber and allows communication with the outside air. The zero reading is thus equal to the ambient pressure, which compensates for variation in atmospheric pressure. The membrane, which is made of a thin transparent silicone rubber, is replaceable and has a 3 mm diameter ring to indicate the desired area of contact. The small and constant area of contact minimizes interference with blood flow.

The instrument is mounted directly on a slit-lamp. The eye is anesthetized and the area of contact with the globe is adjusted to coincide with the indicator ring on the membrane so that both are in focus. The observer slowly increases the pressure by turning the dial until the selected episcleral vein is half blanched. The slit-lamp is retracted, the pressure is read from the scale, and the dial is reset to zero. The reproducibility of this instrument was evaluated by 5 consecutive measurements on each of 30 eyes and was found to be between ±0.7 and

±1.0 mm Hg. The mean interobserver difference was 0.7 ± 1.2 mm Hg.[37]

Air Jet Method

Krakau et al.[14] developed a procedure that employs an air jet to produce the pressure necessary to deform the episcleral veins (Fig. 11-3), thereby avoiding contact with the eye. A diaphragm pump is used to create a stream of air of variable pressure. After being moistened in a water flask, the air passes through a needle valve, which regulates the flow. The air is warmed and exits through a mouthpiece 0.5 mm in diameter and situated 3 mm from the eye. The instrument is mounted on the slit-lamp for stereoscopic viewing. The reproducibility of the method varies between ±0.7 and ±1.1 mm Hg.

Indirect Method

Stepanik[28] measured episcleral venous pressure indirectly by compressing the eye with an impression tonometer. The compression rapidly decreased intraocular pressure to a level below episcleral venous pressure. Subsequently, intraocular pressure reached a level that was assumed to be equal to episcleral venous pressure.

Comparison of Methods

An ideal comparison that applies all of the different methods to the same eye is not available. Only one published study, performed by Brubaker[6] on rabbits, compared the force and pressure chamber methods with direct cannulation. The end points were broad and difficult to reproduce with the force method, even with the most careful practice and under ideal experimental conditions. The standard deviations were ±2.94 mm Hg for the force method, ±0.57 mm Hg for the pressure chamber method, and ±0.13 mm Hg for direct cannulation. Episcleral venous pressure values were 12.4 ± 2.6, 10.8 ± 1.9, and 10.1 ± 2.5 for each method, respectively. The results of the pressure chamber and direct cannulation methods were similar, whereas those of the force method were higher. Moreover, the agreement was more dependent on the selection of the proper end point for the force method.

THE NORMAL EPISCLERAL VENOUS PRESSURE

Episcleral venous pressure has been measured in normal subjects by many authors using the different methods described. Table 11-1 summarizes some of the studies, providing the average, stan-

Table 11-1 Episcleral venous pressure (EVP) in normal eyes

Authors	No. of eyes	EVP, mm Hg (Mean ± SD)	Method
Seidel (1923)[26]	?	7 to 11	Pressure chamber
Samojloff (1927)[25]	15	10.9 ± 1.6	Pressure chamber
Thomassen (1947)[32]	?	up to 65	Pressure chamber
Linner (1949)[18]	24	14.3 ± 1.02	Pressure chamber
Goldmann (1950)[13]	20	9.7 ± 2.2	Force
Rickenbach (1950)[24]	10	11.4 ± 1.5	Force
Linnér (1950)[20]	38	10.0 ± 2.6	Force
Weigelin (1952)[35]	103	9.7 ± 2.5	Pressure chamber
Linnér (1956)[19]	28	11.0 ± 1.4	Pressure chamber
Leith (1963)[17]	20	10.4 ± ?	Pressure chamber
Kupfer (1968)[16]	21	8.3 ± 1.1	Pressure chamber
Podos (1968)[23]	39	9.0 ± 1.4	Force
Stepanik (1969)[28]	16	10.4 ± 4.1	Indirect
Krakau (1973)[14]	6	10.4 ± 0.8	Air jet
Azuma (1973)[4]	450	8.3 ± 2.0	Pressure chamber
Gaasterland (1975)[9]	7	9.4 ± 0.4	Pressure chamber
Phelps (1978)[22]	56	9.0 ± 1.6	Pressure chamber
Talusan (1981)[30]	40	10.1 ± 2.9*	Pressure chamber
Zeimer (1983)[37]	122	7.6 ± 1.3	Pressure chamber

*The points of the authors' Fig. 11-3 with an intraocular pressure ≤20 mm Hg have been used for the calculation.

dard deviation, and population size for each method used. Many factors may have caused the different results obtained by the various investigators, such as choice of end points, identification of vessels, and the type of instrument. In addition, other ocular factors may account for the variability in results. Episcleral venous pressure has been found to be 0.97 mm Hg higher when measured in the recumbent compared with the sitting position.[19,20] Moreover, position of gaze, eye movements, and squeezing of eyelids may affect the readings.[23]

From Table 11-1, episcleral venous pressure has an average value of 9.8 ± 1.8 mm Hg for the pressure chamber method, and 10.0 ± 1 mm Hg for the force method. The overall average is 10.1 ± 1.5 mm Hg. The lower values obtained by Zeimer et al.[37] may be the result of the high transparency and small area of contact of the silicone membrane and to the stereoscopic viewing, which allows the operator to detect changes in blood flow rapidly, thus minimizing interference with blood flow. Episcleral venous pressure is not influenced by the age of the patient.[4,8,15,37]

REFERENCES

1. Ascher, KW: The aqueous veins: physiologic importance of the visible elimination of intraocular fluid, Am J Ophthalmol 25:1174, 1942
2. Ascher, KW: Aqueous veins. II. Local pharmacologic effects on aqueous veins. III. Glaucoma and aqueous veins, Am J Ophthalmol 25:1301, 1942
3. Ascher, KW: Aqueous veins: preliminary note, Am J Ophthalmol 25:1301, 1942
4. Azuma, I: Graphic expression of the intraocular pressure dynamics, Jpn J Ophthalmol 17:310, 1973
5. Bain, WES: Variations in the episcleral venous pressure in relation to glaucoma, Br J Ophthalmol 38:129, 1954
6. Brubaker, RF: Determination of episcleral venous pressure in the eye, Arch Ophthalmol 77:110, 1967
7. Brubaker, RF: Computer-assisted instruction of current concepts in aqueous humor dynamics, Am J Ophthalmol 82:59, 1976
8. Gaasterland, D, et al: Studies of aqueous humour dynamics in man. VI. Effect of age upon parameters of intraocular pressure in normal human eyes, Exp Eye Res 26:651, 1978
9. Gaasterland, D, Kupfer, C, and Ross, K: Studies of aqueous humor dynamics in man. IV. Effects of pilocarpine upon measurements in young normal volunteers, Invest Ophthalmol 14:848, 1975
10. Gaasterland, DE, and Pederson, JE: Episcleral venous pressure: a comparison of invasive and noninvasive measurements, Invest Ophthalmol Vis Sci 24:1417, 1983
11. Gartner, S: Blood vessels of the conjunctiva: studies with high speed macrophotography, Arch Ophthalmol 32:464, 1944
12. Goldmann, H: Die Kammerwasservenen und das Poiseuille'sche Gesetz, Ophthalmologica 118:496, 1949
13. Goldmann, H: Der Druck im Schlemmschen Kanal bei Normalen und bei Glaucoma simplex, Experientia 6:110, 1950
14. Krakau, CET, Widakowich, J, and Wilke, K: Measurements of the episcleral venous pressure by means of an air jet, Acta Ophthalmol 51:185, 1973

15. Kupfer, C: Clinical significance of pseudofacility, Am J Ophthalmol 75:193, 1973
16. Kupfer, C, and Sanderson, P: Determination of pseudofacility in the eye of man, Arch Ophthalmol 80:194, 1968
17. Leith, AB: Episcleral venous pressure in tonography, Br J Ophthalmol 47:271, 1963
18. Linnér, E: Measurement of the pressure in Schlemm's canal and in the anterior chamber of the human eye, Experientia 5:451, 1949
19. Linnér, E: Further studies of the episcleral venous pressure in glaucoma, Am J Ophthalmol 41:646, 1956
20. Linnér, E, Rickenbach, C, and Werner, H: Comparative measurements of the pressure in the aqueous veins and the conjunctival veins using different methods, Acta Ophthalmol 28:469, 1950
21. Mims, JL, and Holland, MG: Applanation and Schiøtz tonometer standardizations for the owl monkey eye with a new technique for measuring episcleral venous pressure, Invest Ophthalmol 10:190, 1971
22. Phelps, CD, and Armaly, MF: Measurement of episcleral venous pressure, Am J Ophthalmol 85:35, 1978
23. Podos, SM, Minas, TF, and Macri, FJ: A new instrument to measure episcleral venous pressure, comparison of normal eyes and eyes with primary open-angle glaucoma, Arch Ophthalmol 80:209, 1968
24. Rickenbach, K, and Werner, H: Scheinbarer Abflussdruck, Tension und Druck in Kammerwasservenen, Ophthalmologica 120:22, 1950
25. Samojloff, AJ: Zur Blutdruckmessung in den Augengefassen mittels der Pelottenmethode, Graefes Arch Clin Exp Ophthalmol 119:235, 1927
26. Seidel, E: Weitere experimentelle Untersuchungen uber die Quelle und den Verlauf der Intraokularen Saftstromung. XX. Mitteilung uber die Messung des Blutdruckes in dem episcleralen Venengeflecht, den vorderen Ciliarund den Wirbelvenen normaler Augen, v Graefes Arch Klin Exp Ophthalmol 115:112, 1923
27. Stepanik, J: Der episklerale Venendruck im Liegen und im Stehen, Ophthalmologica 132:98, 1956
28. Stepanik, J: Neues Verfahren zur Bestimmung des extraokularen episcleralen Venendruckes, v Graefes Arch Klin Exp Ophthalmol 177:116, 1969
29. Talusan, ED, Fishbein, SL, and Schwartz, B: Increased pressure of dilated episceral veins with open-angle glaucoma without exophthalmos, Ophthalmology 90:257, 1983
30. Talusan, ED, and Schwartz, B: Fluorescein angiography, demonstration of flow pattern of anterior ciliary arteries, Arch Ophthalmol 99:1074, 1981
31. Talusan, ED, and Schwartz, B: Episcleral venous pressure, differences between normal, ocular hypertensive, and primary open-angle glaucomas, Arch Ophthalmol 99:824, 1981
32. Thomassen, TL: The venous tension in eyes suffering from simple glaucoma, Acta Ophthalmol 25:221, 1947
33. Thomassen, TL, Perkins, ES, and Dobree, JH: Aqueous veins in glaucomatous eyes, Br J Ophthalmol 34:221, 1950
34. Uribe-Troncoso, M: The physiologic nature of the Schlemm canal, Am J Ophthalmol 4:321, 1921
35. Weigelin, E, and Lohlein, H: Blutdruckmessungen an den episcleralen Gefassen des Auges bei kreislaufgesunden Personen, Graefes Arch Clin Exp Ophthalmol 153:202, 1952
36. Widakowich, J: Episcleral venous pressure and flow dynamics, Acta Ophthalmol 54:500, 1976
37. Zeimer, RC, et al: A practical venomanometer: measurement of episcleral venous pressure and assessment of the normal range, Arch Ophthalmol 101:1447, 1983

Chapter 12

The Nervous System and Intraocular Pressure

Richard A. Stone
Yasuaki Kuwayama

The narrow range of intraocular pressure (IOP) in normal individuals has stimulated a search for potential regulatory mechanisms—mechanical, humoral and/or neural. Because the eye comprises such a small portion of total body mass, locally directed and locally acting mechanisms would seem to be an ideal means for integrating its physiology; the peripheral nervous system is designed to affect such local control. Because most available antiglaucoma agents interact with autonomic mechanisms, clinical pharmacology also suggests a role for the nervous system in the regulation of IOP.

Although the relationship of IOP and the nervous system was an early and intense area of investigation, a precise definition of neural mechanisms that regulate IOP has yet to emerge. The application of modern techniques in neurobiology offers the promises of furthering our understanding of this area. In this chapter, we discuss the peripheral innervation of the eye, with emphasis on the innervation of those structures most relevant to the regulation of IOP. Evidence suggesting a possible coordinating function for the central nervous system also is reviewed. Neurotransmitter receptor mechanisms in the eye and their relevance to IOP are discussed in greater detail in Chapters 24, 25, and 28.

NEUROTRANSMITTERS AND NEUROMODULATORS IN OCULAR NERVES

Peripheral nerves to the eye derive from parasympathetic, sympathetic, and sensory sources (Fig. 12-1).[202] In terms of anatomic organization, the parasympathetic innervation is the most complex. The postganglionic nerves of the ciliary ganglion innervate the eye, with important distribution to the ciliary and iris muscles. Some postganglionic nerves from the pterygopalatine ganglion enter the orbit as rami orbitales.[173,175,176,178] As presently understood, those pterygopalatine nerves innervating the eye supply choroidal blood vessels and probably the trabecular meshwork.[174,177] In addition, scattered microganglia and individual ganglion cells occur in the orbit and sometimes within

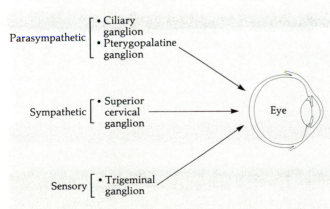

Fig. 12-1 Major sources of ocular innervation. The main peripheral ganglia innervating the eye are indicated.

the eye itself.[27,57] There is marked species and individual variability in the number and precise location of these accessory neurons. The eye's sympathetic innervation derives from the ipsilateral superior cervical ganglion. The trigeminal ganglion provides sensory nerves to the eye, mainly in the ophthalmic nerve. In the monkey and probably in man, the maxillary nerve also contributes to the sensory component of the ciliary nerves.[10,176]

Histochemical methods, complemented by biochemistry, allow description of the distribution of chemically defined nerves within target tissues. Applied to the eye, these methods have provided a detailed knowledge of the intraocular distribution of specific nerve types.

Classic Neurotransmitters

Cholinergic nerves in the eye are believed to derive from parasympathetic sources. The thiocholine technique for visualizing cholinergic nerves localizes not acetylcholine but acetylcholine esterase, the enzyme that metabolizes acetylcholine.[90] Although the issue of its specificity is complex, this histochemical method is the only one used so far to visualize cholinergic nerves in the eye. Because its findings correlate well with biochemical assays of the biosynthetic enzyme choline acetyltransferase[133] and with physiologic responses, it is believed to provide an accurate description of the eye's cholinergic innervation.

Ocular adrenergic nerve fibers derive from the ipsilateral superior cervical ganglion.[44] Their distribution is demonstrated by a specific and sensitive histochemical method in which catecholamines are converted to highly fluorescent chemical derivatives and visualized by fluorescence microscopy.[51] Norepinephrine also has been identified biochemically in the eye.[38,44]

Some peripheral ocular nerve fibers may contain serotonin, another biogenic amine. The histochemical evidence is somewhat indirect, but presumed serotonergic nerve fibers have been identified in the cornea and in the ciliary body.[89,149,150,236] For both tissues, serotonin, its precursor 5-hydroxytryptophan, and its metabolite 5-hydroxyindolacetic acid have been identified biochemically.[89,236] Serotonergic nerve fibers may be sympathetic in origin,[146] and they appear to show considerable species variability.[150]

Dopamine, a precursor in the biosynthesis of norepinephrine, serves as a neurotransmitter in some neurons of the central nervous system, including the retina.[43] DARPP-32, a phosphoprotein in brain neurons containing the D-1 dopamine receptor subtype, also is present in the nonpigmented ciliary epithelium.[211] Dopamine, its agonists, and its antagonists influence IOP,* and a selective dopamine agonist increases ciliary body cyclic AMP.[33] Taken together, these observations raise the question of whether the ciliary processes contain a dopaminergic innervation distinct from its adrenergic innervation. Although peripheral dopaminergic nerves are well known in the kidney,[141] definitive evidence for the eye is not yet available.

Neuropeptides and Co-transmission in the Peripheral Nervous System

In addition to classic neurotransmitters, the peripheral nervous system also contains many biologically active peptides.[92,158] In synthesizing neuropeptides, neurons make large precursor molecules from which are cleaved one or more biologically active peptides, the active forms of which generally contain fewer than 40 amino acids.[46,124] Biologic systems use these peptides for information exchange between cells. A particular peptide may have varied functions, acting as a conventional hormone after release into the bloodstream, as a more locally distributed agent after release from a paracrine cell, or as a neurotransmitter or neuromodulator released from a neuron.[92]

In individual neurons, neuropeptides often coexist with each other or with classic neurotransmitters.[148] A nerve fiber may release coexisting substances simultaneously, or it may release one selectively. The onset of action of neuropeptides often is slower than that of conventional neurotransmitters, and prolonged physiologic effects may result in the target tissue.[79] Further, neuropeptides may alter the responsiveness of peripheral tissues to other neurotransmitters, a phenomenon termed "neuromodulation." Receptors for neuropeptides are just beginning to be found and are not as well understood as those for conventional neurotransmitters. The mechanisms for inactivation of neuropeptides are not well understood either, especially in peripheral tissues. Although some peptides are internalized and degraded after receptor binding, no reuptake mechanisms similar to those for catecholamines have been described. Peptidases are widely distributed throughout the body, but the physiologic role of these enzymes in neuropeptide inactivation is not yet firmly established. Neuropeptides released by peripheral nerves may act at considerable distances from the release site, estimated to be at least tens of micra in sympathetic ganglia.[84]

---

*References 28, 29, 163-165, 189.

The identification of neuropeptides in peripheral tissues like the eye requires both histochemistry and biochemistry. Immunohistochemistry is the basis for the in situ localization of neuropeptides. It uses antibodies to stain neuropeptides in specific structures on tissue sections; fluorescein is a common marker used to visualize the immunohistochemical reaction, but other visualization techniques also are suitable. Because of the potential for antibody cross-reactivity to chemically related antigens, immunohistochemical identification is never absolute and unequivocal identification of a neuropeptide requires biochemical methods. Thus, the suffix "-like immunoreactive" is used commonly in immunohistochemistry. Although biochemistry now has confirmed immunohistochemical findings for several neuropeptides in the eye, the present review still applies the suffix "-like immunoreactive (-LI)" to immunohistochemical results.

In the eye, the study of neuropeptides is revealing a richness and complexity of innervation that was unimagined just a few years ago.[202] Many are now known to be present; more are still being discovered. Nerve fibers containing a particular neuropeptide tend to derive from just one of the main divisions of the peripheral innervation of the eye, but unlike cholinergic and adrenergic nerves, this tendency is not exclusive. The co-localization patterns of neuropeptides with other peptides and with classic neurotransmitters are just now being learned.

Vasoactive intestinal polypeptide and peptide histidine isoleucine

Vasoactive intestinal polypeptide (VIP) was the first neuropeptide identified in ocular autonomic nerve fibers.* As presently understood, nerve fibers containing this peptide are parasympathetic in origin; many, if not all, are likely to be cholinergic as well. VIP-LI ocular nerve fibers largely derive from the pterygopalatine ganglion.[233] In rats, VIP has been identified in the cells of the ciliary ganglion and in its related accessory ganglia.[101,112] The uvea of lower mammals and humans also contains intrinsic VIP-LI neurons.[131,213,223] The specific intraocular distribution of nerves from each of these different parasympathetic sources is not yet well defined.

The protein precursor molecule for VIP, pre-pro-VIP, also contains the sequence for a second biologically active peptide. In lower mammals, this peptide is called peptide histidine isoleucine

(PHI);[220] in humans, the comparable peptide is called peptide histidine methionine (PHM) because of a few amino acid substitutions in its sequence.[80] The cleavage of this precursor results in the co-localization of VIP and PHI in many immunoreactive neurons.[15,50] Consistent with this derivation, PHI-LI nerve fibers also have been observed in the guinea pig choroid[159] and in the rat iris.[16] In the rat iris in particular, the distribution of PHI-LI nerve fibers closely parallels that of nerve fibers containing VIP, suggesting co-localization. Detailed studies of the distribution of PHI in the eye have not yet been reported.

Neuropeptide Y

Neuropeptide Y (NPY) localizes to ocular nerve fibers of many mammalian species,[23,81,207,210,221] including humans;[200] it has been isolated biochemically from rat and guinea pig uvea.[210] With only minor exceptions, the intraocular distribution of NPY-LI nerve fibers closely parallels that of adrenergic nerves.[23,210,221] Superior cervical ganglionectomy causes the disappearance of most ipsilateral NPY-LI ocular nerve fibers and a drop in radioimmunoassay levels of the peptide.[1,23,221,254] Unlike the findings with adrenergic nerves,[44] however, some choroidal NPY-LI nerve fibers persist after sympathectomy. Based on these findings, most but not all NPY-LI ocular nerve fibers derive from the ipsilateral superior cervical ganglion, and NPY likely coexists with norepinephrine in a substantial portion but probably not all ocular sympathetic nerve fibers.

Recently, NPY also has been identified by biochemistry in two cranial parasympathetic ganglia, the pterygopalatine[100] and the otic,[112] and by immunohistochemistry in the ciliary ganglion[112] and its accessory ganglia in the rat.[65] All ciliary ganglion cells in rats are cholinergic[112] and supply the eye. Thus, in addition to colocalizing with norepinephrine in sympathetic nerve fibers, NPY also colocalizes with acetylcholine in some of the eye's parasympathetic nerve fibers. Further complicating these relationships is the observation that superior cervical ganglionectomy enhances the expression of NPY by nonsympathetic neurons with ocular projections.[18] The functional meaning of this dual origin for NPY-LI ocular nerves is far from clear because little is now known about the physiology of NPY in the eye.

Opioid peptides

Many opioid peptides exist in the nervous system, and their biochemistry and neuroanatomy is quite complex.[88] There are three opioid peptide pre-

---

*References 190, 199, 223, 233, 237, 238.

cursor molecules, each derived from different genes: pro-enkephalin, pro-opiomelanocortin, and pro-neoendorphin-dynorphin; the core enkephalin sequence is found in each. There exist fine nerve fibers immunoreactive to leu-enkephalin in the eye of rat[17] and guinea pig (Kuwayama and Stone, unpublished observations). These likely derive from cholinergic parasympathetic neurons of the ciliary ganglion, from accessory ciliary cells and perhaps from other sources.[65] No biochemical analysis of opioid peptides in peripheral ocular tissues has been reported. Another opioid peptide, dynorphin, also has been identified in the guinea pig iris by immunohistochemistry[55] but has not yet been studied more extensively. Opioid mechanisms appear to influence IOP, evidently through effects on outflow.[34] The occurrence of opioid peptides in parasympathetic nerve fibers innervating the eye should stimulate further work with these peptides, including potential cholinergic interactions.

Neuropeptides in ocular sensory nerves

Three neuropeptides have been identified to date in sensory nerve fibers that supply the eye: substance P (SP),* calcitonin gene-related peptide (CGRP),[103,128,206,212,222] and a peptide of the cholecystokinin-gastrin (CCK) family.[151,204]

SP is a member of the tachykinin peptide family.[68,140] Two other tachykinins, substance K and neuromedin K, also have been identified recently in mammalian sensory neurons; only SP has been sought specifically in peripheral ocular nerves by immunohistochemistry. In fact, the field of neuropeptides is developing so rapidly that many of the descriptive studies of SP-LI nerve fibers in the eye were performed before the discovery of these other tachykinins in the mammalian nervous system. Because all three peptides share some similar amino acid sequences, the possibility of antiserum cross-reactivity in the published immunohistochemical studies cannot be excluded at present. Biochemical evidence indicates the presence of true SP in the peripheral nervous system of the eye.[198] More recently, substance K and neuromedin K have been isolated biochemically from the rabbit uvea,[219] and these other tachykinins may also localize to ocular sensory nerves.

The evidence for the occurrence of CGRP and CCK in ocular nerves rests solely on immunohistochemical studies. Two forms of CGRP, products of different genes and differing by only one amino acid, occur in the mammalian nervous system, including the trigeminal ganglion; they have been called alpha-CGRP and beta-CGRP respectively.[2,172] Because of the close sequence homology of these neuropeptides, the antisera available for immunohistochemistry likely do not distinguish between the two forms. Cholecystokinin and gastrin arise from a common phylogenetic precursor and contain the identical C-terminal pentapeptide sequence. Further, both CCK and gastrin are found in multiple molecular forms in the same species, all containing the same C-terminal pentapeptide sequence.[167] Because both CCK- and gastrin-related peptides are found by biochemistry in the peripheral nervous system,[204] there is clear need for direct biochemical characterization of the neuropeptide present in the eye.

Both in the trigeminal ganglion and in ocular nerve fibers, these three classes of neuropeptides demonstrate complex patterns of colocalization.* Interestingly, denervation and colocalization studies in the guinea pig eye indicate that many of the SP-LI iris nerve fibers in this species do not derive from the trigeminal ganglion;[103] but the observation relates primarily to iris physiology, not IOP regulation, and will not be discussed in greater detail in this chapter.

Galanin

Galanin localizes to neurons of the central nervous system, gut and sensory ganglia;[171,192] it recently has been localized to peripheral nerve fibers of the eye.[205,214] Although galanin-LI neurons occur in both the trigeminal and superior cervical ganglia,[171,192] the initial studies suggest a sensory derivation for the immunoreactive ocular nerves. Galanin has physiologic effects on many smooth muscles, including the rabbit iris sphincter muscle;[47] but ocular studies with this peptide are just beginning.

SPECIFIC DISTRIBUTION OF CHEMICALLY DEFINED NERVE TYPES IN THE EYE

Because of the diverse functional nature of intraocular tissues, highly specific descriptions of nerve distributions in the eye are required. The distribution of chemically defined ocular nerve fibers is best studied for the classical neurotransmitters and for the specific neuropeptides VIP,† NPY,‡ SP§ and CGRP.[103,206,212,222] For these peptides, there is striking similarity among different mammalian species, the chief differences relating to

---

*References 45, 111, 130, 190, 201, 209, 223-226, 230.

*References 56, 102, 114, 115, 128, 191.
†References 199, 213, 223, 236, 237.
‡References 23, 81, 200, 207, 210, 211.
§References 45, 111, 130, 201, 209, 223-226, 230.

Table 12-1   Neurotransmitters and biologically active peptides in mammalian ocular nerves

Neurotransmitter/ neuropeptide	Tissue			
	Limbal blood vessels	Drainage angle	Ciliary body blood vessels	Ciliary process
Acetylcholine	?	+	+	+
Norepinephrine *	+	+	+ +	+ + +
Serotonin	?	?	?	+ +
VIP *	+ +	+	+ +	+
Neuropeptide Y *	+ +	+	+ +	+ + +
Substance P *	+ +	+ +	+ +	+ +
CGRP *	+ +	+	+ +	+ +
CCK	+	+	?	+
Galanin	+ +	+ +	+ +	+ +

Arbitrary scale of 1 to 3+ to indicate nerve fiber density, generalized from published reports (see text). Asterisk (*) designates those substances for which human data are available. The distribution of the neuropeptides peptide histidine isoleucine, enkephalin, dynorphin and substance K have not been described in sufficient detail to include in this table. (From Stone, RA, Kuwayama, Y, and Laties, AM: Experientia 43:791, 1987)

nerve fiber density. Whether this generality will hold as more peptides are compared cannot now be known. Where available, findings from human or monkey eyes are discussed; for those neurotransmitters/neuropeptides not yet studied in the human or monkey, results from other species are described when known in sufficient detail. Emphasis is placed on those structures having the greatest relevance to IOP: the ciliary body, drainage angle, and limbal blood vessels (Table 12-1).

Ciliary Body—Blood Vessels and Ciliary Processes

The formation of aqueous humor results from two processes: ultrafiltration and secretion. Ultrafiltration is dependent on the transmural pressure of the ciliary process microvasculature and the functional state of the larger afferent and efferent blood vessels. From microvascular luminal casting, the detailed anatomy of the ciliary process circulation is now known.[54,136-138] In primates, derivative vessels of the "major arterial circle" of the iris radiate into the anterior portions of the ciliary processes and divide to form its capillary net. The circulation of the ciliary process is directed posteriorly and drains into the choroidal veins. Aqueous humor secretion is an active process of the ciliary epithelium. Understanding the control mechanisms governing aqueous humor formation requires definition of those nerves that supply the ciliary body/process blood vessels and those that underlie the ciliary epithelium.

Whereas light microscopic techniques reveal the association of nerve fibers to ciliary body arterioles, the capillary supply in the core of each ciliary process lies so close to the overlying epithelium that the resolution of light microscopy is inadequate to determine whether ciliary process nerve fibers relate primarily to the capillaries, to the overlying epithelium, or to both. For adrenergic nerve fibers, with active reuptake mechanisms for released norepinephrine, this distinction may have functional meaning. Because neuropeptides likely diffuse and act over comparatively long distances, however, distinguishing vascular from epithelial innervation may have less functional importance than learning which specific nerve fiber types are present within a process.

In the studies of choroidal innervation, no efforts have been made to distinguish efferent ciliary process blood vessels from those generally in the choroid. Neither can descriptions of the innervation to the vascular layer beneath pars plana epithelium be related specifically to the efferent blood supply of the ciliary process. Except for important differences in nerve fiber density, the identity of the neurotransmitters and neuropeptides in the choroid generally parallels that of the vascular innervation of the more anterior uvea; the choroidal innervation will not be discussed here in detail.

For parasympathetic nerves in the ciliary body, the density of the cholinergic innervation to the ciliary muscle makes it difficult to distinguish individual nerve fibers on tissue sections stained by the histochemical reaction for acetylcholine esterase.[110] Individual nerve fibers, however, can be seen to enter the ciliary processes with blood vessels. VIP-LI nerve fibers supply the anterior segment,[131,199,213,237] but the nerve fiber density is not as great as that seen in the choroid.[223,233,238] A modest number of immunoreactive nerve fibers supply the arterioles in the anterior ciliary body and also occur within the ciliary processes. Despite the modest number of VIP-LI nerve fibers, many VIP receptors are found in the ciliary body.[134] VIP dilates uveal blood vessels[143,144] and stimulates cyclic AMP production by the ciliary body.[134] These observations suggest an important role for VIP in aqueous humor dynamics; indeed, intracameral or intravenous infusion stimulates aqueous humor formation.[145] Potential interactions of VIP and cholinergic mechanisms in aqueous humor formation remain to be demonstrated.

A plentiful adrenergic innervation to uveal blood vessels and to ciliary processes originates from the superior cervical ganglion.[44,110] Similarly, nerves containing NPY surround anterior ciliary body arterioles and richly innervate the ciliary processes[23,200,207,210] (Fig. 12-2). Interestingly, for cat, monkey, and human, the density of NPY-LI nerve fibers is greater in the anterior than in the posterior region of the ciliary process.[200,210] Although direct confirmation is necessary, these observations suggest that NPY-LI nerves may selectively associate with the afferent rather than the efferent ciliary process circulation. NPY, like norepinephrine, is a uveal vasoconstrictor[142] and it has a "sympathetic-like" neuromodulator role on iris muscles.[156] No studies yet address a possible role for NPY in the regulation of aqueous humor formation. Considering the important role of the sympathetic nervous system in aqueous humor dynamics and the central role of adrenergic agents in clinical glaucoma therapy, such studies are long overdue.

Sensory nerves, immunoreactive to CGRP or SP, surround ciliary body blood vessels and lie within the ciliary processes of many mammalian species,[45,209,224,230] including humans.[201] Studied only in rat and guinea pig, and occurring in low density, CCK-LI nerve fibers similarly surround uveal blood vessels and lie within the ciliary processes.[204] The role of these neuropeptides on aqueous humor formation is not well understood. CGRP, a potent vasodilator,[20] appears to mediate the uveal vasodilation that occurs in the neurogenic ocular injury response,[234] but an ocular role for this peptide under less drastic physiologic conditions is not known. SP has potent effects on fluid flow in the kidney[67] but has not been studied for possible effects on the ciliary processes. The gastrointestinal physiology of the CCK/gastrin family of peptides is well studied; no reports of ocular effects are available. Galanin-LI nerve fibers similarly supply ciliary body blood vessels and the ciliary processes in the porcine eye,[205] and a role for galanin in the regulation of aqueous humor formation also needs to be studied.

Trabecular Meshwork

For almost a century, nerves have been known to be present in the anterior chamber angle.[19,208] In

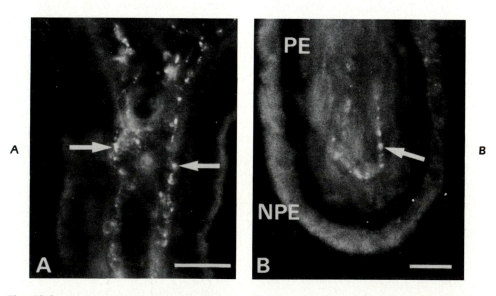

Fig. 12-2 Neuropeptide Y-like immunoreactive fibers are present in the ciliary process of the human eye. **A,** Immunoreactive fibers *(arrows)* between the vascular core and the overlying epithelium. **B,** An immunoreactive nerve fiber *(arrow)* is seen to extend to the tip of the ciliary process. NPE, nonpigmented epithelial layer; PE, pigmented epithelial layer. Fluorescence micrograph; magnification bar, 25 μm. (From Stone, RA: Exp Eye Res 42:349, 1986)

monkeys and humans, these nerves arise from the supraciliary and ciliary plexuses.[52,74,208,246] At the light microscopic level, nerve fibers are found in all regions of the human trabecular meshwork,[74] even in both walls of Schlemm's canal. Among those who have studied this subject, there is general consensus that the nerve fibers in the trabecular meshwork terminate there and are not fibers of passage to the cornea.[52,208] By scanning and transmission electron microscopy, nerve fibers are seen to have varied anatomic relationships to trabecular cells.[52,215] They occur inside the connective tissue core of trabecular sheets, on the surface of trabecular sheets and sometimes crossing intertrabecular spaces. In the monkey, most trabecular nerve fibers are unmyelinated; in humans, some myelinated fibers are found posteriorly near the scleral spur. In monkeys and humans, the Schwann cell coverings sometimes are lost near the nerve terminal. Trabecular axons that have lost their Schwann cell coverings are invested by trabecular endothelial cells in humans and by fibroblast, melanocyte, or endothelial cell processes in the monkey. Parasympathetic, sympathetic, and sensory nerve fibers all contribute to the innervation of the filtration angle.[75,177]

The application of the thiocholine technique for the identification of cholinergic nerves has been limited in the chamber angle because of technical problems. Nevertheless, acetylcholine esterase–positive nerve fibers in modest density have been observed in the chamber angle of such species as rabbit, cat, guinea pig, and, on occasion, in the trabecular meshwork of monkeys.[40,110] No direct studies on humans have been reported. Muscarinic agents lower IOP, primarily by increasing aqueous humor outflow facility. Because most authors suggest that muscarinic agents and parasympathetic stimulation work by mechanically altering the scleral spur and trabecular meshwork through ciliary muscle contraction and not by a direct muscarinic effect on trabecular meshwork cells,[86] the role of these cholinergic nerves remains to be established.

Using immunohistochemical techniques, VIP-LI nerve fibers now have been found in the chamber angle of rat, guinea pig, cat, and human.[199,213] Although not directly studied in denervation experiments, these are likely to be parasympathetic in origin. In humans in particular, a small number of VIP-LI fibers occur primarily in the uveal meshwork. In contrast, none have been found in the trabecular meshwork of the rhesus monkey; other monkey species have not been studied. Intracameral infusion of VIP causes a slight increase in aqueous humor outflow in cynomolgus monkeys, an effect inhibited by atropine.[145] Whether the VIP acts directly on the meshwork or indirectly through the ciliary muscle[216] and other possible interactions of VIP and cholinergic mechanisms in aqueous humor outflow remain to be clarified.

The density of adrenergic innervation to the outflow pathway shows considerable species variation.[39,40-42,110] In humans and monkeys, the trabecular meshwork contains a modest number of adrenergic nerve fibers (Fig. 12-3). In monkeys, the location and number of adrenergic nerve fibers varies with species.[42] Usually, most occur in the posterior uveal trabecular meshwork; nerve fibers also are seen in the middle and sometimes in the anterior portions of the meshwork. In the posterior trabecular region of the cynomolgus monkey, approximately one-third of the nerve terminals are estimated to be adrenergic.[147] In the human eye, adrenergic nerve fibers are demonstrable in tissues from younger individuals, but most specimens from elderly patients studied by the histofluoro-

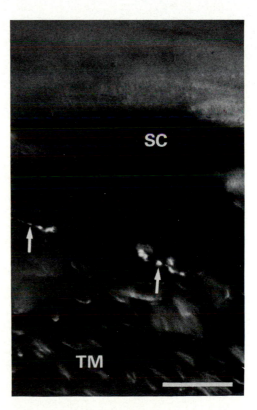

Fig. 12-3 Adrenergic nerve fibers *(arrows)* are illustrated in the trabecular meshwork of the spider monkey. They are revealed by the histofluorometric technique for catecholamines. SC, Schlemm's canal; TM, trabecular meshwork. Fluorescence micrograph; magnification bar, 50 μm. (From Stone, RA, and Laties, AM. In Krieglstein, GK, and Leydhecker, W, editors: Glaucoma update III, Berlin, 1987, Springer-Verlag)

metric method show no adrenergic nerves.[41] The possible loss of adrenergic innervation with age may have relevance to glaucoma, but definitive conclusions are not possible because of the small number of observations and because of aging changes in the human meshwork that interfere with the histochemical evaluation.

NPY-LI nerve fibers, like the adrenergic nerves, show significant species variation in the number and distribution within the chamber angle. For humans and monkeys in particular, trabecular NPY-LI nerve fibers are relatively uncommon.[200,210]

In the rhesus monkey, a few lie in the posterior trabecular meshwork, scleral spur and at the outer wall of Schlemm's canal. In the human, NPY-LI nerve fibers are present in the posterior trabecular meshwork but usually are not seen elsewhere. These NPY-LI nerve fibers have been assumed to be sympathetic in origin, but the recent discovery of NPY in cranial parasympathetic neurons makes uncertain the precise nature of these angle nerves.

Of the sensory nerves in the chamber angle, those containing SP are the most extensively stud-

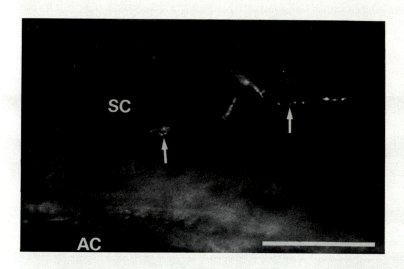

Fig. 12-4 Substance P immunoreactive nerve fibers *(arrows)* are demonstrated by the immunohistochemical technique near the posterior region of Schlemm's canal in the eye of the crab-eating monkey *(Macaca fascicularis)*. AC, anterior chamber; SC, Schlemm's canal. Fluorescence micrograph; magnification bar, 50 μm. (Reproduced with permission from Stone, RA, and Laties, AM. In Krieglstein, GK, and Leydhecker, W, editors: Glaucoma update III, Berlin, 1987, Springer-Verlag)

Fig. 12-5 In the posterior portion of the trabecular meshwork of the human eye are illustrated substance P-like immunoreactive nerve fibers *(arrow)*. AC, anterior chamber; SC, Schlemm's canal. Fluorescence micrograph; magnification bar, 50 μm. (From Stone, RA, and Kuwayama, Y: Arch Ophthalmol 103:1207, 1985. Copyright 1985, American Medical Association.)

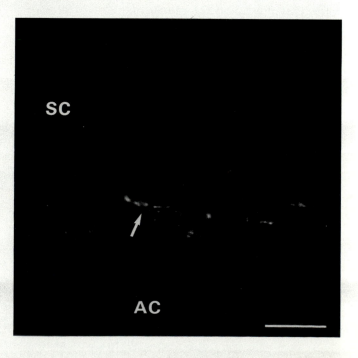

ied. The chamber angle of all mammalian species studied contain SP-LI nerve fibers, and SP-LI nerve fibers represent the densest neuropeptidergic innervation described to date in the trabecular meshwork of humans and monkeys[111,201,209] (Figs. 12-4 and 12-5). Immunoreactive nerve fibers occur in both the uveal and scleral portions of the trabecular meshwork, sometimes extending to its most anterior region. They occur in the juxtacanalicular tissue and on both sides of Schlemm's canal. For CGRP, a small number of immunoreactive nerve fibers are present in the trabecular meshwork of human and rhesus monkey.[212] CCK has been studied only in the chamber angle of the guinea pig, which contains a modest number of immunoreactive nerve fibers.[204]

Many galanin-LI nerve fibers occur in the chamber angle of the porcine eye,[205] and a few enkephalin-like immunoreactive nerve fibers are seen in the drainage angle of rat (Kuwayama, Y, and Stone, RA, unpublished observations).

Limbal Blood Vessels

A highly complex vascular system supplies the corneoscleral limbus.[127] Terminal branches of the anterior ciliary arteries divide into fine capillary arcades that reach the corneal periphery. These fuse into numerous tortuous veins emptying into the episcleral vascular system. The relationship of these vascular channels to the drainage system for aqueous humor is complex and species dependent, even among mammals. In primates and humans, aqueous humor drains from Schlemm's canal into aqueous collector channels and then into aqueous veins; the latter then merge into the limbal vascular system. Dependent on episcleral venous pressure, IOP might also be influenced by alterations of other elements of the limbal circulation.[105] The physiology of this system, however, is not well understood; even the direction of blood flow is controversial.[218]

Despite uncertainties regarding physiology, the limbal and intrascleral vessels are well innervated. While cholinesterase staining for cholinergic nerves has not been reported, the histofluorometric technique for catecholamines has demonstrated adrenergic nerves.[39,40,110] Immunohistochemistry has revealed the occurrence of essentially all the neuropeptides present in perivascular nerves elsewhere in the anterior segment (Fig. 12-6).[202] Because of the difficulty of evaluating this region of the eye in tissue sections, the relations of chemically-defined nerve fibers to arterioles, venules, and aqueous channels is not now known. From a purely anatomic view, however, neural influences on the limbal vasculature may potentially affect the limbal circulation and IOP, but the existence of such mechanisms requires direct study.

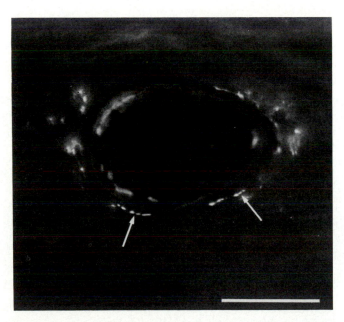

Fig. 12-6 Vasoactive intestinal peptide immunoreactive fibers *(arrows)* surround a blood vessel in the corneoscleral limbus in the rhesus monkey eye. Fluorescence micrograph; magnification bar, 50 μm. (From Stone, RA, Kuwayama, Y, and Laties, AM: Experientia 43:791, 1987)

PARACRINE CELLS IN THE EYE

First noted under the posterior extension of Descemet's membrane,[170] specialized cells cluster in the anterior trabecular meshwork of the rhesus monkey.[166] From their content of a well-developed Golgi apparatus and two types of cytoplasmic inclusions, Raviola[166] has proposed that these meshwork cells are secretory, possibly elaborating a surfactant-like substance.

Based on immunohistochemistry, clustered cells that lie circumferentially in the rhesus monkey trabecular meshwork contain neuron specific enolase (Fig. 12-7), an isomer of the glycolytic enzyme enolase.[203] Based on its histochemical distribution, this enzyme has been proposed as a marker for neurons and neuroendocrine cells.[126] Neuroendocrine cells as a class are called paraneurons, amine precursor uptake and decarboxylation (APUD) cells, or most recently, cells of the diffuse neuroendocrine system. A diverse group of neuroregulatory cells, examples include neurosecretory cells, such as adrenal medullary cells and pancreatic beta-cells, and specialized neuroreceptors, such as the Merkel cell of skin. The localization of neuron specific enolase to discrete trabecular cells suggests that these cells are neuroendocrine in nature and implies the existence of a local neuroregulatory mechanism in this region of the eye. By analogy to other cells containing neuron specific enolase, these immunoreactive trabecular meshwork cells likely contain a peptide hormone, as yet unidentified, and may secrete it directly into the aqueous humor outflow pathway. Alternatively, these cells may constitute a specialized neuroreceptor, per-haps to regulate IOP or aqueous humor composition. These clustered meshwork cells are the only putative neuroendocrine cells so far found in the anterior segment of the eye, and they have not been reported in humans.

THE PERIPHERAL NERVOUS SYSTEM AND INTRAOCULAR PRESSURE

Although the classic concept of opposing cholinergic/parasympathetic adrenergic/sympathetic influences in the eye remains valid, the recent discovery of this vast array of neuropeptides indicates a previously unappreciated heterogeneity and complexity to the peripheral ocular innervation and, by implication, to the mechanisms governing its physiology. In considering effects on IOP, each of these transmitters or modulators may have one or more sites of action: the formation of aqueous humor, the drainage of aqueous humor, and/or the level of episcleral venous pressure. These activities may induce large, small, or undetectable net changes in IOP that do not necessarily reflect the many underlying influences.

In the past, experiments to elucidate the influence of the peripheral nervous system on IOP have been designed either to stimulate or to interrupt each peripheral ganglion or their preganglionic/postganglionic nerves. However, stimulation or denervation does not simply excite or remove one neural activity; it also releases or eliminates coexistent transmitters that may neutralize or potentiate each other. Selective denervations of the eye in particular are now known to enhance the production of neuropeptides in nerves derived from other

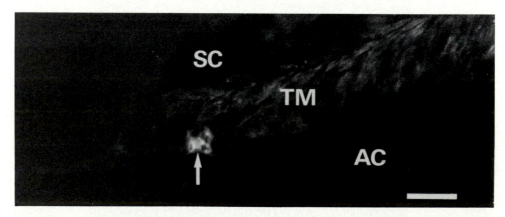

Fig. 12-7 A cluster of cells *(arrow)* in the anterior trabecular meshwork in the rhesus monkey is immunoreactive for neuron-specific enolase. AC, anterior chamber; SC, Schlemm's canal; TM, trabecular meshwork. Fluorescence micrograph; magnification bar, 50 μm. (From Stone, RA, and Laties, AM. In Krieglstein, GK, and Leydhecker, W, editors: Glaucoma update III, Berlin, 1987, Springer-Verlag)

sources. Superior cervical ganglionectomy, for instance, enhances the expression of NPY by parasympathetic neurons[18] and also enhances the expression of several neuropeptides derived from sensory sources.* Whether these chemical changes affect a compensatory homeostatic mechanism with altered release of NPY or other neuropeptides is unknown. Reinnervation of the ciliary muscle after ciliary ganglionectomy is reported,[49] but reinnervation after other denervations has not been clearly demonstrated. These types of observations indicate interactions among the peripheral ganglia serving the eye and a surprising plasticity to its peripheral innervation. Nerve stimulations or denervations may reconstruct or alter the underlying neuronal tone, and these findings make the interpretation of previous experiments more difficult.

A multitude of factors influence both aqueous humor formation, aqueous humor outflow, and hence IOP. The narrow range and stability of normal IOPs suggest that somehow this system is regulated.[91] Such a postulated regulatory system probably would incorporate a "feedback" loop, consisting of a sensory or afferent pathway, a regulatory center presumably in the central nervous system, and an efferent pathway probably through the autonomic nervous systems. Such feedback mechanisms are well established for blood pressure, heart activity, voluntary muscular activity, and other homeostatic mechanisms. Whether IOP, aqueous composition, aqueous secretory rate, and/or aqueous outflow rate might be moderated primarily is not clear even at this time.[25]

Sensory Input

Regarding possible afferent input for a regulatory system, the eye is richly supplied by sensory nerve fibers. In addition to the sensory innervation of the chamber angle and ciliary processes, the uveal tract contains a multitude of sensory nerve fibers, many of which lie on the anterior iris surface. By analogy with the occurrence of free nerve endings in well-established sensory structures, such as the carotid sinus, the rich intraocular distribution of sensory nerve fibers is consistent with the presence of local afferent mechanisms related to IOP, aqueous secretion, or aqueous composition.

The search for specialized sensory receptors in the eye for the regulation of IOP has been without clear result. A possible location for such receptors might be the chamber angle. In this regard, encap-

sulated sensory corpuscles have been found in the chamber angle of sea mammals, such as dolphins and whales,[248,253] and in the chamber angle of some aquatic birds;[247] these are located in sclera, trabecular meshwork, or uveal tissue. The function of these corpuscles is unknown, but they may represent specialized structures for IOP regulation in species that must undergo rapid changes in ambient pressure as they move from aquatic to atmospheric environments. The form and location of these sensory corpuscles varies between species, and they may serve different functions in different animals.[253] No comparable specialized structures have been observed in the eyes of land mammals, including monkeys and man. Many of the terminal nerve fibers in the trabecular meshwork, however, are likely to be sensory in origin, and provocative tissue relationships are present between terminal nerve fibers and the specialized cells of the trabecular meshwork.[208] The possibility of specialized sensory functions within the trabecular meshwork even in primates and humans has been suggested.

In a search for afferent nerve pathways influencing aqueous humor dynamics, afferent impulses in the ciliary nerves of cats and monkeys have been recorded after induced changes in IOP.[13,116,155,243,255] These studies have not demonstrated clearly the existence of a direct afferent pathway relaying information about IOP. In only some animals, the ciliary nerves show afferent impulses after IOP changes. Generally, lowering of IOP reduces spontaneous activity in ciliary nerves; elevation of IOP induces a sudden increase in nerve activity with rapid adaptation of the discharge rate to a somewhat higher rate than the spontaneous one. That impulse frequency is not linearly related to ocular pressure, that the response rate is rapidly adapting, that often no relationship between IOP and sustained discharge rate is demonstrable, and that physiologic responses to physiologic stimuli are only recordable in a small proportion of nerves in some animals create the ambiguity of these experiments. Whether afferent activity in ocular sensory nerves relays information on IOP remains controversial.[23,116,155,255]

If these nerves do not subserve a baroreceptor function, the nature of their stimulus is unclear, especially in response to modest changes in IOP. Very high IOP levels stimulate activity in many ocular sensory nerve fibers, probably because of the mechanical deformation of ocular tissues; here, pain information may well be transmitted.[255] The methods used in most of these studies were best suited for measuring impulses from large sensory

---

*References 31, 87, 102, 181, 234, 254.

nerve fibers. Many small C-type sensory nerve fibers are present in the eye, the activity of which is not likely to have been detected by these recording techniques.

Stimulation of the trigeminal nerve increases IOP of the ipsilateral eye.* The IOP elevation of the ipsilateral eye after antidromic stimulation of the fifth cranial nerve is now recognized as a component of the eye's irritative response to injury, a response that also includes vasodilation, disruption of the blood-aqueous barrier, and miosis. Both neurogenic and prostaglandin-mediated mechanisms have been identified, the relative contribution of each depending on the type of stimulus.[24,35] Although undoubtedly important to the injury response, the role of sensory nerve antidromic activity in the physiologic regulation of IOP has not been demonstrated.

Like direct stimulation, section of the trigeminal nerve in rabbits produces an immediate increase in IOP;[154] but within 1 week, the IOP of the denervated eye is comparable to the normal,[152,154] despite an increase in the facility of aqueous humor outflow.[152]

Only a few clinical reports of IOP after sensory denervation in humans have appeared. IOP decreases in most cases in the days after preganglionic section of the fifth nerve.[69] These changes could be attributable to interruption of the nerve, but they also might arise from irritation of the cut end or from section of sympathetic fibers in the ganglion.[154] Recently, hourly IOP measurements on three patients after surgery of the ophthalmic division of the trigeminal nerve demonstrated inconsistent IOP changes.[129]

Parasympathetic effects

Muscarinic agents, long used for clinical glaucoma therapy, lower IOP primarily by increasing aqueous outflow facility. They are believed to act by contracting the ciliary muscle and mechanically altering the scleral spur and trabecular meshwork[86] and not by a direct muscarinic effect on trabecular meshwork cells.[8] Based on the clinical pharmacology, many studies have sought a role for the parasympathetic nervous system as an efferent pathway regulating IOP.

Oculomotor nerve

Stimulation of the oculomotor nerve causes an immediate rise in IOP[11,113,117,239,252] because of extra-

ocular muscle contraction, a response that must be controlled in studying effects on aqueous humor dynamics.[63,83] Like the muscarinic agents, preganglionic stimulation of the oculomotor nerve increases the facility of aqueous humor outflow in monkeys,[229] in curarized[193] and nonparalyzed rabbits,[235] and in enucleated, arterially perfused cat eyes.[125]

Stimulation of the oculomotor nerve also increases the formation of aqueous humor in nonparalyzed rabbits[235] and in the arterially perfused cat eyes.[125] In curarized rabbits, the increase in aqueous humor formation[193] after preganglionic oculomotor nerve stimulation is not statistically significant. Although the change in aqueous humor inflow in arterially perfused cat eyes results from increased ultrafiltration,[125] the complex and species-dependent effects of oculomotor nerve stimulation on anterior uveal blood flow[194,195] complicate generalization of this interpretation to in vivo studies.

The effects of third nerve stimulation on IOP are much more variable. Stimulation of the ciliary ganglion causes an IOP rise in the dog[53] and rabbit,[179] but a fall in cats with or without prior sympathectomy.[3,4,5] A fall of IOP also occurs in arterially perfused cat eyes after ciliary ganglion stimulation.[116] Stimulation of the preganglionic portion of the oculomotor nerve in rabbits and cats causes an increase in IOP[125,152,235] or a nonsignificant decrease in IOP in curarized rabbits;[193] in monkeys, there is inconsistent variation in IOP.[229] Direct stimulation of the oculomotor nucleus in rabbits[63] and in monkeys[83] does not affect IOP when the influence of the extraocular muscles is eliminated.

Variable effects on IOP also have resulted from surgical interruption of the third nerve. Extirpation of the ciliary ganglion causes an IOP decrease in rabbits.[179] Intracranial or intraorbital section of the preganglionic nerve has caused varied effects on IOP: a fall in rabbits[152] and dogs,[227] an immediate rise in sympathectomized cats,[3] no change in rabbits,[63] and both a rise and fall with an increase in outflow resistance in monkeys.[229]

In summary, these studies of the oculomotor nerve do not provide a coherent mechanism. Stimulation causes complex responses on aqueous humor dynamics, likely increasing aqueous humor outflow facility, but other effects remain somewhat variable and incompletely defined.

Facial nerve

The pterygopalatine ganglion, the other main cranial parasympathetic ganglion that innervates

---

*References 11, 70, 135, 154, 197, 239, 245.

the eye,[101,119,173,174] seems to influence IOP. Clinical reports from the early part of the century indicated that blocking of the pterygopalatine ganglion in glaucoma patients reduces IOP.[123,162] Severance of the preganglionic nerve to the ganglion also reduces IOP in normal subjects.[61,182] In monkeys, interruption of the facial nerve or the pterygopalatine ganglion also reduces IOP.[174] Stimulation of the preganglionic facial nerve causes a moderate IOP rise, accompanied by an atropine-resistant increase of uveal blood flow in rabbits,[59,196] cats[59] and monkeys.[144] These findings suggest that much of the IOP rise is secondary to intraocular vasodilation. The peripheral transmitter of this vasodilation remains to be established, VIP currently being the strongest candidate.[143] Although approximately 15% of the nerve fibers in the trabecular meshwork of the monkey may derive from the pterygopalatine ganglion,[174] a physiologic role for facial parasympathetic nerve fibers in the regulation of IOP remains to be more clearly defined.

Sympathetic Effects

The influence of the sympathetic nervous system on the regulation of IOP has been studied by stimulation or denervation experiments. The clinical use of epinephrine and beta-adrenergic antagonists in glaucoma therapy underscores the clinical relevance of this work. Electrical stimulation of the cervical sympathetic nerves has been studied in cats, dogs,[11,62,70] rabbits,* and monkeys[14,26] to assess the acute effects of sympathetic activity on aqueous humor dynamics. The usual sites of stimulation have been the cervical sympathetic trunk or, less commonly, the superior cervical ganglion.

Generally, stimulation of the cervical sympathetic nerve causes a fall in IOP. This response is preceded by a slight IOP rise in dogs and cats,[11,62,70] but not in rabbits.[62,179,245] The initial rise in pressure is thought to result from contraction of the sympathetically innervated Müller's muscle[36,62,70] and is variably observed because of species differences in the muscle.

Electrical stimulation of the preganglionic cervical sympathetic nerve[62,106] or superior cervical ganglion in rabbits[152,235] decreases IOP because the vasoconstriction of the richly innervated uveal vascular bed reduces ocular volume and because aqueous humor formation is depressed.[106,235] The effect of the stimulation on outflow facility in rabbits is small and varies from a nonsignificant

increase[153] or decrease,[235] to no effect.[106] A greater increase in aqueous humor outflow facility after sympathetic nerve stimulation occurs when the reuptake and binding of neuronally released norepinephrine is prevented by cocaine pretreatment.[153] In the vervet monkey, stimulation of the cervical sympathetic nerves results in a slight increase in the inflow of aqueous humor, presumably mediated by beta-adrenergic receptors,[14] with either no change or a moderate decrease in outflow facility.[26]

Recently, Belmonte et al.[12] implanted a portable electrical stimulator to maintain chronic stimulation of the cervical sympathetic nerve in awake rabbits. Continuous and chronic sympathetic stimulation produces an immediate sharp decrease in IOP followed by a gradual rise to prestimulation values over the next 60 to 90 minutes; a final rebound increase in IOP occurs at the termination of the stimulus. They attributed the immediate sharp decrease and final rebound increase to changes in ocular volume from vasoconstriction and vasorelaxation of uveal blood vessels in response to the onset and cessation of the stimulation respectively. During prolonged sympathetic stimulation, decreased aqueous humor inflow persists but is presumed to be offset by a decrease in outflow to account for the gradual rise of IOP to prestimulation levels. Using selective antagonists, they proposed a series of alpha- and beta-adrenergic mechanisms to interpret these complex responses.

Electrical stimulation of sympathetic nerves excites simultaneously all adrenergic fibers directed to the eye and consequently represents a very complex stimulus. Nevertheless, these studies clearly indicate an influence of the sympathetic nervous system on aqueous humor dynamics.

Interruption of the sympathetic pathway to the eye has been achieved by division of the cervical sympathetic nerve trunk proximal to the superior cervical ganglion (preganglionic sympathectomy) or by excision of the superior cervical ganglion (ganglionectomy). These two procedures produce different results on aqueous humor dynamics.

In acute experiments, preganglionic section of the cervical sympathetic trunk produce varied and conflicting effects on IOP: a fall in rabbits[250] and cats;[77,82] no change in rabbits,[107,121,239] cats[107,121] and monkeys;[26] or variable changes in rabbits.[62]

On the other hand, superior cervical ganglionectomy in rabbits causes a definite, though transient, decrease in IOP.[71,118,120] After ganglionectomy IOP gradually falls to its lowest level in approximately 24 hours and then returns to normal after

---

*References 12, 62, 106, 153, 179, 235, 245.

3 to 4 days.[108,120,184,231] An increase in aqueous humor outflow largely accounts for the IOP fall.[9,108,184] The increase in outflow facility seems to result from norepinephrine release into the anterior chamber from degenerating nerve endings in the uvea and from loss of catecholamine reuptake by degenerated nerves.[37,184]

The changes in aqueous humor outflow after application of topical epinephrine to the eye are consistent with these adrenergic effects on aqueous humor outflow.[105,163,185,187] In this regard, beta-receptors but not alpha-receptors, have been identified in cultured trabecular meshwork cells;[160,161] and epinephrine induces changes in the morphology, phagocytosis, and mitotic activity of cultured trabecular meshwork cells.[232] Taken together, these observations are consistent with an adrenergic influence on aqueous humor outflow and suggest a physiologic role for the sympathetic nerves known to be present in this region of the eye.

On a long-term basis, ocular sympathetic denervation in rabbits does not markedly change aqueous humor dynamics during the light phase of the diurnal cycle. Basal IOP, aqueous humor formation, and outflow facility are essentially the same in innervated and denervated eyes.[64,228] These observations may reflect neuronal plasticity and remodeling after denervation. In contrast, superior cervical ganglionectomy in rabbits eliminates the elevation of IOP at night, indicating that intact ocular sympathetic innervation is required for maintenance of the normal circadian rhythm of IOP in this species.[66] Since preganglionic division of the sympathetic nerve trunk has similar effect, nervous input to the superior cervical ganglion contributes to IOP regulation in the dark.[21]

In cats, the effect of superior ganglionectomy on IOP seems variable.[82,108] Similarly in primates, the results are variable; surgical ganglionectomy has not been seen to lower IOP significantly,[72] but chemical sympathectomy causes up to 35% reduction in IOP and aqueous humor secretion for up to 3 weeks.[73] The data in these species are not sufficient to formulate a coherent hypothesis.

In humans, cervical sympathetic denervation causes the Horner's syndrome of ptosis, miosis, facial anhidrosis, and enophthalmos.[22,30,109,217,240] Several earlier reports found decreased aqueous humor inflow in affected eyes.[22,109,217] More recently, human eyes with Horner's syndrome are found to have a slightly lower mean IOP but also to have values of aqueous humor formation and outflow similar to those of normally innervated contralateral eyes.[251] Blocking the stellate ganglion

by local anesthesia lowers IOP in patients with open-angle glaucoma.[48,132] Cervical sympathetic denervation was practiced at the turn of the century as a therapy for glaucoma,[85] but the procedure has been abandoned[241] because of unpredictable results and side effects. Moreover, as supersensitivity to the IOP lowering effect of epinephrine occurs in denervated eyes of patients with Horner's syndrome[109,183,217] and in ganglionectomized animals,[186] the combined use of chemical sympathectomy (e.g., with 6-hydroxydopamine) and epinephrine has been attempted in the treatment of glaucoma.[76,183] Adverse reactions and the limited period of effectiveness have limited this approach to glaucoma therapy as well.

Although the sympathetic nervous system clearly influences aqueous humor dynamics, the differences between the effects of preganglionic and postganglionic denervations and the species variability in responses is striking. Although species differences in ocular structure and morphology of sympathetic innervation may account for some of the variability,[163] species differences in adrenoreceptor distribution may also need to be considered. The effects on aqueous humor dynamics of NPY, a neuropeptide found in ocular sympathetic as well as in some parasympathetic nerves, are presently unknown and require direct study. Clearly, much more remains to be learned about the role of sympathetic innervation in regulating aqueous humor dynamics.

THE CENTRAL NERVOUS SYSTEM AND INTRAOCULAR PRESSURE

The Optic Nerve

In humans with unilateral optic atrophy, the water drinking test produces a less pronounced rise in IOP on the damaged side,[168] suggesting that a hypothalmic center sensitive to osmotic pressure might influence IOP via efferent nerve fibers in the optic nerve.[78] In experimental animals, unilateral transsection of the optic nerve has been reported to modify the IOP response to water drinking in the ipsilateral eye,[96,98,157] and experimental lesions in the supraoptic hypothalamic nucleus also reduce the water drinking response.[32] However, not all laboratories have been able to repeat these observations,[104,169,188] and a role for efferent optic nerve fibers in IOP regulation currently remains unclear.

The Diencephalon

Many clinical reports have postulated a relationship between the central nervous system and the control of IOP.[249] Patient variability and the complexity of clinical histories render many of these observations inconclusive. Even so, this hypothesis has stimulated a search for a locus in the central nervous system that regulates IOP. Presumably, such a center would serve to integrate sensory input and initiate efferent output to the eye through the autonomic nervous system. Several detailed investigations addressed this issue in the 1950s.* Von Sallmann's comment in 1959 remains as valid now as it was then: "Concrete information, however, remains spotty indeed, and forms nothing more than a feeble framework to which much additional experimental data must be added before a well-grounded hypothesis on the nervous control of IOP can be formulated."[242]

Past workers sought a center in the brain, the stimulation of which would affect IOP selectively. Working mostly in the cat, they measured IOP responses to stereotactic stimulation of discrete brain areas.[58,60,180,244] They particularly tried to stimulate nuclei that would affect IOP without parallel changes in systemic blood pressure or extraocular muscle tone, alterations with secondary IOP effects.

Stimulation in many areas, such as the posterior ventral hypothalamus, induced an IOP change simultaneous with a change in blood pressure. These responses resulted from altered blood flow through intraocular vessels, as part of a generalized vascular response; vascular responses restricted to the eye were not demonstrated clearly in these studies. Stimulation in other areas, such as the dorsal hypothalamus and the ventral thalamus, induced changes in IOP without parallel blood pressure changes.[242] Stimulation in a relatively circumscribed area near the anterior column of the fornix actually tended to change IOP in the direction opposite to the blood pressure.[60] Because of large variability in time of onset, duration, latency, and laterality of IOP responses and because of differences among individual animals, anatomic maps of the physiologic responses in the diencephalon showed marked complexity, and it was not possible to identify distinct nuclei or fiber tracts mediating the IOP responses.[58]

Although these studies failed to identify a discrete diencephalic center regulating IOP, several features are important. First, even within these studies, stimulation over wide areas of the diencephalon affected blood pressure readings. Like the findings for IOP, there was no consistent re-

lationship observed in these studies between the blood pressure response and the region stimulated, both rises and falls being obtained from neighboring points. It is well known that neural reflexes regulate blood pressure. The failure to demonstrate a discrete diencephalic center for regulating IOP, therefore, does not exclude the possibility of a nervous reflex regulating IOP.

Technical limitations also need to be considered in interpreting these studies. The stimulation of fiber tracts would have been affected by their orientation relative to the direction of the stimulating current, technical details not systematically explored at that time. Further, acute IOP changes were studied, using moderately high stimulus intensities of short duration; such stimuli might not uncover steady state control mechanisms or a slowly adapting IOP response. Only a small number of experiments were performed using low-voltage bidirectional wave forms to attempt to minimize tissue damage during relatively long stimulation periods; equivocal effects on IOP resulted. It is important to note that in all these investigations, the measurement parameter was IOP and not aqueous formation or outflow.

In addition, understanding of the anatomy and chemistry of the brain has greatly expanded in the years since these studies were performed. It is now recognized that brain neurons contain multiple neurotransmitters and that one or another of these may be released selectively. Stimulation studies such as those just described may have multiple effects depending on the specific neurons influenced and the neurotransmitter/neuropeptides released under the testing conditions. Considering potential stimulatory and inhibitory influences on a physiologic variable as complex as IOP, it is not surprising that these workers failed to demonstrate a discrete center for IOP regulation.

Despite their limitations, these studies suggested that stimulation of specific brain regions affects IOP independent of or in the opposite direction to blood pressure or extraocular muscle tone. Although not defining specific pathways, these studies nevertheless showed that the brain can influence IOP and are consistent with the hypothesis that neural mechanisms regulate aqueous humor dynamics.

Intraventricular Perfusion Studies

Along similar lines, a number of substances have been introduced into the cerebrospinal fluid by intraventricular perfusion or by single intraventricular injections; effects on IOP have been dem-

---

*References 58, 60, 139, 180, 242, 244.

onstrated, independent of actions on related physiologic parameters, such as blood pressure. Such substances include hypoosmotic agents, hyperosmotic agents, prostaglandins, arachidonic acid, calcium, clonidine, substance P, thyrotropin-releasing hormone and vasopressin.* Administration of agents into the cerebrospinal fluid, however, delivers these agents to wide areas of the brain, and multiple sites of action are possible. Some agents delivered to the cerebrospinal fluid readily cross the blood-brain barrier to the peripheral circulation, and noncentral mechanisms of action also are possible for agents delivered to the cerebrospinal fluid.[6,7] Like the studies with diencephalic stimulation, the intraventricular perfusion studies have not identified a specific brain locus for the regulation of aqueous humor dynamics nor have they defined an integrating neural mechanism for IOP regulation. Nevertheless, the results similarly are consistent with a potential role for the brain in the vegetative processes of the eye.

CONCLUSIONS

Peripheral nerves affect the function of their target tissues by releasing specific neurotransmitters and/or neuromodulators that bind to membrane receptors. These interactions provide the basis for not only normal physiology but also for much clinical ophthalmic pharmacology. Certainly, the extensive use of cholinergic and adrenergic agents in glaucoma therapy underscores the importance of the eye's innervation in clinical ophthalmology.

Histochemical and biochemical research is now defining a complexity to the ocular innervation unimagined only a few years ago. Not only are the classic neurotransmitters norepinephrine and acetylcholine present, but a still expanding array of neuropeptides characterize this innervation. The co-localization of neuropeptides with classic neurotransmitters and with each other is now firmly established in peripheral nerves, including those to the eye.

Both direct and indirect ocular effects ascribed to neuropeptides indicate interactions with autonomic mechanisms. A possible role for neuropeptides in the control of IOP is only beginning to be studied. Even though the neuroanatomic complexity presents a formidable task for ocular physiologists and pharmacologists in the future, novel therapies likely will result from improved understanding of the ocular physiology.

At the level of peripheral ganglia and the central nervous system, our understanding of mechanisms influencing IOP remains fragmentary. Even so, the evidence suggests that neural mechanisms influence aqueous humor dynamics. Whether IOP is regulated directly or whether it is affected only indirectly remains unclear. The now evident complexity of the ocular innervation indicates that considerable work will be necessary to understand the organization of higher neural centers possibly moderating aqueous humor dynamics.

REFERENCES

1. Allen, JM, et al: Reduction of neuropeptide Y (NPY) in the rabbit iris-ciliary body after chronic sympathectomy, Exp Eye Res 37:213, 1983
2. Amara, SG, et al: Expression in brain of a messenger RNA encoding a novel neuropeptide homologous to calcitonin gene-related peptide, Science 229:1094, 1985
3. Armaly, M: Studies on intraocular effects of the orbital parasympathetic pathway. I. Technique and effects on morphology, Arch Ophthalmol 61:14, 1959
4. Armaly, M: Studies on intraocular effects of the orbital parasympathetic pathway. II. Effects on intraocular pressure, Arch Ophthalmol 62:117, 1959
5. Armaly, M: Studies on intraocular effects of the orbital parasympathetic pathway. III. Effect on steady-state dynamics, Arch Ophthalmol 62:817, 1959
6. Banks, WA, and Kastin, AJ: Permeability of the blood-brain barrier to neuropeptides: the case for penetration, Psychoneuroendocrinology 10:385, 1985
7. Banks, WA, and Kastin, AJ: Saturable transport of peptides across the blood-brain barrier, Life Sci 41:1319, 1987
8. Bárány, EH: The mode of action of pilocarpine on outflow resistance in the eye of a primate (Cercopithecus ethiops), Invest Ophthalmol 6:712, 1962
9. Bárány, EH: Transient increase in outflow facility after superior cervical ganglionectomy in rabbits, Arch Ophthalmol 67:303, 1962
10. Beavieux, J, and Dupas, J: Etude anatomo-topographique et histologique du ganglion ophtalmique chez l'homme et divers animaux, Arch Ophthalmol 43:641, 1926
11. Bellarminoff, L: Pflügers Arch 39:449, 1886
12. Belmonte, C, Bartels, SP, Liu, JHK, and Neufeld, AH: Effects of stimulation of the ocular sympathetic nerves on IOP and aqueous humor flow, Invest Ophthalmol Vis Sci 28:1649, 1987
13. Belmonte, C, Simon, J, and Gallego, A: Effects of intraocular pressure changes on the afferent activity of ciliary nerves, Exp Eye Res 12:342, 1971

---

*References 93-95, 97, 99, 122, 179.

14. Bill, A: Effects of norepinephrine, isoproterenol and sympathetic stimulation on aqueous humor dynamics in vervet monkeys, Exp Eye Res 10:31, 1970

15. Bishop, AE, et al: The distributions of PHI and VIP in porcine gut and their colocalization to a proportion of intrinsic ganglion cells, Peptides 5:255, 1984

16. Björklund, H, et al: On the origin and distribution of vasoactive intestinal polypeptide-, peptide HI-, and cholecystokinin-like-immunoreactive nerve fibers in the rat iris, Cell Tissue Res 242:1, 1985

17. Björklund, H, et al: Enkephalin immunoreactivity in iris nerves: distribution in normal and grafted irides, persistence and enhanced fluorescence after denervations, Histochemistry 80:1, 1984

18. Björklund, H, et al: Appearance of the noradrenergic markers tyrosine hydroxylase and neuropeptide Y in cholinergic nerves of the iris following sympathectomy, J Neurosci 5:1633, 1985

19. Boucheron, M: Nerfs de l'hémisphére antérieur de l'oeil, C. R. Soc. Biol. (Paris) 2:71, 1890

20. Brain, SD, et al: Calcitonin gene-related peptide is a potent vasodilator, Nature 313:54, 1985

21. Braslow, RA, and Gregory, DS: Adrenergic decentralization modifies the circadian rhythm of intraocular pressure, Invest Ophthalmol Vis Sci 28:1730, 1987

22. Bron, AJ, and Thomas, J: Sympathetic control of aqueous secretion in man, Br J Ophthalmol 53:37, 1969

23. Bruun, A, et al: Neuropeptide Y immunoreactive neurons in the guinea-pig uvea and retina, Invest Ophthalmol Vis Sci 25:1113, 1984

24. Butler, JM, Unger, WG, and Hammond, BR: Sensory mediation of the ocular response to neutral formaldehyde, Exp Eye Res 28:577, 1979

25. Carlson, KH, McLaren, JW, Topper, JE, and Brubaker, RF: Effect of body position on intraocular pressure and aqueous flow, Invest Ophthalmol Vis Sci 28:1346, 1987

26. Casey, WJ: Cervical sympathetic stimulation in monkeys and the effects on outflow facility and intraocular volume. A study in the East African vervet (Cercopithecus aethiops), Invest Ophthalmol 5:33, 1966

27. Castro-Coreia, J: Studies on the innervation of the uveal tract, Ophthalmologica 154:497, 1967

28. Chiou, GCY: Treatment of ocular hypertension and glaucoma with dopamine antagonists, Ophthalmic Res 16:129, 1984

29. Chiou, GCY, and Chiou, FY: Dopaminergic involvement in intraocular pressure in the rabbit eye, Ophthalmic Res 15:131, 1983

30. Cobb, S, and Scarlett, HW: A report of eleven cases of cervical sympathetic nerve injury causing the oculopupillary syndrome, Arch Neurol Psychiat 3:636, 1920

31. Cole, DF, et al: Increase in SP-like immunoreactivity in nerve fibres of rabbit iris and ciliary body one to

32. Cox, CE, Fitzgerald, CR, and King, RL: A preliminary report on the supraoptic nucleus and control of intraocular pressure, Invest Ophthalmol 14:26, 1975

33. De Vries, GW, Mobasser, A, and Wheeler, LA: Stimulation of endogenous cyclic AMP levels in ciliary body by SK&F 82526, a novel dopamine receptor agonist, Curr Eye Res 5:449, 1986

34. Drago, F, et al: Effects of opiates on intraocular pressure of rabbits and humans, Clin Exp Pharmacol Physiol 12:107, 1985

35. Eakins, KE: Prostaglandin and non-prostaglandin mediated breakdown of the blood-aqueous barrier, Exp Eye Res 25:483, 1977

36. Eakins, KE, and Kats, RL: The effects of sympathetic stimulation and epinephrine on the superior rectus muscle of the cat, J Pharmacol Exp Ther 157:524, 1967

37. Eakins, KE, and Ryan, SJ: The action of sympathomimetic amines on the outflow of aqueous humor from the rabbit eye, Br J Pharmacol 23:374, 1964

38. Edvinsson, L, Owman, C, Rosengren, E, and West, KA: Concentration of noradrenaline in pial vessels, choroid plexus, and iris during two weeks after sympathetic ganglionectomy or decentralization, Acta Physiol Scand 85:201, 1972

39. Ehinger, B: Adrenergic nerves to the eye and its adnexa in rabbit and guinea-pig, Acta Univ Lund, Section II, No 20:1, 1964

40. Ehinger, B: Ocular and orbital vegetative nerves, Acta Physiol Scand 67:1, 1966

41. Ehinger, B: Adrenergic nerves to the eye and to related structures in man and in the cynomolgus monkey (Macaca irus), Invest Ophthalmol 5:42, 1966

42. Ehinger, B: A comparative study of the adrenergic nerves to the anterior eye segment of some primates, Z Zellforsch 116:157, 1971

43. Ehinger, B: Functional role of dopamine in the retina. In Osborne, NN, and Chader, GJ, editors: Progress in retinal research, vol 2, Oxford, 1983, Pergamon Press

44. Ehinger, B, Falck, B, and Rosengren, E: Adrenergic denervation of the eye by unilateral cervical sympathectomy, v Graefes Arch Klin Exp Ophthalmol 177:206, 1969

45. Ehinger, B, et al: Substance P fibres in the anterior segment of the rabbit eye, Acta Physiol Scand 118:215, 1983

46. Eipper, BA, Mains, RE, and Herbert, E: Peptides in the nervous system, Trends in Neuroscience 9:463, 1986

47. Ekblad, E, Håkanson, R, Sundler, F, and Wahlestedt, C: Galanin: neuromodulatory and direct contractile effects on smooth muscle preparations, Br J Pharmacol 86:241, 1985

four months following sympathetic denervation, Exp Eye Res 37:191, 1983

48. Endo, Y: Fluctuation of intraocular pressure by blockage of the stellar ganglion, Acta Soc Ophthalmol Jpn 70:926, 1966

49. Erickson-Lamy, KA, and Kaufman, PL: Reinnervation of primate ciliary muscle following ciliary ganglionectomy, Invest Ophthalmol Vis Sci 28:927, 1987

50. Fahrenkrug, J, Bek, T, Lundberg, JM, and Hökfelt, T: VIP and PHI in cat neurons: co-localization but variable tissue content possible due to differential processing, Regul Pept 12:21, 1985

51. Falck, B, Hillarp, N-Å, Thieme, G, and Torp, A: Fluorescence of catecholamines and related compounds condensed with formaldehyde, J Histochem Cytochem 10:348, 1962

52. Feeney, L: Ultrastructure of the nerves in the human trabecular region, Invest Ophthalmol 1:462, 1962

53. Fink, AE, and Gürber, A: v Graefes Arch Klin Exp Ophthalmol 36:245, 1890

54. Funk, R, and Rohen, JW: SEM studies on the functional morphology of the rabbit ciliary process vasculature, Exp Eye Res 45:579, 1987

55. Gibbins, IL, Furness, JB, and Costa, M: Pathway-specific patterns of the co-existence of substance P, calcitonin gene-related peptide, cholecystokinin and dynorphin in neurons of the dorsal root ganglia of the guinea-pig, Cell Tissue Res 248:417, 1987

56. Gibbins, IL, et al: Co-localization of calcitonin gene-related peptide-like immunoreactivity with substance P in cutaneous, vascular and visceral sensory neurons of guinea pigs, Neurosci Lett 57:125, 1985

57. Givner, I: Episcleral ganglion cells, Arch Ophthalmol 22:82, 1939

58. Gloster, J: Responses of the intra-ocular pressure to diencephalic stimulation, Br J Ophthalmol 44:649, 1960

59. Gloster, J: Influence of facial nerve on intraocular pressure, Br J Ophthalmol 45:259, 1961

60. Gloster, J, and Greaves, DP: Effect of diencephalic stimulation upon intra-ocular pressure, Br J Ophthalmol 41:513, 1957

61. Golding-Wood, J: The ocular effects of autonomic surgery, Proc R Soc Med 57:494, 1964

62. Greaves, DP, and Perkins, ES: Influence of the sympathetic nervous system on the intraocular pressure and vascular circulation of the eye, Br J Ophthalmol 36:258, 1952

63. Greaves, DP, and Perkins, ES: Influence of the third cranial nerve on intra-ocular pressure, Br J Ophthalmol 37:54, 1953

64. Green, K, Elijah, D, and Lollis, G: Drug effects on aqueous humor formation and pseudofacility in sympathectomized rabbit eyes, Exp Eye Res 34:1, 1982

65. Grimes, PA, McGlinn, AM, Kuwayama, Y, and Stone, RA: Peptide immunoreactivity of ciliary and accessory neurons, Invest Ophthalmol Vis Sci 29(suppl):202, 1988

66. Gregory, DS, Aviado, DG, and Sears, ML: Cervical ganglionectomy alters the circadian rhythm of intraocular pressure in New Zealand rabbits, Curr Eye Res 4:1273, 1985

67. Gullner, HG, Campbell, WB, and Pettinger, WA: Role of substance P in water hemeostasis, Life Sci 24:2351, 1979

68. Harmar, AJ: Three tachykinins in mammalian brain, Trends Neurosci 7:57, 1984

69. Hartmann, E: La neurotomie rétrogassérienne. Ses conséquences physiologiques et pathologiques, Paris, 1924, Doin

70. Henderson, EE, and Starling, EH: The influence of changes in the intraocular circulation on the intra-ocular pressure, J Physiol 31:305, 1904

71. Hertel, E: Ueber die Folgen der Exstirpation des Ganglion cervicale superium bei jungen Tieren, v Graefes Arch Klin Exp Ophthalmol 49:430, 1900

72. Hoffman, F: Effect of noradrenalin on intraocular pressure and outflow in cynomolgus monkeys, Exp Eye Res 7:369, 1968

73. Holland, MG, and Mims, JL: Anterior segment chemical sympathectomy by 6-hydroxy-dopamine. I. Effect on intraocular pressure and facility of outflow, Invest Ophthalmol 10:120, 1971

74. Holland, MG, von Sallmann, L, and Collins, EM: A study of the innervation of the chamber angle, Am J Ophthalmol 42:148, 1956

75. Holland, MG, von Sallmann, L, and Collins, EM: A study of the innervation of the chamber angle. II. The origin of trabecular axons revealed by degeneration experiments, Am J Ophthalmol 44:206, 1957

76. Holland, MG, Wei, C-P, and Gupta, S: Review and evaluation of 6-hydroxy-dopamine (6-HD); chemical sympathectomy for the treatment of glaucoma, Ann Ophthalmol 5:539, 1973

77. Höltzke, H: Experimentelle Untersuchungen über den Druck in der Augenkammer, v Graefes Klin Arch Exp Ophthalmol 29:1, 1883

78. Honrubia, FM, and Elliott, JH: Efferent innervation of the retina, Arch Ophthalmol 80:98, 1968

79. Iversen, LL: Amino acids and peptides: fast and slow chemical signals in the nervous system? Proc R Soc Lond 221:245, 1984

80. Itoh, N, Obata, K, Yanaihara, N, and Okamoto, H: Human preprovasoactive intestinal polypeptide contains a novel PHI-27-like peptide, PHM-27, Nature 304:547, 1983

81. Jacobowitz, DM, and Olschowka, JA: Bovine pancreatic polypeptide-like immunoreactivity in brain and peripheral nervous system: coexistence with catecholaminergic nerves, Peptides 3:569, 1982

82. Jaffe, NS: Sympathetic nervous system and intra-ocular pressure, Am J Ophthalmol 31:1597, 1948

83. Jampel, RS, and Mindel, J: The nucleus for accommodation in the midbrain of the macaque, Invest Ophthalmol 6:40, 1967

84. Jan, YN, et al: Peptides in neuronal function: studies using frog autonomic ganglia, Cold Spring Harbor Symp, Quant Biol 48:363, 1983

85. Jonnesco, T: Die Resection des Halssympathicus in der Behandlung des Glaukoms, Wien Klin Wochenschr 12:483, 1899

86. Kaufman, PL, and Bárány, EH: Loss of acute pilocarpine effect on outflow facility following surgical disinsertion and retrodisplacement of the ciliary muscle from the scleral spur in the cynomolgus monkey, Invest Ophthalmol 15:793, 1976

87. Kessler, JA, Bell, WO, and Black, IB: Interactions between the sympathetic and sensory innervation of the iris, J Neurosci 3:1301, 1983

88. Khachaturian, H, Lewis, ME, Schäfer, MK-H, and Watson, SJ: Anatomy of the CNS opioid systems, Trends Neurosci 8:111, 1985

89. Klyce, SD, et al: Neural serotonin stimulates chloride transport in the rabbit corneal epithelium, Invest Ophthalmol Vis Sci 23:181, 1982

90. Koelle, GB, and Friedenwald, JS: A histochemical method for localizing cholinesterase activity, Proc Soc Exp Biol Med 70:617, 1949

91. Krakau, CET: On the regulation of the intraocular pressure, Acta Ophthalmol (Copenh) 47:1069, 1969

92. Krieger, DT: Brain peptides: what, where, and why? Science 222:975, 1983

93. Krupin, T, et al: Increased intraocular pressure and hypothermia following injection of calcium into the rabbit third ventricle, Exp Eye Res 27:129, 1978

94. Krupin, T, et al: Increased intraocular pressure and hypothermia following administration of substance P into rabbit third ventricle, Exp Eye Res 34:319, 1982

95. Krupin, T, Oestrich, CJ, Podos, SM, and Becker, B: Increased intraocular pressure after third ventricle injections of prostaglandin E_1 and arachidonic acid, Am J Ophthalmol 81:346, 1976

96. Krupin, T, Podos, SM, and Becker, B: Effect of optic nerve transection on osmotic alterations of intraocular pressure, Am J Ophthalmol 70:214, 1970

97. Krupin, T, Podos, SM, and Becker, B: Alteration of intraocular pressure after third ventricle injections of osmotic agents, Am J Ophthalmol 76:948, 1973

98. Krupin, T, Podos, SM, Lehman, RAW, and Becker, B: Effect of optic nerve transection on intraocular pressure in monkeys, Arch Ophthalmol 84:668, 1970

99. Krupin, T, et al: Central effects of thyrotropin-releasing hormone and arginine vasopressin on intraocular pressure in rabbits, Invest Ophthalmol Vis Sci 25:932, 1984

100. Kuwayama, Y, Emson, PC, and Stone, RA: Pterygopalatine ganglion cells contain neuropeptide Y, Brain Res 446:219, 1988

101. Kuwayama, Y, Grimes, PA, Ponte, B, and Stone, RA: Autonomic neurons supplying the rat eye and the intraorbital distribution of VIP-like immunoreactivity, Exp Eye Res 44:907, 1987

102. Kuwayama, Y, and Stone, RA: Cholecystokinin-like immunoreactivity occurs in ocular sensory neurons and partially co-localizes with substance P, Brain Res 381:266, 1986

103. Kuwayama, Y, and Stone, RA: Distinct substance P and calcitonin gene-related peptide immunoreactive nerves in the guinea pig eye, Invest Ophthalmol Vis Sci 28:1947, 1987

104. Lam, K-W, Shihab, Z, Fu, Y-A, and Lee, P-F: The effect of optic nerve transection upon the hypotensive action of ascorbate and mannitol, Ann Ophthalmol 12:1102, 1980

105. Langham, ME: The aqueous outflow system and its response to autonomic receptor agonists. In Bito, LZ, Davson, H, and Fenstermacher, JD, editors: The ocular and cerebrospinal fluids, Exp Eye Res Suppl 25:311, 1977

106. Langham, ME, and Rosenthal, AR: Role of cervical sympathetic nerve in regulating intraocular pressure and circulation, Am J Physiol 210:786, 1966

107. Langham, ME, and Taylor, CB: The influence of pre- and post-ganglionic section of the cervical sympathetic on the intraocular pressure of rabbits and cats, J Physiol (Lond) 152:437, 1960

108. Langham, ME, and Taylor, CB: The influence of superior cervical ganglionectomy on intraocular dynamics, J Physiol (Lond) 152:447, 1960

109. Langham, ME, and Weinstein, GW: Horner's syndrome. Ocular supersensitivity to adrenergic amines, Arch Ophthalmol 78:462, 1967

110. Laties, AM, and Jacobowitz, D: A comparative study of the autonomic innervation of the eye in monkey, cat, and rabbit, Anat Rec 156:383, 1966

111. Laties, A, Stone, R, and Brecha, N: Substance P-like immunoreactive nerve fibers in the trabecular meshwork, Invest Ophthalmol Vis Sci 21:484, 1981

112. LeBlanc, GG, Trimmer, BA, and Landis, SC: Neuropeptide Y-like immunoreactivity in rat cranial parasympathetic neurons: coexistence with vasoactive intestinal peptide and choline acetyltransferase, Proc Natl Acad Sci USA, 84:3511, 1987

113. Lederer, R: Der Binnendruck des experimentell and willkürlich bewegten Auges, Arch Augenheilk 72:1, 1912

114. Lee, Y, et al: Coexistence of calcitonin-gene related peptide and substance P-like peptide in single cells of the trigeminal ganglion of the rat: immunohistochemical analysis, Brain Res 330:194, 1985

115. Lee, Y, et al: Distribution of calcitonin gene-related peptide in the rat peripheral nervous system with reference to its coexistence with substance P, Neuroscience 15:1227, 1985

116. Lele, PP, and Grimes, P: The role of neural mechanisms in the regulation of intraocular pressure in the cat, Exp Neurol 2:199, 1960

117. Levinsohn, G: Über den Einfluss der äussern Augenmuskeln auf den intraokularen Druck, v Graefes Arch Klin Exp Ophthalmol 76:129, 1910

118. Lieb, WA, Guerry, D, and Ellis, LJ: Effects of superior cervical ganglionectomy on aqueous humor dynamics, Arch Ophthalmol 60:31, 1958

119. Lin, T, Grimes, PA, and Stone, RA: Nerve pathways between the pterygopalatine ganglion and eye in cat, Anat Rec (In press)

120. Linnér, E, and Prijot, E: Cervical sympathetic ganglionectomy and aqueous flow, Arch Ophthalmol 54:831, 1955

121. Linnér, E, and Prijot, E: Preganglionic cervical sympathectomy and aqueous flow, Arch Ophthalmol 58:77, 1957

122. Liu, JHK, and Neufeld, AH: Study of central regulation of intraocular pressure using ventriculocisternal perfusion, Invest Ophthalmol Vis Sci 26:136, 1985

123. Luedde, WH: Usefulness of the Schiötz tonometer, Am J Ophthalmol 29:289, 1912

124. Lynch, DR, and Snyder, SH: Neuropeptides: multiple molecular forms, metabolic pathways, and receptors, Ann Rev Biochem 55:773, 1986

125. Macri, FJ, and Cevario, SJ: Ciliary ganglion stimulation. I. Effects on aqueous humor inflow and outflow, Invest Ophthalmol 14:28, 1975

126. Marangos, PJ, Polak, JM, and Pearse, AGE: Neuron-specific enolase. A probe for neurons and neuroendocrine cells, Trends in Neuroscience 5:193, 1982

127. Marsh, RJ, and Ford, SM: Blood flow in the anterior segment of the eye, Trans Ophthalmol Soc UK 100:388, 1980

128. Matsuyama, T, et al: Two distinct calcitonin gene-related peptide-containing peripheral nervous systems: distribution and quantitative differences between the iris and cerebral artery with special reference to substance P, Brain Res 373:205, 1986

129. Martin, X: Pression intraoculaire et ganglion trigeminal, Klin Monatsbl Augenheilkd 184:386, 1984

130. Miller, A, Costa, M, Furness, JB, and Chubb, IW: Substance P immunoreactive sensory nerves supply the rat iris and cornea, Neurosci Lett 23:243, 1981

131. Miller, AS, Coster, DJ, Costa, M, and Furness, JB: Vasoactive intestinal polypeptide immunoreactive nerve fibres in the human eye, Aust J Ophthalmol 11:185, 1983

132. Miller, SJH: Stellate ganglion block in glaucoma, Br J Ophthalmol 37:70, 1953

133. Mindel, JS, and Mittag, TW: Choline acetyltransferase in ocular tissues of rabbits, cats, cattle, and man, Invest Ophthalmol 15:808, 1976

134. Mittag, TW, and Tormay, A: Drug responses of adenylate cyclase in iris-ciliary body determined by adenine labelling, Invest Ophthalmol Vis Sci 26:396, 1985

135. Morat, JP, and Doyan, M: Traité de physiologie, vol 2, Paris, 1902, Masson

136. Morrison, JC, deFrank, MP, and van Buskirk, EM: Comparative microvascular anatomy of mammalian ciliary processes, Invest Ophthalmol Vis Sci 28:1325, 1987

137. Morrison, JS, and van Buskirk, EM: Anterior collateral circulation in the primate eye, Ophthalmology 90:707, 1983

138. Morrison, JC, and van Buskirk, EM: Ciliary process microvasculature of the primate eye, Am J Ophthalmol 97:372, 1984

139. Nagai, M, Ban, T, and Kurotsu, T: Studies on the changes of intraocular pressure induced by electrical stimulation of the hypothalamus, Med J Osaka Univ 2:87, 1951

140. Nakanishi, S: Structure and regulation of the preprotachykinin gene, Trends in Neuroscience 9:41, 1986

141. Neff, NH, Hadjiconstantinou, M, and Lackovic, Z: Dopamine. An endogenous peripheral neurotransmitter. p. 179. In Poste, G, and Crooke, ST, editors: Dopamine receptor agonists, New York, 1984, Plenum Press

142. Nilsson, SFE: Effects of NPY on ocular blood flow and local blood flow in some other tissues in the rabbit, J Physiol 390:119P, 1987

143. Nilsson, SFE, and Bill, A: Vasoactive intestinal polypeptide (VIP): effects in the eye and on regional blood flows, Acta Physiol Scand 121:385, 1984

144. Nilsson, SFE, Linder, J, and Bill, A: Characteristics of uveal vasodilation produced by facial nerve stimulation in monkeys, cats and rabbits, Exp Eye Res 40:841, 1985

145. Nilsson, SFE, Sperber, GO, and Bill, A: Effects of vasoactive intestinal polypeptide (VIP) on intraocular pressure facility of outflow and formation of aqueous humor in the monkey, Exp Eye Res 43:849, 1986

146. Neufeld, AH, Ledgard, SE, and Yoza, BK: Changes in responsiveness of the β-adrenergic and serotonergic pathways of the rabbit corneal epithelium, Invest Ophthalmol Vis Sci 24:527, 1983

147. Nomura, T, and Smelser, G: The identification of adrenergic and cholinergic nerve endings in the trabecular meshwork, Invest Ophthalmol 13:525, 1974

148. O'Donohue, TL, et al: On the 50th anniversary of Dale's law: multiple neurotransmitter neurons, Trends Pharmacol Sci 6:305, 1985

149. Osborne, N: The occurrence of serotonergic nerves in the bovine cornea, Neurosci Lett 42:3515, 1983

150. Osborne, NN, and Tobin, AB: Serotonin-accumulating cells in the iris-ciliary body and cornea of various species, Exp Eye Res 44:731, 1987

151. Palkama, A, Uusitalo, H, and Lehtosalo, J: Innervation of the anterior segment of the eye: with special reference to functional aspects. p. 587. In Panula, P, Paivarinta, H, Soinila, S, editors: Neurohistochemistry: modern methods and applications, New York, 1986, Alan R Liss, Inc

152. Palkama, A, Uusitalo, H, and Stjernchantz, J: Some aspects on nervous control of aqueous humor dy-

namics in the rabbit eye, Acta Ophthalmol (Copenh) [Suppl] 123:17, 1974

153. Paterson, CA: The effect of sympathetic nerve on the aqueous humor dynamics of the cocaine pretreated rabbit, Exp Eye Res 5:37, 1966

154. Perkins, ES: Influence of the fifth cranial nerve on the intra-ocular pressure of the rabbit eye, Br J Ophthalmol 41:257, 1957

155. Perkins, ES: Sensory mechanisms and intraocular pressure, Exp Eye Res 1:160, 1961

156. Piccone, M, et al: Effects of neuropeptide Y on the isolated rabbit iris dilator muscle, Invest Ophthalmol Vis Sci 29:330, 1988

157. Podos, SM, Krupin, T, and Becker, B: Effect of small-dose hyperosmotic injections on intraocular pressure of small animals and man when optic nerves are transected and intact, Am J Ophthalmol 71:898, 1971

158. Polak, JM, and Bloom, SR: Regulatory peptides in the autonomic and sensory nervous system, Exp Brain Res 16:11, 1987

159. Polak, JM, and Bloom, SR: Regulatory peptides—the distribution of two newly discovered peptides: PHI and NPY, Peptides 5:79, 1984

160. Polansky, JR, and Alvarado, JA: Isolation and evaluation of target cells in glaucoma research: hormone receptors and drug responses, Curr Eye Res 4:267, 1985

161. Polansky, JR, Weinreb, R, and Alvarado, JA: Studies on human trabecular cells propagated in vitro, Vision Res 21:155, 1981

162. Post, MH, Jr: Glaucoma and the nasal (sphenopalatine [BNA] Meckel's) ganglion, Arch Ophthalmol 50:317, 1921

163. Potter, DE: Adrenergic pharmacology of aqueous humor dynamics, Pharmacol Rev 33:133, 1981

164. Potter, DE, Burke, JA, and Chang, FW: Ocular hypotensive action of ergoline derivatives in rabbits: effects of sympathectomy and domperidone pretreatment, Curr Eye Res 3:307, 1984

165. Potter, DE, and Rowland, JM: Adrenergic drugs and intraocular pressure: effects of selective β-adrenergic agonists, Exp Eye Res 27:615, 1978

166. Raviola, G: Schwalbe line's cells: a new cell type in the trabecular network of Macaca mulatta, Invest Ophthalmol Vis Sci 22:45, 1982

167. Rehfeld, JF: Four basic characteristics of the gastrin-cholecystokinin system, Am J Physiol 240:G255, 1981

168. Riise, D, and Simonsen, SE: Intraocular pressure in unilateral optic nerve lesion, Acta Ophthalmol (Copenh) 47:750, 1969

169. Ringvold, A, and Grofova, I: A study on the postulated transoptic regulation of the intraocular pressure, Acta Ophthalmol (Copenh) 56:201, 1978

170. Rohen, JW, Lütjen, E, and Bárány, E: The relation between the ciliary muscle and the trabecular meshwork and its importance for the effect of miotics on aqueous outflow resistance, v Graefes Arch Klin Exp Ophthalmol 172:23, 1967

171. Rökaeus, Å: Galanin: a newly isolated biologically active neuropeptide, Trends in Neuroscience 10:158, 1987

172. Rosenfeld, MG, et al: Production of a novel neuropeptide encoded by the calcitonin gene via tissue-specific RNA processing, Nature 304:129, 1983

173. Ruskell, GL: The orbital distribution of the sphenopalatine ganglion in the rabbit. In Rohen, JW, editor: The structure of the eye II symposium, Stuttgart, 1965, Schattauer

174. Ruskell, GL: An ocular parasympathetic nerve pathway of facial nerve origin and its influence on intraocular pressure, Exp Eye Res 10:309, 1970

175. Ruskell, GL: The orbital branches of the pterygopalatine ganglion and their relationship with internal carotid nerve branches in primates, J Anat 10:323, 1970

176. Ruskell, GL: Ocular fibres of the maxillary nerve in monkeys, J Anat 118:195, 1974

177. Ruskell, GL: The source of nerve fibres of the trabeculae and adjacent structures in monkey eyes, Exp Eye Res 23:449, 1976

178. Ruskell, GL: Facial nerve distribution to the eye, Am J Optom Physiol Opt 62:793, 1985

179. Schmerl, E, and Steinberg, B: The role of ciliary and superior cervical ganglia in ocular tension, Am J Ophthalmol 32:947, 1949

180. Schmerl, E, and Steinberg, B: Separation of diencephalic centers concerned with pupillary motility and ocular tension, Am J Ophthalmol 33:1379, 1950

181. Schon, F, et al: The effect of sympathectomy on calcitonin gene-related peptide levels in rat trigeminovascular system, Brain Res 348:197, 1985

182. Schuurmans, RP, and Strebel, P: Intraocular pressure and coagulation of the vidian nerve, Klin Monatsbl Augenheilkd 177:459, 1980

183. Sears, ML: The mechanism of action of adrenergic drugs in glaucoma, Invest Ophthalmol 5:115, 1966

184. Sears, ML, and Bárány, EH: Outflow resistance and adrenergic mechanisms, Arch Ophthalmol 64:839, 1960

185. Sears, ML, and Neufeld, AH: Adrenergic modulation of the outflow of aqueous humor, Invest Ophthalmol 14:83, 1975

186. Sears, ML, and Sherk, TE: Supersensitivity of aqueous outflow resistance in rabbits after sympathetic denervation, Nature 197:387, 1963

187. Sears, ML, and Sherk, TE: The trabecular effect of noradrenaline in the rabbit eye, Invest Ophthalmol 3:157, 1964

188. Serafano, DM, and Brubaker, RF: Intraocular pressure after optic nerve transection, Invest Ophthalmol 17:68, 1978

189. Shannon, RP, Mead, A, and Sears, ML: The effect of dopamine on the intraocular pressure and pupil of the rabbit eye, Invest Ophthalmol 15:371, 1976

190. Shimizu, Y: Localization of neuropeptides in the cornea and uvea of the rat: an immunohistochemical study, Cell Mol Biol 28:103, 1982

191. Skofitsch, G, and Jacobowitz, DM: Calcitonin gene-related peptide coexists with substance P in capsaicin sensitive neurons and sensory ganglia of the rat, Peptides 6:747, 1985

192. Skofitsch, G, and Jacobowitz, DM: Immunohistochemical mapping of galanin-like neurons in the rat central nervous system, Peptides 6:509, 1985

193. Stjernschantz, J: Effect of parasympathetic stimulation on intraocular pressure, formation of the aqueous humour and outflow facility in rabbits, Exp Eye Res 22:639, 1976

194. Stjernschantz, J, Alm, A, and Bill, A: Effects of intracranial oculomotor nerve stimulation on ocular blood flow in rabbits: modification by indomethacin, Exp Eye Res 23:461, 1976

195. Stjernschantz, J, and Bill, A: Effects of intracranial oculomotor nerve stimulation on ocular blood flow in monkey, cat and rabbit, Invest Ophthalmol Vis Sci 18:90, 1979

196. Stjernschantz, J, and Bill, A: Vasomotor effects of facial nerve stimulation: noncholinergic vasodilation in the eye, Acta Physiol Scand 109:45, 1980

197. Stjernschantz, J, Geijer, C, and Bill, A: Electrical stimulation of the fifth cranial nerve in rabbits: effect on ocular blood flow, extravascular albumin content and intraocular pressure, Exp Eye Res 28:229, 1979

198. Stjernschantz, J, and Sears, M: Identification of substance P in the anterior uvea and retina of the rabbit, Exp Eye Res 35:401, 1982

199. Stone, RA: Vasoactive intestinal polypeptide and the ocular innervation, Invest Ophthalmol Vis Sci 27:951, 1986

200. Stone, RA: Neuropeptide Y and the innervation of the human eye, Exp Eye Res 42:349, 1986

201. Stone, RA, and Kuwayama, Y: Substance P-like immunoreactive nerves in the human eye, Arch Ophthalmol 103:1207, 1985

202. Stone, RA, Kuwayama, Y, and Laties, AM: Regulatory peptides in the eye, Experientia 43:791, 1987

203. Stone, RA, Kuwayama, Y, Laties, AM, and Marangos, PJ: Neuron-specific enolase-containing cells in the rhesus monkey trabecular meshwork, Invest Ophthalmol Vis Sci 25:1332, 1984

204. Stone, RA, et al: Guinea-pig ocular nerves contain a peptide of the cholecystokinin/gastrin family, Exp Eye Res 39:387, 1984

205. Stone, RA, Kuwayama, Y, and McGlinn, AM: Galanin-like immunoreactive nerves in the porcine eye, Exp Eye Res 46:457, 1988

206. Stone, RA, Kuwayama, Y, Terenghi, G, and Polak, JM: Calcitonin gene-related peptide: occurrence in corneal sensory nerves, Exp Eye Res 43:279, 1986

207. Stone, RA, and Laties, AM: Pancreatic polypeptide-like immunoreactive nerves in the guinea pig eye, Invest Ophthalmol Vis Sci 24:1620, 1983

208. Stone, RA, and Laties, AM: Neuroanatomy and neuroendocrinology of the chamber angle. p. 1. In Krieglstein, GK, and Leydhecker, W, editors: Glaucoma update III. Berlin, 1987, Springer-Verlag

209. Stone, RA, Laties, AM, and Brecha, NC: Substance P-like immunoreactive nerves in the anterior segment of the rabbit, cat and monkey eye, Neuroscience 7:2459, 1982

210. Stone, RA, Laties, AM, and Emson, PC: Neuropeptide Y and the ocular innervation of rat, guinea pig, cat and monkey, Neuroscience 17:1207, 1986

211. Stone, RA, et al: DARPP-32 in the ciliary epithelium of the eye: a neurotransmitter-regulated phosphoprotein of brain localizes to secretory cells, J Histochem Cytochem 34:1456, 1986

212. Stone, RA, and McGlinn, AM: Calcitonin gene-related peptide immunoreactive nerves in human and rhesus monkey eyes, Invest Ophthalmol Vis Sci 29:305, 1988

213. Stone, RA, Tervo, T, Tervo, K, and Tarkkanen, A: Vasoactive intestinal polypeptide-like immunoreactive nerves to the human eye, Acta Ophthalmol (Copenh) 64:12, 1986

214. Strömberg, I, et al: Galanin-immunoreactive nerves in the rat iris: alterations induced by denervations, Cell Tissue Res 250:267, 1987

215. Sugita, A, and Yoshioka, H: Nerve fibers in trabecular meshwork surface, Jpn J Ophthalmol 28:248, 1984

216. Suzuki, R, and Kobayashi, S: Vasoactive intestinal peptide and cholinergic neurotransmission in the ciliary muscle, Invest Ophthalmol Vis Sci 24:250, 1983

217. Swegmark, G: Aqueous humor dynamics in Horner's syndrome, Trans Ophthalmol Soc UK 83:255, 1963

218. Talusan, ED, and Schwartz, B: Fluorescein angiography. Demonstration of flow pattern of anterior ciliary arteries, Arch Ophthalmol 99:1074, 1981

219. Taniguchi, T, Fujiwara, M, Masuo, Y, and Kanazawa, I: Levels of neurokinin A, neurokinin B and substance P in rabbit iris sphincter muscle, Jpn J Pharmacol 42:590, 1986

220. Tatemoto, K: PHI—a new brain-gut peptide, Peptides 5:151, 1984

221. Terenghi, G, et al: Neuropeptide Y-immunoreactive nerves in the uvea of guinea pig and rat, Neurosci Lett 42:33, 1983

222. Terenghi, G, et al: Distribution and origin of calcitonin gene-related peptide (CGRP) immunoreactivity in the sensory innervation of the mammalian eye, J Comp Neurol 233:506, 1985

223. Terenghi, G, et al: Mapping, quantitative distribution and origin of substance P- and VIP-containing nerves in the uvea of guinea pig eye, Histochemistry 75:399, 1982

224. Tervo, K, et al: Immunoreactivity for substance P in the Gasserian ganglion, ophthalmic nerve and anterior segment of the rabbit eye, Histochem J 13:435, 1981

225. Tervo, K, et al: Effect of sensory and sympathetic denervation on substance P immunoreactivity in nerve fibres of the rabbit eye, Exp Eye Res 34:577, 1982

226. Tervo, K, et al: Substance P-immunoreactive nerves in the human cornea and iris, Invest Ophthalmol Vis Sci 23:671, 1982

227. Thomas, RP: Effect of third cranial nerve on intraocular pressure, Arch Ophthalmol 72:529, 1964

228. Tomar, VPA, and Agarwal, BL: Effect of ganglionectomy on intraocular pressure and outflow facility of aqueous humour, Exp Eye Res 19:403, 1974

229. Tornqvist, G: Effect of oculomotor nerve stimulation on outflow facility and pupil diameter in a monkey (Cercopithecus ethiops), Invest Ophthalmol 9:220, 1970

230. Tornqvist, K, et al: Substance P-immunoreactive nerve fibres in the anterior segment of the rabbit eye, Cell Tissue Res 222:467, 1982

231. Treister, G, and Bárány, EH: Mydriasis and intraocular pressure decrease in the conscious rabbit after unilateral superior cervical ganglionectomy, Invest Ophthalmol 9:331, 1970

232. Tripathi, BJ, and Tripathi, RC: Effect of epinephrine in vitro on the morphology, phagocytosis, and mitotic activity of human trabecular endothelium, Exp Eye Res 39:731, 1984

233. Uddman, R, et al: Vasoactive intestinal peptide nerves in ocular and orbital structures of the cat, Invest Ophthalmol Vis Sci 19:878, 1980

234. Unger, WG, et al: Calcitonin gene-related peptide as a mediator of the neurogenic ocular injury response, J Ocular Pharmacol 1:189, 1985

235. Uusitalo, H: Effect of sympathetic and parasympathetic stimulation on the secretion and outflow of aqueous humor in the rabbit eye, Acta Physiol Scand 86:315, 1972

236. Uusitalo, H, et al: Immunohistochemical and biochemical evidence for 5-hydroxytryptamine containing nerves in the anterior part of the eye, Exp Eye Res 35:671, 1982

237. Uusitalo, H, Lehtosalo, JI, and Palkama, A: Vasoactive intestinal polypeptide (VIP)-immunoreactive nerve fibers in the anterior uvea of the guinea pig, Ophthalmic Res 17:235, 1985

238. Uusitalo, H, Lehtosalo, J, Palkama, A, and Toivanen, M: Vasoactive intestinal polypeptide (VIP)-like immunoreactivity in the human and guinea-pig choroid, Exp Eye Res 38:435, 1984

239. von Hippel, A, and Grünhagen, A: Über den Einfluss der Nerven auf die Höhe des intraokularen Druckes, v Graefes Klin Arch Exp Ophthalmol 14:219, 1868

240. von Horner, F: Über eine Form von Ptosis, Klin Monatsbl Augenheilkd 7:193, 1869

241. von Linksz, A: Der Einfluss der Sympathicusaschaltung auf die Blut-Kammerwasserschranke, Klin Wochenschr 10:830, 1931

242. von Sallmann, L: The role of the central nervous system in the regulation of the intraocular pressure, Doc Ophthalmol 13:93, 1959

243. von Sallmann, L, Fuortes, GF, Macri, FJ, and Grimes, P: Study of afferent impulses induced by intraocular pressure changes, Am J Ophthalmol 45:211, 1958

244. von Sallmann, L, and Lowenstein, O: Responses of intraocular pressure, blood pressure and cutaneous vessels to electric stimulation in the diencephalon, Am J Ophthalmol 39:11, 1955

245. von Schultén, MW: Experimentelle Untersuchungen über die Cirkulationsverhältnisse des Auges und über den Zusammenhang zwischen den Cirkulationsverhältnissen des Auges und des Gehirns, v Graefes Klin Arch Exp Ophthalmol 30:1, 1884

246. Vrabec, F: L'innervation du système trabéculaire de l'angle irien, Ophthalmologica 128:359, 1954

247. Vrabec, F: The topography of encapsulated terminal sensory corpuscles of the anterior chamber angle of the goose eye. p. 325. In Smelser, GK, editor: The structure of the eye, New York, 1961, Academic Press

248. Vrabec, F: Encapsulated sensory corpuscles in the sclerocorneal boundary tissues of the killer whale Orcinus orca L, Acta Anat (Basel) 81:23, 1972

249. Waitzman, MB: Hypothalamus and ocular pressure, Surv Ophthalmol 16:161, 1971

250. Wegner, L: Experimentelle Beiträge zur Lehre von Glaucom, v Graefes Klin Arch Exp Ophthalmol 12:1, 1866

251. Wentworth, WO, and Brubaker, RF: Aqueous humor dynamics in a series of patients with third neuron Horner's syndrome, Am J Ophthalmol 92:407, 1981

252. Wessely, K: Über den Einfluss der Augenbewegungen auf den Augendruck, Arch Augenheilkd 81:102, 1916

253. Wickham, MG: Irido-corneal angle of mammalian eyes: comparative morphology of encapsulated corpuscles in odontocete cetaceans, Cell Tissue Res 210:501, 1980

254. Zhang, SQ, et al: Changes in substance P- and neuropeptide Y-immunoreactive fibres in rat and guinea-pig irides following unilateral sympathectomy, Exp Eye Res 39:365, 1984

255. Zuazo, A, Ibañez, J, and Belmonte, C: Sensory nerve responses elicited by experimental ocular hypertension, Exp Eye Res 43:759, 1986

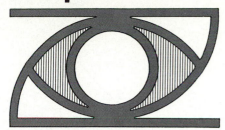

Chapter 13

Ocular Hypotony

Jonathan E. Pederson

Hypotony may be defined statistically as an intraocular pressure below 6.5 mm Hg,[54] but harmful effects on the eye are uncommon with an intraocular pressure above 4 mm Hg.[61] Thus the distinction should be made between "statistical" hypotony and hypotony that leads to visual loss. The box below lists common causes of hypotony, categorized according to mild or profound (see also reference 66).

PATHOPHYSIOLOGY

In the human eye, the rate of aqueous humor formation is approximately 2.5 μl/min.[17] Most of the fluid passes out through the trabecular mesh-work and Schlemm's canal, since the intraocular pressure exceeds the episcleral venous pressure, which is about 9 mm Hg.[73,89] This outflow is highly pressure-dependent. However, there is also a pressure-independent pathway of aqueous outflow, termed *uveoscleral outflow*.[9] This pathway is from the anterior chamber, through the intermuscular spaces of the ciliary muscle, into the suprachoroidal space, and into the choroidal vessels or out through the sclera or emissarial channels (see Chapter 10). The actual percentage of aqueous humor exiting via the uveoscleral route depends on the intraocular pressure.[11,13] In humans, approximately 10% of aqueous outflow passes through this route at a normal intraocular pressure.[14]

In patients with hypotony, the episcleral venous pressure is normal, about 9 mm Hg.[73,89] Thus in the presence of significant hypotony, all aqueous humor must leave the eye by some route other than through Schlemm's canal. There are several "extracanalicular" pathways, such as (1) uveoscleral outflow, (2) wound leak, or (3) posterior flow of aqueous humor through the vitreous and across the retina and choroid (Fig. 13-1). The magnitude of hypotony will depend on the rate of aqueous humor production and the "facility" of extracanalicular outflow. For reduced aqueous humor production to account for hypotony, in the absence of alteration of any other parameter, it must fall to less than 10% of its normal rate.[67] This circumstance is quite unusual and in general both increased extracanalicular outflow and reduced aqueous humor production coexist to produce hypotony.

COMMON FORMS OF HYPOTONY

MILD HYPOTONY

Iridocyclitis
Retinal detachment
Vascular occlusive disease

PROFOUND HYPOTONY

Wound leak
Cyclodialysis
Retinal detachment
Ciliochoroidal detachment
Scleral perforation or rupture

BILATERAL HYPOTONY

Hyperosmolarity
Myotonic dystrophy

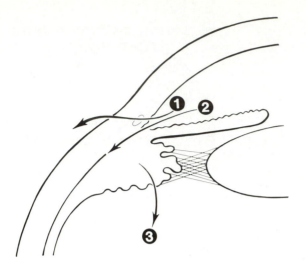

Fig. 13-1 Pathways of aqueous outflow. Trabecular outflow *(1)*; uveoscleral outflow *(2)*; posterior outflow *(3)*.

SPECIFIC CLINICAL DISORDERS

Wound Leak

Wound leak is a common cause of hypotony after anterior segment surgery, but it may go undetected. Its only manifestation may be a low and diffuse filtering bleb that is difficult to distinguish from the normal degree of postoperative chemosis. Occasionally, microcystic subepithelial conjunctival changes are the only telltale sign of a leak through the scleral wound. Excessive filtration after glaucoma filtering surgery represents a special subcategory of hypotony. This is usually self-limited, as further subconjunctival healing proceeds. The management of refractory cases is discussed in Chapter 35.

An external wound fistula may be detected by the Seidel test (Fig. 13-2). Clear aqueous humor streaming into a pool of fluorescein will sometimes produce a dramatic appearance. Failure to detect a positive Seidel test is commonly the result of one of two factors: (1) failure to use a high enough concentration of fluorescein or (2) failure to apply pressure to the globe while inspecting the suspected area. Use of a fluorescein-impregnated paper strip is preferable to using a drop of fluorescein-topical anesthetic solution, because in the latter case, the concentration of fluorescein is often inadequate for detection of a subtle leak. Pressure on the globe is also important, since the leak may be only intermittent if the intraocular pressure is at or close to zero.

In general, external wound leaks should be repaired to prevent endophthalmitis, even if the anterior chamber is formed. Leaks occurring through the conjunctiva at the limbus may not close spontaneously but may be first treated conservatively with a pressure patch plus a carbonic anhydrase inhibitor and a beta-blocker to reduce aqueous humor flow through the fistula. A bandage contact lens or Simmons shell may also tamponade the leak, but the risk of infection must be considered in this circumstance. An inadvertent nonleaking filtering bleb need not be repaired unless it is causing significant patient discomfort or visual impairment secondary to astigmatism or hypotony. Closure of the scleral wound will occasionally result in a dramatic elevation of intraocular pressure until the trabecular meshwork begins to function normally again.

More occult forms of wound leak include scleral rupture from blunt trauma or perforation of the sclera from a retrobulbar needle at the time of intraocular surgery.[79] The latter is more common in eyes with posterior staphylomas. The superior rectus bridle suture needle may also perforate the sclera leading to hypotony from direct filtration across the sclera or secondarily from retinal detachment.[79,83]

Iridocyclitis

Clinicians are familiar with mild hypotony that commonly accompanies acute anterior uveitis.[3] Aqueous humor flow is reduced and the blood-aqueous barrier is abnormal, as manifested by aqueous flare.[62,93,102] These two observations may be interrelated, since the transport processes of the ciliary epithelium do not function efficiently in the presence of an abnormal permeability of the blood-aqueous barrier.[69] If edema of the ciliary body exists, fluid would be expected to move more readily through the edematous tissue from the anterior chamber into the suprachoroidal space (Fig. 13-3).[41] In monkeys with experimentally-induced iridocyclitis and an edematous ciliary body, uveoscleral outflow is markedly increased.[93] In more profound cases of uveitis, ciliary body vasculitis may lead to vascular occlusion and reduced blood flow.[4]

The role of iridocyclitis in the pathogenesis of other forms of ocular hypotony is unclear. Aqueous flare commonly accompanies hypotony and the altered blood-aqueous barrier may be responsible for the observed reduced aqueous flow. An example of this is seen after various types of anterior segment surgery where the intraocular pressure may not return to normal levels for many months. This phenomenon is often referred to as "ciliary body shutdown" or "ciliary body shock." Reduced aqueous humor flow has been noted follow-

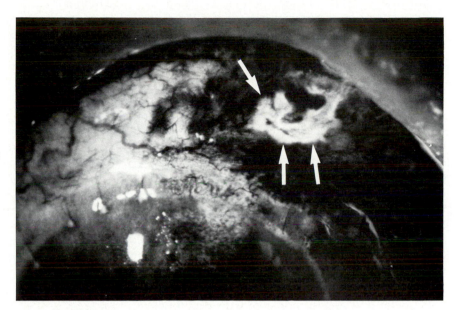

Fig. 13-2 Positive Seidel test in leaking bleb *(arrows)*.

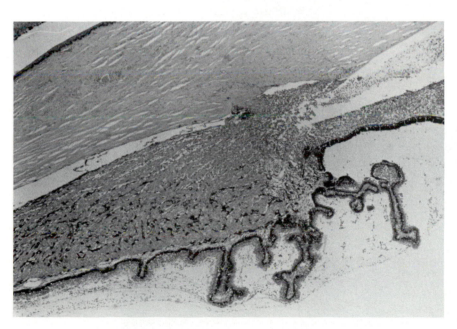

Fig. 13-3 Interstitial ciliary body edema in eye with iridocyclitis enhances uveoscleral outflow. (From Toris, CB, and Pederson, JE: Invest Ophthalmol Vis Sci 28:477, 1978)

ing keratoplasty[8] and glaucoma filtering surgery.[40]

Hypotony and ciliary body detachment have been reported after attempted reopening of an internal sclerostomy site in a patient with a failed filtering bleb.[76] These authors postulated that the YAG energy resulted in "ciliary body shutdown." Removal of a cyclitic membrane may occasionally reverse hypotony, presumably as a result of removing the tractional irritation of the ciliary epithelium. It may also allow reattachment of the ciliary body and a reduction in uveoscleral outflow.

Cyclodialysis

Separation of the ciliary body from the scleral spur is termed *cyclodialysis* (Fig. 13-4). This may occur following cataract surgery,[28,58,86] ocular trauma, or may be intentionally created as a surgical treatment for glaucoma. The popularity of this procedure for the treatment of glaucoma in the United States has waned in recent years, however, because of a high rate of hyphema and unpredictable results, including profound hypotony. Anatomically, cyclodialysis creates free communication between the anterior chamber and suprachoroidal space and would thus be expected to enhance uveoscleral outflow. In monkeys with experimentally-induced cyclodialysis, uveoscleral outflow is markedly enhanced.[91]

It has been argued that cyclodialysis results in reduced aqueous flow.[24] However, aqueous flare is commonly present in eyes with cyclodialysis, especially in the immediate postoperative period.

Eyes with chronic cyclodialysis and *no* aqueous flare have normal aqueous humor flow as measured with fluorophotometry.[71] The logical conclusion is that reduced flow in an eye with cyclodialysis is the result of associated inflammation rather than the cyclodialysis itself. In an effort to evaluate whether increased aqueous outflow can account for hypotony in cyclodialysis, tonography has been employed.[38,39,50] Tonographic data are difficult to interpret in the presence of hypotony, however, and may actually measure extracanalicular rather than trabecular outflow facility. Thus tonographically determined outflow facility in an eye with a cyclodialysis may actually measure the uveoscleral outflow facility.

In the presence of profound hypotony, identification of a cyclodialysis cleft may be difficult as a result of corneal deformation during gonioscopy. If the cyclodialysis cleft is unassociated with significant inflammation, the ciliary body detachment may be so shallow as to be undetectable.

Cyclodialysis creates a dramatic clinical picture. If the cyclodialysis cleft suddenly closes, the intraocular pressure may rise to extreme levels.[50] This is analogous to the rapid pressure rise following closure of a wound leak. If the cleft is reopened with a miotic, the pressure again rapidly falls.[84] The size of the cyclodialysis cleft does not appear to bear any relationship to the degree of hypotony.[24,98] Even a small cleft is capable of carrying the full amount of aqueous humor produced.

Occasionally, exploratory surgery is necessary

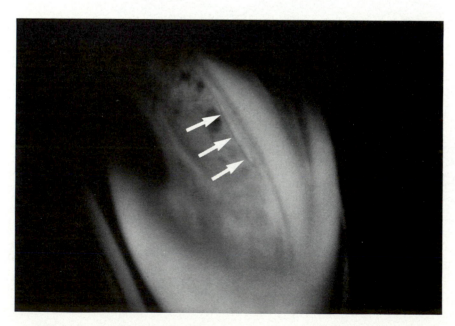

Fig. 13-4 Gonioscopic appearance of inadvertent cyclodialysis cleft (*arrows*).

for identification of the cyclodialysis cleft. If fluorescein-stained balanced salt solution is injected into the anterior chamber, fluorescein-stained fluid will rapidly exit from a supraciliary sclerostomy.[24] Various techniques may be used to close the cleft, including external diathermy,[56] cryotherapy,[5,23] ciliary body suturing,[57,59] external plumbage,[75] and argon laser photocoagulation.[42,48,63] The procedure for surgical closure of the cleft involves localization of the cleft with a diagnostic goniolens (for example, Zeiss four-mirror goniolens), and forceps indentation of the sclera over the cleft to mark the precise site. A partial thickness scleral flap, hinged at the limbus, is prepared over the cleft. A 9-0 or 10-0 nylon suture with a large needle is passed through the scleral bed to reattach the ciliary body. Cryotherapy or diathermy may be placed in the scleral bed to create secure reattachment. The scleral flap is then closed. An excellent summary of various surgical techniques for the closure of cyclodialysis clefts is given elsewhere.[61]

Ciliochoroidal Detachment

Ciliochoroidal detachment commonly occurs in the presence of hypotony (Fig. 13-5). The relationship between ciliochoroidal detachment and hypotony, however, is not clearly understood.[18] It was originally believed that suprachoroidal fluid was derived from aqueous humor, which was then responsible for creating the ciliochoroidal detachment.[35] However, the suprachoroidal fluid protein concentration is much higher than in the aqueous humor, so another mechanism was postulated. Electrophoretic protein analysis of suprachoroidal fluid suggests that the fluid originates from the choroidal vessels with molecular sieving across the capillary endothelium.[25]

Human eyes with suprachoroidal fluid detected on suprachoroidal tap also have stagnation of aqueous humor flow, as estimated following systemic fluorescein administration.[24] Drainage of supraciliary fluid alone reverses hypotony in some eyes. It has been concluded therefore that ciliary body detachment leads to aqueous hyposecretion, which is reversed following drainage. Aqueous humor hyposecretion has been postulated as a fundamental cause of hypotony in this condition.[24] However, it is also known that hypotony is an etiologic factor in the development of ciliochoroidal detachment experimentally.[1,26,43,60,88] In most eyes with ciliochoroidal detachment, aqueous flare is also present[29,90] and breakdown of the blood-aqueous barrier alone may be responsible for the observed hyposecretion.

To evaluate the role of ciliochoroidal detachment on intraocular pressure, a monkey model of ciliochoroidal detachment has been tested.[68] Silicone oil injection into the suprachoroidal space, creating large multilobed billowing choroidal detachments, did not result in any lowering of intraocular pressure. This strongly suggests that mechanical detachment of the ciliary body does not lead to hyposecretion. However, injection of Ring-

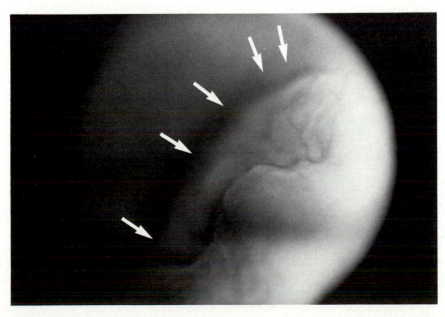

Fig. 13-5 Ciliochoroidal detachment *(arrows)* following glaucoma filtering operation.

er's solution or autologous serum into the suprachoroidal space led to hypotony associated with a normal aqueous humor flow rate. It has been concluded from these studies that uveoscleral outflow is enhanced as a result of the ciliochoroidal detachment and attendant ciliary body edema. Thus hyposecretion seen clinically in humans with ciliochoroidal detachment may be a result of the concurrent iridocyclitis and not the ciliary body detachment per se.

Most patients with ciliochoroidal detachment undergo spontaneous resorption of the suprachoroidal fluid. This may occur by absorption into choroidal vessels or by fluid passing out through emissarial channels.[10,46] A vicious cycle can be induced by hypotony, since this increases transudation across the choroidal vessels and also reduces the pressure drop across the sclera. As a result, the suprachoroidal fluid remains, and contributes to continued hypotony.

Treatment of ciliochoroidal detachment includes the use of cycloplegics and topical steroids. Although cycloplegics increase uveoscleral outflow and theoretically may worsen hypotony, their usefulness in deepening the anterior chamber supercedes any other disadvantage. Occasionally, systemic steroids are employed if the eye is unusually inflamed. Fluid intake may increase aqueous humor production. Acetazolamide may also speed absorption of suprachoroidal fluid by a poorly understood mechanism.[92] Surgical drainage of suprachoroidal fluid is indicated if (1) the anterior chamber is flat with corneal or lenticular decompensation, or (2) peripheral anterior synechiae are forming.[7] Hypotony may improve following drainage of suprachoroidal fluid alone.[24,56] To prevent recurrence of flat anterior chamber, sodium hyaluronate may be injected.[21,33] In more difficult recurrent cases, suturing of the ciliary body to the sclera may be helpful.[85]

In patients after filtering surgery, use of acetazolamide or timolol may result in marked hypotony with ciliochoroidal detachment, which abates after cessation of those agents.[97] Hypotony with ciliochoroidal detachment may also occur for no apparent reason as a late complication of trabeculectomy and may be treated with cycloplegics and topical corticosteroids.[19]

Retinal Detachment

Rhegmatogenous retinal detachment is most commonly associated with mild hypotony, although profound hypotony may occasionally exist.[20,30,53] The level of hypotony is related to the extent of the detachment.[30] Aqueous humor flow was found to be reduced in several studies[30,53,62] but one study revealed a normal flow.[96] The reduced flow may be caused by concurrent iridocyclitis. After repair of the retinal detachment, the intraocular pressure may not immediately return to normal as a result of postoperative iridocyclitis.

In eyes with more profound hypotony, reduced aqueous humor flow alone cannot explain the low intraocular pressure. A number of years ago it was suggested that posterior chamber aqueous humor may be shunted posteriorly through the vitreous, retinal hole, and across the retinal pigment epithelium and choroid, resulting in a type of misdirected posterior aqueous humor flow.[6] It has also been suggested that fluid may exit via the perioptic tissue in eyes with retinal detachment.[80,87] Under this circumstance, the total aqueous production rate could be normal, since methods that measure aqueous humor flow actually measure only anterior chamber flow.

Tonographic outflow facility studies have revealed a normal or reduced outflow facility arguing against a posterior aqueous flow.[30,34,53] However, such a flow would likely be pressure-independent and not detected by tonography.[64] In a monkey model of rhegmatogenous retinal detachment, fluorescein-labeled dextran injected into the vitreous moved into the subretinal space, where it was sequestered for many months.[65] This was interpreted as evidence for flow from the vitreous cavity into the subretinal space. The flow is generated by the retinal pigment epithelium, which pumps fluid from the subretinal space to the choroid and acts as a type of extracanalicular aqueous outflow.[94,95]

The iris retraction syndrome also offers clinical evidence for posterior flow.[22] In an eye with retinal detachment and secluded pupil, administration of acetazolamide causes posterior iris retraction. Presumably, the retinal pigment epithelial fluid removal rate exceeds the aqueous production rate, since the vitreous cavity is a closed system in this circumstance.

Miscellaneous Disorders

Osmotic alterations of the plasma may result in hypotony, as may therapeutically administered hyperosmotic agents. Clinical disorders exemplifying this include dehydration, hyperglycemia, and uremia.[32] Systemic acidosis decreases aqueous humor formation and may result in hypotony.[51] These forms of hypotony are readily reversible by correcting the underlying metabolic defect.

Myotonic dystrophy results in bilateral mild hypotony.[49,101] Several studies have indicated that the outflow facility is increased,[49,78] but a more recent study correcting for ocular rigidity yielded a normal outflow facility.[31] Fluorophotometry yields a normal aqueous flow, but the blood-aqueous barrier is abnormal, and thus aqueous flow may be overestimated.[101] However, if aqueous flow is indeed normal, increased uveoscleral outflow must exist, perhaps as a result of the atrophic ciliary muscle.[100] In general, this form of hypotony is not clinically significant and needs no treatment.

Vascular occlusive disease, such as carotid occlusive disease and temporal arteritis, may cause hypotony.[77] Central retinal vein occlusion may cause prolonged mild hypotony, whereas central retinal artery occlusion may cause more short-lived hypotony.[44]

Other rare causes of mild hypotony are discussed elsewhere.[32,66,81]

DIAGNOSTIC EVALUATION

The box below lists the diagnostic approach to the patient with hypotony.

EFFECT OF HYPOTONY ON VISUAL FUNCTION

Deleterious effects on the eye from hypotony may be divided into two categories: (1) increased transudation of fluid from vessel walls, and (2) breakdown of the blood-ocular barrier with protein leakage. Chronic hypotony in the absence of inflammation may result in no adverse effect on the eye, such as following successful full-thickness glaucoma filtration surgery. More profound hypotony may lead to edema of the optic disc and macula with a marked reduction in visual acuity.[28,36] If inflammation is also present, the eye may become irritated with photophobia, corneal thickening, and aqueous flare and cells. Choroidal thickening may be detected by B-scan ultrasonography.[47] If hypotony is prolonged, a cataract may

form and permanent macular changes may occur. If hypotony is reversed before this time, good vision may return. If not, atrophia bulbi or phthisis bulbi may ensue.

Pathologic studies of hypotony reveal generalized edema of the uvea, retina, and optic nerve with proteinaceous fluid accumulation in the suprachoroidal space.[99]

Hypotony itself may lead to a modest breakdown of the blood-aqueous barrier.[71] This presumably results from release of inflammatory autacoids.[2] If the reduction of intraocular pressure is sudden, such as following paracentesis, a more profound breakdown of the blood-aqueous barrier may occur. The potential for a vicious cycle to develop is apparent, since hypotony leads to breakdown of the blood-aqueous barrier, which leads to hyposecretion, which promotes hypotony.

TREATMENT

Treatment of hypotony is directed toward correction of the underlying abnormality, such as repair of a wound leak, closure of a cyclodialysis cleft, drainage of suprachoroidal fluid, repair of a retinal detachment, or steroid treatment of iridocyclitis. No specific treatment exists for the correction of hypotony itself. Several drugs cause a transient elevation of intraocular pressure but are associated with toxic side effects; these include sodium azide,[52] sodium nitroprusside,[52] cation ionophores,[74] and parasympathomimetics.[15,55,70] The latter agents are known to stimulate aqueous production,[70] reduce uveoscleral outflow,[15] and reverse experimental hypotony.[70] They may also benefit patients with traumatic hypotony.[16,45] In a clinical setting, the use of miotics in an eye with inflammation may be uncomfortable, which commonly precludes their use. Acetazolamide may enhance suprachoroidal fluid absorption in patients with choroidal detachment,[92] but it also has the undesired effect of reducing aqueous secretion.

In difficult cases, exploratory surgery may be necessary to examine for wound leak, cyclodialysis cleft, or the presence of supraciliary fluid. Fluorescein-stained balanced salt solution may be injected into the anterior chamber and, when accompanied by supraciliary sclerotomy, will help identify a wound leak, cyclodialysis cleft, or presence of supraciliary fluid.[24] Release of ciliary body traction caused by a cyclitic membrane may result in reversal of hypotony. Similarly, ciliary body traction from lenticular remnants may be released by posterior capsulotomy, with dramatic reversal of hypotony.[37]

DIAGNOSTIC EVALUATION OF HYPOTONY

1. History of trauma or surgery
2. Seidel test
3. Gonioscopy for cyclodialysis cleft
4. Ophthalmoscopy for retinal or choroidal detachment
5. Ultrasonography[47] or CT scan[72] for poor media
6. Exploratory surgery

REFERENCES

1. Aaberg, TM: Experimental serous and hemorrhagic uveal edema associated with retinal detachment surgery, Invest Ophthalmol 14:243, 1975
2. Ambache, N, Kavanaugh, L, and Whiting, J: Effect of mechanical stimulation on rabbits' eyes: release of active substance in anterior chamber perfusates, J Physiol (Lond) 176:378, 1965
3. Aronson, SB, and Elliott, JH: Ocular Inflammation, St Louis, 1972, The CV Mosby Co
4. Aronson, SB, et al: Ocular blood flow in experimentally induced immunologic uveitis, Arch Ophthalmol 91:60, 1974
5. Barasch, K, Galin, MA, and Baras, I: Postcyclodialysis hypotony, Am J Ophthalmol 68:644, 1969
6. Beigelman, MN: Acute hypotony in retinal detachment, Arch Ophthalmol 1:463, 1929
7. Bellows, AR, Chylack, LT, Jr, and Hutchinson, BT: Choroidal detachment: clinical manifestation, therapy and mechanism of formation, Ophthalmology 88:1107, 1981
8. Berkowitz, RA, Klyce, SD, and Kaufman, HE: Aqueous hyposecretion after penetrating keratoplasty, Ophthalmic Surg 15:323, 1984
9. Bill, A: The aqueous humor drainage mechanism in the cynomolgus monkey (Macaca irus) with evidence for unconventional routes, Invest Ophthalmol 4:911, 1965
10. Bill, A: Movement of albumin and dextran through the sclera, Arch Ophthalmol 74:248, 1965
11. Bill, A: Conventional and uveo-scleral drainage of aqueous humor in the cynomolgus monkey (Macaca irus) at normal and high intraocular pressures, Exp Eye Res 5:45, 1966
12. Bill, A: The routes for bulk drainage of aqueous humour in rabbits with and without cyclodialysis, Doc Ophthalmol 20:157, 1966
13. Bill, A: Further studies on the influence of the intraocular pressure on aqueous humor dynamics in cynomolgus monkeys, Invest Ophthalmol 6:364, 1967
14. Bill, A, and Phillips, CI: Uveoscleral drainage of aqueous humor in human eyes, Exp Eye Res 12:275, 1971
15. Bill, A, and Wahlinder, DE: The effects of pilocarpine on the dynamics of aqueous humor in a primate (Macaca irus), Invest Ophthalmol 5:170, 1965
16. Boet, DJ: Clinical results with phosphorylcholine chloride, Ophthalmologica 132:150, 1956
17. Brubaker, RF: The physiology of aqueous humour formation. In Drance, SM, and Neufeld, AH, editors: Glaucoma: applied pharmacology in medical treatment, Orlando, 1984, Grune & Stratton, Inc
18. Brubaker, RF, and Pederson, JE: Ciliochoroidal detachment, Surv Ophthalmol 27:281, 1983
19. Burney, EN, Quigley, HA, and Robin, AL: Hypotony and choroidal detachment as late complications of trabeculectomy, Am J Ophthalmol 103:685, 1987
20. Burton, TC, Arafat, NT, and Phelps, CD: Intraocular pressure in retinal detachment, Int Ophthalmol 1:147, 1979
21. Cadera, W, and Willis, NR: Sodium hyaluronate for postoperative aphakic choroidal detachment, Can J Ophthalmol 17:274, 1982
22. Campbell, DG: Iris retraction associated with rhegmatogenous retinal detachment syndrome and hypotony: a new explanation, Arch Ophthalmol 102:1457, 1984
23. Castier, PH, Asseman, PH, and Razemon, L: Evolution d'une hypotonie post-traumatique apres cyclopexie, Bull Soc Ophthalmol Fr 82:261, 1982
24. Chandler, PA, and Maumenee, AE: A major cause of hypotony, Am J Ophthalmol 52:609, 1961
25. Chylack, LT, Jr, and Bellows, AR: Molecular sieving in suprachoroidal fluid formation in man, Invest Ophthalmol Vis Sci 17:420, 1978
26. Cooper, SA, and Leopold, IH: Mechanism of serous choroidal detachment, Arch Ophthalmol 55:101, 1956
27. Davenport, WH, Brown, RH, and Lynch, MG: Hypotony after rotation of an intraocular lens haptic into a cyclodialysis cleft, Am J Ophthalmol 101:736, 1986
28. Dellaporta, A: Fundus changes in postoperative hypotony, Am J Ophthalmol 40:781, 1955
29. Dellaporta, A, and Obear, MF: Hyposecretion hypotony, Am J Ophthalmol 58:785, 1964
30. Dobbie, JG: A study of the intraocular fluid dynamics in retinal detachment, Arch Ophthalmol 69:159, 1963
31. Dreyer, RF: Ocular hypotony in myotonic dystrophy, Int Ophthalmol 6:221, 1983
32. Duke-Elder, S, and Jay, B: System of ophthalmology, vol 11, Diseases of the lens and vitreous: glaucoma and hypotony, St Louis, 1969, The CV Mosby Co
33. Fisher, YL, et al: Use of sodium hyaluronate in reformation and reconstruction of the persistent flat anterior chamber in the presence of severe hypotony, Ophthalmic Surg 13:819, 1982
34. Foulds, WS: Experimental detachment of the retina and its effect on the intraocular fluid dynamics, Mod Probl Ophthalmol 8:51, 1969
35. Fuchs, E: Ablosung der Aderhaut nach Staaroperation, v Graefes Arch Klin Exp Ophthalmol 51:199, 1900
36. Gass, JDM: Hypotony maculopathy. In Bellows, JG: Contemporary Ophthalmology, Baltimore, 1972, Williams & Wilkins
37. Geyer, O, Godel, V, and Lazar, M: Hypotony as a late complication of extracapsular cataract extraction, Am J Ophthalmol 96:112, 1983
38. Gills, JP: Cyclodialysis implants in human eyes, Am J Ophthalmol 61:841, 1966
39. Gills, JP, Paterson, CA, and Paterson, ME: Action of cyclodialysis utilizing an implant studied by manometry in a human eye, Exp Eye Res 6:75, 1967

40. Goldmann, H: Über die Wirkungsweise der Cyclodialyse, Ophthalmologica 121:94, 1951

41. Guyton, AC, Scheel, K, and Murpree, D: Interstitial fluid pressure. III. Its effect on resistance to tissue fluid mobility, Circ Res 19:412, 1966

42. Harbin, TS, Jr: Treatment of cyclodialysis clefts with argon laser photocoagulation, Ophthalmology 89:1082, 1982

43. Hawkins, WR, and Schepens, CL: Choroidal detachment and retinal surgery, Am J Ophthalmol 62:813, 1966

44. Hayreh, SS, March, W, and Phelps, CD: Ocular hypotony after retinal vascular occlusion, Trans Ophthalmol Soc UK 97:757, 1977

45. Hupsel, O, and Henkes, HE: The treatment of ocular hypotonia with phosphorylcholine chloride: report on preliminary experimental and clinical results. In Acta XVII of the International Congress of Ophthalmology, vol 1, Toronto, 1955, University of Toronto Press

46. Inomata, H, and Bill, A: Exit sites of uveoscleral flow of aqueous humor in cynomolgus monkey eyes, Exp Eye Res 25:113, 1977

47. Jalkh, AE, Avila, MP, Trempe, CL, and Schepens, CL: Diffuse choroidal thickening detected by ultrasonography in various ocular disorders, Retina 3:277, 1983

48. Joondeph, HC: Management of postoperative and post-traumatic cyclodialysis clefts with argon laser photocoagulation, Ophthalmic Surg 11:186, 1980

49. Junge, J: Ocular changes in dystrophia myotonica, paramyotonia and myotonia congenita, Doc Ophthalmol 21:1, 1966

50. Kronfeld, PC: The fluid exchange in the successfully cyclodialyzed eye, Trans Am Ophthalmol Soc 52:249, 1954

51. Krupin, T, et al: Acidosis, alkalosis, and aqueous humor dynamics in rabbits, Invest Ophthalmol Vis Sci 16:997, 1977

52. Krupin, T, et al: Increased intraocular pressure following topical azide or nitroprusside, Invest Ophthalmol Vis Sci 16:1002, 1977

53. Langham, ME, and Regan, CDJ: Circulatory changes associated with onset of primary retinal detachment, Arch Ophthalmol 81:820, 1969

54. Leydhecker, W: Zur Verbreitung des Glaucoma simplex in der Scheinbar gesunden, augenarztlich nicht behandelten Bevolkerung, Doc Ophthalmol 13:359, 1959

55. Macri, FJ, and Cevario, SJ: The induction of aqueous humor formation by the use of ACh + eserine, Invest Ophthalmol 12:910, 1973

56. Maumenee, AE, and Stark, WJ: Management of persistent hypotony after planned or inadvertent cyclodialysis, Am J Ophthalmol 71:320, 1971

57. McCannel, MA: A retrievable suture idea for anterior uveal problems, Ophthalmic Surg 7:98, 1976

58. Meislik, J, and Herschler, J: Hypotony due to inadvertent cyclodialysis after intraocular lens implantation, Arch Ophthalmol 97:1297, 1979

59. Naumann, GOH, and Volcker, HE: Direkte Zyklopexie zur Behandlung des persistierenden Hypotonie-Syndroms infolge traumatische Zyklodialyse, Klin Monatsbl Augenheilkd 179:266, 1981

60. O'Brien, CS: Detachment of the choroid after cataract extraction, Arch Ophthalmol 14:527, 1935

61. Ormerod, LD, Baerveldt, G, and Green, RL: Cyclodialysis clefts: natural history, assessment, and management. In Weinstein, GW, editor: Open-angle glaucoma: contemporary issues in ophthalmology, vol 3, New York, 1986, Churchill Livingstone, Inc

62. O'Rourke, J, and Macri, FJ: Studies in uveal physiology. II. Clinical studies of the anterior chamber clearance of isotopic tracers, Arch Ophthalmol 84:415, 1970

63. Partamian, LG: Treatment of a cyclodialysis cleft with argon laser photocoagulation in a patient with a shallow anterior chamber, Am J Ophthalmol 99:5, 1985

64. Pederson, JE: Experimental retinal detachment. IV. Aqueous humor dynamics in rhegmatogenous detachments, Arch Ophthalmol 100:1814, 1982

65. Pederson, JE: Experimental retinal detachment. V. Fluid movement through the retinal hole, Arch Ophthalmol 102:136, 1984

66. Pederson, JE: Hypotony. In Duane, TD, editor: Clinical ophthalmology, vol 3, Philadelphia, 1984, Harper & Row Publishers, Inc

67. Pederson, JE: Ocular Hypotony, Trans Ophthalmol Soc UK 105:220, 1986

68. Pederson, JE, Gaasterland, DE, and MacLellan, HM: Experimental ciliochoroidal detachment: effect on intraocular pressure and aqueous humor flow, Arch Ophthalmol 97:536, 1979

69. Pederson, JE, and Green, K: Solute permeability of the normal and prostaglandin-stimulated ciliary epithelium and the effect of ultrafiltration on active transport, Exp Eye Res 21:569, 1975

70. Pederson, JE, and MacLellan, HM: Medical therapy for experimental hypotony, Arch Ophthalmol 100:815, 1982

71. Pederson, JE, MacLellan, HM, and Gaasterland, DE: The rate of reflux fluid movement into the eye from Schlemm's canal during hypotony in the rhesus monkey, Invest Ophthalmol Vis Sci 17:377, 1978

72. Peyman, GA, Mafee, M, and Schulman, J: Computed tomography in choroidal detachment, Ophthalmology 91:156, 1984

73. Phelps, CD, and Armaly, MF: Measurement of episcleral venous pressure, Am J Ophthalmol 85:35, 1978

74. Podos, SM: The effect of cation ionophores on intraocular pressure, Invest Ophthalmol 15:851, 1976

75. Portney, GL, and Purcell, TW: Surgical repair of cyclodialysis induced by hypotony, Ophthalmic Surg 5:30, 1974

76. Prywes, AS, and LoPinto, RJ: Temporary visual loss with ciliary body detachment and hypotony after attempted YAG laser repair of failed filtering surgery, Am J Ophthalmol 101:305, 1986

77. Radda, TM, Bardach, H, and Riss, B: Acute ocular hypotony: a rare complication of temporal arteritis, Ophthalmologica 182:148, 1981

78. Raitta, C, and Karli, P: Ocular findings in myotonic dystrophy, Ann Ophthalmol 14:647, 1982

79. Ramsay, RC, and Knobloch, WH: Ocular perforations following retrobulbar anesthesia for retinal detachment surgery, Am J Ophthalmol 86:61, 1978

80. Ringvold, A: Evidence that hypotony in retinal detachment is due to subretinal juxtapapillary fluid drainage, Acta Ophthalmol 58:652, 1980

81. Roy, RH: Ocular differential diagnosis, Philadelphia, 1975, Lea & Febiger

82. Savir, H: Scleral perforation during cataract surgery, Ann Ophthalmol 15:247, 1983

83. Seelenfreund, MH, and Freilich, DB: Retinal injuries associated with cataract surgery, Am J Ophthalmol 89:654, 1980

84. Shaffer, RN, and Weiss, DI: Concerning cyclodialysis and hypotony, Arch Ophthalmol 68:25, 1962

85. Shea, M, and Mednick, EB: Ciliary body reattachment in ocular hypotony, Arch Ophthalmol 99:278, 1981

86. Slusher, MM: Pseudophakic choroidal detachment with cyclodialysis cyst, Ophthalmic Surg 18:191, 1987

87. Solberg, T, Ytrehus, T, and Ringvold, A: Hypotony and retinal detachment, Acta Ophthalmol 64:26, 1986

88. Spaeth, EB, and DeLong, P: Detachment of the choroid: a clinical and histopathologic analysis, Arch Ophthalmol 32:217, 1944

89. Stepanik, J: Die Tonographie und der episklerale Venendruk, Ophthalmologica 133:397, 1957

90. Streeten, BW, and Belkowitz, M: Experimental hypotony with Silastic, Arch Ophthalmol 78:503, 1967

91. Suguro, K, Toris, CB, and Pederson, JE: Uveoscleral outflow following cyclodialysis in the monkey eye using a fluorescent tracer, Invest Ophthalmol Vis Sci 26:810, 1985

92. Thorpe, HE: Diamox in the treatment of nonleaking flat interior chamber after cataract extraction and associated with choroidal detachment. Proceedings of the XVII International Congress of Ophthalmology, vol 3, Toronto, 1955, University of Toronto Press

93. Toris, CB, and Pederson, JE: Aqueous humor dynamics in experimental iridocyclitis, Invest Ophthalmol Vis Sci 28:477, 1987

94. Tsuboi, S: Measurement of the volume flow and hydraulic conductivity across the isolated dog retinal pigment epithelium, Invest Ophthalmol Vis Sci, 28:1776, 1987

95. Tsuboi, S, Pederson, JE, and Toris, CB: Measurement of the volume flow across the isolated retinal pigment epithelium in cynomolgus monkey eyes with retinal detachments, Invest Ophthalmol Vis Sci 28 (suppl):205, 1987

96. Tulloh, GG: The aqueous flow and permeability of the blood-aqueous barrier in retinal detachment, Trans Ophthalmol Soc UK 92:585, 1972

97. Vela, MA, and Campbell, DG: Hypotony and ciliochoroidal detachment following pharmacologic aqueous suppressant therapy in previously filtered patients, Ophthalmology 92:50, 1985

98. Viikari, K, and Tuovinen, E: On cyclodialysis surgery in the light of follow-up examination, Acta Ophthalmol 35:528, 1957

99. Volcker, HE, and Naumann, GOH: Morphology of uveal and retinal edemas in acute and persisting hypotony, Mod Probl Ophthalmol 20:34, 1979

100. Vos, TA: 25 years dystrophia myotonica (D.M.), Ophthalmologica 141:37, 1961

101. Walker, SD, Brubaker, RF, and Nagataki, S: Hypotony and aqueous dynamics in myotonic dystrophy, Invest Ophthalmol Vis Sci 22:744, 1982

102. Weekers, R, and Delmarcelle, Y: Hypotonie oculaire par reduction du debit de l'humeur aqueuse, Ophthalmologica 125:425, 1953

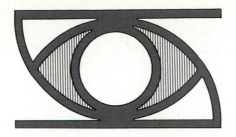

PART TWO

DETERMINATION OF FUNCTIONAL STATUS IN GLAUCOMA

14

Tonography

15

Intraocular Pressure

16

Circadian Variations in Intraocular Pressure

17

Measurement of Aqueous Flow by Fluorophotometry

18

Gonioscopy

19

Exploring the Normal Visual Field

20

Glaucomatous Visual Field Defects

21

Automated Perimetry

22

*Clinical Evaluation of the Optic Disc
and Retinal Nerve Fiber Layer*

23

Quantitative Measurements of the Optic Nerve Head

Chapter 14

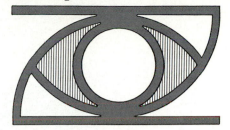

Tonography

John A. McDermott

HISTORICAL BACKGROUND

In the latter part of the nineteenth century, ophthalmologists were aware that external pressure, in the form of digital massage, would decrease the intraocular pressure. Schiøtz observed that repeated tonometry within a relatively short period of time resulted in a lower intraocular pressure.[27] The rate at which intraocular pressure was reduced seemed to be slower in the glaucomatous than in the normal eye.

Subsequent study has provided some explanations for these early observations. When external pressure is applied to the eye, aqueous humor outflow increases, resulting in a lowering of intraocular pressure. This occurs more slowly in the glaucomatous eye as a result of increased resistance to aqueous outflow. In 1950, Grant described a technique, *tonography*, to measure and evaluate the decrease in intraocular pressure associated with the application of an external weight on the eye. He derived the formulas that quantified the rate at which aqueous humor could be forced through the outflow channels by applying external pressure. Grant called this newly derived characteristic of the eye the *facility of aqueous outflow*.[18]

MATHEMATICAL BASIS OF TONOGRAPHY

Before Grant described tonography, many attempts were made to measure the external pressure-induced softening of the globe. Several methods involved placing a Schiøtz tonometer on the eye and intermittently recording, at fixed intervals, the scale readings.[5,20,33] Grant ingeniously used a paper strip recorder (such as that used in the electrocardiograph) connected to an electronic tonom-

eter to obtain a continuous tracing of the change in scale units that occurred while the tonometer was resting on the eye (Fig. 14-1).[18]

For the normal eye, there is a gradual but steady decrease in the intraocular pressure, resulting in a tracing with a gentle downward slope. In the glaucomatous eye, which has increased resistance to the expression of fluid through the outflow channels, there is less change in the intraocular pressure (and, thus a smaller change in the Schiøtz scale units) recording a tracing with a flatter slope (Fig. 14-2). Grant's tonography equations are used to determine the value of the facility of aqueous outflow based on the information on the tracing. The derivation of the equation follows, in a somewhat simplified form.

The globe softens as a certain volume of fluid is expressed from the eye, ΔV. The greater the pressure, P, applied to the eye, and the longer the time interval during which pressure is applied, T, the greater the value of ΔV. Mathematically:

$$\Delta V \propto \Delta P \times T$$

This proportion becomes a mathematical equation by adding a *proportionality constant* that Grant called C, or the facility of aqueous outflow.

$$\Delta V = C \times \Delta P \times T$$

Solving for C:

$$C = \frac{\Delta V}{\Delta P \times T}$$

To understand the derivation of ΔV and ΔP from the tracing, one must appreciate the mechanics by which intraocular pressure is measured with

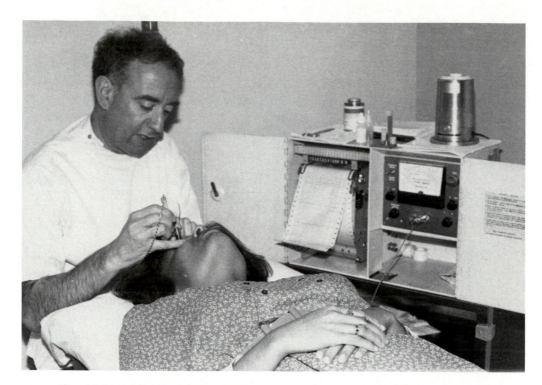

Fig. 14-1   Typical tonography unit with electronic tonometer and paper strip recorder.

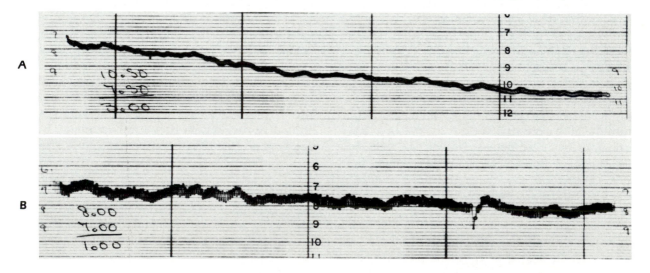

Fig. 14-2   **A,** Normal tonogram: intraocular pressure of 17 mm Hg with facility of aqueous outflow of 0.36 μl/min/mm Hg. **B,** "Flat" tonogram: elevated intraocular pressure (27 mm Hg) with facility of aqueous outflow of 0.02 μl/min/mm Hg.

a Schiøtz tonometer. When the tonometer is placed on the eye, the plunger indents the cornea, and the weight of the instrument distends the globe. The intraocular pressure is raised from the steady-state, pretonometric value, P_o, to a higher pressure induced by the tonometer, P_t. For each Schiøtz reading, Friedenwald had manometrically determined the values of P_o and P_t.[14,15] Friedenwald also measured the volume of the corneal indentation and the volume of the distention of the globe. As the tonometer rests on the eye, the intraocular pressure gradually decreases, the corneal indentation increases, and the distention of the ocular coats decreases. The value of ΔV (the amount of fluid expressed from the eye at the end of time T) is the difference between the volume of corneal indentation and the volume of ocular distention at time T. From Friedenwald's data, Grant devised tables indicating the value of ΔV, based on the initial and the final Schiøtz scale readings recorded during the tracing.

Friedenwald's work enables one to determine P_o and P_t for any scale reading. Thus, ΔP, or the pressure above the steady-state induced by the tonometer, is equal to $P_t - P_o$. But since the intraocular pressure decreases during the tracing, ΔP is constantly changing. Grant determined that this changing ΔP could be represented, for practical purposes, by averaging the values of ΔP (i.e., $P_t - P_o$) at each half minute of the tracing. In the standard tonographic tracing, T is equal to 4 minutes. With values for ΔP, ΔV, and T, C can therefore be determined in $\mu l/min/mm$ Hg. In practice, one does not use Grant's formula since standard tonography tables have been formulated that allow the determination of C based on the initial and the final Schiøtz scale readings, and on the tonometer weight applied during the 4-minute tracing.

FACTORS INFLUENCING TONOGRAPHIC RESULTS

Ocular Rigidity

What has been described, so far, is an oversimplification of what actually occurs in the eye when the tonometer is placed on the cornea. Besides the loss of aqueous humor through the outflow channels, several other phenomena take place that affect the change in volume and the change in pressure during the tracing and, thus, the value of C. The distention of the ocular coats during tonography is not uniform for all eyes. The degree of resistance of an eye to distention, or *ocular rigidity*, will affect the scale reading of the Schiøtz tonometer for any given intraocular pressure. For each

eye, a coefficient of ocular rigidity can be determined that relates ocular distention to pressure changes within the eye. Tonography tables are based on a normal coefficient of ocular rigidity of 0.0215. With lower ocular rigidity (e.g., high myopia) Schiøtz tonometry underestimates the true intraocular pressure, and the resultant tonographic C value is falsely low. Routinely, however, applanation tonometry is performed just before applying the Schiøtz tonometer, during tonography. Applanation tonometry is unaffected by ocular rigidity, and a discrepancy in the intraocular pressure readings, as compared with the Schiøtz tonometer readings, alerts the examiner to abnormal ocular rigidity. In this situation, the value of C can still be determined from the tracing by using a Friedenwald nomogram instead of the standard tonography tables.

Episcleral Venous Pressure

During tonography, the weight of the tonometer increases the episcleral venous pressure.[32] Modern tonography tables are corrected for this increase. The external force of the tonometer also decreases ocular blood flow and actually forces blood from the eye. This effect on C is uncertain.[12]

Pseudofacility

Another phenomenon thought to occur during tonography is pseudofacility: a decrease in the rate of aqueous humor production secondary to the Schiøtz tonometer–induced increase in intraocular pressure. The decreased rate of aqueous humor production increases the value of ΔV. The C value, therefore, is the sum of true facility (flow of aqueous humor through the outflow channels) and pseudofacility (the apparent flow secondary to a reduced rate of aqueous humor formation). Pseudofacility may account for up to 20% of total C.[24]

Intraocular Pressure

Finally, many studies have demonstrated that C depends on the level of intraocular pressure.[11,28] Outflow facility is reduced when intraocular pressure is elevated. Independent of the multiple variables that influence tonography, the calculated C provides invaluable information concerning the means by which drugs affect intraocular pressure. However, as cautioned by Spaeth, calling the C value the "coefficient of aqueous outflow" is an oversimplification and may be misleading.[40]

NORMAL TONOGRAPHIC VALUES

In Grant's initial paper, C values, based on repetitive examination of normal eyes, ranged from

0.15 to 0.34 μl/min/mm Hg with a mean of 0.243. Although the range of normal values varied somewhat, subsequent studies confirmed this mean C value for normal eyes.[3,8,42] Population studies have established that outflow facility is fairly consistent in a given eye, and values compare favorably to those obtained by intracameral perfusion in enucleated eyes.[4,21] There appears to be a gradual decrease in C with aging, but no sex differences have been detected.[25]

TEST PERFORMANCE

A detailed discussion of the specific steps required to perform accurate tonography is beyond the scope of this chapter, but there are several manuals that can help one avoid the abundant sources of error inherent in performing the test.[10,16] Possible technical difficulties range from improperly calibrated equipment to poor patient cooperation. Briefly, in most settings, after applanation tonometry has been performed, the patient lies supine in a quiet setting. After both eyes are anesthetized, the electronic Schiøtz tonometer, which has been checked and calibrated, is applied to one eye while the patient fixates on a ceiling target with the other eye. The Schiøtz weight used during tonography is determined by the initial applanation reading, and a standard 4-minute tracing is obtained.

An acceptable tracing (see Fig. 14-2) has a smooth gradual slope with small oscillations indicating the ocular pulse and somewhat less obvious cycles, of greater duration, caused by respirations. Obviously, if the patient coughs, sneezes, or squeezes his eye, the resulting Valsalva maneuver may invalidate the tracing. After obtaining an acceptable test result, the technician draws a line through the tracing, approximating its slope. Using this line, the examiner reads the scale units at time zero and at 4 minutes and determines C from tonography tables or from the Friedenwald nomogram, based on these readings.

CLINICAL RELEVANCE

Shortly after describing the technique of tonography, Grant reported his results of over 1000 tonograms on 600 normal and glaucomatous eyes.[19] His findings finally resolved the issue of whether the elevated pressure in glaucoma was caused by increased aqueous production or by decreased aqueous outflow. Without exception, he found that reduced outflow facility accounted for the elevation of intraocular pressure in the glaucomatous eye. The lowest C values, some of which were 0.0, occurred during attacks of angle-closure glaucoma.

When the attack was terminated, either surgically or medically, normal C values were restored. In eyes with chronic angle-closure glaucoma, the C values decreased proportionately to the degree of synechial closure of the angle. Successful filtration surgery markedly increased C values. Administration of topical miotics increased outflow facility, establishing the mechanism of action of these drugs.

Tonography initially was thought to demonstrate a marked separation in C values between normal and glaucomatous eyes. The C value in normal eyes ranged from 0.11 to 0.44 μl/min/mm Hg, and in glaucomatous eyes C ranged from 0.0 to 0.11. Tonography appeared to be a test that could distinguish normal from glaucomatous eyes. If one assumes that diminished C values precede elevated intraocular pressure and optic nerve damage, then any glaucoma suspect (i.e., with normal optic nerves and visual fields) with C values in the glaucomatous range would be especially prone to develop optic nerve damage, and thus would be a candidate for early intervention.

Unfortunately, follow-up studies failed to find this clear cut distinction between glaucoma suspects and normal eyes. The two groups overlapped for values between 0.10 and 0.20 μl/min/mm Hg. Kronfeld found that the C value in 14 of 40 normal eyes and 16 of 34 glaucomatous eyes overlapped in this range.[27] Scheie also reported the lower limit of normal as 0.11, but 23% of glaucomatous eyes had a value greater than 0.16 and one third of these C values were greater than 0.21. In Becker's study of 1379 eyes, only 2.5% of normal subjects had C values less than 0.18 μl/min/mm Hg; however, 35% of the glaucomatous eyes had values above 0.18. It became apparent that the C value would not provide the diagnosis for glaucoma.

In an attempt to separate normal patients from glaucoma patients, both Leydecker and Becker suggested using a ratio of the intraocular pressure to the C value.[2,31] The higher the intraocular pressure and the lower the C value, the greater the Po/C ratio. In a series of over 1100 eyes, the average Po/C in normal subjects was 56. Although an overlap between normal eyes and glaucomatous eyes still occurred, compared with the overlap observed using only the C value, the Po/C overlap was smaller. With a Po/C of 100 as the demarcation, 71% of glaucoma patients exceeded this value, whereas only 2% of normal patients fell within this range.[2] Several subsequent studies confirmed the usefulness of Po/C but cautioned that this only reduced and did not eliminate the tonographic overlap.[6,34,37,39] Po/C ratios usually are included in the standard tonographic report.

A further modification of the use of tonography involved combining it with the water-drinking provocative test for open-angle glaucoma. Instead of merely recording intraocular pressure before and 1 hour (later changed to 45 minutes) after consuming a liter of water, as in the simple provocative test, preingestion and postingestion tonography was performed. Patients fasted for 9 to 12 hours before the test, and both C and Po/C were calculated from the tonography tracings. Becker found that the mean C for a normal population of 175 eyes was 0.31 µl/min/mm Hg and was unchanged by water drinking. In his glaucoma population of 153 patients, the mean C decreased from 0.17 to 0.12. More impressive figures, however, were calculated for Po/C.[3] Again, in his extensive test population of 1379 eyes, only 2.5% of normal eyes exceeded a Po/C value of 100, and 95% of glaucomatous eyes were correctly identified.[2] Other studies confirmed Becker's finding that tonography was more useful when combined with water-drinking,[23,43] but several studies concluded that the technique was inferior to water-drinking combined with tonometry using the Goldmann applanation tonometer.[17,29,30,41]

Many longitudinal studies investigated tonography as a prognostic test in glaucoma suspects to predict optic nerve or visual field damage, and to identify eyes in which intraocular pressure would increase over time. Again, tonography fell short of expectations. There was a poor correlation between C values and the degree to which intraocular pressure increased.[17] In individual patients, neither the magnitude of the diurnal fluctuation nor the peak of the diurnal curve could be predicted from C values.[9,22,34,35]

There have been conflicting results regarding the ability of tonography to identify those patients who would develop future optic disc or visual field damage. Kass et al.[26] reported a prospective follow-up of 40 "normal" eyes, followed for 4 years, in which the only abnormality was a Po/C greater than 100. Five eyes, a surprisingly large number, developed visual field defects. However, many of these "normal" patients had visual field defects in the other eye or were relatives of glaucoma patients, making them a rather "select" normal population. DeRoetth followed glaucoma suspects and treated glaucoma patients and found no correlation between C and the development of new, or the deterioration of existing, visual field defects.[7] Armaly reported a 10-year follow-up of over 3000 subjects unselected for intraocular pressure with normal examinations and visual fields. Four patients developed visual field loss during the study. Although these patients had "abnormal" tonographic values at the time visual field loss was discovered, tonograms performed before the onset of damage could not distinguish them from the rest of the population sample.[1]

Pohjanpelto grouped 367 eyes by intraocular pressure and by the presence or absence of optic nerve damage. Although C values were slightly lower in the group with damage, considerable overlap negated any clinical usefulness for individual eyes. The intraocular pressure peak on a diurnal curve was a better predictor of optic nerve damage than the C value.[36] In another study of 50 patients with ocular hypertension followed prospectively for at least 5 years, Po/C >100 and C <0.15 µl/min/mm Hg were very sensitive in detecting patients who would develop visual field loss (4 of 4 for Po/C >100, and 3 of 4 for C <0.15) but were not very specific (prevalence in the total group of Po/C >100 was 75 of 100 eyes, and C <0.15 occurred in 34 of 100 eyes).[44] Similarly Kass, in a 3- to 5-year follow-up of fellow eyes of 31 patients with visual field defects in one eye, found no significant difference in the number of Po/C's >100, or in C values ≤0.11 in those who developed visual field defects in the fellow eye compared with those who did not.[26] Apparently tonography alone cannot be used to diagnose glaucoma.

Examiners also hoped that tonography would help manage established glaucoma cases. In an early study, Roberts found that continued visual field deterioration in patients treated for glaucoma correlated better with a poor C value than with a particular intraocular pressure reading.[38] In a later study with a follow-up of 10 years, the same author found Po/C values were a helpful prognosticator of further deterioration.[39] Only 1 of 38 eyes with progressive visual field defects had a Po/C <100. However, in the 56 patients without visual field deterioration, 60% had Po/C values >100. Again, a disturbing overlap exists between the "controlled" versus "uncontrolled" glaucoma patients. Tonography, however, was still a better prognosticator than intraocular pressure. Other studies, conversely, concluded the opposite: that tonography added nothing to tonometry alone when attempting to predict which eyes would progressively deteriorate.[12,13]

Interest in tonography waned as it became apparent that it offered no "magic number" to determine which glaucoma suspects would develop visual field defects. At best, tonographic results can caution the clinician as to which patients will require careful observation. As far as its use in managing documented glaucoma cases, with the advent of beta-blockers as the drug of choice (medication that does not affect outflow), the importance of tonography has greatly diminished. In addition, it has become apparent that the susceptibility of the optic nerve to a given pressure varies among eyes, and tonography as a measure of aqueous humor dynamics does not address that susceptibility. Glaucoma research has turned toward the posterior segment to define new guidelines for treatment. Although the use of tonography has decreased, it remains a key research tool, especially in defining the mechanism of action of new pharmacologic agents in the treatment of glaucoma.

REFERENCES

1. Armaly, MF: Ocular pressure and visual fields: a ten-year follow-up study, Arch Ophthalmol 81:25, 1969
2. Becker, B: Tonography in the diagnosis of simple (open-angle) glaucoma, Trans Am Acad Ophthalmol Otolaryngol 65:156, 1961
3. Becker, B, and Christensen, RE: Water-drinking and tonography in the diagnosis of glaucoma, Arch Ophthalmol 56:321, 1956
4. Becker, B, and Constant, MA: The facility of aqueous outflow: a comparison of tonography and perfusion measurements in vivo and in vitro, Arch Ophthalmol 55:305, 1956
5. Boeck, J, Kronfeld, PC, and Stough, JT: Effect on intraocular tension of corneal massage with the tonometer of Schiøtz, Arch Ophthalmol 11:796, 1934
6. Cameron, D, Finlay, ET, and Jackson, CRS: Tonometry and tonography in the diagnosis of chronic simple glaucoma, Br J Ophthalmol 55:738, 1971
7. DeRoetth, A: Clinical evaluation of tonography, Am J Ophthalmol 59:169, 1965
8. DeRoetth, A, and Knighton, US: Clinical evaluation of the aqueous flow test: a preliminary report, Arch Ophthalmol 48:148, 1952
9. Drance, SM: Diurnal variation of intraocular pressure in treated glaucoma, Arch Ophthalmol 70:62, 1963
10. Drews, RW: Manual of tonography, St. Louis, 1971, The CV Mosby Co
11. Ellingsen, BA, and Grant, WM: Influence of intraocular pressure and trabeculotomy on aqueous outflow in enucleated monkey eyes, Invest Ophthalmol 10:705, 1971
12. Fisher, RF: Value of tonometry and tonography in the diagnosis of glaucoma, Br J Ophthalmol 56:200, 1972
13. Fisher, RF, Carpenter, RG, and Wheeler, C: Assessment of established cases of chronic simple glaucoma, Br J Ophthalmol 54:217, 1970
14. Friedenwald, JS: Contribution to the theory and practice of tonometry, Am J Ophthalmol 20:985, 1937
15. Friedenwald, JS: Tonometer calibration: an attempt to remove discrepancies found in the 1954 calibration scale for Schiøtz tonometers, Trans Am Acad Ophthalmol Otolaryngol 61:108, 1957
16. Garner, LL: Tonography and the glaucomas, Springfield, IL, 1965, Charles C Thomas, Publisher
17. Graham, PA: The definition of pre-glaucoma: a prospective study, Trans Ophthalmol Soc UK 89:153, 1969
18. Grant, WM: Tonographic method for measuring the facility and rate of outflow in human eyes, Arch Ophthalmol 44:204, 1950
19. Grant, WM: Clinical measurements of aqueous outflow, Arch Ophthalmol 46:113, 1951
20. Grant, WM: Tonography: past, present, and future, Ophthalmology 85:252, 1978
21. Grant, WM, and Trotter, RR: Tonographic measurements in enucleated eyes, Arch Ophthalmol 53, 191, 1955.
22. Gloster, J: Tonometry and tonography, Ophthalmol Clinics 5:911, 1965
23. Greinecker, O: Tonography as a method of examination and its combination with water-drinking test, Am J Ophthalmol 56:492, 1963
24. Hetland-Eriksen, J, and Odhers, T: Experimental tonography on enucleated human eyes. I. The validity of Grant's tonography formula, Invest Ophthalmol 14:199, 1975
25. Johnson, LV: Tonographic survey, Am J Ophthalmol 61:680, 1966
26. Kass, MA, Kolker, AE, and Becker, B: Prognostic factors in glaucomatous visual field loss, Arch Ophthalmol 94:1274, 1976
27. Kronfeld, PC: Tonography, Arch Ophthalmol 48:393, 1952
28. Kronfeld, PC: Some basic statistics of clinical tonography, Invest Ophthalmol 7:319, 1968
29. Kronfeld, PC: Water-drinking and outflow facility, Invest Ophthalmol 14:49, 1975
30. Leighton, DA, and Phillips, CI: Provocative test combining water-drinking and homatropine eye drops: applanation versus tonography, Br J Ophthalmol 55:619, 1971
31. Leydhecker W: Tonography in the early diagnosis of simple glaucoma, Trans Ophthalmol Soc UK LXXVIII:533, 1958
32. Linnér E: Episcleral venous pressure during tonography, Acta XVII Cong Ophthalmol 3:1532, 1955
33. Moses, RA, and Bruno, M: The rate of outflow of fluid from the eye under increased pressure, Am J Ophthalmol 33:389, 1950
34. Newell, FW, and Krill, AE: Diurnal tonography in normal and glaucomatous eyes, Am J Ophthalmol 59:840, 1965
35. Phelps, CD, Woolson, RF, Kolker, AE, and Becker, B: Diurnal variation in intraocular pressure, Am J Ophthalmol 77:367, 1974

36. Pohjanpelto, PEJ: Tonography and glaucomatous optic nerve damage, Acta Ophthalomol 52:817, 1974

37. Portnoy, GI, and Krohn, M: Tonography and projection perimetry: relationship according to receiver operating characteristic curves, Arch Ophthalmol 95:1353, 1977

38. Roberts, RW: Tonography in the management of glaucoma, Trans Am Acad Ophthalmol Otolaryngol 64:163, 1961

39. Roberts, RW: Long-term handling of open-angle glaucoma: tonography and other prognostic aids, Ann Ophthalmol 9:577, 1977

40. Spaeth, GL: Tonography and tonometry. In Duane, TD, editor: Clinical ophthalmology, vol 3, Philadelphia, 1986, Harper & Row

41. Spaeth, GL, and Vacharat, N: Provocative tests and chronic simple glaucoma, Br J Ophthalmol 56:205, 1972

42. Stephanik, J, and Kemper, RA: Outflow aqueous humor, Arch Ophthalmol 51:671, 1954

43. Suzuki, Y, Takenchi, T, and Kitazawa, Y: Use of water-drinking tonography in mass screening for glaucoma, Am J Ophthalmol 61:847, 1966

44. Wilensky, JT, Podos, SM, and Becker, B: Prognostic indicators in ocular hypertension, Arch Ophthalmol 91:200, 1974

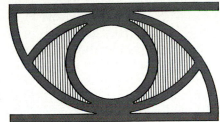

Chapter 15

Intraocular Pressure

Edwin M. Schottenstein

INTRAOCULAR PRESSURE

From a functional standpoint, a "normal" intraocular pressure is one that does not result in glaucomatous optic nerve head damage. Because not all eyes respond similarly to a particular intraocular pressure level, a normal pressure cannot be represented as a specific measurement. Therefore, the most that we can expect is to determine the relative chance of developing glaucoma at different pressure levels given the knowledge of the distribution of intraocular pressure in general populations and in populations of individuals with glaucomatous damage.

Virtually all studies of intraocular pressure distribution demonstrate a correspondence with a normal (Gaussian) bell-shaped curve up to a pressure of 21 mm Hg followed by a skewness toward higher intraocular pressures.* A skewed frequency distribution indicates that 95% of the area under the distribution curve does not lie within two standard deviations of the mean. Therefore, the upper limit of "normal" intraocular pressure is not necessarily 20.5 mm Hg, which is two standard deviations above the mean intraocular pressure of 15.5 ± 2.6 mm Hg, nor is the eye with a "normal" intraocular pressure immune to glaucomatous damage. Consequently, the idea of a maximum "normal" intraocular pressure must be considered as only an estimation.[28]

Some investigators have explained skewness of the intraocular pressure distribution to higher levels as representing two overlapping Gaussian distributions, one of a normal population and the other of a population of glaucomatous subjects.[107,108,154] From a statistical perspective, it is difficult to distinguish between two overlapping Gaussian curves and a single curve with a skewed deviation. In either case, a "normal" pressure is an arbitrary designation, and no specific intraocular pressure can differentiate "normal" eyes from those that will not develop glaucomatous damage.

Factors Influencing Intraocular Pressure

The skewness of the distribution toward higher intraocular pressures does not occur until around 40 years of age. Between ages 20 and 40, the intraocular pressure distribution is Gaussian in the general population.[5] After age 40, the mean intraocular pressure and standard deviation increase.[5] Some think this increase in intraocular pressure is directly associated with increasing age.[5,74,95] However, others have proposed that it is secondary to other influences, such as pulse rate,[24] obesity, or blood pressure.[160,161] It appears to be associated with a reduced facility of aqueous outflow,[14] despite an equivalent drop in aqueous production.[14,22,58] Recent studies have found the intraocular pressure in the Japanese population to decrease with age in both sexes, but more markedly in men.[160-162]

Aside from age, other factors influence the intraocular pressure over a long-term basis. Some studies have shown a more marked skewness and higher mean levels for women compared with

---

*References 5, 10, 16, 63, 76, 77, 86, 107, 108.

men, but others report no sex differences. Women demonstrate a greater increase in mean intraocular pressure with age beginning with the onset of menopause.[5] Some studies have found blacks to have a higher mean intraocular pressure than whites, but these studies were not well controlled or the sample size was small.[88,174] Individuals with a family history of glaucoma tend to have higher intraocular pressures.[5,156] In fact, intraocular pressure has been shown to have hereditary influences.[6,7,106] There is significant association between intraocular pressure and axial length, myopes tending to have higher intraocular pressures.[36,170] Myopia is more common among patients with open-angle glaucoma than among normals, and consequently, it is hard to differentiate whether the higher intraocular pressures in myopes are a manifestation of early open-angle glaucoma or a genuinely higher intraocular pressure distribution in the myopic population. One study of anisometropic myopia did not detect a significant difference in intraocular pressure between the two eyes.[19]

Other factors induce temporary fluctuations in the pressure. For example, the intraocular pressure cyclically fluctuates through the day. Some investigators have related this cycle to cyclic fluctuations of blood levels of adrenocortical steroids.[21,93] Interference with the diurnal variation of corticosteroid levels has been shown to modify the diurnal curve of the intraocular pressure.[21,176] A reported association between serum osmolality and daily intraocular pressure fluctuations[80] has not been confirmed. One study showed an inverse relationship between intraocular pressure and outflow facility,[21] but another showed no correlation.[125]

Generally, the intraocular pressure rises from 0.3 to 6.0 mm Hg when reclining from a sitting to a supine position.[3,5,8,82,97,175] However, this has not been confirmed by some investigators.[94,179] A supine position appears to have a greater influence on the intraocular pressure in eyes with glaucoma,[3,82] particularly low-tension glaucoma[171] or retinal vein obstruction.[179] Patients with systemic hypertension have a significantly higher intraocular pressure elevation after 15 minutes of reclining in the supine position than do their normotensive counterparts.[180] The mechanism by which the intraocular pressure increases in the supine position is not clear.

The inverted position has an even greater likelihood of raising the intraocular pressure. In one study, after 5 minutes of total body inversion, the mean intraocular pressure rose from 16.8 ± 2.8 to 32.9 ± 7.9 mm Hg in nonglaucomatous eyes and from 21.3 ± 2.3 to 37.6 ± 5 mm Hg in glaucomatous eyes.[29]

Depending on the type of physical activity, the intraocular pressure may rise or fall. Extended exercise, such as jogging or bicycling, has been shown to lower the intraocular pressure[105,157] an average of 24% in normal individuals[169] and 30% in patients with open-angle glaucoma.[101] It has been postulated that the intraocular pressure drops as a result of increased serum osmolarity[169] or metabolic acidosis,[101] although the exact mechanism has not yet been elucidated.

Straining, as with a Valsalva maneuver[17] or electroshock therapy[46] has been reported to increase intraocular pressure, most likely by increasing episcleral venous pressure, or orbicularis oculi tone. Blinking increases intraocular pressure 10 mg Hg, and hard lid squeezing may increase it as high as 90 mm Hg.[27] Repeated lid squeezing leads to a modest decrease in intraocular pressure in normal individuals with less of an effect on glaucomatous patients.[66] Conflicting results exist as to whether a diminished orbicularis tone, as with Bell's palsy or a local facial nerve block, lowers the intraocular pressure.[110,165]

Intraocular pressure may rise in response to ACTH, glucocorticoids, and growth hormone and drop in response to progesterone, estrogen, chorionic gonadotropin, and relaxin.[89] It appears to be unrelated to the menstrual cycle in women.[47]

Aside from trichlorethylene[152] and ketamine,[4,113,153] which cause an intraocular pressure elevation, most general anesthetics reduce the intraocular pressure.[1,42] This is particularly important when examining infants under anesthesia for suspected congenital glaucoma. During intraocular surgery, depolarizing muscle relaxants, such as succinylcholine[126] and suxamethonium,[20] should be avoided, because a sudden elevation in intraocular pressure, most likely as a result of a combination of extraocular muscle contraction and intraocular vasodilation, may lead to extrusion of intraocular contents. Succinylcholine causes less rise when given intramuscularly than intravenously.[62] Pretreatment with nondepolarizing muscle relaxants, such as d-tubocurarine and gallamine, do not seem to prevent an intraocular pressure rise during endotracheal intubation,[20,126] unlike pretreatment with diazepam,[33] or the use of fazadinium.[32] Increased P_{CO_2}[92,137,150] results in an intraocular pressure elevation, which is not suppressed by pretreatment with acetazolamide,[137] and an elevated P_{O_2} has an intraocular pressure–lowering effect.[57]

Aside from antiglaucoma medications, many

other drugs affect intraocular pressure. The oral administration of ethyl alcohol lowers intraocular pressure by mechanisms relating to hyperosmotic agents.[79,133] Heroin[65] and marijuana lower the intraocular pressure, but tobacco smoking appears to induce a transient rise in the intraocular pressure.[118,158] In one study, smoking one cigarette was associated with an increase in the intraocular pressure of greater than 5 mm Hg in 37% of open-angle glaucoma patients and 11% of nonglaucomatous individuals.[118] Caffeine appears to cause a slight, transient elevation of intraocular pressure, although the amount consumed with ordinary coffee drinking does not cause a significant, sustained rise.[132] Ingestion of d-lysergic acid diethylamide (LSD) results in an elevated intraocular pressure.[65] Systemic anticholinergics, such as atropine[103,104] and propantheline[73] have no effect on the intraocular pressure in normal or glaucomatous eyes with open iridocorneal angles, particularly when administered for a short time. However, topical cyclopentolate will elevate intraocular pressure in some patients with open-angle glaucoma,[103,172] and it has been suggested that these patients may also manifest a slight intraocular rise in response to long-term administration of systemic anticholinergics.[104] Topical, periocular, and systemically administered corticosteroids[93] can elevate intraocular pressure in susceptible patients (see Chapter 64).

Tonometers and Tonometry

Clinical measurement of intraocular pressure is performed by deforming the globe and correlating the force responsible for the deformation to the pressure within the eye. Both indentation and applanation tonometers effect a deformation of the globe, but the magnitude of the deformation varies.[112] A third type of tonometer, the noncontact tonometer, measures the time required to deform the corneal surface in response to the force produced by a jet of air.

Schiøtz indentation tonometry

The Schiøtz tonometer (Fig. 15-1) consists of a concave footplate attached to a shaft enclosing a freely sliding plunger. The instrument is placed on the anesthetized cornea of a subject in the supine position. The extent to which the cornea is indented by the plunger is measured as the distance from the footplate curve to the plunger base, and a simple lever system moves a needle on a calibrated scale, indicating a scale reading that is converted to an intraocular pressure measurement.

Originally, the tonometer was manufactured in

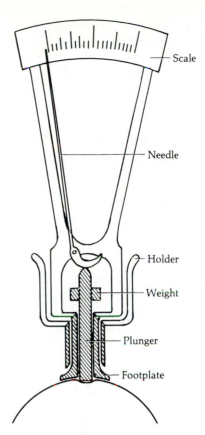

Fig. 15-1 Cut-away view showing basic features of Schiøtz-type indentation tonometer. (From Shields, MB: Textbook of glaucoma, ed 2, Baltimore, 1986, Williams & Wilkins)

Norway under Schiøtz's supervision. As it became popular, other manufacturers produced imitation Schiøtz tonometers, which often gave readings different from the bona fide one and from each other.

A committee appointed by the American Academy of Ophthalmology and Otolaryngology to standardize the manufacturing of Schiøtz tonometers elucidated several critical design standards.[54] The footplate should have a concavity of 15 mm radius of curvature, and its framework should weigh 11 g. The plunger should be 3 mm in diameter and weigh a total of 5.5 g, including the force of the lever resting on top of the plunger. Additional weights can be added to the plunger to increase it to 7.5, 10, or 15 g. The lever magnifies the plunger's movement by 20 times. The tonometer needle is lined up with the scale reading of zero when the plunger extends 0.05 mm beyond the footplate curve. To compensate for the displacement, a test block with a radius of curvature flatter than the footplate is provided. Finally, a 0.025 mm radius of plunger edge curvature was found to be crucial to the scale measurement and reduced the occurrence of corneal abrasions.

The weight of the tonometer on the eye raises the actual intraocular pressure (P_o) to a higher level (P_t). The change in pressure from P_o to P_t is an expression of the resistance of the eye to the displacement of fluid.

Determination of P_o from a scale reading P_t requires conversion. In 1937, Friedenwald[52] attempted to mathematize the extrapolation from the scale reading P_t to the intraocular pressure P_o. He generated an empirical formula for the linear relationship between the log function of the intraocular pressure and the ocular distention. This formula has a numerical constant, the coefficient of ocular rigidity (E), which is roughly an expression of the distensibility of the eye. He developed a nomogram for estimating the value of E based on two tonometric readings with different weights.[52] Subsequent studies using applanation tonometry with different sizes of applanating areas corroborated his formulations.[55] Friedenwald[55] originally calculated the average E to be 0.0245 and used this numerical value to develop a set of conversion tables in 1948 but later revised the average value of E to be 0.025 and developed a new set of conversion tables in 1955.[100] Subsequent studies demonstrate that the 1948 tables agree more closely with measurements by Goldmann applanation tonometry.[2,13]

For Schiøtz tonometry, the patient should be in the supine position looking up at a fixation target while the examiner separates the eyelids and lowers the tonometer footplate to rest on the anesthetized cornea, so that the plunger is free to move vertically. With the tonometer properly positioned, the examiner will observe a fine movement of the indicator needle on the scale in response to ocular pulsations. The scale reading should be noted as an average of the extremes of these excursions. Usually, the 5.5 g weight is initially used, but if the scale reading is 4 or less, additional weight starting with the 7.5 g weight should be added to the plunger. The precision with which the scale reading can be evaluated on the tonometer is limited by oscillations of the indicator needle caused by the ocular pulse.

Limitations on the accuracy of the Schiøtz tonometer are caused by the fact that the ocular rigidity is variable from eye to eye. Because the conversion tables are established on an average coefficient of ocular rigidity, eyes that digress significantly from this E value will give erroneous intraocular pressure measurements. A high E will give a falsely

high intraocular pressure, whereas a low E value will indicate a falsely low measurement. Most hyeropes have a high E value, and high myopes have a low E value.[41] However, one study showed an increasing E value with extreme myopia.[52] An elevated intraocular pressure is associated with a diminished E value,[37] which may be why lower E values are seen during water-provocative testing.[37,41,173] Miotics, particularly strong cholinesterase inhibitors, decrease ocular rigidity.[41] Vasodilators may also reduce it, but vasoconstrictors may increase it.[52] Ocular rigidity is reduced subsequent to retinal detachment surgery,[71,134] and the intravitreal injection of a compressible gas.[9] Keratoconus was once considered to be associated with an abnormally low ocular rigidity. However, this may be an artifact of a thin cornea because it is not low subsequent to keratoplasty.[51]

Other sources of error with Schiøtz tonometry also exist. The variable expulsion of intraocular blood during Schiøtz tonometry may influence the intraocular pressure measurement.[72] Finally, either a steeper or thicker cornea will cause greater displacement of fluid during Schiøtz tonometry, giving a falsely high intraocular measurement.[53]

Many studies have shown the Schiøtz tonometer to give lower intraocular pressure estimates than the Goldmann applanation tonometer,[15,96,163] even when the postural influences on intraocular pressure are compensated for by performing both measurements in the supine position.[8,53,155] Because the Schiøtz tonometer is subject to errors related to ocular rigidity and corneal curvature,[53] it is thought to be of limited value even for screening purposes.[15,96,166] In situations such as retinal detachment surgery[37,134] or eyes containing compressible gas,[134] in which the ocular rigidity is known to be altered, it is particularly unsuitable. Also, intraocular pressure measurements on eyes with irregularly contoured corneas are subject to great variability and inaccuracy.[90]

Applanation tonometry

Applanation tonometry measures intraocular pressure by subjecting the eye to a force that flattens the cornea. Two types have been devised. In the first, the area of the cornea being applanated is held constant, and a variable force is applied. In the second, the force applied to the cornea is held constant, and the area applanated varies.

Variable force applanation tonometry

Goldmann tonometer. Goldmann applanation tonometry is the prime example of variable force applanation tonometry. It is based on the Imbert-Fick law,[60] which states that the pressure within a sphere (P) is roughly equal to the external force (f) needed to flatten a portion of the sphere divided by the area (A) of the sphere which is flattened,

$$(1) \qquad P = f/A \text{ or } PA = f$$

This law applies to spheres that are perfectly spherical, dry, and flexible and infinitely thin. Because the cornea does not satisfy these requirements, this formula becomes somewhat more complicated. A finite force independent of the intraocular pressure is required to distort the cornea from its dome shape to a plane. Therefore, this force (N), tending to push the applanating surface away from the eye, must be added to PA. Second, the tear film creates a surface tension that pulls the applanating surface toward the cornea, and consequently a force (M) must be added to applanating force. The pressure formula then becomes

$$(2) \qquad PA + N = f + M$$

or

$$P = \frac{f + M - N}{A}$$

In addition, because the central thickness of the cornea is approximately 0.55 mm, the outer area of flattening (A) differs from the inner area that is flattened (A_1). It is this inner area with which we are concerned; thus, the formula becomes $P = f + M - N/A_1$. When A_1 is equal to 7.35 mm^2, the opposing forces of corneal inflexibility (N) and surface tension (M) counterbalance each other, and

$$(3) \qquad P = \frac{f}{7.35 \text{ mm}^2}$$

This internal area of applanation is achieved when the diameter of the external area of corneal applanation is around 3.06 mm, although an area of 3.53 mm has reportedly produced comparable intraocular pressures in the human.[167] The same diameter is not suitable for use in animal eyes, presumably because of the difference in structure of the cornea. When developing the fixed area applanation tonometer, Goldmann and Schmidt[60,61] determined that the force required to distort the cornea from its domed shape to a flattened plane, which is independent of the internal pressure, equaled the surface tension of the tear film meniscus for applanation tonometers with diameters between 2.5 and 4 mm in diameter. However, an applanation diameter of 3.06 mm was selected because, when using this diameter, grams force times

10 is directly converted to mm Hg. It is estimated that the volume displaced by the Goldmann applanator is 0.05 μl, and the measured pressure is about 3% greater than the intraocular pressure before application of the instrument. However, the intraocular pressure measured by the Goldmann applanation tonometry is usually recorded without this correction.

The Goldmann applanation tonometer is mounted on the end of a lever that is hinged on the slit-lamp (Fig. 15-2). A biprism, which contacts the cornea, creates two semicircles. The edge of corneal contact is made apparent by the instillation of a small amount of fluorescein into the tear film while viewing in a cobalt blue light. By manually rotating a dial calibrated in mm Hg, the force is adjusted by changing the length of a spring within the device.[121] The prisms are calibrated so that the inner margins of the semicircles touch when 3.06 mm of the cornea is applanated.

When one performs applanation tonometry at the slit-lamp, the patient's head and the microscope should be positioned so that the bar is against the patient's forehead and well above the eyebrows, allowing for the maximum separation of the patient's eyelids, which usually requires raising of the eyebrows. A drop of anesthetic is instilled into the lower cul-de-sac, and a fluorescein-impregnated paper strip is touched to the tears there. Alternatively, a 0.25% sodium fluorescein solution[64] may be used, and commercial solutions that combine 0.25% fluorescein with a topical anesthetic are available.[145] The preservatives in these commercial preparations sufficiently prevent bacterial contamination,[26,78,168] especially when a pipette-type dispenser is used; but the cap of a squeeze bottle may be a reservoir for bacterial contamination.[26]

With the cornea and tonometer prisms maximally illuminated by a cobalt blue light from the slit-lamp, the entire tonometry mechanism is moved toward the patient's eye until the front surface of the plastic piece that contains the tonometer prisms gently touches the apex of the cornea. When contact with the eye has been established, the semicircular patterns are observed through the right ocular of the slit-lamp. The slit-lamp is then raised or lowered until the two semicircles are equal in size, and then the tension dial is adjusted so that the inner edge of the upper and lower semicircles become aligned. As with Schiøtz tonometry, the influence of ocular pulsations create excursions of the semicircular tear meniscus, and the pressure is read as the median over which the arcs glide. This is the desired end point at which

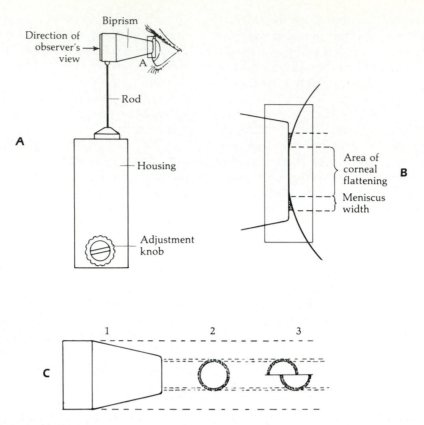

Fig. 15-2 Goldmann-type applanation tonometry. **A,** Basic features of tonometer, shown in contact with patient's cornea. **B,** Enlargement shows tear film meniscus created by contact of biprism and cornea. **C,** View through biprism *(1)* reveals circular meniscus *(2),* which is converted into semicircles *(3)* by prisms. (From Shields, MB: Textbook of glaucoma, ed 2, Baltimore, 1986, Williams & Wilkins)

a reading can be taken from a graduated dial (Fig. 15-3). As mentioned earlier, the reading on the dial indicates grams of force applied to the tonometer, so one must multiply this number by 10 to obtain the intraocular pressure in mm Hg.

The blue central area one observes when performing applanation tonometry is the applanated cornea, and the green semicircles are the fluorescein-stained tears. Without staining the tears, a bright reflection from the air-tear interface is seen. Since the tear meniscus must have a larger diameter than the flattened cornea, when the reflection from its air interface is adjusted to the end point, the flattened cornea must be less than 3.06 mm in diameter. The force required to flatten a smaller area of cornea is less than that for a larger corneal area, and because the applanating force read from the graduated dial is interpreted as one tenth of the intraocular pressure, Goldmann applanation tonometry performed without fluorescein will con-

sistently produce an underestimation of the intraocular pressure and is not recommended.[148]

The width of the tear meniscus may influence the intraocular pressure reading slightly, with wider menisci giving an overestimation of the intraocular pressure.[60] A narrow but adequately stained tear meniscus, as in a dry eye, does not create an error in pressure measurements. Unsatisfactory vertical alignment in which one semicircle is larger than the other produces an erroneously elevated intraocular pressure estimate. The thickness of the cornea has also been shown to influence the intraocular pressure estimate, thin corneas producing lower readings.[45] A thick cornea gives a falsely high reading if the thickness is due to an increased amount of collagen fibrils,[45,85] whereas low readings are produced if the thickness is secondary to corneal edema.[45]

The intraocular pressure is also influenced by corneal curvature, with a rise of approximately 1

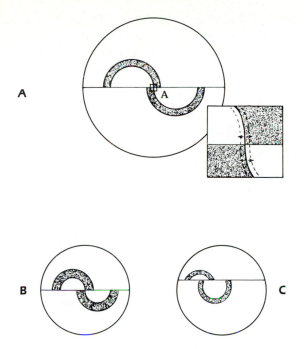

Fig. 15-3   Semicircles of Goldmann-type applanation tonometry. **A,** Proper width and position. Enlargement (A) depicts excursions of semicircles caused by ocular pulsations. **B,** Semicircles are too wide. **C,** Improper vertical and horizontal alignment. (From Shields, MB: Textbook of glaucoma, ed 2, Baltimore, 1986, Williams & Wilkins)

mm Hg for each 3 diopters increase in corneal power.[116] With more than 3 diopters of astigmatism, an elliptical rather than a circular area is produced on the applanated cornea, and this can lead to an erroneous intraocular pressure reading. When the tonometer prisms are in their usual orientation, with the mires displaced horizontally, the intraocular pressure is underestimated by about 1 mm Hg for every 4 diopters of astigmatism for with-the-rule astigmatism and overestimated by about the same amount for the against-the-rule astigmatism.[116] To minimize this error, the tonometer prisms should be rotated so that the axis of least corneal curvature is opposite the red line on the prism holder.[121] Alternatively, an equally accurate method of obtaining the intraocular pressure of an eye with substantial astigmatism is to obtain two intraocular pressure measurements with the mires oriented horizontally and vertically and average these readings.[116] The mires may also be distorted when applanating an irregular cornea, and this may interfere with the accuracy of the intraocular pressure measurement.[121]

Prolonged contact between the cornea and the tonometer prism can damage the corneal epithelium, as revealed by fluorescein staining, making multiple readings in a short time unsatisfactory.[121] Also, prolonged contact can induce an apparent decrease in intraocular pressure over a period of minutes.[121] This seems to be less pronounced in eyes with carotid occlusive disease, suggesting that it may be related to intraocular blood flow.[23]

To diminish the risk of transmitting ocular pathogens that might be present in the tears, care must be taken to sterilize the tonometer tip properly between patients. Hepatitis B surface antigen was detected in the tears of nearly half of carriers and was discovered on the tonometer tip in 25% of them.[120] Likewise, human T-lymphotropic virus type III (HTLV-III) has been detected in the tears of a patient with acquired immune deficiency syndrome (AIDS).[25] However, the chance of developing AIDS through tear transmission appears highly remote. A 10-minute immersion of the tonometer tip under running tap water has been reported to eliminate all detectable hepatitis B surface antigen from contaminated tonometers.[120] When more vigorous sterilization is desired, soaking the tonometer tip in household bleach (sodium hypochlorite)[129] or exposure to ultraviolet light[181] has been suggested. Other recommended precautions include a 5- to 10-minute soak in fresh hydrogen peroxide or 70% ethanol or isopropanol.[25] The tip should be washed under running water and dried before use. To handle large numbers of patient examinations, this approach requires two tips per tonometer.

The Goldmann tonometer is the standard against which other tonometers are measured.[164] However, when two intraocular pressure measurements are taken with the same Goldmann applanation tonometer within a short time of each other, using either one instrument and one examiner[123] or two instruments and two examiners,[138] at least 30% of the two measurements will vary by 2 and 3 mm Hg or more, respectively. This discrepancy may occur as a result of the subjective nature of the optical end point, and consequently, an error of approximately 2 mm Hg must be assumed to be inherent even in the most accurate pressure measuring devices.

Other applanation tonometers

Several variants of the variable force applanation tonometer have been developed.[83] The Perkins (Fig. 15-4) and Draeger (Fig. 15-5) applanation tonometers are two varieties of hand-held tonometers.

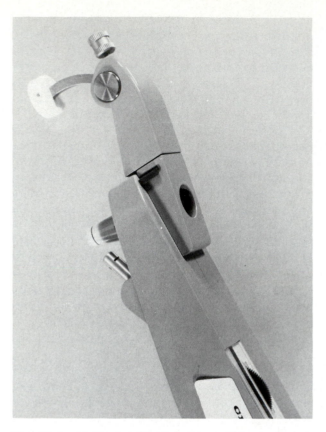

Fig. 15-4 Perkins hand-held tonometer. This tonometer is as accurate but less costly than most other hand-held applanation tonometers. (From Kolker, AE, and Hetherington, J, Jr: Becker-Shaffer's diagnosis and therapy of the glaucomas, St. Louis, 1983, The CV Mosby Co)

Perkins applanation tonometer. The Perkins applanation tonometer uses the same prisms as the Goldmann tonometer, but it is counter balanced so that tonometry can be performed in any position. Illumination of the prism is obtained from four battery-powered bulbs. The force on the prisms is adjusted manually.[135] Its accuracy is comparable with the Goldmann tonometer in both the horizontal and vertical positions.[43,98,147] Being portable, it is particularly practical when measuring the intraocular pressure of infants and children and for use in the operating room for examinations under anesthesia.

Draeger applanation tonometer. The Draeger applanation tonometer is similar to the Perkins but uses a different set of prisms and operates with a motor adjusting the force on these prisms.[38,39] Although it is also portable, there is some disagreement as to its accuracy.[48,98,140] The Perkins and Draeger tonometers are somewhat large; require considerable training to use; and share similar difficulties with the Goldmann tonometer when used on patients with irregular corneas, blepharospasm, and tremors. The Draeger tonometer is somewhat more difficult to use than the Perkins. An inexpensive version has been designed in which Goldmann prisms are mounted on a dynamometer and connected to a blue penlight.[183]

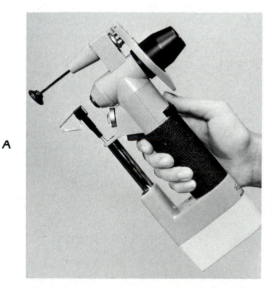

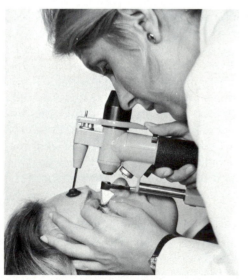

A

B

Fig. 15-5 **A,** Draeger applanation tonometer. **B,** Tonometer in use on a reclining patient. (From Kolker, AE, and Hetherington, J, Jr: Becker-Shaffer's diagnosis and therapy of the glaucomas, St. Louis, 1983, The CV Mosby Co)

Mackay-Marg tonometer. The Mackay-Marg tonometer incorporates a 1.5 mm diameter plunger affixed to a rigid spring that extends 10 μm beyond the plane of a surrounding rubber sleeve. Movement of the plunger is electronically monitored by a transducer and recorded on a moving paper strip.[115] When the tonometer plunger is placed against the cornea, the tracing representing the force against the plunger begins to rise. When an area of 1.5 mm in diameter of the cornea has been applanated, the tracing reaches a peak. At this point, the force against the end of the plunger represents both the intraocular pressure and the force required to deform the cornea. As the tonometer is advanced, the cornea flattens further and the force required to deform the cornea is transferred from the plunger to the surrounding sleeve, creating a dip in the tracing.[111] The trough in the tracing represents the intraocular pressure. With further advance of the tonometer, the area of corneal applanation is increased further, and the force re-corded on the pressure tracing continues to rise again because the intraocular pressure is being artificially elevated[115] (Fig. 15-6). Since the Mackay-Marg tonometer gives instantaneous intraocular pressure recordings, several readings should be averaged in order to account for fluctuation due to ocular pulsations.

The Mackay-Marg tonometer was reported to correlate well with the Goldmann but reads systematically higher.[124] Another study revealed significant disparities between the Mackay-Marg and Goldmann intraocular pressure estimates when a technician was measuring the intraocular pressure with a Mackay-Marg tonometer.[136] In eyes with scarred, edematous, or irregular corneas, the Mackay-Marg tonometer is generally considered to be the most accurate.[91,117] Also, the effects of corneal resistance to deformation and surface tension of tears has less of an influence on the intraocular pressure with a Mackay-Marg tonometer than with a Goldmann tonometer because with the former,

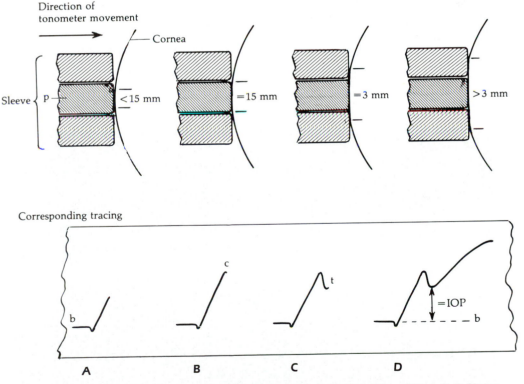

Fig. 15-6   Mackay-Marg tonometry. (Modified from Marg, E, Mackay, RS, and Oechsli, R: Vision Res 1:379, 1962). **A,** As plate (p) contacts cornea, tracing begins to rise. **B,** Crest (c) is reached when diameter of contact equals that of plate surface (1.5 mm). **C,** With further corneal flattening, force of bending cornea is transferred to sleeve, and tracing falls to trough (t) when diameter of contact equals 3 mm. **D,** Still further corneal flattening leads to artificial elevation of intraocular pressure (IOP). Distance from baseline (b) of tracing to trough is read as the IOP. (From Shields, MB: Textbook of glaucoma, ed 2, Baltimore, 1986, Williams & Wilkins)

which applanates a considerably smaller surface area, these effects are greatly minimized.[75] After undergoing epikeratophakia, the intraocular pressure of primate eyes was controlled with a transducer, and the Mackay-Marg tonometer gave reliable intraocular pressure measurements above 20 mm Hg, but was not accurate below this level, whereas the Goldmann tonometer was accurate over the entire pressure range.[131]

Tono-Pen. A number of tonometers similar to the Mackay-Marg performed unsatisfactorily.[12,18,59,109] Because it was not widely used, the Mackay-Marg tonometer is no longer manufactured. A new tonometer, the Tono-Pen (Fig. 15-7), which is portable and battery-operated, uses principles similar to the Mackay-Marg tonometer. The tip has a strain gauge that is activated when it touches the cornea. The built-in microprocessor logic circuit senses a trough force similar to the one measured with a Mackay-Marg tonometer and registers that until an acceptable measurement has been achieved. If the logic circuit does not sense a proper shape to the force curve, that particular measurement is rejected. Four to ten acceptable measurements are averaged to give a final intraocular pressure, which is displayed as a digital readout. The number of measurements necessary to achieve an average reading varies depending on how close the individual measurements are to each other. An indication of the variability and reliability of these measurements, the standard error of the mean, is reported as a percentage of the average.

The probe tip is applied perpendicularly to the cornea until the cornea is just indented. An audible click indicates that the measurement is acceptable. This process is repeated two to ten times until a beep indicates that enough data have been collected to determine a statistically valid average reading. The end point is determined electronically, not optically, and the average of the measurements is displayed in a quartz crystal digital display. An indicator of the reliability and variability of the individual measurements is reported as a standard deviation in terms of the percentage of the displayed average pressure reading. This is displayed by a bar over the 5, 10, 15, or 20 percent markings. The tip of the tonometer is protected by a disposable latex cover.

For pressures of 6 to 24 mm Hg, the Tono-Pen measured on the average 1.7 mm Hg higher than the Goldmann tonometer. In the range above 24 mm Hg, no significant difference was found in the pressures measured with the two instruments.[119]

Pneumatonometer. The pneumatonometer is similar to the Mackay-Marg tonometer in that a core sensing mechanism measures the intraocular

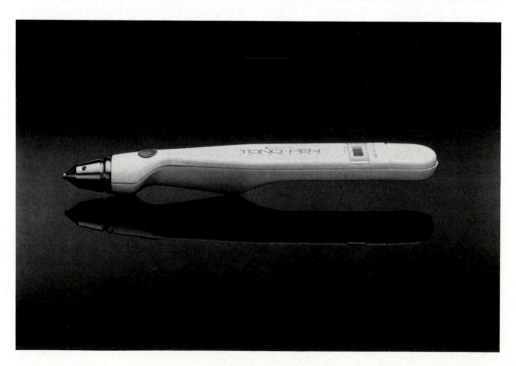

Fig. 15-7　Tono-Pen.

pressure while the force required to bend the cornea is transferred to a surrounding structure. However, unlike the Mackay-Marg tonometer, which has an electronically controlled plunger, the sensor in a pneumatonometer is air pressure.[44,102]

The pneumatonometer is composed of four major components. A sensing unit responds to intraocular pressure when applied to the eye. A pneumatic-to-electric transducer converts the pneumatic signal from the sensor to an electrical signal. A combined amplifier and recording unit processes the signal and provides a visual readout from which the intraocular pressure can be determined. Finally, an air supply unit provides compressed air to operate the sensor. At the end of the sensing unit is a sensing nozzle, which has an outer diameter of approximately 6 mm and a central chamber of 2 mm. The nozzle is covered with a Silastic diaphragm, and a constant flow of pressurized air is expelled through an opening in the central chamber between the nozzle and the diaphragm. The air pressure is dependent on the resistance to the exhaust, and the pneumatic-to-electronic transducer and the combined amplifier and recording unit converts the air pressure to a tracing on a strip of paper.[44] The pneumatonometer can also be used for continuous intraocular pressure monitoring.

Measurements with the pneumatonometer correlate well with those made with the Goldmann applanation tonometer,[81,146] even when the pneumatonometer is operated by a technician.[96] However, it gives significantly higher intraocular pressure estimates.[81,146] The pneumatonometer is useful in eyes with scarred, edematous, and irregular corneas;[99,177] in one study involving cannulated eye bank eyes with abnormal corneas, it yielded more consistent and objective measurements than the Mackay-Marg.[51]

The Mackay-Marg,[127] pneumatonometer,[99] and Tono-Pen can measure the intraocular pressures through a soft contact lens with satisfactory accuracy. However, applanation tonometry on contact lenses with high water content is affected by the power of the lens, and correction tables have been developed to compensate for this.[40]

Constant Force Applanation Tonometry

Maklakov applanation tonometer

The Maklakov applanation tonometer is the prime example of constant force applanation tonometry.[114,141] It is based on the principle that the intraocular pressure can be estimated by measuring the diameter of the corneal area flattened by a known weight of the tonometer.

The tonometer is a dumbbell-shaped metal cylinder with end plates of polished glass on either end with diameters of 10 mm. Identical instruments weighing 5, 7.5, 10, and 15 g are used to measure the intraocular pressure. A thin layer of dye is spread onto the bottom of either end plate, and the instrument is allowed to make contact with the anesthetized cornea of a supine patient for 1 second. A circular white imprint on the end plate results, the diameter of which is measured with a transparent plastic measuring scale to 0.1 mm. If the imprint is oval, either the cornea is astigmatic or the tonometer was moved during the applanation. From the formula

$$P = \frac{W}{\pi r^2} \qquad (15.4)$$

P is expressed in terms of grams/mm². By dividing this value by 136, a conversion to mm Hg can be made. Alternatively, conversion tables of different diameters using columns of corresponding weights have been devised.[141,142]

Corrections must be made for ocular ridigity, the force required to bend the cornea, the force of the tear film surface tension, and tear impingement into the thin layer of dye. New conversion tables that provide nomograms allowing for the extrapolation of intraocular pressure when performing tonometry with two or more weights have been developed.[151]

The Maklakov tonometer is quite popular in the Soviet Union and China but has not gained wide popularity in western countries. Several variations to the original design have been described in the American literature,* but none have gained a wide acceptance.

Noncontact tonometer

The noncontact tonometer flattens the corneal apex by means of a jet of air.[69] The force of the air jet, which is generated by a solenoid-activated piston, increases linearly over time. An optoelectronic applanation monitoring system consisting of a transmitter, which directs a collimated beam of light at the corneal apex, and a receiver and detector, which accepts only parallel coaxial rays of light reflected from the cornea, determines the time required to flatten the cornea. When the cornea is flattened, the reflected light is at peak intensity.

---

*References 11, 70, 87, 97, 143, 144.

The time elapsed is directly related to the force of the jet necessary to flatten the cornea and correspondingly to the intraocular pressure. The various time intervals, which have been calibrated against measurements with the Goldmann applanation tonometer, are converted to an intraocular pressure and are displayed on a digital readout in mm Hg.[50,68,159]

Because the time interval for a typical noncontact tonometer measurement is between 1 and 3 msec, which is .002 of a cardiac cycle, any one measurement is random with respect to the phase of the cardiac cycle; and, consequently, the ocular pulse becomes a significant source of variability. Repeated readings on the same eye with a noncontact tonometer produce a variation of 1 to 3 mm Hg.[49,69,128] Furthermore, glaucomatous eyes have a significantly greater range of momentary fluctuations in intraocular pressure.[50] Therefore, because the probability increases with repeated tonometric measurements that an instantaneous pressure measurement will lie within a given range of mean intraocular pressures, it is recommended that consecutive readings are taken for each eye until a cluster of three measurements within 3 mm Hg is obtained. These are averaged as the intraocular pressure estimate.

The noncontact tonometer is accurate if the intraocular pressure is near normal, but its accuracy is diminished with higher intraocular pressures and in eyes with abnormal corneas or poor fixation.[49,69,84,118] One study showed a close correlation between the mean intraocular pressures obtained by the noncontact tonometer and the Goldmann applanation tonometer but also found considerable individual patient variation.[35] Corneal abrasions, reaction to topical anesthetic, and the transmission of infectious agents are eliminated with the use of noncontact tonometers, and because this instrument can be used reliably by paramedical personnel, it is particularly valuable in mass screening of intraocular pressures.

Continuous Intraocular Pressure Measuring Devices

A tonometer is needed that can continuously monitor the intraocular pressure for hours to days without influencing the pressure. A preliminary device has been investigated in which a flush-fitting Silastic gel contact lens instrumented with strain gauges measures changes in the meridional angle of the corneoscleral junction caused by variations in the intraocular pressure.[67] A similar device using a pressure transducer made in the form of a cylindrical guard ring applanation tonometer has been described,[30,31] as well as a device using a strain gauge embedded in an encircling scleral band to measure the distention of the globe.[182] Finally, an instrument using suction cups has been designed to allow for bilateral recording of the intraocular pressure for up to 1 hour in supine subjects.[130]

Home Tonometry

Attempts have been made to have patients or their relatives measure the intraocular pressure at home during various times of the day either to look for elevated intraocular pressures or to assess the quality of intraocular pressure control. In the past, intraocular pressures were measured by a family member using a Schiøtz tonometer; the accuracy of the results were highly variable. A new instrument using the principles of applanation tonometry has been developed and can be used by the patient without assistance.[178,184,185] Attempts have also been made to estimate the intraocular pressure by measuring the duration of contact of a spring-driven hammer with the eye (impact tonometer)[34] or the frequency of a vibrating probe in contact with the cornea (Vibrotonometer).[149]

REFERENCES

1. Adams, AP, Freedman, A, and Henville, JD: Normocapneic anaesthesia for intraocular surgery, Br J Ophthalmol 63:204, 1979
2. Anderson, DR, and Grant, WM: Re-evaluation of the Schiøtz tonometer calibration, Invest Ophthalmol Vis Sci 9:430, 1970
3. Anderson, DR, and Grant, WM: The influence of position on intraocular pressure, Invest Ophthalmol Vis Sci 12:204, 1973
4. Antal, M, Mucsi, G, and Faludi, A: Ketamine anesthesia and intraocular pressure, Ann Ophthalmol 10:1281, 1978
5. Armaly, MF: On the distribution of applanation pressure, Arch Ophthalmol 73:11, 1965
6. Armaly, MF: The genetic determination of ocular pressure in the normal eye, Arch Ophthalmol 78:187, 1967
7. Armaly, MF, Monstavicius, BF, and Sayegh, RE: Ocular pressure and aqueous outflow facility in siblings, Arch Ophthalmol 80:354, 1968
8. Armaly, MF, and Salamoun, SG: Schiøtz and applanation tonometry, Arch Ophthalmol 70:603, 1963
9. Aronowitz, JT, and Brubaker, RS: Effect of intraocular gas on intraocular pressure, Arch Ophthalmol 94:1191, 1976
10. Banks, JLK, et al: Bedford glaucoma survey, Br Med J 1:791, 1968
11. Barraquer, JI: New applanation tonometer for operating room, Ophthalmologica 153:225, 1967

12. Barron, C, and Horn, D: A comparison of the Cavitron biotronics tonometer to the Goldmann tonometer, Am J Optom Physiol Opt 61:698, 1984

13. Bayard, WL: Comparison of Goldmann applanation and Schiøtz tonometer using 1948 and 1955 conversion scales, Am J Ophthalmol 69:1007, 1970

14. Becker, B: The decline in aqueous secretion and outflow facility with age, Am J Ophthalmol 46:731, 1958

15. Bengtsson, B: Comparison of Schiøtz and Goldmann tonometry in a population, Acta Ophthalmol (Copenh) 50:455, 1972

16. Bengtsson, B: Some factors affecting the distribution of intraocular pressure in a population, Acta Ophthalmol (Copenh) 50:33, 1972

17. Biro, I, and Botar, Z: On the behavior of intraocular tension in various sport activities, Klin Monatsbl Augenheilkd 140:23, 1962

18. Blondeau, P: Clinical evaluation of the Dicon CAT 100 applanation tonometer, Am J Ophthalmol 99:708, 1985

19. Bonomi, L, Mecca, E, and Massa, F: Intraocular pressure in myopic anisometropia, Int Ophthalmol 5:145, 1982

20. Bowen, DJ, McGrand, JC, and Hamilton, AG: Intraocular pressures after suxamethonium and endotracheal intubation, Anesthesia 33:518, 1978

21. Boyd, TAS, and McLeod, LE: Circadian rhythms of plasma corticoid levels, intraocular pressure and aqueous outflow facility in normal and glaucomatous eyes, Ann NY Acad Sci 117:597, 1964

22. Brubaker, RF, et al: The effect of age on aqueous humor formation in man, Ophthalmology 88:283, 1981

23. Bynke, H, and Wilke, K: Repeated applanation tonometry in carotid occlusive disease, Acta Ophthalmol (Copenh) 52:125, 1974

24. Carel, RS, Korczyn, AD, Rock, M, and Goya, I: Association between ocular pressure and certain health parameters, Ophthalmology 91:311, 1984

25. Center for Disease Control: Recommendations for preventing possible transmission of human T-lymphotropic virus type III/lymphadenopathy-associated virus in tears. Morbid Mortal Weekly Rep, 34:553, 1985

26. Coad, CT, Osato, MS, and Wilhelmus, KR: Bacterial contamination of eyedrop dispensers, Am J Ophthalmol 98:548, 1984

27. Coleman, DJ, and Trokel, S: Direct-recorded intraocular pressure variations in a human subject, Arch Ophthalmol 82:637, 1969

28. Colton, T, and Ederer, F: The distribution of intraocular pressures in the general population, Surv Ophthalmol 25:123, 1980

29. Cook, J, and Friberg, TR: Effect of inverted body position on intraocular pressure, Am J Ophthalmol 98:784, 1984

30. Cooper, RL, Beale, DG, Constable, IJ, and Grose, GC: Continual monitoring of intraocular pressure: effect of central venous pressure, respiration, and eye movements on continual recordings of intraocular pressure in the rabbit, dog, and man, Br J Ophthalmol 63:799, 1979

31. Cooper, RL, Beale, DG, and Constable, IJ: Passive radiotelemetry of intraocular pressure in vivo: calibration and validation of continual scleral guard-ring applanation transensors in the dog and rabbit, Invest Ophthalmol Vis Sci 18:930, 1979

32. Couch, JA, Eltringham, RJ, and Magauran, DM: The effect of thiopentone and fazadinium on intraocular pressure, Anaesthesia 34:586, 1979

33. Cunningham, AJ, Albert, O, Cameron, J, and Watson, AG: The effect of intravenous diazepam on rise of intraocular pressure following succinylcholine, Can Anaesth Soc J 28:591, 1981

34. Dekking, HM, and Coster, HD: Dynamic tonometry, Ophthalmologica 154:59, 1967

35. Derka, H: The American optical non-contact tonometer and its results compared with the Goldmann applanation tonometer, Klin Monatsbl Augenheilkd 177:634, 1980

36. Deodati, F, Fontan, P, and Moulendous, JM: La tension oculaire du grand myope, Arch d'Ophtalmol (Paris) 34:77, 1974

37. Draeger, J: Die Abhängigkeit des Rigiditätskoeffizienten von der Höhe des intraokularen Druckes, Ophthalmologica 140:55, 1960

38. Draeger, J: Principal and clinical application of a portable applanation tonometer, Invest Ophthalmol Vis Sci 6:132, 1967

39. Draeger, J: Simple hand applanation tonometer for use in the seated as well as on the supine patient, Am J Ophthalmol 62:1208, 1966

40. Draeger, J: Applanation tonometry on contact lenses with high water content: problems, results, correction factors, Klin Monatsbl Augenheilkd 176:38, 1980

41. Drance, SM: The coefficient of scleral rigidity in normal and glaucomatous eyes, Arch Ophthalmol 63:668, 1960

42. Duncalf, D: Anesthesia and intraocular pressure, Trans Am Acad Ophthalmol Otolaryngol 79:562, 1975

43. Dunn, JS, and Brubaker, RF: Perkins applanation tonometer, clinical and laboratory evaluation, Arch Ophthalmol 89:149, 1973

44. Durham, DG, Bigliano, RP, and Masino, JA: Pneumatic applanation tonometer, Trans Am Acad Ophthalmol Otolaryngol 69:1029, 1965

45. Ehlers, N, Bramsen, T, and Sperling, S: Applanation tonometry and central corneal thickness, Acta Ophthalmol (Copenh) 53:34, 1975

46. Epstein, HM, Fagman, W, Bruce, DL, and Abram, A: Intraocular pressure changes during anesthesia for electroshock therapy, Anesth Analg 54:479, 1975

47. Feldman, F, Bain, J, and Matuk, AR: Daily assessment of ocular and hormonal variables throughout the menstrual cycle, Arch Ophthalmol 96:1835, 1978

48. Finlay, RD: Experience with the Draeger applanation tonometer, Trans Ophthalmol Soc UK 90:887, 1970

49. Forbes, M, Pico, G, Jr, and Grolman, B: A noncontact applanation tonometer, Sight Saving Rev 43:155, 1973

50. Forbes, M, Pico, G, and Grolman, B: A noncontact applanation tonometer description and clinical evaluation, Arch Ophthalmol 91:134, 1974

51. Foster, CS, and Yamamoto, GK: Ocular rigidity in keratoconus, Am J Ophthalmol 86:802, 1978

52. Friedenwald, JS: Contribution to the theory and practice of tonometry, Am J Ophthalmol 20:985, 1937

53. Friedenwald, JS: Some problems in the calibration of tonometers, Am J Ophthalmol 31:935, 1948

54. Friedenwald, JS: Standardization of tonometers decennial report, Trans Am Acad Ophthalmol Otolaryngol 1954

55. Friedenwald, JS: Tonometer calibration: an attempt to remove discrepancies found in the 1954 calibration scale for Schiøtz tonometers, Trans Am Acad Ophthalmol Otolaryngol 61:108, 1957

56. Galin, MA, McIvor, JW, and Magruder, GB: Influence of position on intraocular pressure, Am J Ophthalmol 55:720, 1963

57. Gallin-Cohen, PF, Podos, SM, and Yablonski, ME: Oxygen lowers intraocular pressure, Invest Ophthalmol Vis Sci 19:43, 1980

58. Gartner, J: Aging changes in the ciliary epithelium border layers and their significance for intraocular pressure, Am J Ophthalmol 72:1079, 1971

59. Gelatt, KN, Gum, GG, and Barrie, KP: Tonometry in glaucomatous globes, Invest Ophthalmol Vis Sci 20:683, 1981

60. Goldmann, H, and Schmidt, T: Uber Applanationstonometrie, Ophthalmologica 134:221, 1957

61. Goldmann, H, and Schmidt, T: Weiterer Beitrag zur applanations Tonometrie, Ophthalmologica 141:441, 1961

62. Goldstein, JH, Gupta, MK, and Shah, MD: Comparison of intramuscular and intravenous succinylcholine on intraocular pressure, Ann Ophthalmol 13:173, 1981

63. Graham, P, and Hollows, FC: Sources of variation in tonometry, Trans Ophthalmol Soc UK 84:597, 1964

64. Grant, WM: Fluorescein for applanation tonometry. More convenient and uniform application, Am J Ophthalmol 55:1252, 1963

65. Green, K: Ocular effects of diacetyl morphine and lysergic acid diethylamide in rabbits, Invest Ophthalmol Vis Sci 14:325, 1975

66. Green, K, and Luxemberg, MN: Consequences of eyelid squeezing on intraocular pressure, Am J Ophthalmol 88:1072, 1979

67. Greene, ME, and Gilman, BG: Intraocular pressure measurement with instrumented contact lenses, Invest Ophthalmol Vis Sci 13:299, 1985

68. Grolman, B: A new tonometer system, Am J Optom Arch Am Acad Optom 49:646, 1972

69. Grolman, B: Non-contact applanation tonometry, Optician 166:4, 1973

70. Halberg, GP: Hand applanation tonometer, Trans Am Acad Ophthalmol Otolaryngol 72:112, 1968

71. Harbin, TS Jr, et al: Applanation-Schiøtz disparity after retinal detachment surgery utilizing cryopexy, Ophthalmology 86:1609, 1979

72. Hetlind-Eriksen, J: On tonometry. 2. Pressure recordings by Schiøtz tonometry on enucleated human eyes, Acta Ophthalmol (Copenh) 44:12, 1966

73. Hiatt, RL, et al: Systemically administered anticholinergic drugs and intraocular pressure, Arch Ophthalmol 84:735, 1970

74. Hiller, R, Sperduto, RD, and Krueger, DE: Race, iris pigmentation, and intraocular pressure, Am J Epidemiol 115:674, 1982

75. Hilton, GF, and Shafer, RN: Electronic applanation tonometry, Am J Ophthalmol 62:838, 1966

76. Hollows, FC, and Graham, PA: Intraocular pressure glaucoma and suspects in a defined population, Br J Ophthalmol 50:570, 1966

77. Hollows, FC, and Graham, PA: The Ferndale glaucoma survey. In Hunt, LD, editor: Glaucoma epidemiology, early diagnosis and some aspects of treatment, Edinburgh, 1966, E. and S. Livingston Ltd

78. Holtz, SJ: Clinical study of the safety of a fluorescein-anesthetic solution, Ann Ophthalmol 7:1101, 1975

79. Houle, RE, and Grant, WM: Alcohol, vasopressin, and intraocular pressure, Invest Ophthalmol Vis Sci 6:145, 1967

80. Iverson, DG, and Brown, DW: Diurnal variation of intraocular pressure and serum osmolality, Exp Eye Res 6:179, 1967

81. Jain, MR, and Marmion, VJ: A clinical evaluation of applanation pneumatonograph, Br J Ophthalmol 60:107, 1976

82. Jain, MR, and Marmion, VJ: Rapid pneumatic and Mackay-Marg applanation tonometry to evaluate the postural effect on intraocular pressure, Br J Ophthalmol 60:687, 1976

83. Jensen, JB: An ocular tension indicator of the applanation type, Acta Ophthalmol (Copenh) 45:546, 1967

84. Jessen, K, and Hoffman, F: Current standardization of air-pulse tonometers and methods of air-pulse tonometers and methods of testing them, taking the non-contact tonometer II as an example, Klin Monatsbl Augenheilkd 183:296, 1983

85. Johnson, M, Kass, MA, Moses, RA, and Grodzski, WJ: Increased corneal thickness simulating elevated intraocular pressure, Arch Ophthalmol 96:664, 1978

86. Kahn, HA, et al: The Framingham Eye Study. 1. Outline and major prevalence findings, Am J Epidemiol 106:17, 1977

87. Kaiden, JS, Zimmerman, TJ, and Worthen, DM: An evaluation of the Glauco Test screening tonometer, Arch Ophthalmol 92:195, 1974

88. Kashgarian, M, et al: The frequency distribution of intraocular pressure by age and sex groups, JAMA 197:611, 1966

89. Kass, MA, and Sears, ML: Hormonal regulation of intraocular pressure, Surv Ophthalmol 22:153, 1977

90. Kaufman, HE: Pressure measurement: which tonometer? Invest Ophthalmol Vis Sci 11:80, 1972

91. Kaufman, HE, Wind, CA, and Waltman, SR: Validity of Mackay-Marg electronic applanation tonometer in patients with scarred irregular corneas, Am J Ophthalmol 69:1003, 1970

92. Kielar, RA, Teraslinna, P, Kearney, JT, and Barker, D: Effect of changes of PCO_2 on intraocular tension, Invest Ophthalmol Vis Sci 16:534, 1977

93. Kimura, R, and Maekawa, N: Effect of orally administered hydrocortisone on the ocular tension in primary open-angle glaucoma subjects. Preliminary report, Acta Ophthalmol (Copenh) 54:430, 1976

94. Kindler-Loosli, C, and Schmidt, T: Intraocular pressure after changing the patient's position, v Graefes Arch Klin Exp Ophthalmol 194:17, 1975

95. Klein, BE, and Klein, R: Intraocular pressure and cardiovascular risk variables, Arch Ophthalmol 99:837, 1981

96. Krieglstein, GK: Screening tonometry by technicians, v Graefes Arch Klin Exp Ophthalmol 194:221, 1975

97. Krieglstein, GK, Brethfeld, V, and Colani, E: Comparative intraocular pressure measurements with position in dependent and applanation tonometers, v Graefes Arch Klin Exp Ophthalmol 199:101, 1976

98. Krieglstein, GK, and Waller, WK: Goldmann applanation versus hand-applanation and Schiøtz identation tonometry, v Graefes Arch Klin Exp Ophthalmol 194:11, 1975

99. Krieglstein, GK, Waller, WK, Reimers, H, and Langham, ME: Intraocular pressure measurements on soft contact lenses, v Graefes Arch Klin Exp Ophthalmol 199:223, 1976

100. Kronfeld, PC: Tonometer calibration empirical validation. The committee on standardization of tonometers, Trans Am Acad Ophthalmol Otolaryngol 61:123, 1957

101. Kypke, W, and Hermannspann, U: Glaucoma physical activity and sports, Klin Monatsbl Augenheilkd 164:321, 1974

102. Langham, ME, and McCarthy, E: A rapid pneumatic applanation tonometer. Comparative findings and evaluation, Arch Ophthalmol 79:389, 1968

103. Lazenby, GW, Reed, JW, and Grant, WM: Short-term tests of anticholinergic medication in open-angle glaucoma, Arch Ophthalmol 80:443, 1968

104. Lazenby, GW, Reed, JW, and Grant, WM: Anticholinergic medication in open-angle glaucoma, Arch Ophthalmol 84:719, 1970

105. Lempert, P, Cooper, KH, Culver, JF, and Tredici, TJ: The effect of exercise on intraocular pressure, Am J Ophthalmol 63:673, 1967

106. Levene, RZ, Workman, PL, Broder, SW, and Hirschhorn, K: Heritability of ocular pressure in normal and suspect ranges, Arch Ophthalmol 84:730, 1970

107. Leydhecker, W: Zur der Breitung des Glaucoma Simplex in der Scheinbar gesunden Augenartzlich nicht behandelten Bevolkerung, Doc Ophthalmol 13:350, 1959

108. Leydhecker, W, Akiyama, K, and Neumann, HG: Der intraokulare Druck gesender menschlicher Augen, Klin Monatsbl Augenheilkd 133:622, 1958

109. Lim, JI, and Ruderman, JM: Comparison of the challenger digital applanation tonometer and the Goldmann applanation tonometer, Am J Ophthalmol 102:154, 1986

110. Losada, F, and Wolintz, AH: Bell's palsy: a new ophthalmologic sign, Ann Ophthalmol 5:1093, 1973

111. Mackay, RS, and Marg, E: Fast, automatic, electronic tonometers based on exact theory, Acta Ophthalmol (Copenh) 37:495, 1959

112. Macri, FJ, and Brubaker, RF: Methodology of eye pressure measurement, Biorheology 6:37, 1969

113. Maddox, TS Jr, and Kielar, RA: Comparison of the influence of ketamine and halothane anesthesia on intraocular tensions of nonglaucomatous children, J Pediatr Ophthalmol 11:90, 1974

114. Maklakov: L'ophthalmotonometrie, Arch Ophthalmol (Paris) 5:159, 1885

115. Marg, E, Mackay, RS, and Oechsli, R: Trough height, pressure and flattening in tonometry, Vision Res 1:379, 1962

116. Mark, HH: Corneal curvature in applanation tonometry, Am J Ophthalmol 76:223, 1973

117. McMillan, F, and Forster, RK: Comparison of Mackay-Marg, Goldmann, and Perkins tonometers in abnormal corneas, Arch Ophthalmol 93:420, 1975

118. Mehra, KS, Roy, PN, and Khare, BB: Tobacco smoking and glaucoma, Ann Ophthalmol 8:462, 1976

119. Minckler, DS, et al: Clinical evaluation of the Oculab Tono-Pen, Am J Ophthalmol 104:168, 1987

120. Moniz, E, et al: Removal of hepatitis B surface antigen from a contaminated applanation tonometer, Am J Ophthalmol 91:522, 1981

121. Moses, RA: The Goldmann applanation tonometer, Am J Ophthalmol 46:865, 1958

122. Moses, RA, and Arnzen, RJ: Instantaneous tonometry, Arch Ophthalmol 101:249, 1983

123. Moses, RA, and Liu, CH: Repeated applanation tonometry, Am J Ophthalmol 66:89, 1968

124. Moses, RA, Marg, E, and Oechsli, R: Evaluation of the basic validity and clinical usefulness of the Mackay-Marg tonometer, Invest Ophthalmol Vis Sci 1:78, 1962

125. Moses, RA, and Tarkkanen, A: Tonometry: the pressure-volume relationship in the intact human eye at low pressures, Am J Ophthalmol 47:557, 1959

126. Meyers, EF, Krupin, T, Johnson, M, and Zink, H: Failure of nondepolarizing neuromuscular blockers to inhibit succinylcholine-induced increased intraocular pressure, a controlled study, Anesthesiology 48:149, 1978

127. Meyer, RF, Stanifer, RM, and Bobb, KC: Mackay-Marg tonometry over therapeutic soft contact lenses, Am J Ophthalmol 86:19, 1978

128. Myers, KJ, and Scott, CA: The non-contact ("air-puff") tonometer: variability and corneal staining, Am J Optom Physiol Opt 52:36, 1975

129. Nagington, J, Sutehall, GM, and Whipp, D: Tonometer disinfection and virus, Br J Ophthalmol 67:674, 1983

130. Nissen, OI: Bilateral recording of human intraocular pressure with an improved applanating suction cup tonograph, Acta Ophthalmol (Copenh) 58:377, 1980

131. Olson, PF, McDonald, MB, Werblin, TP, and Kaufman, HE: Measurement of intraocular pressure after epikeratophakia, Arch Ophthalmol 101:111, 1983

132. Peczon, JD, and Grant, WM: Sedatives, stimulants and intraocular pressure in glaucoma, Arch Ophthalmol 72:178, 1964

133. Peczon, JD, and Grant, WM: Glaucoma, alcohol, and intraocular pressure, Arch Ophthalmol 73:495, 1965

134. Pemberton, JW: Schiøtz-applanation disparity following retinal detachment surgery, Arch Ophthalmol 81:534, 1969

135. Perkins, ES: Hand-held applanation tonometer, Br J Ophthalmol 49:591, 1965

136. Petersen, WC, and Schlegel, WA: Mackay-Marg tonometry by technicians, Am J Ophthalmol 76:933, 1973

137. Petounis, AD, Chondrel, S, and Vadaluka-Sekioti, A: Effect of hypercapnea and hyperventilation on human intraocular pressure during general anesthesia following acetazolamide administration, Br J Ophthalmol 64:422, 1980

138. Phelps, CD, and Phelps, GK: Measurement of intraocular pressure: a study of its reproducibility, v Graefes Arch Klin Exp Ophthalmol 198:39, 1976

139. Piltz, JR, Starita, R, Miron, M, and Henkind, P: Momentary fluctuations of intraocular pressure in normal and glaucomatous eyes, Am J Ophthalmol 99:333, 1985

140. Pohjola, S, and Niiranen, M: Clinical evaluation of the Draeger tonometer, Acta Ophthalmol (Copenh) 46:1159, 1968

141. Posner, A: An evaluation of the Maklakov applanation tonometer, Ear Nose Throat Monthly 41:377, 1962

142. Posner, A: Practical problems in the use of the Maklakov tonometer, Ear Nose Throat Monthly 42:82, 1963

143. Posner, A: A new portable applanation tonometer, Ear Nose Throat Monthly, 43:88, 1964

144. Posner, A, and Inglima, R: The Tonomat applanation tonometer, Ear Nose Throat Monthly 46:996, 1967

145. Quickert, MH: A fluorescein-anesthetic solution for applanation tonometry, Arch Ophthalmol 77:734, 1967

146. Quigley, HA, and Langham, ME: Comparative intraocular pressure measurements with pneumotomograph and Goldmann tonometer, Am J Ophthalmol 80:266, 1975

147. Richter, RC, Stark, WJ, Cowan, C, and Pollack, IP: Tonometry on eyes with abnormal corneas, Glaucoma 2:508, 1980

148. Roper, DL: Applanation tonometry with and without fluorescein, Am J Ophthalmol 90:668, 1980

149. Roth, W, and Blake, DB: Vibration tonometry principles of the ViBro-tonometer, J Am Optom Assoc 34:971, 1963

150. Samuel, JR, and Beaugie, A: Effect of carbon dioxide on the intraocular pressure in man during general anesthesia, Br J Ophthalmol 58:62, 1974

151. Schmidt, TFA: Calibration of the Maklakoff tonometer, Am J Ophthalmol 77:740, 1974

152. Schreuder, M, and Linssen, GH: Intraocular pressure and anaesthesia. Direct measurement by needling anterior chamber in the monkey, Anaesthesia 27:165, 1972

153. Schutten, WH, and Van Horn, DL: The effects of ketamine sedation and ketamine-pentobarbitol anesthesia upon the intraocular pressure of the rabbit, Invest Ophthalmol Vis Sci 16:531, 1977

154. Schwartz, B: Primary open-angle glaucoma. In Duane, TD, and Jaeger, EA, editors: Clinical ophthalmology, vol 3, Hagerstown, MD, 1986, Harper & Row

155. Schwartz, JT, and Ell'osso, GG: Comparison of Goldmann and Schiøtz tonometry in a community, Arch Ophthalmol 75:788, 1966

156. Seddon, JM, Schwartz, B, and Flowerdew, G: Case-control study of ocular hypertension, Arch Ophthalmol 101:891, 1983

157. Shapiro, A, Shoenfeld, Y, and Shapiro, Y: The effect of standardized submaximal work load on intraocular pressure, Br J Ophthalmol 62:679, 1978

158. Shepard, RJ, Ponsford, E, Basu, PK, and LaBarre, R: Effects of cigarette smoking on intraocular pressure and vision, Br J Ophthalmol 62:682, 1978

159. Shields, MB: The non-contact tonometer. Its value and limitations, Surv Ophthalmol 24:211, 1980

160. Shiose, Y: The aging effect on intraocular pressure in an apparently normal population, Arch Ophthalmol 102:883, 1984

161. Shiose, Y, and Kawase, Y: A new approach to stratified normal intraocular pressure in a general population, Am J Ophthalmol 101:714, 1986

162. Shiose, Y, Kawase, Y, Sato, T, and Nakanishi, N: Multivariate analysis on normal ocular tension, Jpn J Clin Ophthalmol 35:197, 1981

163. Smith, JL, et al: The incidence of Schiøtz-applanation disparity, cooperative study, Arch Ophthalmol 77:305, 1967

164. Starrels, ME: The measurement of intraocular pressure, Int Ophthalmol Clin 19:9, 1979

165. Starrels, ME, Krupin, T, and Burde, RM: Bells' palsy and intraocular pressure, Ann Ophthalmol 7:1067, 1975

166. Stepanik, J: Why is the Schiøtz tonometer not suitable for measuring intraocular pressure? Klin Monatsbl Augenheilkd 176:61, 1980

167. Stepanik, J: Tonometry results using a corneal applanation 3.53 mm in diameter, Klin Monatsbl Augenheidlkd 184:40, 1984

168. Stewart, HL: Prolonged antibacterial activity of a fluorescein anesthetic solution, Arch Ophthalmol 88:385, 1972

169. Stewart, RH, LeBlanc, R, and Becker, B: Effects of exercise on aqueous dynamics, Am J Ophthalmol 69:245, 1970

170. Tomlinson, A, and Phillips, CI: Applanation tension and axial length of the eyeball, Br J Ophthalmol 54:548, 1970

171. Tsukahara, S, and Sasaki, T: Postural change of IOP in normal persons and in patients with primary wide open-angle glaucoma and low-tension glaucoma, Br J Ophthalmol 68:389, 1984

172. Valle, O: Effect of cyclopentolate on aqueous dynamics in incipient or suspected open-angle glaucoma, Acta Ophthalmolgica 51:52, 1973

173. Vucicevic, ZM, and Ralston, J: Influences of the volume and hydration changes on scleral rigidity, Ann Ophthalmol 4:715, 1972

174. Wallace, J, and Lovel, HG: Glaucoma and intraocular pressure in Jamaica, Am J Ophthalmol 67:93, 1969

175. Weber, AK, and Price, J: Pressure differential of intraocular pressure measured between supine and sitting position, Ann Ophthalmol 13:323, 1981

176. Weitzman, ED, Henkind, P, Leitman, M, and Hellman, L: Correlative 24-hour relationships between intraocular pressure and plasma cortisol in normal subjects and patients with glaucoma, Br J Ophthalmol 59:566, 1975

177. West, CE, Capella, JA, and Kaufman, HE: Measurement of intraocular pressure with a pneumatic applanation tonometer, Am J Ophthalmol 74:505, 1972

178. Wilensky, JT, et al: Self-tonometry to manage patients with glaucoma and apparently controlled intraocular pressure, Arch Ophthalmol 105:1072, 1987

179. Williams, BI, and Peart, WS: Effect of posture on the intraocular pressure of patients with retinal vein obstruction, Br J Ophthalmol 62:688, 1978

180. Williams, BI, Peart, WS, and Letley, E: Abnormal intraocular pressure control in systemic hypertension and diabetic mellitus, Br J Ophthalmol 64:845, 1980

181. Wizemann, A: Modified version of UV sterilizer to disinfect Goldmann tonometer heads, gonioscopes and fundus contact lenses, Klin Monatsbl Augenheilkd 181:40, 1982

182. Wolbarsht, ML, Wortman, J, Schwartz, B, and Cook, D: A scleral buckle pressure gauge for continuous monitoring of intraocular pressure, Int Ophthalmol 3:11, 1980

183. Yablonski, ME: A new portable applanation tonometer, Am J Ophthalmol 80:547, 1975

184. Zeimer, RC, et al: Evaluation of a self-tonometer for home use, Arch Ophthalmol 101:1791, 1983

185. Zeimer, RC, et al: Application of a self-tonometer to home tonometry, Arch Ophthalmol 104:49, 1986

Chapter 16

Circadian Variations in Intraocular Pressure

Ran C. Zeimer

Diurnal (circadian) variations in intraocular pressure were first reported by Sidler-Huguenin in 1898.[72] Using digital tonometry, Sidler-Huguenin found that the intraocular pressure of 10 glaucomatous patients peaked at night before sleep and in the morning 30 to 60 minutes after waking. Maslenikow[48] (1904) quantitated these measurements with the Maklakov tonometer and obtained a more precise idea of the variations. The topic has been so widely studied since then that a review in 1961 contained over 300 references.[54] The knowledge of variations in intraocular pressure is important for the diagnosis, treatment, and even prognosis of glaucoma.

Cycles of physiologic rhythms vary from intervals of seconds, as in respiratory and cardiac cycles, to months, such as the menses. It is generally accepted that the intraocular pressure varies over a 24-hour period. Because the term *diurnal* has been used to mean either a day of 24 hours or the hours of daylight, the word circadian (*circa* meaning about; *dies* meaning day) has been introduced to describe continuous oscillations with a frequency of about 24 hours.

This chapter considers the different methods by which the circadian intraocular pressure variations are measured, as well as their characteristics in normal subjects and in patients with ocular hypertension and glaucoma.

CHRONOBIOLOGY OF INTRAOCULAR PRESSURE

If the circadian variations in intraocular pressure were a pure biorhythm, they could be described by the cosine function:

$$IOP = IOP_{av} + A \cos 2\pi (t/T + Fee/T) \qquad (1)$$

where IOP_{av} is the average intraocular pressure, A is the amplitude, t the time of day, T the period of the rhythm, and Fee the phase. A detailed description of the chronobiology methods involved in cosine fitting has already been reported.[52]

A true circadian rhythm has a period T of approximately 24 hours, and it is generally accepted that the intraocular pressure varies with similar periodicity. When Kitazawa and Horie[40] attempted to fit a cosine function to data obtained in 24 normal subjects, they found that the period was 24 ± 4 hours. Ferrario et al.[21] fitted a cosine function with a period of 24 hours to the data obtained in 12 subjects and determined the phase, mean, and amplitude. However, Mercer[50] cautioned that measurements would have to be made at 6-hour intervals continually for a total of 3000 hours to obtain marginally adequate results. Thus the majority of studies of circadian intraocular pressure variations assume a 24-hour period and concentrate on the other variables included in the equation.

The amplitude (A) measured in mm Hg is the simplest parameter to obtain. If the circadian intraocular pressure variation obeyed equation 1 exactly, A would be equal to half the range, which is the difference between the highest and lowest readings in a day. In reality, the circadian intraocular pressure variation only follows equation 1 in average. Noise resulting from the variability of the measurement and short-term intraocular pressure variations are superimposed on this function. It is outside the scope of this chapter to detail the different short-term variations in intraocular pressure, such as the fast oscillations produced by the ocular pulse, pressure decreases caused by relaxation of extraocular and eyelid muscles, changes caused by accommodation, and fluctuations within less than an hour.[31,39,74] Because noise is superimposed on the cosine function, the range exceeds 2A because it is determined by the lowest and highest momentary values and not the averages. This finding is illustrated by the work of Kitazawa and Horie,[40] who obtained a range of 9.9 mm Hg, which exceeded the value of 5.4 mm Hg for 2A. The circadian variations generate a function over time, referred to as the circadian intraocular pressure curve. A small amplitude indicates a small variation in intraocular pressure corresponding to the clinical classification, flat type (see below).[37]

The phase, measured in hours, determines the time of day at which intraocular pressure reaches its maximum value. Different phases can be associated with different circadian curve types that have been identified clinically.

The circadian intraocular pressure curves can be classified into two major groups[37]: *regular* ones with a biorhythm that is generally similar on different days, or *irregular* ones with intraocular pressure peaks that occur at random (Fig. 16-1). Katavisto[37] suggested subdividing the regular circadian intraocular pressure curves into four categories: (1) the *morning type,* in which the intraocular pressure peaks between 4 and 8 AM and is lowest during the day or night (Fig. 16-2, *A*); (2) the *day type,* in which the tension peaks during the day, usually before noon, but sometimes in the afternoon, and the minimum intraocular pressure occurs during the night or evening (Fig. 16-2, *B*); (3) the *night type,* in which the maximum intraocular pressure is recorded between midnight and 4 AM, and the minimum is recorded during the day (Fig. 16-3, *A*); and (4) the *flat type,* in which the circadian intraocular pressure variation is too small to characterize a periodicity or phase (Fig. 16-3, *B*).

A phase of zero indicates that the maximum intraocular pressure is reached around midnight,

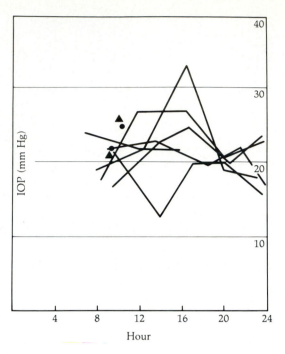

Fig. 16-1 Circadian intraocular pressure curves of varying (irregular) type. Each line represents a different day of testing. Triangles designate applanation tonometry performed in an office.

corresponding to the night type. Phases of 6 and 12 hours indicate the presence of intraocular pressure peaks around 6 AM and noon, respectively, corresponding to the morning and day types. Finally, in cases in which the noise is predominant, the circadian variations are erratic (especially if the measurements are spaced by many hours), causing varying results from day to day. These circadian curves are referred to clinically as the *variable type.*

It appears that the biorhythm expressed by equation 1 provides a theoretical frame that allows us to understand the classification of different types of circadian intraocular pressure curves. Most authors have reported their studies in terms of the mean, the range, and the circadian intraocular pressure curve type rather than the amplitude and the phase.

METHODS OF MEASUREMENT OF CIRCADIAN VARIATIONS IN INTRAOCULAR PRESSURE

In this section, the different protocols of measurements will be critically reviewed. The commercially available tonometers are described in Chapter 15; therefore, only the self-tonometer recently developed by Zeimer et al.[85-87] will be detailed here.

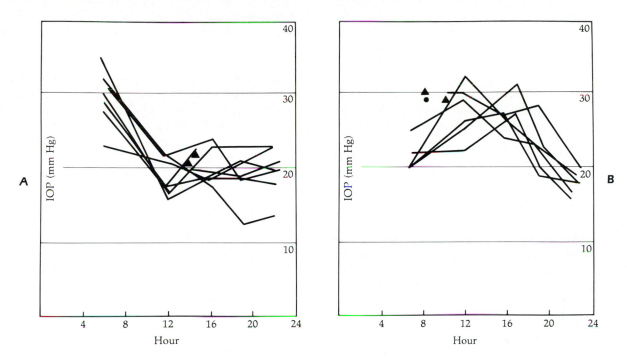

Fig. 16-2 **A,** Circadian intraocular pressure curves of morning type. Symbols are same as in Fig. 16-1. **B,** Circadian intraocular pressure curves of day type. Symbols are same as in Fig. 16-1.

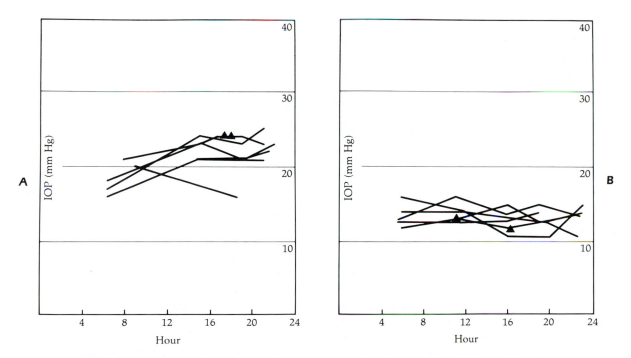

Fig. 16-3 **A,** Circadian intraocular pressure curves of night type. Symbols are same as in Fig. 16-1. **B,** Circadian intraocular pressure curves of flat type. Symbols are same as in Fig. 16-1.

Inpatient Measurements

One method of assessing circadian variation is to hospitalize the patient and repeat intraocular pressure measurements around the clock. The protocols for performing these measurements have differed markedly among clinicians.[61] Around-the-clock evaluations have not proved optimal, since the probability of damaging the corneal epithelium increases. The damaged epithelium also becomes more permeable to drugs, possibly artificially reducing the intraocular pressure. On the other hand, the intraocular pressure must be measured often enough to enhance the probability of detecting peaks, and the number of measurements that can be performed depends on the hospital staff and the comfort of the patient.

In 1965, some glaucoma experts[24] agreed that the preferred schedule was the one developed by Sampaolesi et al.[68] Seven tonometric readings were taken daily: at 6 AM, 9 AM, noon, 3 PM, 6 PM, 9 PM, and midnight. The authors indicated that the 3 AM measurement had no added clinical value and could be omitted. They advocated performing the first measurement while the patient was in bed and in a darkened room.

The obvious advantages of the inpatient procedure are that the intraocular pressure can be measured around the clock and that the patient is under constant medical supervision, which allows a more accurate assessment of the effectiveness of therapy because patient compliance is assured. The major disadvantages of this procedure are its cost, the drastic modification of the patient's normal activities (hospitalization is one of the exogeneous factors that affects circadian variations; see "Stability of the Rhythm"), and the limited number of days during which this procedure can be repeated.

Outpatient-hospital Combination

Many specialists have emphasized that the intraocular pressure should be measured during the patient's usual daily routine. Some centers have introduced a night dispensary system,[60,70] where the intraocular pressure is monitored on an outpatient basis during the day, and the patient is hospitalized only for night recordings. Although the cost is reduced and the patient's activities are less influenced, the activities are not totally normal, since the patient must remain near the clinic. This procedure is also limited by the number of days it can be repeated.

Office Measurements

A widely practiced method of obtaining information on circadian intraocular pressure variations is one in which the patient comes to the physician's office early in the morning and stays there while tonometry is performed numerous times until late afternoon. This procedure is more practical and less expensive than hospitalization. Its disadvantages are that the patient is not performing normal activities (for example, changing the normal sleep cycle to reach the office early), the method is limited to office hours during which the probability of pressure peaks is about 40%, and the number of days it can be repeated is limited. Some ophthalmologists prefer to measure intraocular pressure twice daily over a number of days at different hours each day.[44]

Home Tonometry

Tonometry performed by an assistant

To alleviate some of the disadvantages of methods used to assess the circadian intraocular pressure variations, it has been suggested that the patient be provided with an instrument that would allow the pressure to be measured in the patient's natural environment. Several researchers on the subject have taught a relative of the patient to use a Schiøtz tonometer to take repeated measurements for a number of days[4,19,34,46] Posner[59] replaced the Schiøtz tonometer with his Applanometer, which is a version of the Maklakov tonometer. The advantages of assisted home tonometry are that the circadian intraocular pressure variations are monitored over a number of days, the activities of the patient are not appreciably altered, and the cost of the procedure is minimal. A major drawback, however, is the necessity of a second person's assistance. Typically, patients and relatives are elderly and often are not capable or willing to perform the measurement. In addition, the measurements are limited to a setting in which the assistant is readily available.

Another disadvantage involves the instrumentation. The Schiøtz tonometer's accuracy and reproducibility are questionable, especially when the measurement is performed by a layperson. Complications may occur, such as corneal abrasions.[34] New handheld tonometers are on the market, but no data are available yet on their performance or safety, even by trained professionals.

Self-tonometry

The major limiting factor for the implementation of home self-tonometry appears to have been the lack of an instrument that is accurate, safe, and capable of being used by the patient alone. Zeimer et al.[85-87] have developed a self-tonometer to fill this need (Fig. 16-4).

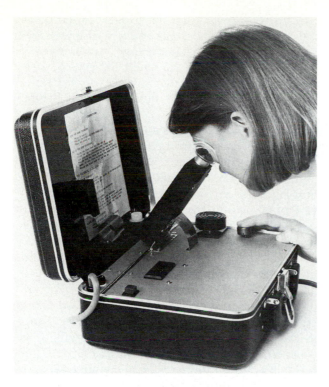

Fig. 16-4 Self-tonometer in use shows patient leaning orbit on eye cup, ready to depress activating knob.

Principle. The self-tonometer is designed to measure the pressure necessary to applanate the cornea. Since pressure rather than force is measured (as with the Goldmann applanation tonometer), it is not necessary to calculate the area of applanation, but only the pressure at which it occurs. The applanation is detected optically by monitoring the amount of light reflected from a flexible membrane that comes in contact with the cornea and to which is applied increasing air pressure. Because the probe must be located at and perpendicular to the apex of the cornea, the instrument is provided with a self-alignment system used by the patient. Finally, to prevent any danger of corneal abrasion, the probe comes in contact with the eye only when the measurement is performed (1.5 seconds) with its axial position automatically adjusted to the position of the eye.

Mode of operation. The patient desensitizes the cornea either by using a drop of topical anesthetic or by wearing a soft bandage contact lens during the one-week period of measurement. The patient places the orbit on an eye cup, views a target through the transparent probe by adjusting a knob, and aligns the orbit on the eye cup until a cross is viewed at the center of a white disc. At this point the patient presses a knob, which activates the au-

tomatically controlled air pressure that moves the probe forward until it touches and applanates the cornea. The probe retracts automatically after the intraocular pressure has been recorded, and the patient is informed if an adequate reading has been obtained. The procedure is repeated until four adequate readings are taken or six attempts have been made. The instrument requires no calibration or maintenance except to periodically wipe the probe's membrane and replace it for use in a different patient.

Performance. Circadian intraocular pressure curves were obtained in 151 individuals (12 normals, 20 ocular hypertensives, and 119 glaucoma patients) using the Goldmann tonometer.[87] About 85% of the subjects were then trained to use the self-tonometer outside the office. These patients had visual acuities ranging between 20/20 and 20/200. The main reasons for inadequate self-tonometry among patients with a visual acuity better than 20/200 were lack of motivation, psychologic problems, heavy blinking, insufficient eyelid clearance, and head instability. The average reproducibility in the patient's natural environment was ±1.4 mm Hg. In general, the patients needed four to five trials to obtain four good readings.[87] The correlation coefficient between the readings of the self-tonometer and those of the Goldmann applanation tonometer was 0.89, and the difference between the readings of the two instruments varied by ±2.5 mm Hg.[86,87] This value was within the range recommended for commercial tonometers and lower than those published for the pneumatonometer (±3.2 mm Hg) and for the noncontact tonometer (±4.6 mm Hg).[35] It was somewhat higher than the variability of ±1.8 mm Hg obtained between two Goldmann applanation tonometers, but equal to the variability of ±2.5 mm Hg in the measurements performed by two experienced ophthalmologists.[56]

Protocol. The patients in this study performed self-tonometry for 5 days, 5 times daily: in the morning when they woke, around noon, in midafternoon, in the evening after supper, and at bedtime. The intraocular pressure and its time of measurement were recorded by the patient. On completion, the patient returned to the clinic, performed self-tonometry, and underwent applanation tonometry. The data were gathered and processed to yield circadian curves, some examples of which are given in Figs. 16-1 to 16-3.

Conclusion. Advantages of the self-tonometer include: the protocol can be made to coincide with the optimal schedule chosen by experts[24]; the circadian curve can be repeated for a number of days;

the measurements are performed under natural conditions, even at the patient's place of work; and the cost of the procedure appears acceptable. However, it is restricted to patients who are motivated to perform the measurements for a few days and who have a visual accuity of 20/200 or better. It is possible that the concentrated attention given by the patient during the course of the measurements may actually enhance short-term compliance to therapy and not necessarily reflect long-term conditions.

CHARACTERISTICS OF CIRCADIAN VARIATIONS IN INTRAOCULAR PRESSURE
Range of Circadian Variations

Most of the published reports have dealt with the range of the circadian intraocular pressure variations rather than the amplitude.

Normals

The maximal ranges of circadian intraocular pressure variations reported by various authors are listed in Table 16-1. In general, most authors found a maximal range of less than 7 mm Hg, but some exceptional cases ranged up to 12 mm Hg. Specific information on the degree of circadian pressure variation in healthy eyes can be gleaned from studies with a large number of subjects and a well-documented methodology. Drance included 404 normal eyes of 220 subjects in an extensive study.[15] Intraocular pressure was measured by Schiøtz tonometry at 6 AM, 9 AM, 11:30 AM, 2 PM, 5 PM, and 10 PM, while the subject was hospitalized. The range of the circadian intraocular pressure varia-

tion was 3.7 ± 1.8 mm Hg. In 84% of the cases, the circadian variation was equal to or lower than 5 mm Hg, and the maximal range was 10 mm Hg. de Venecia and Davis examined 230 eyes of men, 80% of whom were under the age of 40 years.[13] Intraocular pressure was measured with Schiøtz tonometry at 5 AM, 10 AM, 2 PM, 7 PM, and midnight for 3 consecutive days. The range of the circadian variation decreased during the examination. In the first 24 hours it was 5.9 ± 3.0 mm Hg; in the second, 5.0 ± 2.4 mm Hg; and in the third, 4.9 ± 2.2 mm Hg. Katavisto evaluated the intraocular pressure of 50 healthy individuals of 54.1 ± 1.7 years mean age.[37] The pressure measurements were carried out with a Schiøtz tonometer in the hospital at 4 AM, 6 AM, 8 AM, 10 AM, 1 PM, 7 PM, and midnight. The range was similar in men and women: 3.17 ± 1.20 mm Hg. In 82% of the cases the amplitude was from 2 to 4 mm Hg, in 8% it was 5 mm Hg, and in 4% it was 6 mm Hg (the largest range in the series). Kitazawa and Horie[39] studied the circadian intraocular pressure variation in 12 normal subjects, whose measurements were taken in the hospital with a Goldmann applanation tonometer each hour around the clock. The range was 6.5 ± 1.4 mm Hg, with a maximum of 11 mm Hg. Approximately two fifths of the eyes had intraocular pressure ranges over 7.5 mm Hg.[39]

Glaucoma

The majority of the studies of the circadian intraocular pressure in glaucoma patients have been performed either after medical therapy was suspended or before therapy was initiated (Table 16-2). Factors that may have been responsible for the large range of values include differences in instrumentation, number of daily measurements, and the mean intraocular pressure of the glaucoma subjects. The range of circadian intraocular pressure variations is believed to be correlated with the mean intraocular pressure.[12,17,38,40,43]

Table 16-1 Maximal range of circadian intraocular pressure variations in the healthy eye

Maximum variation (mm Hg)	Authors*
3	Hagen (1924),[27] Maslenikow (1904),[48] Pissarello (1915),[58] Sampaolesi (1968)[68]
5	Adler (1959),[1] Agarwal (1959),[2] Duke-Elder (1952),[17] Eggink (1962),[18] Kollner (1916),[42] Matteuci (1953),[49] Radzikhovsky (1963),[62] Sugar (1957), Weinstein (1953)[80]
6	Blaxter (1956),[6] Feigenbaum (1928),[20] Katavisto (1964),[37] Perez-Bufill Pichot (1960),[55] Rohrschneider (1954),[65] Sallmann (1930),[66] Thiel (1924)[77]
7	Dobree (1953),[14] Thomassen (1946)[78]
9	Charbonneau (1954),[8] Cordes (1937)[9]
10	Drance (1960),[15] Kitazawa (1975),[39] Matteucci (1953),[49] Newell (1965),[53] Sallmann (1930)[66]
12	de Venecia (1963)[13]

*Only the first author is identified.

Table 16-2 Mean range of circadian intraocular pressure variations in glaucomatous eyes not receiving therapy

Authors*	No. of eyes	Mean ± SD (mm Hg)
Drance (1960)[15]	138	11 ± 5.7
Katavisto (1964)[37]	329	11.3 ± 4.2
Kitazawa (1975)[39]	27	15.8 ± 8.8
Worthen (1976)[83]	14	18.4 ± 8.4
Greenidge (1983)[25]	32	10.2 ± 4.7
Dannheim (1976)[10]	10	10.6 ± 6.3
Merritt (1979)[51]	20	8.6 ± 3.7
Smith (1985)[73]	800	5.8 ± 3.0

*Only the first author is identified.

Drance[15] examined 138 eyes of 72 primary open-angle glaucoma patients before initiating treatment and found ranges less than 5 mm Hg in 6% of the eyes, 5 to 9 mm Hg in 48%, 10 to 14 mm Hg in 28%, 20 to 24 mm Hg in 5%, and greater than 25 mm Hg in 3%.

Few investigators have reported on the relationship between the range of intraocular pressure in circadian variations and the degree of glaucomatous damage. Drance[15] found a larger variation (mean, 12 mm Hg; standard error of the mean, 0.7 mm Hg) in 81 eyes with glaucomatous optic disc or visual field changes than in 55 eyes without glaucoma damage (mean, 9.5 mm Hg; standard error of the mean, 0.6 mm Hg). In a study of 24 patients who had intraocular pressures ≤22 mm Hg at three consecutive office visits and who then performed self-tonometry, Wilensky et al.[82] found a more significant increase in intraocular pressure peaks in patients with suspected or documented progression of glaucomatous damage than in those patients considered stable. Langley and Swanljung[43] reported that in 26 of 33 patients (79%), the degree of visual field defect increased with the circadian intraocular pressure peak. Airaksinen et al.[3] reported that the range of circadian variations was related more to the occurrence of disc hemorrhages than the mean intraocular pressure. On the other hand, Kitazawa and Horie[40] demonstrated no correlation either between cup/disc ratio or severity of visual field damage and the range of pressure variations. Smith[73] detected no difference between individuals with and without visual field loss measured by computerized perimetry. In a 10-year follow-up by Greve et al.[26] of 29 eyes that underwent surgery, a total of 21 episodes of visual field deterioration occurred in 13 patients. In nine episodes the intraocular pressure peak was equal to or larger than 21 mm Hg, in seven it was between 18 and 21 mm Hg, and in five it was lower than 18 mm Hg. This study was limited by the fact that the intraocular pressure apparently was monitored only during office hours.

There are only a few reports of circadian intraocular pressure measurements in patients receiving their usual therapeutic regimen. Wilensky et al.[82] selected 24 open-angle glaucoma patients with treated pressures ≤22 mm Hg on three consecutive office visits and had them perform home tonometry. Intraocular pressures above 25 mm Hg were observed in one third of the patients, and ranges were up to 17 mm Hg. Drance[16] assessed 133 eyes with primary open-angle glaucoma with apparently controlled pressures (≤19 mm Hg in the office) on medical therapy. In the hospital, one third

of the eyes had intraocular pressure peaks of 24 mm Hg or more. The range of circadian variations was between 1 and 16 mm Hg with a mean of 7.5 ± 3.1 mm Hg. In a similar study (John Cohen, personal communication, 1986), 45 patients with intraocular pressure ≤21 mm Hg at 1 to 12 office visits performed Schiøtz home tonometry. On therapy, 33% had pressures between 21 and 24 mm Hg; 24%, between 24 and 30 mm Hg; and 23%, higher than 30 mm Hg. Even with therapy and with apparently controlled intraocular pressures in the office setting, the range of circadian variations in glaucoma patients may be significantly greater than those found in the normal population.

Ocular hypertension

Little information has been available on circadian intraocular pressure variations in ocular hypertensive patients. Kitazawa and Horie[39] measured intraocular pressure in 14 individuals hourly in the hospital with Goldmann tonometry for at least 24 hours. The mean range of the circadian variation was 8.1 ± 2.6 mm Hg. In 14% of the eyes the range was greater than 11 mm Hg, the maximal value they found in normal subjects. The largest range was 16 mm Hg. The average maximal intraocular pressure was 24 mm Hg, and the average minimal pressure was 16 mm Hg, indicating that this group of patients had an average intraocular pressure around 20 mm Hg. Smith[73] used computerized automated perimetry to examine 400 eyes of subjects without visual field defects and who were diagnosed by referring ophthalmologists as being glaucoma suspects or ocular hypertensives. This group was not necessarily homogeneous and may have included subjects with pathologic clinical findings other than visual field loss. The intraocular pressure, without therapy, was between 8 and 50 mm Hg, with a mean of 21 ± 5.4 mm Hg. The range was between 1 and 19 mm Hg, with a mean of 5.5 ± 2.7 mm Hg.

Time of Intraocular Pressure Peaks and Troughs

Normals

Tables 16-3 and 16-4 and Fig. 16-5 summarize the data on the time of the intraocular pressure peaks and troughs in normal subjects. The data show that the pressure peaks or troughs of different subjects do not occur at the same times but are spread over the hours of the day. This distribution is uneven: normal subjects have an increased probability of low intraocular pressures during the night and elevated pressure early in the morning, with a decline as the day progresses. This pattern was

Táble 16-3 Probability (%) of intraocular pressure peaks during the day in normal eyes

Authors*	No. of eyes	Time					
		4:00	8:00	12:00	16:00	20:00	24:00
Drance (1960)[15]	306	NA†	42	11	27	2	18
de Venecia (1963)[13]	230	NA	38	17	10	9	26
Katavisto (1964)[37]	100	19	25	25	14	5	11
Newell (1965)[53]	60	NA	44	35	NA	24	0
Kitazawa (1975)[39]	24	6	16	28	26	16	6
Average number of eyes		11	30	21	17	10	11

*Only the first author is identified.

†NA (not applicable) indicates that no measurements were made at that time.

NOTE: To standardize the data and compare the results of the different studies, the 24-hour day was divided into six equal time intervals into which the data reported in the literature were fit. Moreover, the distribution has been converted into probability (in %) of obtaining a peak at a given time interval. The average probability has been calculated by averaging the values for each time interval and normalizing the results of the six intervals to yield a total probability of 100% throughout the 24 hours.

Table 16-4 Probability (%) of intraocular pressure troughs over the day in normal eyes

Authors*	No. of eyes	Time					
		4:00	8:00	12:00	16:00	20:00	24:00
Drance (1960)[15]	306	NA†	16	23	33	3	24
de Venecia (1963)[13]	230	NA	9	17	22	34	18
Katavisto (1964)[37]	100	21	14	15	16	15	18
Kitazawa (1975)[39]	24	45	17	7	5	0	22
Average number of eyes		29	12	13	17	11	18

*Only the first author is identified.

†NA (not applicable) indicates that no measurements were made at that time.

NOTE: To standardize the data and compare the results of the different studies, the 24-hour day was divided into six equal time intervals into which the data reported in the literature were fit. Moreover, the distribution has been converted into probability (in %) of obtaining a trough at a given time interval. The average probability has been calculated by averaging the values for each time interval and normalizing the results of the six intervals to yield a total probability of 100% throughout the 24 hours.

reported often in the early literature and concurs with the predominant opinion before 1960 that the intraocular pressure reaches a maximum in the morning. This is only a trend, however, and the intraocular pressure has a significant probability of peaking at any time of the day.

It is instructive to evaluate the occurrence of intraocular pressure peaks between the hours of 8 AM and 6 PM which represent a physician's normal office hours. Since the two center columns in Tables 16-3 and 16-4 refer only to the time between 8 AM and 4 PM some extrapolation is necessary to obtain data for the hours between 4 PM and 6 PM. Half of the probability for the hours listed in column 5 (between 4 PM and 8 PM) yields a 43% probability of obtaining an intraocular pressure peak during office hours. Phelps et al.[57] tested whether the peak intraocular pressure can be predicted without measuring the circadian variations. The peak pressure attained during a 24-hour series of measurements in the hospital was correlated with daytime office tonometry, outflow facility, and intraocular pressure response to dexamethasone. The study was performed on 388 eyes of 204 subjects, including normal controls and individuals referred for elevated intraocular pressure who had no visual field defects. The correlation coefficient between the peak pressure and the office measurement was 0.84, and that between the range of circadian variations and office tonometry was 0.4. These correlations were statistically significant (P < 0.01) as a result of the large population size. However, when a given individual is considered, the prediction error is large. An approximation of the confidence interval indicates that 95% of the predictions would be close to the regression curve to within an interval given by[63]:

$$\text{confidence interval} = \pm 2 S_{peak}(1 - r^2)^{1/2} \tag{2}$$

where S_{peak} is the estimated standard deviation of the peak intraocular pressure (6.1 mm Hg in this study) and r is the correlation coefficient. By sub-

IOP PEAKS IN NORMALS

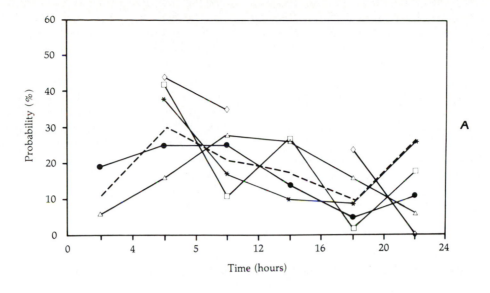

IOP TROUGHS IN NORMALS

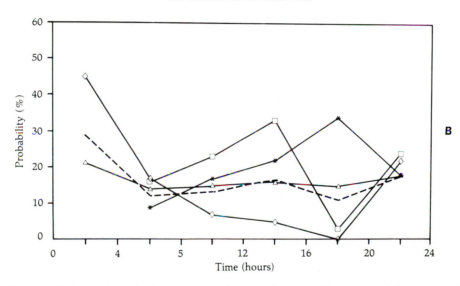

Fig. 16-5 Probability of intraocular pressure peaks, **A,** and troughs, **B,** in hours of day in normal subjects. Results of each author are depicted by different symbols.

stituting the values, the confidence interval was ±6.6 mm Hg. One could predict with 95% confidence that, for an intraocular pressure of 20 mm Hg at the office, the peak would fall between 17 and 30 mm Hg. Such an uncertainty limits the diagnostic value remarkably.

A similar evaluation could be made for the confidence interval in predicting the range of circadian variations from the office intraocular pressure. The correlation coefficient was 0.4, the mean range of circadian variations was 6.3 mm Hg, and the standard deviation was 3.5 mm Hg. The substitution yields a 95% confidence interval between 0 and 13 mm Hg. In conclusion, although there was a statistically significant correlation in a large population between a single office measurement and the peak or range of circadian intraocular pressure variations, the clinical significance of predictions in a single individual was limited for the pressure peak and is essentially null for the range. This was in conflict with the findings of Kitazawa and Horie[40] that office tonometry performed around noon was highly correlated with the intraocular pressure peak (r = 0.98). However, the circadian pressure curves observed by these authors were different from those found by others, in that there was a surprising homogeneity in the ocurrence of peaks around noon (phase of 11.6 ± 3.0 hours). Also, since pressure peaks coincided with the time suggested by them for office tonometry, an enhanced correlation could be anticipated.

Glaucoma

Tables 16-5 and 16-6 and Fig. 16-6 present the intraocular pressure peaks and troughs in glaucomatous eyes. The general impression obtained from Table 16-5 and Fig. 16-6, *A* is that the maxima

can occur, with a significant probability, at all hours of the day. Except for the findings of Kitazawa et al.[39] and Merritt et al.,[51] the probability of pressure peaks being larger in the morning than at other times is similar to that in normal subjects and circadian intraocular pressure variation troughs are relatively distributed evenly over the hours of the day (Table 16-6, Fig. 16-6, *B*). The probability of pressure peaks between the hours of 8 AM and 6 PM is 38%, as determined with the aid of an extrapolation similar to that used in normal subjects. Our own experience with home tonometry[82,87] indicates that about half of the intraocular pressure peaks occur outside of office hours.

Merritt et al.[51] observed that none of 10 juvenile

Table 16-5 Probability (%) of intraocular pressure peaks during the day in glaucomatous eyes

Authors*	No. of eyes	Time					
		4:00	8:00	12:00	16:00	20:00	24:00
Drance (1960)[15]	140	NA†	46	11	21	7	14
Hager (1962)[29]	92	14	45	17	7	6	11
Drance (1963)[16]	133	NA	25	38	4	11	22
Katavisto (1964)[37]	507	19	27	21	12	9	12
Newell (1965)[53]	24	NA	40	30	NA	30	0
Bitran (1968)[5]	200‡	NA	12	55	6	11	15
Kitazawa (1975)[39]	27	21	10	3	0	21	45
Dannheim (1976)[10]	76	NA	36	42	13	5	4
Merritt (1979)[51]	20	NA	8	15	NA	42	35
Average number of eyes		16	24	22	9	14	15

*Only the first author is identified.
†NA (not applicable) indicates that no measurements were made at that time.
‡100 subjects, approximately 200 eyes.
NOTE: To standardize the data and compare the results of the different studies, the 24-hour day was divided into six equal time intervals into which the data reported in the literature were fit. Moreover, the distribution has been converted into probability (in %) of obtaining a peak at a given time interval. The average probability has been calculated by averaging the values for each time interval and normalizing the results of the six intervals to yield a total probability of 100% throughout the 24 hours.

Table 16-6 Probability (%) of intraocular pressure troughs during the day in glaucomatous eyes

Authors*	No. of eyes	Time					
		4:00	8:00	12:00	16:00	20:00	24:00
Drance (1960)[15]	140	NA†	10	20	22	15	33
Katavisto (1964)[37]	507	20	10	10	15	20	25
Bitran (1968)[5]	200‡	NA	6	23	22	20	29
Kitazawa (1975)[39]	20	6	3	14	60	17	0
Merritt (1979)[51]	20	NA	46	25	NA	8	21
Average number of eyes		11	13	16	26	14	19

*Only the first author is identified.
†NA (not applicable) indicates that no measurements were made at that time.
‡100 subjects, approximately 200 eyes.
NOTE: To standardize the data and compare the results of the different studies, the 24-hour day was divided into six equal time intervals into which the data reported in the literature were fit. Moreover, the distribution has been converted into probability (in %) of obtaining a trough at a given time interval. The average probability has been calculated by averaging the values for each time interval and normalizing the results of the six intervals to yield a total probability of 100% throughout the 24 hours.

glaucoma patients had pressure peaks in the early morning, in contrast to patients with other types of glaucoma, and suggested that chronic open-angle glaucoma in the elderly may be different from that in younger patients, Kitazawa and Horie obtained similar findings in 14 primary open-angle glaucoma eyes of patients with a mean age of 33 years.[39] However, the limited population size in these studies precludes well-founded conclusions.

The incidence of circadian intraocular pressure variation troughs found by Katavisto[37] was identical for both male and female patients and for newly diagnosed and advanced cases of glaucoma. In comparison, the circadian pressure variation peaks occurred somewhat later in men than in women. Also, the peaks appeared to take place at an earlier hour in newly diagnosed patients with glaucoma than in glaucoma patients previously receiving treatment.

IOP PEAKS IN GLAUCOMA

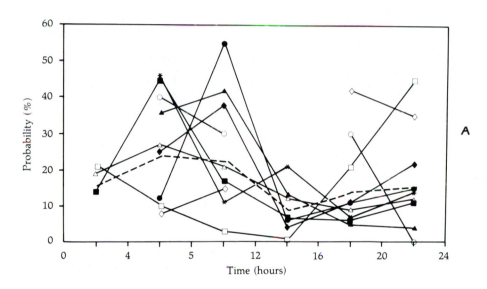

IOP TROUGHS IN GLAUCOMA

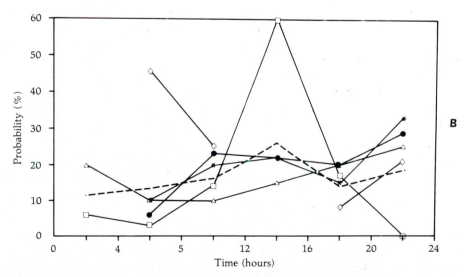

Fig. 16-6 Probability of intraocular pressure peaks, **A,** and troughs, **B,** in hours of day in glaucomatous patients. Results of each author are depicted by different symbols.

Table 16-7   Probability (%) of intraocular pressure peaks during the day in ocular hypertensive patients

Authors*	No. of eyes	Time					
		4:00	8:00	12:00	16:00	20:00	24:00
Kitazawa (1975)[39]	28	39	22	10	3	7	19
Smith (1985)[73]	400	NA†	44	43	13	NA	NA

*Only the first author is identified.
†NA (not applicable) indicates that no measurements were made at that time.
NOTE: To standardize the data and compare the results of the different studies, the 24-hour day was divided into six equal time intervals into which the data reported in the literature were fit. Moreover, the distribution has been converted into probability (in %) of obtaining a peak at a given time interval. The average probability has been calculated by averaging the values for each time interval and normalizing the results of the six intervals to yield a total probability of 100% throughout the 24 hours.

Table 16-8   Probability (%) of intraocular pressure troughs during the day in ocular hypertensive patients

Authors*	No. of eyes	Time					
		4:00	8:00	12:00	16:00	20:00	24:00
Kitazawa (1975)[39]	28	2	9	18	46	23	2
Smith (1985)[73]	400	NA†	46	24	30	NA	NA

*Only the first author is identified.
†NA (not applicable) indicates that no measurements were made at that time.
NOTE: To standardize the data and compare the results of the different studies, the 24-hour day was divided into six equal time intervals into which the data reported in the literature were fit. Moreover, the distribution has been converted into probability (in %) of obtaining a trough at a given time interval. The average probability has been calculated by averaging the values for each time interval and normalizing the results of the six intervals to yield a total probability of 100% throughout the 24 hours.

Ocular hypertension

The information available on ocular hypertension is summarized in Tables 16-7 and 16-8. Although the study by Smith[73] included a large number of eyes, the diagnosis was unclear. The eyes had an elevated intraocular pressure and no visual field defects, but it was not known if they had other signs of glaucoma. Moreover, the circadian variation was monitored only until 3 PM. The study by Kitazawa and Horie[39] measured pressure hourly in a limited number of eyes with ocular hypertension and found a trend toward peaks early in the morning and of troughs in the middle of the day.

Types of Circadian Intraocular Pressure Curves

Normals

The range of circadian intraocular pressure variations in normal patients is about 5 mm Hg. The Schiøtz tonometer was used in many earlier studies and it is difficult to classify the different circadian pressure curves obtained in normal patients using this instrument. Only general impressions can be gleaned from the literature. In 20 hospitalized normal subjects, Kimura[38] found no night type and an even distribution among day, morning, and variable types. Drance[15] indicated that the circadian pressure variations usually showed a marked rhythm. In only 10% of the eyes were there two peaks of intraocular pressure during the same 24-hour period, and the variation was irregular in only 7% of the cases. Katavisto[37] also found that the circadian pressure curve was usually regular, with only one period for each 24 hours. Leikovsky[44] detected double peaks in 25% of cases but used a composite of measurements performed on different days and the reliability was questionable. Ferrario et al.[21] concluded that elderly subjects had curves with peaks delayed by about 2 hours compared with younger subjects, but the number of persons studied (12) did not warrant definite conclusions.

Glaucoma

Table 16-9 includes the probability given by various authors for the different types of circadian intraocular pressure curves in patients with glaucoma. These calculations are only for circadian pressure curves that could be classified; the few

Table 16-9 Probability of different circadian intraocular pressure curve types in glaucoma

Authors*	No. of eyes	Circadian variation types (%)				
		Morning	Day	Night	Flat	Varying
Langley (1951)[43]	72	17	80	NA†	3	NA
Kaneda (1953)[36]	49	20	60	NA	20	NA
MacDonald (1956)[47]	52	NA	biggest	smallest	2nd biggest	NA
Hager (1958)[28]	480	NA	49	10	18	19
Hager (1962)[29]	92	NA	52	2	5	15
Katavisto (1964)[37]	508	24	35	26	2	13
Kimura (1966)[38]	26	65	15	12	8	NA
Average number of eyes		17	50	11	9	12

*Only the first author is identified.

†NA (not applicable) indicates that no measurements were made at that time.

that were reported to be of an "unknown type" are omitted. The dominant curve type appears to be the day type, whereas the night type is the least common. This latter observation coincides well with the probability of peaks showing a decrease at night. On the other hand, the predominance of the day type over the morning type does not concur with the increased probability of intraocular pressure peaks in the morning hours. This may be explained by the fact that in the studies of Hager[28] and Hager and Remischovsky[29] the morning type classification was not used, and some circadian pressure curves of the day type may actually have belonged to the morning type.

Drance[15] showed no difference in the phasic variation of the circadian curves in untreated glaucoma patients with and without visual field changes or cupping. Kimura[38] found the day type most common in primary open-angle glaucoma and the night and morning types in angle-closure glaucoma, but Dannheim[10] found no difference. Henkind and Walsh[32] performed hourly measurements with a Mackay-Marg tonometer on 33 unmedicated hospitalized patients with primary open-angle glaucoma. Approximately 7% of all intraocular pressure readings rapidly rose or fell within an hour, but did not appear to be related to any specific hour of the day.

Stability of the Rhythm

With time

In the few studies in which the circadian intraocular pressure curve was repeated over more than 1 day, there was a general impression that the circadian curve was relatively constant, at least over that period, in normal subjects, ocular hypertensives, and those with open-angle glaucoma.[21,37,43] This confirmed the opinion of many

that the circadian curve is a characteristic of the individual. We have investigated by means of self-tonometry the circadian pressure variations in the natural environment of 133 treated glaucoma patients for 4 to 7 days and found that 80% exhibited a reproducible curve during that period (see Figs. 16-2 and 16-3).

Circadian variations may, however, not be stable if exogenous conditions change. Changing sleep patterns may affect the type of circadian pressure curve. For example, airline pilots flying around the world had curve types that varied significantly with time.[11] Nurses who worked on a night shift for at least 1 year had minimum intraocular pressures at 4 PM, after they had slept for several hours. Sometimes the peak pressure was measured at 4 AM. In contrast, the day personnel showed maximum intraocular pressures at 8 AM and noon, accompanied by a slight, but steady, decrease that reached the minimum value at midnight. Hospitalization can also influence the circadian pressure variations. It has caused a progressive and slow decrease in circadian pressure variations possibly related to a reduction in normal activities.[13,37,69,79] The stability of the circadian intraocular pressure variations over long periods of time is not fully known. Katavisto[37] found no significant alteration in circadian pressure curve types in the darkest and brightest quarters of the year, but Blumenthal et al.[7] reported seasonal changes in intraocular pressure.

With therapy

The circadian pressure curve is usually characteristic for an individual and remains similar even after drug or surgical therapy. However, some patients demonstrate changes. Hager[28] suggested that patients with a varying curve type may convert to a regular type during drug therapy, and Huerkamp[33] reported that with therapy 33% of patients "inverted" their pressure rhythm. In a follow-up of 135 eyes, Katavisto[37] observed that in 20% of patients who were rehospitalized, the curve type had changed from the original classification. The majority of such changes involved day and morning types that became night types and may have corresponded to Huerkamp's "inversion." Katavisto also postulated that in some cases, at the initial phase of glaucoma, the circadian pressure curve is a night or morning type before it becomes a day type. We have repeated (within a year) home tonometry in 35 treated eyes in which therapy had been altered and found that the curve type varied in 37% of the cases.

Numerous studies have assessed the effect of therapy by comparing the average circadian pressure variations of the whole population before and after treatment. Judging by the behavior of the average, the curve remains unchanged and only the mean and the range of the circadian intraocular pressure variations are altered by therapy.[22,25,30,71,83]

Other Characteristics of Circadian Intraocular Pressure Variations

Kitazawa and Horie[39] reported differences between the two eyes of 2 mm Hg or less in 93% and 84% of the measurements for normal patients and those with ocular hypertension, respectively. The difference between the eyes remained remarkably constant for the full 24-hour period. In contrast, Katavisto[37] found that half of the individuals with glaucoma had curve types that differed between the two eyes. Curiously, when they were different, the right eye was of an "earlier" type more often than the left. Our own observations in 133 eyes of glaucoma patients performing home tonometry while receiving therapy indicated that the circadian pressure curve type of the fellow eyes differed in 30% of the cases.

CLINICAL APPLICATION
Diagnosis

Although the exact relationship between intraocular pressure and glaucomatous optic nerve damage has not been defined, the aim of therapy is to "control" the pressure throughout the day. Some investigators have thought that an abnormal intraocular pressure peak or range warrants a diagnosis of glaucoma.* Conversely, Smith[73] found

no direct relationship between abnormal visual fields and intraocular pressure values obtained during part of the day. These different results may be a result of the changing definition of glaucoma over the last few decades illustrated by the introduction of the terms *ocular hypertensive* and *glaucoma suspect*.

Because the intraocular pressure varies during the day, circadian pressure curves provide more information than single measurements. Nonetheless, these measurements are not clinically necessary in all patients. Glaucoma patients who exhibit intraocular pressures above 22 mm Hg in the office are usually considered inadequately controlled. Thus the ophthalmologist does not need circadian pressure curves to decide to alter the therapy until the intraocular pressure reaches lower values.[16] However, once the intraocular pressure has been normalized, circadian pressure curves have been considered of great diagnostic value.* These curves can provide information on both the peak intraocular pressure and the range of circadian pressure variations. Peaks above normal indicate that the intraocular pressure is inadequately controlled.

The necessity and efficacy of circadian pressure curves is especially evident in patients with an apparently controlled intraocular pressure but with progressing glaucomatous damage. Many ophthalmologists have found that abnormal pressure peaks often occur when it is impractical or inconvenient to record on an outpatient basis.† In patients with low-tension glaucoma, only rarely do measurements of daily pressure curves reveal an elevated intraocular pressure.[67,68] Our experience shows a correlation between the number of circadian pressure curve peaks and the progression of glaucomatous damage in patients with apparently controlled intraocular pressures.[82] Moreover, even without abnormal pressure peaks, an abnormal range (Fig. 16-7) can be suspected to cause glaucomatous damage.

Prognosis

Little is known about the relation between the values or types of circadian intraocular pressure variations and prognosis. Katavisto[37] found that 85% to 90% of the eyes with periodic variations obtained in the hospital remained clinically stable for treatment periods of 3 to 6 years. In contrast, eyes with variations of the varying type seemed to

---

*References 5, 17, 23, 37, 45, 68, 80.

*References 15, 16, 19, 34, 41, 43, 57, 64, 75, 79, 81, 84.
†References 16, 41, 59, 64, 75, 81, 82, 87.

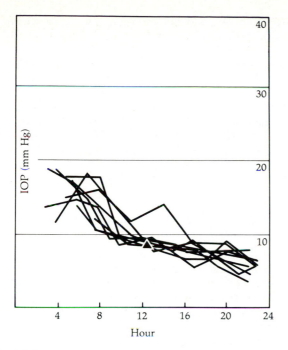

Fig. 16-7 Circadian intraocular pressure curves with normal values but with large range. Symbols are same as in Fig. 16-1.

deteriorate rapidly. In spite of therapy, the deterioration was fastest in eyes with variations with high values; it was evident in 25% of the cases after 2 years and in 50% over a treatment period of 5 years.[37] Sampaolesi[67] obtained circadian pressure curves in 100 hospitalized glaucoma suspects who were followed for 5 to 10 years. He noted that isolated intraocular pressures above 24 mm Hg, means above 19 mm Hg, or variabilities above ±2 mm Hg, always gave rise to damage. Recently, Alpar[4] obtained striking results on the prognostic value of home tonometry. Twenty-one ocular hypertensives who had tonometry readings at home that were 4 to 13 mm Hg higher than the office measurements exhibited progressive glaucomatous damage within 2 years. However, 12 ocular hypertensive patients who had office readings that were always higher than the home readings did not develop damage during a 5-year follow-up. These results indicate that circadian intraocular pressure variations may play a prominent role in the development of glaucomatous damage.

REFERENCES

1. Adler, FH: Physiology of the eye: clinical application, ed. 3, St Louis, 1959, The CV Mosby Co
2. Agarwal, LP, and Saxena, RP: General changes in glaucoma, Ophthalmologica 132:258, 1956
3. Airaksinen, PJ, Mustonen, E, and Alanko, HI: Optic disc hemorrhages: analysis of stereophotographs and clinical data of 112 patients, Arch Ophthalmology 99:1795, 1981
4. Alpar, JJ: The use of home tonometry in the diagnosis and treatment of glaucoma, Glaucoma 5:130, 1983
5. Bitran, D: Evaluacion de la curva de tension diaria, Arch Chil Oftalmol 25:32, 1968
6. Blaxter, PL: The early diagnosis of glaucoma, Trans Ophthalmol Soc UK 76:15, 1956
7. Blumenthal, M, Blumenthal, R, Peritz, E, and Best, M: Seasonal variation in intraocular pressure, Am J Ophthalmol 69:608, 1970
8. Charbonneau, R: Epreuves de provocation dans le glaucome, Union Med Can 83:1004, 1954
9. Cordes, FC: Early simple glaucoma: its diagnosis and management, Arch Ophthalmol 17:896, 1937
10. Dannheim, R: Die Diagnose und Differentialdiagnose des Glaucoma chronicum simplex und des Glaucoma chronicum congestivum, Buch Augenarzt 69:171, 1976
11. Daubs, JG: Patterns of diurnal variation in the intraocular pressure of airline pilots, Aerosp Med 44:914, 1973
12. Davanger, M: Diurnal variations of ocular pressure in normal and in glaucomatous eyes, Acta Ophthalmol 42:764, 1964
13. de Venecia, G, and Davis, MD: Diurnal variation of intraocular pressure in the normal eye, Arch Ophthalmol 69:752, 1963
14. Dobree, JH: Vascular changes that occur during the phasic variations of tension in chronic glaucoma, Br J Ophthalmol 37:293, 1953
15. Drance, SM: The significance of the diurnal tension variations in normal and glaucomatous eyes, Arch Ophthalmol 64:494, 1960
16. Drance, SM: Diurnal variation of intraocular pressure in treated glaucoma: significance in patients with chronic simple glaucoma, Arch Ophthalmol 70:302, 1963
17. Duke-Elder, S: The phasic variations in the ocular tension in primary glaucoma, Am J Ophthalmol 35:1, 1952
18. Eggink, ED: Tonometry as a routine in tracing primary glaucoma, Ophthalmologica 143:113, 1962
19. Epstein, DL: Chandler and Grant's glaucoma, ed. 3, Philadelphia, 1986, Lea & Febiger
20. Feigenbaum, A: Über den Einfluss der Belichtung und Verdunkelung auf den intraokularen Druck normaler und glaukomatoser, Klin Monatsbl Augenheilkd 80:577, 1928
21. Ferrario, VF, Bianchi, R, Giunta, G, and Roveda, L: Circadian rhythm in human intraocular pressure, Chronobiologia 9:33, 1982
22. Fraunfelder, FT, Shell, JW, and Herbst, SF: Effect of pilocarpine ocular therapeutic systems on diurnal control of intraocular pressure, Ann Ophthalmol 8:1031, 1976

23. Goldmann, H: Das Glaukom, in Amsters Lehrbuch der Augenheilkunde, 2 ann. New York, 1954, Karger

24. Goldmann, H: Bericht über das Symposium: Schwierigkeiten und Irrtumer bei Diagnose und Therapie des Glaukoms. In Weigelin, E, editor: Proceedings of the XX International Congress of Ophthalmology, Munich, 1966, Amsterdam, 1967, Exerpta Medica Foundation

25. Greenidge, KC, Spaeth, GL, and Fiol-Silva, Z: Effect of argon laser trabeculoplasty on the glaucomatous diurnal curve, Ophthalmology 90:800, 1983

26. Greve, EL, Leydhecker, W, and Railta, C: Second European Glaucoma Symposium, Helsinki, 1984, The Hague, 1985, Dr W Junk, Publishers

27. Hagen, S: Glaucoma pressure curves, Acta Ophthalmol 2:199, 1924

28. Hager, H: Die Behandlung des Glaukoms mit Miotika, Buch Augenarzt 29:3, 1958

29. Hager, H, and Remischovsky, J: Die Bedeutung der Fruehmessung bei Glaukom und bei Glaukomverdacht, Klin Monatsbl Augenheilkd 140:545, 1962

30. Hass, I, and Drance, SM: Comparison between pilocarpine and timolol on diurnal pressures in open-angle glaucoma, Arch Ophthalmol 98:480, 1980

31. Henkind, P, Leitman, M, and Weitzman, E: The diurnal curve in man: new observations, Invest Ophthalmol 12:705, 1973

32. Henkind, P, and Walsh, JB: Diurnal variations in intraocular pressure: chronic open-angle glaucoma: preliminary report, Trans Ophthalmol Soc NZ 33:18, 1981

33. Huerkamp, B: Über die Auswertung von Augendruckkurven, Klin Monatsbl Augenheilkd 128:394, 1956

34. Jensen, AD, and Maumenee, AE: Home tonometry, Am J Ophthalmol 76:929, 1973

35. Jessen, K, Luebbig, H, and Weigelin, E: Clinical and statistical aspects on standardization of tonometers, v Graefes Arch Klin Exp Ophthalmol 209:269, 1979

36. Kaneda, S, and Kiritoshi, Y: Type of phasic variation of glaucomatous intraocular tension, Acta Soc Ophthalmol Jpn 57:236, 1953

37. Katavisto, M: The diurnal variations of ocular tension in glaucoma, Acta Ophthalmol Suppl 78:1, 1964

38. Kimura, R: Clinical studies on glaucoma, Report I: The diagnostic significance of the diurnal variation of intraocular pressure, Acta Soc Ophthalmol Jpn 70:1326, 1966

39. Kitazawa, Y, and Horie, T: Diurnal variation of intraocular pressure in primary open-angle glaucoma, Am J Ophthalmol 79:557, 1975

40. Kitazawa, Y, and Horie, T: Diurnal variation of intraocular pressure and its significance in the medical treatment of primary open-angle glaucoma. In Krieglstein, GG, and Leydhecker, W, editors: Glaucoma update, Berlin, 1979, Springer-Verlag

41. Kolker, AE, and Hetherington, J, Jr: Becker-Shaffer's diagnosis and therapy of the glaucomas, ed. 5, St Louis, 1983, The CV Mosby Co

42. Kollner, H: Über die regelmassigen taglichen Schwankungen des Augendruckes und ihre Ursache, Arch Augenheilkd 81:120, 1916

43. Langley, D, and Swanljung, H: Ocular tension in glaucoma simplex, Br J Ophthalmol 35:445, 1951

44. Leikovsky, MM: Modification of the method of determining diurnal variations of intraocular pressure, Oftalmol Zh 29:110, 1974

45. Leydhecker, W: The intraocular pressure: clinical aspects, Ann Ophthalmol 8:389, 1976

46. Lynn, JR: Round table discussion on low tension glaucoma and diurnal curve. In Symposium on glaucoma: transactions of the New Orleans Academy of Ophthalmology, St Louis, 1974, The CV Mosby Co

47. MacDonald, DA: Symposium on the clinical assessment of glaucoma with particular reference to diurnal variations in pressure: types of diurnal pressure curves, Trans Can Ophthalmol Soc 7:171, 1956

48. Maslenikow, A: Über Tagesschwankungen des intraokularen Druckes bei Glaukom, Z Augenheilkd 11:564, 1904

49. Matteucci, P: L'aritmia of talmotonica nel glaucoma semplice, Rass Ital Ottal 22:545, 1953

50. Mercer, DMA: Analytical methods for the study of periodic phenomena obscured by random fluctuations. In Biological clocks, CSH symposia on quantitative biology, XXV, Cold Springs Harbor, NY, 1960, The Biological Library

51. Merritt, JC, Reid, LA, Smith R, and Harris, DF: Diurnal intraocular pressure in juvenile open-angle glaucoma, Ann Ophthalmol 11:253, 1979

52. Nelson, W, Tong, YL, Lee, JK, and Halberg, F: Methods for cosinorrhythmometry, Chronobiologia 6:305, 1979

53. Newell, FW, and Krill, AE: Diurnal tonography in normal and glaucomatous eyes, Am J Ophthalmol 59:840, 1965

54. Ourgaud, AG, and Etienne, R: L'exploration fonctionnelle de l'oeil glaucomateux, Paris, 1961, Massin et Cie

55. Perez-Bufill Pichot, J: Tension y campimetria ocular en el glaucoma simple, Arch Soc Oftal Hisp-Amer 20:1171, 1960

56. Phelps, CD, and Phelps, GK: Measurement of intraocular pressure: a study of its reproducibility, v Graefes Arch Klin Exp Ophthalmol 198:39, 1976

57. Phelps, CD, Woolson, RF, Kolker, AE, and Becker, B: Diurnal variation in intraocular pressure, Am J Ophthalmol 77:367, 1974

58. Pissarello, C: La curva giornaliera della tensione nell' occhio normale e nell' occhio glaucomatoso e influenza di fattori diversi (miotici, iridectomia, iridosclerectomia, derivati, pasti) determinata con il tonometro di Schiøtz. Ann Ottal 44:544, 1915

59. Posner, A: Home use of the Applanometer as an aid in the management of glaucoma, Eye Ear Nose Throat Mon 44:64, 1965

60. Poutchkovskaia, N: Ukranian Filatof's Research Institute, eye diseases and tissue therapy, Ophthalmologica 142:328, 1961

61. Radnot, M, and Follmann, P: Diagnosis of primary open-angle glaucoma. In Bellows, JG, editor: Glaucoma: contemporary international concepts, New York, 1979, Masson Publishers

62. Radzikhovsky, BL: A new procedure used to determine 24-hour variations of intraocular pressure and its significance in the diagnosis of glaucoma, Vestn Oftalmol 76:59, 1963

63. Remington, RD, and Schork, MA: Statistics with applications to the biological and health sciences, Englewood Cliffs, NJ, 1970, Prentice-Hall

64. Richardson, KT: Glaucoma and glaucoma suspects. In Heilmann, KK, and Richardson, KT, editors: Glaucoma, conceptions of a disease: pathogenesis, diagnosis, therapy, Stuttgart, 1978, Georg Thieme

65. Rohrschneider, W, and Kuchle, HJ: Die Grosse des "methodischen Messfehlers" der Tonometrie am Auge Kaninchens und des Menschen, Ophthalmologica 128:369, 1954

66. Sallmann, L, and Deutsch, A: Die klinische Bedeutung der Tagesdruckkurve und der Belastungsproben bein Glaukom, v Graefes Arch Klin Exp Ophthalmol 124:624, 1930

67. Sampaolesi, R: Personal interview between the editor and Dr. Roberto Sampaolesi. In Boyd, BB, editor: Highlights of ophthalmology, 1977, Panama

68. Sampaolesi, R, Calixto, N, de Carvalho, CA, and Reca, R: Diurnal variation of intraocular pressure in healthy, suspected and glaucomatous eyes, Mod Probl Ophthalmol 6:1, 1968

69. Scheie, HG: Comments. In Clark, WW, and Carmichael, JM, editors: Symposium on glaucoma: transactions of the New Orleans Academy of Ophthalmology, St Louis, 1957, The CV Mosby Co

70. Schmidt, K: Langjahrige Beobachtungen bei der Diagnose ünter der Behandlung des Glaucoma simplex in der augenarztlichen Praxis, Klin Monatsbl Augenheilkd 141:108, 1962

71. Shapiro, A, and Zauberman, H: Diurnal changes of the intraocular pressure of patients with angle-closure glaucoma, Br J Ophthalmol 63:225, 1979

72. Sidler-Huguenin: Die Spaterfolge der Glaukombehandlung bei 76 Privatpatienten von Prof Haab, Zurich, Beitr Z Augenheilkd 32:1, 1898

73. Smith J: Diurnal intraocular pressure: correlation to automated perimetry, Ophthalmology 92:858, 1985

74. Stamper, RL: Intraocular pressure: measurement, regulation and flow relationships. In Duane, TT, and Jaeger, EA, editors: Biomedical foundations of ophthalmology, Philadelphia, 1982, Harper & Row, Publishers, Inc

75. Starrels, ME: The measurement of intraocular pressure, Int Ophthalmol Clin 19:9, 1979

76. Sugar, HS: The glaucomas, ed 2, New York, 1957, Hoeber-Harper

77. Thiel, R: Klinische Untersuchungen zur Glaukomfrage, v Graefes Arch Klin Exp Ophthalmol 113:329, 1924

78. Thomassen, TL: Experimental investigations into the conditions of tension in normal eyes and in simple glaucoma, particularly performed by subjecting the eyes to weight compressions, Acta Ophthalmol Suppl 27:1, 1946

79. Weekers, R, and Prijot, E: A propos du diagnostic differentiel entre le glaucome chronique simple et le glaucome congestif non inflammatoire, Ann Oculist 186:596, 1953

80. Weinstein, P: Glaucoma: pathology and therapy, St Louis, 1953, The CV Mosby Co

81. Wilensky, JT, and Gieser, DK: Low tension glaucoma. In Weinstein, GG, editor: Open-angle glaucoma, New York, 1986, Churchill Livingstone, Inc

82. Wilensky, JT, et al: Self-tonometry to manage glaucoma patients with apparently controlled intraocular pressure, Arch Ophthalmol 105:1072, 1987

83. Worthen, DM: Effect of pilocarpine drops on the diurnal intraocular pressure variation in patients with glaucoma, Invest Ophthalmol 15:784, 1976

84. Worthen, DM: Intraocular pressure and its diurnal variation. In Heilmann, KK, and Richardson, KT, editors: Glaucoma: conceptions of a disease, pathogenesis, diagnosis, therapy. Stuttgart, 1978, Georg Thieme

85. Zeimer, RC, and Wilensky, JT: An instrument for self-measurement of intraocular pressure, IEEE Trans Biomed Eng 29:178, 1982

86. Zeimer, RC, et al: Evaluation of a self-tonometer for home use, Arch Ophthalmol 101:1791, 1983

87. Zeimer, RC, et al: Application of a self-tonometer to home tonometry, Arch Ophthalmol 104:48, 1986

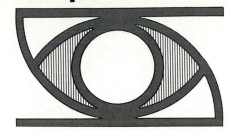

Chapter 17

Measurement of Aqueous Flow by Fluorophotometry

Richard F. Brubaker

Aqueous humor is secreted by the pars plicata of the ciliary body. Most of this aqueous humor flows anteriorly through the pupil into the anterior chamber, where it mixes by convection before draining out of the eye at the iridocorneal angle. The rate of flow of aqueous humor through the anterior chamber is one of the major determinants of the intraocular pressure. This rate of flow can be measured in the living eye in a number of ways. The most direct method is to measure the rate of disappearance of a tracer.

When a high molecular weight tracer such as albumin is injected into the anterior chamber, the tracer mixes readily with the aqueous humor by convection and diffusion. Since the iris and lens form a one-way barrier, the tracer will not enter the posterior chamber. Because of its high molecular weight, albumin will penetrate the corneal endothelium and vascular endothelium rather slowly. Except for what leaves along with the aqueous outflow, the albumin is trapped in the anterior chamber. As a result, the rate of loss of the tracer, which is proportional to its concentration in the aqueous humor, will depend on and will be a measure of the rate of outflow of aqueous humor. It is this principle that is exploited in measuring the rate of aqueous flow by fluorophotometry.

Unlike albumin, fluorescein can penetrate the anterior chamber without being injected and can be detected without a radioactive label. For these reasons, fluorescein is commonly employed as a tracer for the measurement of aqueous humor flow. In this chapter, the corneal depot method of measuring aqueous flow, described originally by Jones and Maurice in 1966,[19] is explained and results of measurements in human eyes are summarized.

APPLICATION OF FLUORESCEIN TO THE EYE

Fluorescein is applied topically to the cornea in a high concentration, sufficient for several hundred nanograms to penetrate the corneal epithelium and enter the corneal stroma, which acts as a reservoir. In normal eyes, penetration can be achieved by instilling 2% fluorescein (2×10^{-2} g/ml) into the cul-de-sac every 5 minutes for a total of four to five applications. The dye distributes itself evenly into the depths of the cornea within 15 or 20 minutes, but uniformity of lateral distribution does not occur for at least 5 to 6 hours after application. Evenness of distribution is a prerequisite for an accurate measurement of flow. If measurements are to begin in the morning, fluorescein can be instilled at bedtime (6 to 8 drops) or between 2 and 3 AM (3 to 5 drops) as recommended by Yablonski et al.[42] With most fluorophotometers, accurate measurements of flow can begin if the stromal concentration of fluorescein is in the range of 10^{-5} to 10^{-6} g/ml. When planning the timing of drop instillation, it is good to keep in mind that the approximate half-life of fluorescein in the normal cornea is 4 hours.

KINETICS OF FLUORESCEIN IN THE EYE

When fluorescein is in the corneal stroma it leaves the stroma by diffusion through the endothelium, the epithelium, and the limbus. Because the endothelium is 1000 times more permeable to fluorescein than the normal epithelium,[25] epithelial loss is negligible, and because the average distance required for diffusion from the stoma to the limbus is so great, the rate of loss from the cornea into limbal vessels is slow. Thus the depot of fluorescein is trapped in the stroma where it leaks slowly into the anterior chamber. Once in the anterior chamber, the tracer cannot escape into the posterior chamber as long as the iris-lens barrier is intact. Furthermore, the rate of loss by diffusion into the vasculature of the iris is slow.[15] The principal route of loss from the anterior chamber and thus from the combined cornea and anterior chamber is the outward flow of aqueous humor. In other words, the reservoir of fluorescein is trapped in a readily observable depot and can escape only by flowing out with the aqueous humor. With this fact in mind, it is easy to see that the rate of flow can be deduced by knowing the rate of loss of fluorescein in proportion to its concentration in the anterior chamber— the clearance of fluorescein.

CALCULATION OF FLOW

Clearance is measured by observing the rate of loss of fluorescein in proportion to the concentration of fluorescein in the anterior chamber.

(1)
$$\text{clearance} = \frac{\text{loss of fluorescein from the eye in a given time interval}}{\text{concentration in chamber} \times \text{time}}$$

The loss of fluorescein from the eye is the combined loss from the cornea and the anterior chamber. At any given time most of the fluorophore is in the stroma. Thus the measurement of corneal fluorescence is the most critical.

If the fluorescein is uniformly distributed in the stroma, its mass can be calculated as the product of its concentration and the volume of the stroma.

(2) mass of fluorescein in stroma =
concentration in stroma × volume of stroma

The mass of fluorescein in the anterior chamber is calculated in the same manner.

(3) mass of fluorescein in anterior chamber =
concentration in chamber × volume of chamber

These relations can be expressed symbolically, as shown in the box at right.

The volume of the stroma (v_c) can be estimated from its central thickness and its horizontal diameter by employing the geometric formula for the volume of a cylinder.

$$v_c = \text{thickness} \times \pi \times (\text{diameter}/2)^2 \qquad (4)$$

The volume of the anterior chamber (v_a) can be estimated from the depth of the central chamber and the diameter of the anterior (h = axial depth of chamber; y = diameter of chamber) by employing the geometric formula for the volume of a spherical segment.

$$v_a = 1/6 \times \pi \times h\,(h^2 + \tfrac{3}{4} \times y^2) \qquad (5)$$

A single measurement of flow requires the measurement of the concentration of fluorescein in the cornea and the anterior chamber at the beginning of an interval of time, $c_c(1)$ and $c_a(1)$ and at the end of the interval, $c_c(2)$ and $c_a(2)$. Since mass equals concentration times volume, the following relations exist.

$$\begin{aligned} m_c(1) &= c_c(1) \times v_c \\ m_a(1) &= c_a(1) \times v_a \\ m_c(2) &= c_c(2) \times v_c \\ m_a(2) &= c_a(2) \times v_a \end{aligned} \qquad (6)$$

The total mass of fluorescein in the eye at the beginning and end of the interval Δt are as follows.

$$\begin{aligned} m(1) &= m_c(1) + m_a(1) \\ m(2) &= m_c(2) + m_a(2) \end{aligned} \qquad (7)$$

The loss of fluorescein during the interval is

$$\Delta m = m(1) - m(2)$$

The rate of loss of fluorescein during the interval is

$$\Delta m / \Delta t$$

The clearance of fluorescein (F) during the interval is

$$F = \Delta m / \Delta t / \bar{c}_a$$

Some of the clearance of fluorescein is the result of diffusion rather than flow. The rate of dif-

---

SYMBOLS AND DEFINITIONS

m_c	Mass of fluorescein in the cornea
m_a	Mass of fluorescein in the anterior chamber
c_c	Concentration of fluorescein in the corneal stroma
c_a	Concentration of fluorescein in the anterior chamber
$\bar{c}_a$	Average concentration of fluorescein in the anterior chamber over an interval of time
$\bar{c}_a$	$= (c_a(1) - c_a(2))/\ln(c_a(1)/c_a(2))$
v_c	Volume of the corneal stroma
v_a	Volume of the anterior chamber
F	Clearance of fluorescein from the anterior chamber

fusional clearance in the normal human eye is approximately 10% of the clearance caused by flow, 0.25 μl/min.[4] Many investigators make allowance for diffusional clearance by subtracting 0.25 μl/min from the measured rate of clearance.

(8) rate of aqueous flow = F − 0.25 μl/min

The interval of time over which paired measurements are made to calculate flow can be varied according to the wishes of the examiner. Ordinarily, this time is 45 to 60 minutes. Approximately 15% of the depot of fluorescein will disappear over 1 hour. Most investigators make several hourly measurements and average them.

FLUOROPHOTOMETRY

The term *fluorophotometry* is used in this chapter to mean the noninvasive determinaiton of the concentration or some other property of fluorescent probes or tracers in living ocular tissues. Fundamental to the method of measuring aqueous flow, as outlined in the preceeding section, is the determination of the concentration of fluorescein in the corneal stroma and the aqueous humor. The determination of concentration in these living tissues, fluorophotometry, can be performed quite reproducibly but is by no means a trivial procedure. To understand fluorophotometry and to perform it accurately, one must have a clear understanding of the measurement of light and the properties of fluorescent materials.

Fluorescence is the property of a material that permits it to absorb and rapidly re-emit light. Fluorophores that are useful as tracers are efficient absorbers at one wavelength and efficient emitters at a longer wavelength. The shift in wavelength, the Stokes' shift, is a property that makes it possible to measure low concentrations of the tracer in ocular fluids and to distinguish fluorescence from scattering. Fluorophores exhibit characteristic properties, but these properties—excitation spectrum, emission spectrum, fluorescent efficiency, Stokes' shift, polarization of fluorescence, or excited state lifetime—vary with the immediate environment of the molecule. These properties can change appreciably with pH or colloid binding. Also, organic molecules such as fluorescein can be metabolized to products with entirely different fluorescent properties. Although fluorescein has been the tracer of choice for many decades in visual science research, carboxyfluorescein, or sulforhodamine B have properties that make them preferable for some measurements, including the measurement of aqueous flow.

Measurement of fluorescein in the eye is much more difficult than measurement under controlled conditions in a cuvet with a fluorometer. The living eye is in constant motion. Thus the measurement must be made quickly. Yet the fluorophotometer must not expose the eye to dangerously intense light. The eye itself has optical properties that affect the measurement. The cornea and, particularly in older persons, the crystalline lens have natural autofluorescence. The distribution of a tracer can be quite irregular in the cornea for many hours after topical administration and persistently uneven after systemic administration. Entry of aqueous humor from the posterior chamber into the anterior chamber can cause relative hypofluorescence in the center of the chamber, the "pupillary bubble." Intense fluorescence in the cornea can interfere with measurements in the anterior chamber because of corneal properties that create an optical boundary function. High concentrations in any layer can affect measurement in deeper layers because of the absorption of light—an inner filter effect. The reflectivity of the iris can affect certain types of measurements. Despite these potential problems, accurate measurements can be made with good fluorophotometers by careful investigators. The most important of these problems are discussed in the sections that follow.

A good fluorophotometer should be able to measure the intensity of fluorescence of fluorescein in the cornea and the anterior chamber. The lower limit of detection of fluorescein, defined as the least signal that is twice the background noise, should be about 10^{-9} g/ml. The instrument should be linear over 4 orders of magnitude, at least to 10^{-5} g/ml. The focal point of the instrument, that is, the intersection between the excitation beam and the acceptance beam of the detector, should be as short as possible along the axis of measurement. Otherwise, corneal fluorescence cannot be measured accurately. The instrument should be able to reject noise from stray background light, permitting it to be used in the presence of modest background illumination. The measurement should be accomplished rapidly—for a single measurement, a fraction of a second; for scanned measurements, a few seconds. The data should be presented in a convenient way, preferably on a computer screen, and should be entered automatically into a computer file. A number of instruments have been described that are satisfactory for measuring aqueous humor flow.*

Having a good fluorophotometer does not assure that accurate measurements of the concentra-

---

*References 4, 24, 26, 27, 36, 40, 43.

tion of fluorescein will be obtained. Some specific sources of error must be avoided.

Corneal Reflectivity

The reflectivity of optical interfaces depends on the angle of incidence, the difference in refractive index between the surfaces, and the polarization of the incident beam. For the air-tear interface, angles of incidence of less than 65 degrees reflect less than 10% of unpolarized light. For greater angles, large fractions of light can be reflected, resulting in large errors. Angles greater than 60 degrees, either of the excitation beam or of the acceptance beam of the detector, should be avoided.

Corneal Optical Boundary Function

Because of the optical properties of the cornea, high concentrations of fluorescein in the stroma can interfere with measurement of low concentrations of fluorescein in the aqueous humor. In the normal human eye, the cornea can generate an apparent signal in the anterior chamber that, even for a well-collimated fluorophotometer, is approximately 1% to 2% of the fluorescent intensity in the cornea.[2,31] The problem is considerably worse if the cornea is hazy or if the optics of the fluorophotometer do not produce sharp images. In the former case, accurate fluorophotometry is not possible. In the latter case, a better instrument should be used. All instruments must be checked and this property measured in subjects with normal corneas. The simplest way to measure this boundary function is to measure the signal originating from the anterior chamber before and 5 to 10 minutes after applying a concentrated drop of fluorescein to the cornea. The boundary function is the ratio of the increment in the signal to the corneal signal after drop application.

For a particular cornea and instrument, the ratio is independent of the concentration of fluorescein. If measurements of flow are to be carried out as described in this chapter, the ratio of fluorescence in the cornea to that in the anterior chamber will seldom be greater than 10:1, and correction for the optical boundary function will be small enough to ignore. However, for eyes with even slightly hazy corneas, the boundary function can be so large that fluorophotometric readings must be corrected. In some corneas, the signal to noise conditions are so poor that fluorophotometry cannot be carried out.

Autofluorescence of the Cornea

Fluorescent materials that excite and emit in the 450 to 550 nm range are present in many ocular tissues, including the cornea and the lens. The autofluorescence can interfere with measurements of low concentrations of fluorescein in the stroma. The degree to which they interfere depends on the wavelengths and bandwidths at which the fluorophotometer operates. It is not uncommon for autofluorescence of the cornea to be equivalent to 8×10^{-9} g/ml fluorescein. Autofluorescence also varies from one person to another. This artifact can be avoided either by measuring autofluorescence in all subjects and subtracting its effects or by simply making measurements when corneal concentrations are much greater than autofluorescence. The autofluorescence of normal aqueous humor is negligible.

Thinness of the Stroma

Measurement of fluorescence in the stroma is particularly difficult because of the thinness of the stroma. This property presents two problems. First, it introduces the possibility that the "to-and-fro" motion of the cornea will blur the measurement unless it is made rather quickly. Second, it introduces uncertainty in the calibration of the measurement unless calibration is made with standard solutions in a chamber of comparable dimensions. A correction must be made to account for the different results obtained in solutions of different thicknesses. The best method is to calibrate each instrument with a chamber the curvature of which is similar to the cornea and the depth of which is continuously variable from zero to several millimeters. Stromal measurements are calibrated according to the measured thickness of the cornea.

Distribution of Fluorescein

As mentioned above, the lateral distribution of fluorescein in the stroma can be quite irregular for many hours after topical administration. Instillation followed by several hours of sleep is the simplest way to avoid erratic results caused by uneven distribution in the cornea.[8] In addition, it is wise not to depend on a stromal measurement at one point, but to measure many points.

Unevenness of distribution can also occur in the anterior chamber, a phenomenon that is unrelated to the time of instillation but depends on the pattern of flow through the pupil in the individual eye. In some eyes, a hypofluorescent area, the "pupillary bubble," persists and causes erratic readings if measurements are made in this area.[16,27] This problem is especially likely to occur when the pupil is small. If such a region is identified, it should be avoided and measurements should be taken from several areas.

Binding of Fluorescein to Albumin

When fluorescein binds to albumin, its spectra are shifted toward longer wavelengths and its fluorescent efficiency is diminished. Both of these effects alter the relation between molarity and fluorescence. The true concentration of fluorescein is underestimated under such conditions unless efforts are made to determine the extent of binding. Binding to albumin and possibly other substances occurs in the corneal stroma, and stromal fluorescence probably underestimates molarity. In the presence of flare in the anterior chamber, a similar problem can exist for cameral measurements. The degree of binding and quenching of albumin varies from one species to another. If stromal fluorescence underestimates molarity of fluorescein, then the published values of the rate of flow of aqueous humor are correspondingly smaller than the true values. Accurate correction of this source of error in the human eye awaits further research into the properties of fluorescence in the stroma. Workers are attempting to quantify this problem by measuring the spectral shift of fluorescein and the polarization of fluorescence in the stroma.

Unaccounted Loss of Fluorescein

In a previous section, it was shown that florophotometric measurement of flow can be carried out only if the major route of loss of the tracer is by means of aqueous outflow. In certain pathologic conditions, this assumption is not valid. Examples are vascularization of the cornea or neovascularization of the iris where diffusional loss of fluorescein directly into the blood can account for a major proportion of its disappearance. Any condition in which the iris-lens diaphragm is disrupted can permit loss of the dye into the posterior segment. In aphakic eyes, pseudophakic eyes, eyes with large iridectomies, or eyes with widely dilated pupils large amounts of fluorescein can enter the posterior chamber and be lost from the system. Fluorescein kinetics in such eyes can be grossly misleading, and calculation of flow from such data is not possible by methods available at the present time.

REPEATABILITY AND ACCURACY

The repeatability of the fluorophotometric method has been determined in two ways. First, the flows have been measured simultaneously in the two eyes of normal subjects. Second, the flow in an eye has been measured on two occasions at the same time of day and the measurements compared. Either method suggests that the repeatability is approximately $\pm$ 16%.[2] The limit of the reproducibility of the technique can be determined from the variance of the measurement of ocular fluorescence for the particular fluorophotometer that is employed. A good fluorophotometer can make repeated measurements of stromal fluorescence in human subjects to $\pm$ 4% and of cameral fluorescence to $\pm$ 6%, limited mainly by the lack of uniformity of the distribution of fluorescence in these tissues.[3] Improvement of the repeatability of measurements of flow is made by making many measurements over a long period of time rather than attempting to measure flow only once over a short interval.

The accuracy of the measurement of flow is more difficult to evaluate. The best that one can do is to compare the results of measurements made by different techniques. O'Rourke has measured the flow of aqueous humor in a small number of human subjects employing a radioactive tracer having a large molecular weight.[30] O'Rourke's method eliminates the possibility of diffusional loss of the tracer and problems associated with the quantification of fluorescence. Holm has employed photogrammetry to measure the volume of the pupillary bubble, which provides direct observation of flow and its calculation by geometric optics.[16] Flows measured by either of these methods are in agreement with flows measured by topical application of fluorescein.

AQUEOUS FLOW IN NORMAL EYES

The average rate of aqueous humor flow in normal persons is approximately 2.5μl/min. In one study of adult subjects aged 20 to 83 years, in which fluorescein was applied by iontophoresis, the rate of flow was 2.4 $\pm$ 0.6 (mean $\pm$ SD) μl/min.[17] In another study of subjects aged 5 to 79 years, in which fluorescein drops were applied, the rate of flow was 2.6 $\pm$ 0.5 μl/min.[18] In neither study was a difference in flow observed between males and females.

There is greater variation in flow from one subject to another than from one eye to the other of a given subject. The rate of flow is similar in all age groups, although a slight regression of flow with age is observed, -0.006 μl/min/yr, or about 20% reduction over a lifetime.[7] Studies of aqueous flow during the first few years of life are lacking.

There is a diurnal variation in the rate of aqueous flow. In the morning, the rate is approximately 3.0 μl/min whereas in the afternoon, it has diminished to 2.4 μm/min. For this reason, comparative studies must be performed at comparable times of the day. At night during sleep, the rate of flow diminishes to its lowest, 1.5 μl/min.[33] Neither lid closure nor reclining during the day mimics this phenomenon. A subject deprived of sleep at night will have a lower flow than during the day, but the lowest flows are seen in sleeping subjects. The mechanism of diurnal changes in the rate of flow is not known. As described below, diurnal changes can be modified by drugs, but no clinically useful drugs for the treatment of glaucoma are able to reduce aqueous flow below the rate observed during sleep.

Though the rate of flow is one of the important determinants of intraocular pressure, flow is relatively unaffected by intraocular pressure except by extremely high pressures. Changes in intraocular pressure brought about by changes in gravity-dependent body position on a tilt table have only a negligible effect on flow.[9] Chronic increases in pressure brought about by application of steroids in steroid responders[1] or by chronic decrease in pressure following laser trabeculoplasty[5] are not accompanied by compensatory changes in flow.

EFFECTS OF DRUGS ON FLOW

As measured by fluorophotometry, many drugs have no appreciable effect on aqueous flow. Among these are topical anesthetics, alpha-adrenergic agonists such as phenylephrine,[22] the alpha-adrenergic antagonist thymoxamine,[23] steroids such as dexamethasone,[34] and a prostaglandin derivative, prostaglandin F_{2a}-isopropyl ester.[20] The cholinergic agonist pilocarpine should probably be included with this group of drugs, since its effect on flow is slight and clinically insignificant.[29]

Three classes of drugs have been found to reduce aqueous flow: carbonic anhydrase inhibitors,[12] beta-adrenergic antagonists,[10,12,32,42] and alpha-2 selective adrenergic agonists.[14] These drugs can reduce flow by one third to one half its

normal rate during the daytime. Interestingly, the beta-blocker timolol has been shown to be ineffective at night during sleep. Timolol suppresses the circadian cycle of the rate of aqueous flow.[37] Chronic treatment with timolol (and probably other beta-blockers) is associated with partial loss of effect of the drug on flow.[6] The rate of flow in the chronically treated eye is midway between the normal daytime rate and the normal nightime rate. Withdrawal from chronic treatment is followed by slow recovery of the flow to its normal rate.[35]

Although the rate of aqueous humor flow can be reduced by several classes of drugs, few drugs increase the rate of flow. One class of drug, the beta-adrenergic agonist, has been shown, under certain circumstances, to stimulate flow in the human eye. Epinephrine,[28,38] salbutamol,[11] isoproterenol,[21] and terbutaline[13] all produce small or moderate increases in flow. These agents are effective mainly at night during sleep when flow is normally slow. This finding has led to the hypothesis that the natural cycle of the rate of flow is driven by endogenous beta-adrenergic tone.

FLUOROPHOTOMETRIC STUDIES IN GLAUCOMA PATIENTS

Fluorophotometry has not been used extensively to study the natural history of glaucoma. The studies that have been done suggest that glaucoma is usually associated with a normal rate of aqueous flow and occasionally associated with reduced aqueous flow. No cases of fluorophotometrically proven hypersecretion glaucoma have been described.

Table 17-1 lists the results of studies in several types of glaucoma, in Horner's syndrome, and in

Table 17-1 Flow studies in abnormal eyes

Disease	N*	Flow (μl/min) Abnormal side	Flow (μl/min) Normal side	Comment	Reference
Steroid-induced glaucoma	5	1.0 times normal	—	Ratio of flow of treated eye to untreated eye	1
Chronic simple glaucoma	9	2.6 ± 0.7	—		Unpublished
	9	2.7 ± 0.9	—		6
Pigmentary glaucoma	3	3.0 ± 0.6	—		6
Unilateral exfoliation syndrome	10	2.0 ± 0.6	2.4 ± 0.7	Difference between eye significant	17
Iridocorneal endothelial syndrome	3	2.4 ± 1.2	1.8 ± 0.2		Unpublished
Fuchs' uveitis syndrome	10	3.2 ± 1.4	3.3 ± 0.8	Iris leakage of fluorescein 5 times normal	18
Horner's syndrome	21	2.2 ± 0.5	2.1 ± 0.6	Difference insignificant	41
Myotonic dystrophy	26	2.5 ± 0.6	—	Blood-ocular barrier leaky	39

*N = Number of eyes

persons with abnormally low intraocular pressure caused by myotonic dystrophy. It is clear that aqueous humor flow is relatively unaffected in all of these syndromes and that the defects responsible for the wide range of pressures found in them must reside in the outflow pathways.

FUTURE ADVANCES IN FLUOROPHOTOMETRY

This chapter has dealt primarily with the measurement of fluorescence to determine the disappearance in vivo of a fluorescent tracer. However, there are other properties of fluorophores that can be exploited for making other physiologic measurements. For example, by measuring either the red shift of the excitation spectrum of fluorescein or by measuring the polarization of fluorescence, it is possible to measure the concentration of albumin in the anterior chamber. The fluorophore resazurin has been shown to be converted to another fluorescent material, resorufin, by the action of ascorbic acid, suggesting that such a reaction could be employed to monitor ascorbate in the living anterior chamber. Pyranine and 2′, 7′-bis(carboxyethyl)-5(6)-carboxyfluorescein are hydrogen ion-sensitive fluorophores that exhibit properties that make them useful as in vivo pH monitors in the cornea and anterior chamber. The fluorescent lifetimes of some fluorophores exhibit sensitivity to oxygen concentration. It is possible that measurement of fluorescent lifetime with an appropriate indicator would permit monitoring of oxygen tension in transparent ocular tissues. All of these uses of fluorophotometry are being developed. Any one of them could bring new applications to the study of ocular disease by means of fluorophotometry.

REFERENCES

1. Anselmi, P, Bron, AJ, and Maurice DM: Action of drugs on the aqueous flow in man measured by fluorophotometry, Exp Eye Res 7:487, 1968
2. Brubaker, RF: The flow of aqueous humor in the human eye, Trans Am Ophthalmol Soc 80:391, 1982
3. Brubaker, RF: Clinical evaluation of the circulation of aqueous humor. In Duane TD, editor: Clinical Ophthalmology, Philadelphia, 1986, Harper & Row, Publishers, Inc
4. Brubaker, RF, and Coakes, RL: Use of a xenon flash tube as the excitation source in a new slit-lamp fluorophotometer, Am J Ophthalmol 86:474, 1978
5. Brubaker, RF, and Liesegang, TJ: Effect of trabecular photocoagulation on the aqueous humor dynamics of the human eye, Am J Ophthalmol 96:139, 1983
6. Brubaker, RF, Nagataki, S, and Bourne WM: Effect of chronically administered timolol on aqueous humor flow in patients with glaucoma, Ophthalmology 89:280, 1982
7. Brubaker, RF, et al: The effect of age on aqueous humor formation in man, Ophthalmology 88:283, 1981
8. Carlson, KH, Bourne, WM, McLaren, JW, and Brubaker, RF: Variations in human corneal endothelial cell morphology and permeability to fluorescein with age, Invest Ophthalmol Vis Sci 28(Suppl):325, 1987
9. Carlson, KH, McLaren, JW, Topper, JE, and Brubaker, RF: Effect of body position on intraocular pressure and aqueous flow, Invest Ophthalmol Vis Sci 28:1346, 1987
10. Coakes, RL, and Brubaker, RF: The mechanism of timolol in lowering intraocular pressure in the normal eye, Arch Ophthalmol 96:2045, 1978
11. Coakes, RL, and Siah, PB: Effects of adrenergic drugs on aqueous humor dynamics in the normal human eye. I. Salbutamol, Br J Ohpthalmol 68:393, 1984
12. Dailey, RA, Brubaker, RF, and Bourne, WM: The effects of timolol maleate and acetazolamide on the rate of aqueous formation in normal human subjects, Am J Ophthalmol 93:232, 1982
13. Gharagozloo, NZ, Larson, RS, Kullerstrand, LJ, and Brubaker, RF: Terbutaline stimulates aqueous humor flow in humans during sleep, Manuscript submitted for publication, 1987
14. Gharagozloo, NZ, Relf, SJ, and Brubaker, RF: Aqueous flow is reduced by the alpha$_2$-adrenergic agonist para-amino-clonidine. Manuscript submitted for publication, 1987
15. Goldmann, H: Über Fluorescein in der menschlichen Vorderkammer. Das Kammerwasser-Minutenvolumen des Menschen, Ophthalmologica 119:65, 1950
16. Holm, O: A photogrammetric method for estimation of the pupillary aqueous flow in the living eye, Acta Ophthalmol 46:254, 1968
17. Johnson, DH, and Brubaker, RF: Dynamics of aqueous humor in the syndrome of exfoliation with glaucoma, Am J Ophthalmol 93:629, 1982
18. Johnson, D., Liesegang, TJ, and Brubaker, RF: Aqueous humor dynamics in Fuchs' uveitis syndrome, Am J Ophthalmol 95:783, 1983
19. Jones, RF, and Maurice, DM: New methods of measuring the rate of aqueous flow in man with fluorescein, Exp Eye Res 5:208, 1966
20. Kerstetter, JR, Brubaker, RF, Wilson, SE, and Kullerstrand, LJ: Prostaglandin F$_{2\alpha}$-1-isopropylester lowers intraocular pressure without decreasing aqueous flow, Am J Ophthalmol, 105:30, 1988
21. Larson, RS, and Brubaker, RF: Isoproterenol stimulates aqueous flow in humans with Horner's syndrome, Invest Ophthalmol Vis Sci 29:621, 1988
22. Lee, DA, Brubaker, RF: Effect of phenylephrine on aqueous humor flow, Current Eye Res 2:89, 1982
23. Lee, DA, Brubaker, RF, and Nagataki, S: Effect of thymoxamine on aqueous humor formation in the

normal human eye as measured by fluorophotometry, Invest Ophthalmol Vis Sci 21:805, 1981

24. Maurice, DM: A new objective fluorophotometer, Exp Eye Res 2:33, 1963

25. Maurice, DM, and Mishima, S: Ocular pharmacokinetics. In Sears, ML, editor: Pharmacology of the eye, Berlin, 1984, Springer-Verlag

26. McLaren, JW, and Brubaker, RF: Light sources for fluorescein fluorophotometry, Applied Optics 22:2897, 1983

27. McLaren, JW, and Brubaker RF: A two-dimensional scanning ocular fluorophotometer, Invest Ophthalmol Vis Sci 26:144, 1985

28. Nagataki, S, and Brubaker, RF: Early effect of epinephrine on aqueous formation in the normal human eye, Ophthalomology 88:278, 1981

29. Nagataki, S, and Brubaker, RF: Effect of pilocarpine on aqueous humor formation in human beings, Arch Ophthalmol 100:818, 1982

30. O'Rourke, J, and Macri, FJ; Studies in uveal physiology. II. Clinical studies of the anterior chamber clearance of isotopic tracers, Arch Ophthalmol 84:415, 1970

31. Pederson, JE, Gaasterland, DE, and MacLellan, HM: Accuracy of aqueous humor flow determination by fluorophotometry, Invest Ophthalmol Vis Sci 17:190, 1978

32. Reiss, GR, and Brubaker, RF: The mechanism of betaxolol, a new ocular hypotensive agent, Ophthalmology 90:1369, 1983

33. Reiss, GR, Lee, DA, Topper, JE, and Brubaker, RF: Aqueous humor flow during sleep, Invest Ophthalmol Vis Sci 25:776, 1984

34. Rice, SW, Bourne, WM, and Brubaker, RF: Absence of an effect of topical dexamethasone on endothelial permeability and flow of aqueous humor, Invest Ophthalmos Vis Sci 24:1307, 1983

35. Schlecht, LP, and Brubaker, RF: The effects of withdrawal of timolol in chronically treated glaucoma patients, 1987 (In review)

36. Smith, AT, et al: An improved objective slit-lamp fluorometer using tungsten-halogen lamp excitation and synchronous detection, Br J Ophthalmol 61:722, 1977

37. Topper, JE, and Brubaker, RF: Effects of timolol, epinephrine, and acetazolamide on aqueous flow during sleep, Invest Ophthalmol Vis Sci 26:1315, 1985

38. Townsend, DJ, and Brubaker, RF: Immediate effect of epinephrine on aqueous formation in the normal human eye as measured by fluorophotometry, Invest Ophthalmol Vis Sci 19:256, 1980

39. Walker, SD, Brubaker, RF, and Nagataki, S: Hypotony and aqueous humor dynamics in myotonic dystrophy, Invest Ophthalmol Vis Sci 22:744, 1982

40. Waltman, DR, and Kaufman, HE: A new objective slit lamp fluorophotometer, Invest Ophthalmol 9:247, 1970

41. Wentworth, WO, and Brubaker, RF: Aqueous humor dynamics in a series of patients with third neuron Horner's syndrome, Am J Ophthalmol 92:407, 1981

42. Yablonski, ME, et al: A fluorophotometric study of the effect of topical timolol on aqueous humor dynamics, Exp Eye Res 27:135, 1978

43. Zeimer, RC, and Cunha-Vaz, JG: Evaluation and comparison of commercial vitreous fluorophotometers, Invest Ophthalmol Vis Sci 21:865, 1981

Chapter 18

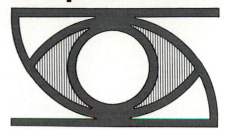

Gonioscopy

Paul Palmberg

Because therapy for each type of glaucoma must be specific to be effective, one needs to determine during the initial evaluation of a glaucoma patient the site at which aqueous flow is impeded and the mechanism responsible. Determining the type of glaucoma requires integrating information obtained from both the history and examination.

Consideration of the ocular and general medical history helps experienced examiners focus on likely glaucoma mechanisms. In addition, the history may prompt special attention to some portions of the examination (e.g., a more systematic search for subtle findings of iridocorneal angle injury in a previously traumatized eye) or it may be the only clue to recognizing the type of glaucoma (e.g., steroid-induced glaucoma).

A complete eye examination is then performed, both to establish the site of aqueous flow impairment and to look for other findings offering clues about the mechanism. Central to the examination is gonioscopy, the visualization of the anterior chamber angle. This is a demanding skill, requiring dexterity to achieve a stable, focused image at the proper viewing angle, a knowledge of how to prevent artifactual observations, and familiarity with a large variety of normal and abnormal findings. The remainder of the ocular examination provides critical information for the diagnosis of many types of secondary glaucoma, such as those associated with retinovascular ischemia, intraocular tumors, lens subluxation, pigment dispersion, exfoliation, inflammatory conditions, corneal endothelial disorders, or increased episcleral venous pressure.

Although we stress the importance of integrating gonioscopic findings with other signs and the history, gonioscopy is the most important factor in making a correct diagnosis. The most common cause of incorrect diagnosis is not the missing of subtle signs of the various secondary glaucomas, but rather the omission of gonioscopy by the clinician who reasons that if the slit-lamp examination does not suggest a narrow angle or ocular inflammation, the patient must have an open-angle mechanism. Chronic angle-closure glaucoma and many types of secondary glaucoma are thereby overlooked. Not only is gonioscopy essential, but it should be repeated periodically to detect the secondary emergence of mixed mechanisms.

Among several excellent discussions of gonioscopy worthy of study are those of Epstein[3] and Shaffer.[7] Excellent gonioscopic photographs are presented in several texts.[3,7,12] The history of gonioscopy is summarized by Gorin.[6]

METHODS OF GONIOSCOPY

To view the anterior chamber angle structures one must overcome an optical problem. Light rays coming from the angle approach the cornea-air interface at an oblique angle that exceeds the critical angle and are totally internally reflected. However, the use of a contact lens to neutralize the corneal refractive power allows visualization of the angle structures either directly (direct gonioscopy) or

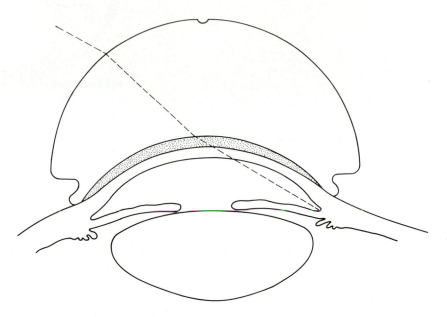

Fig. 18-1 Direct gonioscopy: ray tracing for path of light through anterior chamber, cornea, gonioscopic fluid, Koeppe goniolens, and air.

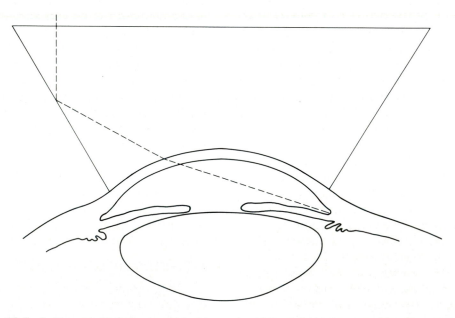

Fig. 18-2 Indirect gonioscopy: ray tracing for path of light through anterior chamber, cornea, tears and Zeiss goniolens, angled reflection from mirror, and path through remainder of lens and air.

through reflection in a mirror mounted in the lens (indirect gonioscopy).[4,7,9]

Direct Gonioscopy

In the technique of direct gonioscopy, a 50-diopter concave goniolens (Koeppe) is placed upon the anesthetized cornea with the patient in a recumbent position (Fig. 18-1). The space between the inner surface of the lens and the cornea is filled with saline or a viscous solution, such as methylcellulose. Viewing is achieved through a binocular magnifier held with one hand while the eye is illuminated by a hand-held light. The heavy viewing device may be suspended on a rope from a pulley mounted on the ceiling and counterbalanced by a weight. Coordination of the patient, lens, viewer, and illuminator requires considerable practice and may require an assistant.[4]

Indirect Gonioscopy

Indirect gonioscopy employs a mirror mounted in a contact lens to visualize the iridocorneal angle (Fig. 18-2). Having thereby converted the vantage point for viewing to straight ahead of the patient, one may conveniently view the iridocorneal angle with the slit-lamp biomicroscope. The viewing angle of the angle recess is adjusted by having the patient adjust his direction of gaze.

Relative Advantages of the Methods and Their Use in Current Practice

The advantages of direct gonioscopy are that (1) it yields a natural view (versus a reflected one) of the meshwork and surrounding tissues, (2) one can adjust the angle of viewing entirely by movement of the examiner, as in looking over a convex iris surface to see if an angle is closed, and (3) by placing a Koeppe lens on each eye, one can rapidly switch back and forth to detect subtle differences in iridocorneal angle depth as evidence for angle recession. Direct gonioscopy is used in the performance of goniotomy for infantile glaucoma and can be used to advantage in goniosynechialysis.

The advantages of indirect gonioscopy are that (1) it offers the advantages of the slit-lamp, such as high magnification (made practical by the stabilization of the patient in the headrest), controlled illumination, and convenience, and (2) it can be used with the Zeiss lens for indentation gonioscopy (discussed later), a crucial technique for assessing angle-closure glaucoma.

Most ophthalmologists do not have the equipment or experience to use direct gonioscopy or prefer the more convenient indirect gonioscopy.

Whether because of choice or lack of familiarity, only 2% of ophthalmologists use direct gonioscopy.*

Goniolenses for Indirect Gonioscopy

Two types of goniolenses, exemplified by the Goldmann and the Zeiss lenses, are in common use (Fig. 18-3). Each has advantages for special applications. About three fifths of ophthalmologists use the Goldmann type of lens, and two fifths use the Zeiss goniolens when examining for the presence of angle closure.† A large majority of glaucoma specialists, however, prefer the Zeiss goniolens.

To use the Goldmann lens, a clear fluid must fill the space between the cornea and goniolens. The lens is prepared for application by holding it corneal side up and placing several drops of a viscous solution of methylcellulose on the concave surface. The lens is then brought near the patient's eye and tipped forward against the cornea quickly enough to entrap the solution. As the lens is pressed against the eye and the pressure then relaxed, a suction-cup effect is created, which keeps the lens centered on the cornea, freeing one's attention for examination of the angle. This is an advantage over the Zeiss lens, which does not create a suction effect and therefore requires continued effort to correct for drift. This difference in ease of use is the primary reason why gonioscopy is taught initially with a Goldmann lens and why many continue to prefer it. The suction-cup effect also allows one to achieve fine focusing of the laser spot on the trabeculum (during laser trabeculoplasty) by pulling the eye to the focus of the beam rather than having to achieve alignment solely by movement of the slit-lamp.

However, the suction effect is not altogether beneficial, since it also distorts the anatomic relationships of the iridocorneal angle and can open a closed angle (discussed later), causing the examiner to miss the diagnosis of angle-closure glaucoma. For this reason, a Zeiss goniolens is preferable for evaluation of patients with narrow angles.

---

*In order to survey the goniolens preference of American ophthalmologists, I conducted informal audience polls at 42 meetings in 24 states between 1984 and 1988. Of the approximately 2000 ophthalmologists participating, about three fifths currently use a Goldmann type of lens, two fifths use a Zeiss type of lens, and only 2% use a Koeppe lens in examining for the presence of angle-closure glaucoma. The results were similar in all regions of the country.

†The *Goldmann* single mirror lens has a corneal contact diameter of 11 mm and a flatter peripheral section, extending to 14 mm, that rests on the sclera. The radius of curvature of the inner surface of the lens is 7.4 mm, so that the lens is more steeply vaulted than the cornea.[10]

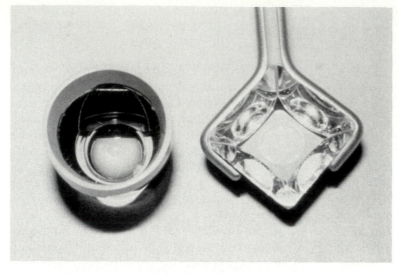

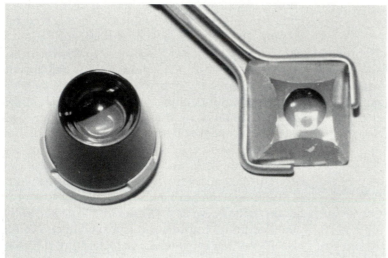

Fig. 18-3 The Goldmann (*left*) and Zeiss (*right*) goniolenses with, **A,** top view and, **B,** bottom view.

The Zeiss four-mirror goniolens comes with a holding fork (see Fig. 18-3), which facilitates application of the lens to the eye. The lens has a 9 mm corneal segment and thus rests solely on the cornea. The radius of curvature of the inner surface of the lens (7.72 mm) closely matches that of the average cornea. The narrow space between the goniolens and the cornea can be adequately filled by either the tear film of the patient or a drop of anesthetic placed on the lens surface.[10] This avoids the need for a viscous goniosolution. No suction-cup effect is created in using this lens.

Gonioscopic Technique

Attention paid to the physical arrangements of patient and examiner can help in avoiding distorting pressures on the eye during assessment for angle-closure and in avoiding tremor that would affect laser beam focusing during anterior segment procedures. The first step is to have the patient sit comfortably erect and to form a base of support for that position by adjustment of the chinrest and table height of the slit-lamp stand. If the slit-lamp is obstructed from sliding forward by the patient's chest, the patient may need to lean forward. The height and position of the examiner's stool should be adjusted to allow the examiner to sit comfortably erect and as far forward as possible.

Goldmann lens

When using a Goldmann type of goniolens, some examiners will be more dexterous using a three-finger technique (thumb, index, and middle fingers) to grasp the lens rim, while others will

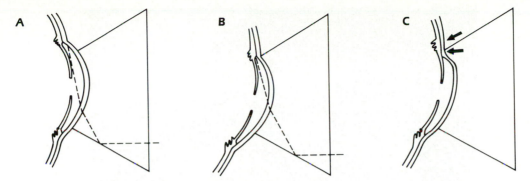

Fig. 18-4 Effect of patient's direction of gaze on view of angle obtained. **A,** With gaze directed ahead one cannot see over convex iris. **B,** With gaze directed toward the mirror one can see "over the hill" to angle structures. Note that a narrow slit-beam of light on iris must intersect eyewall to prove that the deepest open portion of iridocorneal angle is being viewed. **C,** Pressure on lens is shown on corneoscleral junction and artifactually closing a portion of angle *(arrows)*.

prefer a two-finger technique (thumb and index finger). The goniolens is held in the examiner's left hand for examination of a right eye, and right hand for examination of a left eye. To steady the examiner's hand, the fingers not holding the lens are placed either gently on the cheek of the patient or on the vertical bar of the slit-lamp headrest. The wrist should be kept straight and the forearm as vertical as possible. The elbow should be supported either by the tabletop of the slit-lamp if the examiner's forearm is of sufficient length or else by an elbow rest. These measures help the examiner avoid inadvertently resting the weight of the hand and forearm on the goniolens, and they avoid fatigue-related tremor of the muscles of the forearm, arm, shoulder, and back.

The hand not holding the goniolens is used to adjust the slit-lamp microscope so that it is focused on the image of the iridocorneal angle reflected by the goniomirror. Since the sector of angle seen is across the anterior chamber from the mirror, one views, for example, the inferior angle when the mirror is at the top of the lens. The rest of the angle is viewed sequentially by rotating the lens, usually in 90-degree steps for examination, but in more numerous steps during laser trabeculoplasty.

When the view of the iridocorneal angle is obscured by a convex iris, one can "see over the hill" by having the patient look in the direction of the mirror (compare Fig. 18-4, *A* and *B*). In doing so, one must be careful not to allow the rim of the gonioprism to indent the peripheral cornea or limbal sclera, because this would artifactually narrow or even close the iridocorneal angle (Fig. 18-4, *C*). One can avoid this problem by holding the goni-

olens gently and being alert to any sensation of increased pressure of the lens against the fingers holding it.

Having the patient look in the direction of the mirror gives a better view of narrow iridocorneal angles than the frequently recommended procedure of moving the goniolens along the corneal surface toward the angle to be viewed (in the process tilting the mirror). The procedures are not optically equivalent, as might first appear. When the patient's eye is rotated, the light path from the mirror to the examiner remains perpendicular to the goniolens surface, whereas when the lens is tilted, the light path is no longer perpendicular and suffers an astigmatic distortion. Such distortion is particularly a problem during laser trabeculoplasty, because it makes the laser spot into a streak.

Although having the patient look in the direction of the mirror has the advantage of allowing one to see more deeply into the angle recess ("dive bomber" view), it has the disadvantage of making the view of the trabecular meshwork more tangential, foreshortening its image and degrading the image quality. When the iris surface is flat, one can instead have the patient look *away* from the direction of the mirror and thereby obtain a view parallel to the iris and nearly perpendicular to the meshwork ("cruise missile" view), which will yield the optimal image quality (Fig. 18-5). The "cruise missile" view should be used when possible for laser trabeculoplasty, because it allows delivery of a round laser spot rather than the elliptic spot delivered by more tangential views.

When viewing narrow nasal and temporal angles, one needs to align the slit-beam with the view-

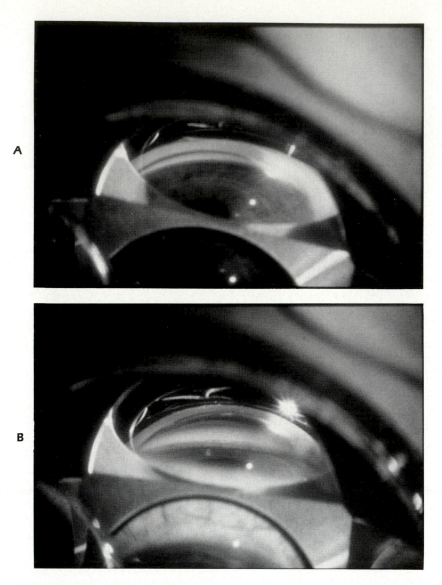

Fig. 18-5 "Dive bomber" view in **A,** clinical view, showing depths of angle but poorly focused and optically truncated view of trabecular meshwork. "Cruise missile" view in **B,** clinical view, showing well-focused perpendicular view of trabecular meshwork.

ing axis in order to illuminate the depths of the angle. With a Zeiss slit-lamp this is straightforward, but with the Haag-Streit instrument one has to tilt the side-arm in order to keep its mirror from obstructing the line of view.

Zeiss goniolens

The Zeiss goniolens may be applied to the eye either in a square or a diamond configuration. For the square configuration, the flat surfaces of the fork are grasped with the thumb on one side and the second and third fingers on the other. The other two fingers rest on the patient's cheek, and the examiner's palm faces the patient. The fork is ori-

ented at a 45-degree angle to the eye. In the diamond configuration, the shaft is oriented horizontally and grasped between the thumb and second finger on the top flat surface and third finger on the bottom flat surface. The backs of the examiner's fingers rest on the patient's cheek.

The square configuration is preferable for several reasons. First, it fits better in the palpebral fissure, and, if contact occurs between the lens and the upper eyelid, the flat surface presented is more comfortable than the corner presented by the diamond configuration. Furthermore, the hand and forearm position used in the square configuration allows one to keep the wrist straight and the forearm vertical for better support and control, whereas the diamond configuration places the wrist in an awkward supinated position and at a mechanical disadvantage for indentation gonioscopy.

To view the undistorted angle configuration, the Zeiss lens should barely touch the corneal surface. This is accomplished by a slight rocking forward of the wrist of the hand holding the lens. This can be done dexterously only if the entire weight of the arm and forearm is supported properly. The position of the lens on the center of the cornea is maintained by the kinesthetic guidance of the two fingers on the patient's cheek. As with the Goldmann lens, one views the depths of narrow angles by having the patient look in the direction of the mirror being viewed. In order to illuminate narrow angles on the nasal or temporal sides, the slit-beam needs to be on the viewing axis.

GONIOSCOPIC ANATOMY AND INTERPRETATION

In a gonioscopic view of an open iridocorneal angle, one can usually identify (from anterior to posterior) the cornea, Schwalbe's line, the anterior (nonpigmented) trabecular meshwork, the filtering portion (often pigmented) of the trabecular meshwork, the scleral spur, the ciliary band, and the iris root (Fig. 18-6). Schwalbe's line is located at the peripheral terminus of the cornea where Descemet's membrane ends in a circumferential ring of collagenous fibers. Sometimes the ring is prominent and protrudes into the anterior chamber. In such cases it is known by the misleading term *posterior embryotoxon* and is often visible through the cornea at the slit-lamp, especially at the temporal limbus. The ring also serves as the anterior attachment site for the sheets of the trabecular meshwork. Even when it does not protrude into the anterior chamber, Schwalbe's line can be identified easily, because first it is the site of transition between the transparent corneal tissue and the off-white, translucent tissue of the trabecular meshwork, and second it is the site of transition from the steeper curvature of the cornea to the flatter curvature of the angle recess and sclera.

The transition between the transparent cornea and translucent trabeculum can be better appreciated when viewed gonioscopically with a thin slit-beam projected into the iridocorneal angle at an oblique angle (Fig. 18-7). The slit of light penetrates the transparent corneal tissues, appearing above Schwalbe's line as a three-dimensional parallelo-

piped of light. At Schwalbe's line the figure of light collapses to a two-dimensional stripe of light on the trabecular surface. In two-dimensional photos or monocular viewing conditions, the transition can still be appreciated, since the light beam on the cornea is distinctly wider than on either the trabecular meshwork or iris. This *parallelopiped method* is an *extremely valuable method of establishing landmarks* when examining an angle that is closed or an angle that is open but has no trabecular pigmentation.

The ridge created by the transition of curvature from cornea to angle recess can be better seen when the patient looks in the direction of the mirror of the goniolens. The ridge acts as a shelf on which pigment particles liberated from the iris pigment epithelium may settle, creating a pigmented line, known as a Sampaolesi line. This line of pigment may mimic the trabecular meshwork in an eye with a closed angle, leading to the erroneous impression that the angle is open. The error can be avoided either by use of the parallelopiped method, in which case the three-dimensional figure of light extends to the false "meshwork," or by opening the iridocorneal angle by indentation gonioscopy (see following discussion) to reveal the true meshwork below the Sampaolasi line.

A Sampaolesi line can also be distinguished from the true pigmented trabecular meshwork by the character and distribution of the pigmentation. The pigment deposited on the shelf at Schwalbe's line resembles salt and pepper. The pigment particles are dark and granular and are deposited in a *discontinuous* fashion. By contrast, the pigment deposited on the trabecular meshwork resembles brown sugar. The pigment particles are finer and deposited for lengthy segments in a *continuous* streak.

The scleral spur is a prominent interior extension of the sclera to which the trabecular beams attach on its anterior edge and to which ciliary muscle fibers attach on its posterior edge. The scleral spur is whiter than the trabecular meshwork and even less translucent, in keeping with its more solid structure.

When the trigonometric angle formed by the surface of the iris and the trabeculum is moderate to wide (20 to 45 degrees), and the filtering portion of the trabecular meshwork can be unequivocally identified, the status of the iridocorneal angle can be assessed by simple inspection. But when the angle is narrow, or the trabeculum is difficult to identify, or both, the supplemental techniques described above must be used.

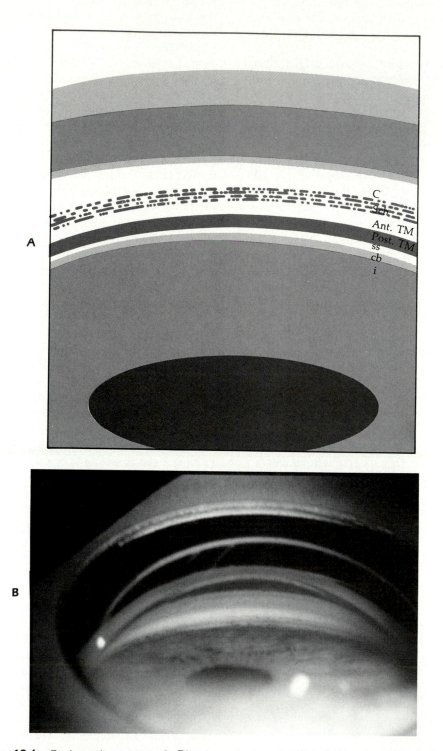

Fig. 18-6   Gonioscopic anatomy. **A,** Diagrammatic view. **B,** Clinical view. Structures include *c,* cornea; *S.1.* Schwalbe's line; *ant TM,* anterior trabecular meshwork, *post TM,* posterior trabecular meshwork; *ss,* scleral spur; *cb,* ciliary band; *i,* iris root.

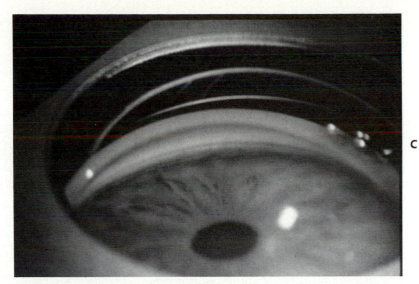

C

Fig. 18-6, cont'd.   C, Injury to opposite eye resulted in an angle recession, with retrodisplacement of iris and underlying ciliary body and exposure of ciliary sulcus.

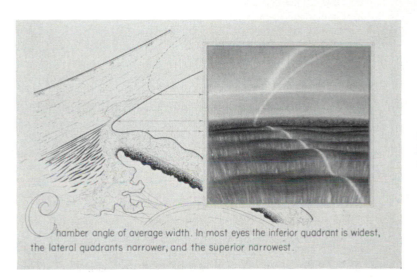

chamber angle of average width. In most eyes the inferior quadrant is widest, the lateral quadrants narrower, and the superior narrowest.

Fig. 18-7 Parallelopiped method of identifying boundary between cornea and trabecular meshwork.

INDENTATION GONIOSCOPY

An invaluable technique in assessing an eye for angle closure is indentation gonioscopy.[5] This technique enables the examiner to alter the position of the iris relative to the trabecular meshwork in a dynamic fashion. It helps distinguish narrow from closed angles and determine whether closed portions of the circumference of the angle are involved only by reversible apposition of the iris to the trabecular meshwork or by peripheral anterior synechiae (PAS).

In this method, the quadrant of the angle to be assessed is first examined with the Zeiss goniolens with no pressure on the cornea and with the patient looking far enough in the direction of the mirror to disclose the line of contact of the iris with the eyewall. A *narrow, short slit-beam* off-axis should be used, in order (1) to assure that the point of contact of the iris with the eyewall is being seen (if one is not seeing adequately "over the hill" into the depths of the angle, the slit beam on the iris surface will not intercept the slit beam on the corneoscleral wall but will end to the side of it); (2) to employ the *parallelopiped method,* and (3) to avoid allowing light to pass through the pupil, because *the pupillary light reflex may result in the opening of a closed angle.*

Next, one applies pressure with the Zeiss lens directly toward the center of the eye, resulting in a deepening of the anterior chamber in the angle

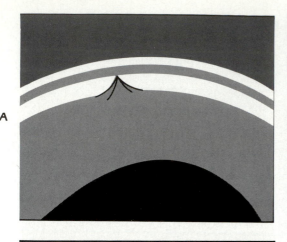

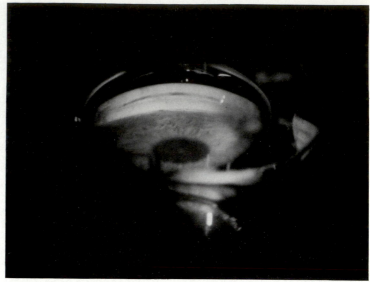

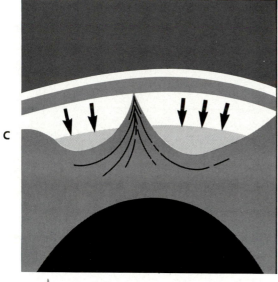

Fig. 18-8 Tethering of iris to eyewall by peripheral anterior synechiae during indentation gonioscopy. **A,** Diagrammatic view before indentation. **B,** Corresponding clinical view. **C,** Diagrammatic view with indentation gonioscopy.

recess. As the iris bows backward, one can see progressively deeper iridocorneal angle structures. If a previously hidden pigmented portion of the trabecular meshwork or peripheral anterior synechiae are thus disclosed, the diagnosis of angle closure is made more certain.

In eyes in which there is considerable iris convexity, the patient should be directed to look far in the direction of the mirror in order to allow the examiner to see over the hill, the area of contact of the Zeiss goniolens may be sufficiently decentered on the cornea that the exertion of direct pressure on the gonioprism causes further rotation of the eye rather than corneal indentation. In such cases, one has to provide both the inward force and a force to prevent rotation (i.e., when viewing the superior iridocorneal angle, with the patient's eye looking down, pressing inward while simultaneously *lifting with the inferior rim* of the goniolens).

In some cases, indentation with the goniolens

buckles the cornea, distorting the view of the iridocorneal angle. Useful information can still be obtained in those cases if the surface of the peripheral iris can be discerned. If peripheral anterior synechiae are present, they will tether the involved portion of the iris, and it will be left in place while adjacent uninvolved portions move posteriorly (Fig. 18-8).

The mechanism by which corneal indentation deepens the peripheral angle is not, as is often supposed, just a reversal of the pressure gradient from the posterior chamber to the anterior chamber, though one generally occurs. Corneal indentation still deepens the angle when a large sector iridectomy is present and no pressure gradient is possible. Rather, the increased intraocular pressure from corneal indentation causes a stretching of the limbal ring of sclera, resulting in a partial straightening of the corneoscleral angle and posterior rotation of the attached iris and ciliary body. A similar deepening of the anterior chamber occurs when the suction cup effect of a Goldmann lens increases the intraocular pressure. Above an intraocular pressure of about 40 mm Hg, little more expansion of the ring can occur, and consequently indentation gonioscopy is often ineffective.

Indentation gonioscopy can be used to advantage in situations other than examining narrow angles. It can be used to bow back the iris in looking for an iridodialysis in an eye with a unilateral glaucoma or in looking for a cyclodialysis cleft.

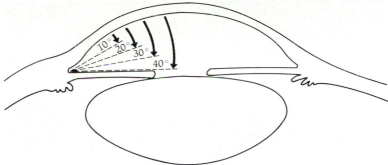

Fig. 18-9   Shaffer grading system for the width of the iridocorneal angle.

GRADING ANGLE DEPTH

It is customary to record the findings of gonioscopy in a standardized fashion. The purpose of such records is to document findings pertinent to the diagnosis of a particular type of glaucoma or to follow changes in the appearance of the iridocorneal angle over time that might signal impending angle closure.

Shaffer System

The most common grading system is that proposed by Shaffer.[7] It is based on an estimate of the geometric angle formed by the iris and the corneoscleral wall at the approach to the trabecular meshwork. The iridocorneal angle is graded on a scale of 0 (closed), slit (open only a few degrees, I (about 10 degrees), II (20 degrees), III (30 degrees) and IV (40 degrees or more) (Fig. 18-9).

Scheie System

It is important in communications between ophthalmologists to specify whether one is using the Shaffer grading system or the rather opposite convention of the Scheie system,[8] in which a grade I angle is widely open, a grade II angle allows one to see just to the scleral spur but not to the ciliary body, a grade III angle allows one to see only to the anterior trabecular meshwork, and a grade IV angle is closed.

It has been found that Shaffer grade slit and I angles are at considerable risk of closure, either spontaneously or with provocative testing. When narrow but open angles are present in eyes with elevated intraocular pressure, one should consider the possibility that the mechanism of pressure elevation is damage to the trabeculum from intermittent closure. Smudges of iris pigment on or above the trabeculum (Fig. 18-10) or small tentlike peripheral anterior synechiae provide strong evidence that such intermittent closure has indeed taken place. Grade II angles bear watching, because

they may become more shallow in the future, and Grade III and IV angles are probably not at risk of primary angle closure.

Quadrants may differ by one or two grades in the same eye, the superior angle generally being the narrowest and the inferior the widest. Eyes that are narrow circumferentially are at greatest risk of acute angle-closure glaucoma attacks, whereas eyes that are narrow in only one or two quadrants are more likely to develop partial angle-closure (with chronic, moderate pressure elevations insufficient to cause pain or corneal edema).

Angle grading is more difficult in those eyes in which the iris side of the angle is not straight but is instead concave or convex, especially when the convexity is in the form of a prominent last roll ("plateau iris" configuration), and in those eyes in which the iris insertion is abnormally located at or even anterior to the scleral spur.

Spaeth System

Spaeth[11] has developed a classification system that expands on the Shaffer grading of angles to include a specification of the shape of the peripheral angle (Fig. 18-11) and site of iris insertion. A concave peripheral iris is denoted q, a regularly straight iris r, and a steeply convex iris s. The implication is that an s configuration of the iris brings iris tissue into closer proximity with the functional trabecular meshwork and thereby increases the risk of angle-closure. Thus even an iridocorneal angle with a grade I to II approach may be at imminent risk of angle-closure when a plateau iris configuration is present. The site of iris insertion in this system is specified as **A** if the insertion is *anterior* to the trabecular meshwork (e.g., synechial closure to Schwalbe's line), **B** if the insertion is just *behind* Schwalbe's line, **C** if the insertion is at the scleral spur, **D** if the angle is *deep* with a visible face of the ciliary body, and **E** if the angle is *extremely* deep.

In primary congenital glaucoma the iris and

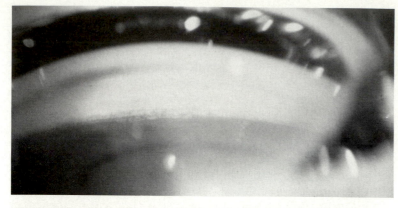

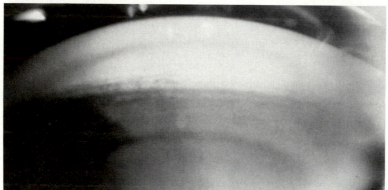

Fig. 18-10 **A,** Smudges of iris pigment above trabecular meshwork appear as three lines, perhaps representing "high tide" lines. **B,** Smudged pigment also is deposited over trabecular meshwork itself, as revealed by indentation gonioscopy of closed angle.

ciliary body fail to migrate posteriorly during development, and the iris commonly inserts into the trabecular meshwork.[1] After cutting of the superficial layers of the trabeculum during a goniotomy operation, the iridocorneal angle usually opens in a fashion resembling the cutting of an accordion strap, the iris then appearing to insert into the now exposed scleral spur.

van Herick Technique

Angle depth also may be estimated from the slit-lamp appearance of the anterior chamber. In the technique described by van Herick,[13] a thin slit-beam is focused on the cornea and anterior chamber at and perpendicular to the temporal limbus, and the optical section viewed at a 60-degree angle. If the iris is seen to touch the corneal endothelium, angle closure is clearly present. A grade I angle corresponds approximately to a peripheral chamber depth less than one-fourth corneal thickness, a grade II angle to a one-fourth corneal thickness depth, a grade III angle to a one-half corneal thickness depth, and a grade IV angle to a corneal thickness depth or greater. Although the van Herick method is useful in cases in which corneal edema, guttata, or scarring preclude a useful gonioscopic view, *it should not be regarded as an adequate substitute for gonioscopy.* Angles estimated to be as deep as

grade II by this method can be closed. Even in eyes with deep anterior chambers, valuable observations (angle recession, inflammatory synechiae, rubeosis, abnormal pigment, tumor, ghost cells) can be missed if gonioscopy is omitted.

GONIOSCOPIC FINDINGS

Peripheral anterior synechiae are adhesions of the iris to the trabecular meshwork (Fig. 18-12). Among the mechanisms leading to their formation are appositional angle closure, inflammation, neovascular membranes, migrating corneal endothelial cells (ICE syndrome), and trauma.

The location and configuration of PAS can be a clue to the mechanism of their origin. In primary angle-closure glaucoma, synechiae typically form first in the superior angle because it is generally the narrowest part. Inflammatory PAS tend to be broad-based and to form preferentially in the inferior angle because of settling of white blood cells. PAS in the ICE syndrome can advance anterior to Schwalbe's line, an unusual finding in other conditions. PAS with a tooth-shaped appearance may form after laser trabeculoplasty.

It is important to distinguish between PAS, which are tented-up portions of the iris held by adhesions to the trabecular meshwork, and iris processes, which are a normal variant, composed of

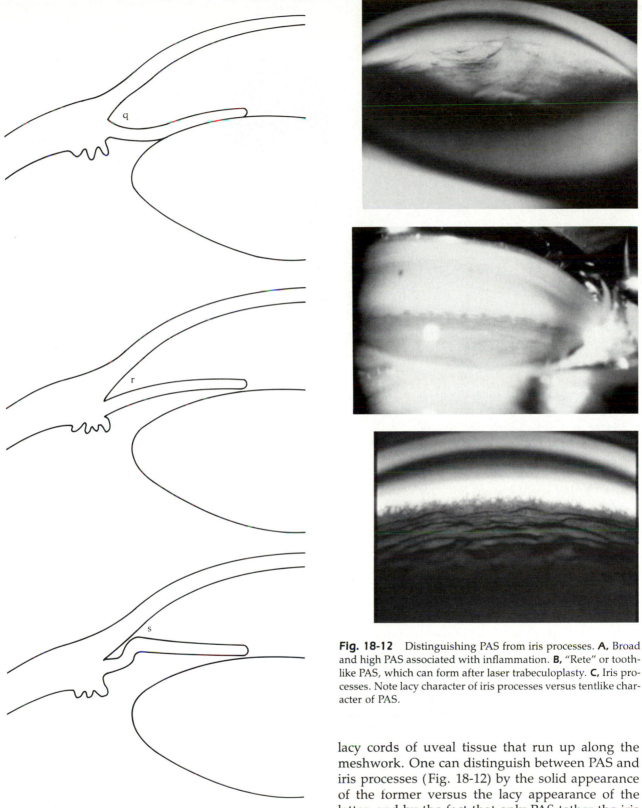

Fig. 18-11 Diagrammatic representation of angle configurations designated in Spaeth system *q* or queer (concave), *r* or regular, and *s* or steep.

Fig. 18-12 Distinguishing PAS from iris processes. **A,** Broad and high PAS associated with inflammation. **B,** "Rete" or toothlike PAS, which can form after laser trabeculoplasty. **C,** Iris processes. Note lacy character of iris processes versus tentlike character of PAS.

lacy cords of uveal tissue that run up along the meshwork. One can distinguish between PAS and iris processes (Fig. 18-12) by the solid appearance of the former versus the lacy appearance of the latter, and by the fact that only PAS tether the iris to the angle wall, preventing backward movement during indentation gonioscopy.

When new vessels in the iris invade the iri-

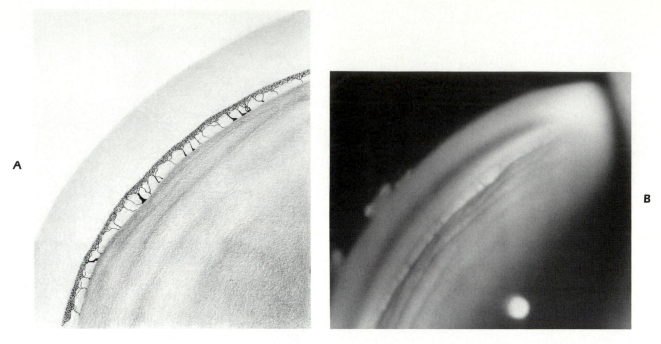

Fig. 18-13 Angle neovascularization in, **A,** diagrammatic and, **B,** clinical views, showing grape-arbor pattern of vessels.

docorneal angle, they form a fibrovascular membrane on the trabecular surface that obstructs aqueous outflow. Only the vessels are visible. Trunk vessels rise across the scleral spur and branch like a grape arbor on the surface of the trabecular meshwork. The vessels are so small that one sees only a red hue to the meshwork at low power, and only the trunk vessels may be resolved at high power (Fig. 18-13).

A number of gonioscopic findings are important in detecting the effects of trauma. Blunt trauma may produce tears in the trabecular meshwork and posterior displacement of the ciliary body, "angle recession" (see Fig. 18-6). It is the tear of the trabecular meshwork that may cause glaucoma, but the tear and subsequent scar of the meshwork may be impossible to detect clinically after healing, while the angle recession remains. Injury may also result in a cyclodialysis cleft (Fig. 18-14), which allows aqueous fluid to exit the eye via the suprachoroidal space, causing hypotony. Other trauma findings of interest are foreign bodies and microscopic hyphemas.

Trabecular pigmentation is generally light in blue-eyed persons and the young, and moderate in brown-eyed persons and the aged. It may be slightly increased in primary open-angle glaucoma but not diagnostically so. It has been reported that the pigmentation of the meshwork may be more

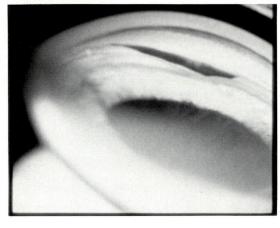

Fig. 18-14 Cyclodialysis cleft. Iris and ciliary body are separated from ciliary sulcus, leaving a deep cleft.

segmental in primary open-angle patients.[2] Trabecular meshwork pigmentation is graded on a scale of 0 (none), 1 (faint), 2 (average), 3 (heavy), and 4 (very heavy). Greater degrees of trabecular pigmentation are generally seen only in conditions in which iris pigment is dispersed abnormally, such as exfoliation syndrome and pigmentary glaucoma. Increased angle pigment may also be seen as a result of an iris melanoma or chafing of the haptic of a posterior chamber lens on the posterior surface of the iris.

REFERENCES

1. Anderson, DR: The development of the trabecular meshwork and its abnormality in primary infantile glaucoma, Trans Am Ophthalmol Soc 79:458, 1981
2. Campbell, DG, Boys-Smith, JW, and Wood, W: Segmentation of trabecular pigmentation in primary open angle glaucoma, Invest Ophthalmol Vis Sci 25(suppl):122, 1984
3. Donaldson, D: Atlas of external diseases of the eye, vol IV. Anterior chamber, iris and ciliary body, St Louis, 1973, The CV Mosby Co
4. Epstein, D, editor: Chandler-Grant's glaucoma, ed 3, Philadelphia, 1986, Lea & Febiger
5. Forbes, M: Gonioscopy with corneal indentation: a method for distinguishing between appositional closure and synechial closure, Arch Ophthalmol 76:488, 1966
6. Gorin, G: Gonioscopy. In Cairns, JE, editor: Glaucoma, vol 1, New York, 1968, Grune & Stratton
7. Kolker, AE and Hetherington, J, Jr., editors: Becker and Shaffer's diagnosis and therapy of the glaucomas, ed 5, St Louis, 1976, The CV Mosby Co
8. Scheie, HG: Width and pigmentation of the angle of the anterior chamber, Arch Ophthalmol 58:510, 1957
9. Shields, MB: Textbook of glaucoma, ed 2, Baltimore, 1987, Williams & Wilkins
10. Smith, R: Bubble-free gonioscopy. In Krieglstein, GK, and Leydhecker, W, editors: Glaucoma update II, 1983, Springer-Verlag
11. Spaeth, GL: The normal development of the human anterior chamber angle: a new system of descriptive grading, Trans Ophthalmol Soc UK 91:709, 1971
12. van Buskirk, EM: Clinical atlas of glaucoma, Philadelphia, 1986, WB Saunders Co
13. van Herick, W: Estimation of width of angle of anterior chamber, Am J Ophthalmol 68:626, 1969

Chapter 19

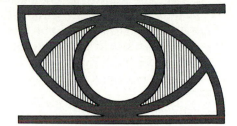

Exploring the Normal Visual Field

John R. Lynn
Ronald L. Fellman
Richard J. Starita

HISTORICAL CONSIDERATIONS

The concept of the visual field dates back to the fifth century B.C. when Hippocrates described hemianopic field defects. As early as 150 BC, Ptolemy attempted to measure and document the visual field. By the seventeenth century, Mariotte found the physiologic blind spot, associated it with the optic nerve head, and thus was the first to describe a scotoma. During the early part of the eighteenth century, Boerhaave investigated scotomas.

In 1801, Thomas Young made the first exact measurements of the visual field.[47] A quarter of a century later, Purkinje further delineated the limits of the normal visual field.[36]

Von Graefe[18] introduced campimetric examinations to the clinical environment. He clearly mapped out the physiologic blind spot, central scotomas, contraction of isopters, and hemianopsias. About the same time, Förster developed the first arc perimeter, extending practical testing beyond 45 degrees.[16] Because the visual angle of the test object remained constant with this method, he gave birth to the more restrictive definition of the term perimetry. Förster's work was a prelude to perimetry, as well as a determination of the outer limit of the visual field and charting of gross defects.

Arc perimetry continued until 1889 when Bjerrum discovered that he could get much more information about glaucomatous fields by using the back of his consulting room door.[5] His work led to the evolution of the Bjerrum or tangent screen and the development of multiple isopter kinetic campimetry. Quantitative campimetry still provides as much precision in central visual field mapping as is available. In the first part of the twentieth century, his method was elaborated in great detail by Rönne,[38] Sinclair and Traquair,[43] and Walker.[44]

In the twentieth century, Ferree and Rand[13] extended the early work of Förster with stimuli of constant visual angles, carrying arc perimetry with solid test objects to its epitomy. Goldmann showed that a 16-fold change in area of the test object is approximately equivalent to a 10-fold change in the intensity of the projected light that forms the test spot.[17] Then he introduced his hemispheric projection perimeter, which became the clinical standard for 30 years.

Louise Sloan first recognized the importance of stationary or static threshold perimetry.[40] Harms and Aulhorn investigated many aspects of perimetry and established static perimetry, supplementing kinetic testing as the highest clinical standard.[20] They designed the Tübinger perimeter for manual testing by both static and kinetic perimetry. Drance[7] documented the important effects of aging on the central and peripheral isopters of the visual field in normal subjects. A few years later, Armaly[1] popularized the concept of suprathreshold screening, emphasizing those areas of the visual field most commonly affected by glaucoma.

Dubois-Poulsen and Magis made the first attempt at automated kinetic perimetry in the early

1960s but were limited by the level of technology available.[9] Lynn and Tate demonstrated the first static automated campimeter in 1969, using a computer and a modified television set.[30] Fankhauser, Koch, Spahr, Heijl, Krakau and others are credited for the rapid development of static automated perimetry.[12,21,25,26,41]

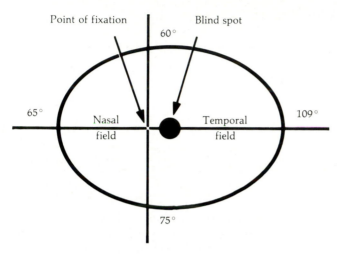

Fig. 19-1 Normal limits of the right eye's visual field: temporally 109 degrees, superiorly 60 degrees, nasally 65 degrees, and inferiorly 75 degrees. Despite voluntary immobility, the eye detects the presence of a large, bright object at any location within the ovoid limiting line (isopter), except inside the normal blind spot. Because the visual field of the left eye is a mirror image of the right, the two blind spots never overlap, so their presence goes unnoticed.

CONCEPT: THE NORMAL GRADIENT OF A VISUAL FIELD

The Visual Field: Definitions, Limits, and Conventions

The visual field of one eye comprises all the space it can see at any given instant. In current clinical testing of a visual field, the eye to be tested must look steadily at a light or other fixation target that is straight ahead. Conventionally, the visual field of each eye is plotted separately as the patient sees it (i.e., objects seen in the right visual space of each eye are plotted on the right side of both visual field charts).

The word perimetry is used almost interchangeably with visual field testing; it means measurement of the periphery. The periphery of the normal visual field varies in radius as shown in Fig. 19-1. Large test objects are seen initially at a perimetric angle of 62 to 65 degrees nasally and between 105 and 109 degrees temporally. All perimetric angles are situated at the center of the pupil where the line that passes through the fixation target crosses those that pass through the objects used to test the visual field (Fig. 19-2). The area available for admission of light is decreased as the test source is moved from a central zone toward the periphery because the pupil appears circular in shape when viewed frontally and progressively elliptical with an enlarging perimetric angle.

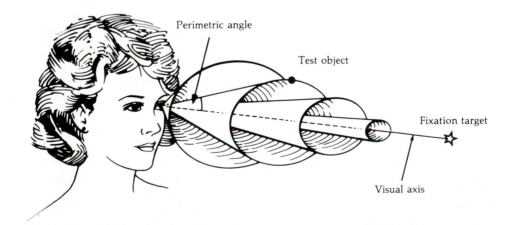

Fig. 19-2 Conoids that share apical peaks in the pupil and a concentric surround of the visual axis. The visual axis is aimed at a fixation point, the object of current interest. In the normal, light-adapted eye, visual sensitivity is maximal at fixation. A line from any of the test objects crosses the visual axis in the pupil center to form that test object's "perimetric angle." The entire 3-D surface of each conoid is equally sensitive to a test object of known visual angle and contrast. Thus, test objects with progressively larger visual angles or more contrast produce a succession of conoids with increasing perimetric angles.

The angular size or visual angle of a test object also is measured at the center of the pupil and relates the lines from the extreme edges of the test object as they converge there. The angular size of a test spot is affected by plus or minus magnification effects of external corrective lenses and by changes in distance between a test object and the eye.

Retinal Anatomic and Functional Significance

Anatomy

Because the specialized sensory cells in the retina are not distributed homogeneously and their neural connections are not disbursed evenly, retinal sensitivity varies significantly from one zone to another. The retina is a layered structure. Light entering the eye must pass successively through transmitting cells (ganglions) and interconnecting cells (bipolar, horizontal, and amacrine) before reaching the photoreceptor cells (rods and cones) (Fig. 19-3).

Polyak has described the form, function, and distribution of photoreceptor cells, which collectively number approximately 126,500,000 in each retina.[35] Of these, about 110 to 125 million are rods and 6.3 to 6.8 million are cones. In Fig. 19-4, the number of rods and the number of cones have been

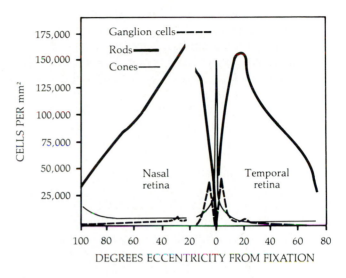

Fig. 19-4   Osterberg's curves: photoreceptor cell count as a function of perimetric angle. These curves reveal the density of rods, cones, and ganglion cells along a horizontal line through the fovea.

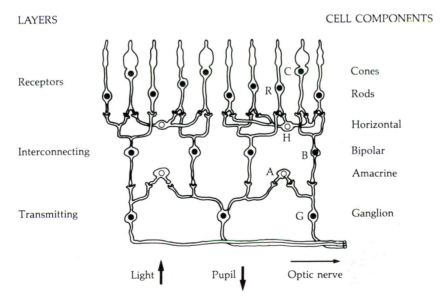

Fig. 19-3   Simplified anatomy of the retina: (1) rods *(R)* and cones *(C)*, the sensory cell components, make up the receptor layer; (2) horizontal *(H)*, bipolar *(B)*, and amacrine *(A)* cells comprise the interconnecting layer; (3) ganglion cells *(G)* are the transmitting layer, for the optic nerve is composed of their axons. The ratio between sensory and transmitting cells in the fovea approaches 1 to 1, whereas the peripheral retina may have as many as 300 receptor cells feeding into a single ganglion cell.

plotted by Osterberg as a function of the perimetric angle in degrees.[33] The number of cones per square millimeter is about 145,000 in the fovea. At an eccentricity or perimetric angle of 10 degrees, the number of cones drops to about 10,000 per square millimeter. Beyond this the count never exceeds 8000 and remains relatively constant to the periphery. On the other hand, there are no rods centrally in the fovea. The number of rods increases to a peak of about 135,000 per square millimeter at approximately 18 degrees nasally and temporally from the fovea. The rod density then gradually falls off to 115,000 per square millimeter at 35 degrees in the temporal retina and at 50 degrees in the nasal retina.

A second major reason for the inherently variable sensitivity of one retinal zone as compared with another is the changing interconnections, manifest as a difference in ratios between receptor cells and their transmitting or ganglion cells. The latter total approximately 1 million per eye, or somewhat less than 1% of the total number of photoreceptors. An intermediate number of interconnecting cells or bipolar cells are present between the receptor cells and the ganglion cells. The numbers tend to suggest an 11:1 ratio between receptor and interconnecting cells and a similar 11:1 ratio between interconnecting and transmitting cells. This "average" system may exist, if at all, only in a small part of the retina. The fact that interconnections are not homogeneous in the retina is best illustrated in the fovea where most of the 115,000 cones are served by their own individual intercon-

necting cells and their own individual ganglion cells.[35] Thus, the ratio between receptor and transmitting cells in the fovea approaches 1:1. In the peripheral retina, this same ratio must be much more than the average 126:1 to make up for the "private line" connections that are so dense in the central field. The disparity in receptor-to-transmitting cell ratios does not have a sharp cutoff but rather a gradual transition from 1:1 centrally to perhaps 300:1 in the periphery. Thus, the central part of the retina is anatomically represented in the brain as individual points, whereas the peripheral retina shows up only as zones.

Function

Several measures of visual physiology parallel the ocular anatomy previously described. Electrophysiologists have studied retinal ganglion cell function in experimental animals, projecting tiny light spots directly onto or near retinal areas called receptive fields. The light spots are capable of stimulating or inhibiting the receptive field's response, depending on its type and whether the light strikes the middle of the receptive field or its periphery. The size of a receptive field is determined when the test lights are barely too far from the center of the field to stimulate or inhibit it. Receptive field sizes are much smaller in the retinal center than in its periphery.

Aulhorn's curves (Fig. 19-5) show the minimal intensities at which normal human subjects respond to the presence of stationary test objects along a horizontal line through fixation with a va-

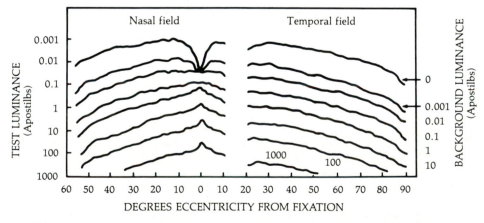

Fig. 19-5 Aulhorn's curves of light sense: average static perimetric thresholds along the horizontal meridian at various background luminances, right eye. The ordinate scale on the left represents the projected intensity of barely visible light (ΔL). The eight different curves are labeled with their background intensities on the right. The background luminances determine both the adaptation state of the retina and the contrasting intensity (L) of the differential light sense.

riety of background light intensities.[42] The three lower curves indicate visual function in bright light, the two upper curves represent light sense in total or subtotal darkness, and the intermediate curves show function in twilight illuminations. Physiologists prefer to call only the uppermost curve in Fig. 19-5 "light sense;" all the others are increment thresholds or differential light sense curves to the purist. A comparison of Fig. 19-4 with Fig. 19-5 suggests correctly that cones are associated with vision in bright light and rods with vision in dim illumination.

When background intensity is high in the lower curves of Fig. 19-5, their shapes show a peak in the central field and a gradual fall off into the periphery, reminiscent of Osterberg's plot of cone distribution. When the background light is dim or absent in the upper curves, the light sense improves far more in the midperiphery than it does in the center, similar to Osterberg's plot of rod distribution. Although rods are much more sensitive to dim light than are cones, the absence of rods in the fovea means the central light sense during deep mesopic and scotopic testing never becomes better or worse than when background or test object light is barely enough to stimulate the cones.

The discipline of photometry provides different units for measuring both the light emitted by point sources, such as a distant star, and the light coming from larger, so-called extended sources. Since point sources would be difficult to obtain and use in perimetry, consideration here is limited to light per unit area of an emitting, transmitting, or reflecting surface. Luminance, so defined, is the physical counterpart of the psychologic term brightness. In perimetry, the most commonly used unit of luminance is the apostilb (asb). The next most commonly used unit, millilambert, is equal to ten apostilbs. The nit, or candela per meter squared, at 3.142 apostilbs, is logarithmically half way between the millilambert and the asb.

The rods begin to function when light from the test surface exceeds 10 millionths (10^{-5}) asb and they continue to operate exclusively as long as the background and stimulus values are less than 0.003 asb.[23] Because the photopigments of rods are bleached by high levels of illumination, the cones function exclusively when the background light exceeds 3 asb.[23] Both types of receptor cells are said to function simultaneously when the background light is between 0.003 and 3 asb.

Night vision is referred to as scotopic; it employs rods only and the background luminance is zero to 0.003 asb. Visual function at twilight is called mesopic; both rods and cones function together and the background measures 0.003 to 3 asb. Daylight vision is termed photopic; it uses cones only and the background intensity must be 3 asb or more. In photopic conditions, the central area of the retina is more sensitive than its surroundings; in mesopic adaptation, the central area is very similar in sensitivity to the nearby retina; and, in scotopic conditions, the central retina is less sensitive than the area immediately surrounding it. The dark adapted eye's conversion to cones requires only a few seconds in the light, whereas the rods do not start working well until at least 10 minutes in the dark. In this way, rods are very slow and cones are fast.

A unique characteristic of the photopic range is rather uniform obedience to Weber's law. This law states that a just noticeable change in stimulus divided by the stimulus is a constant ($\Delta B/B = K$). If we regard the background (L) as the stimulus and the intensity of a projected test light (ΔL) as the change in stimulus when the test is barely seen, we can restate Weber's law as $\Delta L/L = C$. This means in the photopic range, the absolute intensity of both test and background are unimportant as long as their relationship, the ratio of $\Delta L/L$, is known and constant for each test object. This diminishes the need for constant voltage transformers and daily absolute calibration.

Fig. 19-6 shows the visual acuity or "form sense" of the retina as a function of eccentricity or perimetric angle. This curve and Osterberg's representation of the cone distribution (see Fig. 19-4) are both plotted with an arithmetic or linear vertical scale. On the other hand, the light sense curves of Fig. 19-5 are appropriately plotted with a logarithmic ordinate. The basic reason for this geometric scale goes back to Weber's law: a just noticeable change in stimulus divided by the stimulus equals a constant. Here we are discussing the difference between consecutive changes in the stimulus values of barely visible test objects in the various portions of the field. The normal periphery and abnormal defective zones require intense stimuli, which must differ from one another significantly. The normal central field contains zones that reproducibly differ from one another by minute changes in an already small stimulus value. Only a logarithmic scale can encompass all these differences, for a just noticeable change in threshold in the periphery of the field may be 10,000 times as intense as a just noticeable change near the center of the same visual field. Thus, Osterberg's curves (see Fig. 19-4) and the steep manner in which visual

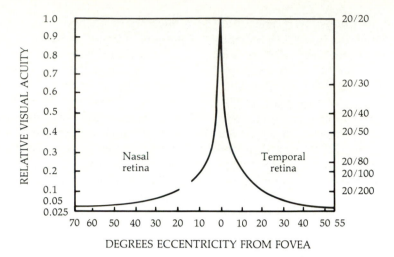

Fig. 19-6 Visual acuity ("form sense") as a function of perimetric angle. Under photopic conditions, visual acuity falls off in a steep manner similar to Osterberg's cone distribution (see Fig. 19-5).

acuity falls (Fig. 19-6) resemble one another more closely than either of them resembles the photopic light sense represented by the three lower curves of Fig. 19-5. If these three lower curves were plotted like Figs. 19-4 and 19-6 on a linear scale, the central slope would become still flatter near the center.

Limit Between the Zones of Sensitivity: the Isopter

The limit between all the visible space and the peripheral area where nothing can be seen is the largest of a whole family of normally ovoid lines called *isopters.* One may test a single member of this family by moving a small test object inward from unseen areas in the periphery until it is just seen centrally. The limits of visibility at which this small test object is seen are properly charted to delineate the visual field. In the mathematical sense, an isopter is the locus of similar visual threshold determinations, or in the ophthalmologic sense, a threshold line joining points of equal sensitivity on a visual field chart.

Conventions and Definitions

At the stage of an examination when only one test object has been used, all marks are recorded on the visual field chart in the same color. Marks are added until the examiner is virtually certain of the visual field limits in each area (Fig. 19-7). The points then may, or as the authors prefer, may not be connected by a line, preferably of the same color as the plotted points. When present, the line allows the interpreter to see the perimetrist's opin-

ion regarding the isopter's shape and location (Fig. 19-7). The original points should always remain visible to show the raw data that support this conclusion.

If a given isopter is large enough to surround the normal blind spot or any pathologic defects, the portion of the isopter immediately surrounding the defect may be plotted with the same test object as the peripheral portion of the isopter. If so, both are charted with the same color pencil and are defined as the same isopter despite the lack of overlap or even contact between the two closed-curve lines. When larger or brighter test objects are used to test the same visual field, these produce larger isopters. Blind or defective areas within the field either disappear or become smaller when they are plotted with larger or brighter test objects. These defective areas are called *scotomas* only if they are totally surrounded by a visual field with greater retinal sensitivity. When the isopter for a given test retains its ovoid shape but contains an area that is closer than normal to fixation, the defect is called a *contraction.* When the isopter shows a concavity, the defective portion of the field may be called a *localized contraction,* a cut or a *step defect.* When half the visual field is not seen, the pattern is often called a *hemianopsia.* True hemianopsias (neurologic) may or may not show half field defects, but they do show defects in the right and/or left visual field of both eyes caused by one lesion at or behind the chiasm.

Isopters are recognized as a group of closely related, nonoverlapping curves that describe the

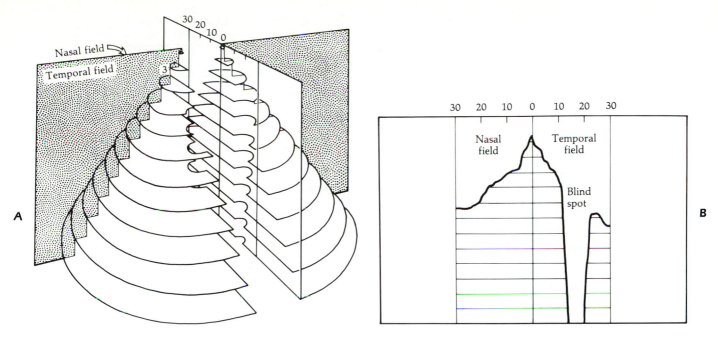

Fig. 19-8 Traquair's hill of vision. **A,** Representation of visual field as pieces of plywood cut in the shapes of isopters and stacked appropriately. Shaded plane separates near temporal field from farther nasal field. Clear plane where plywood has been sectioned vertically and separated corresponds to **B,** a representation of the visual field as a profile, created by testing along a horizontal line through fixation (i.e., a 180 degree meridian by static perimetry). Thus, the hill or island of vision may be visualized from above as kinetic isopters, or its profile may be visualized from any side as static meridians.

TEST PARAMETERS IN PERIMETRY

The size, intensity, duration, and color of test objects are variables, which, when altered, produce definite changes in the visual field. Some of these parameters may not be changed on a given perimeter. However, they should always be stabilized or at least observed and documented. With automated perimetry gaining widespread popularity, some of the parameters of physiologically ideal perimetry may be mismanaged or, more commonly, managed with assumptions that are not always valid. For this reason, a significant part of this section deals with manual settings on the Goldmann perimeter as examples of control devices, each of which has some counterpart in automated perimetry. Description of these manual settings is not as much an advocacy of "old-fashioned" perimetry as an illustration of important principles in the determination of the visual field.

Absolute and Relative Calibration

Manual calibration is vital to proper use of the Goldmann perimeter and a good example of a process that has been incorporated into the automated

perimeters. Calibration of the maximal available test object intensity is not very important if the test background is in the photopic range (Weber's law), as selected by Goldmann. Because the intensity of the light bulb does wane with time, a light meter and rheostat are provided to maintain 1000 asb. This so-called "absolute" calibration should be performed once monthly.

Infinitely more important is calibration of the background relative to an attenuated version of the test object projected just outside the test bowl. This visual comparison should be conducted before each patient's examination during manual control of intensities. This so-called "relative" calibration actually establishes the adaptation and the contrast that controls the visual threshold. Because the sources of background illumination and the projected test object are one light bulb in the Goldmann perimeter, fluctuations in electrical current cannot alter the relationship established by this calibration.

Room lighting must be stabilized before calibration at a level low enough to avoid shadows on the inside of the hemisphere. The patient's clothing and the color and style of the hair are important as absorbers or reflectors of light from and to the background. Alterations of this type are capable of changing the threshold by a decibel or more. The reflective influence of the patient can be stabilized by performing the relative calibration after the subject is in place before the perimeter. This means relative calibration must be performed just before each testing session, not once daily or weekly.

Stimulus Values of a Test Object: Geometric Increases in Size and Brightness

The range of test objects to probe the variable sensitivities within the visual field is large. Differences between test objects are more appropriately created by serial multiplication of sizes and intensities than by serial additions of any specified amount. Serial additions of fixed small amounts require too many stimulus steps when testing dense defects or the normal periphery. Large fixed additions do not permit the exploration and definition of significant relative defects in the central field.

When Goldmann designed his perimeter in the 1940s, the maximal reliable intensity available was 1000 asb. This has subsequently been increased to 10,000 asb. Goldmann chose a background of 31.5 asb, about 10 times the minimum required for the benefits of photopic testing (i.e., rapid clinical adaptation to light and obedience to Weber's law). The maximal contrast ($\Delta L/L$; 1000/31.5 = 31.7) was not enough to probe the depths of many defects when it was combined with a test size small enough to detect tiny scotomas. For this reason, he provided additional stimulus values by optional enlargement of the test object size.

On the Goldmann perimeter, increasing test object intensity is designated by an increase in the Arabic number from 1 to 4, and increasing object size is indicated by an increase in Roman numerals from 0 to V. The standard geometric increase in brightness is obtained by multiplying the former test object's projected intensity by 3.16 or adding 0.5 log unit to the log of its previous brightness increment over background. The standard geometric increase in test object size is obtained by multiplying the former test object's area by four, which is the same as adding 0.6 log units to the log of its former area. The visual angles of Goldmann's test objects (angular size measured at the pupil) are, from 0 to V respectively: 0.054, 0.108, 0.216, 0.431, 0.862, and 1.724 degrees. These stimulus sizes have become the standard for both manual and automated perimeters.

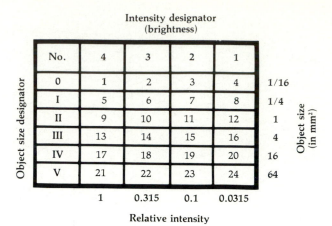

Fig. 19-9 Intensity and size designators of test objects on the Goldmann perimeter. Standard intensities of projected test objects are represented by the Arabic numbers, 1 through 4. By multiplying their relative intensities times 1000, these numbers correspond to 31.5, 100, 315, and 1000 asb respectively. The intensities of adjacent Arabic numbers differ by 0.5 log unit (5 dB). The standard object sizes are represented by Roman numerals 0 through V; their diameters correspond to visual angles of 0.05, 0.11, 0.21, 0.43, 0.86, and 1.72 degrees respectively, and the surface areas of test objects with adjacent Roman numerals differ from one another by 0.6 log unit (6 dB). Using these two parameters, 24 test combinations are possible, covering a range in excess of 4.0 log units (40 dB), which is adequate for clinical purposes.

Preferred Stimulus Values on the Goldmann Perimeter

A choice of six sizes may be selected with any of four intensities; therefore, a total of 24 different combinations is available (Fig. 19-9). Because a single standard change in intensity is regarded approximately the same as a single standard change in size, the Roman and Arabic designators of any test object may be added together to obtain the "stimulus value" of that test. Since the smallest, dimmest test object is designated 0-1 and the largest, brightest test object is V-4, the stimulus values of these unique minimal and maximal tests are 1 (0 + 1) and 9 (5 + 4) respectively. The remaining 22 possible combinations provide two to four alternatives for the seven intervening standard stimulus values. Designation of a standard stimulus value allows the relative worth of an isopter to be estimated. Consecutive standard stimulus values differ in relative value by approximately 0.5 log unit.

Fig. 19-10 shows a normal visual field plotted with the nine "standard" isopters: 0-1, I-1, I-2, I-3, I-4, II-4, III-4, IV-4, and V-4 on the Goldmann perimeter. On the basis of two considerations, these nine spots are used as standards in preference to

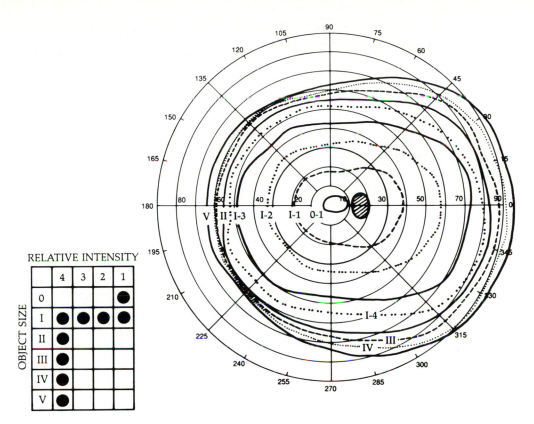

RELATIVE INTENSITY

OBJECT SIZE	4	3	2	1
0				●
I	●	●	●	●
II	●			
III	●			
IV	●			
V	●			

Fig. 19-10 Standard isopters on the Goldmann perimeter from the right eye of a normal 29-year-old patient. The nomenclature for isopters on the Goldmann perimeter consists of three designators: a Roman numeral for size, an Arabic number for standard intensity, and a letter for intermediate intensity. Although the labels on thse standard isopters are abbreviated, their complete designations are 0-1-e, I-1-e, I-2-e, I-3-e, I-4-e, II-4-e, III-4-e, IV-4-e, and V-4-e.

the other 15 possible combinations (Fig. 19-11). First, since the smallest test size (0) is prone to inconclusive results, regardless of the intensity used, this test size fails to yield reproducible isopters. The choice of any test size larger than 0 avoids this problem. Second, the edges of large test objects arrive sooner than the edges of smaller ones. Thus, artifact is introduced because locations are represented where their centers are projected. Also, the overlapping edges of large test objects might not be capable of detecting small dense scotomas. For both reasons, smaller test objects are preferred in manual perimetry, especially when one is trying to find and define small, dense blind spots. Thus, the smaller standard isopters are selected by varying the intensity while retaining the smallest reliable test size, 0.25 mm² (0.108 degrees visual angle or size I). After the intensity reaches a maximum with this size (I-4), it remains at level 4 so the subsequent stronger stimuli may be as small in size as possible (II-4, III-4, IV-4 and V-4). Use of the nine standard isopters in manual perimetry thus improves reli-

Intensity designator

No.	4	3	2	1
0	ESV 4	ESV 3	ESV 2	STD 1
I	STD 5	STD 4	STD 3	STD 2
II	STD 6	ESV 5	ESV 4	ESV 3
III	STD 7	ESV 6	ESV 5	ESV 4
IV	STD 8	ESV 7	ESV 6	ESV 5
V	STD 9	ESV 8	ESV 7	ESV 6

Object size designator

Fig. 19-11 Nine standard test objects. Because a single change in size is approximately equivalent to a single change in standard intensity on the Goldmann perimeter, the 24 possible combinations actually yield a maximal range of only nine different stimulus values. Each of these can be subdivided into five intermediate steps, totalling 45 distinct stimulus values, which differ from one another by 0.1 log unit (1 dB). This table indicates the nine test objects that are "standard" and labels the remaining 15 to show the standards to which they are equivalent. ESV stands for Equivalent Stimulus Value (sum of Roman and Arabic numerals); STD means Standard. (See text for explanation of why the nine standard test objects are preferred over their equivalents.)

ability and sensitivity and is helpful in permitting comparisons of fields tested at different medical facilities.

Between the Standard Isopters: the Intermediate Test Objects

The Goldmann perimeter has the capacity of mapping four additional "intermediate" isopters (*a* through *d*) between any two adjacent "standard" isopters, all of which formally end with the appellation *e* (Fig. 19-12). Like standard settings 1, 2, and 3, the intermediate settings actually insert neutral density filters into the path of the test object projector. When the Goldmann perimeter is set on 4-e, all light is projected; changing the settings from "d" to "a" or "3" to "1" progressively reduces projected light. As previously noted, the projected or added light of the test objects that plot adjacent standard isopters differs by a multiplication factor of 3.16 or its reciprocal, which is an addition or subtraction factor of 0.5 log unit. The projected light (L) of adjacent "intermediate" isopters differs by multiplication factors of about 1.26 or 0.79, which are respectively equivalent to adding or subtracting 0.1 log unit, or subtracting or adding 1 dB.

The Octopus Alternatives

The Octopus was the first commercially available static automated perimeter. The Octopus constituted an early attempt to eliminate variable test sizes, despite its limitation in projected intensity to the same 1000 asb used in the Goldmann perimeter. The first option selected to achieve this goal was a decrease in background intensity to 4 asb. This is near the mesopic limit of 3 asb, which can be reached by many patients when their pupils are pharmacologically constricted. Nevertheless, the background change elevated the maximal contrast, $\Delta L/L$, sometimes called the "Weber fraction," to 1000/4 or 250 from Goldmann's 31.7. This ratio with the size I test object remained insufficient for mapping the depth of many dense scotomas. Thus, the Octopus set on size I would not have been capable of distinguishing most "relative defects" from totally blind or "absolute defects." The lack of information within the dense relative defects would have eliminated the visual field as a means of following local progression or regression of the disease. To solve this problem, a standard test size of 0.431 degrees, equivalent to Goldmann's III, was instituted. Although this test size is incapable of finding tiny defects, it has endured as a minimal standard size for subsequent static automated pe-

Relative intensity designator and multipliers

		a (×0.40)	b (×0.50)	c (×0.63)	d (×0.79)	e (×1.00)
	1 (×0.0316)	19 (0.0125)	18 (0.016)	17 (0.020)	16 (0.025)	15 (0.0316)
	2 (×0.10)	14 (0.040)	13 (0.050)	12 (0.063)	11 (0.079)	10 (0.10)
	3 (×0.316)	9 (0.125)	8 (0.16)	7 (0.20)	6 (0.25)	5 (0.316)
	4 (×1.00)	4 (0.40)	3 (0.50)	2 (0.63)	1 (0.79)	0 (1.00)

Fig. 19-12   Four standard and 16 intermediate intensities on the Goldmann perimeter. The intermediate intensities (a through e) differ from their adjacent table members by 0.1 log unit (1 dB), whereas standard intensities (1 through 4) differ from one another by 5 dB. Standard intensities are so designated by bold print; they are the group of intensities with the suffix "-e." Any of the 20 intensities shown could be presented with any of the six test object sizes on the Goldmann perimeter for a total of 120 possible combinations, but equivalent values make this wide range unnecessary in normal practice. Standard isopters with their intermediates use all 20 intensities shown with size I, the top row with size 0, and the bottom row with sizes II, III, IV, and V.

rimeters because it is less than 0.5 degrees in angular size, routinely spaced at least 4.25 degrees from its neighbors and it never moves. Also, for the scotoma-detecting benefit of the larger-size (III) test to be exhausted, 96 times as many loci would have to be tested and take 96 times as long. Finally, when size III or larger test objects are used, refinement of the refraction can be less precise without an impact on the test results. The persistent clinical need for extra stimulus value in very dense relative defects is satisfied in the Octopus 201 or 2000 by optional use of the size V test object.

Differential Light Sense: a Geometric Progression Plus a Constant

Since the total light of a projected test object is the sum of the projected light ΔL and the light that was already on the background (L), the sequence of the test objects' total intensities is a geometric progression plus a constant. If, for example, the test objects are I-1-c, I-1-d, and I-1-e (see Fig. 19-12), the projected light (ΔL) is respectively 20, 25, and 31.5 asb (and respectively 17, 16, and 15 dB). Because the background intensity (L) is typically 31.5 asb in the Goldmann perimeter, the total intensity (L + ΔL) of each of these three spots is respectively 51.5, 56.5, and 63.5 asb. The contrast of these spots, $\Delta L/L$, is respectively 0.63, 0.79, and 1.00.

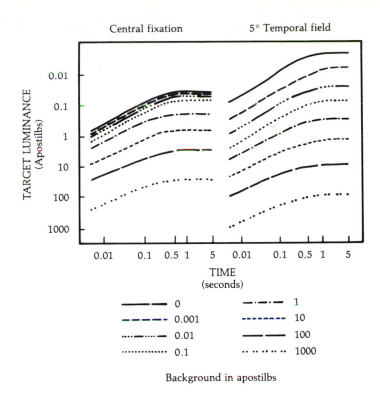

Central fixation   5° Temporal field

TIME
(seconds)

Background in apostilbs

Fig. 19-13   Effect of temporal summation: Increment threshold in apostilbs plotted against exposure time in seconds under different retinal adaptation states. Slope is steep at less than 0.1 second and summation is complete by 0.5 second. (From Aulhorn, E, and Harms, H: In Autrum, J: Handbook of sensory physiology, vol 7, New York, 1972, Springer-Verlag)

Summation: Spatial and Temporal

Summation is the ability of the retina to detect the presence of a large test object of long duration at locations where a smaller test object of short duration would be invisible, given the same contrast or intensity relative to the background, in both tests.[27] Summation is related to the simultaneous or near simultaneous firing of adjacent receptor cells that are interconnected. Summation is purely *spatial* when stationary tests of enlarging sizes are presented for identical brief durations or for times in excess of 500 msec. When the size is held constant and the test presentation is varied in duration (up to 500 msec), the greater visibility of the tests that endure longer is the result of *temporal* summation. Summation that depends on movement within the same time limit to stimulate larger areas of the retina is both temporal and spatial.

Duration of Test in Static Perimetry

Test duration has not been varied systematically in clinical testing of the visual field. However, Aulhorn and Harms have shown (Fig. 19-13) that temporal summation continues to improve sensitivity until the test duration reaches 500 msec.[3] If the time of presentation is less than 500 msec and not the same in successive test sessions, a change should be expected in the reported sensitivity. Comparisons between results of static automated perimeters are made more difficult because manufacturers choose different stimulus durations: Octopus uses 100 msec, Humphrey 200 msec. Fig. 19-13 suggests Humphrey's extra time should result in a 2 to 3 dB apparent improvement in sensitivity over Octopus if other factors are equal.

The Inherent Benefits and Inaccuracies of Kinetic Testing

In kinetic perimetry or campimetry, a compensatory balance exists between summation, which enlarges the field plot, and slow reaction time, which constricts it. This occurs because the stimulus value of a moving test is enhanced to include all the interconnected retina, which is stimulated by the test object within a time period possibly as long as 500 msec.[3] The *visual reaction time* or *la-*

tency period occurs between the instant when a stimulus barely becomes adequate and the response indicating it is present. The duration of a visual reaction time varies between 100 and 1500 msec, depending on retinal location and the patient's general condition. It is not a true function of stimulus movement velocity.

The faster a test object moves (within the limits of clinical visual field testing), the larger the effective local area that is being stimulated as a result of summation. On the other hand, the faster the test object moves inward during the latency period, the smaller the field that is registered. A more slowly moving test object does not stimulate as many receptors within the critical period of ½ sec, so that the slow test object penetrates farther toward the point of fixation than the fast one before the signal starts along the optic nerve toward the brain. During the subsequent latency period, slowly moving test objects do not travel as far into visible space as rapidly moving test objects. As a result of both effects, the recorded locations of both slow and relatively fast moving stimuli are often approximately the same. This compensation for inconstant velocity of test movement is fortunate, for in our relatively crude methods of kinetic visual field testing on manual perimeters, it would be difficult, if not impossible, to eliminate small amounts of variability in the speed of test objects. The theoretical difference in position of an isopter from beginning to end of the reaction period is called the *translocation error*.

Although Goldmann has shown experimentally that there is an optimal speed for kinetic test object movement (5 degrees/sec at 40 to 60 degrees eccentricity),[17] prolonged reaction times in certain patients require some flexibility in test object velocities. Of course, the compensation of summation and reaction time is valid only for a limited range of speeds and reaction times.

Despite the beneficial effect of summation, the latency period between the ocular reception of an adequate visual stimulus and the subjective response to that stimulus makes the outer plotted limits of any isopter smaller than would be the case if perception were signaled instantly (the translocation error). Similarly, reaction time inevitably expands the plotted inner limits of any blind area. This inaccuracy can go unnoticed most of the time, but when the scotoma-plotting inner and periphery-mapping outer parts of the same isopter are close enough to share points or actually overlap, confidence in the testing technique is reduced.

The Inherent Benefits and Inaccuracies of Static Perimetry

The kinetic perimetry paradox of an area where test objects are unseen from two directions yet intuitively known to be visible can be avoided by static perimetry because the recorded position of a stationary test object is independent of reaction time. However, when any of the retina is exposed to light, whether seen or almost seen, the light energy has a bleaching effect on the photopigments of the retina or, more likely because of its brief duration, a neural effect involving inhibition of certain connecting cells in the retina. This phenomenon, called *local retinal adaptation*, poses a limit on static perimetry because the retina needs about two seconds to rest after any test object exposure near or exceeding threshold. By the same token, when an invisibly dim spot in the field gradually brightens, the retina adjusts to the presence of that light, so it requires more light to be seen than if the test had been presented as intermittent flashes of light, each having an intensity greater than the former one.

Lynn and Tate explored the clinical value of moving the test object around the circumference of a small circle as a means of avoiding the effects of local adaptation.[31] Traditional static testing was more sensitive by 3 dB than the same test object continuously applied with various rates of gradually increasing intensity. Unfortunately, when the test object was rotated, it yielded the same threshold as the test object in stationary mode if the intensity in both instances were gradually increased and continuously present. During the last 3 dB of increase in intensity before threshold, movement of the eye in any direction projected the test object onto retina that was not locally adapted, resulting in an easily seen stimulus and very unstable fixation. This differs significantly from the random shifts in fixation during traditional perimetry, which have approximately equal chances of increasing or decreasing the reported threshold. Because of an unacceptable level of scatter, the continuously present stimulus of gradually increasing intensity was abandoned.

Traditional Static Perimetry: the Manual Procedure

Because local retinal adaptation poses rigid requirements for resting the retina between sequential exposures at each site, manual static perimetry is slow. If one idealistically considers manually testing every available point in the entire visual field of both eyes, the time consumed would be about

240 hours. Therefore, because the number of locations to be tested is limited by practical considerations, intelligent choice of proposed test sites is important.

Static test locations may be selected arbitrarily or, preferably, on the basis of previous testing results. If a suspicious area is detected on kinetic testing, a popular manual static pattern choice, termed a meridian, may be selected. Static testing of a *meridian* means the preselected static points are chosen along a test line that passes through the visual field's center and through the suspicious zone (Fig. 19-14). When an isolated defective area or blind spot is found by kinetic testing of the visual field, the depth of that defect should be established by selecting one or more points near the center of the defect for static testing. In the absence of prior information about the field other than suspicion of

glaucoma, static test points are often selected along the circles located 5, 10, and 15 degrees from fixation.

After the locations of proposed static points have been selected, the subject is asked to fixate and respond whenever a stationary test spot blinks on. The subject is shown where the first test object is to appear, and alerted before the presentation of each stimulus. Each test object is initially presented 3 to 7 dB dimmer than the expected threshold. If a meridian is to be tested, the first location selected is the central spot where the subject fixates. If the initial presentation of about ½ to ¾ sec goes undetected (as expected), the test spot is extinguished while filter settings are adjusted to increase the intensity of added light by 1 dB, which is 126% of the former intensity (an addition of 0.1 log unit). The time consumed in filter change should occupy

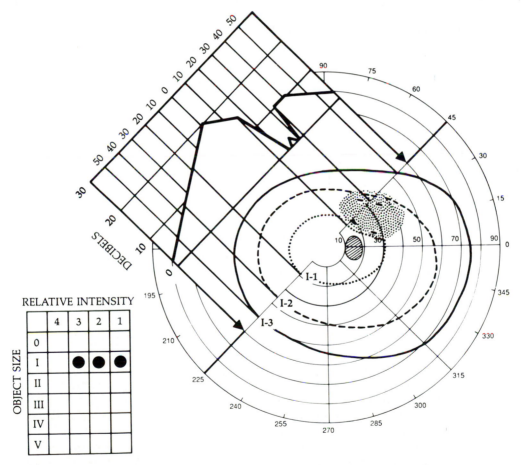

Fig. 19-14   Meridional static cut following kinetic perimetry. The scatter in the I-2 isopter and the slight concavity in the I-1 isopter suggest the presence of a deeper defect superotemporally between the two isopters. The static meridional cut through this area confirms a dense scotoma between 20 and 30 degrees. Thus, static perimetry serves as a valuable adjunct when suspicions are raised by kinetic perimetry.

about 2 sec to allow for recovery of local adaptation of the retina. A brighter but probably still unseen spot is again presented in the same central location. This cycle of test presentation and subsequent filter adjustment continues until the subject sees the test object. The intensity of the first barely visible spot is rechecked, then recorded at zero eccentricity on the static perimetry chart.

The subject is then told or, more likely, shown the location of the second test position on the meridian, usually 1 degree from the fixation point, and spots that are dimmer than the expected threshold are again presented in a repetition of the original cycle.

As the spots along a meridian are tested serially, a profile of the visual island develops on the charting paper (see Fig. 19-8 and upper left portion of Fig. 19-14). The spots are usually presented 1 degree apart in the central 5 degree and progressively less frequently in the periphery. After one limb of the meridian is completed, the test is presented 1 degree to the other side of center; the subject is alerted more specifically than usual; and the other half of the meridian is tested like the first half.

The graphic profile or meridian obtained in this way provides an excellent understanding of the sensitivity along one line that passes through fixation but no data about the rest of the field. This is a traditional plot that is only useful if the perimetrist already knows enough about the patient's field to obtain the profile at the proper angle.

Algorithms: the Basis for Static Automated Perimetry

The manual technique of static perimetry just described was standard until the 1970s. Perimetry was revolutionized when the local adaptation time between consecutive stimuli at a given location could be used for testing of other locations.[30] This was possible because (1) a record-keeping system could remember at several locations the recent history of stimulus strength and associated response type (seen or not), (2) an electronic device could trigger test presentations of specific values at the same preselected locations, and (3) some sort of logic connected these two systems. That original logic was relatively simple in a so-called "real time data acquisition and control" system, a computer.

The logic for conducting any process is its *algorithm*. This term is often applied to one or more parts of the total strategy used in automated perimetry. The first rule of all threshold seeking algorithms is to record the most recent test intensities when the patient both responds and fails to respond to stimuli at a specific location. The second rule specifies the machine's reaction to the most recent patient response when the occasion arises for retesting that spot. By the latter rule, the test intensity is always increased if the most recent response type was "not seen." Conversely, the intensity is decreased if the latest response type was "seen." The third rule is to use 2 sec or more duration before additional stimuli are presented at any one location. The most common algorithms currently used for static automated perimetry are the 4-2 and the region growing programs routinely used by the Humphrey Field Analyzer, the Octopus automated perimeter and others.

The 4-2 and 4-2-2 algorithms

The 4-2 portion of this strategy concerns the sequence of intensities to be presented at each point selected for testing. The magnitude of test intensity change in the 4-2 algorithm is large, whereas the initial response type remains the same. When the response type becomes different, the subsequent intensities are changed by a smaller amount. For example, the step size between initial successive stimuli in the 4-2 algorithm is always 4 dB, a 150% increase or a 60% decrease in projected light. After the initial response type changes, suggesting the threshold is close, the step size between successive stimuli becomes 2 dB, a 59% increase or a 37% decrease. As soon as the response type changes for the second time, the 4-2 algorithm is complete at the location described, where threshold is usually defined as the mean of the final two stimuli. Changing by steps of 4 dB in the initial rough search and by 2 dB in the refinement is the essence of the 4-2 algorithm for determining threshold. If the strategy is allowed to continue until a third reversal, still using 2-dB steps, it is called the 4-2-2 algorithm.

In Fig. 19-15, *A,* the sequential order of events used to obtain threshold exemplifies the 4-2 algorithm and its extension to become and 4-2-2 algorithm. The first three stimuli were not seen so intensity was regularly increased by 4 dB steps until it was seen (test No. 4). Steps of 2 dB were always used after this point and stimulus intensity was progressively decreased until the test object was not seen (test No. 9). At this stage, the 4-2 algorithm was completed and a threshold of 21 dB could be reported as the mean of the last two tests. In this example, however, the stimulus intensity was again increased to complete the 4-2-2 algorithm, still using the 2 dB steps until the test object

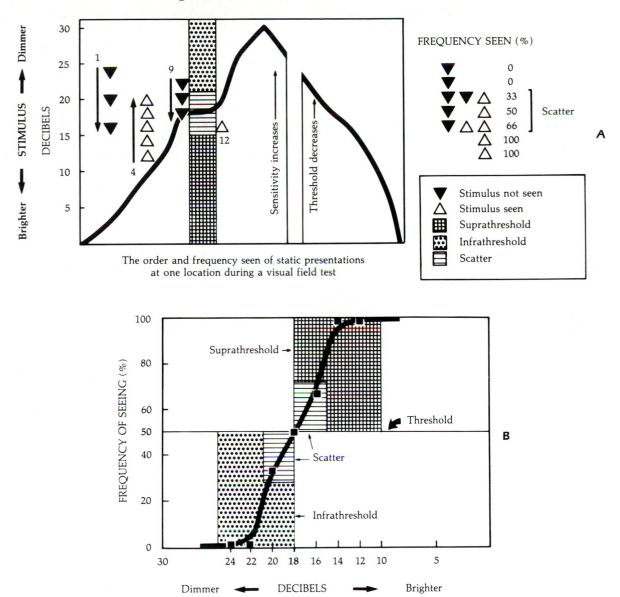

4-2-2 Algorithm and the island of vision

The order and frequency seen of static presentations
at one location during a visual field test

Fig. 19-15 Generating a frequency of seeing curve. **A,** Graphic representation of sequentially presented stimuli at one preselected retinal location showing their order, intensity (dB) and type of response (seen, unseen). **B,** Graphic representation of the percentage of stimuli seen at each intensity tested at the same preselected retinal location. The thresholds to the 4-2 algorithm, the 4-2-2 algorithm, and the frequency of seeing curves are 21, 17, and 18 dB respectively. (See text for derivation of these values.)

was seen once more (test No. 12). The 4-2-2 threshold could then be reported as the average of the last two stimuli presented, or 17 dB. Discrepancies of 4 dB between thresholds from these two algorithms are not uncommon though results are identical in about three eighths of the thresholds traced in glaucoma patients.[29] If one asks which threshold is correct, a third measure is available within the same data. By definition, threshold is the dimmest light seen 50% of the time. This value can be determined directly from the frequency of seeing curve shown in Fig. 19-15, *B*, a graph plotting the percentage of stimuli seen at each intensity level tested. In this example, calculated threshold is 18 dB. Thus, the 4-2 algorithm is obviously faster, but the longer 4-2-2 is a little more accurate.

The region growing algorithm

Valuable time is wasted in patients with defects if all tests start at predetermined intensities, even if the test values correspond to expected normals. When a given patient's results obtained on a different day are available, these may be used as starting points for a new test. This strategy saves some time but the results are not quite the same. In the Octopus perimeters, "region growing" has supplanted the option of starting from prior thresholds.

In region growing, a limited number of spots (usually one per quadrant) are tested to full thresholds before any other stimuli are presented. Results of these tests are then used as starting points for adjacent locations. These, in turn, finish their thresholding before another adjacent growth region receives starting instructions. Growth finally extends to include all of the quadrant where it began but not the adjacent ones. The algorithm can conform to the hill of vision or not, and it can attempt to start at threshold, below it, or as Lynn and Fellman showed best, above threshold.[29] It is most valuable in cases with significant field defects.

Algorithm for Kinetic Perimetry

To date, kinetic perimetry has only been automated in a primitive way, not including any real test of scotomas. Using the Perimetron field machine, Parrish et al.[34] found a standard deviation (SD) of 2.6 to 5.5 degrees in isopter position during automated kinetic perimetry. The greatest variation appeared in the temporal field where the slope is normally flattest.

A major current problem in kinetic perimetry, not seen in static automated perimetry, is the need for a human examiner to make important decisions during kinetic perimetry. The decisions include which track is to be tested next, how fast to move the test, whether to accept a given patient response as seen or not, where to place the accepted response on the test chart, the locations and methods for supplementary testing, and where the isopter lines are to be drawn. The speed of test object movement should be regulated for precise knowledge regarding the effects of temporal and spatial summation. The speed of test object movement should also be inversely proportional to the subject's reaction time. Because reaction time varies markedly from subject to subject and moderately from moment to moment in a given subject, its repeated measurement should be required periodically during the field test. The direction of movement of kinetic test objects should be perpendicular to the expected isopter. Direction of movement in the normal field, therefore is almost radial, but this is not the case in defective visual fields with cuts or scotomas.

Table 19-1 *The relationship of Octopus decibels* and Humphrey decibels to luminance*

Relative values		Absolute luminance values		
Humphrey decibels	Octopus decibels	Apostilbs	Decalamberts	Lamberts
50	40	0.1	.0001	.00001
40	30	1.0	.001	.0001
30	20	10.0	.01	.001
20	10	100.0	.10	.01
19	9	125	.125	.0125
18	8	159	.159	.0159
17	7	200	.20	.020
16	6	250	.25	.025
15	5	316	.316	.0316
14	4	400	.40	.040
13	3	500	.50	.050
12	2	631	.63	.063
11	1	794	.79	.079
10	0	1000	1.00	.10
5	−5	3160	3.16	.316
0	−10	10,000	10.0	1.0

*The decibel, a *relative* unit for comparing intensities in any system, is minus 10 times the logarithm of the maximal intensity or luminance of the projected test object. One bel is a 10-fold change in stimulus intensity or one logarithmic unit. The decibel (dB) is .1 of a bel. An increase of one dB is a 20% reduction in stimulus luminance; a decrease of one dB is a 25% increase in projected test object intensity. Log of .001 = −3; log of .01 = −2; log of .1 = −1; log of 1 = 0; log of 10 = 1.

If the decisions of a kinetic perimeter were well automated, scatter might exceed that found by competent manual perimetrists; but studies involving these parameters should help provide better methods of quantitating scatter.

Kinetic Versus Static: Comparisons and Ideal Relationships

On the static automated systems like Octopus, which share with the Goldmann perimeter a maximal test object intensity of 1000 asb, the projected luminances of 1000, 315, 100, and 31.5 asb are represented as 0, 5, 10 and 15 dB respectively. The Goldmann perimeter would report these as -4-e, -3-e, -2-e and -1-e (Table 19-1). Six locations on the field profile in Fig. 19-14 are appropriately intersected near the 5, 10, and 15 dB levels by projections from the 45 degree meridian where the I-3-e, I-2-e and I-1-e kinetic isopters cross the meridian in the lower part of the figure. This comparison reveals the degree to which static and kinetic thresholds have long been regarded as equivalent.

Fankhauser and Schmidt[11] investigated more formally the difference in threshold values found in normal subjects with static and kinetic perimetry (Fig. 19-16). Peripheral retinal locations are not as sensitive to static as they are to kinetic techniques so they require more light to reach threshold. The larger receptive fields in the retinal periphery with their associated summation, both temporal and spatial, probably account for the increased sensitivity found near the fovea, which presumably explains why tiny stationary test objects that are visible in this area disappear with any movement.

Kinetic perimetry is nicely complemented by static perimetry when the latter is used at reproducible locations within defective areas. This combination is especially beneficial in follow-up testing because the depth of a scotoma may change without any alteration in the pattern of the isopters surrounding it. In cooperative patients, closely spaced static perimetry of well-chosen meridia is generally more accurate than kinetic perimetry in measuring the depth, slope, and extent of any demonstrated defect (Fig. 19-17); whereas kinetic perimetry has the advantages of rapid, comprehensive coverage of the entire field and production of recognizable isopter patterns. Kinetic isopter

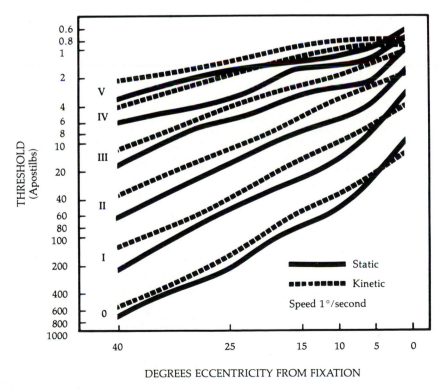

Fig. 19-16 Difference in sensitivity found in normal subjects with six different test sizes, comparing static and kinetic perimetry. Kinetic sensitivities are higher throughout the visual field except very near the center where static sensitivities are higher. (From Fankhauser, F, and Schmidt, T: Ophthalmologica 139:409, 1960)

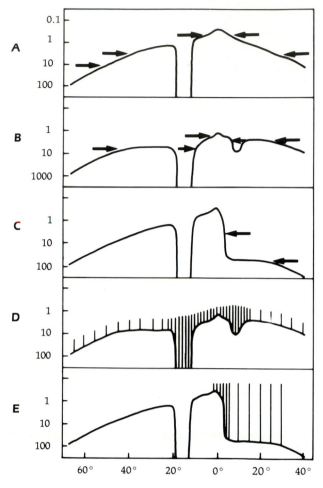

Fig. 19-17 Evaluation of slopes and scotomas by traditional manual and kinetic perimetry. **A,** Flat slope defects and shallow scotomas are more difficult to map kinetically than with closely spaced meridians by static perimetry. **B,** The shallow scotoma may be easily missed by kinetic techniques, but **D,** static perimetry easily reveals the defect. **C,** The steepness of the slope is not well demonstrated kinetically, but in **E,** the steep slope is easily seen on a static meridional profile. (See text for discussion of precision and value of profiles.) (From Aulhorn, E, and Harms, H: In Autrum, J: Handbook of sensory physiology, vol 7, New York, 1972, Springer-Verlag)

patterns reveal areas of uncertainty or suspicion, thereby indicating where to test further for scotomas by static testing.

Precision in perimetry depends on the amount of data collected. Maximal information comes as shown in Fig. 19-17 with nearly adjacent static tests. Multiple isopter kinetic testing can gather a great deal of data, faulted though it be by translocation error. Static automated perimetry is less precise than these two manual quantitative tests

except when extra testing of suspected regions is available on the automated instrument and requested by the operator.

Although static automated perimetry can be programmed to test meridia and thus plot profiles, this test format has been partially abandoned in recent years for several reasons. First, the computer can keep track of many more points than the human perimetrist, so there is no problem in managing data from locations off the meridian. Second, most automated perimetry does not currently include any form of kinetic testing to help decide which meridian or meridia should be tested so exhaustively. Third, there is an urgent need for comprehensive coverage of the entire field, which was formerly provided by kinetic testing. As this need has become obvious, a time limit has also become evident, especially in glaucoma patients.[28]

The resultant compromise in static automated perimetry is an array of 100 test spots or less, generally spaced at visual angles of 6 to 8.5 degrees from one another in the central 25 to 30 degrees of the field. With a similar time investment, one may obtain a more widely spaced test of the field outside 30 degrees or a supplemental grid of test locations inside 30 degrees, which may or may not be merged with the initial test data. If the two central patterns are merged, the resultant intertest visual angles are never closer than 4.25 degrees nor greater than 6 degrees. Thus, the visual angle between adjacent static automated test locations is much larger than the translocation error due to reaction time in kinetic perimetry.

The output of most static automated perimeters is currently dual; numbers, which are the raw data, and the interpolated gray scale. The numbers are the sensitivities discovered at the locations printed. The gray scale interpolation is an excellent immediate overview suitable for orienting patients about their problem: "Where it's dark it means you can't see as well." Also, it quickly guides the physician to the numbers he needs for accurate interpretation. The gray scale printout is only an interpolation, calculated from relatively widespread data. Because the junctions of different gray intensities do not represent measured isopters, they usually differ significantly from directly determined kinetic isopters.

INTERPRETATION OF RESULTS
Visual Threshold Versus Sensitivity

In the frequency of seeing curve that portrays the classic visual threshold (see Fig. 19-15, *B*), three zones are observable: a luminance or brightness range where the stimulus is always seen (probability of being seen = 100%), a range where the test spot is too dim and never seen (probability of being seen = 0%), and a range between these extremes where the spot is seen some of the time. *Threshold* is usually defined as the brightness of a test that has a 50% probability of being seen. *Suprathreshold* implies that a light stimulus will be seen greater than 50% of the time because the stimulus is larger and/or brighter than threshold. *Infrathreshold* implies a light stimulus will be seen less than 50% of the time because it is smaller and/or dimmer than threshold (see Fig. 19-15, *B,*). The minimal amount of light required for visualization is directly proportional to threshold. These terms are clinically applied to static testing of the visual field.

As noted earlier in this chapter, each isopter obtained by kinetic testing represents the visual threshold locations for the particular test object used to outline it. The abstract three-dimensional shape, which represents the composites of visual thresholds from all the space before a subject, is often compared to "the surface of the visual island," where the hard rock and stone of the island correspond to areas that are seen and the air surrounding the island in all directions corresponds to stimuli that are not seen.

As one climbs up the island of vision, sensitivity increases so that the amount of light required for barely seeing the test object decreases, along with threshold. Conversely, when one goes back down the visual island, the more light is needed for visualization, the worse that area sees, and the higher the threshold. The height at any location on the island of vision is directly proportional to retinal sensitivity and inversely proportional to threshold. Thus, threshold and sensitivity are the reciprocals of one another. The term threshold is rooted in psychophysics where a 50% response has real meaning because 20, 30, or even more tests of a given stimulus value are presented so that true percentages can be calculated. In reporting threshold results, stimulus intensity is plotted versus location. In this realm, the terms suprathreshold (above threshold) and infrathreshold (below it) mean respectively above and below the plotted 50% line on a frequency of seeing curve. On the visual island, the opposite holds, for above threshold means under the island surface and below threshold means the air over the island.

Sensitivity is important to the clinician, for lack of sensitivity implies some pathologic process. An increase in sensitivity may imply that a previously pathologic area is improving. We are accustomed psychologically to seeing good things going up on graphs and bad things coming down. The visual island, use of decibels, and the plotting of sensitivity augment this tendency.

Decibels Versus Apostilbs: Relative Versus Absolute

The decibel scale is a logarithmic or geometric system used to represent the relative sensitivity of the island of vision. One bel is equivalent to one log unit of change in sensitivity or a 10-fold change in light sense. One decibel is a change equivalent to .1 of a log unit. If the change is a decrease by 1 dB, it represents a 26% increase in projected test object light. A 1dB increase is equivalent to a 20% decrease in projected test object light (see Table 19-1).

Unlike apostilbs or millilamberts, the decibel scale is not an absolute measurement of luminance but rather serves as an expedient relative measurement. It varies from one manufacturer's perimeter to another, depending on the maximal available stimulus intensity. For example, the Octopus perimeter has a maximal stimulus intensity of 1000 asb, which is equal to .1 of a large luminance unit, the lambert, or to 1 decalambert. In the Octopus, decibels are −10 times the logarithm of the projected test intensity as measured in decalamberts (see Table 19-1). Zero decibels represents 1000 asb, 10 dB equals 100 asb, 20 dB equals 10 asb, 30 dB equals 1 asb, and the relative log scale continues. In the Humphrey visual field analyzer, the decibel signifies −10 times the log of the projected test intensity as measured in Lamberts. Zero decibels on this instrument corresponds to the maximal stimulus intensity of 10,000 asb or one Lambert. A decrease of 20 dB on either instrument from 10 asb to 1000 asb at a given retinal location means that area's sensitivity is diminished because 100 times more added light is required to reach a higher threshold. Table 19-1 shows that even a 1 dB decrease corresponds to a 26% increase in light added to the test object's projected intensity. A 1 dB increase represents an improvement in sensitivity with a 20% decrease in intensity of projected light.

Suprathreshold Screening

As noted earlier, the more presicion required in perimetry, the more data are required and, it follows, the more time. The intratest deterioration of threshold in glaucoma patients by a phenomenon other than ordinary fatigue is a good reason for limiting time. Another is that time equals money, a factor well recognized in clinical practice. In this vein, there is a definite need for brief tests that can be performed on patients or subjects who have no known visual field loss. Population studies by public health personnel and nonspecific tests by general ophthalmologists are the kinds of utilization that make screening important.

Screening fields by the modified technique of Armaly have been tested on a population containing normals and known glaucoma patients to determine the selectivity and sensitivity of the method.[37] Although the quite favorable measurements of false-positive and false-negative conclusions certainly justify use of screening fields, the technique, originally manual, has been extended to automated instruments, and both have been used inappropriately to follow patients with established glaucoma.

Screening fields are diverse in programming content, but most of them attempt to probe each test location once at an intensity 4 to 6 dB brighter than the calculated threshold. If the spots are seen, the subject is regarded as having no significant pathology. Any missed test objects can be presented a second time at the same stimulus value or a still brighter one. Results of originally seen, secondarily seen, and always unseen tests must be coded differently. If the results are shown symbolically, this has the advantage of avoiding confusion with truly thresholded tests. An expected disadvantage of symbolic coding is the future absence of any information about the decibel value of tests presented only once and seen in the past.

Because screening static fields use locations similar to full threshold fields, significant intertest space is never tested. Because response to a given test may be "incorrect" with respect to threshold more than 20% of the time,[29] single tests may be missed or seen inappropriately. Conclusions about function from a static screening field also may be incorrect because the most damaged locations were never tested, but the untried slope of surrounding areas could not even suggest the need to retest any area. Certainly, no valid statistical tests that deal with thresholds can simultaneously use data from screening fields.

INTERPRETING VARIABILITY IN THE VISUAL FIELD: SCATTER VERSUS FLUCTUATION

Visual threshold is a statistical concept; it means the test was seen 50% of the times it was exposed at the stimulus value called threshold. It is naive to assume that all tests brighter than threshold will be seen and all those dimmer than

threshold will be invisible, though these are the implications of a sharp limit on visibility and the basis for isopter lines.

When the points determining an isopter do not agree and retesting to determine the accuracy of points finds that many are inconsistent, the problem is called *scatter*. The counterpart of this kinetic perimetry phenomenon in static automated perimetry is called *fluctuation*. Since the results of static perimetry are expressed in decibels, which are integers between 0 and 45, fluctuation is easier to quantitate than scatter. When applied to visual threshold, the term fluctuation means an estimation of the variability in results if the measurement were repeated. One refers to the variability in repeated measurements in the same testing session as *short-term fluctuation* (SF) and to the changes between different testing sessions as *long-term fluctuation* (LF). The *total fluctuation* (TF) that occurs at any given set of test locations over time is a result of both SF and LF. These three terms (TF, SF, LF) are related mathematically by their variance. *Variance* is the square of a given fluctuation, and the variance equation states TF^2 is equal to the sum of SF^2 and LF^2. Clinically, SF and TF can be estimated by repeating measurements in each session and over time. LF is not estimated directly but calculated by factoring out SF from TF using the variance equation.[15]

By understanding fluctuations one can answer with a specified degree of confidence whether a given location in the visual field conforms to normal values, whether it represents a defective portion of the field, and whether it has grown better or worse over the time since previous similar tests were conducted.

The Value of Measuring Fluctuation

The classic frequency of seeing curve relates the percentage of tests seen on the ordinate and the intensity of the test spot on the abscissa. When the data used to calculate the 50% limit are tightly clustered, the S-shaped cumulative frequency curve rises steeply. This frequency of seeing curve has a small standard deviation (SD), a function which applies to measurements of all sorts, provided the data fit the bell-shaped or "normal" distribution. The implications of normally distributed data having a measured threshold of 19 dB and a standard deviation of 1.0 dB are (1) a 99% chance that the actual threshold is between 16 dB and 22 dB ($\pm$ 3SD), (2) a 95% change that the actual threshold is between 17 dB and 21 dB ($\pm$ 2SD), and (3) an 83% chance that the actual threshold is between 18 dB and 20 dB ($\pm$ 1SD). This range of visual performance data can be shown in very alert normal subjects.

In the glaucoma patient, a threshold of 19 might also prevail, but a standard deviation of 3 dB is the rule at a randomly selected location. In such a case the range in decibel values and their corresponding chances of visual perception are (1) a 99% chance that the actual threshold is between 10 dB and 28 dB, (2) a 95% chance that the actual threshold is between 13 dB and 25 dB, and (3) an 83% chance that the actual threshold is between 16 dB and 22 dB. This example demonstrates that any tested point within a single session has a level of uncertainty that depends on its reproducibility.

Static automated perimeters calculate a statistical function that is used like the standard deviation. This is called root mean square (RMS) or short-term fluctuation (SF). The data for calculating this function are collected by measuring thresholds at 10 preselected locations twice. The differences between the paired values are squared, summed, and divided by 20 before the square root is extracted. For each pair that is totally blind, the number 20 is reduced by 2. Although the test takes extra time, the resultant number allows one to evaluate all the decibel data regarding this patient on this date. If, for example, fluctuation is found to be 1.3 dB in a patient with glaucoma, it means the range of clinically insignificant change (1% confidence) is only $\pm$ 3.9 dB, which is 3 times the fluctuation found. A change of 4 dB or more is then significant at the 1% confidence level. If fluctuation testing were omitted in this case, a change of 9 dB, (3 $\times$ 3) would have been required to achieve this level of significance.

When an RMS of 4.3 dB is tripled in another glaucoma patient, the insignificant range is extended to $\pm$ 12.9 dB, so defects or change less than 13 dB could occur by chance alone in more than 1% of cases. Reliance on the average value of 9 in this case would lead to the incorrect conclusion that an isolated change of 10 to 12 dB was clinically significant.

Knowledge of the reproducibility of a measurement is as critical as the precision with which it is determined. Clinical decisions are based on change in the visual field. The earliest significant change in a computerized field is not consistent. Fluctuations may help distinguish early defects before definite loss can be documented. Although normal subjects show variability, the features that set the abnormal field apart are clustered defects within an arcuate distribution, a quadrant or hem-

ifield, especially when much of the remaining field is stable or fluctuating upward. The impression of abnormality is solidified when the field is repeated on another date and defects are still present in the same suspected group of locations. Familiarity with expected variability facilitates interpretation of such changes.

Global Indices

When the perimetric computer contains a database generated from sufficient numbers of age-matched controls, calculations of *mean defect* (MD) are possible. MD is the overall mean deviation of the tested eye from age corrected normal values. It is an index for diffuse change indicating generalized depression or elevation in measured threshold. In normals it usually ranges from 0 to $\pm$2 dB. The calculation of a second "global index" called short-term fluctuation (SF) is of approximately the same value as RMS and in normals ranges from 1 to 2 dB. When both MD and SF are available, a third "visual field index" called *corrected loss variance* (CLV) can be calculated.[14] CLV is an index of the local nonuniformity of a visual field defect. It can be estimated by adjusting the hill of vision for MD and factoring out SF.[2] CLV is sensitive to real, local defects and in normals ranges from 1 to 2 dB.

MD, SF, and CLV are referred to as global vision field indices. They are statistical representations of the entire tested visual field. This type of data reduction allows examination of overall trends that could otherwise be missed.

Generalized loss of sensitivity (MD), increased fluctuation (SF), and localized loss of sensitivity (CLV) are known characteristics of the glaucomatous field. An increase in any or all of these three global indices over normal values should alert the clinician to the possibility of glaucomatous damage. Global indices are most useful in detecting the barely damaged patient to help establish an early diagnosis of glaucoma. They are much less helpful in following patients for progressive damage over time, so the clinician should not rely on global indices as accurate indicators of progressive visual field damage.

Internal Inconsistency

When the ordered intensity-response steps of static testing to threshold are available for review as in Fig. 19-15, *A*, internal inconsistencies are likely to become evident. The two types of inconsistencies are tests not seen at intensities brighter than the calculated threshold (misses) and tests reported seen at intensities dimmer than threshold (false alarms). Since internal inconsistency cannot occur during the first 3 steps of a 4-2 algorithm, the more tests of threshold one performs, the less immunity there is from inconsistency. For example, Lynn and Fellman[29] showed the internal inconsistency rate of the 4-2 algorithm in 98 glaucomatous eyes was 6.3% on the first trial at each of 10 preselected locations. Extending the same tests to a third reversal of response type (the 4-2-2 algorithm) yielded a 10.0% internal inconsistency rate. When all the data from these same 4-2-2 thresholds were combined with one repeated 4-2-2 threshold at these same locations, the rate was 20.2%. Although the *internal inconsistency rate* (IIR) does not correlate well with measurement of fluctuation, individual thresholds showing apparently significant change are viewed differently when they contain large inconsistencies as compared to none. Also, the IIR covers all the test locations in the field, yet it is free of the time tax required by repeated threshold measurements at 10 spots during the collection of data for calculation of fluctuation.

The Effects of Age

Several investigators have studied the effect of age on the central and peripheral visual thresholds of normal subjects. Early work by Goldmann[17] established the most common standard isopters for an average normal subject of 20 to 30 years. His data, in the form of isopters to the I-1-e, I-2-e, I-3-e, and I-4-e test objects plotted on a transparent plastic sheet, has long been distributed with the Goldmann perimeter. Goldmann also indicated the isopters were in the same locations for a normal subject of 60 to 70 years, but the test objects then were increased by one standard step to I-2-e, I-3-e, I-4-e, and II-4-e. This implies normal subjects have an evenly distributed 5 dB decrease in visual sensitivity over 40 years when testing is performed kinetically.

Drance et al.[8] suggested that generalized change is a continuous process starting in youth and going on to senescence. They further determined that the rate of change was linear and independent of senile miosis but partly affected by senile ptosis.

Haas et al.[19] reemphasized the point that all psychophysical tests are age dependent. They evaluated 203 normal eyes by static automated perimetry (Octopus) and found sensitivity decreases markedly with age, starting at the age of 20 years or less. Age influenced the upper half of the visual field to a larger extent than the lower half, with an average decrease in the visual field of 0.58 dB per decade.

Katz and Sommer[24] described the asymmetry and variation in the field of vision in 146 normal eyes using the Humphrey Visual Field Analyzer. As expected, the sensitivity among older eyes was lower at every point tested within the central 30 degrees. Generalized reduction in retinal sensitivity with aging was not uniform. The average number of decibels decreased by 2.3 from the center to midcentral periphery and an additional 1.6 from the midcentral periphery out to 30 degrees. The greatest drop in decibels, 5.3, occurred from the center to the superior periphery.

Jaffe et al.[22] found a substantial effect of eccentricity on the rate of age-related decline in the normal visual field, as tested on the Octopus automated perimeter. Near fixation, sensitivity declined approximately 0.5 dB per decade, and, at 27 degrees eccentricity, the average decline was 1 dB per decade. Dolman et al.[6] demonstrated a quantitative decrease in optic nerve axons with age, which indicates that age-related visual field decay may represent a progressive loss of neurosensory structures.

A thorough understanding of age-related changes in the visual field is necessary before attempting to determine visual field change due to glaucoma.

PHYSIOLOGIC BASIS FOR PERIMETRY

Various physiologic factors can cause psychophysical alterations that influence the patient's response to visual field examination. Recognition of these factors is important because the induced alterations can be falsely interpreted as pathologic change. Many ophthalmologists have succumbed to a numbers game, accepting the output of their visual field instruments as dogma; however, this approach is not valid. The generated data must be understood to properly describe, quantitate, and evaluate the visual field, thereby enhancing care of the glaucoma patient.

Refractive Status

Changing the refractive status of the eye can alter the visual threshold dramatically in the central 30 degrees of the field, whether testing is performed by kinetic or static techniques (Fig. 19-18). If light from the test object is not well focused on the retina, the result is a *refractive scotoma*. Weinreb and Perlman[45] recently demonstrated the effect of refraction on automated perimetric thresholds.

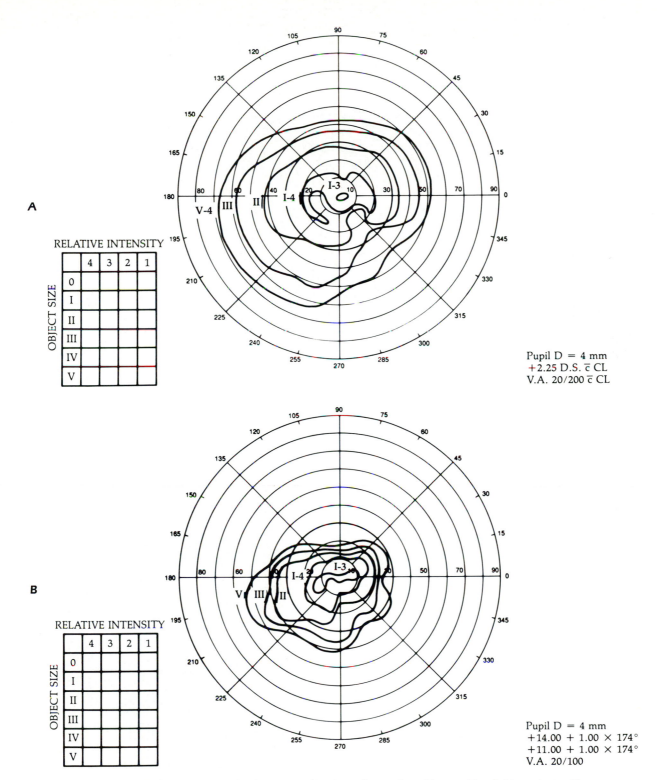

A

RELATIVE INTENSITY

OBJECT SIZE

	4	3	2	1
0				
I				
II				
III				
IV				
V				

Pupil D = 4 mm
+2.25 D.S. c̄ CL
V.A. 20/200 c̄ CL

B

RELATIVE INTENSITY

OBJECT SIZE

	4	3	2	1
0				
I				
II				
III				
IV				
V				

Pupil D = 4 mm
+14.00 + 1.00 × 174°
+11.00 + 1.00 × 174°
V.A. 20/100

Fig. 19-18   The effect of refraction on kinetic perimetry in a 24-year-old aphakic patient with glaucoma. **A,** Visual field in the left eye performed with the appropriate contact lens and near add shows glaucomatous loss inferiorly. **B,** Visual field in same eye using the appropriate spectacle correction and near add demonstrates glaucomatous progression.

Continued.

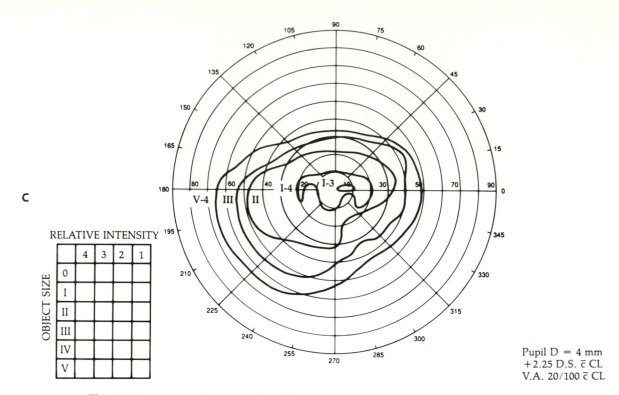

RELATIVE INTENSITY

OBJECT SIZE	4	3	2	1
0				
I				
II				
III				
IV				
V				

Pupil D = 4 mm
+2.25 D.S. c̄ CL
V.A. 20/100 c̄ CL

Fig. 19-18 cont'd   C, A repeat visual field using the previous contact lens and near add shows a return to the previous examination in **A**.

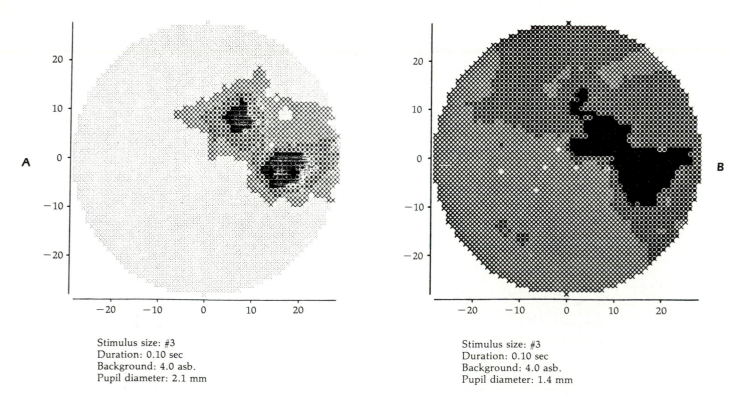

Stimulus size: #3
Duration: 0.10 sec
Background: 4.0 asb.
Pupil diameter: 2.1 mm

Stimulus size: #3
Duration: 0.10 sec
Background: 4.0 asb.
Pupil diameter: 1.4 mm

Fig. 19-19   Effect of pupil size on static perimetry. **A,** Quantitative static visual field on the right eye of an elderly patient with glaucoma demonstrates a paracentral scotoma in the superior temporal quadrant (pupil diameter = 2.1, RMS = 1.9). **B,** Repeat visual field on same eye after the use of a miotic shows nonuniform reduction in retinal sensitivity, the paracentral scotoma being most affected (pupil diameter = 1.4, RMS = 2.8).

They found that for each diopter of uncorrected refractive error, there was a 1.26 dB decrease in visual sensitivity within the central 6 degrees of the visual field. The effect of blur on threshold may simulate important pathology, for it often appears as a paracentral scotoma. Benedetto and Cyrlin also studied the effect of refractive state on static thresholds. With small amounts of blur ($\pm$ 2 diopters of sphere), they found a slight reduction in central sensitivity.[4] They considered this to be clinically insignificant in normals, but the effect in diseased eyes was exaggerated by comparison. With blur in excess of 2 diopters, they found a generalized reduction in retinal sensitivity, especially marked in the central field. Several other investigators have demonstrated similar reductions in threshold with an increase in refractive error.[10]

Perimetry should routinely be performed with an accurate distance refraction combined with appropriate additional correction for the patient's age and the perimeter radius. The refraction in the perimeter should be refined each time by checking and changing the prescription in accordance with the patient's preference for 0.5 diopter more or less of sphere. The final refractive prescription in the perimeter should be recorded after each visual field test.

Pupil Size

The amount of light entering the eye is proportional to the square of the diameter of the pupil or to its area. A decrease in the pupil diameter from 4.75 to 1.5 mm causes a 10-fold (1 log unit) reduction in the amount of light arriving at the retina. This degree of change in retinal illumination often alters the level of dark adaptation of the retina, from photopic to mesopic. A pupil diameter of less than 2.4 mm also decreases the resolving power of the eye due to diffraction at the edge of the pupil. All of these factors alter the shape of the island of vision and have a deleterious effect on threshold (Fig. 19-19).

McCluskey et al.[32] evaluated the effect of pilocarpine on the kinetic visual field in normals. Using the Goldmann perimeter, they found a 65% reduction in the I-2-e isopter area 30 minutes after instillation of pilocarpine. After 2 hours, there persisted a 56% reduction in isopter area. Theoretically, the threshold values should not be affected by pupil size if the contrast between the stimulus intensity ($\triangle L$) and the background intensity (L) remain in a fixed ratio (Weber's law says $\triangle L/L = C$ under photopic conditions). However, the work of LeGrand[27] suggests that retinal adap-

tation is in the mesopic range when the pupil is 2 mm or less, despite a background of 31.5 asb, so Weber's law may not apply.

Stimulus Size

Visual field changes caused by variation in test object size are explained by spatial summation.[46] A stimulus size III on a Goldmann perimeter occupies 4 mm^2, whereas a stimulus size V covers 64 mm^2, a 16-fold difference in size. This amount of change in spot size is roughly equivalent to a 10-fold change in stimulus intensity. Changes in spot size alter spatial summation and lead to differences in visual thresholds (Fig. 19-20). Summation is a reciprocal function of the amount of light to which the retina is adapted, with scotopic vision producing the greatest summation and photopic least.

Background Luminance

Aulhorn[3] has demonstrated the relationship of threshold to multiple retinal adaptation levels. With a background luminance of 100 asb, the center of the field has a threshold of approximately 5 asb. By decreasing the background luminance to 10 asb, threshold at the fovea is about 0.8 asb, and at a background of 1 asb, the foveal threshold is roughly 0.16 asb (see Fig. 19-5). Further evaluation of this figure reveals a change in the shape of the island of vision for each background luminance investigated and a dramatic lack of increase in central retinal sensitivity when backgrounds are less than 0.1 asb. Clinically, a decrease in background luminance enhances both the contrast and, via its adaptation state, the sensitivity of the retina (Fig. 19-21). As a result, the reported number of decibels is larger with lower background intensities and smaller when the background is brighter. Controversy surrounds the optimal background luminance to separate normal from abnormal.

Psychologic Effects

Psychologic effects must be considered when evaluating a psychologic function, such as the visual field. Stress, anxiety, systemic medications, training, and fear of blindness can influence the patient's response during perimetry. Many patients are aware that a worsening visual field may require surgical intervention with its attendant risk. Thus, patients may become extraordinarily motivated during visual field testing, and this psychologic effect on the visual field may result in increased scatter, more false positives, and decreased response time. These changes may make the visual field appear improved, all because of a

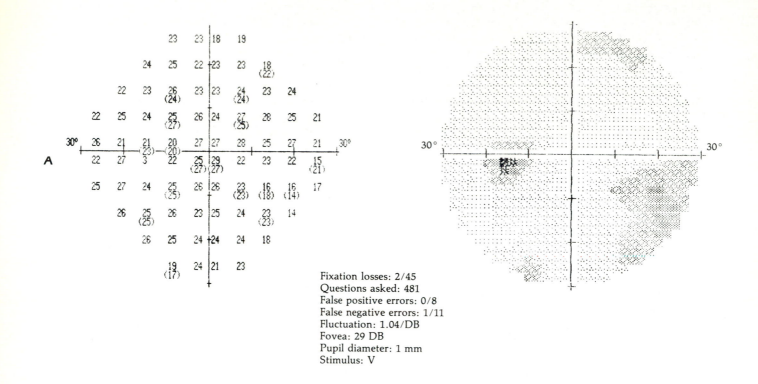

Fixation losses: 2/45
Questions asked: 481
False positive errors: 0/8
False negative errors: 1/11
Fluctuation: 1.04/DB
Fovea: 29 DB
Pupil diameter: 1 mm
Stimulus: V

Pupil diameter: 1 mm
Stimulus: III

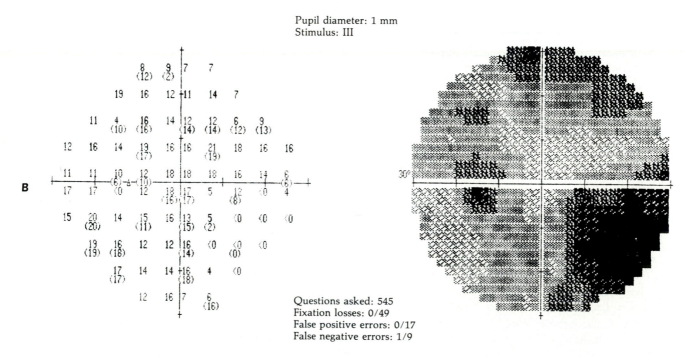

Questions asked: 545
Fixation losses: 0/49
False positive errors: 0/17
False negative errors: 1/9

Fig. 19-20 Effect of stimulus size on static perimetry. **A,** Visual field in the left glaucomatous eye shows a relative defect, an inferior nasal step (stimulus size = V, pupil diameter = 1.0). **B,** repeat visual field on same eye shows a nonuniform reduction in retinal sensitivity, the inferior arcuate area and periphery being most affected (stimulus size = III, pupil diameter = 1.0).

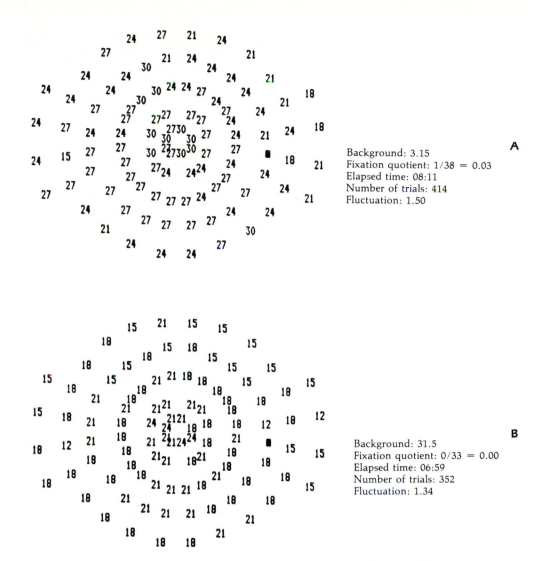

Background: 3.15
Fixation quotient: 1/38 = 0.03
Elapsed time: 08:11
Number of trials: 414
Fluctuation: 1.50

Background: 31.5
Fixation quotient: 0/33 = 0.00
Elapsed time: 06:59
Number of trials: 352
Fluctuation: 1.34

Fig. 19-21   The effect of background luminance in static perimetry. **A,** Visual field examination on the right eye of a glaucoma suspect shows an abnormal point in the inferior nasal step area (background = 3.15 asb). **B,** Repeat visual field performed at a higher background luminance (31.5 asb) shows a generalized decrease in retinal sensitivity and confirms the suspicious defect in the inferior nasal step area.

greater willingness to say yes to a test object being seen. Simply stated, the stimulus strength that a subject is willing to report as "seen" is influenced by the psychologic factors that affect the patient's perception of how important it is to see the test spot.

Training is another factor that has a profound influence on perimetric threshold. The amount of feedback given a patient during and after a visual field exam will have a psychologic impact and may speed learning and improve performance. Aulhorn and Harms studied the influence of training on perimetric threshold and found there may

be up to a 10-fold change (1 log unit) in threshold with practice.[2] They found this improvement greatest in early trial sessions, and it was maintained in subsequent tests.

REFERENCES

1. Armaly, MF: Ocular pressure and visual fields, Arch Ophthalmol 81:25, 1969
2. Aulhorn, E, and Harms, H: Early visual field defects in glaucoma, Glaucoma symposium, Tutzing Castle 1966, Basel, 1967, Karger
3. Aulhorn, E, and Harms, H: Visual perimetry. In: Handbook of sensory physiology, vol 7, New York, 1972, Springer-Verlag

4. Benedetto, MD, and Cyrlin, MN: The effect of blur upon static perimetric thresholds. In Heijl, A, and Greve, EL, editors: Documenta Ophthalmologica proceedings Series 42. Sixth International Visual Field Symposium. Dordrecht, 1985, Junk Publishers

5. Bjerrum, JP: Om en tilfojelse til saedvanlige syns-feltundersogelse samt om synfeltet ved glaukom, Nord Ophth Tidsskr, Kjobenh 2:144, 1889

6. Dolman, CL, McCormick, AO, and Drance, SM: Aging of the optic nerve, Arch Ophthalmol 98:2053, 1980

7. Drance, SM: The early field defects in glaucoma, Invest Ophthalmol 8:84, 1969

8. Drance, SM, Berry, V, and Hughes, A: Studies in the reproducibility of visual field areas in normal glaucoma subject, Can J Ophthalmol 1:14, 1966

9. Dubois-Poulson, A, and Magis, C: Premieres applications a l'ophthalmologie des techniques modernes d' automation et d'analyse de l'information, Bull Mem Soc Fr Ophthalmol 79:576, 1966

10. Frankhauser, F, and Enoch, JM: The effects of blur upon perimetric thresholds; a method for determining a quantitative estimate of retinal contour, Arch Ophthalmol 68:240, 1962

11. Fankhauser, F, and Schmidt, T: Die optimalen bedingungen fur die Untersuchung der raumlichen Summation mit stehender Reizmarke nach der Methode der quantitativen Lichtsinn Perimetrie, Ophthalmologica 139:409, 1960

12. Fankhauser, F, Spahr, J, and Bebie, H: Some aspects of the automation of perimetry, Surv Ophthalmol 22:131, 1977

13. Ferree, CE, and Rand, G: An illuminated perimeter with campimeter features, Am J Ophthalmol 5:455, 1922

14. Flammer, J, et al: Quantification of glaucomatous visual field defects with automated perimetry, Invest Ophthalmol Vis Sci 26:176, 1985

15. Flammer, J, Drance, SM, and Zulauf, M: Differential light threshold: short- and long-term fluctuation in patients with glaucoma, normal controls, and patients with suspected glaucoma, Arch Ophthalmol 102:704, 1984

16. Förster, R: Vorzeigung des Perimeter, Klin Monatsbl Augenheilk 7:411, 1869

17. Goldmann, H: Grundlagen exakter Perimetrie, Ophthalmologica 109:57, 1945

18. Graefe, A von: Über die Untersuchung des gesichtsfeldes bei amblyopischen Affectionen, Graefes Arch Klin Exp Ophthalmol 2:258, 1856

19. Haas, A, Flammer, J, and Schneider, U: Influence of age on visual fields of normal subjects, Am J Ophthalmol 101:199, 1986

20. Harms, H, and Aulhorn, E: Vergleichende Untersuchungen uber den Wert der quantitativen Perimetrie, Skiaskotometrie und Verschmelzungsfrequenz fur die Erkennung beginnender Gesichtsfeldstorungen beim Glaukom, Doc Ophthalmol 13:303, 1959

21. Heijl, A, and Krakau, CET: An automatic perimeter for glaucoma visual field screening and control, v Graefes Arch Klin Exp Ophthalmol 197:13, 1975

22. Jaffe, GJ, Alvarado, JA, and Juster, RP: Age-related changes of the normal visual field, Arch Ophthalmol 104:1021, 1986

23. Jayle, GE, Ourguard, AG, and Baisinger, LF: Night vision, Springfield, IL, 1959, Charles C Thomas

24. Katz, J, and Sommer, A: Asymmetry and variation in the normal hill of vision, Arch Ophthalmol 104:65, 1986

25. Koch, P, Roulier, A, and Fankhauser, F: Perimetry-information theoretical basis for its automation, Vision Research 12:1619, 1972

26. Krakau, CET: Aspects on the design of an automatic perimeter, Acta Ophthalmol 56:389, 1978

27. LeGrand, Y: Light, contour, and vision, ed 2, London, 1968, Chapman and Hall

28. Lynn, JR, Batson, E, and Fellman, RL: Internal inconsistency versus root mean square as measures of threshold variability. Documenta Ophthalmologica Proceedings, Series 42, Sixth International Visual Field Symposium, Santa Margherita Ligure, Italy, 1984. Dordrecht, The Netherlands, Dr. W. Junk Publishers

29. Lynn, JR, Fellman, RL, and Starita, RJ: New contingent algorithm for static automatic perimetry based upon chain pattern analysis, Documenta Ophthalmologica Proceedings, Series 43, Seventh International Visual Field Symposium, Amsterdam, The Netherlands, 1986. Dordrecht, The Netherlands, 1986, Dr. W. Junk Publishers

30. Lynn, JR, and Tate, GW: Computer controlled apparatus for automatic visual field examination, US patent 3,883,234, issued May 1975

31. Lynn, J, Tate, G: Unpublished data

32. McCluskey, DJ, et al: The effect of pilocarpine on the visual field of normals, Ophthalmology 93:843, 1986

33. Osterberg, G: Topography of the layer of rods and cones in the human retina, Acta Ophthalmol Suppl 6, 1935

34. Parrish, RK, Schiffman, J, and Anderson, DR: Static and kinetic visual field testing, Arch Ophthalmol 102:1497, 1984

35. Polyak, SL: The retina. Chicago, 1941, University of Chicago Press

36. Purkinje, JE: Beobachtungen und Versuche zur physiologie der sinne, Berlin, G. Reimer, 2:6, 1825

37. Rock, WJ, Drance, SM, and Morgan, RW: Visual field screening in glaucoma. An evaluation of the Armaly technique for screening glaucomatous visual fields, Arch Ophthalmol 89:287, 1973

38. Rönne, H: Ueber des Gesichtfeld beim Glaukom, Klin Monatsbl Augenheilk 47:12, 1909

39. Scott, GI: Traquair's clinical perimetry, ed 7, London, 1957, Henry Kimpton

40. Sloan, LL: Instruments and technics for the clinical testing of light sense III—an apparatus for studying regional differences in light sense, Arch Ophthalmol 22:233, 1939

41. Spahr, J, and Fankhauser, F: On automation of perimetry—problems and solutions. Nl'anne-Therapeutique et Colineque en Ophthalmolgie, Tome XXV, Marseille, 1974, Librairie Fueri Lami

42. Tate, GW: The physiological basis for perimetry. In Drance, SM, and Anderson, DA, editors: Automatic perimetry in glaucoma, Grune & Stratton, 1985, Orlando

43. Traquair, HM: Introduction to clinical perimetry, London, 1927, Kimpton

44. Walker, CB: Some new instruments for measuring visual field defects, Arch Ophthalmol 42:577, 1913

45. Weinreb, RN, and Perlman, JP: The effect of refractive correction on automated perimetric thresholds, Am J Ophthalmol 101:706, 1986

46. Wilensky, JT, Mermelstein, JR, and Siefel, HG: The use of different-sized stimuli in automated perimetry, Am J Ophthalmol 101:710, 1986

47. Young, T: The Bakerian Lecture. On the mechanism of the eye. Philos Trans R Soc Lond [Biol] 91:23, 1801

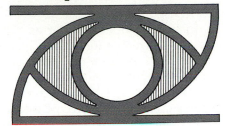

Chapter 20

Glaucomatous Visual Field Defects

Stephen M. Drance

HISTORICAL BACKGROUND

The concept of localized visual field defects for which boundaries could be defined began with Mariotte's discovery of the blind spot as early as 1668. By 1708, Boerhaave was already aware of the existence of scotomas. Thomas Young (1801) made exact measurements of the normal visual field and the physiologic blind spot. von Graefe first described contraction of the visual field and paracentral defects in glaucoma. The introduction of the perimeter by Förster (1869) confirmed the peripheral visual field changes of glaucoma. Bjerrum (1889), using the technique of campimetry, paved the way for the discovery of early central glaucomatous visual field defects and made possible the first attempts at quantitative perimetry. The excellent studies of Rönne, Traquair, and Peters characterized the different patterns of the localized visual field disturbances characteristic of glaucoma.

Goldmann (1945) introduced his perimeter, which standardized the target size, brightness, and background illumination, paving the way for the development of more accurate methods of evaluation of the visual field in the modern era. The description of static perimetry by Sloan (1939) and the practical introduction of the static perimeter by Harms and Aulhorn (1962) led to reevaluation of the earliest glaucomatous defects. Isolated paracentral scotomas were shown by Aulhorn and Harms as well as Drance[5,7] to be the common early visual field defects in glaucoma. Central and pe-

ripheral nasal steps were found to occur in the absence of paracentral scotomas but were more often associated with the paracentral defects. It was then realized that isolated peripheral defects, particularly nasally but occasionally temporally, could occur and were sometimes the earliest localized visual field defects. The studies of Aulhorn et al.,[5,6] Armaly[3] and Phelps et al.[13] showed that the defects occurred more frequently in the upper part of the visual field and were also closer to fixation in the upper fields. Generalized contraction of the isopters and generalized enlargement and baring of the blind spot had been previously emphasized, but the lack of specificity of such changes because of altered transparency of the media, miosis, refractive errors, and aging made them difficult to interpret.

Werner et al. (1977) showed that localized scatter in both kinetic and static responses was a precursor to subsequent localized visual field defects in glaucomatous patients.[17] With the introduction of the automated perimeter (see Chapter 21) in the 1970s by Lynn, Fankhauser, and others, it became clear that generalized changes in the differential light threshold and increased localized scatter occur before nerve fiber bundle visual field defects. By the same token, other psychophysical disturbances including disturbances of color vision, contrast sensitivity, and receptive field–like disturbances can occur before localized nerve fiber bundle damage in the field.

Generalized Changes in the Differential Light Sense

In 1966 Aulhorn and Harms[5] reported on 2684 eyes of glaucoma patients and glaucoma suspects who had been examined with static perimetry. Thirty-one percent had normal visual fields and of the remainder, 38% had a generalized contraction of the isopters. Armaly[3] found that 6 of 100 patients with elevated intraocular pressure who were examined by his method of selective perimetry had a contraction of isopters. In addition, he found that 6 of 100 patients with elevated intraocular pressure had a contraction of isopters that was pressure dependent.

Drance and Lakowski examined asymmetric patients in whom one eye had a nerve fiber bundle field defect. The central isopters of that eye were contracted compared with the fellow eye without a defect in only about 30% of the cases.[8] Werner et al. independently reported similar findings.[18]

If a generalized isopter contraction always precedes a localized nerve fiber bundle defect, one would expect the isopters of the damaged eyes always to be contracted compared with the undamaged fellow eye. This is not the case. Hart and Becker[11] found that 35.6% of eyes that went on to develop localized field defects showed blind spot enlargement and 31% showed central isopter constriction. Therefore, in all of these studies, approximately two thirds of the patients did not demonstrate a generalized contraction of the isopters associated with the development of a classic nerve fiber bundle defect.

Hart and Becker found that isopter contraction occurred significantly more frequently during the year before the onset of the definitive field defects when compared with a control group who did not subsequently develop field defects. It can be concluded that, although contraction of the central isopters commonly occurs in eyes that subsequently develop localized visual field defects, the majority of localized defects are not preceded or accompanied by such an isopter contraction.

The interest in generalized isopter contraction was rekindled by quantitative studies of optic nerve axons. Quigley et al.[14] showed that up to 40% to 50% of nerve fibers could be lost in the absence of a field defect. Airaksinen and Tuulonen[1] showed that localized nerve fiber bundle loss and diffuse loss of nerve fibers in the retina precedes visual field defects. The abnormalities of other psychophysical functions such as foveal function,[2] color sense,[8] temporal[4] and spatial[16] contrast sensitivity, and receptive field–like functions[9] occurred before the development of visual field defects, further suggesting that these are preceded by generalized disturbances.

Localized Nerve Fiber Bundle Defects

The features of paracentral scotomas along the course of the arcuate nerve fibers, the associated or independent central and peripheral nasal steps, the classic arcuate nerve fiber bundle defects, and the temporal and other sector-shaped defects are well known. To identify the earliest visual field defects, we studied a group of 35 eyes with previously normal visual fields that developed reproducible nerve fiber bundle field defects.[17] Visual fields were plotted every 4 months. The appearance of the first reproducible defect therefore denoted an early visual field defect but did not imply early disease. In 51% the first visual field disturbance was a paracentral scotoma with a nasal step. An additional 26% had a paracentral scotoma alone, whereas 20% showed only nasal steps, two thirds of which were in the central isopters and one third only in the peripheral isopters. The remaining 3% first developed sector-shaped defects in other quadrants. The upper and lower hemifields could become involved at almost the same time, and although scotomas were often initially relative, they could also be dense from the beginning.

In 1982 Hart and Becker[11] studied the initial glaucomatous defects of 98 eyes of 72 patients and reported that 54% had nasal steps, 41% had paracentral or Bjerrum scotomas, 30% had arcuate blind spot enlargement, 90% had isolated arcuate scotomas separated from the blind spot, and 3% had temporal defects. The upper visual field was more commonly involved than the lower in a ratio of 3 to 2. In some eyes, the nasal steps involved both the central and peripheral isopters, but others had only a peripheral or central nasal step. The most common area of paracentral disturbance was adjacent to the superior nasal pole of the blind spot (Fig. 20-1).

Phelps et al.[13] illustrated the location of paracentral defects of varying severity (Fig. 20-2). Werner et al.[17] found a localized scatter of both static and kinetic responses that preceded the subsequent development of visual field defects. Studies using quantitative threshold perimetry showed an increased short-term fluctuation in areas without an increased threshold to be present in early glaucoma.[10,15] Flammer et al.[10] showed the sequence of

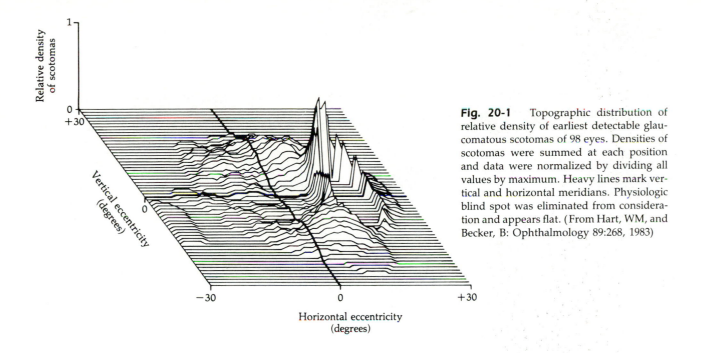

Fig. 20-1 Topographic distribution of relative density of earliest detectable glaucomatous scotomas of 98 eyes. Densities of scotomas were summed at each position and data were normalized by dividing all values by maximum. Heavy lines mark vertical and horizontal meridians. Physiologic blind spot was eliminated from consideration and appears flat. (From Hart, WM, and Becker, B: Ophthalmology 89:268, 1983)

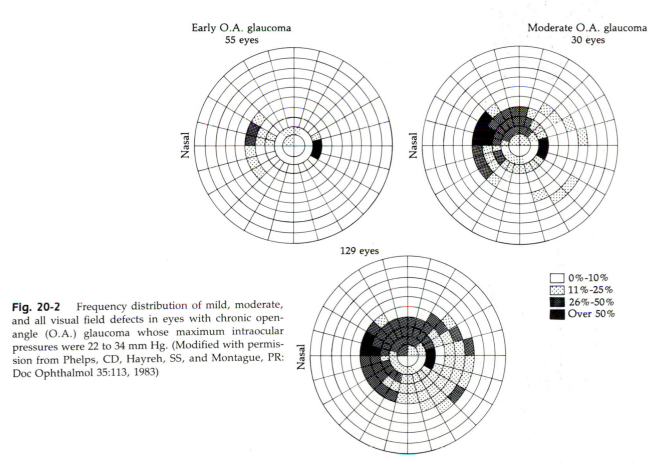

Fig. 20-2 Frequency distribution of mild, moderate, and all visual field defects in eyes with chronic open-angle (O.A.) glaucoma whose maximum intraocular pressures were 22 to 34 mm Hg. (Modified with permission from Phelps, CD, Hayreh, SS, and Montague, PR: Doc Ophthalmol 35:113, 1983)

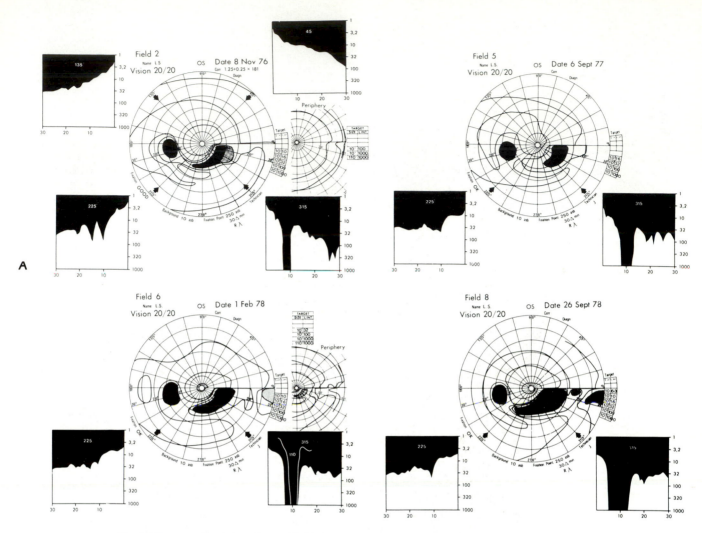

Fig. 20-3 **A** and **B,** Selected visual field showing continuous progression of scotoma in the inferior hemifield. The intervening fields, not illustrated, confirm the continuous progression.

early glaucomatous disturbances to begin with an increase of localized short-term fluctuation with a normal threshold. Increased fluctuation with a reduction in sensitivity (increased threshold) was the the next stage of the visual field disturbance. This was followed by a relative scotoma in an area where the threshold was difficult to determine because of the increased fluctuation and that was felt, therefore, not to be a clearly demarcated disturbance, as had been previously suggested by kinetic perimetry.

It would not appear, judging from longitudinal studies, that the nature, location, density, and frequency of the earliest localized defects have been described. These disturbances are preceded by increase in the short-term fluctuation in the area in which a defect subsequently develops.

Progression of Glaucomatous Damage

The manner in which the progression occurs has not been fully explored, apart from the well-known sequence of an arcuate scotoma breaking through to the periphery in the upper and lower field and gradually leading to a central island of vision and/or a peripheral temporal island. The manner in which the progression occurs has not been fully explored, but at least four ways have been identified.

1. Scotomas can continuously increase in size and depth (Fig. 20-3).
2. Scotomas can become larger and/or deeper in an episodic manner (Fig. 20-4).
3. Fresh scotomas or sector-shaped defects may develop (Fig. 20-5).
4. There may be generalized loss of retinal sen-

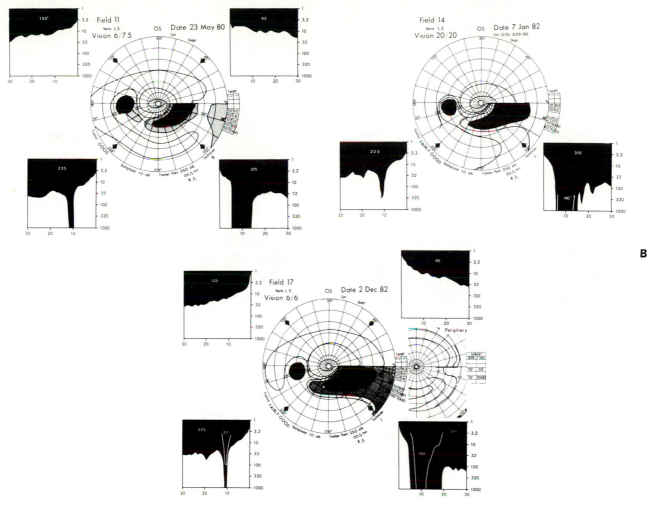

Fig. 20-3, cont'd   For legend see opposite page.

sitivity as manifested by a gradual constriction of all isopters not accounted for by opacities of the media (Fig. 20-6). In addition, there may be improvement in the visual field.

Hart and Becker[11] described the chronology of 98 eyes developing field defects in which the initial defects were relative. Twenty-two eyes showed a disappearance of the early scotoma after medical therapy. The disappearance was not related to intraocular pressure reduction and in all of the 22 eyes the defects recurred and were denser within 5 years in the territory of the nerve fiber bundle originally disturbed. Sixty-seven of the eyes showed a similar gradual onset but had no temporary improvement, and in the remaining 9 eyes there was a relatively abrupt onset followed by rapid progression in the size and density of the

defect. Although the onset of the defects appeared to be gradual, the progression of established defects seemed to occur episodically. Following an increase in size and density, eyes remained without further progression. Sixty-three of the eyes were observed for at least a decade and 13 involved both hemifields from the outset, whereas in the remaining 50, the defects were confined to either the superior or inferior hemifield. Twenty-two percent of those 50 eyes showed defects in the other hemifield at the end of the decade, whereas in the other 78% the defect remained confined to the same hemifield. All showed marked progression over the 10 years, so that in 72% of them the loss was marked and dense, and in 6% the loss was absolute, while only 4% were left with a shallow relative defect. In those 13 eyes in whom both hemifields were initially involved, the progression was even more

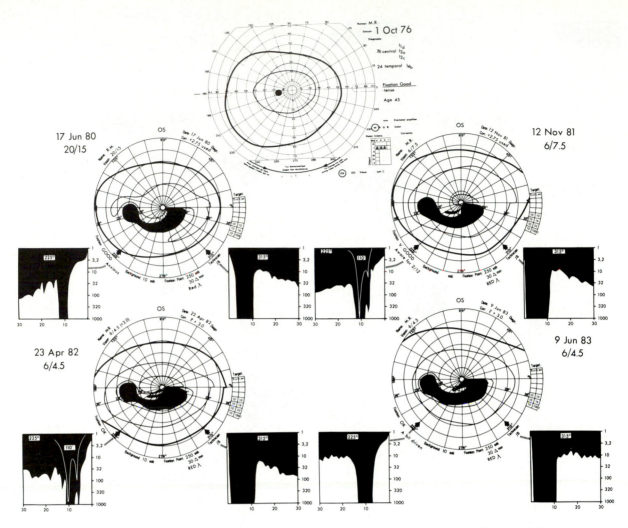

Fig. 20-4 Visual fields indicating sudden onset of scotoma noticed by patient (17 June 1980). Occurrence of fresh episode shown statically and kinetically (12 Nov 1981) with subsequent lack of damage.

marked, so that 54% developed absolute field loss in the decade. There was no significant difference in the mean intraocular pressure or age that could be related to the degree of progression. Most of the eyes had well-controlled intraocular pressures. The mean pressures were slightly but not significantly lower in the group of eyes suffering the greatest extent of field loss.

Some questions should be addressed to progression of the defect. Do scotomas increase in size and density at the same time? How often do fresh scotomas occur? Is there a diffuse change in the sensitivity of the visual field? Is it greater or smaller than the changes in the scotoma? Is there always change in the central field when the peripheral field changes? Is the rate of loss related to intraocular pressure? Can rate of progression be affected by therapy?

To try to answer some of these questions, 48 eyes of 48 patients with chronic open-angle glaucoma and an accurate perimetric follow-up for a number of years, of which at least 2 must have been with a scotoma, were studied.[12] The initial visual acuity was 20/30 or better, and the final acuity was 20/40 or better. Planimetry was carried out on all scotomas as was planimetry of the static profiles of the island of vision through the scotoma. The central sensitivity of each field was known. The mean duration of follow-up was 8 ± 3½ years with a median of 7½ years and ranged from 2 to 15 years. Forty-two (87.5%) of the eyes showed progression, five (10.4%) remained stable, and one

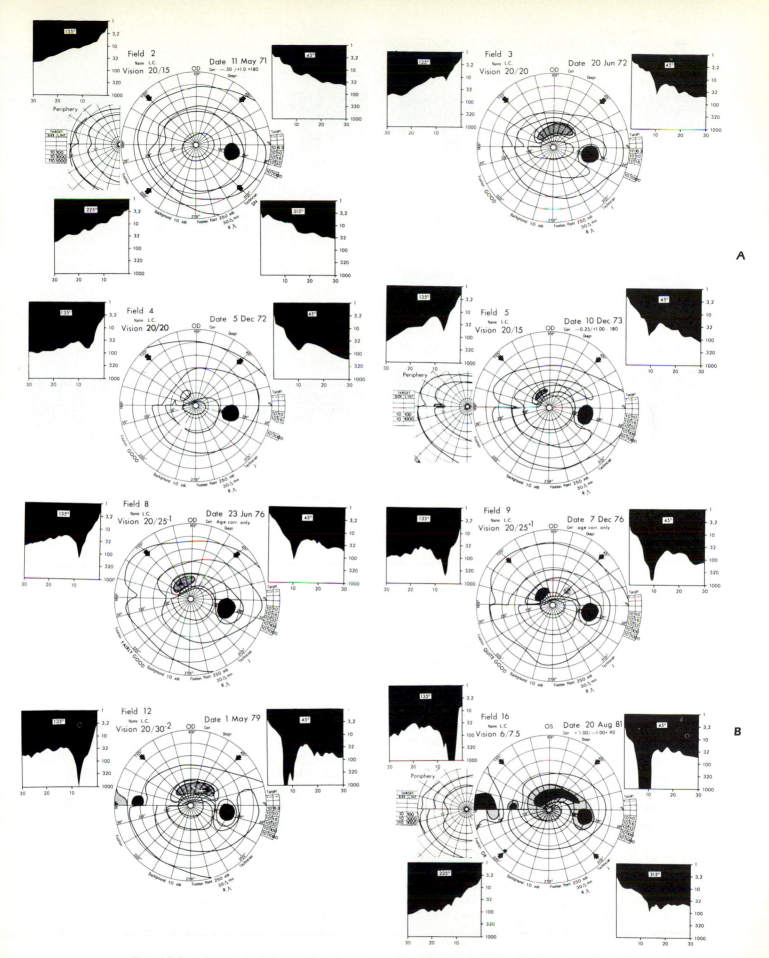

Fig. 20-5 **A** and **B,** Selected visual fields to illustrate development of a fresh scotoma, which shows progression and appearance of a new scotoma or inferior hemifield (field 16).

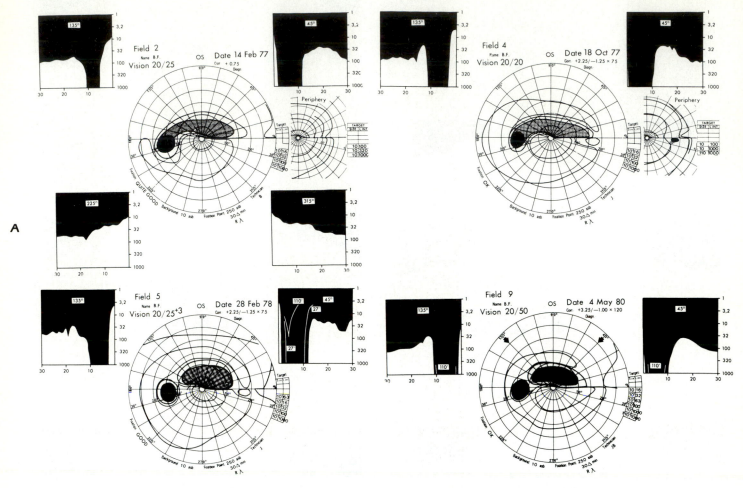

Fig. 20-6 **A** and **B,** Selected visual fields showing increase in size and density of scotoma in upper hemifield but with decreased vision because of lens opacity and overall loss of sensitivity.

(2.1%) improved. An increase in density of a scotoma was the most common mode of progression and occurred in 78% of progressing defects, whereas an increase in the size of the scotoma occurred in 52%, and a new scotoma appeared in 49% of eyes showing progression. Of 45 eyes that had only 1 hemifield involved by the scotoma at the onset, 22 (63%) remained in that hemifield, whereas 13 (37%) showed involvement of the other hemifield over the period of observation. Many of the eyes showed combinations of all three modes of progression. The duration of follow-up was related to the chance of developing a new scotoma and the involvement of the second hemifield. The age at diagnosis and the intraocular pressure were not significantly related to qualitative progression. The study of the relationship of rates of progression to intraocular pressure may be rewarding in the future.

It would appear that most scotomas progress by increasing in depth, a smaller number increase in size, and about half of eyes develop a new scotoma. One third of those eyes with a single hemifield involvement develop involvement of the other half. Progression appears to be related to the length of follow-up and not to the age at the time of diagnosis or to the level of intraocular pressure. Most studies show that the majority of patients with field loss progress over time.

The implications for perimetry of visual field defects in glaucoma are that threshold information of disturbed points in a scotoma or its quantification with kinetic perimetry are necessary if the most common mode of progression, which indicates deterioration of the disease, is to be detected. Careful delineation of the area of scotomas and examination of the unaffected field are necessary because these types of change can also occur as

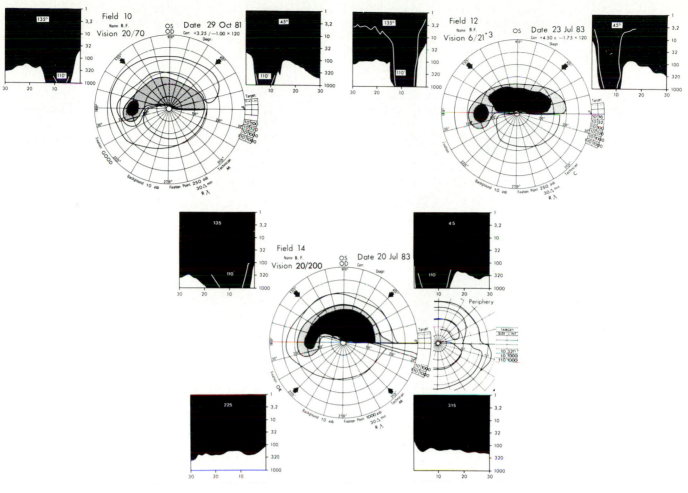

Fig. 20-6, cont'd   For legend see opposite page.

isolated signs of progression.

It is essential that further work be done to elucidate whether intraocular pressure reduction is important in determining the course and rate of the progression of glaucomatous visual field defects.

REFERENCES

1. Airaksinen, PJ, and Tuulonen, A: Early glaucoma changes in patients with and without an optic disc hemorrhage, Acta Ophthalmol (Copenh) 62:197, 1984.
2. Anctil, JL, and Anderson, DR: Early foveal involvement and generalized discussion of the visual field in glaucoma, Arch Ophthalmol 102:363, 1984
3. Armaly, MF: Selective perimetry for glaucomatous defects in ocular hypertension, Arch Ophthalmol 87:518, 1972
4. Atkin, A, et al: Abnormalities of central contrast sensitivity in glaucoma, Am J Ophthalmol 88:205, 1979
5. Aulhorn, E, and Harms, H: Early visual field defects in glaucoma. In Leydhecker, W, editor: Glaucoma; Tützing Symposium 1966, Basel, 1967, Karger
6. Aulhorn, E, and Karmeyer, H: Frequency distribution in early glaucomatous visual field defects, Doc Ophthalmol 14:75, 1976
7. Drance, SM: The early field defects in glaucoma, Invest Ophthalmol 8:84, 1969
8. Drance, SM, and Lakowski, R: Early psychophysical disturbances in chronic open angle glaucoma. In Transactions of the New Orleans Academy of Ophthalmology, St. Louis, 1981, The C.V. Mosby Co
9. Enoch, JM, and Campos, EC: Analysis of patients with open angle glaucoma using perimetric techniques reflecting receptive field like proportion, Doc Ophthalmol Proc Series 19:137, 1978
10. Flammer, J, Drance, SM, and Zulauf, M: The short and long term fluctuation of the differential light threshold in patients with glaucoma, normal controls and glaucoma suspects, Arch Ophthalmol (In press)

11. Hart, WM, and Becker, B: The onset and evolution of glaucomatous visual field defects, Ophthalmology 89:268, 1982

12. Mikelberg, F, and Drance, SM: The mode of progression of visual field defects in glaucoma, Am J Ophthalmol 98:443, 1984

13. Phelps, CD, Hayreh, SS, and Montague, PR: Visual fields in low tension glaucoma, primary open angle glaucoma and anterior ischemic optic neuropathy, Doc Ophthalmol Proc Series 35:113, 1983

14. Quigley, HA, Addicks, EM, and Green, WR: Optic nerve damage in human glaucoma. III. Quantitative correlation of nerve fiber loss and visual field defect in glaucoma, ischemic neuropathy, papilledema and toxic neuropathy, Arch Ophthalmol 100:135, 1982

15. Sturmer, J, Gloor, B, and Tobler, HJ: Wie Sehen Glaukomgesithtsfelder Wirklich Aus, Graefes Arch Clin Exp Ophthalmol (In press)

16. Tyler, CW: Specific defects of flicker sensitivity in glaucoma and ocular hypertension, Invest Ophthalmol Vis Sci 20:202, 1981

17. Werner, EB, Drance, SM, and Schulzer, M: Early visual field defects in glaucoma, Arch Ophthalmol 95:1173, 1977

18. Werner, EB, Saheb, N, and Patel, S: Lack of generalized constriction of affected visual field in glaucoma patients with defects in one eye, Can J Ophthalmol 17:53, 1982

Chapter 21

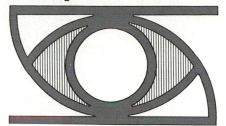

Automated Perimetry

Marshall N. Cyrlin

HISTORY

For many years manual kinetic perimetry with either a tangent screen, arc, or Goldmann-type bowl perimeter represented the primary method of examination of the visual field in patients with glaucoma. Before the introduction of computerized automated perimetry, manual static perimetry with the Tübinger or Goldmann perimeter was employed in research settings or in the clinical evaluation of specific areas of the visual field in patients. Manual static perimetry was too tedious and time consuming for the routine testing of the entire visual field. The current widespread availability of economically priced automated perimeters capable of both screening and full thresholding examinations has resulted in the ability to perform high-quality, reproducible visual field testing in routine patient evaluation. The concept of thresholding and the decibel unit nomenclature for the description of visual field sensitivity are discussed in Chapter 19.

GOALS OF AUTOMATED PERIMETRY

Standardization of Test Conditions

Automated perimeters allow standardization of test conditions in several ways. After ambient room illumination has been set to a prespecified standard, the perimeter may be calibrated or may autocalibrate before the initiation of testing. The testing strategy program selected by the operator is performed by the computerized perimeter following a preprogrammed, reproducible algorithm. Specifically, any given program number or test will always be performed in exactly the same manner.

This eliminates perimetrist bias, which has been a long-standing source of variability in manual perimetry. Nevertheless, the operator still plays an important role in instructing the patient, selecting the test strategy, applying the appropriate near correction for central visual field examinations, and monitoring the patient during the course of the test. With some patients, the operator may need to interrupt the examination to reinstruct the patient or readjust the seat or head position for greater comfort. Rarely, the entire examination may need to be discontinued if the patient is unable to perform the test properly. For these reasons, the patient should not be left unattended once the test has begun.

Estimation of Patient Reliability

Estimation of patient reliability is an important aspect of automated perimetry. This is accomplished with various perimeters by recording fixation losses, false positive or false negative responses, and fluctuation rate.

Fixation losses (movement of the eye away from the fixation target) are recorded by perimeters that intermittently perform blind spot monitoring. This method does not continuously monitor fixation. Stimuli can be presented when fixation is not maintained. A patient with a high number of fixation losses would have a generally unreliable visual field.

False positive responses are recorded when a patient elicits a response to the sound of a projection perimeter at a time when no visual stimulus is presented. *False negative responses* are recorded when a patient does not respond to a maximal visual stimulus at a point that was seen earlier during the examination. As a general rule, false positive or false negative rates greater than 20% indicate unreliability.

Fluctuation rate, also reported as SF (short-term fluctuation) or RMS (root mean square), is a measure of intraexamination reproducibility. The details of the mathematical calculation are discussed in Chapter 19. It is derived from the statistical analysis of the amount of variation determined at 10 or more points that are retested during the same examination and is reported in decibels (dB). A hypothetical RMS of 0 dB would indicate perfect reproducibility. As a general rule, in patients with a normal to a moderately damaged visual field, an RMS under 1.5 dB is excellent, 1.5 to 2.0 dB is very good, 2.0 to 3.0 dB is good, 3.0 to 3.5 dB is fair, and 3.5 to 4.5 dB is poor. Rates higher than 4.5 may indicate a totally unreliable examination. The greater the damage to the visual field, the higher is the expected fluctuation rate.[7] Higher than expected fluctuation in a normal field may be an indication of early glaucomatous visual field loss rather than unreliability.[8]

Computerized Analysis of Test Results

Automated perimetry is ideally suited for computerized analysis of test results either by the perimeter itself or by an external computer. Analysis may consist of comparison of an individual examination with a stored data base of predicted normal values, statistical data reduction or calculation of visual field indices, or evaluation of serial examinations. With appropriate hardware and software, the test results may be transmitted to a mainframe computer for analysis of data from a single center or for data analysis in multicenter studies.

METHODS OF AUTOMATED PERIMETRY

Types of Automated Perimeters

The distinction between kinetic and static perimetry has been discussed in Chapter 19. Most automated perimeters in use today employ automated static testing methods. Automated perimeters employing kinetic testing, such as the Perimetron, have not proved useful for testing all the patterns of visual field loss.[4,12] Recently available instruments may combine central static testing with a peripheral kinetic strategy. Because most perimeters currently available use static strategies, the remainder of this chapter is devoted to this method.

The greatest distinction in automated perimeter design is between projection instruments, such as the Octopus and Humphrey Visual Field Analyzer, and LED (light emitting diode) instruments, such as the Dicon and Digilab perimeters. Other perimeters employ fiberoptic bundles rather than LEDs.

Projection perimeters offer the advantages of unlimited possible test strategies, either programmed by the manufacturer or by the user, and the potential for varying the size or the color of the stimulus. Potential disadvantages are the greater possibility of mechanical breakdown, including the need to replace lamps, and the accompanying audible sounds, which may confuse some patients.

Advantages of LED instruments are economy, less potential for breakdown, quiet operation, and the possibility of multiple simultaneous stimulus presentation. Potential disadvantages are limitations of the number of test patterns and the size or color of stimuli. Possible visual cueing of the patient by the LED openings in the perimeter bowl may be eliminated by rear projection systems, as found in the Digilab instrument.

Fixation monitoring during automated perimetry may be accomplished by direct viewing with a telescope or video camera, blind spot monitoring, or by video monitoring of the pupil position and eyelid closure. Combinations of these may also be used. Blind spot monitoring is commonly achieved by the Heijl-Krakau method. The method first determines the blind spot. The perimeter than periodically presents a stimulus to the blind spot area. If the patient perceives the stimulus, a fixation loss is recorded. The disadvantage of this technique is that a significant portion of the total testing time must be devoted to blind spot monitoring. Fixation may also be lost between blind spot testing if this method is not also combined with direct viewing. The Octopus perimeter employs a video system that monitors fixation by determining the position of the pupil relative to the surrounding iris. An advantage to this system is that a fixation loss or closure of the eyelid may be automatically discarded and the point retested. Some patients with dark irides may be difficult to monitor by this method.

Instrument Variables

Instrument variables include background illumination, stimulus intensity, stimulus size, stimulus color, presentation time, interstimulus time, and cupola distance.

Background illumination is typically fixed at 4 apostilbs (asb), as in the Octopus perimeter, or at 31.5 asb (equivalent to the Goldmann manual perimeter), as in the Humphrey perimeter. Some instruments, such as the Squid or Digilab 750, have user selectable background illumination. Perimeters with 31.5 asb background illumination test in a slightly more photopic range and provide brighter stimuli. The physiologic consequences of the state of adaptation and background illumination are discussed in Chapter 19.

Stimulus intensity is controlled by the perimeter or set by the operator for single- or multiple-level testing. In threshold testing, the perimeter automatically changes the intensity of the stimulus to bracket the patient's threshold at each test location.

Stimulus size may be set by the operator in projection perimeters such as the Octopus or Humphrey perimeters. This is a potential advantage in patients with advanced visual field loss or extremely low threshold sensitivities. *Stimulus color* may be changed on some projection perimeters. This may be useful for research purposes but is not routinely employed in the testing of glaucoma patients. LED or fiberoptic perimeters typically do not have variable stimulus size or color. The stimulus color in many LED perimeters is light green (570 nm), which corresponds to peak visual sensitivity.

Presentation time is fixed by the perimeter, lasting 0.1 second in the Octopus perimeter and 0.2 second in the Humphrey perimeter, and is based on the visual physiology described in Chapters 7 and 19. *Interstimulus time* is the time between presentations and may be varied to adapt to the speed of the patient's responses.

The *cupola distance* varies from 30 to 51 cm in the different models of automated perimeters. The operator must know the exact distance in order to use the appropriate correcting lens for testing the central field. The manufacturer usually provides a chart of the correct "add for age" for each model.

TEST STRATEGIES

Test strategies incorporate both the pattern and number of spots tested and the method by which each of these determinations is made.

Typical patterns of examinations are the central 10, 12, 24, or 30 degrees (Fig. 21-1), portions of the field such as from 30 to 60 degrees (Fig. 21-2, *A*), the nasal step area (Fig. 21-2, *B*) or the entire visual field (Fig. 21-2, *C*). The manufacturer may provide programs designed to test at points particularly susceptible to glaucomatous damage (Fig. 21-3).

The perimeter may allow the operator to design user-defined test strategies (Fig. 21-4).

The simplest level of testing is the single- or multiple-level screening examination. The single level test consists of a single suprathreshold stimulus, derived from a predicted value or from testing by the perimeter, which is used for the entire examination. A variation of this is the threshold-related examination in which the single stimulus intensity is increased as testing approaches further into the periphery. In either case, the results consist solely of a pattern of seen or unseen points.

Multiple level tests, such as the Octopus program 03 or 07, distinguish normal points from relative and absolute scotomas (Fig. 21-5). Examinations such as the Dicon Two Zone Program perform stepped suprathreshold testing by retesting missed points at increasing intensities (Fig. 21-6). Screening tests can also be performed in which missed points are completely thresholded, such as when the "Quantify Defects" option on the Humphrey perimeter is selected (Fig. 21-7). The advantage of screening tests is their ability to rapidly identify an abnormal visual field and to give some information regarding the location and depth of scotomas. They are not as valuable for following glaucoma patients as the partial or full-thresholding strategies.

The principle of bracketing and determining the threshold of any given test point is discussed in Chapter 19. Full-thresholding strategies, such as Octopus program 32, determine the exact threshold at each point (Fig. 21-8). Fast (partial) thresholding programs, such as Octopus program 34, perform complete thresholding only on abnormal points. This shortens testing time in an individual with a basically normal field by not determining the exact sensitivities at each point. However, this method may lead to false interpretation in the follow-up of a patient with an initial full field that develops gradual diffuse or localized loss of sensitivity. This loss may remain undetected until it has fallen below the predetermined sensitivity level. The full-thresholding strategy is the most accurate for following glaucoma patients and glaucoma suspects with normal visual fields.

Full-thresholding examinations may also provide information concerning patient reliability by performing double determinations (repeat thresholding), such as in Octopus program 32 (Fig. 21-8) or Humphrey program 30-2 with the fluctuation on (Fig. 21-9). The importance of these measurements has already been noted. The Humphrey perimeter performs additional multiple determinations on test points that fall below expected values.

Text continued on p. 414.

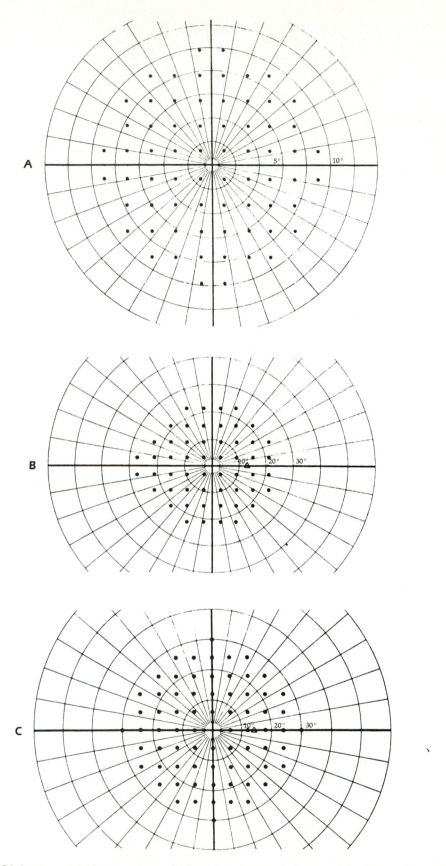

Fig. 21-1 Central field test patterns. **A,** Central 10 degrees (2 degrees of resolution). **B,** Central 24 degrees (6 degrees of resolution). **C,** Central 30 degrees (6 degrees of resolution). (Reproduced with permission from The Field Analyzer Primer, Allergan Humphrey, 1987)

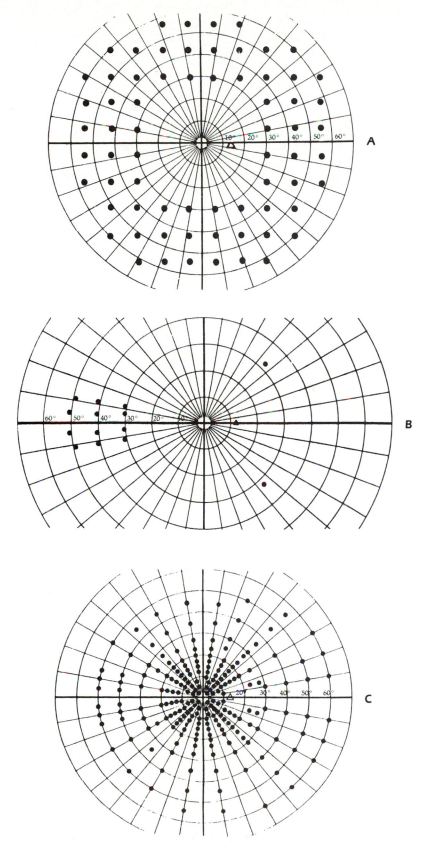

Fig. 21-2   Visual field test patterns. **A,** Mid-field examination from 30 to 60 degrees. **B,** Test for nasal defects. **C,** Full field examination. (Reproduced with permission from the The Field Analyzer Primer, Allergan Humphrey, 1987)

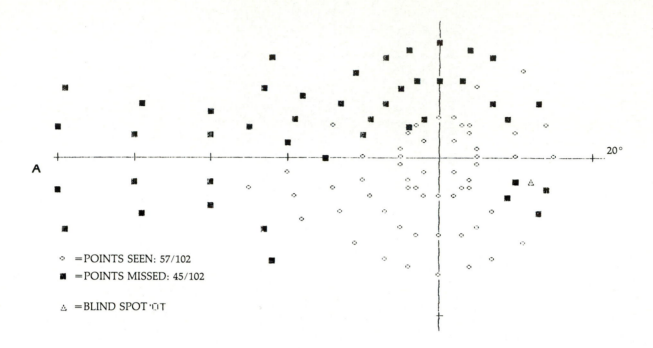

A

☌ =POINTS SEEN: 57/102

▨ =POINTS MISSED: 45/102

△ =BLIND SPOT·⊡T

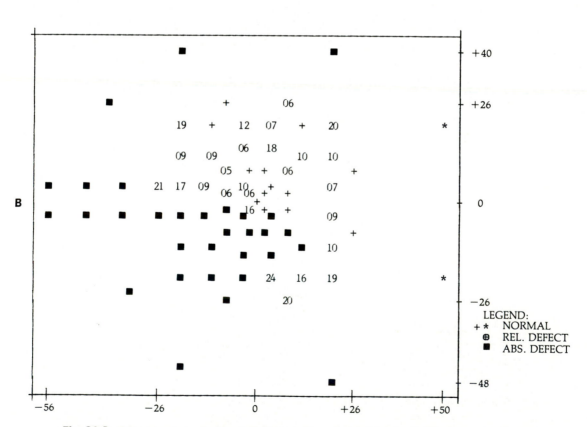

B

LEGEND:
+ ✶   NORMAL
⊕   REL. DEFECT
■   ABS. DEFECT

Fig. 21-3 Glaucoma tests. **A,** Armaly pattern on Humphrey perimeter. **B,** G1 program on Octopus perimeter. Both tests concentrate on paracentral and arcuate areas as well as nasal step.

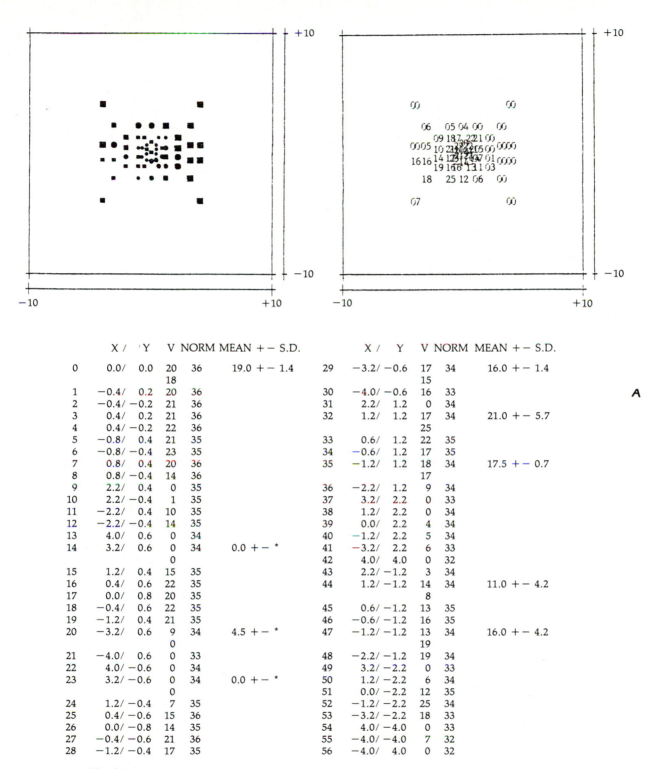

#	X / Y	V	NORM	MEAN + − S.D.	#	X / Y	V	NORM	MEAN + − S.D.
0	0.0/ 0.0	20	36	19.0 + − 1.4	29	−3.2/ −0.6	17	34	16.0 + − 1.4
		18					15		
1	−0.4/ 0.2	20	36		30	−4.0/ −0.6	16	33	
2	−0.4/ −0.2	21	36		31	2.2/ 1.2	0	34	
3	0.4/ 0.2	21	36		32	1.2/ 1.2	17	34	21.0 + − 5.7
4	0.4/ −0.2	22	36				25		
5	−0.8/ 0.4	21	35		33	0.6/ 1.2	22	35	
6	−0.8/ −0.4	23	35		34	−0.6/ 1.2	17	35	
7	0.8/ 0.4	20	36		35	−1.2/ 1.2	18	34	17.5 + − 0.7
8	0.8/ −0.4	14	36				17		
9	2.2/ 0.4	0	35		36	−2.2/ 1.2	9	34	
10	2.2/ −0.4	1	35		37	3.2/ 2.2	0	33	
11	−2.2/ 0.4	10	35		38	1.2/ 2.2	0	34	
12	−2.2/ −0.4	14	35		39	0.0/ 2.2	4	34	
13	4.0/ 0.6	0	34		40	−1.2/ 2.2	5	34	
14	3.2/ 0.6	0	34	0.0 + − *	41	−3.2/ 2.2	6	33	
		0			42	4.0/ 4.0	0	32	
15	1.2/ 0.4	15	35		43	2.2/ −1.2	3	34	
16	0.4/ 0.6	22	35		44	1.2/ −1.2	14	34	11.0 + − 4.2
17	0.0/ 0.8	20	35				8		
18	−0.4/ 0.6	22	35		45	0.6/ −1.2	13	35	
19	−1.2/ 0.4	21	35		46	−0.6/ −1.2	16	35	
20	−3.2/ 0.6	9	34	4.5 + − *	47	−1.2/ −1.2	13	34	16.0 + − 4.2
		0					19		
21	−4.0/ 0.6	0	33		48	−2.2/ −1.2	19	34	
22	4.0/ −0.6	0	34		49	3.2/ −2.2	0	33	
23	3.2/ −0.6	0	34	0.0 + − *	50	1.2/ −2.2	6	34	
		0			51	0.0/ −2.2	12	35	
24	1.2/ −0.4	7	35		52	−1.2/ −2.2	25	34	
25	0.4/ −0.6	15	36		53	−3.2/ −2.2	18	33	
26	0.0/ −0.8	14	35		54	4.0/ −4.0	0	33	
27	−0.4/ −0.6	21	36		55	−4.0/ −4.0	7	32	
28	−1.2/ −0.4	17	35		56	−4.0/ 4.0	0	32	

A

Fig. 21-4   User-defined tests. **A,** High-resolution central examination written with Octopus Sargon program. Beneath graphic displays is a value table illustrating all test points and their thresholds.

Continued.

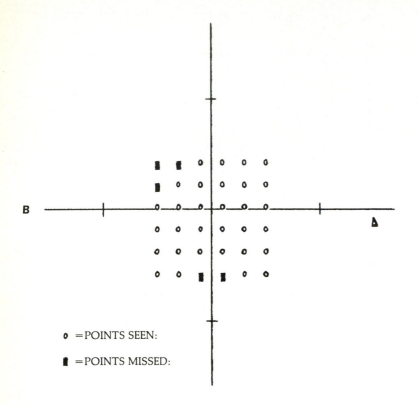

B

Fig. 21-4, cont'd B, User-defined test of central 5 degrees on Humphrey perimeter. This is an example of a single-intensity screening test.

o = POINTS SEEN:

◼ = POINTS MISSED:

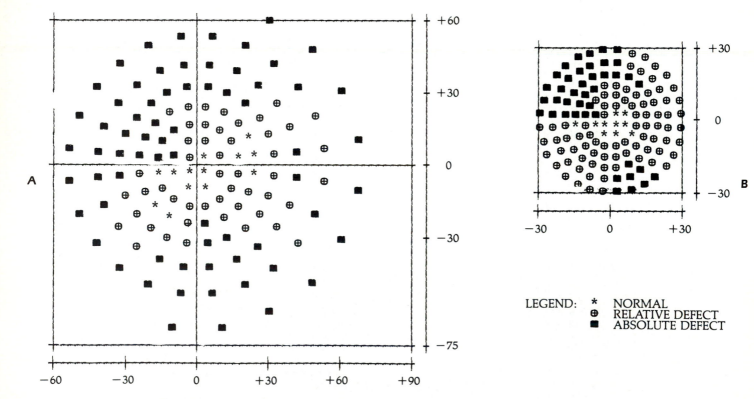

LEGEND: * NORMAL
⊕ RELATIVE DEFECT
◼ ABSOLUTE DEFECT

Fig. 21-5 Multiple-level tests. Octopus program 07 full-field examination, **A,** and Octopus program 03 central 30 degree examination, **B.** These tests both illustrate diffuse depression of sensitivity and a superior nasal step.

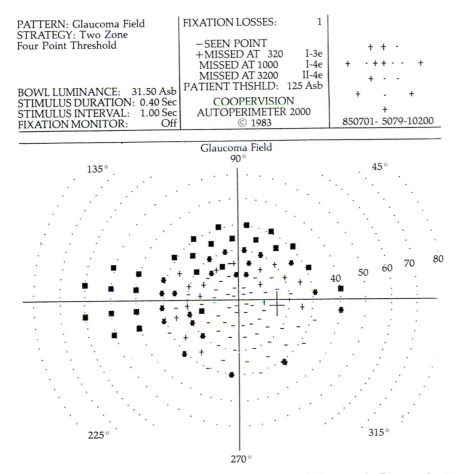

PATTERN: Glaucoma Field
STRATEGY: Two Zone
Four Point Threshold

FIXATION LOSSES: 1

−SEEN POINT
+MISSED AT   320   I-3e
 MISSED AT 1000   I-4e
 MISSED AT 3200   II-4e

BOWL LUMINANCE: 31.50 Asb
STIMULUS DURATION: 0.40 Sec
STIMULUS INTERVAL: 1.00 Sec
FIXATION MONITOR: Off

PATIENT THSHLD: 125 Asb

COOPERVISION
AUTOPERIMETER 2000
© 1983

850701- 5079-10200

Fig. 21-6 Stepped suprathreshold test. Two-zone glaucoma field test on the Dicon perimeter tests missed points at three stimulus intensities.

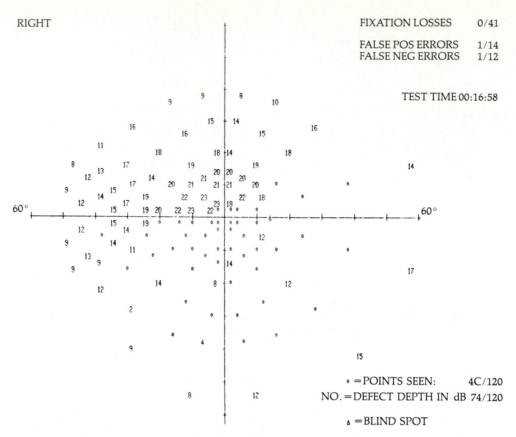

RIGHT

FIXATION LOSSES   0/41

FALSE POS ERRORS   1/14
FALSE NEG ERRORS   1/12

TEST TIME 00:16:58

○ =POINTS SEEN: 4C/120
NO. =DEFECT DEPTH IN dB 74/120

▲ =BLIND SPOT

Fig. 21-7 "Quantify defects" screening test. This option on Humphrey perimeter completely thresholds all missed points and is most useful for screening on patients with generally normal fields.

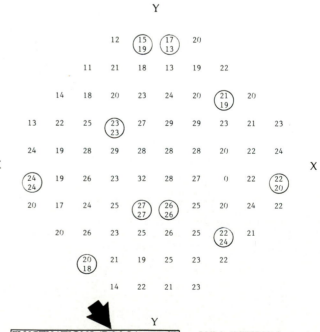

Fig. 21-8 Full-thresholding central 30 degree test. Octopus program 32 calculates threshold of sensitivity at each test location. Circled numbers are repeat threshold points that are used for calculation of fluctuation rate *(arrow)*.

FLUCTUATIONS (R.M.S.): 1.5 dB   LUM. INTERVAL: 4

CENTRAL 30 — 2 THRESHOLD TEST

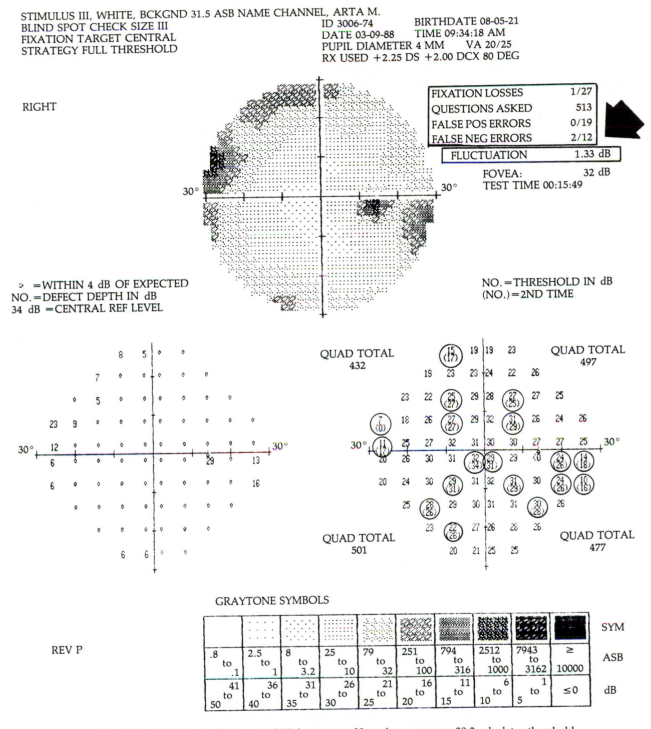

Fig. 21-9 Full-thresholding central 30 degree test. Humphrey program 30-2 calculates threshold of sensitivity at each test location. Circled numbers are repeat thresholded points that are used for calculation of fluctuation rate *(arrow)*. Fixation losses and false responses are indicated above fluctuation rate *(box)*.

DATA PRESENTATION

The printouts from an automated perimeter provide several categories of information regarding the patient, test conditions, reliability, and sensitivity of the test points examined.

Patient data and test conditions include patient name, identification number or birth date, test date, eye tested, program type, test strategy, pupil size, correction used, and vision. Information may also be provided as to the number of questions, repetitions, or test time.

Reliability factors previously mentioned include fixation losses, false positive responses, false negative responses, and fluctuation rate (SF or RMS) (see Fig. 21-9 and 21-10).

The sensitivity of test points may be indicated by seen or not seen symbols in the case of single-level tests (Fig. 21-11, *A*) or by several symbols in multiple-level tests (Fig. 21-11, *B*). Examinations that perform full-thresholding can present data in various formats. The absolute threshold values of the points tested may be presented on a grid of the test pattern or may be presented compared with or subtracted from age predicted or estimated normal values (Fig. 21-12). The thresholds may also be displayed in a value table or listing (Fig. 21-13). A hill of vision or "static profile cut" are other graphic modes of display (Fig. 21-14).

A popular mode of display of thresholds is the gray scale printout available on many perimeters

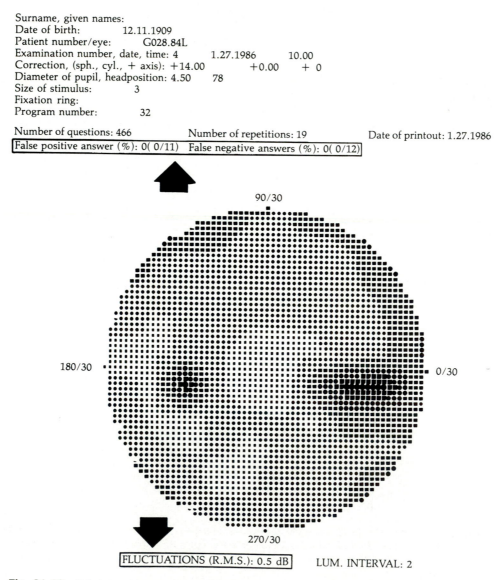

Surname, given names:
Date of birth: 12.11.1909
Patient number/eye: G028.84L
Examination number, date, time: 4   1.27.1986   10.00
Correction, (sph., cyl., + axis): +14.00   +0.00   + 0
Diameter of pupil, headposition: 4.50   78
Size of stimulus: 3
Fixation ring:
Program number: 32

Number of questions: 466   Number of repetitions: 19   Date of printout: 1.27.1986
False positive answer (%): 0(0/11) False negative answers (%): 0(0/12)

90/30

180/30   0/30

270/30

FLUCTUATIONS (R.M.S.): 0.5 dB   LUM. INTERVAL: 2

Fig. 21-10 Reliability factors. This glaucoma patient with a nasal field defect has excellent test reliability with no false answers and an extremely low fluctuation rate *(arrows).*

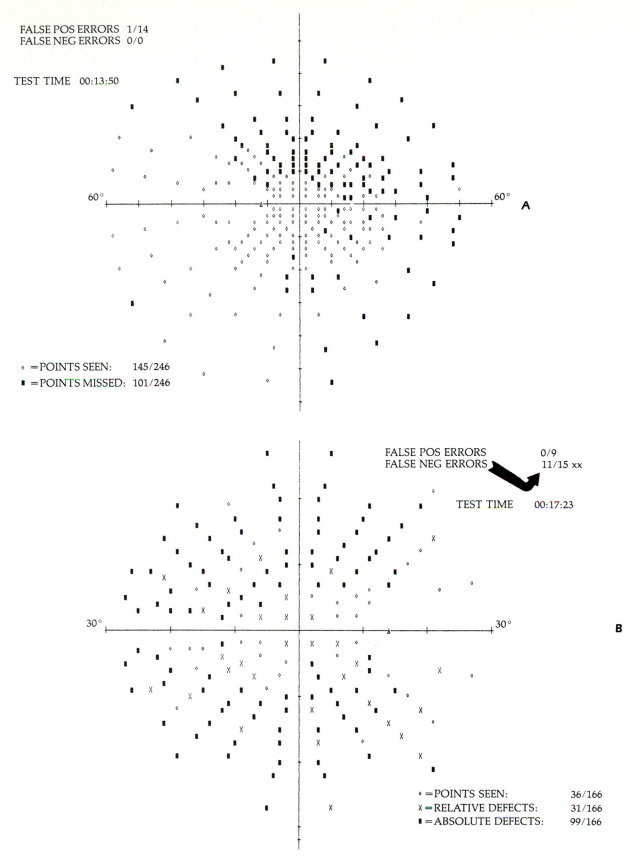

Fig. 21-11   Screening tests. **A,** Single-level test. There is extensive superior field loss in this single level screening test, which does not distinguish relative from absolute scotomas. **B,** Multiple-level test. There is extensive diffuse field loss consisting mostly of absolute scotomas. The extremely high false negative error rate *(arrow)* indicates poor patient reliability.

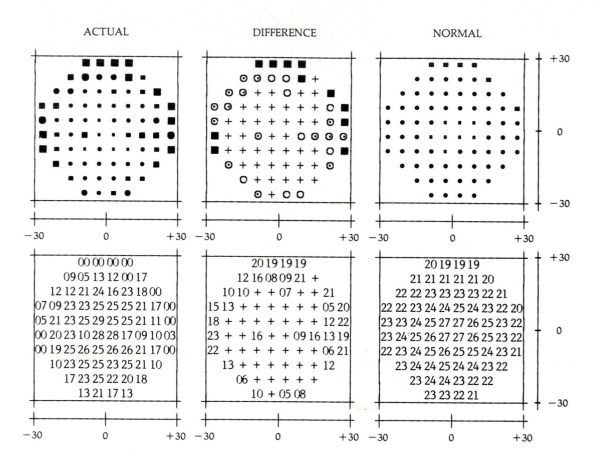

DIFFERENCE TABLE (NORMAL MINUS ACTUAL):

+   DEVIATION < =4 dB
O   DEVIATION 5....9 dB
⊙   DEVIATION 10...19 dB
⊗   DEVIATION > 19 dB
■   ABS. DEFECT   FLUCTUATIONS (R.M.S.): 2.1 dB   LUM. INTERVAL: 2

Fig. 21-12   Normal value comparison. This printout from an Octopus program 32 displays predicted "age-corrected" normal values *(lower right)* for comparison with the patient's actual threshold results *(lower left)*. The difference plot *(lower center)* indicates the depth of the defect compared with the predicted normal at each test position.

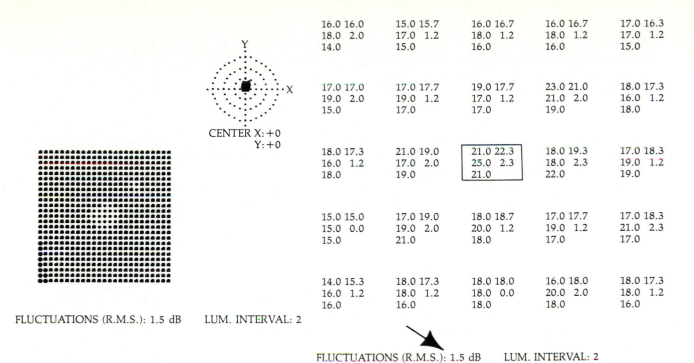

16.0 16.0	15.0 15.7	16.0 16.7	16.0 16.7	17.0 16.3
18.0 2.0	17.0 1.2	18.0 1.2	18.0 1.2	17.0 1.2
14.0	15.0	16.0	16.0	15.0
17.0 17.0	17.0 17.7	19.0 17.7	23.0 21.0	18.0 17.3
19.0 2.0	19.0 1.2	17.0 1.2	21.0 2.0	16.0 1.2
15.0	17.0	17.0	19.0	18.0
18.0 17.3	21.0 19.0	21.0 22.3	18.0 19.3	17.0 18.3
16.0 1.2	17.0 2.0	25.0 2.3	18.0 2.3	19.0 1.2
18.0	19.0	21.0	22.0	19.0
15.0 15.0	17.0 19.0	18.0 18.7	17.0 17.7	17.0 18.3
15.0 0.0	19.0 2.0	20.0 1.2	19.0 1.2	21.0 2.3
15.0	21.0	18.0	17.0	17.0
14.0 15.3	18.0 17.3	18.0 18.0	16.0 18.0	18.0 17.3
16.0 1.2	18.0 1.2	18.0 0.0	20.0 2.0	18.0 1.2
16.0	16.0	18.0	18.0	16.0

CENTER X: +0
Y: +0

FLUCTUATIONS (R.M.S.): 1.5 dB   LUM. INTERVAL: 2

FLUCTUATIONS (R.M.S.): 1.5 dB   LUM. INTERVAL: 2

Fig. 21-13   Value table. This program, Octopus 61, consists of 25 test points that may be placed by perimetrist at any coordinate in field of vision. Plot on left indicates that the test was centered as fixation (X = 0, Y = 0). An interpolated gray scale is also displayed. Value table on right lists threshold sensitivity at each test point. At each point the three leftmost numbers are the results of three separate threshold determinations, and the two rightmost numbers are the mean and fluctuation for these individual values *(box)*. Fluctuation rate is also calculated for entire examination *(arrow)*. This test covers an area of 12 square degrees and has 3 degrees of resolution. It is an excellent test for evaluating central islands, or it can be moved to another point for detailed examination of other areas.

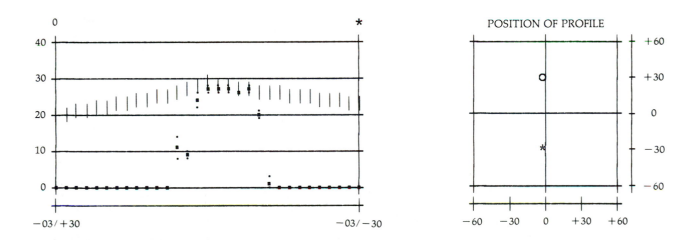

POSITION OF PROFILE

STRATEGY: UP-DOWN (NORMAL)
LENGTH OF PROFILE (DEG)   : 60.0
NUMBER OF TEST LOCATIONS   : 31
RESOLUTION (DEG)   : 02.0
NUMBER OF REPETITIONS   : 02
R.M.S. FLUCTUATION (dB)   : 02.1

· SINGLE DETERMINATION
▪ LOCAL MEAN
| NORMAL

Fig. 21-14   Profile cut. This graphic display is a static profile cut on vertical meridian from 30 degrees above fixation to 30 degrees below fixation as generated by F program on Octopus perimeter. Each point displayed is fully thresholded, and a value table can be printed. Profile displays can also be derived from central field test results on many perimeters, but actual number of test points comprising the profile are therefore limited.

(Fig. 21-15). This printout assigns different density symbols to thresholds within fixed ranges, usually every 5 dB. An absolute scotoma is assigned a totally black symbol with progressively smaller symbols assigned to regions of high sensitivity (Fig. 21-16). This results in a reduction of the data because similar but not equal points are assigned identically. To increase the graphic impact, the computer interpolates sensitivities for the area between the actual test points and displays symbols for these (Fig. 21-17). This can artifactually make steep scotomas, such as the edge of the blind spot, appear more shallow. The gray scale printout is helpful to quickly identify areas of similar sensitivity that appear in an "isopter" pattern (Fig. 21-18). This display is useful for identifying areas of pathology or possible change. It should not be relied on without also evaluating the actual numerical thresholds for making a clinical decision.

EXAMINATION FOR GLAUCOMA

Commonly a full or central screening program is performed as the initial test in the evaluation of glaucoma (Fig. 21-19, *A*). It can be debated as to whether it is necessary to perform an examination of the peripheral field, because the accuracy of testing is less, and it is not common to find an isolated peripheral defect without a central extension.[14,15,17] Nonetheless, it is often helpful to have at least one initial determination, a measurement of the entire visual field. This can provide information on the visual function of patients with severe defects and can confirm the presence of a questionable defect at the edge of a central field examination (Fig. 21-19, *B*).

After an initial screening field that does not threshold the abnormal points, a decision must be made as to what type of follow-up examination should be performed. For patients with an appreciable amount of remaining central field, a central 30-degree thresholding program, such as Octopus 32 or Humphrey 30-2, is typically obtained. This type of examination consists of 76 test points, spaced with 6-degree resolution, offset from the horizontal and vertical meridians by 3 degrees. This strategy, which straddles the horizontal meridian, may better isolate superior and inferior arcuate scotomas than one that tests on axis, such as Octopus 31 or Humphrey 30-1 programs (Fig. 21-20). If additional resolution of the entire central 30 degrees is desired, the latter programs may also be obtained and the results combined for a resultant 4.2 degrees of resolution of field (Fig. 21-21). An alternative to

separate initial screening and thresholding tests is a first examination that may serve both functions, such as a Humphrey screening with "Quantify Defects" (Fig. 21-22, *A*) or an Octopus G1 glaucoma program, which screens peripherally and thresholds centrally (Fig. 21-22, *B*). The latter program may also be repeated on follow-up examinations and the visual field indices (discussed later) compared.

Performing a screening examination as the first test may also serve two additional purposes: (1) It allows a patient unfamiliar with automated perimetry to become accustomed to this type of examination, which may result in more reliable responses on subsequent examinations. It has been well documented that a "learning curve" exists and that some patients will require several testing sessions until consistently reliable results are obtained (Fig. 21-23). (2) It permits the clinician or operator the opportunity to select the most appropriate follow-up thresholding test; for example, a glaucoma patient with a 10-degree or smaller remaining central island would be tested with an Octopus program 61 or 64 or a Humphrey central 10-2 program.

The aforementioned central programs increase the resolution from the 6 degrees obtained in the central 30-degree programs to 3 or 2 degrees, respectively. This has the advantages of providing more information in the patient's remaining field and of reducing patient anxiety by spending more of the testing time on the seeing rather than the nonseeing areas (Fig. 21-24). The increased resolution of the central programs can be helpful even in patients where the field loss may be limited to one quadrant (Fig. 21-25). If the remaining area of visual field is not centered at fixation, programs such as the Octopus 61 or 64 can be shifted off axis (Fig. 21-26). It is often possible to obtain a more meaningful examination by changing from a standard stimulus size to a larger one on a projection perimeter (Fig. 21-27). Finally, it may be possible to custom design a "user defined" program and save it for reuse on an individual patient or for a different patient with similar patterns of field loss. Examples of this are the Custom Test option on the Humphrey or the Sargon programs on the Octopus (Fig. 21-28).

The limiting factor in visual field evaluation is the ability of the patient to perform the appropriate examination reliably and without fatigue. The problem is similar to that described by a wise professor who correctly noted, "The mind can only absorb what the seat can endure!"

Text continued on p. 432.

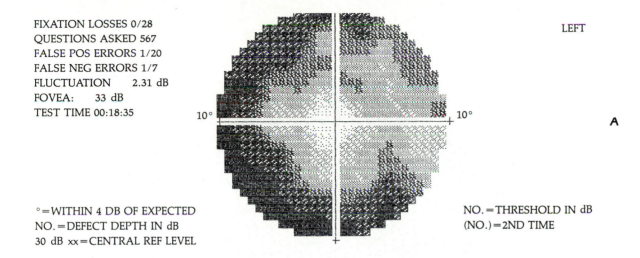

FIXATION LOSSES 0/28
QUESTIONS ASKED 567
FALSE POS ERRORS 1/20
FALSE NEG ERRORS 1/7
FLUCTUATION   2.31 dB
FOVEA: 33 dB
TEST TIME 00:18:35

LEFT

A

° = WITHIN 4 DB OF EXPECTED
NO. = DEFECT DEPTH IN dB
30 dB xx = CENTRAL REF LEVEL

NO. = THRESHOLD IN dB
(NO.) = 2ND TIME

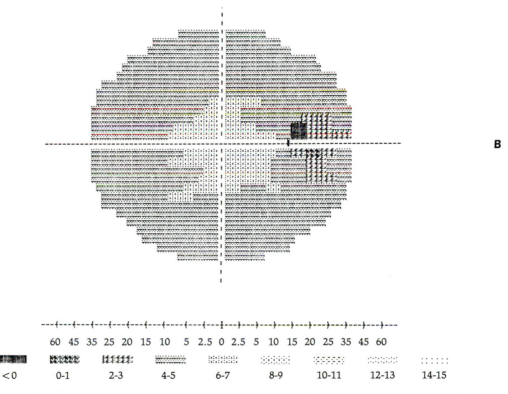

B

| 60 | 45 | 35 | 25 | 20 | 15 | 10 | 5 | 2.5 | 0 | 2.5 | 5 | 10 | 15 | 20 | 25 | 35 | 45 | 60 |

| <0 | 0-1 | 2-3 | 4-5 | 6-7 | 8-9 | 10-11 | 12-13 | 14-15 |

Fig. 21-15   Gray scales. **A,** Central 10 degree test (10-2) on Humphrey perimeter on a patient with a small central island of remaining vision. **B,** Central 30 degree test on Cambridge perimeter on a patient with diffuse depression of sensitivity.

Continued.

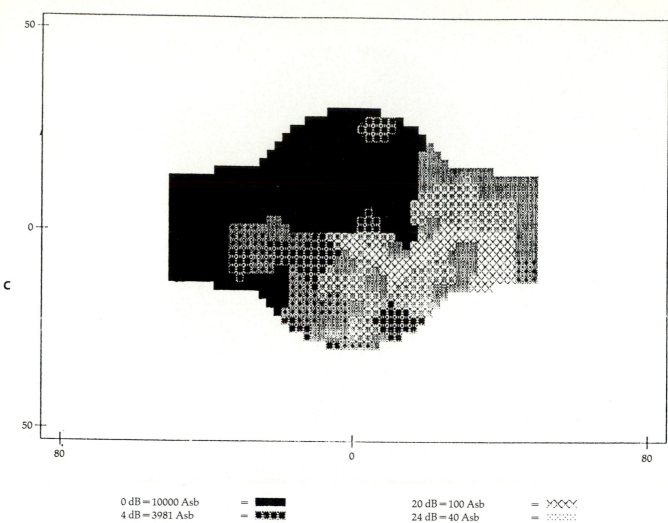

0 dB = 10000 Asb	= ▬▬▬	20 dB = 100 Asb	= ✕✕✕✕
4 dB = 3981 Asb	= ▓▓▓▓	24 dB = 40 Asb	= ⬚⬚⬚⬚
8 dB = 1585 Asb	= ▒▒▒▒	28 dB = 16 Asb	= ⁖⁖⁖⁖
12 dB = 631 Asb	= ▒▒▒▒	32 dB = 6 Asb	= ∴∴∴∴
16 dB = 251 Asb	= ✕✕✕✕	36 dB = 2 Asb	= · · · ·

Fig. 21-15, cont'd **C,** Central test with peripheral extension on Fieldmaster perimeter on patient with severe superior and nasal loss.

Symb.	⁚⁚⁚	⁚⁚⁚	⦙⦙⦙	●●●	▪▪▪	●●●	▪▪▪	✖✖	■
dB	51-36	35-31	30-26	25-21	20-16	15-11	10-6	5-1	0
asb	0,008- 0,25	0,31- 0,8	1- 2,5	3,1- 8	10- 25	31- 80	100- 250	315- 800	1000

A

1 asb = 0,318 cd/m²

SYM.									
ASB	.8 to .1	2.5 to 1	8 to 3.2	25 to 10	79 to 32	251 to 100	794 to 316	2512 to 1000	7943 to 3162	≥ 10000
DB	41 to 50	36 to 40	31 to 35	26 to 30	21 to 25	16 to 20	11 to 15	6 to 10	1 to 5	≤ 0

B

Fig. 21-16 Gray scale symbols. The gray scale symbols from Octopus perimeter, **A,** and Humphrey perimeter, **B,** include equivalent decibel ranges. Apostilb values differ because of the different ratio of stimulus to background illumination in these instruments.

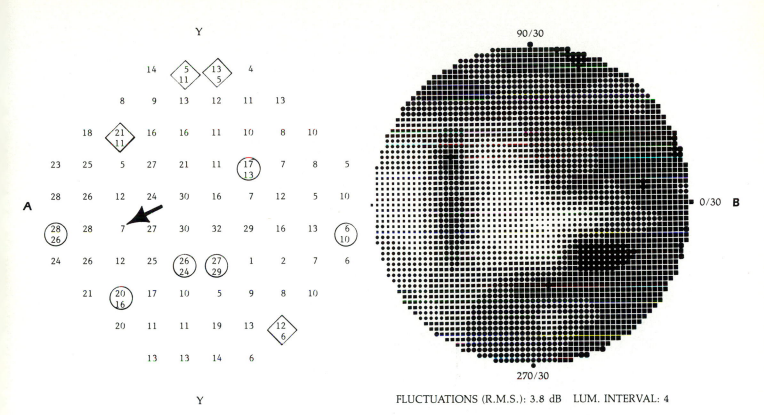

FLUCTUATIONS (R.M.S.): 3.8 dB   LUM. INTERVAL: 4

Fig. 21-17 Interpolated values. Symbols on gray scale, **B,** are interpolated from actual thresholds, **A.** Blind spot *(arrow)* is not an absolute scotoma in this patient, because test point did not correspond with center of blind spot. Dense or absolute scotomas, such as the blind spot, located within relatively strong surrounding areas will appear to have diffuse rather than steep borders on gray scale. Large difference of two threshold values in four of the double thresholded points *(diamonds)* skew the fluctuation rate to a more unreliable level than would be predicted from the more central points *(circles).*

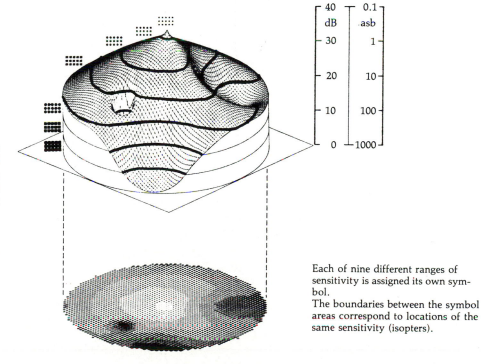

Fig. 21-18 Isopters. Gray scale boundaries between symbol areas correspond to isopters on kinetic perimetry. (Reproduced with permission from Perimeter Digest, Interzeag AG, 1983)

Each of nine different ranges of sensitivity is assigned its own symbol.
The boundaries between the symbol areas correspond to locations of the same sensitivity (isopters).

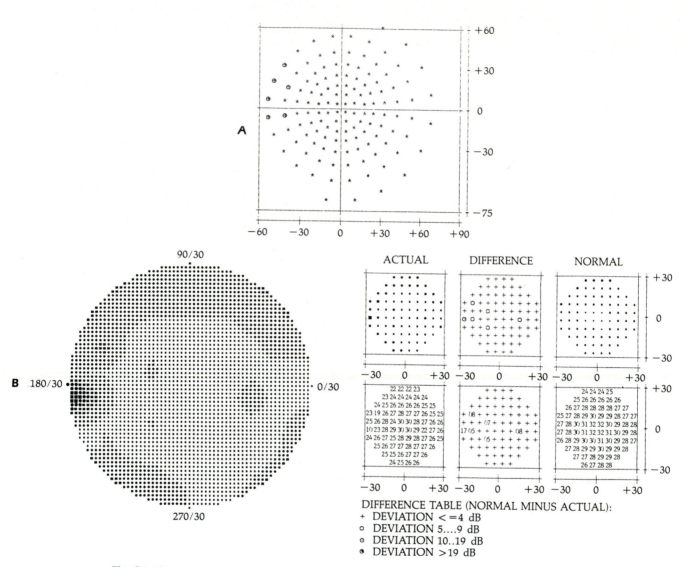

Fig. 21-19 Comparison of full-field with central-only tests. **A,** Octopus program 07, full screening program *(top)* suggests presence of a peripheral nasal step with no evidence of central extension on this test. **B,** Octopus central 30 degree test performed on same patient on same day suggests a peripheral nasal step extending centrally *(bottom)*. Although many or most glaucomatous nerve fiber bungle defects can be detected with the central 30 degree field alone, combined evaluation of peripheral and central fields is often beneficial.

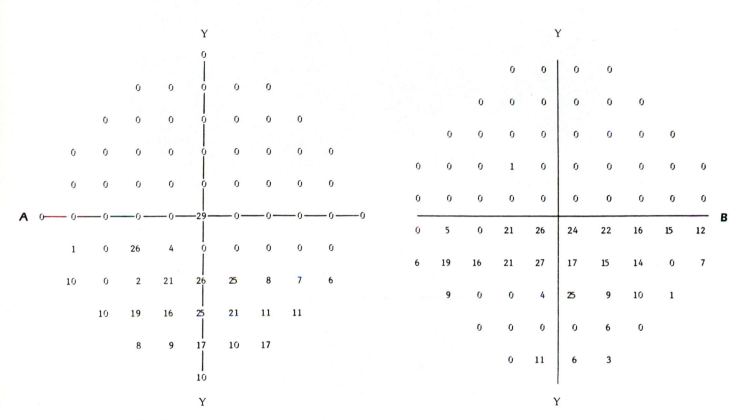

Fig. 21-20 Comparison of central 30 degree programs. Central program, **A,** with points on axis, such as the Humphrey 30-1 or the Octopus 31 and, **B,** with points 3 degress off axis, such as Humphrey 30-2 and Octobus 32.

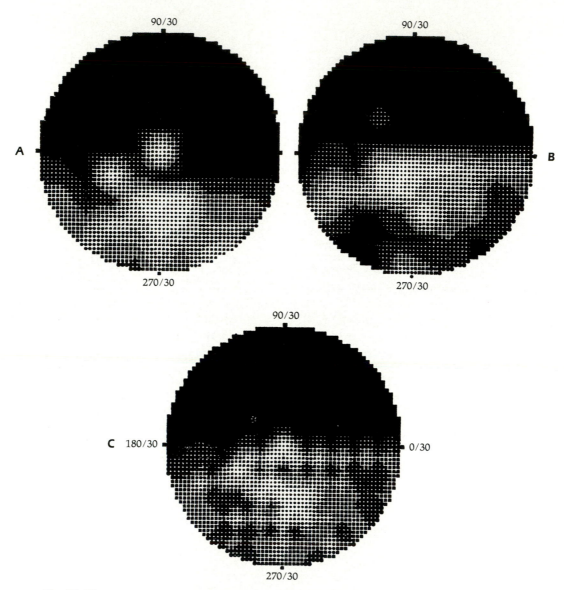

Fig. 21-21 Combined examinations. Gray scale of Octopus program 31, **A,** merged with program 32, **B,** to give combined gray scale printout with greater resolution, **C.**

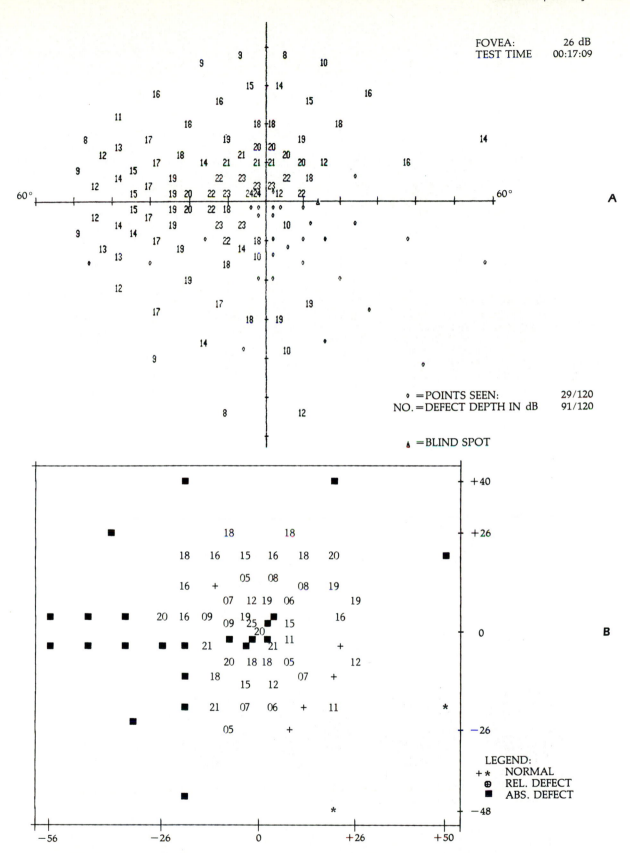

FOVEA: 26 dB
TEST TIME 00:17:09

∘ =POINTS SEEN: 29/120
NO. =DEFECT DEPTH IN dB 91/120

▲ =BLIND SPOT

LEGEND:
+ * NORMAL
⊕ REL. DEFECT
■ ABS. DEFECT

Fig. 21-22 Screening with thresholding. **A,** Humphrey 120 full-field screening program with "Quantify the defects" option to threshold all abnormal points. **B,** Octopus program performs screening of peripheral points and nasal step with three-zone strategy and performs thresholding of central 30 degrees.

	EX1	EX2	EX3	EX4	SUMMARY
DATE OF EXAM: DAY	08.22	03.06	08.08	04.09	
YEAR	1984	1985	1985	1986	
PROGRAM / EXAMINATION	34/02	32/03	32/04	32/05	
TOTAL LOSS (WHOLE FIELD)	1541	1452	1023	899	1228±157
MEAN LOSS (PER TEST LOC)					
WHOLE FIELD	20.8	19.6	13.8	12.1	16.6±2.1
QUADRANT UPPER NASAL	20.5	19.2	13.7	11.7	16.3±2.1
LOWER NASAL	22.0	20.1	14.9	11.2	17.1±2.5
UPPER TEMP.	20.9	20.4	14.2	14.3	17.5±1.9
LOWER TEMP.	19.9	18.8	12.4	11.4	15.6±2.2
ECCENTRICITY 0-10	14.9	13.9	9.5	10.8	12.3±1.3
10-20	21.3	18.5	11.8	10.8	15.6±2.5
20-30	22.3	21.6	15.8	13.0	18.2±2.2
MEAN SENSITIVITY					
WHOLE FIELD (N: 24.1)	*	4.5	10.3	11.9	*±*
QUAD. UPP. NAS. (N: 23.4)	*	4.3	9.7	11.7	*±*
LOW. NAS. (N: 24.4)	*	4.3	9.5	12.9	*±*
UPP. TMP. (N: 23.5)	*	3.1	9.3	9.2	*±*
LOW. TMP. (N: 25.1)	*	6.3	12.6	13.6	*±*
ECC. 0-10 (N: 26.9)	*	13.0	17.4	16.1	*±*
10-20 (N: 24.9)	*	6.4	13.1	14.1	*±*
20-30 (N: 23.0)	*	1.3	7.1	9.8	*±*
NO. OF DISTURBED POINTS	74	74	74	73	74±0
R.M.S. FLUCTUATION	*	1.8	2.7	2.8	2.4
TOTAL FLUCTUATION					4.9

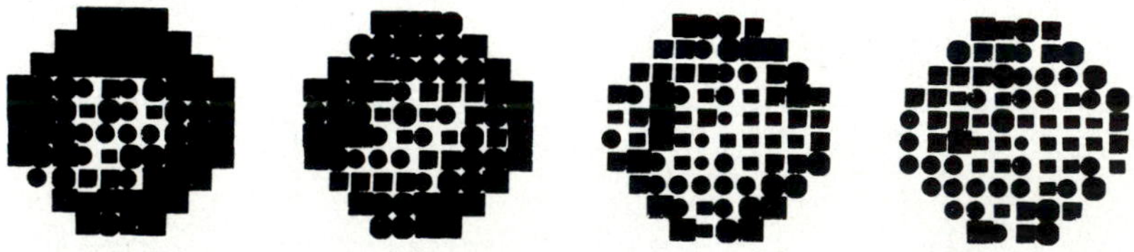

Fig. 21-23 Learning curve. Octopus Delta analysis of serial program 32 illustrating dramatic improvement in performance in patient with stable glaucoma.

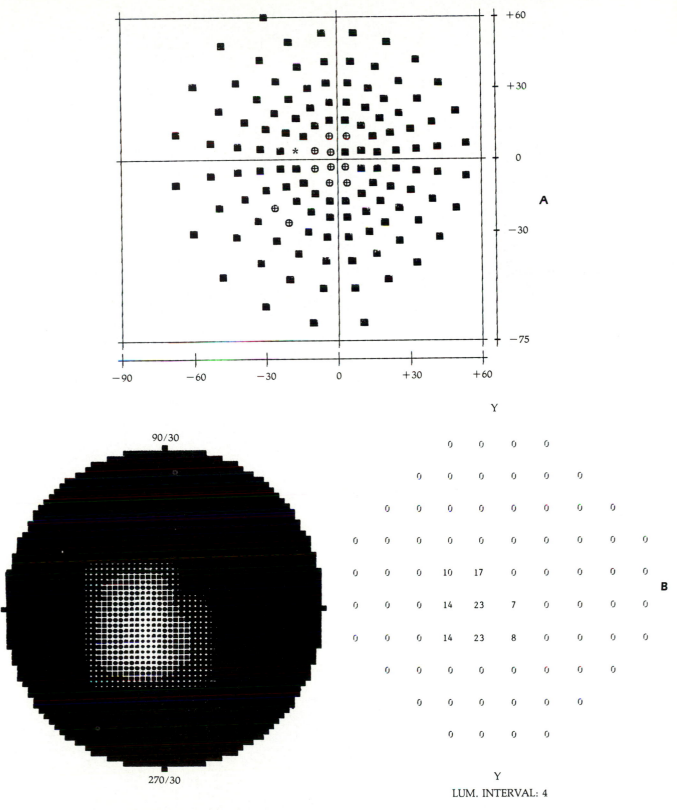

Fig. 21-24 Screening fields in advanced glaucoma. **A,** Screening fields reveals loss to central 10 degrees. **B,** Based on information from the screening test, perimetrist should not have proceeded with central 30 degree field as next examination.

Continued.

CENTER X: −6
Y: −6

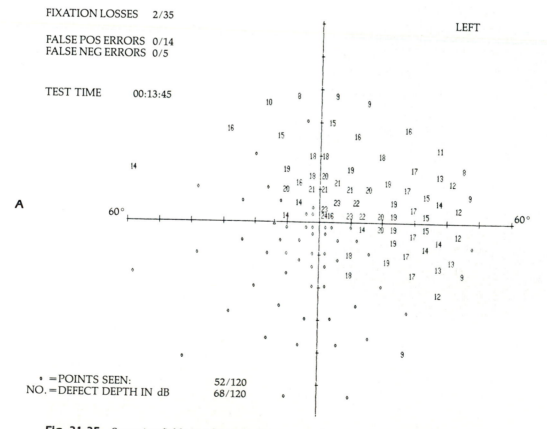

CENTER X: −6
Y: −6

```
11.5  11.2     1.5   7.2      7.5   8.8      4.5   3.2      1.5   1.2
 8.5   2.5    18.5   9.8     13.5   4.2      3.5   1.5      0.5   0.6
13.5           1.5           5.5             1.5            1.5

16.5  18.2    17.5  17.5     18.5  18.8     15.5  15.2      5.5   4.2
18.5   1.5    18.5   1.0     16.5   2.5     16.5   1.5      1.5   2.3
19.5          16.5           21.5           13.5            5.5

16.5  17.8    20.5  18.8     11.5  15.2      1.5  10.5      7.5   4.8
18.5   1.2    20.5   2.9     12.5   5.5     17.5   8.2      3.5   2.3
18.5          15.5           21.5           12.5            3.5

10.5  12.2    19.5  19.5     13.5   9.8     18.5  18.8      1.5   7.5
12.5   1.5    16.5   3.0      4.5   4.7     17.5   1.5     19.5  10.4
13.5          22.5           11.5           20.5            1.5

 2.5   3.5     8.5  11.2      0.5   7.5      0.5   4.5      0.5   0.5
 4.5   1.0    12.5   2.3      7.5   7.0     12.5   6.9      0.5   0.0
 3.5          12.5           14.5            0.5            0.5
```

FLUCTUATIONS (R.M.S.): 4.5 dB   LUM. INTERVAL: 2

FLUCTUATIONS (R.M.S.): 4.5 dB   LUM. INTERVAL: 2

Fig. 21-24, cont'd   C, High-resolution central field testing is the appropriate examination and yields more information with less patient frustration.

FIXATION LOSSES   2/35

FALSE POS ERRORS 0/14
FALSE NEG ERRORS 0/5

TEST TIME   00:13:45

LEFT

A

60°   60°

∘ = POINTS SEEN: 52/120
NO. = DEFECT DEPTH IN dB 68/120

Fig. 21-25 Screening fields in advanced glaucoma. **A,** Screening field illustrating severe superior and nasal field loss.

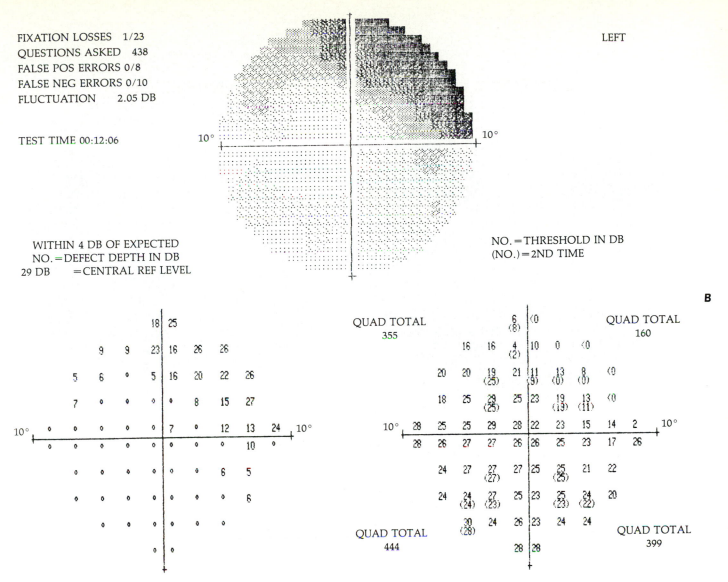

FIXATION LOSSES 1/23
QUESTIONS ASKED   438
FALSE POS ERRORS 0/8
FALSE NEG ERRORS 0/10
FLUCTUATION   2.05 DB

TEST TIME 00:12:06   10°   10°   LEFT

WITHIN 4 DB OF EXPECTED
NO.=DEFECT DEPTH IN DB   NO.=THRESHOLD IN DB
29 DB   =CENTRAL REF LEVEL   (NO.)=2ND TIME

B

```
            18│25                    QUAD TOTAL          6      ⟨0        QUAD TOTAL
                                        355             (8)                  160
       9   9  23│16  26  26                    16   16   4  │10   0   ⟨0
                                                          (2)
     5   6   0   5│16  20  22  26         20   20   19  21│11  13   8    ⟨0
                                                        (25)  (9) (0)  (0)
       7   0   0   0│0   8  15  27              18   25   28  25│23  19  13   ⟨0
                                                        (25)      (19)(11)
10°  0   0   0   0   0│7   0  12  13  24  10°  10° 28  25  25  29  28│22  23  15  14   2  10°
     0   0   0   0   0│0   0   0  10   0       28   26   27  27│26  26  25  23  17  26
       0   0   0   0   0│0   0   6   5              24   27   27  27│25  25  21  22
                                                        (27)      (25)
       0   0   0   0   0│0   0   6              24   24   27  25│23  25  24  20
                                                    (24)(23)      (23)(22)
         0   0   0│0   0   0   0    QUAD TOTAL          30  24  26│23  24  24  QUAD TOTAL
                                      444             (28)                       399
            0│0                                      28│28
```

Fig. 21-25, cont'd   B, Central 10 degree field provides more information in area above fixation than screening field or central 30 test.

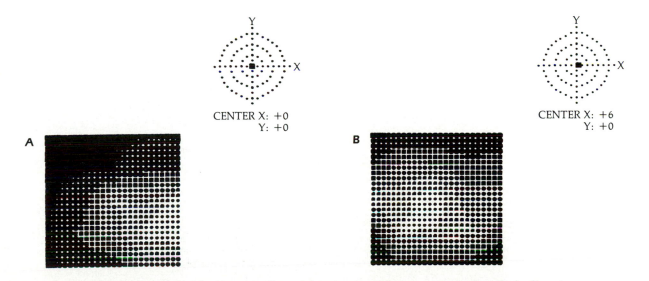

CENTER X: +0   CENTER X: +6
       Y: +0   Y: +0

A   B

Fig. 21-26 Movable programs. Gray scale printout of Octopus program 61 shifted off center, x = +6 y = +0, B, illustrates better positioning of test than one centered at fixation, x = +0 y = +0, A.

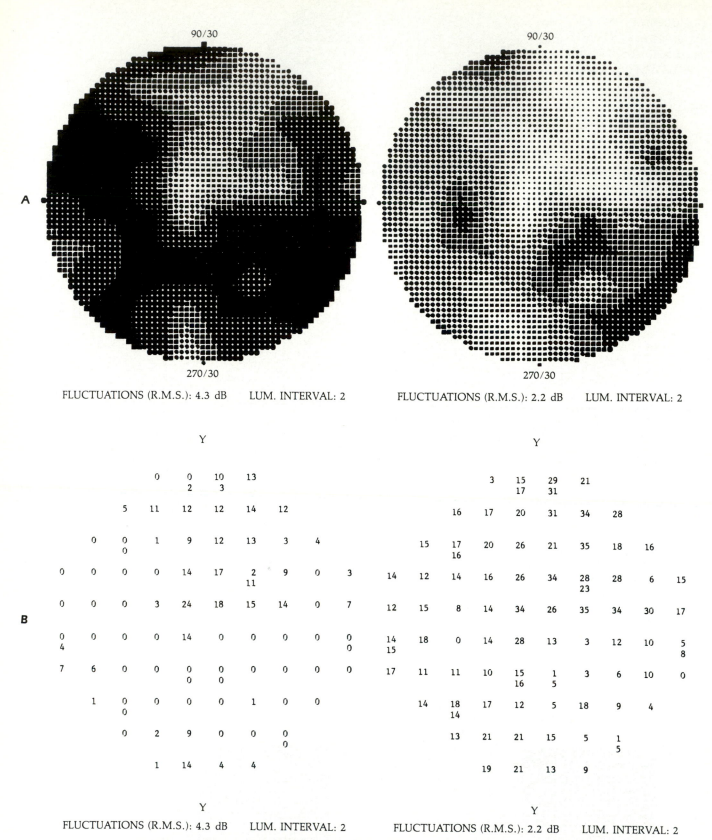

90/30

270/30

FLUCTUATIONS (R.M.S.): 4.3 dB   LUM. INTERVAL: 2

90/30

270/30

FLUCTUATIONS (R.M.S.): 2.2 dB   LUM. INTERVAL: 2

A

B

Y

Left printout (A):

			0	0	10	13			
				2	3				
		5	11	12	12	14	12		
	0	0	1	9	12	13	3	4	
		0							
0	0	0	0	14	17	2 / 11	9	0	3
0	0	0	3	24	18	15	14	0	7
0 / 4	0	0	0	14	0	0	0	0	0 / 0
7	6	0	0	0 / 0	0 / 0	0	0	0	0
	1	0 / 0	0	0	0	1	0	0	
		0	2	9	0	0	0 / 0		
		1	14	4	4				

Y

FLUCTUATIONS (R.M.S.): 4.3 dB   LUM. INTERVAL: 2

Y

Right printout (B):

			3	15	29	21			
				17	31				
		16	17	20	31	34	28		
	15	17 / 16	20	26	21	35	18	16	
14	12	14	16	26	34	28 / 23	28	6	15
12	15	8	14	34	26	35	34	30	17
14 / 15	18	0	14	28	13	3	12	10	5 / 8
17	11	11	10	15 / 16	1 / 5	3	6	10	0
	14	18 / 14	17	12	5	18	9	4	
		13	21	21	15	5	1 / 5		
		19	21	13	9				

Y

FLUCTUATIONS (R.M.S.): 2.2 dB   LUM. INTERVAL: 2

Fig. 21-27 Effect of stimulus size. **A,** A larger number of test points may be evaluated with a greater ability to detect future progression when stimulus size is increased from size 3 (*left*) to size 5 (*right*) on Octopus program 32. **B,** Threshold values for above gray scale printouts.

USER-DEFINED PROGRAM

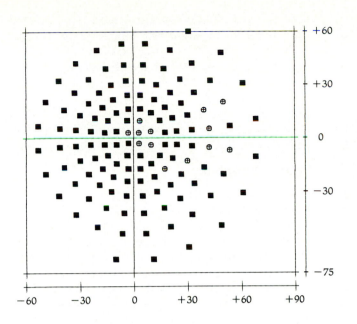

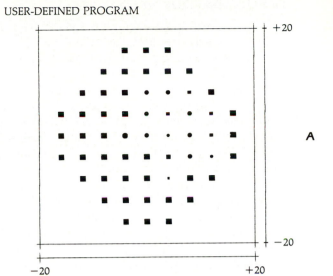

A

USER-DEFINED PROGRAM. LABEL: C16   (DATE OF PROGRAM: 05 10 1983)

	X /	Y	V	NORM	MEAN + − S.D.
0	− 4.0/	16.0	0	28	
1	0.0/	16.0	0	28	
2	4.0/	16.0	0	27	
3	− 8.0/	12.0	0	29	
4	− 4.0/	12.0	0	29	
5	0.0/	12.0	0	29	
6	4.0/	12.0	0	28	
7	8.0/	12.0	0	28	
8	−12.0/	8.0	0	29	
9	− 8.0/	8.0	0	30	
10	− 4.0/	8.0	0	30	
11	0.0/	8.0	13	30	
12	4.0/	8.0	14	29	
13	8.0/	8.0	18	29	
14	12.0/	8.0	0	29	
15	−16.0/	4.0	0	29	
16	−12.0/	4.0	0	30	
17	− 8.0/	4.0	0	31	
18	− 4.0/	4.0	0	31	0.0 + − *
			0		
19	0.0/	4.0	13	32	13.5 + − 0.7
			14		
20	4.0/	4.0	14	31	15.5 + − 2.1
			17		
21	8.0/	4.0	15	30	
22	12.0/	4.0	18	29	
23	16.0/	4.0	0	28	
24	−16.0/	0.0	0	30	
25	−12.0/	0.0	0	31	
26	− 8.0/	0.0	0	32	
27	− 4.0/	0.0	6	33	3.5 + − 3.5
			1		
28	0.0/	0.0	8	35	15.0 + − 9.9

	X /	Y	V	NORM	MEAN + − S.D.
			22		
29	4.0/	0.0	21	32	20.5 + − 0.7
			20		
30	8.0/	0.0	13	31	
31	12.0/	0.0	16	30	
32	16.0/	0.0	0	29	
33	−16.0/ −	4.0	0	29	
34	−12.0/ −	4.0	0	30	
35	− 8.0/ −	4.0	0	31	
36	− 4.0/ −	4.0	0	32	0.0 + − *
			0		
37	0.0/ −	4.0	0	32	0.0 + − *
			0		
38	4.0/ −	4.0	12	31	6.0 + − *
			0		
39	8.0/ −	4.0	12	31	
40	12.0/ −	4.0	21	30	
41	16.0/ −	4.0	0	29	
42	−12.0/ −	8.0	0	30	
43	− 8.0/ −	8.0	0	30	
44	− 4.0/ −	8.0	0	30	
45	0.0/ −	8.0	0	31	
46	4.0/ −	8.0	26	31	
47	8.0/ −	8.0	0	31	
48	12.0/ −	8.0	0	30	
49	− 8.0/ −12.0		0	29	
50	− 4.0/ −12.0		0	29	
51	0.0/ −12.0		0	30	
52	4.0/ −12.0		0	30	
53	8.0/ −12.0		0	30	
54	− 4.0/ −16.0		0	29	
55	0.0/ −16.0		0	29	
56	4.0/ −16.0		0	29	

B

Fig. 21-28 User-defined (custom) programs for advanced field loss. **A,** User-defined test of central 16 degrees (Octopus Sargon program C16 by William Whalen, MD) symbol plot performed after screening field 07 *(right)*. **B,** Number table of thresholds for above test points. A printout with numbers rather than symbols on above plot can also be obtained.

GLAUCOMATOUS FIELD DEFECTS

The nature of glaucomatous field defects and their characteristic patterns as established by manual kinetic and static perimetry are discussed in Chapter 20. As a general rule, the typical glaucomatous findings with automated perimetry parallel the diffuse depressions and localized nerve fiber layer defects[5] detected by previous methods. Specifically, they consist of focal or diffuse depression (Fig. 21-29, *A*), focal paracentral scotomas (Fig. 21-29, *B*), nasal steps (Figs. 21-29, *C* and *D*), Seidel scotomas (Fig. 21-29, *E*), arcuate or Bjerrum scotomas (Figs. 21-29, *F* and *G*), or combinations of these (Figs. 21-29, *H* to *K*). Advanced glaucomatous findings consist of central and temporal islands (Figs. 21-29, *L* and *M*).

Visual field abnormalities in patients with low-tension glaucoma have been found by some investigators to be steeper with focal paracentral scotomas located closer to fixation (Fig. 21-30), when compared with patients with high-tension glaucoma.[1,6] This has not been found in other studies[11,13] and may be explained by differences in selection criteria, method of testing, or method of analysis.

As we gain more experience with automated perimetry, new and better methods of testing and interpretation will continue to evolve.

INTERPRETATION OF AUTOMATED PERIMETRY

The proper interpretation of automated fields includes a determination of the validity of the data based on test conditions, the elimination of artifact, assessment of patient reliability, and consideration of pitfalls in evaluation physiologic or other pathologic conditions. Interpretation of a reliable field includes a determination of the existence of a glaucomatous defect and an evaluation of the probability of progression in the visual field over time.

Test Conditions

For the results of automated perimetry to be meaningful and reproducible, the examination must be carried out in a standardized manner each time. Variability may be introduced into the examination by failure of the perimetrist to calibrate the instrument at the beginning of the testing session. Some perimeters have an automatic prompt message regarding calibration. Calibration errors are more likely to arise secondary to variation in the lighting in the examination area. It is essential that room illumination not change once calibration is performed.

The perimetrist must provide the patient with a current refractive correction and near add each time the examination is performed. Uncorrected refractive errors may affect the results of the examination.[3,10] The correcting lens may be a potential source of test artifact by obstructing the patient's vision at the edge of the lens (Fig. 21-31). This "lens rim artifact" is characterized by its location in the outer row of the central 30-degree field or in this area in the full screening field. Typically it is dense and does not extend to contiguous areas.

Patient Reliability

Patient reliability is an important factor to consider in avoiding erroneous interpretation of test results. The operator should note the patient's mental status and level of comfort and cooperation during the examination.

Evaluation of the false positive (FP) and false negative (FN) responses, the root mean square (RMS) or short-term fluctuation (SF), and the number of repetitions can help detect those examinations that are of limited or no diagnostic value. An artifactual "normal" visual field may be detected in a patient with a high FP score or high RMS (Fig. 21-32).

Another factor to be considered is the patient's prior experience with visual field testing. The initial test on an automated perimeter, even for the patient previously tested by manual perimetry, may be difficult or stressful for the patient. This can produce a first examination that is less reliable or exhibits greater defects than are actually present (Fig. 21-33). This "learning curve" effect may be reduced by running a screening program before testing with the thresholding examination.

Physiologic Conditions

Ptosis or marked dermatochalasis can cause artifactual loss of the superior field that must be distinguished from lens rim artifact or true glaucomatous loss (Fig. 21-34).

Cataract, other media opacities, and miotic pupils are the primary physiologic conditions that can result in an artifactual decrease in the threshold sensitivity. Lens opacities typically result in a diffuse loss of sensitivity, which is found to improve following cataract extraction (Fig. 21-35). Even in the absence of severe lens opacities the miotic pupil can cause a significant diminution of sensitivity (Fig. 21-36).

Whenever possible, it is desirable for the pupils to be at least 2.5 to 3.0 mm before testing the visual field in order to obtain the most accurate results. It is also helpful to allow the patient to adapt to the illumination of the perimeter before beginning the examination. *Text continued on p. 448.*

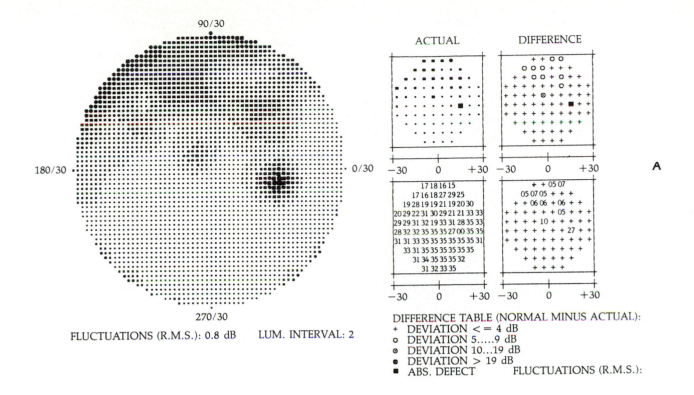

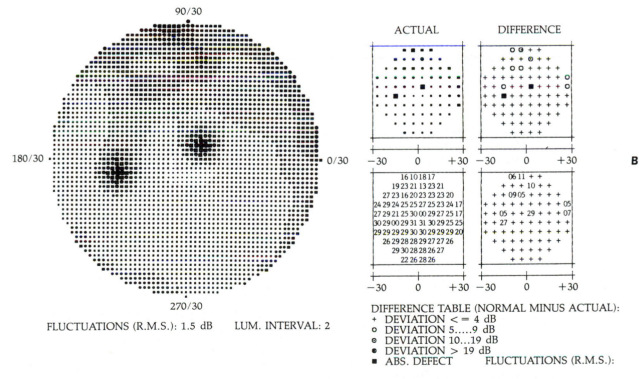

Fig. 21-29 Glaucomatous visual field defects. **A,** Early superior arcuate and focal paracentral depression of threshold sensitivity. **B,** Dense paracentral scotoma with superior arcuate loss of sensitivity.

Continued.

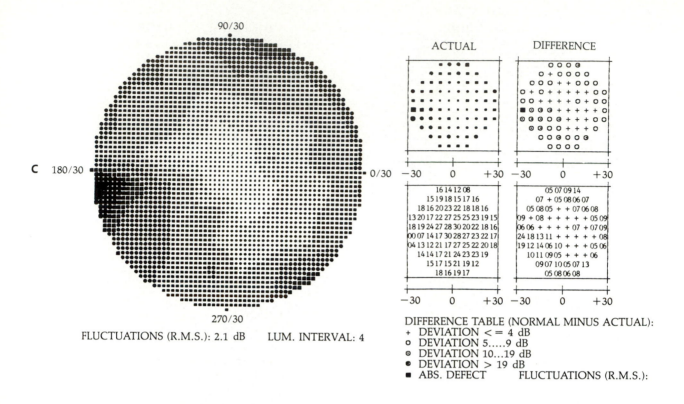

FLUCTUATIONS (R.M.S.): 2.1 dB   LUM. INTERVAL: 4

DIFFERENCE TABLE (NORMAL MINUS ACTUAL):
+ DEVIATION < = 4 dB
o DEVIATION 5.....9 dB
⊙ DEVIATION 10...19 dB
● DEVIATION > 19 dB
■ ABS. DEFECT   FLUCTUATIONS (R.M.S.):

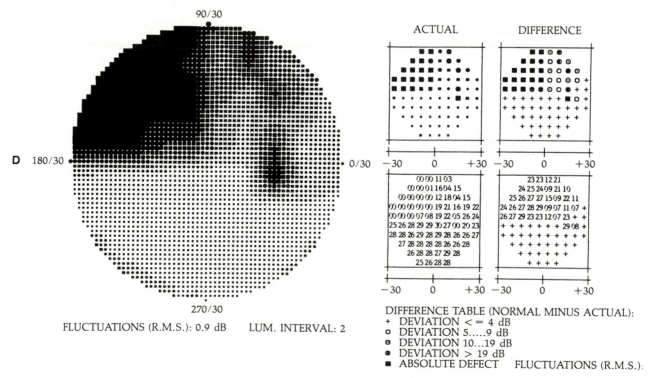

FLUCTUATIONS (R.M.S.): 0.9 dB   LUM. INTERVAL: 2

DIFFERENCE TABLE (NORMAL MINUS ACTUAL):
+ DEVIATION < = 4 dB
o DEVIATION 5.....9 dB
⊙ DEVIATION 10...19 dB
● DEVIATION > 19 dB
■ ABSOLUTE DEFECT   FLUCTUATIONS (R.M.S.):

Fig. 21-29, cont'd **C,** Small nasal step with diffuse central loss of sensitivity. **D,** Large, dense superior nasal step with superotemporal loss of sensitivity.

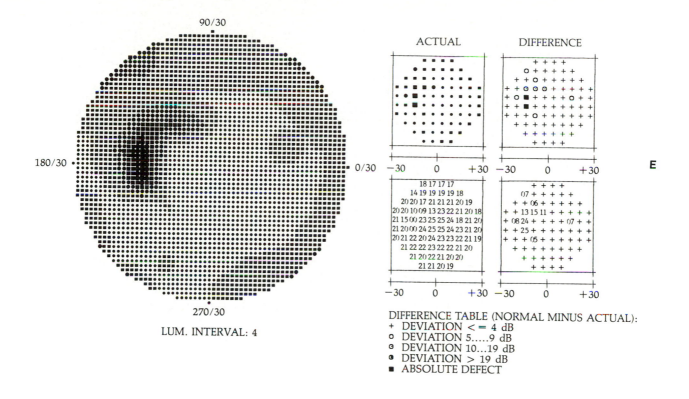

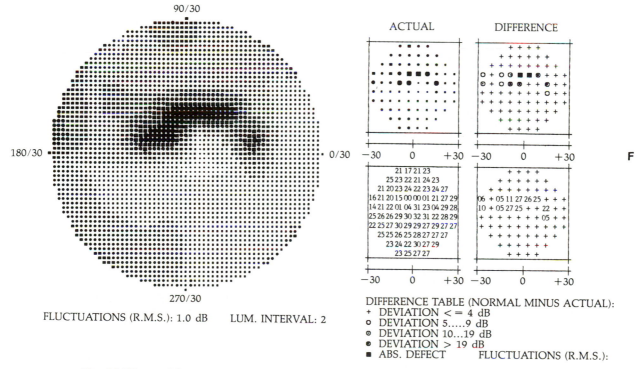

Fig. 21-29, cont'd **E,** Seidel scotoma extends from blind spot into superior arcuate region. **F,** Dense superior Bjerrum scotoma with nasal step.

Continued.

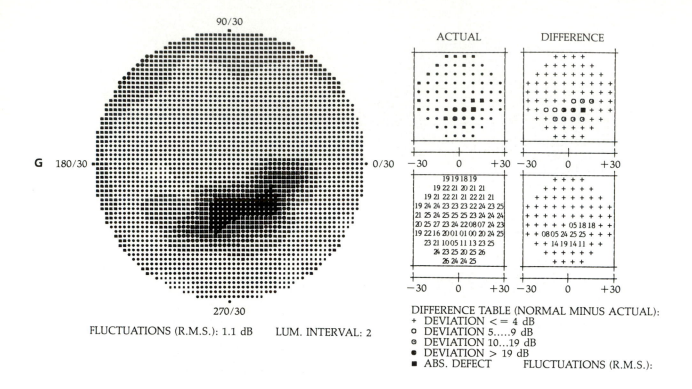

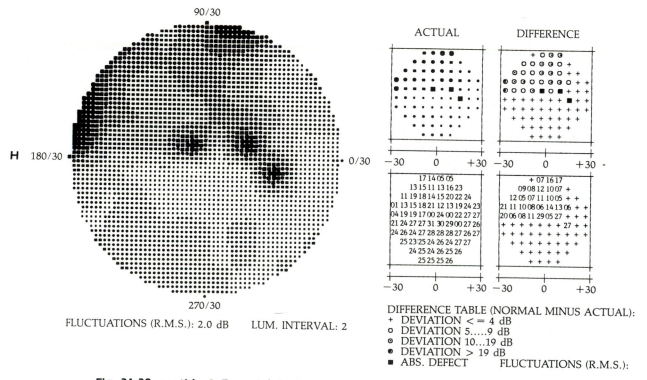

Fig. 21-29, cont'd **G,** Dense inferior Bjerrum scotoma. **H,** Nasal step, dense paracentral and arcuate scotomas.

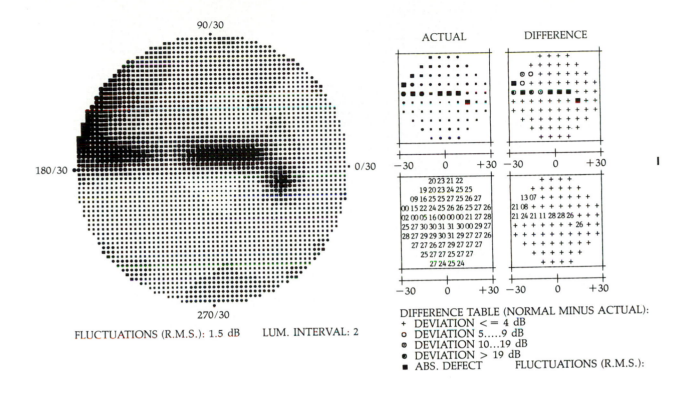

FLUCTUATIONS (R.M.S.): 1.5 dB   LUM. INTERVAL: 2

ACTUAL   DIFFERENCE

                                          I

```
      20 23 21 22                       + + + +
   19 20 23 24 25 25                  + + + + + +
   09 16 25 25 27 25 26 27          13 07 + + + + +
00 15 22 24 25 26 26 25 27 26      21 08 + + + + + +
02 00 05 16 00 00 00 21 27 28      21 24 21 11 28 28 26 + + +
25 27 30 30 31 31 30 00 29 27      + + + + + + + 26 + +
28 27 29 29 30 31 29 27 27 26      + + + + + + + + +
   27 27 26 27 29 27 27 27           + + + + + + + +
   25 27 27 25 27 27                  + + + + + + +
      27 24 25 24                       + + + +
```

DIFFERENCE TABLE (NORMAL MINUS ACTUAL):
+   DEVIATION < = 4 dB
o   DEVIATION 5.....9 dB
⊙   DEVIATION 10...19 dB
●   DEVIATION > 19 dB
■   ABS. DEFECT   FLUCTUATIONS (R.M.S.):

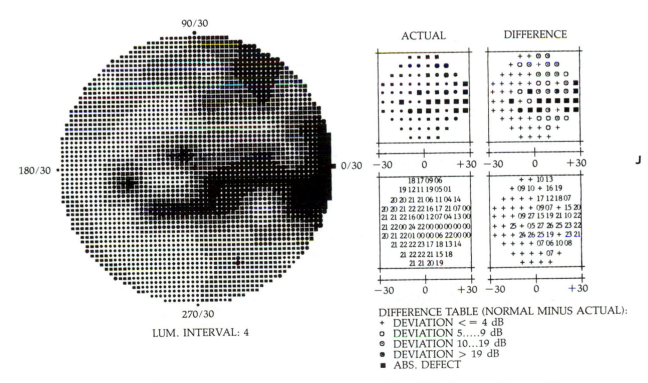

LUM. INTERVAL: 4

ACTUAL   DIFFERENCE

                                          J

```
      18 17 09 06                       + + 10 13
   19 12 11 19 05 01                  + 09 10 + 16 19
   20 20 21 21 06 11 04 14          + + + + 17 12 18 07
20 20 21 22 22 16 17 21 07 00      + + + + + 09 07 + 15 20
21 21 22 16 00 12 07 04 13 00      + + + 09 27 15 19 21 10 22
21 22 00 24 22 00 00 00 00 00      + + + 25 + 05 27 26 25 23 22
20 21 22 01 00 00 06 22 00 00      + + + 24 26 25 19 + 23 21
   21 22 22 23 17 18 13 14           + + + + 07 06 10 08
   21 22 22 21 15 18                  + + + + + 07 +
      21 21 20 19                       + + + +
```

DIFFERENCE TABLE (NORMAL MINUS ACTUAL):
+   DEVIATION < = 4 dB
o   DEVIATION 5.....9 dB
⊙   DEVIATION 10...19 dB
●   DEVIATION > 19 dB
■   ABS. DEFECT

Fig. 21-29, cont'd   I, Nasal step contiguous with arcuate defect. **J,** Nasal step contiguous with inferior arcuate defect with associated superior loss of sensitivity.

Continued.

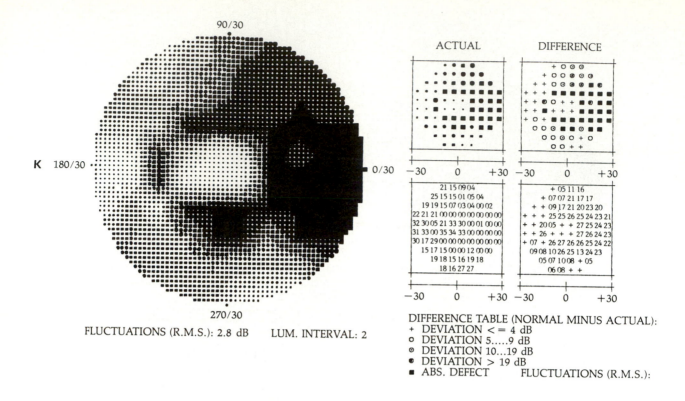

90/30

K 180/30 · · · · · 0/30

270/30

FLUCTUATIONS (R.M.S.): 2.8 dB   LUM. INTERVAL: 2

ACTUAL   DIFFERENCE

−30   0   +30   −30   0   +30

```
 21 15 09 04               + 05 11 16
25 15 15 01 05 04        + 07 07 21 17 17
19 19 15 07 03 04 00 02     + + 09 17 21 20 23 20
22 21 21 00 00 00 00 00 00 00   + + + 25 25 26 25 24 23 21
32 30 05 21 33 30 00 01 00 00   + + 20 05 + + 27 25 24 23
31 33 00 35 34 33 00 00 00 00   + + 26 + + + 27 26 24 23
30 17 29 00 00 00 00 00 00 00   + 07  + 26 27 26 26 25 24 22
15 17 15 00 00 12 00 00          09 08 10 26 25 13 24 23
19 18 15 16 19 18                05 07 10 08 + 05
18 16 27 27                       06 08 + +
```

−30   0   +30   −30   0   +30

DIFFERENCE TABLE (NORMAL MINUS ACTUAL):
+ DEVIATION < = 4 dB
o DEVIATION 5.....9 dB
⊙ DEVIATION 10...19 dB
◉ DEVIATION > 19 dB
■ ABS. DEFECT   FLUCTUATIONS (R.M.S.):

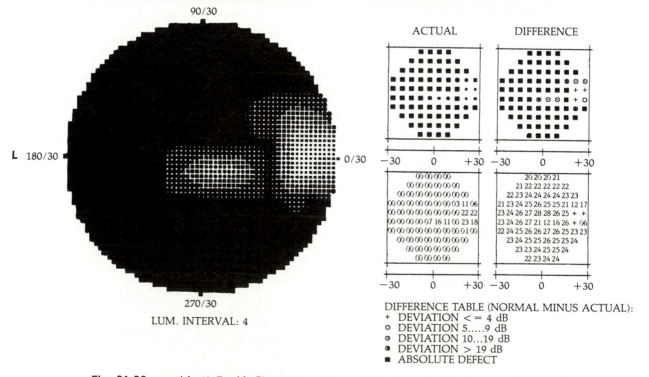

90/30

L 180/30 · · · · · 0/30

270/30

LUM. INTERVAL: 4

ACTUAL   DIFFERENCE

−30   0   +30   −30   0   +30

```
 00 00 00 00               20 20 20 21
00 00 00 00 00 00         21 22 22 22 22 22
00 00 00 00 00 00 00 00     22 23 24 24 24 24 23 23
00 00 00 00 00 00 00 00 03 11 06   21 23 24 25 26 25 25 21 12 17
00 00 00 00 00 00 00 22 22   23 24 26 27 28 28 26 25 + +
00 00 00 00 00 07 16 11 00 23 18   23 24 26 27 21 12 16 26 + 06
00 00 00 00 00 00 00 00 01 00   22 24 25 26 26 27 26 25 23 23
00 00 00 00 00 00 00          23 24 25 25 26 25 25 24
00 00 00 00 00 00             23 23 24 25 25 24
00 00 00 00                   22 23 24 24
```

−30   0   +30   −30   0   +30

DIFFERENCE TABLE (NORMAL MINUS ACTUAL):
+ DEVIATION < = 4 dB
o DEVIATION 5.....9 dB
⊙ DEVIATION 10...19 dB
◉ DEVIATION > 19 dB
■ ABSOLUTE DEFECT

Fig. 21-29, cont'd   K, Double Bjerrum (superior and inferior arcuate) scotoma. **L,** Central and temporal islands of vision in end stage glaucoma (right eye).

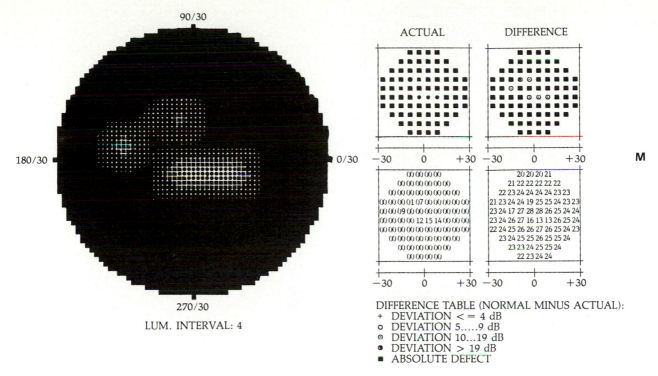

Fig. 21-29, cont'd **M,** Central and temporal islands of vision in end stage glaucoma (left eye).

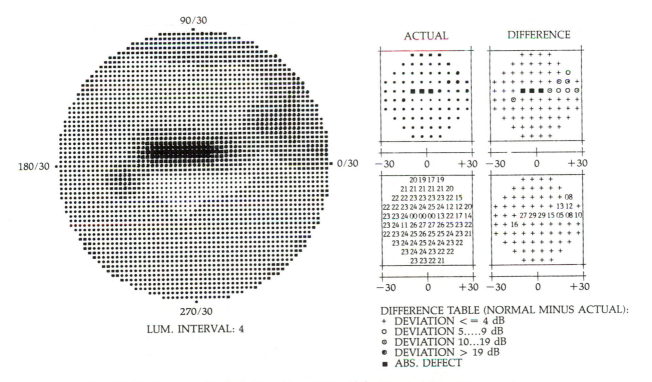

Fig. 21-30 Dense paracentral scotoma in patient with low-tension glaucoma.

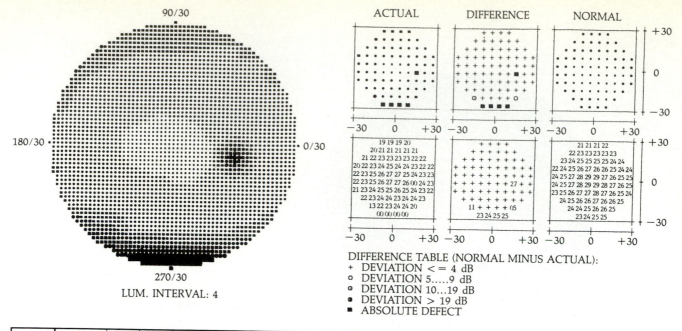

ACTUAL DIFFERENCE NORMAL

DIFFERENCE TABLE (NORMAL MINUS ACTUAL):
+ DEVIATION < = 4 dB
o DEVIATION 5.....9 dB
⊙ DEVIATION 10...19 dB
● DEVIATION > 19 dB
■ ABSOLUTE DEFECT

90/30

180/30 · · · · · · 0/30

270/30

LUM. INTERVAL: 4

Symb.	⠿	⠿	⠿	⠿	⠿	⠿	⠿	⠿	■
dB	51-36	35-31	30-26	25-21	20-16	15-11	10-6	5-1	0
asb	0,008-0,25	0,31-0,8	1-2,5	3,1-8	10-25	31-80	100-250	315-800	1000

1 asb = 0,318 cd/m²

Fig. 21-31 "Lens rim artifact" caused by positioning of correcting for central 30 degree field.

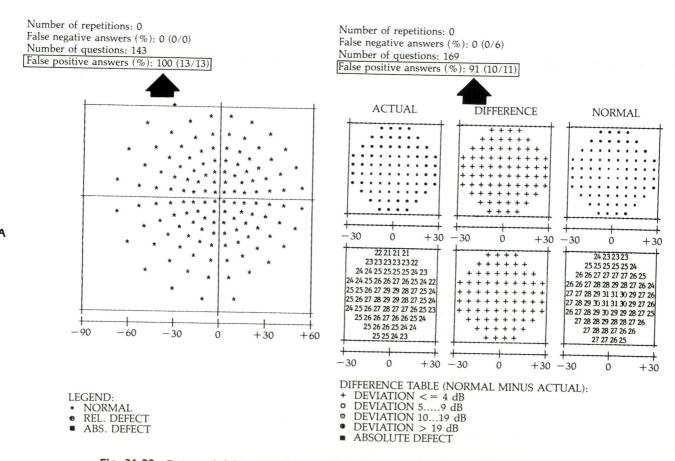

Number of repetitions: 0
False negative answers (%): 0 (0/0)
Number of questions: 143
False positive answers (%): 100 (13/13)

Number of repetitions: 0
False negative answers (%): 0 (0/6)
Number of questions: 169
False positive answers (%): 91 (10/11)

ACTUAL DIFFERENCE NORMAL

A

LEGEND:
★ NORMAL
● REL. DEFECT
■ ABS. DEFECT

DIFFERENCE TABLE (NORMAL MINUS ACTUAL):
+ DEVIATION < = 4 dB
o DEVIATION 5.....9 dB
⊙ DEVIATION 10...19 dB
● DEVIATION > 19 dB
■ ABSOLUTE DEFECT

Fig. 21-32 Patient reliability. **A,** Both screening field *(left)* and central field *(right)* show no loss of sensitivity. These are not normal examinations, as evidenced by the high false positive rates *(arrows)*, and should be considered totally unreliable.

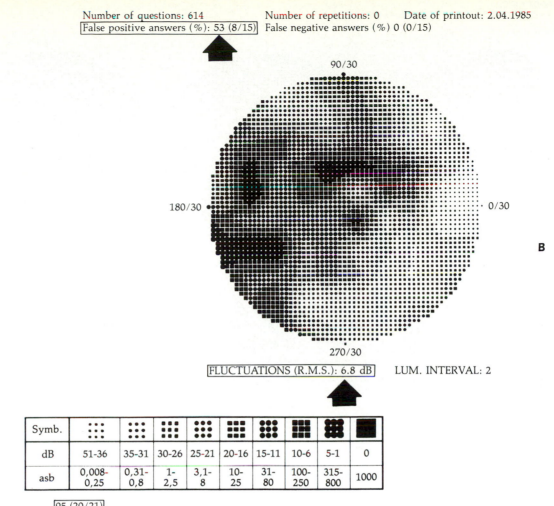

90/30

180/30 •   • 0/30

B

270/30

FLUCTUATIONS (R.M.S.): 6.8 dB   LUM. INTERVAL: 2

Symb.	⠿	⠿	▦	▦	▦	▦	▦	▦	■
dB	51-36	35-31	30-26	25-21	20-16	15-11	10-6	5-1	0
asb	0,008-0,25	0,31-0,8	1-2,5	3,1-8	10-25	31-80	100-250	315-800	1000

95 (20/21)
False positive answers (%):

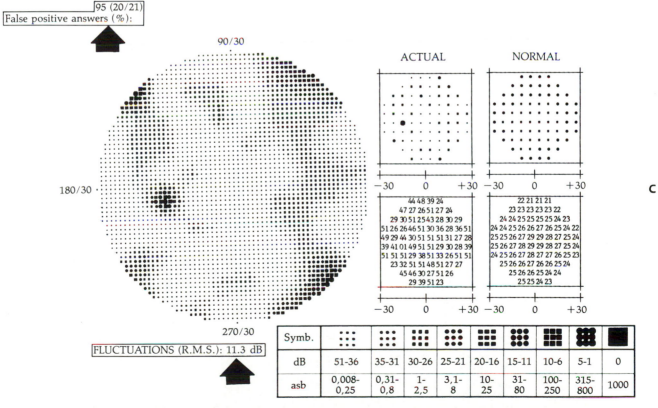

90/30

ACTUAL   NORMAL

180/30 •

C

44 48 39 24   22 21 21 21
47 27 26 51 27 24   23 23 23 23 23 22
29 30 51 25 43 28 30 29   24 24 25 25 25 25 24 23
51 26 26 46 51 30 36 28 36 51   24 24 25 26 26 27 26 25 24 22
49 29 44 30 51 51 51 31 27 28   25 25 26 27 29 29 28 27 25 24
39 41 01 49 51 51 29 30 28 39   25 26 27 28 29 29 28 27 25 24
51 51 51 29 38 51 33 26 51 51   24 25 26 27 28 27 27 26 25 23
23 32 51 51 48 51 27 27   25 26 26 27 26 26 25 24
45 46 30 27 51 26   25 26 26 25 24 24
29 39 51 23   25 25 24 23

270/30

FLUCTUATIONS (R.M.S.): 11.3 dB

Symb.	⠿	⠿	▦	▦	▦	▦	▦	▦	■
dB	51-36	35-31	30-26	25-21	20-16	15-11	10-6	5-1	0
asb	0,008-0,25	0,31-0,8	1-2,5	3,1-8	10-25	31-80	100-250	315-800	1000

Fig. 21-32, cont'd **B,** Results of this examination are of little value because of high false positive and fluctuation rates. **C,** This usually reliable patient was treated after a fatiguing day at work. Threshold values in this patient with true glaucomatous field defects were much better than predicted normal values because of total lack of reliability *(arrows).*

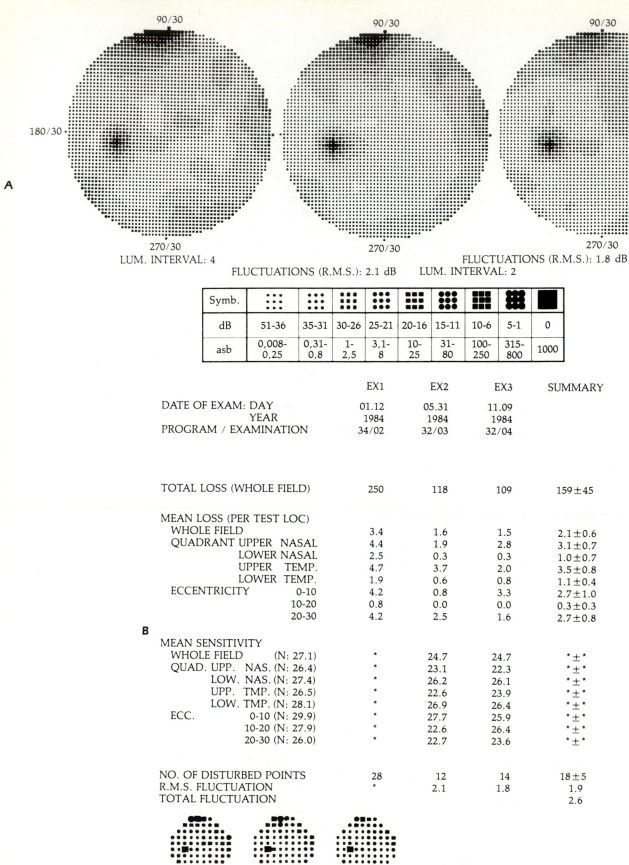

Symb.	⠿	⠿	⠿	⠿	⠿	⠿	⠿	⠿	■
dB	51-36	35-31	30-26	25-21	20-16	15-11	10-6	5-1	0
asb	0,008-0,25	0,31-0,8	1-2,5	3,1-8	10-25	31-80	100-250	315-800	1000

	EX1	EX2	EX3	SUMMARY
DATE OF EXAM: DAY	01.12	05.31	11.09	
YEAR	1984	1984	1984	
PROGRAM / EXAMINATION	34/02	32/03	32/04	
TOTAL LOSS (WHOLE FIELD)	250	118	109	159±45
MEAN LOSS (PER TEST LOC)				
WHOLE FIELD	3.4	1.6	1.5	2.1±0.6
QUADRANT UPPER NASAL	4.4	1.9	2.8	3.1±0.7
LOWER NASAL	2.5	0.3	0.3	1.0±0.7
UPPER TEMP.	4.7	3.7	2.0	3.5±0.8
LOWER TEMP.	1.9	0.6	0.8	1.1±0.4
ECCENTRICITY 0-10	4.2	0.8	3.3	2.7±1.0
10-20	0.8	0.0	0.0	0.3±0.3
20-30	4.2	2.5	1.6	2.7±0.8
MEAN SENSITIVITY				
WHOLE FIELD (N: 27.1)	*	24.7	24.7	*±*
QUAD. UPP. NAS. (N: 26.4)	*	23.1	22.3	*±*
LOW. NAS. (N: 27.4)	*	26.2	26.1	*±*
UPP. TMP. (N: 26.5)	*	22.6	23.9	*±*
LOW. TMP. (N: 28.1)	*	26.9	26.4	*±*
ECC. 0-10 (N: 29.9)	*	27.7	25.9	*±*
10-20 (N: 27.9)	*	22.6	26.4	*±*
20-30 (N: 26.0)	*	22.7	23.6	*±*
NO. OF DISTURBED POINTS	28	12	14	18±5
R.M.S. FLUCTUATION	*	2.1	1.8	1.9
TOTAL FLUCTUATION				2.6

Fig. 21-33   Learning curve. **A,** Gray scale printout of serial visual fields in a patient with stable glaucoma demonstrating improvement with repeat testing. **B,** Octopus Delta series printout of above. Note decrease in loss values from first to second examination.

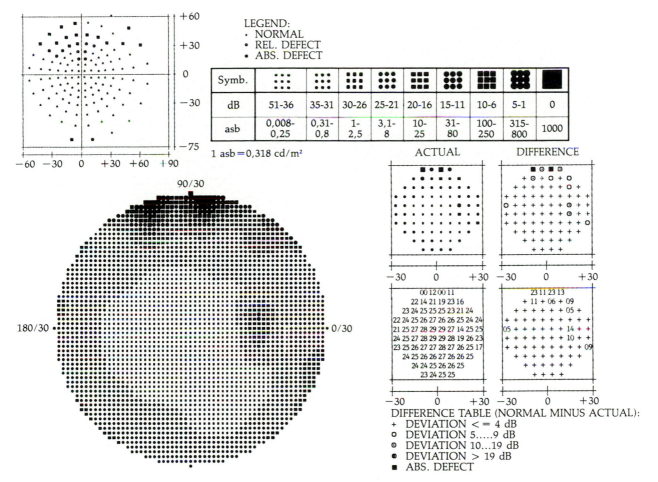

LEGEND:
- NORMAL
- REL. DEFECT
- ABS. DEFECT

Symb.	⁖⁖⁖	⁘⁘⁘	⁙⁙⁙	⠿	⣏	⬤⬤⬤	▦	✱✱	■
dB	51-36	35-31	30-26	25-21	20-16	15-11	10-6	5-1	0
asb	0,008-0,25	0,31-0,8	1-2,5	3,1-8	10-25	31-80	100-250	315-800	1000

1 asb = 0,318 cd/m²

ACTUAL

```
        00 12 00 11
      22 14 21 19 23 16
    23 24 25 25 23 21 24
 22 24 25 26 27 26 26 25 24 24
 21 25 27 28 29 29 27 14 25 25
 24 25 27 28 29 28 19 26 23
 23 25 26 27 27 28 27 26 25 17
    24 25 26 26 27 26 26 25
      24 24 25 26 26 25
        23 24 25 25
```

DIFFERENCE

```
           23 11 23 13
         + 11 + 06 + 09
       + + + + + + 05 +
     + + + + + + + + + +
   05 + + + + + + + 14 + +
     + + + + + + + 10 + +
     + + + + + + + + + 09
       + + + + + + + +
         + + + + + + +
           + + + +
```

DIFFERENCE TABLE (NORMAL MINUS ACTUAL):
- \+ DEVIATION < = 4 dB
- o DEVIATION 5.....9 dB
- ⊙ DEVIATION 10...19 dB
- ● DEVIATION > 19 dB
- ■ ABS. DEFECT

Fig. 21-34 Nonglaucomatous field loss. This superior field defect is result of ptosis in this patient, normal-appearing optic nerve, and elevated intraocular pressure.

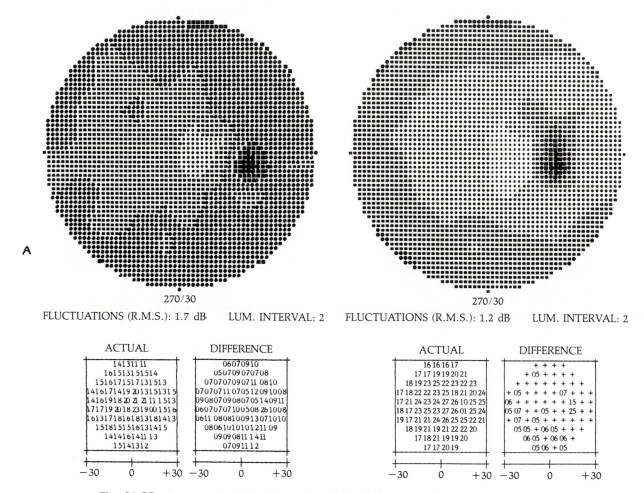

FLUCTUATIONS (R.M.S.): 1.7 dB   LUM. INTERVAL: 2   FLUCTUATIONS (R.M.S.): 1.2 dB   LUM. INTERVAL: 2

Fig. 21-35 Cataract. **A,** Diffuse loss of sensitivity *(left)* improves following cataract extraction *(right).*

	EX1	EX2	EX3	EX4	SUMMARY
DATE OF EXAM: DAY	04.05	11.19	04.23	04.15	
YEAR	1985	1985	1986	1987	
PROGRAM / EXAMINATION	34/02	32/03	32/04	32/05	
TOTAL LOSS (WHOLE FIELD)	45	198	634	112	247±132
MEAN LOSS (PER TEST LOC)					
WHOLE FIELD	0.6	2.7	8.6	1.5	3.3±1.8
QUADRANT UPPER NASAL	0.5	3.6	7.6	0.8	3.1±1.6
LOWER NASAL	0.7	1.8	8.2	3.5	3.6±1.7
UPPER TEMP.	0.6	4.2	8.5	0.4	3.4±1.9
LOWER TEMP.	0.7	1.1	10.1	1.2	3.2±2.3
ECCENTRICITY 0-10	0.9	1.3	7.5	0.4	2.5±1.7
10-20	0.8	1.6	9.2	1.3	3.2±2.0
20-30	0.5	3.5	8.6	1.9	3.6±1.8
MEAN SENSITIVITY					
WHOLE FIELD (N: 24.1)	*	19.4	15.5	21.0	*±*
QUAD. UPP. NAS. (N: 23.4)	*	18.1	15.8	20.1	*±*
LOW. NAS. (N: 24.4)	*	20.5	16.2	19.7	*±*
UPP. TMP. (N: 23.5)	*	17.8	15.0	21.9	*±*
LOW. TMP. (N: 25.1)	*	21.1	15.0	22.4	*±*
ECC. 0-10 (N: 26.9)	*	23.1	19.4	24.9	*±*
10-20 (N: 24.9)	*	20.8	15.8	22.1	*±*
20-30 (N: 23.0)	*	17.8	14.3	19.5	*±*
NO. OF DISTURBED POINTS	8	30	74	20	33±14
R.M.S. FLUCTUATION	*	0.9	1.7	1.2	1.3
TOTAL FLUCTUATION					3.3

B

Fig. 21-35, cont'd   B, Octopus Delta series analysis documents increasing loss of sensitivity as cataract becomes more dense (EX1 to EX3). Sensitivity improves following cataract extraction (EX4).

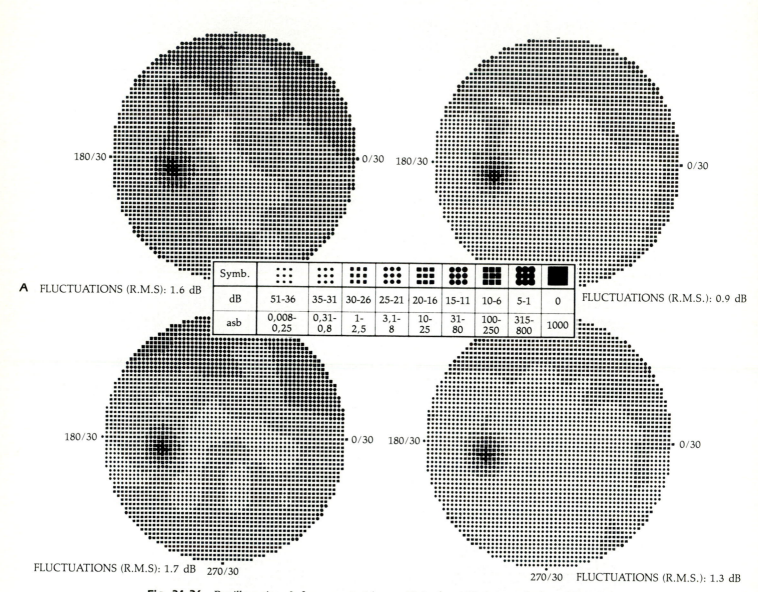

Symb.	⠿	⠿	⠿	⠿	⠿	⠿	⠿	⠿	■
dB	51-36	35-31	30-26	25-21	20-16	15-11	10-6	5-1	0
asb	0,008-0,25	0,31-0,8	1-2,5	3,1-8	10-25	31-80	100-250	315-800	1000

A FLUCTUATIONS (R.M.S): 1.6 dB

FLUCTUATIONS (R.M.S.): 0.9 dB

FLUCTUATIONS (R.M.S): 1.7 dB

FLUCTUATIONS (R.M.S.): 1.3 dB

Fig. 21-36 Pupillary size. **A,** Improvement in sensitivity from dilating pupils from 1.5 to 4 mm *(upper)* reproduced again at later date *(lower).*

	EX1	EX2	EX3	EX4	SUMMARY
DATE OF EXAM: DAY	01.06	01.06	05.26	05.26	
YEAR	1983	1983	1983	1983	
PROGRAM / EXAMINATION	32/02	32/03	32/05	32/06	
TOTAL LOSS (WHOLE FIELD)	432	53	391	52	232 ± 103
MEAN LOSS (PER TEST LOC)					
WHOLE FIELD	5.8	0.7	5.3	0.7	3.1 ± 1.4
QUADRANT UPPER NASAL	7.7	1.2	7.3	1.6	4.4 ± 1.8
LOWER NASAL	4.2	0.0	4.1	0.0	2.1 ± 1.2
UPPER TEMP.	6.3	1.4	5.7	0.6	3.5 ± 1.5
LOWER TEMP.	5.1	0.3	3.9	0.6	2.5 ± 1.2
ECCENTRICITY 0-10	6.6	0.9	5.9	1.8	3.8 ± 1.4
10-20	6.3	1.2	5.3	0.3	3.3 ± 1.5
20-30	5.5	0.5	5.1	0.6	2.9 ± 1.4
MEAN SENSITIVITY					
WHOLE FIELD (N: 24.1)	17.7	21.0	18.1	21.3	19.6 ± 0.9
QUAD. UPP. NAS. (N: 23.4)	15.5	19.5	16.1	19.6	17.7 ± 1.1
LOW. NAS. (N: 24.4)	19.4	22.0	19.4	22.1	20.7 ± 0.8
UPP. TMP. (N: 23.5)	16.8	20.1	17.1	20.9	18.7 ± 1.0
LOW. TMP. (N: 25.1)	19.3	22.7	20.1	22.7	21.2 ± 0.9
ECC. 0-10 (N: 26.9)	20.1	23.4	20.7	23.4	21.9 ± 0.9
10-20 (N: 24.9)	18.3	21.4	19.0	22.0	20.2 ± 0.9
20-30 (N: 23.0)	16.9	20.3	17.1	20.5	18.7 ± 1.0
NO. OF DISTURBED POINTS	63	10	59	10	36 ± 15
R.M.S. FLUCTUATION	1.6	0.9	1.7	1.3	1.4
TOTAL FLUCTUATION					2.2

B

Fig. 21-36, cont'd **B,** Octopus Delta series analysis of above examinations documenting improvement from EX1 to EX2 performed on same day and from EX3 to EX4 4 months later.

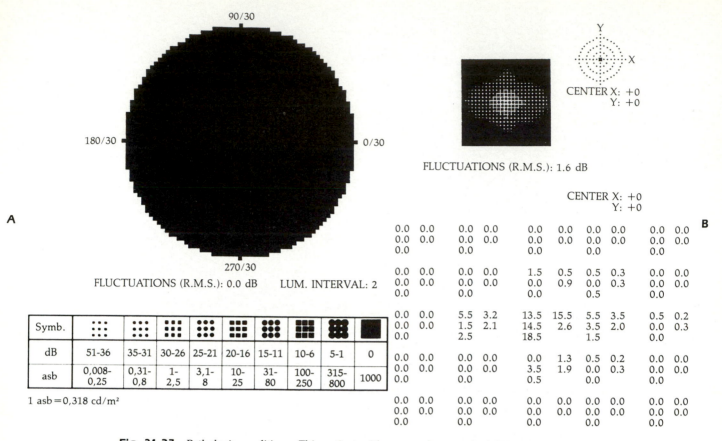

A

90/30

180/30

0/30

270/30

FLUCTUATIONS (R.M.S.): 0.0 dB   LUM. INTERVAL: 2

Symb.	⁚⁚⁚	⁚⁚⁚	⁝⁝⁝	⁞⁞⁞	▦	●●●	▦	✖	■
dB	51-36	35-31	30-26	25-21	20-16	15-11	10-6	5-1	0
asb	0,008-0,25	0,31-0,8	1-2,5	3,1-8	10-25	31-80	100-250	315-800	1000

1 asb = 0,318 cd/m²

B

Y
X
CENTER X: +0
Y: +0

FLUCTUATIONS (R.M.S.): 1.6 dB

CENTER X: +0
      Y: +0

```
0.0 0.0   0.0 0.0    0.0  0.0  0.0 0.0   0.0 0.0
0.0 0.0   0.0 0.0    0.0  0.0  0.0 0.0   0.0 0.0
0.0       0.0        0.0       0.0       0.0

0.0 0.0   0.0 0.0    1.5  0.5  0.5 0.3   0.0 0.0
0.0 0.0   0.0 0.0    0.0  0.9  0.0 0.3   0.0 0.0
0.0       0.0        0.0       0.5       0.0

0.0 0.0   5.5 3.2   13.5 15.5  5.5 3.5   0.5 0.2
0.0 0.0   1.5 2.1   14.5  2.6  3.5 2.0   0.0 0.3
0.0       2.5       18.5       1.5       0.0

0.0 0.0   0.0 0.0    0.0  1.3  0.5 0.2   0.0 0.0
0.0 0.0   0.0 0.0    3.5  1.9  0.0 0.3   0.0 0.0
0.0       0.0        0.5       0.0       0.0

0.0 0.0   0.0 0.0    0.0  0.0  0.0 0.0   0.0 0.0
0.0 0.0   0.0 0.0    0.0  0.0  0.0 0.0   0.0 0.0
0.0       0.0        0.0       0.0       0.0
```

Fig. 21-37 Pathologic conditions. This patient with severe glaucoma had 20/40 vision but total absense of visual fields as routinely tested with central 30 degree examination, **A.** This obvious paradox occurred because central island of vision was completely located between four central test points. High-resolution central field testing, **B,** is more appropriate in this situation.

Pathologic Conditions

Correct interpretation of visual fields often depends on knowledge and integration of the patient's ocular and medical history, vision, and eye examination (Fig. 21-37). It is important to remember that other conditions can produce glaucoma-like visual field abnormalities (Fig. 21-38). In addition, glaucoma patients can and will have other diseases that result in accompanying visual field defects (Fig. 21-39).

Evaluation of the Glaucomatous Defect

When an automated static perimetry field is evaluated, it should be kept in mind that the limited number of points tested represents only a small sampling of all the retinal locations that comprise the entire field. Therefore, an examination should be chosen that has a reasonable probability of detecting a defect if one truly exists. Each individual point tested must be further evaluated for "abnormality" by suprathreshold or preferably threshold determination. An individual point may be considered to be "abnormal" if it deviates from an expected value derived from an age-corrected normal population or one derived from the relationship of sensitivity to surrounding points, modal values, or a predicted hill of vision. The amount of deviation necessary to constitute abnormality varies with individual perimeters. As a generalization, a point depressed 5 dB or more from its expected value may be considered to be statistically significantly abnormal. For a 2.0 dB fluctuation rate, this represents greater than a 2–standard deviation depression. A single minimally depressed point, even in a characteristic location for glaucoma, does not necessarily constitute a scotoma. The depth of any scotoma and values of its neighboring points also aid in interpretation. The greater the magnitude of a defect and the more contiguously abnormal points are present, the greater the likelihood that any given area represents a true glaucomatous defect.

Program number: 34

Number of questions: 217   Number of repetitions: 0   Date of printout: 1.14.1985
False positive answers (%): 0 (0/11)   False negative answers (%): 8 (1/12)

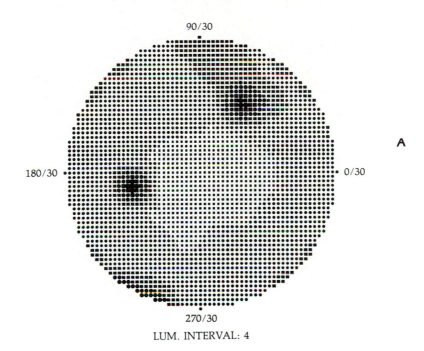

LUM. INTERVAL: 4

Program number: 34

Number of questions: 150   Number of repetitions: 0   Date of printout: 1.30.1985
False positive answers (%): 0 (0/12)   False negative answers (%): 0 (0/3)

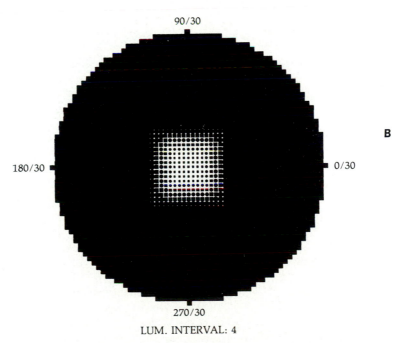

LUM. INTERVAL: 4

Fig. 21-38 Pathologic conditions. **A,** Dense scotoma in superior arcuate area in this patient was found to correlate with chorioretinal scar found on funduscopic examinations **B,** This small residual central island vision resulted from retinitis pigmentosa—not from advanced glaucoma.

Program number: 32

Number of questions: 473   Number of repetitions: 3   Date of printout: 3.27.1984
False positive answers (%): 9 (1/11)   False negative answers (%): 0 (0/12)

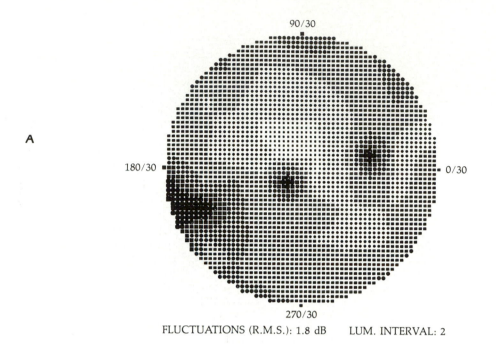

FLUCTUATIONS (R.M.S.): 1.8 dB   LUM. INTERVAL: 2

Program number: 32

Number of questions: 477   Number of repetitions: 0   Date of printout: 4.07.1987
False positive answers (%): 0 (0/11)   False negative answers (%): 0 (0/12)

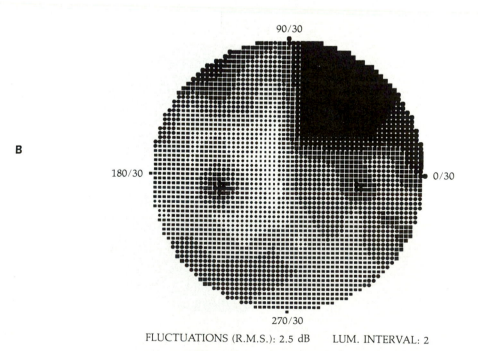

FLUCTUATIONS (R.M.S.): 2.5 dB   LUM. INTERVAL: 2

Fig. 21-39 Pathologic conditions. **A,** Inferior paracentral defect in visual field of this glaucomatous patient resulted from a macular lesion. **B,** Superonasal field defect in this glaucomatous patient resulted from an acute cerebrovascular accident.

An example of minimum criteria for a glaucomatous defect, as defined by one national collaborative study of glaucoma,[9] is two contiguous points in the central 20 degrees on the Octopus 32 program that have threshold values 5 dB or more below the age-adjusted normal values, or three contiguous points in the central 30 degrees that have threshold values 5 dB or below the age-adjusted normal values. For the purposes of this study, the four superiormost, four inferiormost, and four points surrounding the blind spot on this program are excluded from consideration because of their lesser reliability. Although these criteria have proved useful for this study, they may be too strict considering the variability in visual field examination. Some ophthalmologists use the criteria of two contiguous "nonrim" points that are depressed at least 8 dB to indicate an abnormal finding.

In the evaluation of any field, knowledge of the appearance of the optic nerve is helpful. One should expect to find cupping or notching of the nerve corresponding to a dense focal or diffuse defect. Part of the interpretation of the field should be, "Does this correlate to the clinical findings?"

Visual Field Indices and Evaluation of Change

An important function of visual field examination is the evaluation of whether progression or change has occurred over time. As a general rule, most glaucomatous fields either remain stable or worsen. However, there is evidence that some patients may actually exhibit an improvement following regulation of the intraocular pressure. Methods for evaluating change include point-by-point analysis, either directly or by statistical analysis, by the calculation of "visual field indices," by regression analysis, by graphic representation, or by a combination of the above. Many of these methods depend on software supplied by the manufacturer of the perimeter and rely on an inboard or external computer to perform the calculations or comparisons.

Visual field indices reduce the data from a large number of test points and double determinations to a few numbers that summarize the characteristics of the field. The indices of primary interest in the Octopus program G1 are the mean defect (MD), its inverse the mean sensitivity (MS), the loss variation (LV), and the corrected loss variation (CLV). The MD is a measure of diffuse loss and minimizes the effect of localized defects. The CLV, on the other hand, emphasizes the significance of focal scotomas. A calculation of the short-term fluctuation is

also provided (Figs. 21-40 and 21-41). The STATPAC software package for the Humphrey perimeter also calculates the MD as well as *pattern standard deviation* (PSD), *corrected pattern standard deviation* (CPSD), short-term fluctuation (SF), and probability analyses (Fig. 21-42). The PSD is a measurement of the degree to which the shape of the measured field departs from the normal, age-corrected reference field. A low PSD signifies a smooth hill of vision. A high PSD signifies an irregular hill and results from actual field irregularities or variability in patient response. The CPSD is a measure of how much the total shape of the patient's hill of vision deviates from the shape of the hill of vision normal for the patient's age, corrected for intratest variability. The hill of vision may be irregular in shape because of actual field loss, unreliable patient responses, or a combination of both. Probability analysis is also reported. For an in-depth discussion of these indices, the reader is referred to the manufacturers' manuals.[2,16]

Change or progression of defects can be determined visually by point-by-point analysis or by computerized analysis with some perimeters. An example of the criteria for progression, as defined by one national collaborative study of glaucoma[9] is a change in each of two spots in the central 30 degrees of field on Octopus 32 that have any of the following characteristics: (1) a threshold value 7 dB or more below the threshold value of an abnormal spot on the field of reference (deepening of an existing scotoma), or (2) a threshold value 9 dB or more below the threshold value of a normal spot adjacent to an abnormal point on the field of reference (enlargement of an existing scotoma), or (3) a threshold value 11 dB or more below the threshold value of a normal spot on the field of reference (new scotoma). Additional rules define an abnormal spot to take into consideration the variability of the threshold of any given point from one examination to the next caused by fluctuation. The complexity of manually applying arbitrary rules such as these underscores the utility of computerized analysis of visual fields.

One example of computerized visual field analysis is the Octopus DELTA program, which employs a series analysis with data reduction and a change mode that performs a point-by-point evaluation with a paired t-test analysis to indicate any statistically significant change in either the whole field or in areas found to be pathologic (Figs. 21-43 and 21-44). Another example is the Humphrey STATPAC software, which offers a series overview printout (Figs. 21-45, *A* and 21-46, A) and a change

Text continued on p. 466.

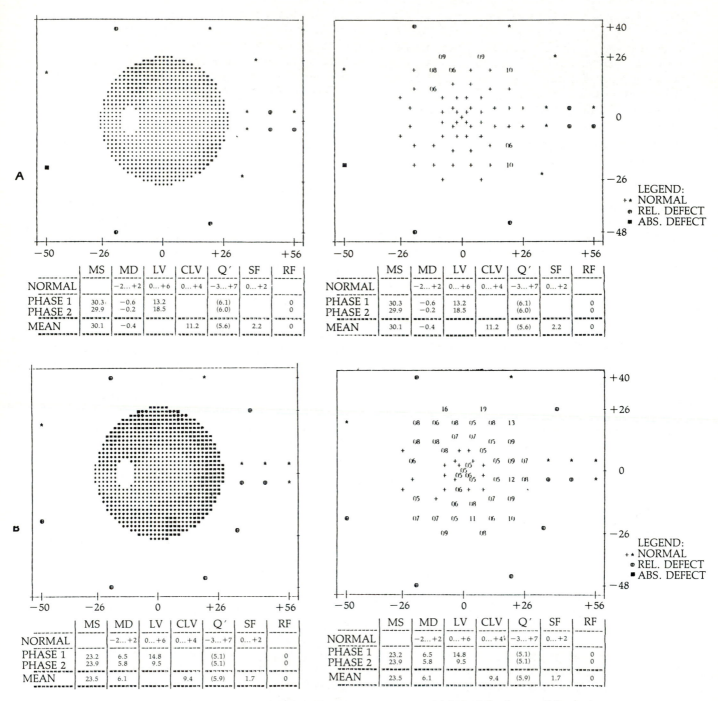

Fig. 21-40   Octopus visual field indices. **A,** Program G1 visual field with focal areas of depression is characterized by normal MS, minimal MD, and high CLV. **B,** Program G1 visual field with diffuse depression is characterized by low MS and moderately increased MD and CLV.

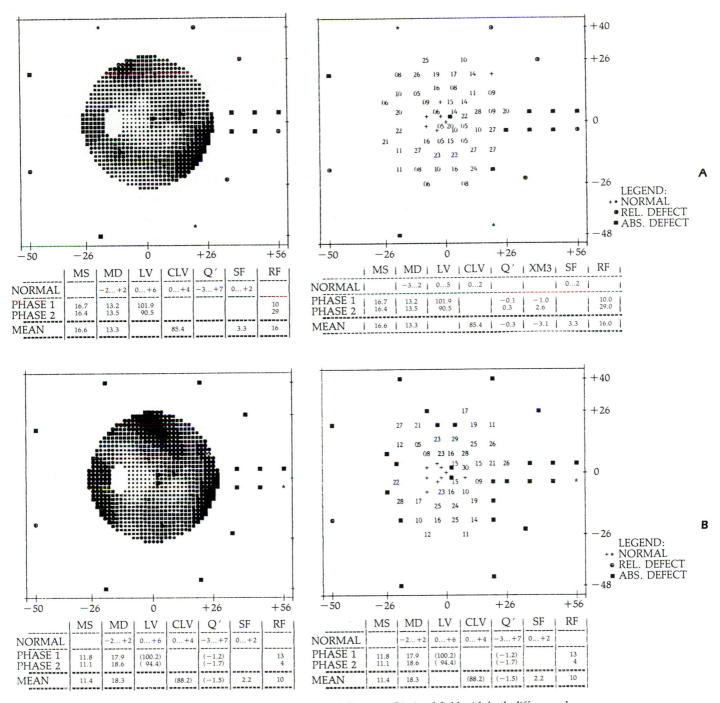

Fig. 21-41   Octopus visual field indices. **A,** Program G1 visual field with both diffuse and severe focal scotomas characterized by low MS and MD with extremely high CLV. **B,** More advanced glaucomatous field damage than above with a further worsening of field indices.

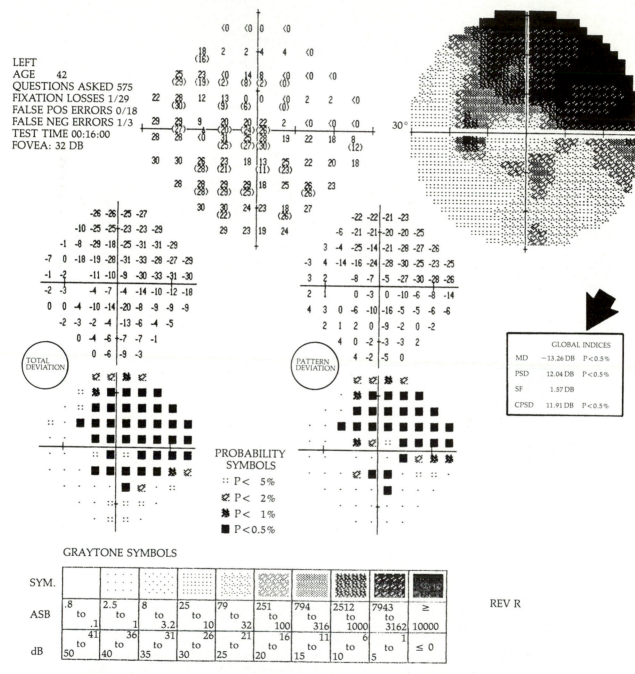

Fig. 21-42 Humphrey visual field indices. Single-field analysis printout from Humphrey STATPAC presents actual threshold determinations *(upper left)* and gray scale printout *(upper right)*. Total deviation plot *(circled, middle left)* presents difference from normal values and is adjusted for diffuse alterations in sensitivity in pattern deviation plot *(circled, middle right)*. Below these are corresponding probability values and short-term fluctuation are also provided *(box)*.

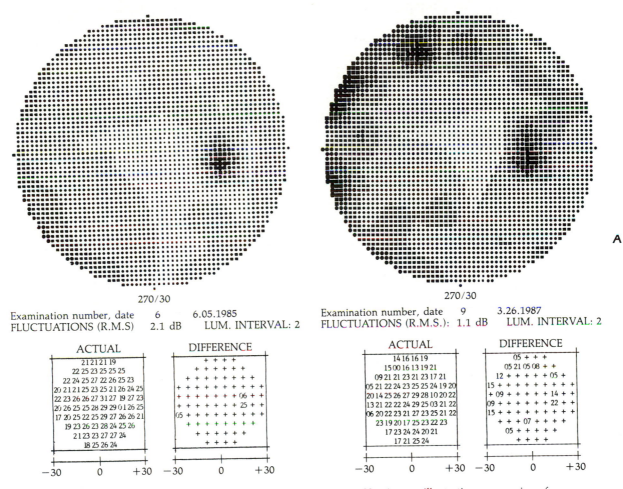

270/30   270/30

Examination number, date 6 6.05.1985	Examination number, date 9 3.26.1987
FLUCTUATIONS (R.M.S) 2.1 dB LUM. INTERVAL: 2	FLUCTUATIONS (R.M.S.): 1.1 dB LUM. INTERVAL: 2

Fig. 21-43 Octopus Delta Analysis. **A,** Standard program 32 printouts illustrating progression of glaucomatous defects from 6/05/85 to 3/26/87.

Continued.

	EX1	EX2	EX3	SUMMARY
DATE OF EXAM: DAY	06.05	09.18	03.26	
YEAR	1985	1986	1987	
PROGRAM / EXAMINATION	32/06	32/08	32/09	
TOTAL LOSS (WHOLE FIELD)	5	92	121	72±34
MEAN LOSS (PER TEST LOC)				
WHOLE FIELD	0.1	1.2	1.6	1.0±0.5
QUADRANT UPPER NASAL	0.0	1.1	3.8	1.6±1.1
LOWER NASAL	0.3	3.8	1.9	2.0±1.0
UPPER TEMP.	0.0	0.0	0.7	0.2±0.2
LOWER TEMP.	0.0	0.0	0.0	0.0±0.0
ECCENTRICITY 0-10	0.0	1.3	0.0	0.4±0.4
10-20	0.0	0.3	0.4	0.2±0.1
20-30	0.1	1.6	2.6	1.4±0.7

B

MEAN SENSITIVITY	EX1	EX2	EX3	SUMMARY
WHOLE FIELD (N: 23.7)	24.1	21.6	20.6	22.1±1.1
QUAD. UPP. NAS. (N: 23.1)	23.4	21.1	18.0	20.8±1.6
LOW. NAS. (N: 24.0)	22.8	19.2	19.7	20.6±1.1
UPP. TMP. (N: 23.2)	24.4	22.9	21.2	22.9±0.9
LOW. TMP. (N: 24.7)	26.1	23.3	23.4	24.3±0.9
ECC. 0-10 (N: 26.6)	27.0	24.0	25.5	25.5±0.9
10-20 (N: 24.6)	24.7	22.9	22.7	23.4±0.6
20-30 (N: 22.6)	23.1	20.4	18.3	20.6±1.4

	EX1	EX2	EX3	SUMMARY
NO. OF DISTURBED POINTS	1	13	13	9±4
R.M.S. FLUCTUATION	2.1	1.1	1.1	1.4
TOTAL FLUCTUATION				2.7

Fig. 21-43, cont'd   **B**, Series printout presenting total loss, mean loss per test location (mean defect), mean sensitivity, number of disturbed points, and fluctuation rates for examinations performed over above time period. In addition to means for entire field, calculations are also provided by quandrant and degrees of eccentricity.

```
                         - 7.  - 5:    5:    0:

                  - 7.  -25.  - 7.  -12.  - 6:  - 4:

           -13.  - 3:  - 4:  - 4:  - 1:  - 3:  - 8.  - 2:

    -15.    0:    1:  - 1:    0:    0:    4:  - 2:  - 5:  - 5:

     - 2:  - 9.  - 1:    0:    0:  - 2:    1:        - 7:  - 1:

     - 7.  - 5:  - 3:  - 3:  - 4      0:  - 4:        - 5:  - 3:

    -11     0:  - 3:    1:  - 4:  - 2:  - 4:  - 1:  - 5:    1:

            4:  - 4:  - 6:  - 6.  - 3:  - 1:  - 3.    3:

                  - 4.    0:    1:  - 3:  - 7:  - 3:

                         - 1:  - 4:  - 1:    0:
```

DIFFERENCE TABLE: MEAN B MINUS MEAN A (NEGATIVE VALUES: DECREASED SENSITIVITY)
0-0 ALL RESULTS ZERO   < > LOW NORMAL VALUES
DOTS INDICATE THAT SOME (.) OR ALL (:) RESULTS ARE IN NORMAL RANGE (FULLY VALID)

CONFIDENCE INTERVAL FOR MEAN DIFFERENCE / T-TEST
(1) PATHOL, AREA (UNDOTTED)   NOT CARRIED OUT (NOT ENOUGH DATA)
(2) WHOLE FIELD   −3.6+1.0 (T-TEST: ALTERATION IS INDICATED)

C

PROGRAM/EXAM/DATE	SUMMARY A 32/06/06.05.85	SUMMARY B 32/09/03.26.87	DIFF (B MIN A)
TOTAL LOSS (WHOLE FIELD)	5±*	121±*	+116±*
MEAN LOSS (PER TEST LOC)			
WHOLE FIELD	0.1±*	1.6±*	+ 1.6±*
QUADRANT UPPER NASAL	0.0±*	3.8±*	+ 3.8±*
LOWER NASAL	0.3±*	1.9±*	+ 1.6±*
UPPER TEMP.	0.0±*	0.7±*	+ 0.7±*
LOWER TEMP.	0.0±*	0.0±*	0.0±*
ECCENTRICITY 0-10	0.0±*	0.0±*	0.0±*
10-20	0.0±*	0.4±*	+ 0.4±*
20-30	0.1±*	2.6±*	+ 2.5±*
MEAN SENSITIVITY			
WHOLE FIELD (N: 23.6)	24.1±*	20.6±*	− 3.6±*
QUAD. UPP. NAS. (N: 22.9)	23.4±*	18.0±*	− 5.4±*
LOW. NAS. (N: 23.9)	22.8±*	19.7±*	− 3.1±*
UPP. TMP. (N: 23.0)	24.4±*	21.2±*	− 3.2±*
LOW. TMP. (N: 24.6)	26.1±*	23.4±*	− 2.6±*
ECC. 0-10 (N: 26.4)	27.0±*	25.5±*	− 1.5±*
10-20 (N: 24.4)	24.7±*	22.7±*	− 2.1±*
20-30 (N: 22.5)	23.1±*	18.3±*	− 4.8±*
NO. OF DISTURBED POINTS	1±*	13±*	+12±*
R.M.S. FLUCTUATION	2.1	1.1	
TOTAL FLUCTUATION	*	*	

Fig. 21-43, cont'd **C,** Changed printout calculates difference of mean values between selected examinations *(left)* and point-by-point analysis displayed in difference table *(right)*. Results of paired t-test analysis are also presented.

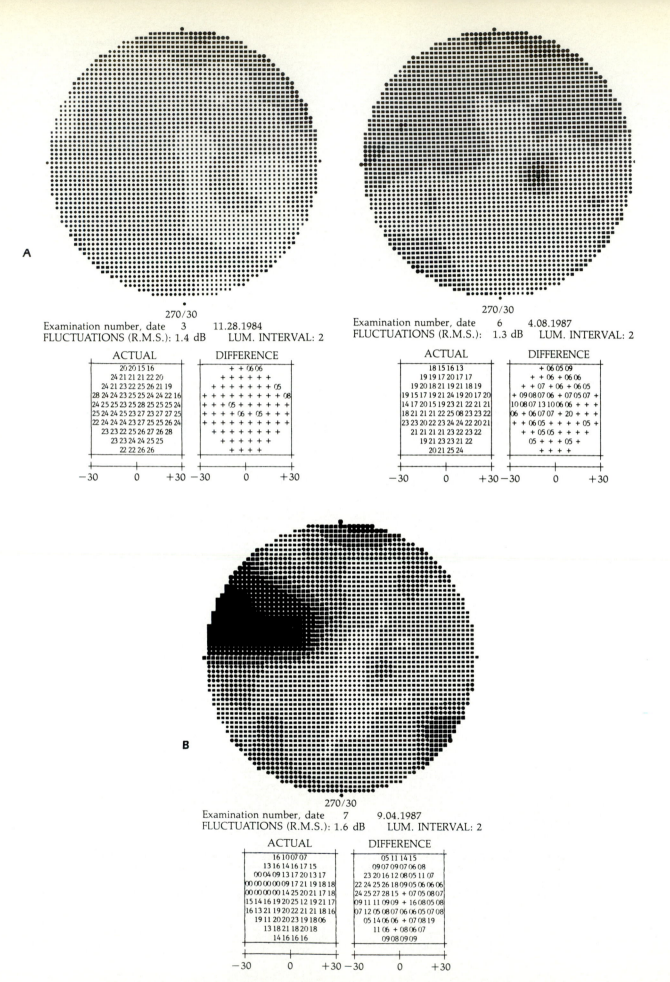

270/30
Examination number, date   3   11.28.1984
FLUCTUATIONS (R.M.S.): 1.4 dB   LUM. INTERVAL: 2

ACTUAL

```
        20 20 15 16
       24 21 21 21 22 20
      24 21 23 22 25 26 21 19
    28 24 24 23 25 25 24 24 22 16
    24 25 25 23 25 28 25 25 25 24
    25 24 24 25 23 27 23 27 27 25
    22 24 24 24 23 27 25 25 26 24
       23 23 22 25 26 27 26 28
         23 23 24 24 25 25
           22 22 26 26
```

DIFFERENCE

```
         + + 06 06
        + + + + + +
       + + + + + + 05
     + + + + + + + + + 08
     + + + 05 + + + + + +
     + + + 06 + 05 + + +
     + + + + + + + + + +
        + + + + + + + +
          + + + + + +
            + + + +
```

−30   0   +30 −30   0   +30

270/30
Examination number, date   6   4.08.1987
FLUCTUATIONS (R.M.S.): 1.3 dB   LUM. INTERVAL: 2

ACTUAL

```
        18 15 16 13
       19 19 17 20 17 17
      19 20 18 21 19 21 18 19
    19 15 17 19 21 24 19 20 17 20
    14 17 20 15 19 23 21 22 21 21
    18 21 21 21 22 25 08 23 23 22
       23 23 20 22 23 24 24 22 20 21
         21 21 21 21 23 22 23 22
           19 21 23 23 21 22
             20 21 25 24
```

DIFFERENCE

```
          + 06 05 09
         + + 06 + 06 06
        + + 07 + 06 + 06 05
      + 09 08 07 06 + 07 05 07 +
      10 08 07 13 10 06 06 + + +
      06 + 06 07 07 + 20 + + +
        + + 06 05 + + + + 05 +
          + + 05 05 + + + +
            05 + + + 05 +
              + + + +
```

−30   0   +30 −30   0   +30

B

270/30
Examination number, date   7   9.04.1987
FLUCTUATIONS (R.M.S.): 1.6 dB   LUM. INTERVAL: 2

ACTUAL

```
        16 10 07 07
       13 16 14 16 17 15
      00 04 09 13 17 20 13 17
    00 00 00 00 09 17 21 19 18 18
    00 00 00 00 14 25 20 21 17 18
    15 14 16 19 20 25 12 19 21 17
    16 13 21 19 20 22 21 21 18 16
       19 11 20 20 23 19 18 06
         13 18 21 18 20 18
           14 16 16 16
```

DIFFERENCE

```
         05 11 14 15
        09 07 09 07 06 08
       23 20 16 12 08 05 11 07
     22 24 25 26 18 09 05 06 06 06
     24 25 27 28 15 + 07 05 08 07
     09 11 11 09 09 + 16 08 05 08
     07 12 05 08 07 06 06 05 07 08
        05 14 06 06 + 07 08 19
          11 06 + 08 06 07
            09 08 09 09
```

−30   0   +30 −30   0   +30

Fig. 21-44 Octopus Delta Analysis. **A,** Standard program 32 printouts illustrating progression of glaucomatous defects from 11/28/84 to 4/8/87. **B,** Additional loss has occurred with formation of a dense nasal defect by 9/4/87, despite attempts to lower intraocular pressure.

	EX1	EX2	EX3	EX4	SUMMARY
DATE OF EXAM: DAY	11.28	12.22	04.08	09.04	
YEAR	1984	1985	1987	1987	
PROGRAM / EXAMINATION	32/03	32/04	32/06	32/07	
TOTAL LOSS (WHOLE FIELD)	41	191	253	768	313±157
MEAN LOSS (PER TEST LOC)					
WHOLE FIELD	0.6	2.6	3.4	10.4	4.2±2.1
QUADRANT UPPER NASAL	0.3	1.8	5.1	18.2	6.3±4.1
LOWER NASAL	0.3	2.8	2.7	8.1	3.5±1.6
UPPER TEMP.	1.4	3.9	4.1	7.5	4.2±1.3
LOWER TEMP.	0.3	1.8	1.7	7.4	2.8±1.6
ECCENTRICITY 0-10	1.3	4.5	6.3	10.3	5.6±1.9
10-20	0.0	2.6	4.1	10.2	4.2±2.2
20-30	0.6	2.1	2.4	10.5	3.9±2.2
MEAN SENSITIVITY					
WHOLE FIELD (N: 25.1)	23.6	20.8	20.1	14.5	19.7±1.9
QUAD. UPP. NAS. (N: 24.4)	23.3	20.4	18.0	6.2	17.0±3.7
LOW. NAS. (N: 25.4)	23.4	21.2	21.2	17.1	20.7±1.3
UPP. TMP. (N: 24.5)	22.1	19.3	19.2	16.8	19.4±1.1
LOW. TMP. (N: 26.1)	25.7	22.5	21.9	18.2	22.1±1.5
ECC. 0-10 (N: 27.9)	24.9	21.9	20.5	16.9	21.1±1.7
10-20 (N: 25.9)	24.3	21.6	20.6	15.5	20.5±1.8
20-30 (N: 24.0)	23.0	20.3	19.7	13.4	19.1±2.0
NO. OF DISTURBED POINTS	7	29	36	70	36±13
R.M.S. FLUCTUATION	1.4	2.2	1.3	1.6	1.6
TOTAL FLUCTUATION					3.7

C

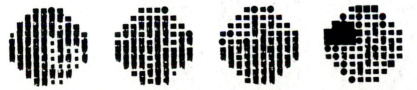

Fig. 21-44, cont'd   C, Series printout of visual fields in **A** and **B.**

Continued.

```
                       - 2:  - 5.    1   - 3

                  - 5:  - 2:  - 4.  - 1:  - 5.  - 3.

             - 5:  - 1:  - 5.  - 1:  - 6.  - 5:  - 3.    0

        - 9:  - 9.  - 7.  - 4.  - 4.  - 1:  - 5.  - 4.  - 5.    4.

       -10.  - 8.  - 5.  - 8   - 6.  - 5.  - 4.        - 4:  - 3:

        - 7.  - 3:  - 3.  - 4.  - 1   - 2:  -15         - 4:  - 3:

          1:  - 1:  - 4.  - 2.    0:  - 3:  - 1:  - 3:  - 6.  - 3:

             - 2:  - 2:  - 1.  - 4.  - 3:  - 5:  - 3:  - 6:

                - 4.  - 2:  - 1:  - 1:  - 4.  - 3:

                   - 2:  - 1:  - 1:  - 2:
```

DIFFERENCE TABLE: MEAN B MINUS MEAN A (NEGATIVE VALUES: DECREASED SENSITIVITY)
0-0 ALL RESULTS ZERO   < > LOW NORMAL VALUES
DOTS INDICATE THAT SOME (.) OR ALL (:) RESULTS ARE IN NORMAL RANGE (FULLY VALID)

CONFIDENCE INTERVAL FOR MEAN DIFFERENCE / T-TEST
(1) PATHOL, AREA (UNDOTTED) −4.3±6.4 (T-TEST: DATA DO NOT PROVE ALTERATION)
(2) WHOLE FIELD   −3.6±0.6 (T-TEST: ALTERATION IS INDICATED)

D

PROGRAM/EXAM/DATE	SUMMARY A 32/03/11.28.84	SUMMARY B 32/06/04.08.87	DIFF (B MIN A)
TOTAL LOSS (WHOLE FIELD)	41±*	253±*	+212±*
MEAN LOSS (PER TEST LOC)			
WHOLE FIELD	0.6±*	3.4±*	+ 2.9±*
QUADRANT UPPER NASAL	0.3±*	5.1±*	+ 4.8±*
LOWER NASAL	0.3±*	2.7±*	+ 2.4±*
UPPER TEMP.	1.4±*	4.1±*	+ 2.7±*
LOWER TEMP.	0.3±*	1.7±*	+ 1.4±*
ECCENTRICITY 0-10	1.3±*	6.3±*	+ 4.9±*
10-20	0.0±*	4.1±*	+ 4.1±*
20-30	0.6±*	2.4±*	+ 1.8±*
MEAN SENSITIVITY			
WHOLE FIELD (N: 25.1)	23.6±*	20.1±*	− 3.6±*
QUAD. UPP. NAS. (N: 24.4)	23.3±*	18.0±*	− 5.3±*
LOW. NAS. (N: 25.4)	23.4±*	21.2±*	− 2.3±*
UPP. TMP. (N: 24.5)	22.1±*	19.2±*	− 2.9±*
LOW. TMP. (N: 26.1)	25.7±*	21.9±*	− 3.8±*
ECC. 0-10 (N: 27.9)	24.9±*	20.5±*	− 4.4±*
10-20 (N: 25.9)	24.3±*	20.6±*	− 3.8±*
20-30 (N: 24.0)	23.0±*	19.7±*	− 3.2±*
NO. OF DISTURBED POINTS	7±*	36±*	+29±*
R.M.S. FLUCTUATION	1.4	1.3	
TOTAL FLUCTUATION	*	*	

Fig. 21-44, cont'd   D, Change printout illustrating moderate loss from 11/28/84 to 4/8/87.

```
                     - 4.  -10.  - 8   - 9

                -11.  - 5.  - 7.  - 5.  - 5.  - 5.

           -24.  -17.  -14.  - 9.  - 8.  - 6.  - 8.  - 2

      -28.  -24.  -24.  -23.  -16.  - 8.  - 3.  - 5.  - 4.    2

      -24.  -25.  -25.  -23   -11.  - 3:  - 5.        - 8.  - 6.

      -10.  -10.  - 8.  - 6.  - 3   - 2:  -11         - 6.  - 8.

      - 6.  -11.  - 3.  - 5.  - 3.  - 5.  - 4.  - 4.  - 8.  - 8.

            - 4.  -12.  - 2.  - 5.  - 3:  - 8.  - 8.  -22.

                  -10.  - 5.  - 3:  - 6.  - 5.  - 7.

                        - 8.  - 6.  -10.  -10.
```

DIFFERENCE TABLE: MEAN B MINUS MEAN A (NEGATIVE VALUES: DECREASED SENSITIVITY)
0-0 ALL RESULTS ZERO   < > LOW NORMAL VALUES
DOTS INDICATE THAT SOME (.) OR ALL (:) RESULTS ARE IN NORMAL RANGE (FULLY VALID)

CONFIDENCE INTERVAL FOR MEAN DIFFERENCE / T-TEST
(1) PATHOL, AREA (UNDOTTED) -7.7 ± 7.5 (T-TEST: ALTERATION IS INDICATED)
(2) WHOLE FIELD -9.1 ± 1.6 (T-TEST: ALTERATION IS INDICATED)

E

PROGRAM/EXAM/DATE	SUMMARY A 32/03/11.28.84	SUMMARY B 32/07/09.04.87	DIFF (B MIN A)
TOTAL LOSS (WHOLE FIELD)	$41 \pm *$	$768 \pm *$	$+727 \pm *$
MEAN LOSS (PER TEST LOC)			
WHOLE FIELD	$0.6 \pm *$	$10.4 \pm *$	$+ 9.8 \pm *$
QUADRANT UPPER NASAL	$0.3 \pm *$	$18.2 \pm *$	$+ 17.9 \pm *$
LOWER NASAL	$0.3 \pm *$	$8.1 \pm *$	$+ 7.7 \pm *$
UPPER TEMP.	$1.4 \pm *$	$7.5 \pm *$	$+ 6.1 \pm *$
LOWER TEMP.	$0.3 \pm *$	$7.4 \pm *$	$+ 7.2 \pm *$
ECCENTRICITY 0-10	$1.3 \pm *$	$10.3 \pm *$	$+ 9.0 \pm *$
10-20	$0.0 \pm *$	$10.2 \pm *$	$+ 10.2 \pm *$
20-30	$0.6 \pm *$	$10.5 \pm *$	$+ 9.9 \pm *$
MEAN SENSITIVITY			
WHOLE FIELD (N: 25.1)	$23.6 \pm *$	$14.5 \pm *$	$- 9.1 \pm *$
QUAD. UPP. NAS. (N: 24.4)	$23.3 \pm *$	$6.2 \pm *$	$- 17.1 \pm *$
LOW. NAS. (N: 25.4)	$23.4 \pm *$	$17.1 \pm *$	$- 6.3 \pm *$
UPP. TMP. (N: 24.5)	$22.1 \pm *$	$16.8 \pm *$	$- 5.3 \pm *$
LOW. TMP. (N: 26.1)	$25.7 \pm *$	$18.2 \pm *$	$- 7.5 \pm *$
ECC. 0-10 (N: 27.9)	$24.9 \pm *$	$16.9 \pm *$	$- 8.0 \pm *$
10-20 (N: 25.9)	$24.3 \pm *$	$15.5 \pm *$	$- 8.8 \pm *$
20-30 (N: 24.0)	$23.0 \pm *$	$13.4 \pm *$	$- 9.5 \pm *$
NO. OF DISTURBED POINTS	$7 \pm *$	$70 \pm *$	$+63 \pm *$
R.M.S. FLUCTUATION	1.4	1.6	
TOTAL FLUCTUATION	*	*	

Fig. 21-44, cont'd   E, Change printout illustrating severe loss of 11/28/84.

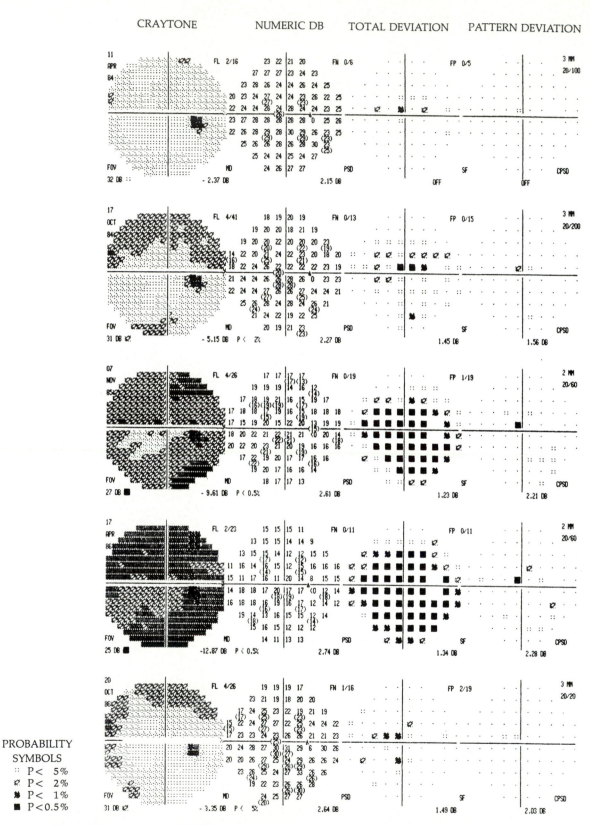

Fig. 21-45 Humphrey STATPAC analysis. **A,** Series overview printout illustrating loss of sensitivity caused by progressive cataract and improvement following surgery. Pattern deviation plots indicate that the loss of sensitivity represents diffuse change without focal scotoma formation. (Reproduced with permission from STATPAC User's Guide, Allergan Humphrey, 1986).

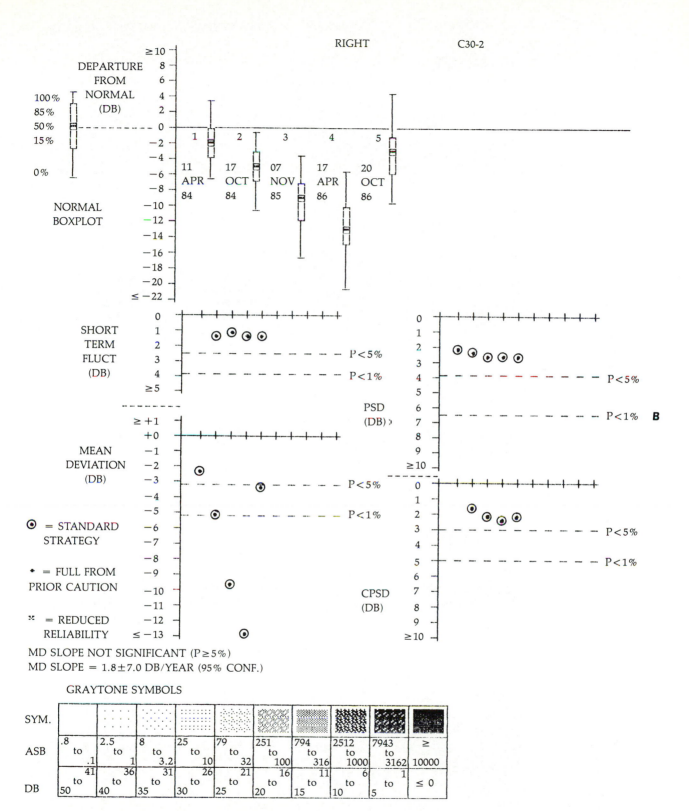

Fig. 21-45, cont'd   B, Change analysis printout with box plot histogram and linear regression analysis of **A.** There is no significant change in field indices. (Reproduced with permission from STATPAC User's Guide, Allergan Humphrey, 1986)

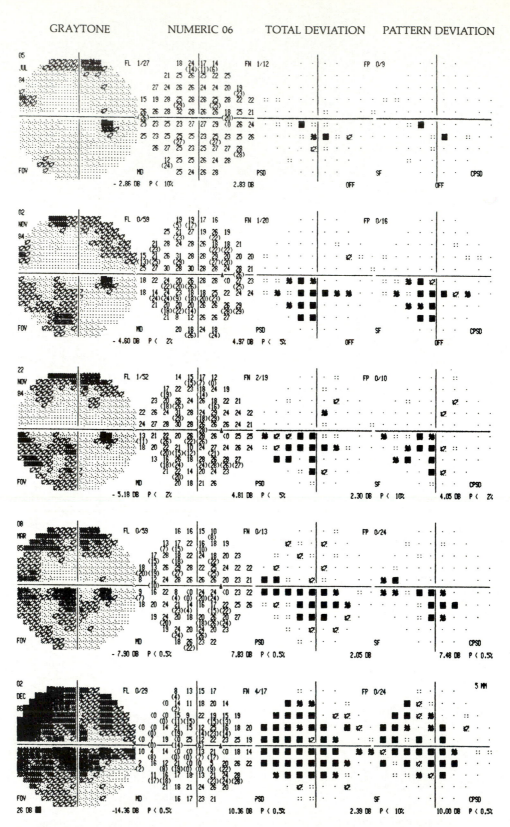

Fig. 21-46 Humphrey STATPAC analysis. **A,** Series overview printout illustrating loss of sensitivity caused by progressive glaucoma. (Reproduced with permission from STATPAC User's Guide, Allergan Humphrey, 1986)

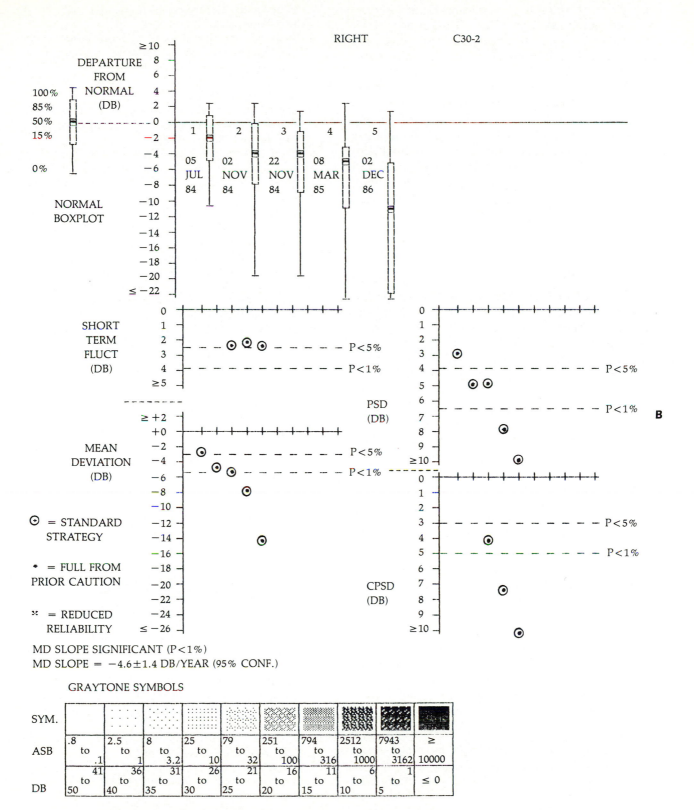

Fig. 21-46, cont'd   B, Change analysis printout with box plot histogram and linear regression analysis of **A.** There is significant change in field indices. (Reproduced with permission from STATPAC User's Guide, Allergan Humphrey, 1986)

analysis with a graphic box plot histogram and linear regression analysis (Figs. 21-45, *B* and 21-46, *B*). For an in-depth discussion of these programs, the reader is referred to the manufacturers' manuals.[2,16]

No single method of serial field analysis, either visual or sophisticated computerized program, is completely satisfactory. It is necessary for the clinician to realize that statistically significant changes in the visual field may not be of any clinical significance when considering their magnitude and the clinical picture of the patient. Regardless of the method employed, it is important to evaluate fields serially to minimize alterations caused by long-term fluctuation and to lessen the likelihood of missing small changes that may occur over time.

THE FUTURE

The hardware component of automated perimeters is already quite refined. Future perimeters may be hybrids combining accurate kinetic testing of peripheral isopters with static testing of the central field. Greater advances will probably occur in the development of more specific or efficient test strategies and more meaningful data analysis as we gather additional knowledge of the pathophysiology of glaucoma and glaucomatous field defects. Eventually "smart" perimeters employing artificial intelligence algorithms may determine both the type of examination and the appropriate data analysis for the clinician. However, visual field examination will always remain an important part of, not a computerized solution to, the clinical decision process regarding the diagnosis and management of glaucoma.

REFERENCES

1. Anderton, S, and Hitchings, RA: A comparative study of the visual fields of patients with low-tension glaucoma and those with chronic simple glaucoma. In Greve, EL, and Heijl, A, editors: Fifth International Visual Field Symposium, The Hague, Netherlands, 1983, Dr W Junk Publishers
2. Bebie, H, and Fankhauser, F: Program DELTA (Handbook for operation and application of the Octopus DELTA program), Schlieren, Switzerland, 1981, Interzeag AG
3. Benedetto, MD, and Cyrlin, MN: The effect of blur upon static perimetric thresholds. In Heijl, A, and Greve, EL, editors: Sixth International Visual Field Symposium, Dordrecht, Netherlands, 1985, Dr W Junk Publishers
4. Brusini, P, and Tosoni, C: Two years experience with the Perimetron automatic perimeter in glaucoma patients. In Heijl, A, and Greve, EL, editors: Sixth International Visual Field Symposium, Dordrecht, Netherlands, 1985, Dr W Junk Publishers
5. Caprioli, J, Sears, M, and Miller, JM: Patterns of early visual field loss in open angle glaucoma, Am J Ophthalmol 103:512, 1987
6. Caprioli, J, and Spaeth, GL: Comparison of visual field defects in the low-tension glaucomas with those in the high-tension glaucomas, Am J Ophthalmol 97:730, 1984
7. Flammer, J, Drance, SM, Fankhauser, F, and Augustiny, L: Differential light threshold in automated static perimetry, factors influencing short-term fluctuation, Arch Ophthalmol 102:876, 1984
8. Flammer, J, Drance, SM, and Zulauf, M: Short- and long-term fluctuation in patients with glaucoma, normal controls and patients with suspected glaucoma, Arch Ophthalmol 102:704, 1984
9. GLT Handbook: GLT Study Group, Springfield, Virginia, National Technical Information Service, Accession # PB 86-101037.
10. Goldstick, B, and Weinreb, RN: The effect of refractive error on automated global analysis program G1, Am J Ophthalmol 104:229, 1987
11. Greve, EL, and Geijssen, C: Comparison of glaucomatous visual field defects in patients with high and low intraocular pressure. In Greve, EL, and Heijl, A, editors: Fifth International Visual Field Symposium, The Hague, Netherlands, 1983, Dr W Junk Publishers
12. Heijl, A, and Drance, SM: A clinical comparison of three computerized automatic perimeters in the detection of glaucoma defects, Arch Ophthalmol 199:832, 1981
13. King, D, et al: Comparison of visual field defects in normal-tension glaucoma and high-tension glaucoma, Am J Ophthalmol 101:204, 1986
14. LeBlanc, RP, Lee, A, and Baxter, M: Peripheral nasal defects. In Heijl, A, and Greve, EL, editors: Sixth International Visual Field Symposium, Dordrecht, Netherlands, 1985, Dr W Junk Publishers
15. Mills, RP: Usefulness of peripheral testing in automated screening perimetry. In Heijl, A, and Greve, EL, editors: Sixth International Visual Field Symposium, Dordrecht, Netherlands, 1985, Dr W Junk Publishers
16. STATPAC User's Guide: San Leandro, California, 1986, Allergan Humphrey
17. Wirtschafter, JD: Examination of the peripheral visual field, Arch Ophthalmol 105:761, 1987

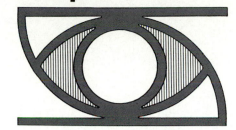

Chapter 22

Clinical Evaluation of the Optic Disc and Retinal Nerve Fiber Layer

P. Juhani Airaksinen
Anja Tuulonen
Elliot B. Werner

HISTORY

The invention of the ophthalmoscope[121] made it possible to observe the interior of the eye and soon led to the recognition of glaucomatous optic disc changes by von Jaeger[102,103] and von Graefe[82-84] in the middle of the nineteenth century. This was followed by the histopathologic studies of Müller in 1856.[135] Although von Jaeger and von Graefe at first believed that the glaucomatous disc was swollen, von Graefe soon realized that it was excavated.[17,63,83] This observation was confirmed by Weber and later described in detail by von Jaeger.[64,103,224]

Extensive descriptions of normal and pathologic discs were given by Elschnig in 1907.[70] In 1917 Elliot[66] was the first to differentiate between cupping and pallor of the disc. Cupping was usually associated with elevated intraocular pressure, but probably the first description of low-tension glaucoma was given by von Graefe in 1857.[84]

The large majority of early optic disc descriptions dealt with advanced glaucoma. Some of the first descriptions of an originally normal disc and its glaucomatous progression were provided by Elschnig,[70] Fuchs,[75] Elliot,[66,67] Müller,[135] and Pickard.[151] Pickard also developed a technique of quantitating changes in the optic disc over time.[152] The history of the clinical recognition of the glau-comatous optic nerve has been reviewed by Kronfeld[119,120] and Greve.[87]

EVALUATION OF THE OPTIC DISC

A variety of signs of glaucomatous optic nerve damage detectable with the ophthalmoscope have been described.[209] Observation of these signs requires the detection of changes in the normal ophthalmoscopic appearance of the optic disc. The features of the optic nerve head that can be evaluated are listed in the box below.

At the optic nerve head, or optic disc, the axons of the retinal ganglion cells are gathered together and exit from the eye through a scleral opening approximately 1 to 4 mm^2 in area (Fig. 22-1). This

---

**FEATURES OF THE OPTIC NERVE HEAD
USED IN OPTIC DISC EVALUATION**

1. Size and shape of the optic cup
2. Cup to disc ratio
3. Visibility of the lamina cribrosa
4. Configuration of the disc rim
5. Pallor of the optic disc
6. Configuration of the retinal blood vessels at the optic disc
7. Peripapillary atrophy

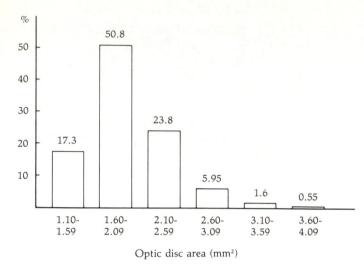

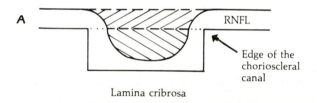

Fig. 22-1 Frequency distribution of optic disc areas in mm² (corrected for magnification of individual's eye) in 173 eyes of 173 individuals.

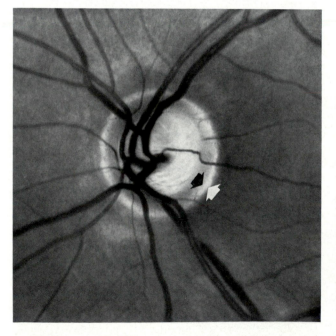

Fig. 22-2 A, Schematic drawings of optic disc showing optic disc margin formed by edge of chorioscleral canal. *RNFL,* retinal nerve fiber layer. **B,** Optic disc photograph showing margin of optic disc *(black arrow).* White arrow points to edge of retinal pigment epithelium. White ring between arrows represents physiologic scleral rim or Elschnig ring surrounding optic disc.

opening, the scleral canal, forms the optic disc margin (Fig. 22-2). The bundles of the ganglion cell axons bend approximately 90 degrees backward at the level of the scleral opening. The area of the bending axons from the disc margin to the edge of the optic cup is known as the disc rim or the neuroretinal rim. In addition to nerve fibers, the optic nerve head contains glial tissue, blood vessels, capillaries, and extracellular space (see Chapter 4).

The optic cup is an excavation inside and below the disc rim to the level of the lamina cribrosa, which forms the bottom of the cup. The lamina cribrosa consists of collagenous connective tissue stretched across the scleral canal. There are openings in the lamina cribrosa through which the nerve fiber bundles exit. These perforations may be visible normally, or they may be covered by the nerve fibers.

Newer methods of quantitative evaluation of the optic disc in glaucoma are covered in Chapter 23. This chapter will discuss more traditional clinical techniques and findings.

THE OPTIC DISC

Normal Anatomy

Recognition of the pathologic changes in the glaucomatous optic disc requires the examiner to be thoroughly familiar with the range of appearance of normal optic discs. There is considerable variation in the size of the so-called physiologic cup

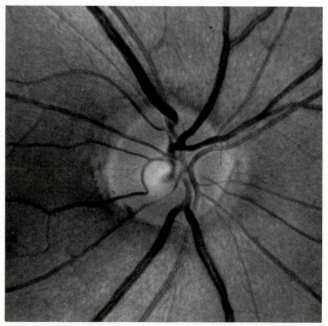

Fig. 22-3 A small optic disc (1.4 mm²) with small optic cup.

among normal individuals. The number of ganglion cell axons varies between about 1.0 and 1.3 million among normal individuals,[28] whereas the size of the scleral opening may vary from 0.7 to 4.4 mm^2.[36,43,44,106,107] Variation in the size of optic discs leads to different-sized optic cups (see Plate II, Figs. 4 through 8). When 1.2 million nerve fibers pass through a small scleral opening, a small cup remains in the center of the disc (Fig. 22-3). When 1.2 million fibers pass through a large scleral canal, a large cup is formed (Fig. 22-4). Because the number of nerve fibers is the same in these two examples, the disc rim area will be approximately the same despite a considerable difference in the appearance of the optic discs. It is the large optic disc that causes difficulty in the diagnosis of glaucoma (Fig. 22-5).

The results of semiquantitative analysis of the retinal nerve fiber layer have correlated well with disc rim area measurements.[6] It has therefore been of interest to determine the area of the disc rim and correct the measurements for the individual magnification of the patient's eye using the method described by Littmann.[125] Corrected values show good correlation with disc area measurements from enucleated eyes.[106]

Analysis of the relationship between the disc, cup, and disc rim is complicated by the fact that the disc rim area and the optic cup actually tend to be larger in larger discs.[36,43-44] Thus, use of the cup/disc ratio or disc-rim area alone will not clearly separate the normal from the glaucomatous population. These parameters can, however, be useful in raising the suspicion of glaucoma and in following changes over time in glaucoma patients.

A number of studies of the distribution of the cup/disc ratio in the population have been conducted. Pickard[151,152] developed a technique of quantitating the amount of cupping relative to the area of the disc using drawings and a transparent grid. Cup sizes were expressed as a percent of the total disc. He noted that glaucoma is sometimes seen in the presence of relatively small cups, whereas very large cups may be seen in an otherwise normal eye, a finding subsequently confirmed by Armaly.[23]

Armaly[24] introduced the modern concept of the cup/disc ratio as a ratio of disc diameter to cup diameter expressed as a decimal fraction. He found that less than 10% of the normal population had a cup/disc ratio of 0.5 or greater. He also found that the cup/disc ratio was genetically determined, a finding later confirmed by Bengtsson.[39] He noted that cup size alone was inadequate for the diagnosis of glaucoma and that other criteria would have to be developed. Subsequent studies have

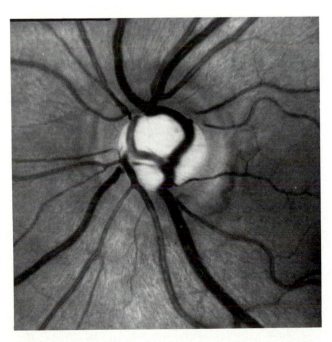

Fig. 22-4   A large optic disc (3.41 mm^2) with large physiologic cup.

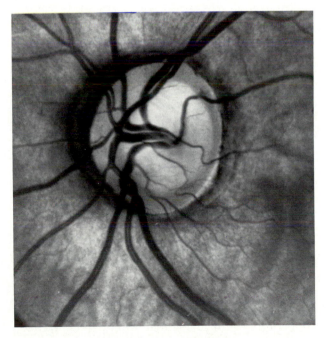

Fig. 22-5   A large optic disc with large, suspicious cup. Optic disc size is 3.58 mm^2, and neuroretinal rim area is 1.40 mm^2, which is within normal range. Optic disc has remained unchanged during 11-year follow-up with normal intraocular pressure, normal visual fields, and normal retinal nerve fiber layer.

shown that even in apparently normal eyes, there is a relationship between age, the level of intraocular pressure, and the size of the cup.[26,192]

The Framingham eye study[109,122] screened 5053 persons and found the vertical cup/disc ratio was 0.5 or greater in 550, or approximately 11%. The horizontal cup/disc ratio was 0.5 or greater in 587 of the subjects, or approximately 11.5%. Recent evidence indicates that blacks tend to have larger optic cups than whites.[30,46a]

The normal optic disc has a vertically oval appearance. The cup is normally near the center of the disc and is either round or slightly vertically oval. A cup that is much larger vertically than horizontally is unusual in a nonglaucomatous eye.[46,122] The technique used to examine the optic disc can affect the estimate of cup/disc ratio. Cup/disc ratios generally appear larger when the disc is viewed stereoscopically.[46,192]

The disc rim consists of ganglion cell axons, glial tissue, and blood vessels. The normal disc rim appears as a donut of tissue surrounding the cup. It has a pink color and appears slightly elevated above the disc margin. The superior and inferior portions of the disc rim are usually equal in width, although the temporal aspect of the rim is often thinner than elsewhere. The appearance of the disc rim varies tremendously in the normal population, especially in myopic eyes. The apparent color of the disc rim is affected by the clarity of the optical media, especially by the presence of a cataract or in aphakia.

Glaucomatous Changes

The essential pathologic process in glaucoma is loss of ganglion cell axons. As axons are lost, the amount of neural tissue in the disc rim decreases, resulting in alterations in the appearance of the disc rim and configuration of the optic cup (see Plate II, Fig. 9). A descriptive classification of the ophthalmoscopic signs of glaucomatous damage to the optic disc is shown in the box above.

Enlargement of the optic cup

The optic cup enlarges in glaucoma as a result of loss of retinal nerve fibers.[9,159] This loss occurs in two distinct patterns, localized and diffuse. In any individual patient, one or the other pattern may predominate, or both patterns may occur. The appearance of the glaucomatous cup in an individual patient will depend on the dominant pattern of the nerve fiber loss.[21,110,210] In experimental glaucoma in monkey eyes, large fibers atrophy more

---

OPTIC DISC CHANGES IN GLAUCOMA

I. Enlargement of the optic cup
  A. Generalized
  B. Local
  C. Vertical-horizontal disproportion
  D. Asymmetry between the two eyes
  E. Baring of the lamina cribrosa
II. Loss of disc rim
  A. Diffuse thinning
  B. Localized notching
III. Increased pallor of the optic disc
  A. Central area of pallor
  B. Pallor of the neuroretinal rim
  C. Global analysis of pallor
IV. Vascular changes
  A. Change in configuration of retinal vessels on the disc
    1. Nasalization
    2. Bayonetting
    3. Baring of circumlinear vessel
  B. Flame-shaped hemorrhages
V. Peripapillary atrophy

---

rapidly, although no fiber size is spared from damage.[167]

Because of the large variation in the appearance of the optic disc in the population, generalized, concentric enlargement of the cup may be difficult to distinguish from an otherwise normal but large physiologic cup; however, generalized enlargement of the glaucomatous cup is characterized by concentric thinning of the disc rim. Although the rim may be somewhat thinner in some areas than others, striking loss of disc rim in one area only is not prominent (Fig. 22-6).

In a longitudinal study Pederson and Anderson[148] found that generalized expansion of the optic cup was the most common type of progressive optic disc change in glaucoma. These disc changes have been noted to precede development of visual field defects.[134,207,228] In earlier cross-sectional studies such optic discs may have been regarded as having large physiologic cups because of the absence of visual field defects. This type of cupping has frequently been reported.[96,101,200,210] Concentric optic disc cupping is also common in childhood glaucoma.[194,195]

Localized loss of disc rim. When the localized pattern of nerve fiber loss predominates, small notches appear in the disc rim (Fig. 22-7). These notches appear as well-defined areas of thinning or complete loss of the rim and extension of the cup in one area only. Small notches at the superior and inferior poles of the disc should be looked for

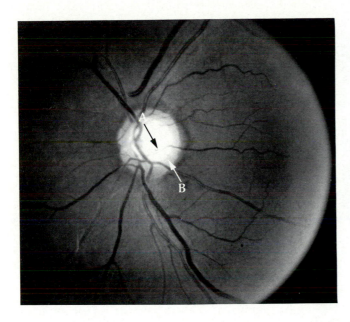

Fig. 22-6 Generalized enlargement of cup in patient with glaucoma. Central cup and area of pallor are large. Disc rim is uniformly thin and does not demonstrate areas of focal narrowing. This disc also demonstrates baring of circumlinear vessel along inferior disc rim margin. There is an area of pallor between circumlinear vessel (A) and disc rim (B).

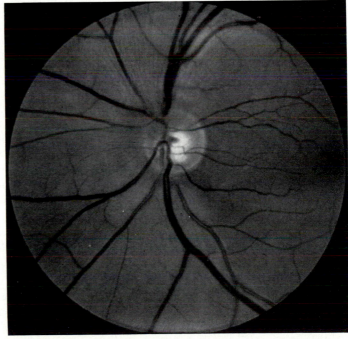

Fig. 22-7 Localized notching of disc rim. Between 5 and 6 o'clock position disc rim is thinner than elsewhere because of loss of neural tissue and subsequent extension of cup in this area.

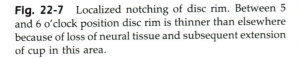

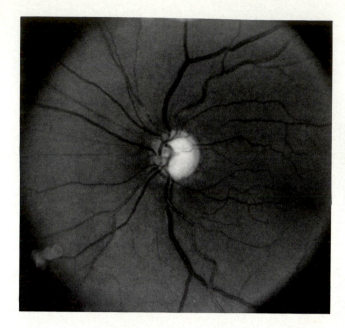

Fig. 22-8 Vertically oval cup. There has been greater loss of disc rim superiorly and inferiorly giving cup vertically oval appearance compared with configuration of entire disc. This disc also demonstrates *bayonetting* of vessels near inferior pole where artery and vein bend sharply as they cross disc margin.

in glaucoma patients. Notching of the rim occurs more often in the lower than in the upper pole.[96,110,200,210] Localized notching may sometimes be so deep as to resemble a congenital pit.[170]

It is not clear why some patients show localized loss of neural tissue at the vertical poles, whereas others show either diffuse loss of fibers or a combination of the two patterns. Structural variability in the lamina cribrosa has been proposed to explain the vulnerability of the vertical poles to glaucomatous damage.[160a] The superior and inferior poles appear to contain larger pores and thinner connective tissue support for the passage of nerve fiber bundles than do the nasal and temporal parts of the lamina. Some authors have found focal fiber loss to be more common in eyes with moderate to low intraocular pressure and concentric cupping more common in eyes with high intraocular pressure.* However, Pederson and Anderson[148] did not find such an association. They thought that these two patterns of optic nerve damage occur successively during disease progression in a given eye, so that cupping is initiated with diffuse fiber loss and followed by small, focal fiber losses. On the other hand, Quigley et al.[162,165] presented histologic evidence that damage starts with focal nerve fiber loss and is later succeeded by diffuse loss of fibers.

Vertical enlargement of the cup. Since early localized loss of nerve fibers and rim tissue tends to occur mainly at the superior and inferior poles

of the disc, the cup is most likely to enlarge more vertically than horizontally (Fig. 22-8). A vertically oval appearance of the optic cup is a frequently reported feature of the glaucomatous disc.[31,41,110,172,225] Tomlinson and Phillips[219] pointed out, however, that the optic disc normally is vertically oval, and therefore a normal optic cup is also vertically oval and may not be indicative of glaucoma. Gloster[78] stated that the shape of the cup should be considered only in relation to the shape of the disc. When the vertical dimension of the cup is much larger than one would expect based on the shape of the disc, one should suspect glaucomatous damage.

Asymmetry of cupping. In the absence of a congenital anomaly of the optic nerve or a significant degree of anisometropia, the left and right optic discs of a normal individual resemble each other closely. An easily detectable difference in the size of the cup between the two eyes of an otherwise normal individual is unusual.[24,37,46,192] In the Framingham study, an asymmetry of cup/disc ratio of greater than 0.1 was found in less than 7% of the population. One of the most common features in glaucoma patients, however, is asymmetry between the two optic cups[24,71,173] (Fig. 22-9).

Baring of the lamina cribrosa

The retinal nerve fibers leave the eye by passing through the openings of the lamina cribrosa. Normally, these openings are not well seen with the ophthalmoscope because they are obscured by the overlying nerve fibers. As nerve fibers are lost

*References 45, 58, 86, 101, 104, 201, 210.

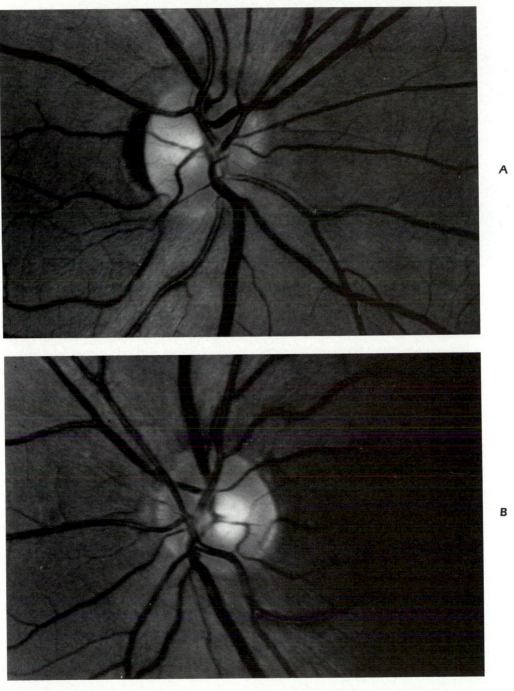

Fig. 22-9 Asymmetry of cupping and pallor. Right disc **A,** shows a significantly smaller cup and area of pallor than left disc, **B.**

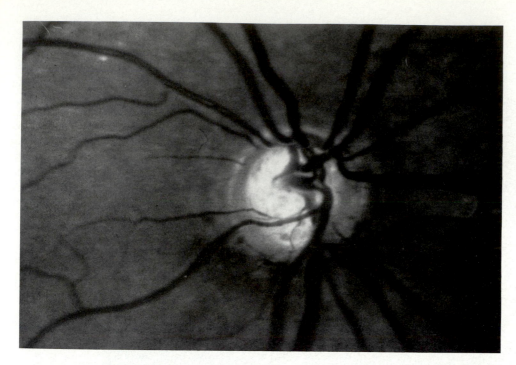

Fig. 22-10 Baring of lamina cribrosa. Openings in lamina cribrosa are easily visible in areas where neural tissue has been lost. This has been called *laminar dot sign.*

in glaucoma, however, the openings of the lamina cribrosa are more easily seen.[172,211] This has been termed the *laminar dot sign*[172] and is one of the most readily detectable signs of glaucomatous optic nerve damage (Fig. 22-10). In one study patients with more advanced glaucomatous damage were found to have larger laminar openings [130] (see Plate II, Fig. 9).

Pallor of the optic disc

Optic disc pallor is an important indicator of glaucomatous optic nerve damage,[67] and it is important to separate pallor from cupping. However, this distinction is often not made. Many investigators have not reported accurately whether they have defined the margins of the optic cup according to central area of pallor or by the bend of the small vessels across the disc rim[186] (Fig. 22-11). Cupping is a three-dimensional structure that must be assessed using the contour, not the color, of the optic disc and, therefore, can be accurately estimated only stereoscopically, whereas pallor can be measured using two-dimensional methods.

Schwartz[187] suggested that pallor represents the area of avascularity of glial tissue within which the vascular elements may lie. However, Quigley et al.[163,164] showed that pallor is not a result of a decrease in capillary density (number per unit area) but rather a thinning of the neural tissue of the rim

of the optic disc and consequent change in tissue composition and transparency. Thinning of the rim decreases the total volume of capillaries and allows a more direct reflection from the collagenous portion of the nerve head, making the returning light white in color. Fluorescein angiography may show small blood vessels in pale optic discs.[88]

The measurement of pallor is difficult because disturbances of the ocular media may significantly alter the measurements of the changes of pallor during follow-up. Variation in photographic techniques and film development is another source of error if the measurements are taken from optic disc photographs. With the use of photogrammetry, several colorimetric or densitometric methods were developed to measure the pale area of the optic disc.[50,77,147,189] The relative reflectance of light in the different points of the optic disc can be measured at a few single points or by scanning using devices with linear or rotatory systems.

The techniques of measuring the pallor can be divided into techniques that:

1. Delineate the boundary of the central area of pallor and calculate its ratio to the size of the optic disc.[136,137,179,190]
2. Measure the pallor in a few selected points on the neuroretinal rim.[127,175]
3. Record a pallor value for all points of the optic disc with a global analysis.[129]

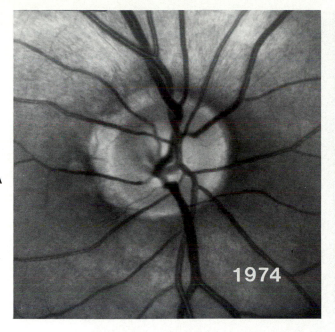
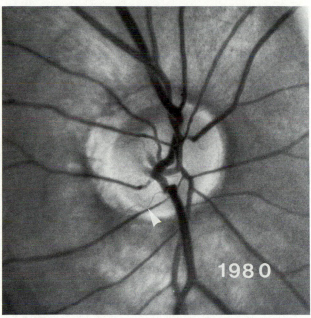

Fig. 22-11   Optic disc photographs of 60-year-old patient with ocular hypertension who developed glaucoma during 6-year follow-up. **A,** In 1974, central area of pallor had normal appearance. Inferotemporal neuroretinal rim was paler and more translucent than corresponding area superiorly. **B,** In 1980, a rim notch has developed inferotemporally indicated by shifting of small vessel *(arrow)*. Pallor area has changed less indicating discrepancy between the appearance of the cup by color and by contour.

Central area of pallor.   Schwartz[187] defined pallor as the area of maximum color contrast within the optic disc. This more or less centrally located pale area represents the bottom of the physiologic cup, which is covered by a thin layer of neuronal and glial tissue over collagenous lamina cribrosa. After delineating the central area of pallor, either with manual planimetric systems[190] or computerized devices,[136] the boundary of the optic disc is marked on the image. Pallor is expressed as a percentage of the total disc area.

In normal eyes there is an increase of pallor area with age,[190] and the maximal color contrast generally coincides with the degree of cupping; in glaucomatous eyes the latter is no longer true.[186] The area of pallor tends to be smaller than the area of cupping in early glaucoma.[110,186]

In cross-sectional[185] and follow-up studies[220] the area of pallor has correlated well with visual field changes. In ocular hypertensive patients the increase in area of pallor is greater than that in normal patients during a follow-up of 2 to 9 years[136,188,220] and correlates with changes in fluorescein angiography.[221]

Neuroretinal rim pallor.   In addition to the number of functioning nerve fibers that form the neu-

roretinal rim, the color of the rim is also important.[96,97] The normal pink color of the neuroretinal rim is displaced by pale and translucent atrophic tissue in the glaucomatous optic disc. In some cases this rim color change may occur without a change in the central area of pallor, or they may occur simultaneously.

Marre et al.[127] and Robert and Hendrickson[175] measured a relative pallor value of a few points on the disc rim. The pallor value is strongly dependent on the location of the points measured. Patient follow-up may be difficult using this method. The rim may initially be broad enough at the chosen location to allow a proper measurement, but a development of glaucomatous notching necessitates shifting the measurement site.

Acute elevation of intraocular pressure causes pallor of the optic disc.[74] Robert et al.[177,178] measured the change of pallor during artificially raised intraocular pressure and found that the response to artificial elevation in normal patients is different from that in glaucoma patients.[177] They interpreted this to be a sign of healthy autoregulatory mechanisms in normal patients, whereas the vascular bed of the glaucomatous optic disc suffers from autoregulatory failure. To avoid problems associated with

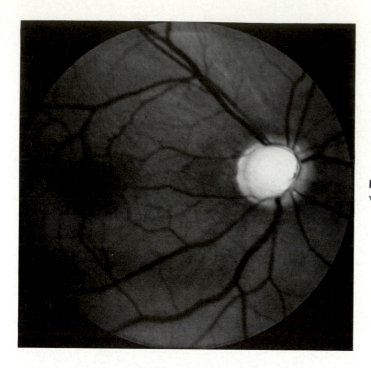

Fig. 22-12 Nasalization of vessels in optic disc with advanced cupping.

photography, they further improved their method by making continuous measurements directly from the ophthalmoscopic image of the optic disc with simultaneous intraocular pressure recordings.[92,176]

Global analysis of pallor. The Rodenstock Optic Disc Analyzer measures a relative pallor value for approximately 1000 points within the optic disc[129] (see Plate II, Fig. 2). The data of these points are used to form a cumulative pallor histogram, and the program constructs a pallor map of the entire optic disc, including points within both the central area of pallor and neuroretinal rim. Therefore, the values obtained with this method do not show a good correlation to those obtained with the computerized boundary analysis, simply because of the different techniques of measurement and definition of pallor.[129]

Vascular changes

Configuration of vessels. As the optic cup enlarges in glaucoma, the normal course and pattern of the retinal vessels on the disc may be altered. Characteristic changes in the configuration of the vessels have been described in glaucoma and serve as ophthalmoscopic clues to the presence of cupping.[172,210]

Nasalization of the vessels is thought to be a sign of glaucomatous cupping (Fig. 22-12). The retinal vessels normally enter the eye along the nasal border of the cup. If the cup is large, either physiologically or as a result of glaucoma, the vessels will appear to be displaced nasally as a result of the normal anatomic configuration. Nasalization of the vessels is not specific for glaucoma.[25]

In areas where the disc rim is absent or very thin, a retinal vessel may pass under the overhanging edge of the cup and make a sharp bend as it crosses the cup margin (see Fig. 22-8). This has been termed *bayonetting* because of the resemblance of the sharply angled vessel to the sharp angle of a rifle bayonet. This configuration is rarely seen in normal discs, even in the presence of a large physiologic cup.

Circumlinear vessels are small branches of the central retinal artery or vein that follow a curved path along the margin of the optic cup.[93] If the cup enlarges, the cup margin will recede from the circumlinear vessel, and an area of pallor will appear between the vessel and the cup margin (see Fig. 22-6). This has been called *baring of the circumlinear vessel* and is often present in glaucoma.[29] The sign, however, is not specific for glaucoma and may be seen in other optic nerve disease and in large physiologic cups.[145,213]

Hemorrhage. In 1970, Drance and Begg[56] reported a small, flame-shaped hemorrhage in the anterior optic nerve head of a 56-year-old woman with glaucomatous optic disc and visual field changes that progressed after the hemorrhage had disappeared. Subsequent reports have confirmed this initial observation.[32,33] Splinter hemorrhages had been described by Bjerrum[42] in 1889 and

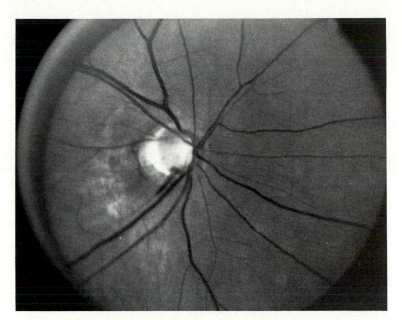

Fig. 22-13 Splinter hemorrhage extending from inferotemporal portion of optic disc onto retina in patient with primary open-angle glaucoma.

Schnabel[184] in 1908, but their possible association with progression of glaucoma had not been appreciated.

It has now become apparent that splinter hemorrhages on the optic disc are a common finding in patients with glaucoma (Fig. 22-13).* Hemorrhages are more prevalent in manifest open-angle glaucoma than in ocular hypertension,[212] but they are frequently found also in low-tension glaucoma (see Chapter 44). Disc hemorrhages are quite unusual in normal, nonglaucomatous individuals.[2,40,111] The reported prevalence of optic disc hemorrhages in high-tension glaucoma patients has varied from 4.2% to 7%, whereas a higher prevalence has been reported in low-tension glaucoma patients.[80,111] In a population survey, Bengtsson found a disc hemorrhage in 80% of glaucoma patients.[40] Women are affected by disc hemorrhages more often than men.[40]

Disc hemorrhages are usually found in the inferotemporal sector of the optic nerve head,† where they are twice as frequent as those located superiorly. This distribution correlates with the distribution of glaucomatous visual field defects, which are found more often in the superior than in the inferior visual field.[76,85,112,138,199]

Disc hemorrhages in glaucoma usually appear as splinter or flame-shaped hemorrhages in the superficial nerve fiber layer on the optic disc surface. Sometimes they extend into the peripapillary ret-

ina, but the major portion of the hemorrhage is always on the disc surface and not in the retina. Sometimes the hemorrhage occurs deeper in the neural tissue, in which case it has a more round appearance.

The patients are asymptomatic, and there is no edema of the optic disc.[32] Hemorrhages are transient but may recur,[38,89] and they are usually visible from 1 to 35 weeks.[33,89,111] It has been reported that 92% of disc hemorrhages are present for at least 4 weeks.[111] Bilateral disc hemorrhages occur in 6.3% to 29% of cases.[1,40,59,198] Recurrent hemorrhages have been reported in 12% to 62% of patients.[40,111,198]

Optic disc hemorrhages are often associated with disc rim notching at the site of the bleeding,[16,38,198,222] and they have been reported to predict the site of the retinal nerve fiber layer defect.[13]

The relationship between intraocular pressure and disc hemorrhages is unclear. Several authors have reported hemorrhages to be more prevalent in glaucoma patients with relatively low intraocular pressures.[80,111,118,202] However, Drance et al.[59] did not find any statistically significant difference in the mean intraocular pressures of patients with and without hemorrhages. Tuulonen et al.[222] reported that the smaller the variation in the intraocular pressure, the more probable the occurrence of a hemorrhage. Airaksinen,[12] however, reported diurnal variation of more than 5 mm Hg in 77% of eyes with a hemorrhage and found that the higher the intraocular pressure, the greater the risk of bleeding in the horizontal disc area. The inferior sector,

---

*References 4, 12, 38, 40, 80, 212.
†References 12, 33, 40, 124a, 198, 216.

on the other hand, was at risk even at low levels of intraocular pressure, and the superior sector was at risk at intermediate levels of intraocular pressure.

The prognostic significance of a disc hemorrhage in glaucoma has been the subject of controversy. Some authors have reported that the presence of a disc hemorrhage is a significant risk factor for future progressive optic nerve damage.[60,61] Others have not been able to confirm this finding. In glaucomatous eyes which have an optic disc hemorrhage, the incidence of visual field progression has been reported to be higher when compared either to control patients with similar visual fields[59] or to fellow eyes without a hemorrhage.[198] Ocular hypertensive patients with an optic disc hemorrhage develop glaucomatous damage more often than ocular hypertensives without a hemorrhage.[16] Multivariate analyses[60,61] have shown that a disc hemorrhage is a risk factor increasing the probability of glaucomatous damage. Tuulonen et al.,[222] however, found no statistically significant differences between patients with an optic disc hemorrhage and those without one in the rate of change of optic disc cupping and pallor when measured quantitatively with stereophotogrammetry and computerized image analysis.

Some investigators have reported that the probability of finding a disc hemorrhage increases with the number of examinations.[40,80] A hypothesis that hemorrhages occur in all glaucoma patients has also been presented.[40] Conversely, it has been suggested that patients with and without hemorrhages represent different glaucoma populations,[4,111] and that those patients who do not show a hemorrhage at one or two random examinations probably will not show one on follow-up examinations.[4] It is also possible that disk hemorrhages in glaucoma patients occur more frequently during certain phases of the disease and are rare at other times.

According to some investigators,[153,222] diabetes mellitus increases the probability of a disc hemorrhage. However, Kottler and Drance[115] reported systemic hypertension, not diabetes mellitus, to be the only systemic disorder occurring more often in glaucoma patients with disc hemorrhages.

Disc hemorrhages are regarded as a sign of the ischemic nature of glaucomatous optic neuropathy.[31,33] Quigley,[160] however, proposed a mechanical origin for the glaucomatous optic disc hemorrhage, suggesting that hemorrhages might be caused by stretching and rupture of the optic nerve capillaries in association with cupping of the disc, or by pinching of the vessels at the lamina cribrosa

in association with pressure-induced distortion of the sheets of the lamina. A venous origin of the hemorrhages has also been proposed.[40]

When a disc hemorrhage is detected, one should eliminate other ocular causes, including posterior vitreous detachment, systemic diseases, and the use of systemic drugs, such as anticoagulants. An isolated disc hemorrhage is a sign of an active process at the disc, which may lead to other glaucomatous damage over time and, therefore should be regarded as an indication of early and possibly progressive glaucomatous damage.

Peripapillary atrophy

Peripapillary atrophy is a frequently observed finding in glaucoma patients. Nevertheless, little information is available on the significance of peripapillary atrophy in the development and progression of glaucoma. Primrose[156,157] suggested that a peripapillary halo may be an early sign of glaucoma. Wilensky and Kolker[226] graded peripapillary halos and atrophies and found that the degree of halo was virtually identical in patients with or without glaucoma, but the degree of atrophy was significantly greater in glaucomatous eyes. More recently, Anderson[20,22] suggested a possible association between localized glaucomatous optic disc changes and peripapillary atrophy. He thought that a crescent may mark a sector that is anatomically weak and particularly susceptible to glaucomatous damage and suggested that peripapillary atrophy might account for the development of low-tension glaucoma.

Heijl[90] found a highly significant correlation between location of peripapillary atrophy and visual field defects. Airaksinen et al.,[10] however, found only a weak correlation between the increase in areas of peripapillary atrophy and the decrease of disc rim area during a follow-up of 9 years. The presence or absence of peripapillary atrophy did not seem to influence the rate of change of disc rim area either in low- or high-tension glaucoma.

The optic nerve head is the only location in the central nervous system where there is a physiological window in the blood-brain barrier. Extracellular substances diffuse into the optic disc. It is possible that vasoactive substances in the blood, such as angiotensin, come into contact with optic nerve head vessels causing vasospasm and ischemia.[22] In peripapillary atrophy, this window is enlarged because of lack of pigment epithelium, and therefore the area of diffusion may be greater. This could explain the correlation between the locations of peripapillary atrophy and glaucomatous optic disc damage in some eyes.

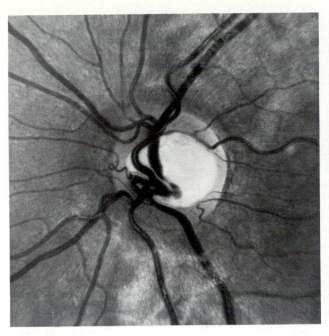

Fig. 22-14 Healthy optic disc of 8-year-old boy. Pigment epithelium reaches to edge of chorioscleral canal. There is absence of physiologic scleral rim and peripapillary atrophy.

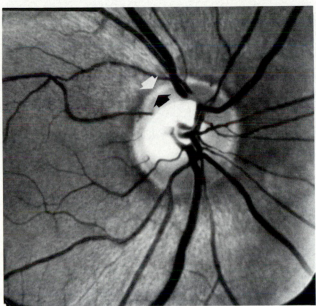

Fig. 22-15 Normal optic disc with physiologic scleral ring or Elschnig ring surrounding optic disc. Scleral rim is limited centrally to edge of chorioscleral canal *(black arrow)* and peripherally to edge of retinal pigment epithelium *(white arrow)*.

Around the optic disc there is usually a well-defined white or yellowish-white ring, the outer border formed by the edge of pigment epithelium and the inner border formed by the edge of the scleral canal. This zone is called the *scleral rim* or the *Elschnig ring.*[68,69] Around this fairly uniform physiologic scleral rim there can be at least two different types of very irregularly shaped atrophic areas with variously distinct borders. In the inner atrophic area bare sclera is visible, sometimes partly covered by choroid, with choriocapillaris and retinal pigment epithelium missing. Around this inner or more central zone there is often a more peripheral atrophic area with disorganization of the pigment and partial atrophy of the choriocapillaris and retinal pigment epithelium. These observations have led to the following classification[10]:

1. No atrophy and no physiological scleral rim (Fig. 22-14)
2. Physiologic scleral rim but no atrophy (Fig. 22-15)
3. Total atrophy of the retinal pigment epithelium and choriocapillaris, inner zone (Fig. 22-16)
4. Partial atrophy of peripapillary layers peripherally adjacent to the inner zone (Fig. 22-17)

This classification has been slightly modified by Jonas et al.[105]

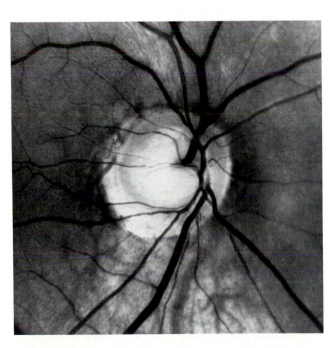

Fig. 22-16 Glaucomatous optic disc with diffuse thinning of neuroretinal rim inferiorily with corresponding total atrophy of retinal pigment epithelium and choriocapillaris.

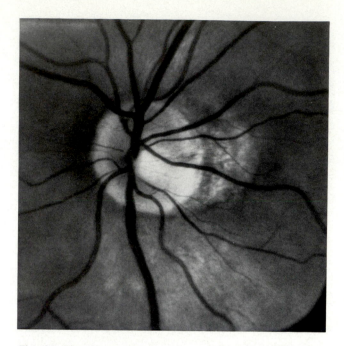

Fig. 22-17 Partial atrophy of peripapillary layers with disorganization, hypopigmentation, and hyperpigmentation of retinal pigment epithelium. Small disc hemorrhage is located at 3 o'clock position.

Examination Techniques and Documentation of Changes

Clinical techniques

Traditionally, the evaluation of the optic disc in glaucoma has relied on the ability of the experienced clinician to detect the signs of glaucomatous damage by examination of the ophthalmoscopic or photographic image of the optic disc.[203] Recently, several more objective and quantitative techniques of optic disc evaluation have been developed. These are discussed in detail in Chapter 23.

The oldest and most widely used method of optic disc examination is the direct ophthalmoscope. This method is easy to use and requires little time. The image is highly magnified, and the disc can often be seen well despite a small pupil. Because of the lack of stereopsis, subtle changes in the contour of the surface of the disc can easily escape detection. For this reason the direct ophthalmoscope should be used only for quick screening and not for careful analysis of the disc.

A variety of devices that allow stereoscopic viewing of the optic disc through the slit-lamp optics include fundus contact lenses such as the Goldmann lens, noncontact concave lenses such as the Hruby lens, and high-power 90 diopter convex lenses. These lenses provide an excellent, stereoscopic view of the disc and are the preferred clinical method of examination. The examination is more time-consuming and requires greater patient cooperation than the direct ophthalmoscope. It is also more difficult to visualize the disc through a small pupil.

Photographic techniques

Descriptions and drawings of the optic disc have been used to record the results of examinations of the optic nerve. These techniques, however, have proven less than satisfactory, and optic disc photography is now considered an indispensable adjunct to the clinical evaluation.[197]

Fundus photography was made possible by the development of reflexless ophthalmoscopy in the late nineteenth century.[217] The first practical fundus cameras were developed by Nordenson in the early part of the twentieth century.[63,139] Techniques for obtaining stereoscopic fundus photographs followed shortly thereafter.[140,217]

Whereas monoscopic photographs of the disc can be useful for recording the disc appearance, more information is obtained from stereoscopic photographs, which have become the standard method for recording the glaucomatous optic disc. Stereoscopic disc photographs should be obtained at regular intervals whenever possible on glaucoma patients.[57,91,141] Some authors, however, have claimed that monoscopic photographs can be as useful as stereoscopic photographs in detecting and following glaucomatous damage.[79,196]

Stereoscopic photographs may be obtained with techniques that produce either true stereo or a pseudostereo effect. True stereo is obtained by taking simultaneous photographs of the optic disc using the principle of stereoscopic indirect ophthalmoscopy[53,54] or beam splitters.[116,128,174,180,181] Pseudostereo effects are obtained by taking 2 consecutive photographs of the disc from different angles by shifting the camera slightly between the two photographs[18] or using the Allen stereoseparator.[19] Although pseudostereoscopic photographs are probably adequate for routine clinical evaluation, reproducible and quantitative analysis of the contour and volume and depth of the optic nerve head require true, simultaneous stereoscopic photography.[187] Pseudostereoscopy does not influence lateral measurements, which, unlike the depth of the cup, are not sensitive to changing the stereobase.

A large number of investigations have been performed in the field of ophthalmic photogrammetry.* The majority of these studies were aimed at measuring the depth and volume of the optic cup either in relative or absolute measures. Takamoto and Schwartz[214] have reported good reproducibility for cup volume and cup depth measurements in glaucomatous eyes.

The cup volume and cup depth are usually measured from the top of the nerve fiber layer (see Fig. 22-2). The thickness of the nerve fiber layer decreases with progression of glaucoma.[171] Therefore the superficial nerve fiber layer is not a stable reference level. Depending on the extent of changes above and below the level of the edge of the chorioscleral canal (Fig. 22-2), the cup volume may remain unchanged, increase, or decrease with progression of glaucoma. The edge of the chorioscleral canal might be clinically the most stable level of reference for cup volume and cup depth measurements.

Reproducibility of clinical optic disc evaluation

Despite efforts to quantitate the subjective clinical evaluation of the optic disc, it has become apparent that there are many difficulties in developing a technique that gives reproducible results that can be compared when a patient is examined at different times or by different clinicians. All the subjective methods of evaluating glaucomatous optic disc changes depend on the observer, who estimates the location of the disc margin, cup margin, depth of the cup, the margin of the area of maximum color contrast (pallor), and contour of the disc rim.

Probably the most common method of evaluating glaucomatous changes of the optic disc has been estimation of the vertical and horizontal cup/disc ratio. Pickard[151,152] and later authors† used printed grids or circles to aid in the estimation of the cup/disc ratio. The clinical use of the cup/disc ratio became popular after 1967 when Armaly defined the cup/disc ratios in normal and glaucomatous populations.[24-26]

Clinically, the cup/disc ratio estimation is usually performed with an ophthalmoscope in white light. The estimates of cup/disc ratio by different clinicians may vary greatly.[108] In a now classic study, Lichter[124] sent 20 optic disc photographs to several well-known glaucoma clinicians. Both intraobserver and interobserver variability in estimating cup/disc ratios were astonishingly high. Subsequent authors have used various techniques to reduce the variability of cup/disc estimates with better reproducibility.*

Large methodologic or definitional differences in different studies and among clinicians are such that high variability in the estimation of the cup/disc ratio continues to be a practical problem. It should be noted that the principle of cup/disc ratio measurement in glaucoma follow-up in itself is not faulty; it is just a question of choosing an appropriate method of measurement. In a routine clinical setting, cup/disc ratio estimation may be useful, but it does not meet the requirements of an accurate biometric measurement.

The percentage of pallor is typically estimated subjectively by visual inspection through an ophthalmoscope. Clinical estimation of the extent of pallor seems to be subject to the same high variability and lack of reproducibility as the estimation of cup/disc ratio.[48,123] This is mostly attributable to the limitations of the human visual system in making accurate assessments. Subjective methods are thus inexact. Manual planimetric measurements involve a subjective, time-consuming, and laborious determination of the optic disc measurement and depend on the experience of the planimetrist but do show good intraobserver reproducibility.[9,136,137]

RETINAL NERVE FIBER LAYER

In recent years much work has been done to improve the ability of clinicians to observe and quantitate optic nerve damage in glaucoma. It has become important to improve examination techniques for detection of glaucomatous damage very early in the disease process, preferably at a stage when changes might even be reversible.

Observation of the optic nerve head and testing of the visual field remain the most important clinical examinations for glaucoma suspects and patients with glaucoma. Recently, however, it has become apparent that examination of the retinal nerve fiber layer may provide information about the extent of glaucomatous damage not otherwise available through traditional techniques of perimetry and optic nerve evaluation.[158,193]

Normal Anatomy

The optic nerve head can be regarded as a bulk representation of the ganglion cell axons in the eye. The rim of the optic disc is formed by axons converging from the retina to the scleral canal. In the

---

*References 18, 19, 49, 53, 55, 98, 104, 117, 155, 180, 182, 183, 191, 215.
†References 47, 94, 113, 146, 185, 203.

*References 65, 81, 95, 113, 114, 123, 218.

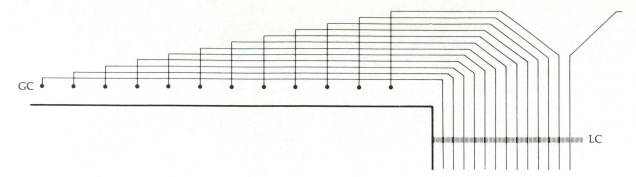

Fig. 22-18 Schematic drawing showing probable retinotopic organization of retinal nerve fibers. More peripherally originating fibers are situated deep in retina and are covered by increasing number of more proximally originating nerve fibers. Ganglion cells (GC) and lamina cribrosa (LC).

retina the axons are spread out in a thin layer; and therefore, even minor losses of axons probably can be observed in the retinal nerve fiber layer when appropriate techniques are used.

There has been some confusion about the organization of the fibers in the retinal nerve fiber layer. In 1950, Wolff and Penman[227] concluded that the nerve fibers which lie peripherally in the nerve head originate from the periphery of the retina. Later studies[132,168] showed that nerve fibers from the peripheral retina are located deep in the retinal nerve fiber layer, furthest away from the vitreous, and are also located peripherally in the anterior optic nerve head. Fibers that originate closer to the optic disc traverse the more peripheral fibers obliquely and assume a superficial position closer to the vitreous. In the optic nerve head they are located more centrally. Ogden[142-144] could not confirm this. His work suggests that the location of nerve fibers is related more to their size than their origin in the retina, but that differences are found in different primate species. Airaksinen and Alanko,[5] however, made some clinical observations that seem to support the retinotopic organization of nerve fibers presented in Figure 22-18.

In primate eyes Quigley and Addicks[161] found that 2 disc diameters from the optic nerve head the nerve fiber layer is less than 40 μm thick. Closer to the optic disc the nerve fiber layer thickness rapidly increases, up to 200 μm thick superiorly and inferiorly. In the nasal area and the papillomacular bundle area, the nerve fiber layer thickness is approximately 60 μm.

In a healthy eye the retinal nerve fiber layer appears slightly opaque with radially oriented striations. The striations have been described as resembling horsehair.[154] The normal arcuate pattern of the fibers above and below the macula is often easily seen (Fig. 22-19).

Histologic studies have shown that the striations are formed by bundles of axons compartmentalized in glial tunnels formed by Müller cell processes.[169] In the temporal and nasal peripapillary retina, the striations are fine stripes consisting of one fiber bundle per stripe, but in the thicker, arcuate areas, the striations are broader and there are several bundles per stripe.[161] In good quality photographs the retinal nerve fibers can be followed into the periphery where the fibers form the temporal horizontal raphe (Fig. 22-19). The small retinal vessels normally have a blurred and cross-hatched appearance because they are buried in the retinal nerve fiber layer (Fig. 22-20).

Classification of Retinal Nerve Fiber Layer Abnormalities

Retinal nerve fiber layer abnormalities can be separated into three groups by their appearance:

1. Slitlike or groovelike defects (Fig. 22-21) are often difficult to separate from the grooves that frequently can be seen in the healthy nerve fiber layer, particularly in the arcuate nerve fiber bundle area approximately 3 to 4 disc diameters away from the optic nerve head. In many cases these slitlike defects probably are not a sign of an abnormality. There are, however, grooves that extend all the way to the optic disc margin. These types of defects are likely to be abnormal; however, optic disc and visual field abnormalities are usually not detected.

2. Wedge-shaped defects are the easiest to detect (Figs. 22-22 and 22-23). They are located in the superior and inferior arcuate nerve fiber bundle areas and are usually well outlined against the surrounding healthy areas. They are often observed in eyes with an optic disc hemorrhage that later develop notching of the disc rim and small scotomas in the central visual field nasally.

3. Diffuse or generalized loss of nerve fibers is

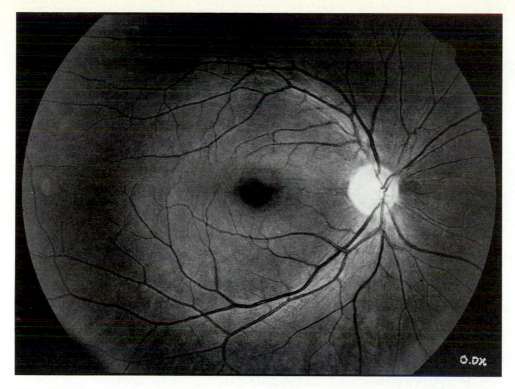

Fig. 22-19 Monochromatic blue-light photograph of normal retinal nerve fiber layer. Nerve fiber bundles curve around macula and form temporal raphe.

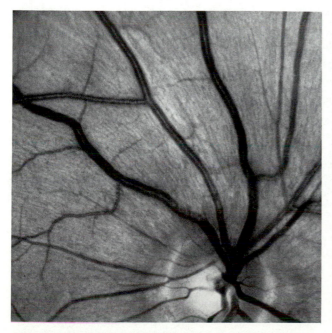

Fig. 22-20 Normal retinal nerve fiber layer with poor visibility and blurred, cross-hatched appearance of small vessels buried in nerve fiber layer with large number of axons crossing on top of them.

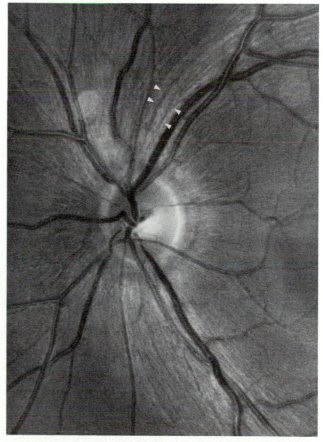

Fig. 22-21 Slitlike defects *(arrows)* in superior arcuate nerve fiber bundle area extending close to optic disc, arousing suspicion of abnormality. Otherwise, nerve fiber layer is normal.

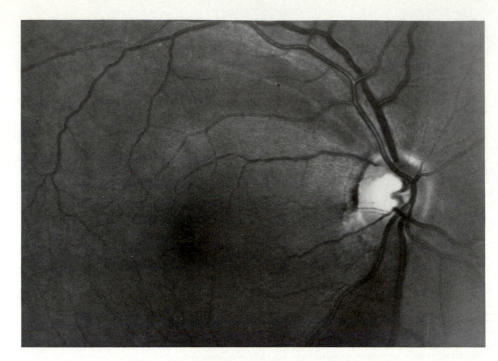

Fig. 22-22 A dense but strictly localized superior nerve fiber layer defect next to papillomacular bundles.

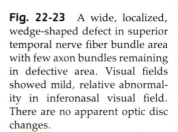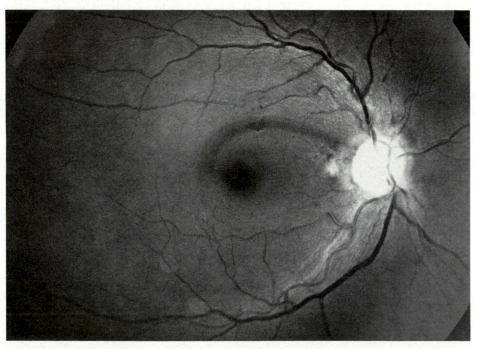

Fig. 22-23 A wide, localized, wedge-shaped defect in superior temporal nerve fiber bundle area with few axon bundles remaining in defective area. Visual fields showed mild, relative abnormality in inferonasal visual field. There are no apparent optic disc changes.

the most difficult type of abnormality to detect (Fig. 22-24). The visibility of the vessels, particularly the small capillaries buried in the nerve fiber layer, provides valuable clues when the amount of nerve fibers is assessed. Furthermore, one has to estimate the amount of fundus pigmentation in relationship to the visibility of the nerve fibers because the nerve fiber layer visibility is poorer in slightly pigmented eyes. It is helpful if a normal or clearly abnormal fellow eye can be used for comparison. It is not unusual to find generalized reduction of fibers combined with an even more profound localized fiber loss, often situated in the arcuate nerve fiber bundle areas (Fig. 22-25).

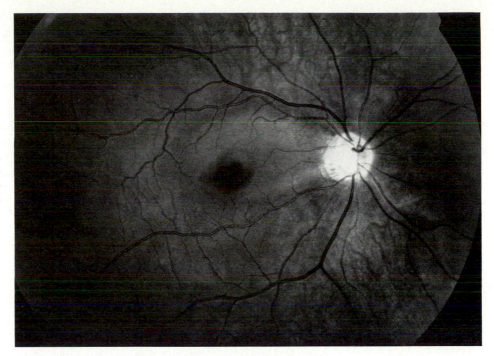

Fig. 22-24 Marked generalized atrophy of retinal nerve fiber layer. Only part of papillomacular bundles have remained intact.

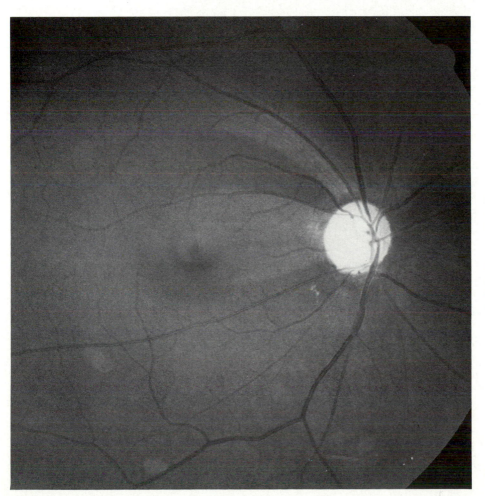

Fig. 22-25 Marked diffuse atrophy of retinal nerve fiber layer, particularly in inferior area, with dense, localized, wedge-shaped defect superotemporally. Note preserved arcuate fibers and papillomacular bundles adjacent to wedge-shaped defect superiorly.

Observation and assessment of the retinal nerve fiber layer can be affected by the pupil size, clarity of the ocular media, and pigmentation of the fundus. A large interobserver variation in retinal nerve fiber layer assessment has been observed,[208] but intraobserver results are consistent.[7] A major problem is that evaluation of photographs is subjective and requires much experience. It is hoped that computerized image analysis might provide possibilities for further development of retinal nerve fiber layer assessment and quantification of the findings.

Glaucomatous Changes

Hoyt et al.[99,100] were the first to report the significance of narrow, slitlike defects and large wedge-shaped defects of the retinal nerve fiber layer in glaucoma. They also noted diffuse loss of the nerve fibers in some patients. In a retrospective study, Sommer et al.[206] estimated that retinal nerve fiber layer abnormalities may precede visual field damage by as much as 5 years and that detectable nerve fiber layer defects were present in almost all eyes that developed visual field defects, but were unusual in ocular hypertensive eyes that did not lose visual field.

Quigley et al.[165] found that nerve fiber layer defects were generally present in eyes with glaucomatous visual field loss and were rarely seen in normal eyes. They concluded that examination of the nerve fiber layer was as sensitive in detecting eyes with visual field loss as was the optic disc configuration. Subsequent studies confirmed the correlation between the location of the nerve fiber loss and the visual field defects, but loss of a large number of axons (up to 40%) is possible in the presence of normal visual fields examined manually with a Goldmann perimeter.[162] Histologic studies in an animal model showed that clinical detection of nerve fiber layer atrophy was possible after loss of 50% of the neural tissue in a given area.[161]

Airaksinen et al.[13] showed that small splinter hemorrhages often preceded the development of nerve fiber layer defects, and the location of the defect was accurately predicted by the location of the hemorrhage.[2] In many of these patients visual fields were normal despite the presence of a clearly outlined, wedge-shaped area of nerve fiber loss in the retina. These same patients were later examined by Airaksinen and Heijl[3] with high resolution automated perimetry. By specifically targeting the examination to the areas of damage seen in the photographs, visual field defects could be demonstrated in the majority of cases. This technique, however, was very time consuming and not practical in the routine clinical setting. Airaksinen and Alanko[5] further showed that nerve fiber layer defects developed before detectable enlargement of the cup/disc ratio in ocular hypertensive patients following the appearance of a disc hemorrhage.

It has been recognized that the damage seen in the nerve fiber layer in glaucoma may be either diffuse or localized. Although both types occur in advanced glaucoma, early cases often tend to demonstrate one type or the other. Diffuse damage is somewhat more difficult to detect than localized damage, but it seems to be more common in patients with other signs of glaucomatous damage, whereas localized defects are more common in patients thought to have ocular hypertension.[7] The diffuse type of retinal nerve fiber layer abnormality often goes along with concentric enlargement of the optic cup,[6] generalized reduction of retinal sensitivity,[8] and disturbances of color vision.[11]

In a large prospective study, Sommer et al.[108] found that the detection of nerve fiber layer defects was a highly sensitive and specific way to identify glaucomatous eyes. They also showed that focal slitlike defects were much less specific and likely to be normal.

Histologic studies have shown that the pattern of nerve fiber layer loss is different in glaucoma when compared to other optic neuropathies.[162,166,167] This finding has been interpreted as indicating a different mechanism for the damage seen in glaucoma.

Evaluation of the nerve fiber layer offers the possibility of improved early detection of glaucomatous damage. The technique is still qualitative and requires subjective interpretation by the clinician. Quantitative and objective methods for evaluating the nerve fiber layer are being developed.

Examination Techniques

Clinical techniques

It is possible to see the retinal nerve fiber layer through a dilated pupil with an ophthalmoscope using white or green light, but a much better view can be achieved when a contact or Hruby lens is used together with a green filter in front of the slit-lamp light source. A wide slit-beam provides even illumination of the fundus. With these methods, most sector-shaped retinal nerve fiber layer defects can be detected, but some will be visible only in good photographs. On the other hand, all the defects visible by clinical examination can generally be demonstrated with photographs.

The normal crosshatched and blurred appearance of small retinal vessels is an important and useful sign in a retinal nerve fiber layer examination. With a decreasing number of fibers, the small vessels become more and more clearly visible and eventually lie totally naked on the retina, covered only by the internal limiting membrane. In areas where the nerve fiber layer has been lost, the small retinal vessels appear unusually sharp, clear, and well focused (Fig. 22-26).

The background color of the fundus also provides a clue to the state of the nerve fiber layer. In defective areas, particularly in areas of localized nerve fiber loss, ophthalmoscopic or contact lens observation reveals, in white light, a darker and deeper red color of the defective area in contrast to the more silvery or opaque hue of the intact nerve fiber layer. With green light, the defective areas appear to be considerably darker green than the surrounding normal areas. Additionally, in defective areas the bared retinal pigment epithelium has a mottled appearance (see Fig. 22-21).

Photographic techniques

In 1917, Vogt[223] introduced retinal nerve fiber layer evaluation in red-free light into ophthalmology, but it was not until 50 years later that monochromatic light was used in ophthalmic photography by Behrendt and Wilson.[35] They used interference filters and black-and-white film and noticed that although the retinal nerve fiber layer was invisible in red light, its visibility was enhanced in green-blue and blue light. Blue light does not penetrate beyond the retinal nerve fiber layer and is reflected from the superficial nerve fiber layer back to the camera except in areas where the nerve fiber layer is destroyed and the light is absorbed by the underlying pigment epithelium. This provides the contrast between normal and degenerated areas.[34]

Mizuno et al.[133] found that the visibility of nerve fibers was better in the dark-adapted than in the light-adapted retina. Delori and Gragoudas[51] found wave lengths from 475 to 520 nanometers (nm) best suited for retinal nerve fiber layer photography. Later Ducrey et al.[62] settled on 495 nm for clear optic media and 545 nm for turbid media. Miller and George[131] achieved best results with a 540 nm filter and black-and-white film, a result confirmed by other authors.[126]

Sommer et al.[204] could improve the nerve fiber

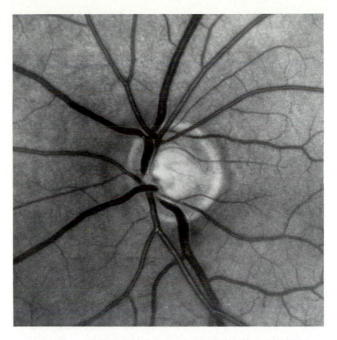

Fig. 22-26 Marked diffuse thinning of retinal nerve fiber layer in association with concentrically enlarged optic cup. Note good visibility of vessels, including small capillaries. Atrophy of retinal nerve fiber layer has unmasked mottled appearance of retinal pigment epithelium.

visibility using a 566 nm short-pass cut-off filter. They also found that polarizing light may add to the visibility of the nerve fibers.[205] Airaksinen[15] and later Peli et al.[149] reported easier detection of nerve fiber layer defects with a wide angle fundus camera, using high-resolution, fine-grain, black-and-white film with a blue monochromatic interference filter (wave length 495 nm). This technique was published in detail by Airaksinen and Nieminen.[14] Peli et al.[150] have used computerized image enhancement to improve analysis of the nerve fiber layer photographs.

In another method the nerve fiber layer is first photographed on color film using white light, and then the color slide is reproduced on black-and-white film through a green filter to eliminate the disturbing image of deeper retina and choroid.[72,99] With proper laboratory techniques and some special methods, good results can be achieved.[73] Delori et al.[52] reported, however, that with monochromatic light, nerve fibers can be observed 2 to 3 times further away from the optic disc than with white light. In part this is also caused by the higher resolving power of low-sensitive, black-and-white films in contrast to that of the color films.[62,72]

REFERENCES

1. Airaksinen, PJ: Fellow eyes of glaucomatous patients with uniocular optic disc hemorrhage, Acta Opthalmol 59:231, 1981
2. Airaksinen, PJ: Early glaucomatous changes after an optic disc hemorrhage. In Lütjen-Drecoll, E, editor: Basic aspects of glaucoma research, Stuttgart, New York, 1982, FK Schattauer Verlag
3. Airaksinen, PJ, and Heijl, A: Visual field and retinal nerve fiber layer in early glaucoma after optic disc hemorrhage, Acta Ophthalmol 61:186, 1983
4. Airaksinen, PJ: Are optic disc hemorrhages a common finding in all glaucoma patients? Acta Ophthalmol 62:193, 1984
5. Airaksinen, PJ, and Alanko, HI: Effect of retinal nerve fiber loss on the optic nerve head configuration in early glaucoma, v Graefe's Arch Klin Exp Ophthalmol 220:193, 1983
6. Airaksinen, PJ, and Drance, SM: Neuroretinal rim area and retinal nerve fiber layer in glaucoma, Arch Ophthalmol 103:203, 1985
7. Airaksinen, PJ, et al: Diffuse and localized nerve fiber loss in glaucoma, Am J Ophthalmol 98:566, 1984
8. Airaksinen, PJ, et al: Visual field and retinal nerve fiber layer comparisons in glaucoma, Arch Ophthalmol 103:205, 1985
9. Airaksinen, PJ, Drance, SM, and Schulzer, M: Neuroretinal rim areas in early glaucoma, Am J Ophthalmol 99:1, 1985
10. Airaksinen, PJ, et al: Change of peripapillary atrophy in glaucoma. In Krieglstein, GK, editor: Glaucoma update III, Berlin, 1987, Springer-Verlag
11. Airaksinen, PJ, et al: Color vision and retinal nerve fiber layer in early glaucoma, Am J Ophthalmol 101:208, 1986
12. Airaksinen, PJ, Mustonen, E, and Alanko, HI: Optic disc hemorrhages: analysis of stereophotographs and clinical data of 112 patients, Arch Ophthalmol 99:1795, 1981
13. Airaksinen, PJ, Mustonen, E, and Alanko, HI: Optic disc hemorrhages precede retinal nerve fiber layer defects in ocular hypertension, Acta Ophthalmol 59:627, 1981
14. Airaksinen, PJ, and Nieminen, H: Retinal nerve fiber layer photography in glaucoma, Ophthalmol 92:877, 1985
15. Airaksinen, PJ, Nieminen, H, and Mustonen, E: Retinal nerve fiber layer photography with a wide angle fundus camera, Acta Ophthalmol 60:362, 1982
16. Airaksinen, PJ, and Tuulonen, A: Early glaucoma changes in patients with and without an optic disc hemorrhage, Acta Opthalmolo 62:197, 1984
17. Albert, DM: Jaeger's atlas of diseases of the ocular fundus, Philadelphia, 1972, WB Saunders Co
18. Allen, L: Ocular fundus photography, Am J Ophthalmol 57:13, 1964
19. Allen, L, Kirkendall, WM, Snyder, WB and Frazier, O: Instant positive photographs and stereograms of ocular fundus fluorescence, Arch Ophthalmol 75:192, 1966
20. Anderson, DR: Correlation of the peripapillary anatomy with the disc damage and field abnormalities in glaucoma. In Greve, EL and Heijl, A, editors: Fifth International Visual Field Symposium, The Netherlands, 1983, Dr W Junk Publishers
21. Anderson, DR: What happens to the optic disc and retina in glaucoma? Ophthalmol 90:766, 1983
22. Anderson, DR: Relationship of peripapillary haloes and crescents to glaucomatous cupping. In Krieglstein, GK, editor: Glaucoma update III, Berlin, 1987, Springer-Verlag
23. Armaly, MF: Lessons to be learned from a glaucoma surgery, J Iowa Med Soc 50:501, 1960
24. Armaly, MF: Genetic determination of cup/disc ratio of the optic nerve, Arch Ophthalmol 78:35, 1967
25. Armaly, MF: The optic cup in the normal eye. I. Cup width, depth, vessel displacement, ocular tension, and outflow facility, Am J Ophthalmol 68:401, 1969
26. Armaly, MF, and Sayegh, NE: The cup/disc ratio, Arch Ophthalmol 82:191, 1969
27. Balazsi, AG, Drance, SM, Schulzer, and Douglas, GR: Neuroretinal rim area in suspected glaucoma and early chronic open-angle glaucoma: correlation with parameters of visual function, Arch Ophthalmol 102:1011, 1984
28. Balazsi, AG, et al: The effect of age on the nerve fiber population of the human optic nerve, Am J Ophthalmol 97:760, 1984
29. Balazsi, G, and Werner, EB: Relationship between baring of circumlinear vessels of the optic disc and glaucomatous visual field loss, Can J Ophthalmol 18:333, 1983
30. Beck, RW, et al: Is there a racial difference in physiologic cup size? Ophthalmology 92:873, 1985
31. Begg, IS, Drance, SM, and Goldman, H: Fluorescein angiography in the evaluation of focal circulatory ischemia of the optic nerve head in relation to the arcuate scotoma in glaucoma, Can J Ophthalmol 7:68, 1972
32. Begg, IS, Drance, SM, and Sweeney, VP: Hemorrhage on the disc: a sign of acute ischaemic optic neuropathy in chronic simple glaucoma, Can J Ophthalmol 5:321, 1970
33. Begg, IS, Drance, SM, and Sweeney, VP: Ischaemic optic neuropathy in chronic simple glaucoma, Br J Ophthalmol 55:73, 1971
34. Behrendt, T, and Duane, TD: Investigation of fundus oculi with spectral reflectance photography. I. Depth and integrity of fundal structures, Arch Ophthalmol 75:375, 1966
35. Behrendt, T, and Wilson, LA: Spectral reflectance photography of the retina, Am J Ophthalmol 59:1079, 1965
36. Bengtsson, B: The variation and covariation of cup and disc diameters, Acta Ophthalmol 54:804, 1976

37. Bengtsson, B: The alteration and asymmetry of cup and disc diameters, Acta Ophthalmol 58:726, 1980

38. Bengtsson, B: Findings associated with glaucomatous visual field defects, Acta Ophthalmol 58:20, 1980

39. Bengtsson, B: The inheritance and development of cup and disc diameters, Acta Ophthalmol 58:733, 1980

40. Bengtsson, B, Holmin, C, and Krakau, CET: Disc hemorrhage and glaucoma, Acta Ophthalmol 59:1, 1981

41. Betz, P, et al: Biometric study of the disc cup in open-angle glaucoma, v Graefe's Arch Klin Ophthalmol 218:70, 1982

42. Bjerrum, F: Om en tilfojelse til den saedvanlige synfletsundersogelse samt om synsfeltet ved glaucom, Nord Ophthalmol Tidsskr 2:141, 1889

43. Britton, RJ, et al: The area of the neuroretinal rim of the optic nerve in normal eyes, Am J Ophthalmol 103:497, 1987

44. Caprioli, J, and Miller, JM: Optic disc rim area is related to disc size in normal subjects, Arch Ophthalmol 105:1683, 1987

45. Caprioli, J, and Spaeth, GL: Comparison of the optic nerve head in high- and low-tension glaucoma, Arch Ophthalmol 103:1145, 1985

46. Carpel, EF, and Engstrom, PF: The normal cup-disk ratio, Am J Ophthalmol 91:588, 1981

46a. Chi, T, et al: Racial variation in optic disc parameters, Invest Ophthalmol Vis Sci 29:134, 1988

47. Colenbrander, MC: Measurement of optic disc excavation, Ophthalmologica 139:491, 1960

48. Cooper, RL, Alder, VA, and Constable, IJ: Measurement vs. judgement of cup-disc ratios: statistical evaluation of intraobserver and interobserver error, Glaucoma 4:169, 1982

49. Crock, G: Stereotechnology in medicine, Trans Ophthalmol Soc UK 90:577, 1970

50. Davies, EWG: Colorimetric measurement of the optic disc, Exp Eye Res 9:106, 1970

51. Delori, FC, and Gragoudas, ES: Examination of the ocular fundus with monochromatic light, Ann Ophthalmol 8:703, 1976

52. Delori, FC, et al: Monochromatic ophthalmoscopy and fundus photography: the normal fundus, Arch Ophthalmol 95:861, 1977

53. Donaldson, DD: A new camera for stereoscopic fundus photography, Trans Am Ophthalmol Soc 62:429, 1964

54. Donaldson, DD: A new camera for stereoscopic fundus photography, Arch Ophthalmol 73:253, 1965

55. Dowman, IJ, and Elkington, AR: Photogrammetric measurement of the retina of the eye. In Proceeding of the Symposium of Commission V International Society for Photogrammetry, Biostereometrics 74:972, 1974

56. Drance, SM, and Begg, IS: Sector hemorrhage: a probable acute ischemic disc change in chronic simple glaucoma, Can J Ophthalmol 5:137, 1970

57. Drance, SM, and Airaksinen, PJ: Signs of early damage in open-angle glaucoma. In Weinstein, GW, editor: Open-angle glaucoma: contemporary issues in ophthalmology, New York, 1986, Churchill Livingstone

58. Drance, SM, et al: Diffuse visual field loss in chronic open-angle and low-tension glaucoma, Am J Ophthalmol 104:577, 1987

59. Drance, SM, et al: The importance of disc hemorrhage in the prognosis of chronic open-angle glaucoma, Arch Ophthalmol 95:226, 1977

60. Drance, SM, et al: Use of discriminant analysis. II. Identification of persons with glaucomatous visual field defects, Arch Ophthalmol 96:1571, 1978

61. Drance, SM, et al: Multivariate analysis in glaucoma: use of discriminant analysis in predicting glaucomatous visual field damage, Arch Ophthalmol 99:1019, 1981

62. Ducrey, NM, Delori, FC, and Gragoudas, ES: Monochromatic ophthalmoscopy and fundus photography. II. The Pathological Fundus, Arch Ophthaomol 97:288, 1979

63. Duke-Elder, S: The foundations of ophthalmology: heredity, pathology, diagnosis, and therapeutics. In System of ophthalomolgy, vol 7, St Louis, 1962, The CV Mosby Co.

64. Duke-Elder, S: Diseases of the lens and vitreous: glaucoma and hypotony. In System of ophthalmology, vol 11, London, 1969, Henry Kimpton

65. Eiden, SB, et al: Interexaminer reliability of the optic cup to disc ratio assessment, Am J Optom Physiol Opt 63:753, 1986

66. Elliot, RH: Glaucoma: a handbook for the general practitioner, London, 1917, HK Lewis & Co, Ltd

67. Elliot, RH: A treatise on glaucoma, ed 2, London, 1922, Fraude, Hodder and Stoughton

68. Elschnig, A: Das Colobom am Sehnerveneintritt und der Conus nach unten, Archiv für Augenheilkunde 51:391, 1900

69. Elschnig, A: Der normale Sehnerveneintritt des menschlichen Auges. Denkschrift der Kaiserlichen Akademie der Wissensschaften. In Wien, Mathematisch-naturwissenschaftliche Klasse, Band 70: 219, 1901

70. Elschnig, A: Über physiologische, atrophische und glaukomatöse Excavation, Ber Dtsch Ophthalmol 34:2, 1907

71. Fishman, RS: Optic disc asymmetry: a sign of ocular hypertension, Arch Ophthalmol 84:590, 1970

72. Frisen, L: Photography of the retina nerve fiber layer: an optimised procedure, Br J Ophthalmol 64:641, 1980

73. Frisen, L, and Hoyt, WF: Unsharp masking in fundus photography, Invest Ophthalmol 12:461, 1973

74. Fritz, A: Physiopathologie de la circulation capillaire et veineuse retinienne, Doc Ophthalmol 7:265, 1954

75. Fuchs, E: Über die Lamina cribrosa, v Graefe's Arch Ophthalmol, 91:435, 1916

76. Furuno, F, and Matzuo, H: Early stage progression in glaucomatous visual field changes, Doc Ophthalmol Proc Ser 19:247, 1979

77. Gloster, J: The colour of the optic disc, Doc Ophthalmol 26:155, 1969

78. Gloster, J: Vertical ovalness of glaucomatous cupping, Br J Ophthalmol 59:721, 1975

79. Gloster, J: The value of optic disc photography in the diagnosis and management of glaucoma. In Rehak, S, Krasnov, MM, and Paterson, GD, editors, Prague, Avicenum/Berlin, 1977, Springer-Verlag

80. Gloster, J: Incidence of optic disc hemorrhages in chronic simple glaucoma and ocular hypertension, Br J Ophthalmol 65:452, 1981

81. Good, GW, and Quinn, TQ: Component evaluation of cup/disk ratio estimation, J Am Optometric Assoc 55:889, 1984

82. von Graefe, A: Vorläufige Nortiz über das Wesen des Glaucoma, v Graefe's Arch Ophthalmol 1:371, 1954

83. von Graefe, A: Mitteilungen vermischten Inhalts, v Graefe's Arch Ophthalmol 2:187, 1855

84. von Graefe, A: Amaurose mit Sehnervenexcavation, v Graefe's Arch Ophthalmol 3:484, 1857

85. Gramer, E, Gerlach, R, Krieglstein, GK, and Leydhecker, W: Zur Topographie früher glaukomatöser Gesichtsfeldausfälle bei der Computerperimetrie, Klin Mbl Augenheilk 180:515, 1982

86. Greve, EL, and Geijssen, C: Comparison of glaucomatous visual field defects in patients with high and with low intraocular pressures. In Greve, EL, and Heijl, A, editors: Fifth International Visual Field Symposium, Dordrecht, 1983, Dr. W Junk Publishers

87. Greve, R: Zur Geschichte des Glaukoms, Klin Mbl Augenheilk 188:167, 1986

88. Hayreh, SS: Colour and fluorescence of the optic disc, Ophthalmologica 165:100, 1972

89. Heijl, A: Frequent disc photography and computerized perimetry in eyes with optic disc hemorrhage: a pilot study, Acta Ophthalmol 64:274, 1986

90. Heijl, A, and Samander, C: Peripapillary atrophy and glaucomatous visual field defects. In Greve, EL, and Heijl, A, editors: Sixth International Visual Field Symposium, The Netherlands, 1985, Dr W Junk Publishers

91. Heilmann, K, and Richardson, KT: Clinical value of photography. In Glaucoma: conceptions of a disease, Stüttgart, Germany, 1978, Georg Thieme Verlag

92. Hendrickson, P, Robert, Y, and Stöckli, HP: Principles of photometry in the papilla, Arch Ophthalmol 102:1704, 1984

93. Herschler, J, and Osher, RH: Baring of the circumlinear vessel: an early sign of optic nerve damage, Arch Ophthalmol 98:865, 1980

94. Hitchings, RA, Brown, DB, and Anderson, SA: Glaucoma screening by means of an optic disc grid, Br J Ophthalmol 67:352, 1983

95. Hitchings, RA, et al: An optic disc grid: its evaluation in reproducibility studies on the cup-disc ratio, Br J Ophthalmol 67:356, 1983

96. Hitchings, RA, and Spaeth, GL: The optic disc in glaucoma. I. Classification, Br J Ophthalmol 60:778, 1976

97. Hitchings, RA, and Spaeth, GL: The optic disc in glaucoma. II. Correlation of the appearance of the optic disc with the visual field, Br J Ophthalmol 61:107, 1977

98. Holm, O, and Krakau, CET: Photographic method for measuring the volume of papillary excavations, Ann Ophthalmol 1:327, 1970

99. Hoyt, WF, Frisen, L, and Newman, NM: Funduscopy of nerve fiber layer defects in glaucoma, Invest Ophthalmol 12:814, 1973

100. Hoyt, WF, and Newman, NM: The earliest sign of glaucoma, Lancet 1:692, 1972

101. Iwata, K: Topographical analysis on the genesis of glaucomatous cupping, Glaucoma 1:16, 1979

102. von Jaeger, E: Über Staar und Staaroperationen, Vienna, 1854, LW Seidel

103. von Jaeger, E: Ophthalmoskopischer Handatlas, Vienna, 1869, Druck und Verlag der KK Hof und Staatsdruckerei

104. Jönsas, CH: Stereophotogrammetric techniques for measurements of the eye ground, Acta Ophthalmol 117(Suppl):1, 1972

105. Jonas, JB, Airaksinen, PJ, and Robert, Y: Definitionsentwurf der intra- und para-papillären Parameter fur die Biomorphometrie des Nervus Optikus, Klin Mbl Augenheilk (In press)

106. Jonas, JB, Gusek, GC, Guggenmoos-Holzmann, I, and Naumann, GOH: Size of the optic nerve scleral canal and comparison with intravital determination of optic disc dimensions, v Graefe's Arch Klin Exp Ophthalmol 226:213, 1988

107. Jonas, JB, Händel, A, and Naumann, GOH: Tatsächliche Masse der Vitalen Papilla Nervi Optici dei Menschen, Fortschr Ophthalmol 84:356, 1987

108. Kahn, HA, et al: Standardizing diagnostic procedures, Am J Ophthalmol 79:768, 1975

109. Kahn, HA, and Milton, RC: Alternative definitions of open-angle glaucoma: effect on prevalence and associations in the Framingham eye study, Arch Ophthalmol 98:2172, 1980

110. Kirsch, RE, and Anderson, DR: Clinical recognition of glaucomatous cupping, Am J Ophthalmol 75:442, 1973

111. Kitazawa, Y, Shirato, S, and Yamamoto, T: Optic disc hemorrhage in low-tension glaucoma, Ophthalmol 93:853, 1986

112. Kitazawa, Y, Takahashi, O, and Ohiva, Y: The mode of development and progression of field defects in early glaucoma: a follow-up study Doc Ophthalmol Proc Ser 19:211, 1979

113. Klein, BEK, et al: Quantitation of optic disc cupping, Ophthalmol 92:1654, 1985

114. Klein, BEK, et al: Optic disc cupping as clinically estimated from photographs, Ophthalmology 94:1481, 1987

115. Kottler, MS, and Drance, SM: Studies of hemorrhage on the optic disc, Can J Ophthalmol 11:102, 1976

116. Kottler, MS, Drance, SM, and Schulzer, M: Simultaneous stereophotography: its value in clinical assessment of the topography of the optic cup, Can J Ophthalmol 10:453, 1975

117. Kottler, MS, Rosenthal, AR, and Falconer, DG: Digital photogrammetry of the optic nerve head, Invest Ophthalmol 13:116, 1974

118. Krakau CET: Disc hemorrhages: forerunners of chronic glaucoma. In Krieglstein, GK, and Leydhecker, W, editors: Glaucoma update II, Heidelberg, 1983, Springer-Verlag

119. Kronfeld, PC: History of ophthalmology, Surv Ophthalmol 19:154, 1974

120. Kronfeld, PC: Glaucomatous cupping: the history of its recognition. In Symposium on glaucoma, Springfield, IL, 1976, Charles C Thomas, Publisher

121. Law, FW: The origin of the ophthalmoscope, Ophthalmology 93:140, 1986

122. Leibowitz, HM, et al: The Framingham eye study monograph, Surv Ophthalmol 24:335, 1980

123. Leydhecker, W, Krieglstein, GK, and Collani, E: Observer variation in applanation tonometry and estimation of the cup disk ratio. In Krieglstein, GK, and Leydhecker, W, editors: Glaucoma update, Berlin, 1979, Springer-Verlag

124. Lichter, PR: Variability of expert observers in evaluating the optic disc, Trans Am Ophthalmol Soc 74:532, 1976

124a. Lichter, PR and Henderson, JW: Optic nerve infarction, Trans Am Ophthalmol Soc 75:103, 1977.

125. Littmann, H: Zür Bestimmung der wahren Grösse eines Objektes auf dem Hintergrund des lebenden Auges, Klin Mbl Augenheilkd 180:286, 1982

126. Manor, RS, et al: Narrow-band (540-NM) green-light stereoscopic photography of the surface details of the peripapillary retina, Am J Ophthalmol 91:774, 1981

127. Marre, E, Mierdel, P, and Zenker, HJ: Farbwerte ausgewählter Papillenareale beim Glaukom, Klin Mbl Augenheilk 185:388, 1984

128. Matsui, M, Pare, J-M, and Norton, EWD: Simultaneous stereophotogrammetric and angiographic fundus camera, Am J Ophthalmol 85:230, 1978

129. Mikelberg, FS, et al: Measurement of optic nerve head pallor with a video-ophthalmograph and with computerized boundary analysis, Can J Ophthalmol 23:120, 1988

130. Miller, KM, and Quigley, HA: The clinical appearance of the lamina cribrosa as a function of the extent of glaucomatous optic nerve damage, Ophthalmology 95:135, 1988

131. Miller, NR, and George, TW: Monochromatic (red-free) photography and ophthalmoscopy of the peripapillary retinal nerve fiber layer, Invest Ophthalmol Vis Sci 17:1121, 1978

132. Minckler, DS: The organization of nerve fiber bundles in the primate optic nerve head, Arch Ophthalmol 98:1630, 1980

133. Mizuno, K, et al: Red-free light fundus photography: photographic optogram, Invest Ophthalmol 7:241, 1968

134. Motolko, M, and Drance, SM: Features of the optic disc in preglaucomatous eyes, Arch Ophthalmol 99:1992, 1981

135. Müller, H: Glaukom und Excavation des Sehnerven. I. Über Glaukom. Sitz Ber d Phys Med Ges zu Würzburg p 26, 1856

136. Nagin, P, and Schwartz, B: Detection of increased pallor over time: computerized image analysis in untreated ocular hypertension, Ophthalmology 92:252, 1985

137. Nagin, P, Schwartz, B, and Nanba, K: The reproducibility of computerized boundary analysis for measuring optic disc pallor in the normal optic disc, Ophthalmology 92:243, 1985

138. Nicholas, SP, and Werner, EB: Location of early glaucomatous visual field defects, Can J Ophthalmol 15:131, 1980

139. Nordenson, JW: Om centrisk fotografering au ogonbotten, Hygea 77:1538, 1915

140. Nordenson, JW: Stereoskopische Ophthalmographie durch einfache Aufnahmen, Upsala Lak Forh 78:338, 1927

141. Odberg, T, and Riise, D: Early diagnosis of glaucoma: the value of successive sterophotography of the optic disc, Acta Ophthalmol 63:257, 1985

142. Ogden, TE: The nerve fiber layer of the primate: an autoradiographic study, Invest Ophthalmol 13:95, 1974

143. Ogden, TE: Nerve fiber layer of the macaque retina: retinotopic organization, Invest Ophthalmol Vis Sci 24:85, 1983

144. Ogden, TE: Nerve fiber layer of the owl monkey retina: retinotopic organization, Invest Ophthalmol Vis Sci 24:265, 1983

145. Osher, RH, and Herschler, J: The significance of baring of the circumlinear vessel: a prospective study, Arch Ophthalmol 99:817, 1981

146. Parr, JC: Clinical estimation of optic disc cupping with a description of a graticule, Trans Ophthalmol Soc NZ 18:93, 1966

147. Pe'er, J, and Zajicek, G: Computer image analysis of the optic disc, Ophthalmologica 181:266, 1980

148. Pederson, JE, and Anderson, DR: The mode of progressive disc cupping in ocular hypertension and glaucoma, Arch Ophthalmol 98:490, 1980

149. Peli, E, et al: Nerve fiber layer photography: a comparative study, Acta Ophthalmol 65:71, 1987

150. Peli, E, Hedges, TR, and Schwartz, B: Computerized enhancement of retinal nerve fiber layer, Acta Ophthalmol 64:113, 1986

151. Pickard, R: A method of recording disc alterations and a study of the growth of normal and abnormal disc cups, Br J Ophthalmol 7:81, 1923

152. Pickard, R: The alteration in size of the normal optic disc cup, Br J Ophthalmol 32:355, 1948

153. Poinoosawmy, D, Gloster, J, Nagasubramanian, S, and Hitchings, RA: Association between optic disc hemorrhages in glaucoma and abnormal glucose tolerance, Br J Ophthalmol 70:599, 1986

154. Pollock, SC, and Miller, NR: The retinal nerve fiber layer, Int Ophthalmol Clin 26:201, 1986

155. Portney, GL: Photogrammetic categorial analysis of the optic nerve head, Trans Am Acad Ophthalmol Otol 78:275, 1974

156. Primrose, J: The incidence of the peripapillary halo glaucomatosus, Trans Ophthalmol Soc UK 89:585, 1969

157. Primrose, J: Early signs of the glaucomatous disc, Br J Ophthalmol 55:820, 1971

158. Quigley, HA: Better methods in glaucoma diagnosis, Arch Ophthalmol 103:186, 1985

159. Quigley, HA: Early detection of glaucomatous damage. II. Changes in the appearance of the optic disk, Surv Ophthalmol 30:111, 1985

160. Quigley, HA: The pathogenesis of optic nerve damage in glaucoma. In Beckman, H, Campbell, DG, L'Esperance, FA, et al, editors: Symposium on the laser in ophthalmology and glaucoma update, St Louis, 1985, The CV Mosby Co

160a. Quigley, HA, and Addicks, EM: Regional differences in the structure of the lamina cribrosa and their relation to glaucomatous optic nerve damage, Arch Ophthalmol 99:137, 1981

161. Quigley, HA, and Addicks, EM: Quantitative studies of retinal nerve fiber layer defects, Arch Ophthalmol 100:807, 1982

162. Quigley, HA, Addicks, EM, and Green, WR: Optic nerve damage in human glaucoma. III. Quantitative correlation of nerve fiber loss and visual field defect in glaucoma, ischemic neuropathy, papilledema, and toxic neuropathy, Arch Ophthalmol 100:135, 1982

163. Quigley, HA, Hohman, RM, and Addicks, EM: Quantitative study of optic nerve head capillaries in experimental optic disc pallor, Am J Ophthalmol 93:689, 1982

164. Quigley, HA, et al: Blood vessels of the glaucomatous optic disc in experimental primate and human eyes, Invest Ophthalmol Vis Sci 25:918, 1984

165. Quigley, HA, Miller, NR, and George, T: Clinical evaluation of nerve fiber layer atrophy as an indicator of glaucomatous optic nerve damage, Arch Ophthalmol 98:1564, 1980

166. Quigley, HA, Miller, NR, and Green, WR: The pattern of optic fiber loss in anterior ischemic optic neuropathy, Am J Ophthalmol 100:796, 1985

167. Quigley, HA, et al: Chronic glaucoma selectively damages large optic nerve fibers, Invest Ophthalmol Vis Sci 28:913, 1987

168. Radius, RL, and Anderson, DR: The course of axons through the retina and optic nerve head, Arch Ophthalmol 97:1154, 1979

169. Radius, RL, and Anderson, DR: The histology of retinal nerve fiber layer bundles and bundle defects, Arch Ophthalmol 97:948, 1979

170. Radius, RL, Maumenee, AE, and Green, WR: Pit-like changes of the optic nerve head in open-angle glaucoma, Br J Ophthalmol 62:389, 1978

171. Radius, RL, and Pederson, JE: Laser-induced primate glaucoma. II. Histopathology, Arch Ophthalmol 102:1693, 1984

172. Read, RM, and Spaeth, GL: The practical clinical appraisal of the optic disc in glaucoma: the natural history of cup progression and some specific disc-field correlations, Trans Am Acad Ophthalmol Otolaryngol 78:255, 1974

173. Richardson, KT: Optic cup symmetry in normal newborn infants, Invest Ophthalmol 7:137, 1968

174. Riedel, H: Photography. In Heilmann, K and Richardson, KT, editors: Glaucoma: conceptions of a disease, Stüttgart, Germany, 1978, Georg Theime Verlag

175. Robert, Y, and Hendrickson, P: Color appearance of the papilla in normal and glaucomatous eyes: a photopapillometric study, Arch Ophthalmol 102:1772, 1984

176. Robert, Y, Hendrickson, P, and Best, R: Dynamic provoked circulatory response (DPCR) of the papilla, New Trends in Ophthalmology 1:253, 1986

177. Robert, Y, and Maurer, W: Pallor of the optic disc in glaucoma patients with artificial hypertension, Doc Ophthalmol 57:203, 1984

178. Robert, Y, Niesel, P, and Ehrengruber, H: Measurement of the optical density of the optic nerve head. I. The pallor of the papilla in artificial ocular hypertension, v Graefe's Arch Klin Exp Ophthalmol 219:176, 1982

179. Rosenthal, AR, Falconer, DG, and Barret, P: Digital measurement of pallor-disc ratio, Arch Ophthalmol 98:2027, 1980

180. Saheb, NE, Drance, SM, and Nelson, A: The use of photogrammetry in evaluating the cup of the optic nerve head for a study in chronic simple glaucoma, Can J Ophthalmol 7:466, 1972

181. Schirmer, KE: Instamatic photogrammetry, Can J Ophthalmol 9:81, 1974

182. Schirmer, KE: Simplified photogrammetry of the optic disc, Arch Ophthalmol 94:1997, 1976

183. Schirmer, KE, and Kratky, V: Photogrammetry of the optic disc, Can J Ophthalmol 8:78, 1973

184. Schnabel, WJ: Klinische Daten zur Entwicklungsgeschichte der glaukomatösen Exkavation, Zeitschr Augenheilk 19:335, 1908

185. Schwartz, B: Correlation of pallor of the optic disc with asymmetrical visual field loss in glaucoma. XXII Concilium Ophthalmologicum, Paris, 1976, Masson Publishers

186. Schwartz, B: Cupping and pallor of the optic disc, Arch Ophthalmol 89:272, 1973

187. Schwartz, B: New techniques for the examination of the optic disc and their clinical application. Symposium: the optic disc in glaucoma, Trans Am Acad Ophthalmol Otolaryngol 81:227, 1976

188. Schwartz, B: Optic disc changes in ocular hypertension, Surv Ophthalmol 25:148, 1980

189. Schwartz, B, and Kern, J: Scanning microdensitometry of optic disc pallor in glaucoma, Arch Ophthalmol 95:2159, 1977

190. Schwartz, B, Reinstein, NM, and Lieberman, DM: Pallor of the optic disc: quantitative photographic evaluation, Arch Ophthalmol 89:278, 1973

191. Schwartz, B, and Takamoto, T: Biostereometrics in ophthalmology for measurement of the optic disc in glaucoma. Proc SPIE 166, NATO Symposium on Applications of Human Biostereometrics, p 251, 1978

192. Schwartz, JT, Reuling, FH, and Garrison, RJ: Acquired cupping of the optic nerve head in normotensive eyes, Br J Ophthalmol 59:216, 1975

193. Sears, ML: Clinical and scientific basis for the management of open-angle glaucoma, Arch Ophthalmol 104:191, 1986

194. Shaffer, RN: The role of the astroglial cells in glaucomatous disc cupping, Doc Ophthalmol 26:516, 1969

195. Shaffer, RN, and Hetherington, J, Jr: The glaucomatous disc in infants: a suggested hypothesis for disc cupping, Trans Am Acad Ophthal Otolaryngol 73:929, 1969

196. Sharma, NK, and Hitchings, RA: A comparison of monocular and 'stereoscopic' photographs of the optic disc in the identification of glaucomatous visual fields defects, Br J Ophthalmol 67:677, 1983

197. Shields, MB: Textbook of Glaucoma (Formerly a Study Guide for Glaucoma), ed 2 Baltimore, 1987, Williams & Wilkins

198. Shihab, ZM, Lee, PF, and Hay, P: The significance of disc hemorrhage in open-angle glaucoma, Ophthalmology 89:211, 1982

199. Shinzato, E, Suzuki, R, and Furuno, F: The central visual field changes in glaucoma using Goldmann perimeter and Friedmann visual field analyser. In Greve, EL, editor: Second international visual field symposium, The Hague, 1977 Dr W Junk Publishers

200. Shiose, Y: Quantitative disc pattern as a new parameter for glaucoma screening, Glaucoma 1:41, 1979

201. Shiose, Y, et al: Glaucoma and the optic disc. I. Studies on cup and pallor in the optic disc, Jpn J Clin Ophthalmol 32:51, 1978

202. Slight, JR: The significance of disk hemorrhages: a red flag sign, Trans Pacific Coast Oto-Ophthalmological Soc 62:25, 1981

203. Snydacker, D: The normal optic disc: ophthalmoscopic and photographic studies, Am J Ophthalmol 58:958, 1964

204. Sommer, A, et al: High-resolution photography of the retinal nerve fiber layer, Am J Ophthalmol 96:535, 1983

205. Sommer, A, et al: Cross-polarization photography of the nerve fiber layer, Arch Ophthalmol 102:864, 1984

206. Sommer, A, et al: The nerve fiber layer in the diagnosis of glaucoma, Arch Ophthalmol 95:2149, 1977

207. Sommer, A, Pollack, I, and Maumenee, AE: Optic disc parameters and onset of glaucomatous field loss, Arch Ophthalmol 97:1444, 1979

208. Sommer, A, et al: Evaluation of nerve fiber layer assessment, Arch Ophthalmol 102:1766, 1984

209. Spaeth, G: Morphological damage of the optic nerve. In Heilmann, K and Richardson, KT, editors: Glaucoma: conceptions of a disease, Stüttgart, Germany, 1978, Georg Thieme Verlag

210. Spaeth, G, Hitchings, RA, and Sivalingam, E: The optic disc in glaucoma: pathogenetic correlation of five patterns of cupping in chronic open-angle glaucoma, Symposium on Glaucoma, Trans Am Acad Ophthalmol Otolaryngol 81:217, 1976

211. Susanna, R: The lamina cribrosa and visual field defects in open-angle glaucoma, Can J Ophthalmol 18:124, 1983

212. Susanna, R, Drance, SM, and Douglas, GR: Disc hemorrhages in patients with elevated intraocular pressure, Arch Ophthalmol 97:284, 1979

213. Sutton, GE, Motolko, MA, and Phelps, CD: Baring of a circumlinear vessel in glaucoma, Arch Ophthalmol 101:739, 1983

214. Takamoto, T, and Schwartz, B: Reproducibility of photogrammetric optic disc cup measurements, Invest Ophthalmol Vis Sci 26:814, 1985

215. Takamoto, T, Schwartz, B, and Marzan, G: Stereomeasurement of the optic disc, Photogram Eng Remote Sensing 45:79, 1979

216. Tamada, Y, Sasamori, H, and Ishikawa, Y: Splinter hemorrhage of the optic disc in glaucoma, Folia Ophthalmol Jpn 30:1713, 1979

217. Thorner, W: Die Stereoskopische Photographie des Augenhintergrundes, Klin Monatsbl Augenheilk 47:481, 1909

218. Tielsch, JM, et al: Intraobserver and interobserver agreement in measurement of optic disc characteristics, Ophthalmology 95:350, 1988

219. Tomlinson, A, and Phillips, CI: Ovalness of the optic cup and disc in the normal eye, Br J Ophthalmol 58:543, 1974

220. Tuulonen, A, et al: Comparison of the changes in the area of optic disc pallor and visual fields: a 9-year follow-up study. In Greve, EL, and Heijl, A, editors: International visual field symposium, Dordrecht, 1987, Martinus Nijhoff/Dr W Junk Publishers

221. Tuulonen, A, Nagin, P, Schwartz, B, and Wu, D-C: Increase of pallor and fluorescein-filling defects of the optic disc in the follow-up of ocular hypertensives measured by computerized image analysis, Ophthalmology 94:558, 1987

222. Tuulonen, A, Takamoto, T, Wu, D-C, and Schwartz, B: Optic disk cupping and pallor measurements of patients with a disk hemorrhage, Am J Ophthalmol 103:505, 1987

223. Vogt, A: Die Nervenfaserstreifung der menschlichen Netzhaut mit besonderer Berücksichtigung der Differential-Diagnose gegenuber pathologischen streifenförmigen Reflexen (präretinalen Fältelungen), Klin Mbl Augenheilkd 58:399, 1917

224. Weber, A: Ein Fall von partieller Hyperämie der Choroidea bei einem Kaninchen, Arch Ophthalmol 2:133, 1855

225. Weisman, RL, et al: Vertical elongation of the optic cup in glaucoma, Trans Am Acad Ophthalmol Otolaryngol 77:157, 1973

226. Wilensky, JT, and Kolker, AE: Peripapillary changes in glaucoma, Am J Ophthalmol 81:341, 1976

227. Wolff, E, and Penman, GG: The position occupied by the peripheral retinal fibers in the nerve fiber layer and at the nerve head, Acta XVI Concilium Ophthalmologicum 1:625, 1950

228. Yablonski, ME, Zimmerman, TJ, Kass, MA, and Becker, B: Prognostic significance of optic disc cupping in ocular hypertensive patients, Am J Ophthalmol 89:585, 1980

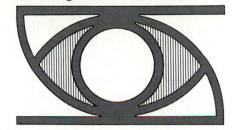

Chapter 23

Quantitative Measurements of the Optic Nerve Head

Joseph Caprioli

Helmholtz first viewed the ocular fundus in 1850 with the aid of parallel reflecting glass plates. Modified versions of this first ophthalmoscope were soon used to examine the optic nerve in patients with glaucoma. In 1858 Müller[64] described glaucomatous cupping and atrophy of the optic nerve. Important clinical observations and contributions were later made by Elschnig, Elliot, Kronfeld, Pickard, and others. More recently, Armaly[6] correlated the appearance of the optic nerve head and the visual field abnormalities of glaucoma. The availability of improved techniques with which to assess the optic nerve head and quantify the visual field has shifted the diagnostic emphasis from the measurement of intraocular pressure to the structural and functional abnormalities of glaucoma. Although progressive cupping of the optic nerve head may precede measurable visual field defects,* perimetric abnormalities have remained the major criteria used in following glaucomatous optic nerve damage, partly because of the inability, until recently, to make reliable quantitative observations about the optic nerve head.

Several retrospective studies performed with serial stereoscopic disc photographs revealed that changes in disc contour usually occur before visual field defects are manifest.[70,98] Odberg and Riise[69] prospectively studied 46 patients with ocular hypertension. Sequential stereophotography of the optic disc revealed increased cupping as the first pathologic sign in 19 patients, while only one developed a measurable visual field defect without an observable disc change. Quigley et al. estimated, from histologic examination, the number of nerve fibers in five optic nerves of normal subjects and in three of glaucoma suspects. The latter group had normal visual fields, tested with the Goldmann perimeter. The mean number of axons in the control group was 964,000; the 95% confidence limits for this measurement were 827,000 to 1,000,100. Estimates of axon numbers for the glaucoma suspects were 848,000, 808,000, and 577,000; two of these estimates were smaller than the lower confidence boundary and one value was only 60% of the normal average. When making quantitative comparisons, one must consider the sensitivity of the methods used to detect abnormalities of the optic disc and visual field and the effects of possible age-related changes.

The optic disc can be described by its topography and color. Time-honored clinical estimates of the cup-disc ratio used to estimate changes in topography of the nerve head are of little or no value in detecting the earliest optic nerve changes in patients with glaucoma.[55] Detailed drawings of the disc offer considerably more than do estimates of the cup-disc ratio because details of rim abnormalities, sloping margins, extent of visible lamina, and estimations of pallor can be indicated.[71,97] Bedell[9] was the first to write of the advantage of fundus photography over sketches or descriptions of the optic disc in patients with glaucoma. Serial

---

*References 6, 7, 68, 70, 71, 79, 98.

stereophotography of the optic nerve seems to be the best routine method with which to detect small changes in the optic disc over time.[68,70,98]

The history of fundus photography has been summarized by Donaldson.[29] In 1909, Thorner[107] described a method for taking stereoscopic fundus photographs, but the method was cumbersome and ill suited for routine clinical work. Six years later, Nordenson[68] reported the design of his fundus camera. It was the Zeiss-Nordenson camera that was used routinely for many years to obtain stereoscopic photographs of the ocular fundus. Stereoscopic effects were obtained by having the patient change fixation or by shifting the camera position. Allen et al.[5] introduced a stereo image separator, which allowed sequential photographs to be taken of the optic disc at a prescribed stereoscopic base. However, there is variability in the depth effects produced by nonsimultaneous stereoscopic methods. Small shifts of fixation cause the stereoscopic base to be uncertain. Donaldson[29] described a camera that allowed simultaneous stereoscopic photographs to be taken on adjacent frames of film. Later, a twin-prism separator was introduced in front of the objective lens of the fundus camera.[49,88,90] The twin prisms were placed apex to apex and provided separate stereoscopic images on a single frame of film with a stereoscopic base determined by the power of the prism. Matsui et al.[58] recorded simultaneous stereoscopic fundus photographs with an image-separating prism placed behind the objective lens.

Imaging of the ocular fundus has been achieved with high sensitivity video cameras.[40] Early attempts at video fundoscopy failed because of the low sensitivities of the instruments.[75,80] Advances in television technology have provided high resolution, high sensitivity cameras. Images can be rapidly processed with computerized digital analysis. Video techniques and image intensification offer the advantages of viewing and recording images in real time, of being many times more sensitive than film, and of avoiding the inconsistencies of film exposure and development.

TOPOGRAPHIC MEASUREMENTS OF THE OPTIC NERVE SURFACE

Routine clinical comparisons of optic nerve topography are best achieved by carefully comparing sequential sets of stereophotographs, or by comparing a previous stereophotograph to a stereoscopic view of the optic disc. The qualitative and subjective nature of these comparisons has sparked a search for more sensitive and quantitative methods.

Stereochronoscopy was first described by Schirmer[89] and further developed by Goldmann and Lotmar.[37-39] Photographs of the optic disc taken at different times at a fixed and reproducible angle with respect to the eye are paired and viewed stereoscopically. Changes in the structure of the disc appear as stereoscopic effects. Fixed-angle photographs are taken with the aid of a small auxiliary lens placed in front of the objective lens, which serves to focus the corneal reflex on an eyepiece reticule.[38] Goldmann and Lotmar presented several cases of chronic open-angle glaucoma in which disc changes detected by stereochronoscopy were not detected by comparison of ordinary stereo pairs. The technique has not found widespread clinical use because it is qualitative and subjective.

Bengtsson and Krakau[12] used rapid alternate projection of optic disc transparencies to make comparisons of sequential photographs. Changes in structure appear as lateral image shifts between alternate projections. Such comparisons seem to be no more sensitive than careful observation of sequential stereoscopic pairs.

Electronic subtraction has been applied to the detection of two-dimensional changes of the optic disc.[4] The methods employed were originally developed for the study of roentgenograms. Sequential black and white negatives of the optic nerve are electronically scanned, digitized, subtracted from each other, and displayed on a television screen. Image shifts become apparent as areas of high contrast. Under optimal photographic conditions, the technique can resolve lateral changes of 25 μm.[3] Electronic subtraction within two dimensions does not provide any information about depth.

Bengtsson[11] observed the diameter of the optic cup to be dependent on the size of the disc. The absolute width of the disc rim, however, is less variable than the size of the cup and is less dependent on disc diameter. The area of the disc rim may be better correlated to the total number of ganglion cell axons traversing the disc than is cup size, although recent evidence obtained with both manual and computerized techniques suggests that the disc rim area is not independent of disc size.[17,20] Narrowing of the disc rim occurs in patients with visual field defects from glaucoma.[14]

Planimetric measurements of the area of the disc rim have been used to study photographs retrospectively and semiquantitatively. Balazsi et al.[8] made absolute measurements of the disc rim (which the authors term "neuroretinal rim") corrected for magnification induced by the optical components of the eye.[56] The positions of the disc rim and disc edge were determined by tracing projected images while viewing a corresponding stereoscopic pair. The area of the traced disc rim was measured with a computerized planimeter. Enlarged black and white stereoscopic prints were used to make similar measurements in normal, ocular hypertensive, and glaucoma patients.[2] Normal subjects had the largest measured disc rim areas (1.40 ± 0.19 mm[2]), whereas glaucoma patients with visual field loss had the smallest rim areas (0.89 ± 0.28 mm[2]). The method is a simple way to assess early diffuse loss of nerve fibers. However, determining the position of the rim edge is subjective and may be difficult and poorly reproducible when no perceptible change in slope of the rim occurs.

Photogrammetry

Multiple, absolute measurements of depth across the surface of the optic nerve head represent the best way to define its contour. Ideally, such an approach would be as effective for discs with various morphologic characteristics, such as steep rim margins, as those with shallow, sloping rim margins. Stereophotogrammetry, the science of making three-dimensional measurements from stereophotographs, was first applied to the study of the ocular fundus by Crock.[25,26] Height measurement from aerial photographs is given by the general formula:

$$h = \frac{H^2}{FB}(\triangle p_1 + \triangle p_2)$$

where h equals the height of the object being measured, H equals the height from which the object is photographed, F equals the focal length of the camera, B equals the stereoscopic base (separation of the optical centers of the cameras) and $\triangle p_1$ and $\triangle p_2$ refer to the distances from the base to the top of the object on the photographs. This formula can be adapted for ocular fundus photography as follows:[30]

$$d = \frac{ff'}{FB}(\triangle p_1 + \triangle p_2)$$

where d equals the depth of the cup, f is the distance from the optical center of the camera to the principal plane of the eye, and f' is the distance from the principal plane of the eye to the surface of the fundus (Fig. 23-1). When f and f' are not known, depth can be measured in arbitrary units. Under these situations, quantitative comparisons between eyes would not be useful, but relative comparisons of the same eye over time can be

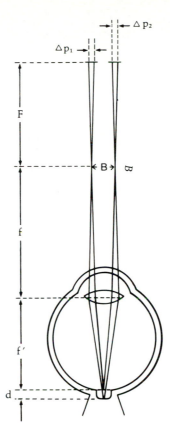

Fig. 23-1   Mathematic basis for photogrammetric measurements of depth in the ocular fundus. See text for explanation of symbols.

made. Reliable estimates of f and f' can be made if the refractive error, corneal curvature, and the axial length of the eye are known.[56]

Analog stereophotogrammetry employs a trained photogrammetrist and stereoscopic plotter to make depth measurements directly from stereophotographs. The results are a function of the skill and stereoacuity of the operator. Accurate measurements are possible only when the stereoscopic base is precisely known. Therefore, the use of nonsimultaneous stereophotography can lead to significant errors because of fixation shifts.[86,87] Reproducibility is increased with the use of the twin prism separator or the Donaldson fundus camera; the latter provides the most consistent results.[86] Multiple depth measurements of the optic nerve surface can be used to define quantitatively the position of the cup rim. Parameters such as cup-disc ratio, cup volume, cup area, and disc rim area can then be calculated. A contour map of theoptic nerve head can be constructed (Fig. 23-2). Analog photogrammetry has been used to study the three-dimensional structure of the op-

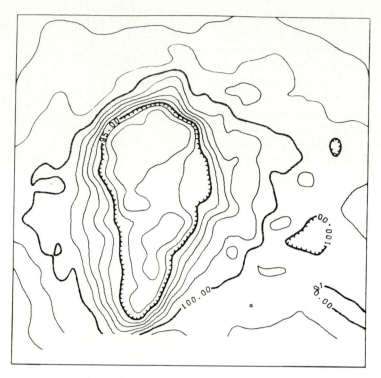

Fig. 23-2 Topographic map of optic nerve head derived from analog stereophotogrammetry. (From Johnson, CA, Keltner, JL, Krohn, MA, and Portney, GL: Invest Ophthalmol Vis Sci 18:1252, 1979)

tic nerve head in normal, ocular hypertensive, and glaucomatous eyes.* Quantitative comparison of serial contour measurements standardized to an appropriate reference plane probably represents the best approach for recognizing small changes.

The reproducibility of analog stereophotogrammetry was reported by Krohn et al.[50] who used a combination of cameras and films. The best results were obtained with the Donaldson fundus camera. Eight eyes of five patients were photographed six to eight times, and the three clearest photographs were studied. The coefficient of variation (standard deviation/mean) for volume, area, and depth ranged from 2% to 12%. Takamoto and Schwartz[104] performed a systematic study of the reproducibility of their analog stereophotogrammetric technique. With a Kern PG-2 stereo plotter and an experienced photogrammetrist (Takamoto), stereophotographs taken with a Donaldson fundus camera were measured. One eye each of 10 normal subjects, 10 ocular hypertensives, and 10 patients with glaucoma were photographed three times and analyzed. An average of 300 points on the surface of the optic nerve head were digitized for depth.

*References 45, 72, 73, 88, 92, 104.

Table 23-1 *Reproducibility of stereophotogrammetric measurements of the optic nerve head**

	Normals (n = 10)	Ocular hypertensives (n = 10)	Glaucoma (n = 10)
Cup volume/disc area	7.7	7.9	4.5
Cup depth/disc area	4.6	6.7	6.1
Cup area/disc area	5.2	7.6	4.7

Modified from Takamoto, T, and Schwartz, B: Invest Ophthalmol Vis Sci 26:814, 1985
*Values represent the median coefficient of variation (%).

Measurements of cup area, cup depth, and cup volume were normalized to the disc area. The median coefficient of variation ranged from 4.5% to 7.9% (Table 23-1).

It has been suggested that analog stereophotogrammetry could be used to make quantitative measurements of stereochronoscopic effects.[103] As in stereochronoscopy, two photographs taken at fixed and reproducible angles with respect to the optic nerve are viewed simultaneously in a stereoscopic plotter and the apparent depths measured. The measured depths represent change of contour over time. Preliminary experiments were performed with a model eye, which indicate the feasibility of the technique.[103] No systematic studies have been performed in patients.

Patterns projected onto the optic nerve through an entrance pupil and viewed through a separate exit pupil have been used to provide landmarks on the optic nerve head to help gauge depth measurements. Holm and Krakau[44] projected stripes on the optic nerve and used planimetry to develop depth profiles. Cohan[23] used multiple slit illumination of the optic nerve head from a modified Zeiss photographic slit-lamp to assist recognition of the optic nerve surface structure. Although a qualitative technique was described, the author pointed out that boundaries created by the projected stripes add features to the disc surface that assist the photogrammetrist to make depth determinations on otherwise featureless areas of the disc.

Computerized Image Analysis

Digital processing of scanned stereoscopic photographs has been used to make photogrammetric measurements.[48] Computer algorithms designed to duplicate the operation of the analog stereoscopic plotter[26] were used to create topographic maps of the nerve head. An important difference is that the digital technique does not require a trained photogrammetrist for analysis. A comparison of the reproducibility of analog and digital photogrammetry for topographic measurements initially indicated superiority of the digital method,[49] but refinements in technique and analysis have since increased the sensitivity of analog methods.[102]

Computerized image analysis of simultaneous stereoscopic video images of the optic nerve head has been described by Cornsweet et al.[24] The prototype instrument has been further developed by Rodenstock Instruments (Munich, West Germany).[18,61] To make depth measurements, simultaneous stereoscopic pairs of video images are recorded while a set of vertical stripes is projected on the surface of the disc. This technique provides features (the stripes) on areas of the disc that may be featureless and facilitates image analysis. The deformations of the striped pattern contain the depth information. A computer algorithm selects corresponding segments from the stereoscopic images and computes their cross-correlation function. Depth calculations are made along each of the stripes, about 10 of which traverse an optic disc of average size. There is considerably greater resolution along the stripes (vertically) than between the stripes (horizontally). The display provides a color-coded depth map of the optic nerve head (Fig. 23-3 and Plate II, Fig. 2), profile sections

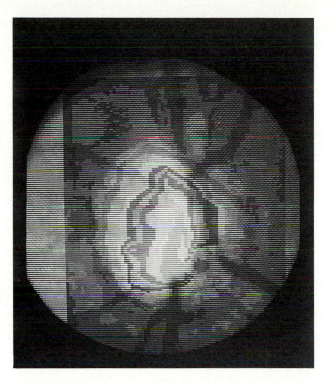

Fig. 23-3   Black and white photograph of color-coded contour map of optic nerve head derived from digital image analysis of simultaneously recorded striped video images. Distance between adjacent colors indicated on scale is 100 μm.

through the optic nerve head (Fig. 23-4), and a listing of parameters such as cup-disc ratio, disc rim area, and cup volume. The depth measurements can be further processed on an external computer to provide local averages calibrated in microns from a standard retinal reference plane, to provide an absolute depth matrix of the fundus centered at the optic nerve (Caprioli and Miller, unpublished data) (Fig. 23-5). Such an approach may prove to be more useful than the analysis of structural parameters (e.g., cup-disc ratio, disc rim area), which were originally derived from ophthalmoscopic descriptions and which may not use the available contour information to greatest advantage.

Reproducibility of such topographic parameters as linear measurements of disc diameter, cup-disc ratio, disc area, disc rim area, and volume of the optic nerve cup with the Rodenstock system has been measured.[18,51] Improvements in analytic algorithms have decreased the variability of more recent results. The median coefficient of variation of 10 repeated measurements in seven normal eyes and seven glaucomatous eyes had a range of 1.4% to 7.9% (Table 23-2). Subsequent studies have found similar results for variability of these standard disc parameters, have found no influence of

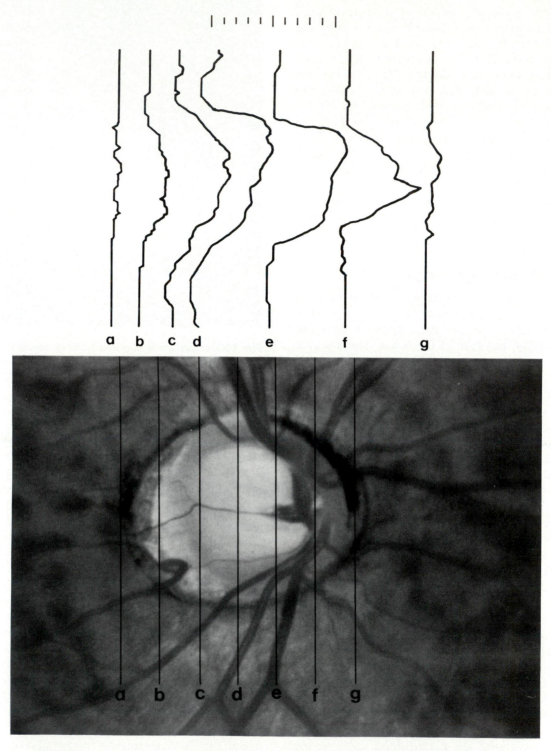

Fig. 23-4 Corresponding cross-sectional depth profiles of optic nerve head redrawn from the computer display derived from digital image analysis of simultaneously recorded striped video images. Scale at top indicates 1.0 mm in depth. See also Plate II, Fig. 3.

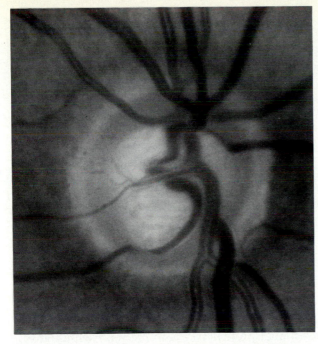

A

B

Fig. 23-5 **A,** A 25 × 25 magnification-corrected depth matrix of the fundus, centered at the optic nerve head. **B,** Data have been derived from digital image analysis of simultaneously recorded striped video images of optic nerve head. Numbers represent distance in microns above (−) or below (+) a standard retinal reference plane. Underlined values lie on edge of optic disc.

10	-6	-19	-23	-29	-36	-41	-39	-20	-4	-13	-33	-58	-77	-80	-32	56	296	312	182	63
9	-6	-19	-22	-29	-37	-42	-37	3	37	6	-26	-56	-84	-96	-41	53	285	301	175	60
7	-12	-25	-25	-36	-52	-48	-26	-10	8	37	21	-26	-48	-42	-12	57	287	302	175	59
7	-10	-23	-26	-39	-55	-41	-2	18	48	133	119	32	-35	-72	-37	35	237	255	150	54
6	-11	-22	-17	-22	-30	-18	15	52	81	50	20	-3	-17	-25	-37	-43	-15	8	25	38
6	-9	-21	-19	-6	9	21	36	73	_119_	_188_	_180_	_118_	_78_	_58_	_44_	31	23	25	32	37
0	-16	-20	0	29	60	100	140	_130_	_156_	399	420	269	139	57	_102_	_149_	135	105	71	38
3	6	16	39	79	124	174	_223_	_234_	275	483	496	362	196	65	169	_269_	_222_	146	65	-2
11	9	22	65	115	166	_242_	_348_	473	596	675	626	493	447	438	310	201	_257_	_224_	127	41
-4	-1	20	79	139	200	_371_	602	633	647	677	655	595	613	654	538	406	296	_194_	100	22
6	11	32	83	152	227	_393_	605	627	637	681	675	632	663	719	632	499	247	_114_	66	27
7	22	45	86	154	230	_347_	494	580	658	709	689	622	658	723	575	403	245	_156_	112	71
19	33	53	88	154	230	_302_	389	530	661	686	670	633	600	548	408	264	168	_110_	74	45
20	34	51	75	127	186	_237_	307	483	651	688	674	634	532	394	317	238	140	_85_	60	40
15	24	34	52	100	156	_239_	_355_	490	618	666	660	623	515	364	272	181	_90_	_47_	36	26
1	17	33	51	88	132	175	_241_	_398_	558	645	619	_522_	396	257	162	_73_	_7_	-9	3	14
-6	17	35	42	53	66	98	163	_282_	_419_	580	562	420	306	211	_106_	_2_	-73	-77	-35	3
-22	-3	13	24	35	47	81	148	268	_404_	_566_	_525_	_341_	207	_116_	_54_	-17	-136	-141	-73	-10
-17	-26	-23	2	15	24	45	89	172	259	321	288	189	147	135	60	-33	-173	-181	-106	-36
-30	-40	-47	-46	-28	-5	24	63	115	164	180	153	100	87	89	25	-63	-215	-223	-140	-61
-36	-38	-42	-47	-36	-20	4	36	66	91	81	65	49	37	24	-15	-76	-209	-211	-127	-50
-22	-31	-32	-18	-14	-12	-3	14	33	50	42	35	29	26	18	-13	-72	-228	-232	-137	-50
-15	-11	-9	-13	-14	-13	4	32	27	18	11	1	-11	-1	19	2	-53	-259	-273	-158	-54
-6	12	24	18	3	-15	-3	27	15	-1	-12	-10	0	17	29	4	-58	-262	-275	-160	-56

the size of the cup on variability,[77] and have predicted upper limits of random variability in normals at the 99% level of 0.05 for cup-disc ratio, 0.18 mm² for disc rim area, and 0.06 mm³ for cup volume.[15] Mikelberg et al.[59,60] and Caprioli and Miller[19] reported the relationship between measurements with the Rodenstock analyzer and manual analysis of stereoscopic photographs. Correlation coefficients for vertical cup-disc ratio, horizontal cup-

disc ratio, disc rim area, and optic disc area were highly significant.

PAR Microsystems Corporation (New Hartford, NY) has developed and marketed an image analysis system for the ocular fundus. Videographic image acquisition can be obtained directly through a Topcon simultaneous stereoscopic fundus camera interfaced to two charge-coupled device (CCD) video cameras, or from color transparencies projected on a screen. Images are digitized, and a cross-correlation algorithm calculates depth data for conjugate image points of the stereoscopic pair. Because no pattern is projected on the fundus, the technique depends on inherent image contrast to determine the depth of conjugate image points. Structural parameters may then be extracted from the depth data. Depth data are displayed as cross-sectional profiles or a graphic representation of a three-dimensional contour map (Fig. 23-6). The reproducibility of these parameters (average coefficient of variation) have been reported by Varma et al. as 2.4% for cup-disc ratio, 5.5% for disc rim area, and 5.2% for cup volume.[109]

Spaeth et al.[101] used computerized image anal-

Table 23-2 *Reproducibility of stereophotogrammetric measurements of the optic nerve head with videographic digital image analysis*

	Normals (n = 7)	Glaucomas (n = 7)
Disc area	3.1	1.9
Vertical cup/disc	5.8	3.9
Horizontal cup/disc	7.9	3.3
Rim area	5.6	7.5
Cup volume	7.1	7.6

Modified from Caprioli, J, et al: Arch Ophthalmol, 104:1035, 1986
*Values represent the median coefficient of variation (%).

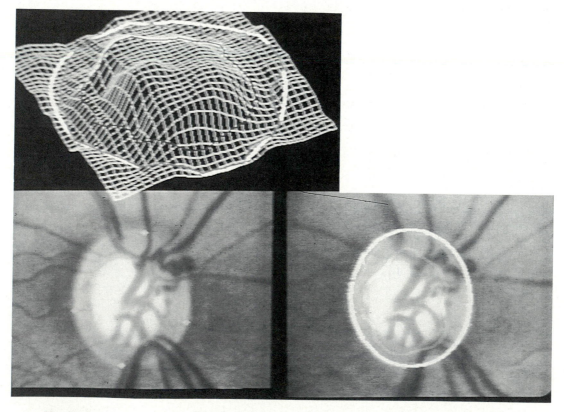

Fig. 23-6 Computer display of depth information obtained from simultaneously recorded video images of optic nerve head. Location of disc edge and cup edge are indicated on a three-dimensional display.

ysis (PAR system) to study optic disc vessel shifts in glaucoma. Stereoscopic disc photographs of 34 eyes of 19 glaucoma patients followed for 10 years or more were analyzed retrospectively. Assuming that a shift in the position of blood vessels is a pathologic change in glaucomatous optic discs, the image analyzer seemed to be more sensitive in detecting such shifts than was the clinical examination of photographs. Fixed-angle photography of the optic disc may be required to avoid apparent shifts in disc vessels caused by parallax, which could limit the usefulness of the technique.

Accuracy

The accuracy of photogrammetric techniques is an issue separate from reproducibility. A method of measurement may be highly reproducible, yet inaccurate. Although accuracy is probably not too important when comparative measurements are made in the same eye over time, inaccuracy will introduce error when comparing eyes of different patients or groups of patients. The resolution of the fundus image on photographs taken with the Zeiss fundus camera is approximately 7 to 8 μm.[32,52] Linear lateral measurements of fundus features can be quite accurate if the appropriate corrections for magnification of the optical system of the eye are made.[1,56]

The accuracy of depth measurements is not as good. Rosenthal et al.[85] made measurements of artificial cup depth in a model eye with digital photogrammetry. Most measurements were within 10 to 80 μm of the actual cup depth. However, model eyes imitate only poorly the conditions of the human fundus because variations of contour, color, tissue reflectance, and optical qualities cannot be reproduced. Accurate contour measurements depend on the accurate identification of the internal surface of the nerve fiber layer of the optic nerve head and surrounding retina. Light penetrates this nearly transparent layer to different degrees depending on its wavelength and on the density and color of the tissue. It has not yet been established with certainty that any photogrammetric contour measurements actually measure the very surface of the nerve fiber layer.

MEASUREMENTS OF OPTIC NERVE COLOR

Although changes in cupping of the optic nerve head are often paralleled by changes in pallor, they are not necessarily interdependent parameters. In normal eyes, the location of the maximum color contrast of the optic disc usually coincides with the margin of the disc rim. However, in certain diseases of the optic nerve, including glaucoma, this relationship no longer holds.[91] One retrospective study of ocular hypertensive eyes, which used subjective techniques, showed an increase in pallor but not in cupping over time when compared to normal eyes.[93] Another retrospective study of optic disc pallor performed with computerized image analysis demonstrated greater progression of pallor over time in ocular hypertensives compared to controls.[65]

Attempts to quantify the color of the optic disc date to Bock,[16] who in 1950 compared the color of the optic disc with shades of oil paints by viewing them simultaneously through a modified indirect ophthalmoscope. Kestenbaum[47] advocated the grading of optic atrophy by counting the number of small vessels on the disc rim. Gloster[34] developed a technique to estimate the oxygen saturation of blood with fundus reflectometry. Colorimetric estimates of the optic disc were also made by measuring the relative amounts of magenta- and yellow-filtered light required to match the color of the disc while it was viewed simultaneously through a modified indirect ophthalmoscope.[13]

Pallor Measurements from Photographs

Microdensitometric measurements of photographs to develop color contour maps of the disc have been made using shades of red standardized to carboxyhemoglobin solutions[27] and of high contrast black and white negatives of the optic disc.[92,94]

Because of variations in flash intensity, which occur with standard fundus cameras, exposures were standardized by diverting light from the illumination source through a neutral density step wedge onto an adjacent area of film. Optical density measurements of the optic disc could then be standardized against the step wedge function. Frequency distribution curves of optical density can be developed to facilitate quantitative analysis. Unevenness of flash illumination may reduce the reliability of the technique if it is not taken into account.[33,42]

To minimize problems with inconsistencies of the illumination source, film, exposure, and development of film, a boundary technique was developed to identify the area of greatest contrast on the optic disc.[95] The area of pallor within the boundary of greatest contrast is measured by planimetry to obtain a pallor-disc ratio. In a series of 140 normal subjects, the median value for this ratio was 19%; the ratio increased with age.

Digital measurements of pallor with an electronic scanner have also been reported.[85] Red and green portions of the image on color film are extracted by copying transparencies through the appropriate filters onto black and white film. A red filtered image provides the greatest contrast for identification of the disc edge. A green filtered image provides the greatest contrast of areas within the disc, from which the pallor boundary is identified with the help of a computer algorithm. Nagin et al.[66] reported a technique of computerized image analysis for quantifying pallor from photographs. Video images are made of a color slide through red and green filters and are digitized. Image analysis algorithms are used to track the edge of the disc (with the red filtered image) and the boundary of maximum contrast within the disc (with the green filtered image). The relative area within the boundary is calculated. Not infrequently the automatic algorithm breaks down, and the operator must assist the computer by specifying "plan" points through which the boundary must be drawn. Under optimal photographic conditions, the error of the method that measures the area of pallor with this technique approaches 2%.

Reflectometry

Fundus reflectometry uses direct measurements of light reflected from an external source by the ocular fundus. The procedure avoids problems with variation of film, its exposure, and development. Light (usually monochromatic) is optically collected from the fundus and measured with a photomultiplier tube or photosensitive diode. The color of the optic disc is not only dependent on the reflectance of the components of the optic nerve head (i.e., axons, glia, blood, and collagen) but also on light reflected from the surrounding fundus, especially the choroid.[36] Light of different wavelengths penetrates the eye to various degrees. Red light traverses the retina and choroid and is reflected by the sclera. Blue light is more highly scattered by the crystalline lens and inner retina and penetrates little into the choroid.[28,35] For this reason, blue light is useful to visualize the nerve fiber layer of the retina, and red light is helpful to visualize the choroid. Bleaching of visual pigments may also affect continuous measurements of reflectance from portions of the fundus.[110]

Photopapillometry is a term applied to measurements of selected wavelengths of light reflected from the optic disc. Measurements are made with a silicone diode incorporated into the image plane of a fundus camera or a Haag-Strait 900 slit-lamp. Earlier use of an electronic flash as the illumination source has been replaced by the use of greater signal amplification and a stabilized incandescent light source. The reflectance from small,

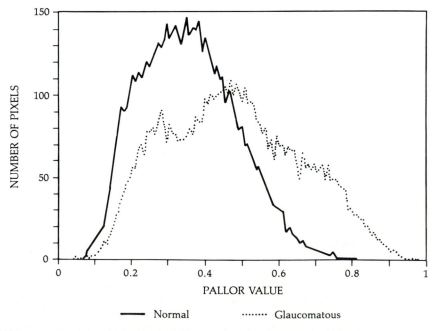

Fig. 23-7 Frequency distribution of pallor values of all pixels derived from video images of optic nerve in red and green light. A pallor value of 0 indicates a pure red pixel; a value of 1 indicates a white pixel.

selected areas of the optic disc can be measured instantaneously or continuously.

Videographic techniques have been applied to optic disc reflectometry.[24] Monochromatic video images made with green and red light are recorded and digitized. The "pallor value" at each picture element (pixel) is calculated as:

$$p = \frac{2 \times (\text{green reflectance})}{\text{green reflectance} + \text{red reflectance}}$$

With this scheme, a value of 0 indicates a pure red pixel, and a value of 1 indicates a white pixel. By computing the values of all the pixels within the margin of the optic disc, a frequency distribution of pallor can be constructed (Fig. 23-7) or a pallor map generated (Fig. 23-8; see also Plate II, Fig. 2).

The reproducibility of pallor measurements was investigated in seven normal eyes and seven glaucomatous eyes.[62] Each eye in the study was imaged nine separate times. Pallor values were ordered and means were calculated for the largest 5% of the values (h1), second 20% (h2), third and fourth 30% (h3, h4), fifth 20% (h5), and smallest 5% (h6). The average standard deviation of the means expressed as a percentage of full pallor scale was 4.3% in normal eyes and 6.6% in glaucomatous eyes. A measure of distribution width (h2 – h5) reflects the contrast between vessels and pale portions of the disc and is larger in patients with glaucoma. The mean reproducibility of this measure was 3.3% for normal eyes and 3.4% for glaucomatous eyes. This measure may be affected relatively little by changes in ocular media and may provide a useful clinical measurement of optic disc pallor in longitudinal studies.

MEASUREMENTS OF OPTIC DISC ANGIOGRAMS

Fluorescein angiography has been used to study the vascular perfusion of the optic nerve head and surrounding choroid.* Perfusion defects in the anterior optic nerve head occur more frequently in ocular hypertensives than in controls.[31] In glaucoma patients, areas of perfusion defects correspond to areas of visual field loss.[57] Spaeth[100] demonstrated increased perfusion of the optic nerve head after lowering intraocular pressure in some patients with glaucoma. Talusan et al.[106] found in a retrospective study that the development of new visual field defects in glaucoma patients was associated with the development of new absolute filling defects or areas of hypofluorescence of the optic nerve head. The prognostic value of vascular filling defects of the optic nerve head with fluorescein angiography has not been determined prospectively.

Rosen and Boyd[84] made densitometric measurements of fluorescein angiograms to measure peak choroidal, retinal, and optic disc fluorescence. The peak choroidal fluorescence occurred before or with the retinal peak fluorescence in normal patients. In glaucoma patients, peak choroidal fluorescence occurred after peak retinal fluorescence. Estimates of retinal blood flow in humans have been made by applying digital image processing methods to videographically recorded fluorescein angiograms.[46,76] The reliability of these techniques has yet to be established. Nagin et al.[67] have used computerized image analysis to quantify fluorescein angiograms of the optic disc, peripapillary choroid, and retina. Angiograms were analyzed to measure the fluorescein filling rate of the optic disc and to quantify the area of fluorescein filling defects.

QUANTITATIVE STUDIES IN GLAUCOMA

Topography

Holm et al.[43] studied the cup-disc ratio and volume of disc excavation in patients with glaucoma. Subjects were classified by their intraocular pressure response to topical corticosteroids and the

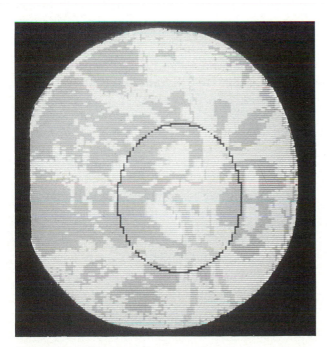

Fig. 23-8 "Pallor map" of optic nerve head derived from video images in red and green light. Colors toward right of scale indicate increasing value for pallor. See also Plate II, Fig. 2.

---

*References 10, 41, 51, 84, 96, 99.

presence of visual field defects. Cup volumes greater than 1.0 mm³ were nearly always present in patients with visual field loss. The cup volume varied directly with the degree of visual field loss and generally correlated with the cup-disc diameter. Cup volume asymmetry between eyes of the same patient occurred more frequently in patients with glaucoma and was usually associated with asymmetry of visual field defects. Optic nerve cup volume asymmetry greater than 0.20 mm³ was also found by Portney[73] to be a sign of glaucoma.

The three-dimensional geometry of normal and glaucomatous optic cups was studied with analog photogrammetry.[74] An attempt was made to reconsruct sequential optic nerve changes in glaucoma by analyzing patients in different stages of disease. Topographic measurements indicated deepening and vertical elongation of the cup in early phases of the disease. Johnson et al.[45] found depth, area, and volume of the optic nerve head to be progressively larger for normals, ocular hypertensives, and glaucoma patients; but considerable overlap of the values prevented accurate separation of the diagnostic groups based on topographic parameters alone.

Measurements of the deformation of the optic nerve head with increases of intraocular pressure have been made to estimate its mechanical compliance. If mechanical factors are operative in glaucomatous nerve damage, then the mechanical properties of the nerve head under increased pressure may determine which patients are at greatest risk. For instance, patients with low optic nerve head compliance (little or no posterior deformation at an elevated intraocular pressure) may be at less risk than patients who have a high compliance (larger posterior deformation at an elevated intraocular pressure). Levy et al.[54] studied movements of the lamina cribrosa with acute pressure elevation in primate eyes by positioning a fine platinum wire in the lamina and measuring its displacement roentgenographically. Posterior displacement of the wire varied from 40 to 80 μm at increases of intraocular pressure from 15 to 60 mm Hg above baseline. Investigations in enucleated human eyes produced similar findings.[53] Zeimer et al.[112] made measurements of optic nerve head compliance with laser Doppler velocimetry in enucleated human eyes and in a live rabbit eye. Retrodisplacement of a single point on the optic nerve head of 1 to 7 μm/cm H₂O occurred. The Doppler measurements were subsequently shown to correlate well with mechanical measurements of optic nerve head displacement.[111] It may be difficult to apply this technique to regional measurements of optic nerve compliance.

Caprioli and Sears measured acute regional conformational changes of the optic nerve head with the Rodenstock analyzer in human subjects.[22] Acute elevation of the intraocular pressure 20mm Hg above baseline was produced with a suction cup ophthalmodynamometer in six normal patients and in four patients with primary open-angle glaucoma. Significant increases in cup volume were caused by deepening of the cup in four of six normal eyes and three of four glaucomatous eyes. The largest changes in cup volume occurred in eyes with low ridigity (myopes). Distinct notches of the disc rim developed with increased pressure in glaucomatous eyes and reversed with normalization of intraocular pressure. The compliance of the supporting structure of the optic nerve head varied among individuals and varied regionally within single nerves.

Topographic measurements of the optic nerve head corrected for the optical dimensions of individual eyes were made with computerized videographic image analysis (Rodenstock Analyzer) in 22 normal controls, 51 glaucoma suspects, and 47 glaucoma patients.[19] Glaucoma suspects had elevated intraocular pressures and normal visual fields in both eyes (Octopus program 32). Glaucoma patients had typical visual field defects. There were significant differences among the patient groups for cup-disc ratio ($P = 0.005$), disc rim area ($P = .0006$), and cup volume ($P = .002$). Mean ($\pm$ SEM) disc rim area was 1.6 $\pm$ 0.07 mm² for controls, 1.06 $\pm$ 0.04 mm² for glaucoma suspects, and 0.87 $\pm$ 0.05 mm² for glaucoma patients. Mean ($\pm$ SEM) optic nerve cup volume was 0.33 $\pm$ 0.4 mm³ for controls, 0.46 $\pm$ 0.04 mm³ for glaucoma suspects, and 0.60 $\pm$ 0.05 mm³ for glaucoma patients. There was a large degree of overlap of the values for the structural parameters among the patient groups. It was concluded that single measurements of such parameters offer little diagnostic help in glaucoma and that quantitative comparisons of sequential optic nerve measurements are required to detect early structural damage from glaucoma.

Measurable structural alterations in the optic nerve head may precede visual field abnormalities in early open-angle glaucoma. The optic nerve heads of 10 patients with unilateral visual field loss from primary open-angle glaucoma, and 12 age- and sex-matched normal subjects were studied with computerized image analysis (Rodenstock Analyzer).[21] In patients with asymmetric primary open-angle glaucoma, eyes with normal visual fields had only a slightly larger (mean $\pm$ SEM) disc rim area ($0.90 \pm .04$ mm^2) than eyes with glaucomatous visual field defects ($0.78 \pm .05$ mm^2). However, both sets of eyes in the asymmetric primary open-angle glaucoma patients had smaller mean disc rims areas ($P < .0007$) than did the control group ($1.27 \pm .09$ mm^2). These findings support the hypothesis that loss of the optic disc rim can be detected before perimetric abnormalities develop in primary open-angle glaucoma.

The clinical usefulness of quantitative measurements of optic nerve topography in glaucoma patients seems promising. Answers must come from prospective, longitudinal studies of patients with glaucoma and glaucoma suspects who undergo sequential quantitative perimetry and parallel measurements of optic nerve topography.

Pallor

The clinical usefulness of quantitative measurements of optic disc pallor also awaits verification by prospective, longitudinal studies. There is some evidence that changes in pallor may occur at an early stage of glaucomatous optic nerve damage. In a cross-sectional study, Schwartz[93] subjectively evaluated cupping and pallor in a group of ocular hypertensive patients. Although the frequency distribution of pallor in this group was skewed to the right compared with controls (more pale than controls), there was no significant difference in the frequency distribution of cupping in this group compared to controls. Computerized image analysis was subsequently used to measure the area of pallor of the optic disc in a retrospective study of normals and low risk ocular hypertensives.[65] Although no significant changes over time were observed for the normal group, the ocular hypertensive group showed significant increases in pallor for most quadrants of both eyes over a 2-year period.

Robert and Hendrickson[81] used photopapillometry to assess the brightness of the optic disc in young normals, elderly normals, and glaucoma patients. Sites of the nasal and temporal disc rim were measured. No differences among the three groups of patients were evident, but a distinct difference in the brightness of the nasal and temporal disc occurred in the right eyes of patients and not in the left eyes. There was little difference in the brightness of the two sites measured in left eyes, but the brightness of the temporal site was greater than the nasal site in right eyes. The red content of the rim of the disc is partly a manifestation of the blood contained within it and is partly caused by light scattered into it by the large vessels and surrounding choroid. The closer the retinal vessels are to the measured site on the disc rim, the greater the light scattered by them contributes to the color of the adjacent disc rim. In left eyes, the retinal vessels emanate from the disc in a symmetric pattern. In right eyes the retinal vessels exit closer to the nasal margin of the disc. The difference in vascular patterns was thought to cause the apparent differences in brightness of the temporal and nasal areas of the right and left eyes.

Increased pallor with acute elevation of intraocular pressure has been documented by microdensitometry of black and white negatives[83] and by photopapillometry.[42] Robert and Maurer[82] evaluated the effect of acutely elevated intraocular pressure on optic disc pallor in normal and glaucomatous eyes. The results suggest that autoregulation of blood flow with incremental increases of intraocular pressure is present in normal patients but not in glaucoma patients. However, it is not entirely clear that changes in pallor of the optic nerve head are due solely to changes in its blood volume. A decrease of choroidal blood volume with elevated intraocular pressure is well known to occur, and reflectance of light from the choroid through the optic nerve head represents a significant component of disc color.[36] The effect of sustained elevations of intraocular pressure on the color of the optic nerve head is an issue about which little is currently known.

Fluorescein Angiograms

There is limited experience with computerized image analysis of fluorescein angiograms of the optic disc in patients with glaucoma. Nagin et al.[67] reported retrospective analyses of fluorescein angiograms of two patients. The first patient was a 16-year-old with juvenile glaucoma and a normal visual field at the time of the first angiogram who developed field loss at the time of a second angiogram 4 years later. The area of filling defect on the initial angiogram was 8% compared with 30% on the second angiogram. The second patient was a 55-year-old ocular hypertensive with an initial filling defect of 15%, which increased to 20% 4 years later; the visual field remained normal. Tuulonen et al.[108] studied sequential angiograms in 24 glaucoma suspects an average of 3.9 years apart. An increase in the area of fluorescein filling defects and a slowed filling rate correlated with glaucomatous optic disc and visual field progression. The reproducibility of this technique is unknown.

FUTURE RESEARCH

Computerized image analysis is a rapidly expanding technology. Further improvements in image acquisition, recording, and analysis will undoubtedly occur in the near future. Such improvements can provide increased accuracy and reproducibility of quantitative measurements of the optic nerve. The resolution of high sensitivity video cameras and charge-coupled devices continues to increase, and image enhancement techniques may provide means to detect changes in contour and color of the optic nerve head that are not presently possible.

The clinical usefulness of the techniques used to quantify the contour and color of the optic nerve head awaits the results of prospective, longitudinal evaluations of these methods in glaucoma suspects and patients with glaucoma. Considerable evidence suggests that changes in the structure and color of the optic disc may precede measurable visual field disturbances. Quantitative measurements of the thickness of the nerve fiber layer of the retina may provide another way to assess early structural damage.[105] Early attempts to extract descriptive numerical parameters from the depth data have conformed to our previous clinical descriptions of the optic nerve head derived from ophthalmoscopy. To make additional progress in this area, it may be necessary to abandon certain clinical notions and prejudices concerning optic nerve structure so that the newer quantitative depth measurements may be used to best advantage. Good correlations with visual function may not be uncovered until structural parameters are identified that accurately reflect the number of retinal ganglion cell axons entering the optic nerve head. An alternate approach would be to evaluate the entire topography of the optic nerve head and surrounding nerve fiber layer with respect to a reproducible and constant reference plane, such as at the level of the internal opening of the scleral canal, or at the level of the retina some distance from the optic nerve head where the nerve fiber layer is thin and remains fairly constant even with progressive glaucomatous loss of fibers. Such measurements made sequentially could provide important information regarding the rate of axonal death in glaucoma. Of course, control data for senescent ganglion cell death would also be required. Additional work in this area, as well as some innovative thinking, will be needed to develop more meaningful approaches to the measurement of neural tissue at the optic nerve head and its rate of change with age and disease.

The physical, chemical, and electrical responses of ganglion cells to mechanical deformation, pressure gradients, and hypoxia at the optic nerve head are not yet known. The degree of insult required to cause damage is not known. There is little information concerning the rates of death of retinal ganglion cells in noxious environments. The rate of axonal death and the point of irreversible damage bears directly on the issue of functional loss versus gross structural damage as early measurable signs of glaucoma. Additional information in these areas will provide clues concerning the best ways to detect early glaucomatous optic nerve damage.

REFERENCES

1. Airaksinen, PJ, Alanko, HI, and Juvala, PA: Magnification corrected measurements in the fundus of the eye, Invest Ophth Vis Sci 26(Suppl):223, 1985
2. Airaksinen, P, Drance, SM, and Schulzer, M: Neuroretinal rim area in early glaucoma, Am J Ophthalmol 99:1, 1985
3. Alanko, HI, and Airaksinen, PJ: Sensitivity of the electronic subtraction method in evaluation of simulated optic disc changes, Acta Ophthalmol (Copenh) 60:293, 1982
4. Alanko, H, Jaanio, E, Airaksinen, PJ, and Nieminen, H: Demonstration of glaucomatous optic disc changes by electronic subtraction, Acta Ophthalmol (Copenh) 58:14, 1980
5. Allen, L, Kirkendall, WM, Snyder, WB, and Frazier, O: Instant positive photographs and stereograms of ocular fundus fluorescence, Arch Ophthalmol 75:192, 1966
6. Armaly, MF: The correlation between appearance of the optic cup and visual function, Trans Am Acad Ophthalmol Otolaryngol 73:898, 1969
7. Aulhorn E, and Harms, H: Papillenveranderung und Gesichtsfeldstorung beim Glaukom, Ophthalmologica 139:279, 1960
8. Balazsi, GA, Drance, SM, Schulzer, M, and Douglas, G: Neuroretinal rim area in suspected glaucoma and chronic open-angle glaucoma, Arch Ophthalmol 102:1011, 1984
9. Bedell, AJ: Photographs of the fundus oculi, normal and pathological conditions, with case histories, single and stereoscopic views, NY J Med 27:951, 1927
10. Begg, IS, and Goldmann, H: The development of a technique for the densitometric analysis of fluorescein angiograms, Can J Ophthalmol 7:63, 1972
11. Bengtsson, B: The variation and covariation of cup and disc diameters, Acta Ophthalmol (Copenh) 54:804, 1976
12. Bengtsson, B, and Krakau, CT: Flicker comparison of fundus photographs, Acta Ophthalmol (Copenh) 57:503, 1979

13. Berkowitz, JS, and Balter, S: Colorimetric measurement of the optic disk, Am J Ophthalmol 69:385, 1970

14. Betz, PH, et al: Biometric study of the disc cup in open-angle glaucoma, Graefe's Arch Clin Exp Ophthalmol 218:70, 1982

15. Bishop, K, et al: Variability of optic disc topography measurements on the Rodenstock optic disc analyzer (RODA). Invest Ophthalmol Vis Sci 28(Suppl): 188, 1987

16. Bock, RH: Zur klinischen Messung der Papillenfarbe, Ophthalmologica 120:174, 1950

17. Britton, RJ, et al: The area of the neuroretinal rim of the optic nerve in normal eyes, Am J Ophthalmol 103:497, 1987

18. Caprioli, J, Klingbeil, U, Sears, M, and Pope, B: Reproducibility of optic disc measurements with computerized analysis of stereoscopic video images, Arch Ophthalmol 104:1035, 1986

19. Caprioli, J, and Miller, JM: Topographic measurements of the optic nerve head in glaucoma. Invest Ophthalmol Vis Sci 28(Suppl):188, 1987

20. Caprioli, J, and Miller, JM: Optic disc rim area is related to disc rim in normal subjects, Arch Ophthalmol 105:1683, 1987

21. Caprioli, J, Miller, JM, and Sears, M: Quantitative evaluation of the optic nerve head in patients with unilateral visual field loss from primary open-angle glaucoma, Ophthalmology 94:1484, 1987

22. Caprioli, J, and Sears, M: Acute conformational changes of the human optic nerve head, Invest Ophthalmol Vis Sci 27(Suppl):41, 1986

23. Cohan, B: Multiple-slit illumination of the optic disc, Arch Ophthalmol 96:497, 1978

24. Cornsweet, TN, et al: Quantification of the shape and color of the optic nerve head, Advances in diagnostic visual optics, New York, 1983, Springer-Verlag Inc, p 141

25. Crock, G: Stereotechnology in medicine, Trans Ophthalmol Soc UK 90:577, 1970

26. Crock, G, and Parel, JM: Stereophotogrammetry of fluorescein angiographs in ocular biometrics, Med J Aust 586, 1969

27. Davies, EG: Quantitative assessment of colour of the optic disc by a photographic method, Exp Eye Res 9:106, 1970

28. Delori, FC, Gragoudas, ES, Francisco, R, and Pruett, RC: Monochromatic ophthalmoscopy and fundus photography, Arch Ophthalmol 95:861, 1977

29. Donaldson, DD: A new camera for stereoscopic fundus photography, Arch Ophthalmol 73:253, 1965

30. Ffytche, TJ, Elkington, AR, and Dowman, IJ: Photogrammetry of the optic disc, Trans Ophthalmol Soc UK 93:251, 1973

31. Fishbein, SL, and Schwartz, B: Optic disc in glaucoma. Topography and extent of fluorescein filling defects, Arch Ophthalmol 95:1975, 1977

32. Flower, RW, and Hochheimer, BF: A clinical technique and apparatus for simultaneous angiography of the separate retinal and choroidal circulations, Invest Ophthalmol 12:248, 1973

33. Fonda, S, Gatti, AM, and Vecchi, D: Reliability of photometric measurements with the Zeiss fundus camera, Acta Ophthalmol (Copenh) 61:58, 1983

34. Gloster, J: Fundus oximetry, Exp Eye Res 6:187, 1967

35. Gloster, J: A new method of studying the vascular circulation of the human eye. Trans Ophthalmol Soc UK 88:477, 1968

36. Gloster, J: Colorimetry of the optic disc, Trans Ophthalmol Soc UK 93:243, 1973

37. Goldmann, H: On stereochronoscopy, Doc Ophthalmol 51:269, 1981

38. Goldmann, H, and Lotmar, W: Rapid detection of changes in the optic disc: stereo-chronoscopy, Graefes Arch Clin Exp Ophthalmol 202:87, 1977

39. Goldmann, H, and Lotmar, W: Rapid detection of changes in the optic disc: stereochronoscopy. Evaluation technique, influence of some physiologic factors, and follow-up of a case of choked disc, Graefes Arch Ophthalmol 205:263, 1978

40. Haining, WM: Video funduscopy and fluoroscopy, Br J Ophthalmol 65:702, 1981

41. Hayreh, SS, and Walker, WM: Fluorescent fundus photography in glaucoma, Am J Ophthalmol 6:982, 1967

42. Hendrickson, P, Robert, Y, and Stockli, HP: Principles of photometry of the papilla, Arch Ophthalmol 102:1704, 1984

43. Holm, OC, Becker, B, Asseff, CF, and Podos, SM: Volume of the optic disk cup, Am J Ophthalmol 73:876, 1972

44. Holm, OC, and Krakau, CT: A photographic method for measuring the volume of papillary excavations, Ann Ophthalmol 1:327, 1969

45. Johnson, CA, Keltner, JL, Krohn, MA, and Portney, GL: Photogrammetry of the optic disc in glaucoma and ocular hypertension with simultaneous stereo photography, Invest Ophthalmol Vis Sci 18:1252, 1979

46. Jung, F, et al: Quantification of characteristic blood-flow parameters in the vessels of the retina with a picture analysis system for video-fluorescence angiograms: initial findings, Graefes Arch Clin Exp Ophthalmol 221:133, 1983

47. Kestenbaum, A: Clinical methods of neuro-ophthalmologic examination, ed 2, New York, 1961, Grune & Stratton, p 147

48. Kottler, MS, Rosenthal, AR, and Falconer, DG: Digital photogrammetry of the optic nervehead, Invest Ophthalmol 13:116, 1974

49. Kottler, MS, Rosenthal, AR, and Falconer, DG: Analog vs. digital photogrammetry for optic cup analysis, Invest Ophthalmol 15:651, 1976

50. Krohn, MA, Keltner, JL, and Johnson, CA: Comparison of photographic techniques and films used in stereophotogrammetry of the optic disk, Am J Ophthalmol 88:859, 1979

51. Laatikainen, L: Fluorescein angiographic studies of the peripapillary and perilimbal regions in simple, capsular and low tension glaucoma, Acta Ophthalmol [Suppl] (Copenh) 111:1, 1971

52. Laing, RA, and Danisch, LA: An objective focusing method for fundus photography, Invest Ophthalmol 14:329, 1975

53. Levy, NS, and Crapps, EE: Displacement of optic nerve head in response to short-term intraocular pressure elevation in human eyes, Arch Ophthalmol 102:782, 1984

54. Levy, NS, Crapps, EE, and Bonney, RC: Displacement of the optic nerve head, Arch Ophthalmol 99:2166, 1981

55. Lichter, PR: Variability of expert observers in evaluating the optic disc, Trans Am Ophthalmol Soc 74:532, 1976

56. Littmann, H: Zur Bestimmung der wahren Grösse eines Objektes auf dem Hintergrund des lebenden Auges, Klin Mbl Augenheilk 180:286, 1982

57. Loebl, M, and Schwartz, B: Fluorescein angiographic defects of the optic disc in ocular hypertension, Arch Ophthalmol 95:1980, 1977

58. Matsui, M, Parel, JM, and Norton, ED: Simultaneous stereophotogrammetric and angiographic fundus camera, Am J Ophthalmol 85:230, 1978

59. Mikelberg, FS, et al: The correlation between optic disk topography measured by the video-ophthalmograph (Rodenstock Analyzer) and clinical measurement, Am J Ophthalmol 100:417, 1985

60. Mikelberg, FS, et al: The correlation between cup-disk ratio, neuroretinal rim area, and optic disk area measured by the video-ophthalmograph (Rodenstock analyzer) and clinical measurement, Am J Ophthalmol 101:7, 1986

61. Mikelberg FS, et al: Reliability of optic disk topographic measurements recorded with a video-ophthalmograph, Am J Ophthalmol 98:98, 1984

62. Miller, JM, and Caprioli, J: Videographic measurements of optic disc pallor, Invest Ophthalmol Vis Sci 28(Suppl):188, 1987

63. Miller, JM, and Caprioli, J: Videographic quantification of optic disc pallor, Invest Ophthalmol Vis Sci 29:320, 1988

64. Müller, H: Anatomische Beitrage zur Ophthalmologie: Uber Nerven-Veranderungen an der Eintrittsstelle des Sehnerven, Arch Ophthalmol 4:1, 1858

65. Nagin, P, and Schwartz, B: Detection of increased pallor over time, Ophthalmology 91:252, 1984

66. Nagin, P, Schwartz, B, and Ninba, K: The reproducibility of computerized boundary analysis for measuring disc pallor in the normal optic disc, Ophthalmology 92:243, 1985

67. Nagin, P, Schwartz, B, and Reynolds, G: Measurement of fluorescein angiograms of the optic disc and retina using computerized image analysis, Ophthalmology 92:547, 1985

68. Nordenson, JW: Om centrisk fotografering av Ogonbottnen, Hygea 77:1538, 1915

69. Odberg, T, and Riise, D: Early diagnosis of glaucoma, Acta Ophthalmol (Copenh) 63:257, 1985

70. Pederson, JE, and Anderson, DR: The mode of progressive disc cupping in ocular hypertension and glaucoma, Arch Ophthalmol 98:490, 1980

71. Pickard, R: A method of recording disc alterations and a study of the growth of normal and abnormal disc cups, Br J Ophthalmol 7:81, 1923

72. Portney, GL: Photogrammetric categorical analysis of the optic nerve head, Trans Am Acad Ophthalmol Otolaryngol 78:275, 1974

73. Portney, GL: Photogrammetric analysis of volume asymmetry of the optic nerve head cup in normal, hypertensive, and glaucomatous eyes, Am J Ophthalmol 80:51, 1975

74. Portney, GL: Photogrammetric analysis of the three-dimensional geometry of normal and glaucomatous optic cups, Trans Am Acad Ophthalmol Otolaryngol 81:239, 1976

75. Potts, AM, and Brown, MC: A color television ophthalmoscope, Trans Am Acad Ophthalmol Otolaryngol 62:136, 1958

76. Preussner, PR, et al: Quantitative measurement of retinal blood flow in human beings by application of digital image-processing methods to television fluorescein angiograms, Graefe's Arch Clin Exp Ophthalmol 221:110, 1983

77. Prince, AM, et al: Reproducibility of Rodenstock optic nerve analysis in eyes with different cup-disc ratios, Invest Ophthalmol Vis Sci 28(Suppl):188, 1987

78. Quigley, HA, Addicks, EM, and Green, WR: Optic nerve damage in human glaucoma, Arch Ophthalmol 100:135, 1982

79. Read, RM, and Spaeth, GL: The practical clinical appraisal of the optic disc in glaucoma: the natural history of cup progression and some specific disc-field correlations, Trans Am Acad Ophthalmol Otolaryngol 78:255, 1974

80. Ridley, H: Television in ophthalmology, Proceedings of the 16th International Congress of Ophthalmology, London, 2:1397, 1950

81. Robert, Y, and Hendrickson, P: Color appearance of the papilla in normal and glaucomatous eyes, Arch Ophthalmol 102:1772, 1984

82. Robert, Y, and Maurer, W: Pallor of the optic disc in glaucoma patients with artificial hypertension, Doc Ophthalmol 57:203, 1984

83. Robert, Y, Niesel, P, and Ehrengruber, H: Measurement of the optical density of the optic nerve head. I. The pallor of the papilla in artificial ocular hypertension, Graefe's Arch Clin Exp Ophthalmol 219:176, 1982

84. Rosen, ES, and Boyd, TS: New method of assessing choroidal ischemia in open-angle glaucoma and ocular hypertension, Am J Ophthalmol 70:912, 1970

85. Rosenthal, AR, Falconer, DG, and Barrett, P: Digital measurement of pallor-disc ratio, Arch Ophthalmol 98:2027, 1980

86. Rosenthal, AR, Falconer, DG, and Pieper, I: Photogrammetry experiments with a model eye, Br J Ophthalmol 64:881, 1980

87. Rosenthal, AR, Kottler, MS, Donaldson, DD, and Falconer, DG: Comparative reproducibility of digital photogrammetric procedure utilizing three methods of stereophotography, Invest Ophthal Vis Sci 16:54, 1977

88. Saheb, NE, Drance, SM, and Nelson, A: The use of photogrammetry in evaluating the cup of the optic nervehead for a study in chronic simple glaucoma, Can J Ophthalmol 7:466, 1972

89. Schirmer, KE: Simplified photogrammetry of the optic disc, Arch Ophthalmol 94:1997, 1976

90. Schirmer, KE, and Kratky, V: Photogrammetry of the optic disc, Can J Ophthalmol 8:78, 1973

91. Schwartz, B: Cupping and pallor of the optic disc, Arch Ophthalmol 89:272, 1973

92. Schwartz, B: New techniques for the examination of the optic disc and their clinical application, Trans Am Acad Ophthalmol Otolaryngol 81:227, 1976

93. Schwartz, B: Optic disc changes in ocular hypertension, Surv Ophthalmol 25:148, 1980

94. Schwartz, B, and Kern, J: Scanning microdensitometry of optic disc pallor in glaucoma, Arch Ophthalmol 95:2159, 1977

95. Schwartz, B, Reinstein, NM, and Lieberman, DM: Pallor of the optic disc, Arch Ophthalmol 89:278, 1973

96. Schwartz, B, Rieser, JC, and Fishbein, SL: Fluorescein angiographic defects of the optic disc in glaucoma, Arch Ophthalmol 95:1961, 1977

97. Shaffer, RN, Ridgway, WL, Brown, R, and Kramer, SG: The use of diagrams to record changes in glaucomatous disks, Am J Ophthalmol 80:460, 1975

98. Sommer, A, Pollack, I, and Maumenee, AE: Optic disc parameters and onset of glaucomatous field loss, Arch Ophthalmol 97:1444, 1979

99. Spaeth, GL: Pathogenesis of visual loss in patients with glaucoma. Pathologic and sociologic considerations, Trans Am Acad Ophthalmol Otolaryngol 75:296, 1971

100. Spaeth, GL: Fluorescein angiography: its contributions towards understanding the mechanisms of visual field loss in glaucoma, Trans Am Ophthalmol Soc 73:491, 1975

101. Spaeth, GL, et al: Optic disc vessel shift in glaucoma: image analysis versus clinical evaluation. Invest Ophthalmol Vis Sci 28(Suppl):188, 1987

102. Takamoto, T, and Schwartz, B: Photogrammetric measurement of the optic disc cup in glaucoma, Intl Arch Photogrammetry, 23:732, 1980

103. Takamoto, T, and Schwartz, B: Stereochronometry: quantitative measurement of optic disc cup changes, Invest Ophthalmol Vis Sci 26:1445, 1985

104. Takamoto, T, and Schwartz, B: Reproducibility of photogrammetric optic disc cup measurements, Invest Ophthalmol Vis Sci 26:814, 1985

105. Takamoto, T, and Schwartz, B: Three dimensional mapping of retinal vessels in ophthalmology, Intl Arch Photogrammetry Remote Sensing 26:349, 1986

106. Talusan, ED, Schwartz, B, and Wilcox, LM: Fluorescein angiography of the optic disc, a longitudinal follow-up study, Arch Ophthalmol 98:1579, 1980

107. Thorner, W: Die stereoskopische Photoghraphie des Augenhintergrundes, Klin Mbl Augenheilk 47:481, 1909

108. Tuulonen, A, Nagin, P, Schwartz, B, and Wu, D-C: Increase of pallor and fluorescein-filling defects of the optic disc in the follow-up of ocular hypertensives measured by computerized image analysis, Ophthalmology 94:558, 1987

109. Varma, R, Spaeth, GL, Steinmann, WC, and Wilson, RP: Variability in digital analysis of optic disc topography, Arch Ophthalmol (In press)

110. Weale, RA: Photochemical reactions in the living cat's retina, J Physiol (London) 121:322, 1953

111. Zeimer, RC, and Chen, K: Comparison of a noninvasive measurement of optic nervehead mechanical compliance with an invasive method, Invest Ophthalmol Vis Sci 128:1735, 1987

112. Zeimer, R, Wilensky, JT, Goldberg, MF, and Solin, SA: Noninvasive measurement of optic nerve-head compliance by laser doppler velocimetry, J Opt Soc Am 71:499, 1981

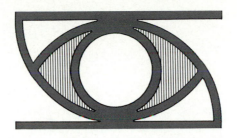

PART THREE

PHARMACOLOGY

24

Ocular Cholinergic Agents

25

Adrenergic and Dopaminergic Drugs in Glaucoma

26

Carbonic Anhydrase Inhibitors

27

Hyperosmotic Agents

28

Alternative and Future Medical Therapy of Glaucoma

Chapter 24

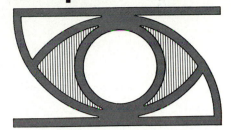

Ocular Cholinergic Agents

George F. Nardin
Thom J. Zimmerman
Alan H. Zalta
Kathy Felts

Ocular cholinergic agents are a group of medications used topically in the treatment of glaucoma for the purpose of lowering intraocular pressure. Members of this group of medications have been the mainstay for the medical management of most types of primary and secondary glaucoma since the discovery of their ocular hypotensive effect in the latter half of the nineteenth century. In the course of their extensive use, a number of different agents have been developed. The mechanism by which these agents act seems to be quite similar, though their actual site of activity in the autonomic nervous system varies considerably.

On the basis of this differing site of action the ocular cholinergic agents can be divided into two groups. Direct-acting drugs function directly at the neuromuscular junction of the parasympathetic nervous system, thereby directly stimulating the effector muscle. Members of this group include pilocarpine, the oldest and most widely used cholinergic agent, and carbachol, a more potent, less commonly used medication. The second class of cholinergic agents is the indirect-acting parasympathomimetics. This group of medications, also known as anticholinesterase agents, acts to stimulate the parasympathetic nervous system by binding the enzymes acetylcholinesterase and butyrylcholinesterase, thereby preventing them from hydrolyzing acetylcholine at the neuromuscular junction. The inhibition of these enzymes allows a dramatic buildup of acetylcholine at the neuromuscular junction, resulting in the profound stimulation of the parasympathetic nervous system at sites where this block has taken place. Included in this class of medications are demecarium bromide (Humorsol), echothiophate iodide (Phospholine Iodide), and diisopropyl fluorophosphate (DFP or Floropryl). Though much less commonly used than pilocarpine or carbachol in the treatment of glaucoma, these agents have very potent pressure lowering effects on the eye. The anticholinesterase agents are further subdivided into two groups: those that are considered reversible (carbamate inhibitors), which include demecarium bromide, distigmine bromide, physostigmine, neostigmine, and pyridostigmine; and relatively irreversible cholinesterase inhibitors, including echothiophate and diisopropyl fluorophosphate. Although all these medications may effectively lower intraocular pressure, only echothiophate, and to a somewhat lesser extent, demecarium bromide (DFP) are actually used in the treatment of glaucoma.

DIRECT-ACTING PARASYMPATHOMIMETIC AGENTS

Pilocarpine

Pilocarpine became available in the Western Hemisphere in the 1870s when a Brazilian physician (Coutinbou) first brought pilocarpine to Paris from Pernambuco where it had been used by the natives.[19] Its primary use at that time was to induce sweating and salivation, which it certainly did at the dose recommended (60 to 90 grains). Five years later, Gerrard and Hardy isolated pilocarpine, after which a number of European physicians set about finding a use for its diaphoretic properties.[15] Mar-

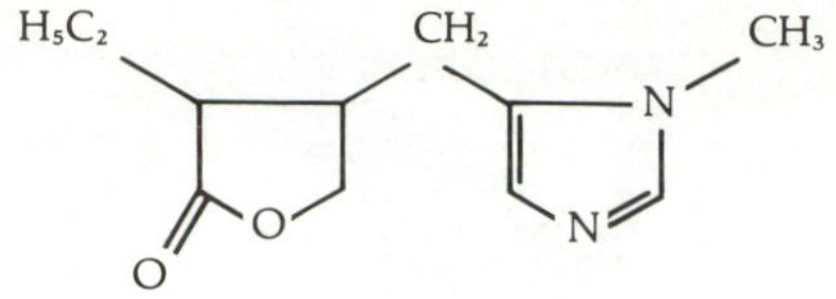

Fig. 24-1 Pilocarpine.

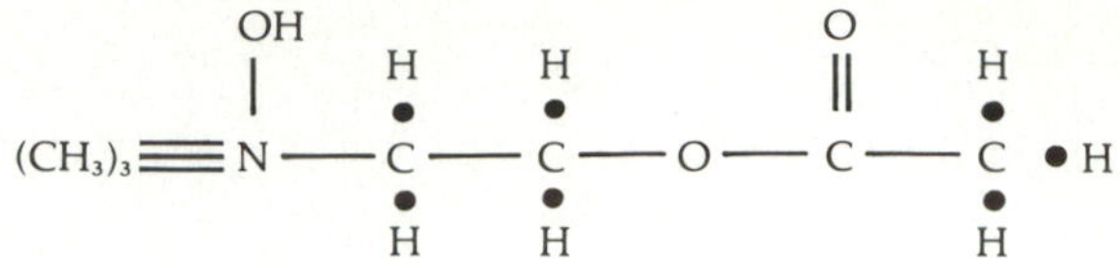

Fig. 24-2 Acetylcholine.

tindale noted that pilocarpine caused an accommodative spasm and what was felt to be a slight mydriasis, later noted to be a slight miosis of the pupils.[20] Several German physicians explored the uses of this medication and noticed its ocular effects, including intraocular pressure reduction.[23]

A chief source of pilocarpine today is the plant *Pilocarpus microphyllus*, where it occurs as the isomer isopilocarpine (Fig. 24-1).

The purified compound is either a colorless liquid or a needle-like crystal and is soluble both in water and in alcohol. Its pKa in aqueous solution is 6.87, a value too low for a sufficient degree of dissociation to penetrate the lipid-aqueous barrier of the cornea. For this reason, the hydrochloride form or the nitrate salt with pKa values of 12.75 and 7.15 respectively are used for ophthalmic preparations. Though somewhat different in structure from acetylcholine (Fig. 24-2), pilocarpine's positively charged center acts in a similar manner to acetylcholine at the postganglionic parasympathetic receptor site.

Unlike acetylcholine, pilocarpine stimulates only the muscarinic receptors located in the smooth muscle.[4,8] Systemically, it causes increased lacrimation and sweating, an occasional marked decrease in blood pressure, and a slowing of the pulse similar to acetylcholine. Pilocarpine stimulates the pupillary sphincter and the ciliary muscle causing miosis and accommodative spasm.[4]

Preparations of pilocarpine for use in ophthalmology are available as solutions, ointments, powders, and controlled-release systems (Ocusert). The solutions are available in concentrations ranging from 0.25% to 10%. Ocuserts, which release 20 or 40 μg/hr, are available, as is 4% aqueous gel in a synthetic polymer acrylic acid (Table 24-1).

Most available preparations of pilocarpine contain the hydrochloride salt, though the nitrate is also available. In addition to the active ingredient, various buffers, preservatives, and viscolysing agents are also included.

Mechanism of action

Pilocarpine acts at the parasympathetic muscarinic receptor site, as does the physiologic me-

diator, acetylcholine. Stimulation of the parasympathetic nerve ending causes constriction of the pupillary sphincter and miosis. Contraction of the ciliary muscle produces tension on the scleral spur, to which the ciliary muscle is attached. This posterior stretching of the scleral spur is thought to produce traction on the trabecular meshwork, pulling it open and facilitating the outflow of aqueous humor and the lowering of intraocular pressure. The same effects have been noted to occur with posterior movement of the lens, which, because of its zonular attachments in the ciliary body, also produces posterior traction on the scleral spur and stretching of the trabecular meshwork.[21] This suggests that the actual effect of pilocarpine is not directly related to any physiologic change in Schlemm's canal, as had earlier been suggested.[9] Additional evidence for this mechanism of action was provided by Kaufman and Barany,[13] who showed that when the ciliary muscle is disinserted from its attachment to the scleral spur, miotic agents have no effect on the trabecular meshwork or on the intraocular pressure.

Clinical uses

Although a wide range of concentrations of pilocarpine is available, the most commonly used are the 1% to 4% solutions. Concentrations greater than 4% do not generally augment the ocular hypotensive effect,[9] though some darkly pigmented individuals may show an added benefit from these higher doses.[8] Original dose-response studies demonstrated a duration of action of 6 to 8 hours. Customarily, pilocarpine is given every 6 or 8 hours.[9] More recent investigations have shown that increasing ocular contact time by employing nasolacrimal occlusion and simple eyelid closure increases both the duration of action and the effect of lower concentrations.[24] It is important to keep in mind that the dosage and frequency of these drugs should be individually titrated for each patient. It seems wise to start with the lowest concentration and increase the dose until the desired pressure-lowering effect is obtained.

Pilopine HS Gel slowly releases the medication. It is recommended that this medication be

Table 24-1   Formulations of pilocarpine

Trademark, manufacturer	Form, concentrations	Vehicle	Buffering agents	Preservatives, surfactants, and counterirritants
Adsorbocarpine Alcon Laboratories	Solution pilocarpine HCL 1%, 2%, 4%	Adsorbobase (providone and water soluble polymers)		Benzalkonium chloride 0.004% edetate disodium 0.1%
Isopto Carpine Alcon Laboratories	Solution pilocarpine HCL 0.25%, 0.5%, 1%, 2%, 3%, 4%, 5%, 6%, 8%, 10%	Hydroxypropyl methylcellulose 0.5%	Boric acid, sodium chloride, sodium citrate, hydrochloric acid and/or sodium hydroxide, citric acid, hydrochloric acid and/or sodium hydroxide, hydrochloric acid and/or sodium hydroxide	Benzalkonium chloride
Pilocar IO Lab Pharmaceuticals	Solution pilocarpine HCL 0.5%, 1%, 2%, 3%, 4%, 6%	Hydroxypropyl methylcellulose	Potassium chloride, boric acid, sodium carbonate	Benzalkonium chloride 0.01%, edetate disodium
Pilocel Professional Pharmacal	Solution pilocarpine HCL 0.25%, 0.5%, 1%, 3%, 4%, 6%	Hydroxypropyl methylcellulose 0.25%	Boric acid, sodium citrate	Benzalkonium chloride
Ocusert Alza Corporation	Controlled-release pilocarpine system 20 μg/hr, 40 μg/hr	None	None	None
Pilopine HS Gel Alcon Laboratories	Controlled-release pilocarpine aqueous gel	Carbopol 940	Hydrochloric acid and sodium chloride	Benzalkonium chloride

administered on a once-a-day basis, preferably at bedtime because the blurriness caused by the pilocarpine and the ointment vehicle are less bothersome to the patient. The Ocusert Pilo 20 and Pilo 40 have a much more prolonged duration of action than Pilopine HS Gel. Customarily, these are administered weekly, though there is some individual variation in the duration of response. For this reason, it is advisable to monitor intraocular pressure frequently during their use. Though the Ocusert system has been shown to be very effective, it has never gained wide acceptance. It offers several theoretic advantages and may be preferred by younger patients in whom miosis and ciliary spasm remain fairly constant and therefore less bothersome.

Side effects

The most common ocular side effects of pilocarpine are decreased vision in low illumination secondary to pupillary miosis, and induced myopia and supraorbital and temporal headaches attributable to stimulation of the ciliary muscle. Instillation of 2% pilocarpine causes an average accommodative myopia of 5.8 diopters in patients between the ages of 20 and 40 years, 5.0 diopters in

persons between the ages of 40 and 60, and an insignificant shift in patients over the age of 60. As a result, pilocarpine is often poorly tolerated in younger patients and much better tolerated in elderly patients, who have little residual accommodative ability. The miosis can be particularly detrimental in those patients who have central lens opacities. Miosis may be less with the Ocusert system and, therefore, useful in patients with lens opacities.[2,3] Headaches and blurred vision are likely to be worse at the onset of therapy, and with continued application, the browache may disappear completely and visual functioning may improve.

Other side effects include sensitization of the eyelids and conjunctiva, vascular injection, retinal detachment, lens opacities, iris cysts, and precipitation of angle-closure glaucoma.[5] The increase in permeability of the blood-aqueous barrier from the use of pilocarpine can result in severe inflammation when the drug is used postoperatively and in other inflammatory conditions.

Systemic side effects result from muscarinic receptor and smooth muscle stimulation. In particular, stimulation of smooth muscle of the gastrointestinal tract, pulmonary system, urinary tract, and sweat glands with the administration of large dose of pilocarpine may occur,[4] and result in nausea, vomiting, diarrhea, sweating, bronchial spasm, pulmonary edema, and slowing of the heart. Only rarely do these more severe side effects occur after topical administration and usually in doses in excess of 100 mg (far more than delivered with the recommended regimen).

Low-dose pilocarpine used in conjunction with other ocular hypotensive agents, such as acetazolamide, hyperosmotic agents, and beta-blockers, usually constitutes the initial treatment for acute angle-closure glaucoma. Often, the high intraocular pressure encountered in this condition is sufficient to cause ischemia of the sphincter muscle to the degree that it is unresponsive to pilocarpine. Lowering of the intraocular pressure with the concomitant use of other hypotensive agents often restores circulation of the iris and ciliary body, allowing pilocarpine to constrict the pupil and pull the iris out of the angle, thereby breaking the attack. Doses of 1% to 2% pilocarpine are usually sufficient for this purpose. Higher doses and more frequent applications may actually result in worsening of the condition by causing further anterior displacement of the lens-iris diaphragm and greater compromise of the angle.[2,3]

Pilocarpine shows an additive hypotensive effect when used in conjunction with other agents in the therapy of open-angle glaucoma. It is commonly used with one or more of these medications when intraocular pressure is not adequately maintained on one agent alone.

CARBACHOL

In an attempt to find more therapeutically useful acetylcholine-like compounds, carbachol was first synthesized in 1932.[14] Of the drugs investigated at that time, carbachol alone met the criteria for use in the treatment of glaucoma because of its resistance to hydrolysis by the cholinesterases and its suitable specificity.[18,22] Carbachol differs structurally from acetylcholine in that it possesses a carbamyl group rather than an acetyl group. Pharmacologically, this difference is manifest by the relative inability of cholinesterases to degrade carbachol. Though pilocarpine and carbachol differ significantly in their structure (Fig. 24-3), their actions greatly resemble each other.

A significant difference between the two drugs is that carbachol contains a quaternary nitrogen, which gives the molecule a polar charge. This polar area renders it relatively insoluble in lipid solution, which in turn limits its corneal permeability. The

$$(CH_3)_3N + {-\!\!-} CH_2 {-\!\!-} CH_2 {-\!\!-} O {-\!\!-} \overset{\displaystyle O}{\overset{\|}{C}} {-\!\!-} NH_2 \bullet Cl^-$$

Fig. 24-3 Carbachol.

fact that it is resistant to hydrolysis by the cholinesterases, however, does make it a more potent agent than pilocarpine and gives it a longer duration of action. Like pilocarpine, carbachol reduces intraocular pressure by increasing aqueous outflow. The action seems to be direct stimulation of postsynaptic receptors at the neuromuscular junction of the ciliary muscle and at the presynaptic receptor to release acetylcholine. Additionally, the carbamyl group on this compound may provide some anticholinesterase effect, thereby giving it three sites for cholinergic stimulation.

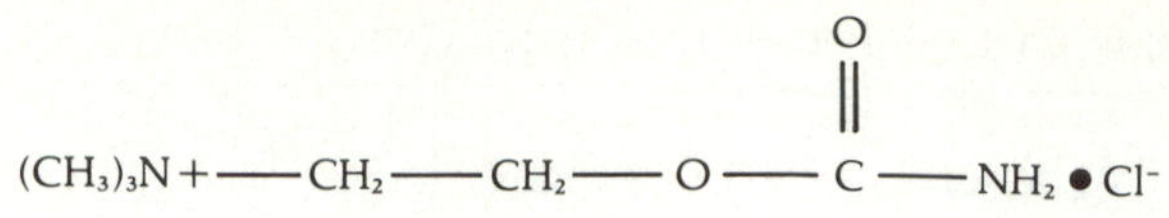

Carbachol is available in concentrations of 0.75%, 1.5%, 2.25%, and 3%. The perservative, benzalkonium chloride, is used in all formulations to enhance its corneal permeability. Typically, the drug is given three times daily. Carbachol has most of the same local side effects as the other parasympathomimetics, though they are somewhat more severe and more common than those caused by pilocarpine. Accommodative spasm, pupillary miosis, dimming of vision, headaches, and conjunctival hyperemia are very common with the use of this medication. Because of the greater miosis and accommodative spasm, carbachol is often less well tolerated than pilocarpine. Despite this, however, it is often very useful in patients in whom pilocarpine is either poorly tolerated or ineffective or when less frequent application of a miotic is desirable. Carbachol causes a more marked increase in vascular permeability than does pilocarpine, making its use even more undesirable in the face of ocular inflammatory conditions.[20] Additionally, because of its strong stimulation of the ciliary muscle, there seems to be a greater tendency for this medication to displace the lens-iris diaphragm anteriorly, which may further compromise the angle in an eye with a preexisting narrow or closed angle. For these two reasons, it is not recommended for use in the treatment of angle-closure glaucoma.

Systemic side effects are encountered somewhat more frequently with the use of carbachol than with pilocarpine, particularly increased salivation, gastric secretion, perspiration, vomiting, diarrhea, bradycardia, and bronchial constriction.

Table 24-2 Commercial preparations of anticholinesterase agents

Generic name	Trade name	Concentration	Container size	Vehicle
Demecarium bromide	Humorsol (Merck, Sharp, & Dohme)	0.125% and 0.25% solutions	5 ml	Sodium chloride, Benzalkonium chloride
Echothiophate iodide	Phospholine Iodide (Ayerst)	Lyophilized powder 1.5 mg, 3.0 mg, 6.25 mg and 12.5 mg with 5 ml. dilutent for preparation of 0.03%, 0.06%, 0.125% and 0.25% solutions		
Diisopropyl fluorophosphate (DFP)-Isofluorophate	Floropryl (Merck, Sharp, & Dohme)	0.025% gel 0.1% solution	3.5 g 5 ml	Mineral oil gel Anhydrous peanut oil

Because of its side effects, the use of carbachol is relatively contraindicated in patients with severe respiratory, cardiovascular, or gastrointestinal tract disease.

ANTICHOLINESTERASE AGENTS

The anticholinesterase organophosphates are a group of compounds initially synthesized in the early years of World War II when scientists were searching for a substance useful in chemical warfare.[16] Many of the agents that were synthesized were later produced commercially as insecticides, some of which are still in common use today. It was not until the 1950s that these agents began to be used in the treatment of glaucoma. It was noted at that time that they had very strong parasympathomimetic activity and a much longer duration of action in their intraocular pressure lowering abilities than either pilocarpine or carbachol.[9]

Three anticholinesterase agents are available for commercial use today. Echothiophate iodide (Phospholine Iodide) is available in four concentrations, 0.03%, 0.06%, 0.125%, and 0.25%. It is extremely sensitive to degradation and must be prepared fresh just before dispensing and then must be kept refrigerated. Prepared and kept this way, the solution is stable for about a year. Diisopropyl fluorophosphate, another "irreversible" inhibitor, is also an extremely potent parasympathomimetic agent but is rarely used today because of its marked susceptibility to hydrolysis. It is so easily hydrolyzed to an inactive form that it must be prepared in mineral oil or gel, which greatly impedes its tolerability because of the blurriness resulting from ocular instillation. In addition, contamination of the solution, with even a small amount of tear fluid or any other water-containing substance, is enough to inactivate the entire con-

tents of the bottle. Demecarium bromide (Humorsol) is the only "reversible" anticholinesterase agent presently used in ophthalmology. This drug is a very stable compound, being relatively insensitive to heat and hydrolysis and, therefore, is formulated or constituted in an aqueous solution and dispensed similarly to other eye drops. It is available in concentrations of 0.125% and 0.25% (Table 24-2).

Though the direct-acting and indirect-acting anticholinesterase agents differ significantly in their chemical structure, both types of compounds appear to function by inactivating acetylcholinesterase and butyrylcholinesterase. Inactivation by reversible inhibitors results from binding of the drug to the cholinesterase enzyme, which is then only slowly reversed by hydrolysis. The irreversible anticholinesterase agents, DFP and echothiophate, bind with acetylcholinesterase by alkyl phosphorylation of the enzyme to form a stable drug/enzyme complex, which is only minimally reversible. The binding of cholinesterase, either reversibly or irreversibly, prevents hydrolysis of acetylcholine. The transmitter then accumulates in large quantities at the neuromuscular junction, strongly stimulating the parasympathetic nerve ending.

Much less is known about the dose-response and duration of action of these anticholinesterase agents than is known about pilocarpine and carbachol. Extreme miosis occurs within half an hour of administration and maximum intraocular pressure reduction occurs within 24 hours.[9] Pressure reduction is of extremely long duration, lasting anywhere from several days to 2 weeks. Though commonly administered twice daily, adequate pressure reduction may be maintained with instillation once daily and sometimes as infrequently as twice a week. As with other miotics, the patient's sensitivity to these medications may diminish with time.

Local ocular side effects of anticholinesterase agents are similar to those of other miotics, but in many cases are more profound. Often side effects are severe enough to warrant discontinuation of the drug. Proliferation of the pigment epithelium resulting in iris cyst formation is fairly common.[9] The cysts usually disappear with discontinuation of the medication, and simultaneous instillation of phenylephrine may reduce their occurrence. Formation of cataracts is a well-documented effect of drugs that inhibit lens cholinesterase. Acetylcholinesterase is present in the lens capsule. Inhibition of this enzyme increases hydration of the lens and may upset the ionic balance and oxygen consumption of the lens, resulting in anterior subcapsular lens opacities.[7,17] Allergic contact dermatitis is not infrequent. Theoretically, because of the strong stimulation of the ciliary muscle, retinal detachment is thought to be more common with anticholinesterases than with other miotics.

Systemic side effects are similar to those of pilocarpine but may also be more marked. These include nausea, vomiting, diarrhea, hyperperistalsis, dizziness, and hypotension.[4,9] It is important to be aware of the occurrence of the systemic side effects with these agents, in particular, the gastrointestinal problems and diarrhea, for which a number of patients have had extensive medical workups before the offending agent has been found. A significant inhibition of plasma cholinesterase levels has been noted within 3 to 4 weeks of the onset of administration of a 0.25% solution of echothiophate iodide twice daily.[1] Investigators have also noted a decrease in red blood cell cholinesterase though not as often or as dramatically as a decrease in plasma levels.[10,11] Because of the possible bradycardia and bronchial smooth muscle stimulation, the use of these agents may be contraindicated in the presence of heart disease and restrictive airway disease. This possible exacerbation of restrictive airway disease, particularly asthma or emphysema, is often overlooked in these patients.

Because of their interference with the function of acetylcholinesterase and butyrylcholinesterase, certain drug interactions are more likely to occur and should be avoided.[10] In particular, certain anesthetics, including chloroprocaine, procaine, tetracaine, and dibucaine rely on plasma cholinesterase for their hydrolysis.[12] Inhibition of this enzyme by cholinergic inhibitors may result in the potentiation of pharmacologic effects of these anesthetics, increasing not only their desired effects but also their toxicities. Additionally, the commonly used muscle relaxant in the induction of general anesthesia, succinylcholine, is inactivated by cholinesterases. With the decrease in plasma cholinesterase levels brought about by the use of anticholinesterase agents, the effects of succinylcholine in paralyzing the patient is markedly potentiated, resulting in the need for lengthy respiratory support after surgery. For this reason, it is important to inform the patient and the anesthesiologist about the side effects of these medications in the event that general anesthesia is required.

In general, the use of anticholinesterase medications for the treatment of open-angle glaucoma is reserved for cases in which the patient has become intolerant to pilocarpine or carbachol or when the pressure lowering effect of these medications is inadequate. Like other miotic agents, these drugs can be used in conjunction with beta-blockers and with epinephrine compounds, as well as carbonic anhydrase inhibitors. Conditions, such as cataractous lens changes and peripheral retinal pathology may be relative contraindications to the use of these drugs. However, these agents are very effective in aphakic or pseudophakic glaucoma. Because of the degree of miosis and accommodative spasm, their use in younger patients is often not possible. The use of anticholinesterase agents in the treatment of acute angle-closure glaucoma is contraindicated. Extreme caution should be used in patients with narrow angles. With the intense stimulation of the ciliary muscle, these agents may actually narrow the angle further and precipitate or perpetuate angle-closure. Additionally, the vasodilatory effects of these medications result in a marked increase and permeability of the blood-aqueous barrier, which often greatly intensifies the inflammation accompanying angle-closure glaucoma and worsens synechiae formation.

REFERENCES

1. de Roetth, A, et al: Blood cholinesterase activity in glaucoma patients treated with Phospholine Iodide, Am J Ophthalmol 62:834, 1966
2. François, J, and Goes, F: Comparative ultrasonographic study of the effect of pilocarpine 2% and Ocusert P20 on the eye components, Am J Ophthalmol 86:233, 1978
3. François, J, and Goes, F: Ultrasonographic study of the effect of different miotics on the eye components, Ophthalmologica 175:328, 1977
4. Goodman, LS, and Gilman, A, editors: The pharmacological basis of therapeutics, ed 5, New York, 1985, Macmillan

5. Grant, WM: Toxiocology of the eye: drug, chemicals, plants, venoms, ed 2, Springfield, IL, 1974, Charles C Thomas

6. Hallett, M, and Cullen, RF: Intoxication with echothiophate iodide, JAMA 222:1414, 1972

7. Harkkonen, M, and Tarkkannen, A: Effect of Phospholine Iodide on energy metabolites of the rabbit lens, Exp Eye Res 10:1, 1970

8. Harris LS, and Galin, MA: Dose response analysis of pilocarpine induced ocular hypotension, Arch Ophthalmol 93:42, 1975

9. Havener, WH: Ocular pharmacology, ed 4, St. Louis, 1978, The CV Mosby Co

10. Hiscox, PEA, and McCulloch, C: The effect of echothiophate iodide on systemic cholinesterase, Can J Ophthalmol 1:274, 1966

11. Humphreys, JA, and Holmes, JH: Systemic effects produced by echothiophate iodide in treatment of glaucoma, Arch Ophthalmol 69:737, 1963

12. Kalow, W: Hydrolysis of local anesthetics by human serum cholinesterase, J Pharmacol Exp Ther 104:122, 1952

13. Kaufman, PL, and Bárány, EH: Loss of acute pilocarpine effect on outflow facility following surgical disinsertion and retrodisplacement of the scleral spur in the cynomolgus monkey, Invest Ophthalmol Vis Sci 15:793, 1976

14. Kreitmair, H: Die Papavarinwirkung eine Benzylreaktion, Arch F Path u Pharmakol 164:509, 1932

15. Manse, RHG, and Holmes, HL: The alkaloids: chemistry and physiology, New York, 1953, Academic Press

16. McCombie, H, and Saunders, BC: Alkyl fluorophosphonates: preparation and physiological properties, Nature 157:287, 1946

17. Michon, J, and Kinoshita, JH: Experimental miotic cataract, Arch Ophthalmol 79:79, 1968

18. Militor, H: A comparative study of the effects of five choline compounds used in therapeutics: acetylcholine chloride, acetyl-beta-methylcholine chloride, carbaminoyl choline, ethyl ether beta-methylcholine chloride, carbaminoyl beta methycholine chloride, J Pharmacol Exp Ther 58:337, 1936

19. Ringer, S, and Gould, AP: On Jabornadi, Lancet 157-59, 1875.

20. Stocker, FW: Experimental studies on the blood-aqueous barrier, Arch Ophthalmol 37:583, 1947

21. Van Buskirk, EM, and Grant, WM: Lens depression and aqueous outflow in enucleated primate eyes, Am J Ophthalmol 76:632, 1973

22. Velhagen, K: Die Grundlager der okularen Pharmakologie und Toxikologie des Carbaminocholins, Arch Augenheilk 107:319, 1933

23. Weber, A: Die Ursache des Glaukoms, von Graefe's Arch Ophthalmol 23:91, 1877

24. Zimmerman, TJ, Kendall, KS, Mundorf, TK, and Nardin, GF: Pilocarpine: a re-look at dose response and duration of action, Invest Ophthalmol Vis Sci 28 (suppl): 377, 1987

Chapter 25

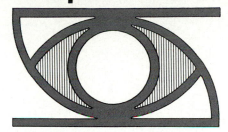

Adrenergic and Dopaminergic Drugs in Glaucoma

Thomas W. Mittag

The adrenergic pharmacology of aqueous humor dynamics has been reviewed from both a clinical and basic science perspective.[45,52,59,64,76] Frequent review of this area is warranted because of changing ideas on the physiologic regulation of intraocular pressure and its pharmacologic manipulation. The present decade has been an era of rapid change in our concept of the physiologic regulation of intraocular pressure and its pharmacologic manipulation. The potential impact of the application of biochemical and molecular methods on the drug therapy of glaucoma is enormous. The recent successful cloning and sequencing of several adrenergic receptor subtypes[20,35] is a dramatic illustration of this. This brief review will update some of the concepts relating to catecholamine receptor systems and provide a framework for a more specific discussion of the effects on intraocular pressure of a variety of drug types. For the purposes of this review the term *catecholamine* includes systems affected by the endogenous transmitters norepinephrine (NE), epinephrine (E), and dopamine (DA). Metabolic events relating to the biosynthesis and metabolism of these transmitters are covered in standard textbooks.

CATECHOLAMINE RECEPTORS: GENERAL CONCEPTS

Basic Definitions

The receptor concept is fundamental to pharmacology. The relatively new technique of ligand-binding has helped redefine our concepts of the physical nature of a receptor, which now refers to the macromolecule containing the recognition domain (binding sites) for a specific endogenous hormone (signal) that initiates a chain of events (signal transduction) resulting in specific cellular responses.

The signal transduction system, which is directly coupled to a receptor, involves other macromolecular components, which can generate a *second messenger* molecule from endogenous precursors. This complex of macromolecules associated with the receptor protein may be termed a *receptor system.* There has been a spectacular increase in our understanding of signal transduction through the discovery of G-proteins,[83] and in many cases the biochemical consequences of the hormone-receptor interaction can now be directly correlated with the classic pharmacology of drug response. Simplified schemes for three signal transduction systems involving catecholamine receptors are shown in Fig. 25-1.

It is now 40 years since Ahlquist[1] proposed the subdivision of adrenergic recognition sites into alpha and beta subclasses. Since then, on the basis of examination of many thousands of adrenergic drugs, each subclass has been further divided into at least two subtypes. In addition, there may even be a third subclass of receptor for NE.[10] The currently accepted existence of four types of adrenergic receptors for NE and two for DA has been corroborated by ligand-binding studies and by molecular differences in amino acid sequence of the

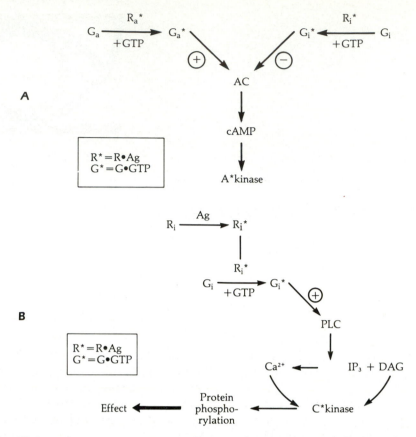

Fig. 25-1 Simplified schemes depicting some presently known signal transduction systems for adrenergic and for dopaminergic receptors. **A,** Dual regulation of adenylate cyclase via activatory receptors (R_a, e.g., beta-adrenergic or DA_1) and inhibitory receptors (R_i, e.g., alpha$_2$-adrenergic, DA_2), which control in part the concentration of the second messenger cAMP, and the activity of cAMP-dependent protein kinase (A* kinase). **B,** Scheme for activation of protein kinase C (C* kinase) by receptors (R_i, e.g., alpha$_1$-adrenergic) involved in the generation of inositol polyphosphates *(IP$_3$* and diacylglycerol *(DAG)* second messengers via G-protein regulation of phospholipase C *(PLC)*. *R**, Receptor activated by agonist (Ag) binding; *G**, G-protein activated by GTP binding to the alpha-subunit.

receptor proteins in the case of adrenergic receptors.[35]

The binding of a certain class of ligand (agonists) catalyzes a change of state in the receptor from the ground state (R) to the activated state (R*), whereas binding of another class of ligand (antagonists) does not catalyze this change and may in fact stabilize the ground state. Agonist activation of R to R* initiates the signal transduction process as depicted in Fig. 25-1. For all four adrenergic receptors and the two DA receptors, the next step involves activation of coupling proteins (G-proteins) by R*. The G-proteins are regulators of specific cellular enzymes or ion channels. At least three different G-proteins are associated with adrenergic receptor subtypes: beta$_1$- and beta$_2$-receptors are associated with the activation of G_s, which is a stimulatory regulator of adenylyl cyclase (Fig. 25-1, *A*). This generates the second messenger cyclic AMP (cAMP), resulting in protein phosphorylation via activated cAMP-dependent protein kinase (A* kinase). Alpha$_2$-receptors are associated with another G protein, G_i, which inhibits adenylyl cyclase (Fig. 25-1, *A*), whereas alpha$_1$-receptors are associated with a G-protein, which also seems to be G_i, and which activates a specific, regulated phospholipase C (PLC) enzyme (Fig. 25-1, *B*). PLC produces two second messengers from polyphosphoinositide lipid precursors, namely inositol triphosphate (IP$_3$) and diacylglycerol (DAG). Ca^{2+} mobilization via IP$_3$ in the presence of DAG is the signal required to activate another protein kinase

(PKC). Dopamine receptors are similarly associated with G_s (DA_1) or G_i proteins (DA_2).

The G-protein family of coupling proteins are capable of binding guanyl nucleotides, have GTPase enzymatic activity, and have a similar three-component structure. Two of these subunits may be identical for many G-proteins, which appear to differ only in their alpha-component.[17] It thus seems that the alpha-component determines not only with which receptor a particular G-protein can be associated, but also the specific enzyme or channel that it can regulate.

The interaction between receptors and G-proteins is fairly well understood. When receptors are in the activated R* state, they can catalyze the exchange of guanosine diphosphate (GDP) bound to the G-protein for cytoplasmic glutamyl transpeptidase (GTP). This binding of GTP causes dissociation of the G-protein into its subunits, the alpha-portion carrying the GTP (G*) and functioning as a specific regulator of cellular processes. However G* is transitory because its GTPase activity converts it into an inactive GDP complex that reassociates with the other subunits to reform the ground state G-protein (G) (Fig. 25-1).

The association of receptors with G-proteins can be identified by the binding behavior of agonists.[51] In the absence of Mg^{+2} and GTP the high affinity binding of agonists likely reflects binding to a [receptor + G-protein] complex. The addition of Mg^{+2} and GTP to the binding reaction permits agonist activation of G by the GDP/GTP exchange process and dissociates it from the receptor protein. The shift to low affinity binding of agonists under these binding reaction conditions likely reflects binding to R alone.

At the present time, only four physiologic substances are unequivocally considered to act as second messengers by virtue of being able to elicit cellular responses, namely cAMP, Ca^{+2}, inositol triphosphate (IP_3), and cGMP. The first three of these have been associated with adrenergic or DA receptors/G-proteins, and their analytic determination represents a biochemical measurement of drug response at such receptors. Subsequent steps of signal transduction beyond the second messenger level are complex, and in many cases the details are unknown. For example, it is unclear how a single second messenger molecule such as Ca^{+2}, which has many cellular effects, is restricted to a particular response in a particular cell type. However, one general mechanism that is recognized as a major element of second messenger function is regulation of protein phosphorylation. The post-translational modification of proteins with respect to the degree and site of phosphorylation plays a role in many cellular responses and can cause the following effects: (1) changes in metabolic or other enzymatic activity, (2) changes in sensitivity to hormone signals, (3) changes in ion and other transport processes, (4) changes in cellular surface properties/cell shape, or (5) changes in the interactions between cells and their extracellular matrix.

Receptor Regulation of Tissue Function

The validity of the ligand-binding method for receptor identification in tissue homogenates is confirmed by the classic pharmacology of the intact tissue response. However, to understand the relationship between receptors and cellular physiology or biochemistry, the gross presence of receptors in a tissue is insufficient information, and their cellular and even subcellular location needs to be known. Histologic and immunocytochemical methods are important for this purpose.

Tracing of nerves by methods that visualize a transmitter substance or the enzymes involved in its biosynthesis can indicate which cells are likely to have receptors for the transmitter. The elegant studies by Laties and Jacobowitz[42] and by Ehinger,[21] among others, during the 1960s used the Falk-Hillarp method to map adrenergic nerves in the anterior uvea. The presence of such nerves in the trabecular region, in ciliary processes, and associated with the vascular system is especially relevant to the use of adrenergic drugs in glaucoma. These techniques are still undergoing refinements to improve specificity and resolution of very fine nerve fibers and to define their cellular destination.[62]

Histochemical approaches that use neuronal transmitter markers, however, are biased toward the detection of synaptic contacts between nerves and their target cell. More recent physiologic studies have indicated that other modes of intercellular communication may be at least as important in the regulation of relatively slow autonomic functions. Thus nerves need not specifically make synaptic contact with particular cells but may affect many neighboring cells by a neurosecretory mechanism.

Another nonsynaptic form of intercellular communication is the paracrine system, in which a transmitter or hormone substance is released locally from certain secreting cells and affects neighboring cells. The release of the local hormone from the paracrine cell could be controlled by synaptic transmission onto the cell by a neurohormone different from that released by the paracrine cell itself. Paracrine cells containing catecholamines have been identified in several autonomic tissues and in epithelial tissues.[57,84] These nonsynaptic mechanisms are by definition more diffuse because many cells within a reasonable diffusional distance can respond. The tracing of nerves does not indicate the location of cells responsive to neurosecretory or paracrine communication nor the type of receptors on them. These receptors are thus often termed *extrajunctional* to distinguish them from the junctional receptors associated with synapses and nerve endings.

More recently, the ligand-binding method has been adapted to the histochemical level,[38] and it is now possible to identify receptors on cells directly. Such studies in ocular tissues were performed first using fluorescent antagonists,[43] and more recently tritium-labeled ligands and autoradiography.[23] In this way beta-adrenergic receptor sites have been identified on nonpigmented ciliary epithelial cells and on human trabecular meshwork cells.[31] These studies complement results obtained with cultures of these cell types showing the presence of beta$_2$-adrenergic receptors.[63] The presence of one subtype of adrenergic receptor on these cells does not preclude the possible occurrence of other catecholamine receptors such as alpha-adrenergic or DA-receptors on the same cells.

Further refinements and resolution of receptor-site visualization methods are needed to provide information on the subcellular or regional membrane location of receptors. The location of receptors at this level of resolution is important in isotropic cells that have "sidedness," such as epithelial cells. The apical side of such cells could have a different set of receptors/signal transduction systems than the basolateral side. Such a differential distribution of receptors is suggested in some histochemical studies and also by the finding that in the isolated rabbit ciliary body, catecholamines affect electrical properties only from the blood (stromal) side.[15]

Another important regional localization of receptors is on the presynaptic membrane of nerve terminals. The function of these receptors in a physiologic situation has been difficult to demonstrate, but their role as a feedback inhibitor of transmitter release can be readily shown pharmacologically. The presence of such receptors has been demonstrated in iris–ciliary body preparations by measuring the evoked (by field stimulation) release of NE from tissues preloaded with labeled NE. Evoked release is decreased in the presence of alpha$_2$-adrenergic agonists.[33] Although presynaptic adrenergic receptors seem to be generally of the alpha$_2$-subtype, the postsynaptic receptor can be either the same or a different subtype.

It is inferred that the physiologic role of presynaptic autoinhibition is to ensure that when the release of NE reaches a certain level it becomes self-limiting and shuts off further release. If feedback autoinhibition is physiologically relevant, then it is a possible site of drug action and therefore complicates the conventional interpretation of drug effects based on responses in intact animals. This can be illustrated by considering a synapse with alpha$_2$-presynaptic and beta$_2$-postsynaptic receptors in a physiologic situation (i.e., with existing tone). Treatment with a selective alpha$_2$-agonist will decrease NE release and decrease the post-synaptic beta$_2$-receptor-mediated response. This result is functionally equivalent to using a beta$_2$-adrenergic blocker. Conversely, treatment with a selective alpha$_2$-blocker could enhance the release of transmitter (by preventing endogenous feedback inhibition) and increase the postsynaptic response without changing the level of neuronal activity.

Basis for Differential Receptor-Initiated Responses

Structural differences in drugs and receptors

The major factor determining selective responses to adrenergic drugs with different structural characteristics are the molecular differences in the recognition component of receptors. The exploitation of these differences has been the driving force for much of modern drug development. It is also in part the basis of organ-specific therapy, giving rise to the terminology for beta$_1$-selective drugs as "cardioselective" and beta$_2$-selective agents as "bronchoselective." However, the association of receptor subtype and a specific organ or tissue is not a constant, and the preceding organ-based division of beta-receptor drugs holds for humans but not other species. Thus, the same function in a particular tissue can be regulated via a different receptor in different species. A variant of this species difference is that the same function may be regulated by two or more receptor systems, but the normal degree of control exerted via each of these systems can vary between species. An example of this may be the responsiveness of primates but lack of response in other species to beta-blockers with respect to intraocular pressure: Primates appear to have an appreciable level of endogenous regulation of aqueous humor dynamics mediated via beta-receptors, whereas rabbits have little.

It is also worth considering that the degree of control of a particular response can vary with state of the tissue, such as in neonatal, geriatric, or pathologic situations. All these factors contribute to some of the problems in glaucoma research, such as the risk of extrapolating experimental findings to different mammalian species, and major disappointments in antiglaucoma drug development where the drug in clinical trials fails to live up to expectations indicated by preclinical studies.

Receptor distribution and number

Another basis for differential drug response is a nonuniform regional distribution of subtypes of a receptor (qualitative) as well as the number of receptors (quantitative) in a tissue. The importance of these factors is most clearly seen in the vascular system. With regard to the qualitative factor, extensive studies have shown that postsynaptic alpha$_1$-receptors generally predominate in peripheral arterial regulation, whereas postsynaptic alpha$_2$-receptors predominate in the venous system.[73] There is also evidence suggesting that blood vessels may have two variants of the alpha-receptor type differentially located at presynaptic and postsynaptic sites. This may eventually lead to designation of an "alpha$_3$" receptor if molecular structural differences from the established alpha$_2$-subtype are shown.[35] Additionally, the degree of presynaptic autoinhibitory control varies according to the distribution of presynaptic receptors. There is also a differential distribution in various vascular beds of extrajunctional receptors that are not directly associated with nerve endings.

The quantitative factor may be an important determinant of response when there are significant regional variations in receptor density. The number of agonist-occupied receptors needed to elicit the maximal response to NE may be a small fraction of the available alpha-receptors, as in some peripheral arterioles (about 10%) or there may be too few receptors to give a response, as in cerebral microvessels. These extremes of responsiveness may have ocular counterparts in the uveal and retinal vasculature respectively.

The role of effective receptor number can be illustrated by considering a blood vessel in which one region has 3 times the receptor density of another region. For an equivalent degree of sympathetic tone (same amount and concentration of NE release), according to the law of mass action, the number of occupied receptors (and hence activated signal transduction systems) will be approximately threefold greater in one region of the vessel causing vasoconstriction; whereas the lower density region of the vessel might give only a threshold response.

Based on similar quantitative considerations, when these two regions of the blood vessel are at an equivalent vasoconstrictive response level, they will be differentially sensitive to the same antagonist drug concentration.

The role of endothelial cells is another recently recognized factor in the pharmacology of blood vessels. These cells are responsive to a range of transmitter substances and hormones and can change their shape, contact with adjacent cells, or interaction with the extracellular matrix, all of which affect endothelial permeability. Endothelial cells can also behave as a paracrine signal system by releasing substances that affect the function of adjacent cells. Some of these substances have been characterized, such as those derived from arachidonic acid, but the chemical identity of others, such as endothelium-derived relaxing factors, are not yet fully known.[24] Endothelial cells represent a potentially important and not fully understood target for drug modulation of the microvasculature.

Some or all of the preceding factors may be directly relevant to glaucoma therapy because most glaucoma drugs affecting catecholamine receptors will cause vascular changes. There is also evidence that the pathology of glaucoma has a vascular component.[40]

Signal coupling efficiency/use-dependent changes in receptor function

The concept of "spare" receptors referred to here has important consequences at the molecular level. Response depends on receptors capable of activating the signal transduction system, but the "spare" receptors may or may not be coupled to the signal transduction system. However, even at the maximal cellular response level, additional occupancy of coupled receptors can cause the level of second messenger to increase further. Persistent overstimulation of the signal transduction system, which decreases responsiveness and the efficiency of transduction, is variously termed desensitization, subsensitivity, tachyphylaxis, or refractoriness.

Several mechanisms seem to control the efficiency of signal transduction. Modification of G-proteins by phosphorylation may decrease either their activation by R* or the capability of G* to regulate an enzyme or channel protein (see Fig. 25-1). This is thought to be the general mechanism for heterologous desensitization, so-called because all the receptor proteins (R) that couple to that particular G-protein will show hyporesponsiveness. The other form of desensitization (homologous) is receptor-specific because only the receptor activated by the specific agonist is desensitized. In this case, the receptor protein itself has a decreased ability to generate G*, and additional receptors may be removed from the cell membrane by internalization. It is thought that these changes in the receptor protein are brought about by phosphorylation by a specific kinase (R-kinase), which can phosphorylate receptors in the active state (R*) but not in the ground state. The R-kinases for beta-adrenergic receptors[5] and for rhodopsin[4] have been identified, and these enzymes are partly cross-reactive for the respective activated receptor proteins.

It is clear that, as a consequence of decreased signal transduction efficiency by either mechanism, more receptors must be occupied, requiring higher concentrations of agonist, to reach the same level of response as in the nondesensitized state. The practical result of desensitization is that greater drug doses are required to reach the initial response level. With repeated dosing the maximal response level may decline.

From the foregoing discussion it is clear that the relationship of cellular responsiveness to the number and state of receptors present is complex and variable. Not only is the total density important in determining supersensitive or subsensitive responses, but redistribution of receptors from coupled to uncoupled states may be the major determinant in the late response phase of treatment with agonist drugs. For example, the induction of the desensitized state of a receptor in a physiologic situation can be functionally equivalent to specific blockade of that receptor by antagonist drugs. The concepts of spare receptors (receptor reserve) and desensitized (uncoupled) receptors may have application for mechanisms of adrenergic drug effects in the eye.

Pharmacokinetics

The topical ocular application of drugs to determine quantitative relationships between dose and intraocular responses has special difficulties. In general, the comparative value of such data applies to different doses of the same agent, but it is often very misleading when comparing drugs of differing chemical structure. The major reason for this is the wide range of conjunctival and corneal permeability exhibited by compounds of varying structure. A better comparison of drugs with respect to their in vivo receptor specificity and potency would be obtained at equivalent intraocular concentrations, data that are rarely available. Even

after accounting for corneal permeability, the time-action curves of different agents may not be comparable because of differences in intraocular pharmacokinetics and the amount of drug retained by various intraocular tissues.[48] The capture efficiency of cells for drugs depends on many factors including lipid/aqueous solubility (partition coefficient), pH trapping (drug pKa), metabolic trapping (e.g., prodrugs) and protein binding (e.g., melanin binding), all of which depend on drug structure.

As a result, it seems that for some adrenergic agents used topically in the eye the absolute potency at the receptor level can be of lesser importance compared to the drugs' pharmacokinetics. A case in point is the epinephrine prodrug dipivefrin, made by esterifying epinephrine with pivalic acid. An order of magnitude increase in apparent potency results mainly from a more favorable partition coefficient and metabolic trapping by hydrolysis of the prodrug by intracellular esterases. Pharmacokinetic factors are similarly important for the three beta-blockers used clinically at comparable dosages (timolol, levbunolol, and betaxolol), all of which have a high capture efficiency by ocular tissues but differ by more than two orders of magnitude with respect to their absolute potency at beta$_2$-adrenergic receptors.

DRUGS AFFECTING INTRAOCULAR PRESSURE

Catecholamines affect function in all the structures involved in aqueous humor dynamics: trabecular outflow, aqueous production, uveoscleral outflow, and the intraocular microcirculation. There are probably several different cell types and several different receptors associated with each of the above components that determine intraocular pressure.

Catecholamine drug action in the eye is highly complex. A single agent may affect both inflow and outflow in several ways. The contribution of each of these elements to the overall effect can change from the early phase to the late phase of response and also depends on whether an acute dose or repeated chronic doses are given. In many cases the only available data on drug mechanisms are from animal studies where the contribution of various mechanisms can differ significantly from humans.

Discussion of the ocular actions and mechanisms of catecholamines is a highly speculative undertaking, often made more difficult because of the large body of contradictory literature on the subject. Nevertheless, it is worthwhile to establish a hypothetical framework for adrenergic mechanisms and aqueous humor dynamics, and it is preferable to merely listing all the agents and their reported effects.

Agents Affecting Catecholamine Synthesis Storage, Release, and Metabolism

Denervation

The investigations of aqueous humor dynamics in subjects with unilateral Horner's syndrome is important from a conceptual point of view. Such subjects have normal intraocular pressure and aqueous flow[90] and do not have an increased prevalence of glaucoma in the absence of sympathetic tone from the superior cervical ganglion. Thus adrenergic regulation appears not to be essential for the maintenance of normal intraocular pressure, although the diurnal variation of intraocular pressure in experimental animals does depend on an intact superior cervical ganglion.[26] Evidence for diurnal sympathetic regulation of aqueous flow in humans is provided by fluorophotometric studies showing greater responses to blockers of beta-adrenergic receptors during the day and to agonists at night.[88]

It is not known whether other regulatory mechanisms take over in Horner's syndrome or the ganglionectomized situation. Such subjects, however, do show supersensitivity to exogenous epinephrine. This observation gave rise to the concept of *chemical sympathectomy*, which combined subconjunctival injections of 6-hydroxydopamine to induce increased sensitivity, together with topical epinephrine for the treatment of refractory glaucoma.[75] The increased response to epinephrine is mostly the result of elimination of the uptake system by destruction of the nerve terminal, which prevents rapid transmitter loss, but is also partly caused by postsynaptic adaptation of the receptor systems into hyperresponsive states.

The presynaptic component of the sympathectomy response can be achieved without causing degeneration of the nerve terminal by the use of a number of drugs. These include inhibitors of the major NE metabolizing enzymes; monamine oxidase or catecholamine methyltransferase; blockers of NE uptake systems, such as cocaine or protriptyline; or by agents that interfere with granule storage of NE, such as reserpine or guanethidine. In some cases, these treatments can give a direct early response caused by release of endogenous catecholamine stores. Subsequent to this phase, when

nerve terminal function is blocked, there is potentiation and/or prolongation of responses to exogenous epinephrine or NE.

The possibility of using sympathetic nerve terminals for false transmitter therapy has also been evaluated. Both alpha-methyl tyrosine and alpha-methyldopa, if taken up by nerve terminals, could function as precursors for the neuronal synthesis of alpha-methylnorepinephrine, which could be released as a false transmitter, replacing NE. Because this transmitter analog has less alpha$_1$-adrenergic receptor activity and less neuronal reuptake compared with NE,[39] responses would be shifted to mechanisms involving alpha$_2$- and beta-receptors and would also be prolonged relative to endogenous NE.

None of these approaches based on altering nerve terminal function has progressed beyond the experimental stage. However, other presynaptic nerve terminal mechanisms such as inhibition of transmitter release (autoinhibition) or blockade of transmitter synthesis may be components in the clinical action of epinephrine, alpha$_2$-adrenergic agonists (clonidine), and DA$_2$-agonists.

Agonists

Nonselective agonists

Epinephrine remains an important drug in the therapy of open-angle glaucoma. Because the selectivity ratio of epinephrine for adrenergic receptor subtypes is too low to be significant at the dosages used in glaucoma treatment, actions at all receptor types and all possible mechanisms may influence its effect on intraocular pressure.

Thus it is not too surprising that no principal mechanism of action has emerged, and epinephrine affects aqueous flow, trabecular outflow, and uveoscleral outflow. It is thus likely that all mechanisms affecting aqueous humor dynamics are components of the exogenous epinephrine or NE response, and their relative importance depends on such variables as dose, time, and species, giving rise to many apparently contradictory findings. In addition, the dosages of epinephrine that are used clinically are likely in the range of physiologic overdosage at some receptor/signal transduction systems. The development of desensitization has been documented in experimental animals.[54] Accordingly, changes in signal-coupling efficiency, such as desensitization, must be seriously considered for the late phase therapeutic responses of epinephrine in humans. All of these considerations also apply to the prodrug form of epinephrine (dipivalyl epinephrine or dipivefrin) because even though the administered dosages are lower, the level of epinephrine present in intraocular tissues may be higher than when epinephrine itself is administered topically.

Beta-adrenergic selective agonists

Agonists that have a high selectivity for the beta$_2$-receptor subtype have been developed more recently. Topical application of isoproterenol in normal subjects and in patients with ocular hypertension was found to decrease intraocular pressure.[25] The drug was thought to reduce aqueous humor formation, but a subsequent study in normal subjects showed no effect of isoproterenol on intraocular pressure or on aqueous humor flow.[11] Similarly, findings on isoproterenol in rabbits are also contradictory, but in this case are related to the drug's effects on outflow facility.[41]

The most consistent findings regarding beta-adrenergic agonists responses suggest that isoproterenol and the beta$_2$-subtype selective agents salbutamol and terbutaline lower intraocular pressure in primates principally by reducing aqueous humor formation.[91] However, beta-adrenergic agonists can also increase the rate of aqueous formation in primates.[7] Differences may occur in the primary site of action of these drugs as a function of time. Although it has been reported that the intraocular arterial vascular beds in rabbits and monkeys lack a beta-receptor-mediated relaxation response,[6] relaxation of vascular smooth muscle could increase intraocular blood volume and ciliary perfusion rate, which may possibly cause an increase in aqueous formation and raise intraocular pressure. Such responses to beta-agonists have been reported.[60] If, on the other hand, vasodilation were to occur predominantly in the venous circulation, then increases in outflow facility might be anticipated.

Vascular endothelial cells are also a potential site for beta-adrenergic agonist effects.[82] The fenestrated ciliary capillaries are permeable to plasma proteins, and estimates of the plasma protein concentration in the ciliary extravascular space (stroma) range up to 70% of the plasma concentration. Colloid osmotic pressure will cause a backflow of water from the posterior chamber into the stroma until balanced by a rise in solute concentration of the nascent aqueous humor.[18] As discussed previously, endothelial cells are pharmacologically reactive and their permeability properties may determine stromal oncotic pressure. An increase in stromal plasma protein content would increase the backflow of fluid from the aqueous to the stromal side and be perceived as a net decrease in aqueous formation. This action of beta-adrenergic agonists might be difficult to demonstrate experimentally in fenestrated ciliary vessels, but it has been reported for nonfenestrated iris vessels that respond with an increase in permeability to macromolecules.[85]

Nonvascular mechanisms for beta-agonist effects include direct actions on trabecular cells and on nonpigmented ciliary epithelial cells, both of which bear beta$_2$-adrenergic receptors.[22,23] Trabecular endothelial cells could respond with an increase in permeability similar to the postulated response of ciliary vascular endothelial cells, resulting in improved outflow. The beta-receptor/adenylate cyclase system may directly regulate the ion transport functions of the nonpigmented ciliary epithelial cells, which may be shut down by activation of beta-receptors.[77] At the present time, it is not clear whether the shutdown of transport in nonpigmented epithelial cells is directly caused by increases in cAMP or to decreased cAMP levels. The decreased levels could occur as a result of desensitization and uncoupling of the cAMP generating system from receptors caused by overstimulation by exogenous beta-agonist. In this state the second messenger system is hyporesponsive to endogenous receptor signals and behaves as if a beta-receptor blocker were present. This hypothesis predicts that a reversal of response will be seen between the early direct phase of drug action and the later indirect (desensitized) phase. Thus, depending on time and dosage, increases or decreases in aqueous humor formation may be observed, as have been reported for beta-agonist responses.

As with the actions of epinephrine, the confusion relating to beta-agonist effects on intraocular pressure results from the fact that for almost every set of data on a particular mechanism there are equally reliable data for the opposite effect of that mechanism.

The inconsistent findings reported for beta-agonists together with side effects such as ocular pain and systemic cardiovascular effects have discouraged studies on the beta-selective agonists as potential antiglaucoma agents.

Alpha-adrenergic selective agonists

Early studies used phenylephrine, a relatively selective alpha$_1$-agonist. It is an effective mydriatic with minimal intraocular pressure effects in humans[2] but may either elevate or reduce intraocular pressure in animals.[72] Methoxamine behaves similarly. The hypertensive effects in animals may be related to the contraction of extraocular muscles[71] and the hypotensive responses to ocular arterial vasoconstriction, causing a reduced ocular blood volume. Because both of these mechanisms are undesirable for a glaucoma therapeutic agent, the alpha$_1$-subclass of adrenergic agonist does not seem to be a promising area for new drugs.

The development of relatively selective alpha$_2$-agonists began with clonidine. This agonist is somewhat alpha$_2$-selective and is a potent hypotensive drug with both systemic and central nervous system sites of action. Low topical ocular doses (0.125%) in humans cause a significant fall in intraocular pressure along with some effect on pupil size, but only minimal effects on systemic blood pressure.[29] At higher doses, systemic hypotension also contributes to the lowering of intraocular pressure. The decrease in intraocular pressure is associated with a lowering of episcleral venous pressure, increased facility of outflow, and a decrease in aqueous humor formation in experimental animals.[13] The drug also has a significant contralateral effect in the untreated eye, which may be caused by drug crossover, a consensual response, or drug reaching the brain and affecting central nervous system regulation of intraocular pressure.

Several more selective alpha$_2$-agonists have been developed. These include BHT-920, p-aminoclonidine, and UK-14301. Low topical doses (0.1%) of BHT-920 to one eye lower intraocular pressure in both eyes of experimental animals, including monkeys,[30] show little pupillary effect, and cause small changes in ocular and systemic blood flow.[86] It is unlikely that the reduced intraocular blood volume is responsible for the intraocular pressure effect, which is most likely caused by a reduction of aqueous humor formation.[86] Other selective alpha$_2$-agonists give a similar response pattern.

Based on earlier concepts that alpha$_2$-adrenergic receptors were mostly located presynaptically, it might be supposed that the alpha$_2$-agonists affect intraocular pressure by decreasing NE release presynaptically. This should cause vasodilation in the ocular circulation. However, this has not been observed for BHT-920, and furthermore, rabbit eyes decentralized by transsection of the superior cervical postganglionic nerve trunk have enhanced ocular responses to systemic BHT-920, suggesting postsynaptic supersensitivity.[86] For these reasons the main effect of BHT-920 cannot be ascribed to presynaptic receptors.

These results strongly suggest that postsynaptic alpha$_2$-adrenergic receptors are partly in-

volved in the ocular responses to alpha$_2$-agonists. Ligand-binding studies show that the majority of adrenergic receptors in rabbit ciliary processes are of the alpha$_2$-subtype,[56] and their number is not significantly decreased by sympathectomy.[61] These postsynaptic alpha$_2$-receptors show negative coupling to adenylate cyclase and can block the increase in cAMP levels induced by beta-agonist activation (isoproterenol) in rabbit ciliary body.[55] The same effect on cAMP levels is achieved by blockade of beta-receptors using beta-blockers.[58] Therefore, it may not be merely coincidental that both alpha$_2$-agonists and beta$_2$-blockers lower intraocular pressure principally by reducing aqueous humor formation and that both types of drug can decrease ciliary body cAMP levels.

The alpha$_2$-agonist drugs are extremely effective ocular hypotensive agents in lower animals and in primates. Intraocular pressure can be maximally reduced by these agents to as low as 8 to 10 mm Hg, which is close to the episcleral venous pressure. One of these drugs, p-aminoclonidine, has undergone clinical trials[70] and is now available as an ocular hypotensive agent in the United States. Clonidine has been available for this use in Europe for some time.

Dopaminergic agonists

Dopamine, in addition to activating DA receptors, has an appreciable affinity for alpha-adrenergic receptors (alpha$_2$ more than alpha$_1$). Investigations in animals show that dopamine itself decreases intraocular pressure with a significant contralateral effect, causes vasodilation without mydriasis, and lowers aqueous humor formation.[79] This pattern of effects is similar to that of alpha$_2$-agonists. Indeed, the effects of DA are blocked in part by alpha$_2$-adrenergic antagonists in addition to DA-receptor antagonists,[47] similar to the effect of these blockers on alpha$_2$-agonist responses.[86]

Noncatecholamine selective agonists for the DA$_2$-receptor subtype are more effective than DA itself in lowering intraocular pressure. These drugs include hydroxyaminotetralin derivatives[87] and the ergot derivatives pergolide, lergotrile,[65] bromocryptine,[50] and LY-141865.[66] However, some ergot derivatives are also active at alpha$_2$-adrenergic receptors,[49] and conversely many alpha$_2$-agonists are active at DA$_2$-receptors. Yet another similarity between alpha$_2$ and DA$_2$-receptors is their negative coupling to adenylate cyclase.[34]

The mechanism of action of the DA$_2$-selective agonists seems to be primarily a decrease of aqueous formation.[80] In rabbits, superior cervical ganglionectomy reduces or eliminates the intraocular pressure response to DA$_2$-agonists in the treated eye, suggesting that sympathetic function is essential for the action of these drugs.[68] Potter and Burke[67] have suggested that the DA$_2$-agonists lower intraocular pressure by presynaptic inhibition of NE release. However, a postsynaptic site of action could also be compatible with these findings because, if the DA$_2$-agonists act to lower the increased cAMP levels caused by sympathetic tone (mediated by beta-adrenergic receptors), then their effect will not be seen when the sympathetic tone is eliminated by ganglionectomy.

There are many similarities and cross-reactivities between drug types classified as agonists at alpha$_2$-adrenergic or at DA$_2$-receptors. Until more information on the separate roles of these receptors in intraocular pressure regulation becomes available, the similarity between the alpha$_2$- and DA$_2$-agonist effect is sufficiently close for agonist drugs belonging to these groups to be considered together.

A few selective DA$_1$-receptor agonist drugs have been reported. This subtype of DA-receptor causes activation of adenylate cyclase and is present in human and bovine ciliary processes.[19] One such drug, the selective DA$_1$-agonist fenoldapam, raised intraocular pressure in humans when given by intravenous infusion.[36] Since DA$_1$ agonists cause vasodilation, the intraocular pressure effect may be the result of increased ocular blood volume.

Antagonists

Beta-adrenergic antagonists

Drugs in this class have become major therapeutic agents for primary open-angle glaucoma.[9] Their primary mechanism of action in humans is a reduction of aqueous humor formation.[16] Their main site and mechanism of action are thought to be mediated by blockade of beta$_2$-adrenergic receptors on nonpigmented epithelial cells.

Many beta-blockers of differing structure reduce intraocular pressure, but for the most effective agents pharmacodynamic factors seem more important than their beta$_2$/beta$_1$ selectivity ratio or absolute receptor affinity. Timolol has high potency but is not selective. Levobunolol is more beta$_2$-selective, whereas betaxolol is somewhat beta$_1$-selective with a relatively low beta-receptor affinity. All of these drugs have a high capture ratio in ocular tissues, which contributes to their superiority for topical therapy compared with many other beta-blocking drugs that have been evaluated.

Receptor selectivity and affinity of individual beta-blockers seems to have a greater bearing on the degree of side effects. Cardiac side effects are more prominent for beta$_1$-selective drugs, whereas pulmonary and vascular effects are more prominent for beta-$_2$ selective agents. It must be remembered that overdoses of drugs with high receptor affinity may carry a greater risk of side effects because their systemic concentration threshold is much lower than drugs with a lower receptor affinity.

Some important questions remain to be resolved. One of these relates to the presence of beta-adrenergic receptors on primate trabecular cells and the apparent lack of an outflow effect in response to beta-adrenergic drugs, both agonists and antagonists. The second question concerns the confusion about the molecular mechanism by which this class of drug reduces intraocular pressure. Because agents that raise cellular cAMP levels (beta-receptor agonists, cholera toxin,[78] forskolin[12]) lower intraocular pressure, Sears and Mead[77] proposed that increases in ciliary process cAMP levels directly mediate the fall in net aqueous humor formation. This hypothesis is incompatible with the concept that blocking beta-receptors to prevent increased cAMP levels in ciliary processes causes the decrease in net aqueous formation.

Two suggestions have been put forward to try to resolve this contradiction. One is that agents initially raising cAMP levels cause a hyporesponsive state by molecular desensitization and uncoupling of beta-receptors,[8] and a second proposes that beta-blockers lower intraocular pressure by mechanisms independent of either beta-receptors or cAMP.[27] Evidence that may support the latter idea is that the doses and intraocular concentrations of particular beta-blockers,[74] their beta-receptor affinity and steric configuration[46]—factors that determine their ability to specifically block beta-receptors—do not correlate with their effectiveness on intraocular pressure. Another explanation that has been proposed is that beta-adrenergic receptor agonist and antagonist effects have different origins, with agonists acting on the ciliary epithelium and antagonists on the ciliary microvasculature.[3]

However, there are discrepancies relating to the current hypotheses. The finding that the intraocular pressure effect of forskolin (a direct activator of the adenylate cyclase enzyme in ciliary processes that also potentiates transmitter release[32]) is abolished by sympathectomy is not consistent with the hypothesis that the increased cAMP in ciliary processes directly causes decreased aqueous formation. Similarly, the reported intraocular pressure lowering effects of cholera toxin, an irreversible activator of adenylate cyclase, is difficult to rationalize in terms of the desensitization hypothesis. The lack of response to beta-adrenergic receptor drugs of ocular blood flow does not support a microvascular hypothesis. Clearly the relationship of beta-receptors and cAMP to the ocular hypotensive response is poorly understood and requires further investigation.

Alpha-adrenergic antagonists

Some alpha-adrenergic antagonists lower intraocular pressure in animals and in humans, as do the alpha$_2$-agonists, creating a paradox analogous to that relating to beta-receptors.[53] However, in this case the available evidence, at least for the alpha$_2$-receptor selective drugs, suggests that agonists and antagonists may act at different sites in experimental animals. The alpha$_2$-agonists primarily affect aqueous formation, whereas the alpha$_2$-antagonists do not seem to affect either inflow or conventional outflow.[78] This finding suggests that they may alter uveoscleral outflow, although this has not been directly demonstrated.

Antagonists that are highly selective for alpha$_1$-receptors (prazosin) as well as those selective for alpha$_2$-receptors (rauwolscine) can be effective ocular hypotensive agents, but there can be large species differences in response. Their intraocular pressure effect appears largely independent of systemic vascular effects, which requires somewhat higher doses, and these drugs likely have a direct site of action in the eye.

One unexpected finding, particularly with alpha$_1$-blockers is that typical alpha-blockade effects such as miosis and hyperemia may be observed without the expected rise in intraocular pressure, which should result from vasodilation and increased ocular blood volume. Thymoxamine, an alpha$_1$-selective blocker, shows this behavior with no effect on intraocular pressure and has been proposed as a diagnostic agent in angle-closure glaucoma.[44]

However, other antagonists also classified as alpha$_1$-selective, such as prazosin, have little pupillary effect but can significantly lower intraocular pressure in animals, though less so in primates.[81] Prazosin is a potent hypotensive agent in the peripheral circulation in humans, causing arterial vasodilation. Prazosin seems to decrease aqueous hu-

mor secretion,[37] but the involvement of functional postsynaptic alpha$_1$-adrenergic receptors is not supported by the findings that sympathectomy does not eliminate the response and that it can be antagonized with another nonselective alpha-blocker, phentolamine. These latter results suggest that extrajunctional rather than junctional (postsynaptic) alpha$_1$-receptors are involved in the action of prazosin and that the effect on intraocular pressure may be caused by a shift of the balance between extrajunctional alpha$_1$- and alpha$_2$-receptor-mediated tone toward the alpha$_2$-side.

The findings with various alpha-receptor-blocking drugs suggest important concepts about ocular alpha$_1$-receptors. There may be molecular differences between alpha$_1$-receptors in the iris dilator muscle and the alpha$_1$-receptors in arterial or venous microcirculations. Thus the ocular vascular beds may contain a variant of the alpha-receptor similar to that proposed in the peripheral circulation as the "vascular" or "alpha$_3$-receptor." These receptors exhibit drug binding and response properties between those of the conventional alpha$_1$ and alpha$_2$ receptors.[89] Additionally, there may be important regional differences in the proportions of junctional and extrajunctional alpha-receptors in the ocular microcirculation.

Vascular mechanisms may also be involved in the ocular hypotensive responses to alpha$_2$-blockers. These drugs can have effects on either arterial or venous vessels that could decrease intraocular pressure. On the arterial side, blockade of presynaptic alpha$_2$-receptors could increase vasoconstrictor tone, and similarly blockade of endothelial alpha$_2$-receptors might prevent the release of endothelial relaxing factors, which will also increase vasoconstrictive tone. Ocular blood volume will be reduced by these arterial effects. Alternatively, the ocular vascular beds may have a similar regional distribution of postsynaptic receptors, as has been found in the peripheral circulation, with the result that alpha$_2$-receptors play a more important functional role in veins than in arteries. The consequence of this would be that alpha$_2$-antagonists would reduce venous tone and could selectively decrease venous pressure. Such an effect on intrascleral venous vessels could contribute to increased outflow via the uveoscleral route.

The preceding discussion on possible mechanisms for alpha-antagonist effects is highly speculative because much basic information regarding location and subtypes of alpha-receptors is still lacking. However, it indicates that this area of ocular pharmacology could provide antiglaucoma drugs, particularly if the action of these drugs were to be relatively selective for the venous microcirculation, or they were to affect the uveoscleral outflow pathway.

Dopamine receptor antagonists

Relatively few studies on DA antagonists have been performed in the eye. Haloperidol, which does not distinguish between DA-receptor subtypes, has been reported to cause an initial rise in intraocular pressure followed by a fall.[14] Systemic domperidone, a DA_2 antagonist, blocks the hypotensive responses of DA_2-agonists but has little effect on its own.[68] As noted previously for drugs that are DA_2- or alpha$_2$-receptor agonists, DA-antagonist compounds may also have appreciable affinity for ocular alpha$_2$-adrenergic receptors. Until the specificity of a particular drug has been established in ocular tissues, it is risky to deduce receptor mechanisms based exclusively on the response to that drug. These cautions should apply not only to future studies on the selective DA-receptor blockers that are now becoming available, but to all agents for which affinity for catecholamine receptor subtypes has not been experimentally established, preferably in ocular tissues.

GENERAL CONCLUSIONS AND FUTURE DIRECTIONS

An attempt to summarize the preceding discussion on selective catecholamine receptor drugs is presented in Table 25-1. Many of the drug mechanisms that have been proposed may eventually prove incorrect. The reasoning behind these concepts of drug mechanisms is the more important part of this discussion.

It is abundantly clear that much basic information is lacking regarding the adrenergic pharmacology of aqueous humor dynamics particularly at the cellular and molecular levels.

Among the catecholamine agonists, epinephrine is still the drug with the most prominent effect on trabecular outflow. There is a great need to find a more selective agent that acts in the same way but without the vascular effects of epinephrine. The effectiveness of some agonists in the alpha$_2$/ DA_2-receptor selective group suggests that it may be worthwhile to extend studies on these drugs to humans. These agents generally act to reduce aqueous formation, as do the beta-blockers, and they could be useful as an adjunct to beta-blocker therapy or in refractory cases. There may be some reluctance to seriously consider alpha$_2$-agonists because their perceived vasoconstrictor properties could be inherently dangerous because of the possible association of increased arterial resistance with glaucoma. However, epinephrine is a good vasoconstrictor and yet has had wide clinical use in glaucoma therapy. Furthermore, the more recent knowledge on regional distribution of alpha$_2$-receptors in the vascular system and at presynaptic or endothelial cell locations precludes generalizations. These drugs can sometimes have little vasoconstrictive effect and may well do the opposite in specific vascular beds. They warrant further investigation.

Among antagonist drugs, further development

Table 25-1 Proposed mechanisms for IOP active catecholamine drug subtypes acting at intraocular sites

Drug type/ receptor specificity	IOP effect	Aqueous humor dynamics	Site and mechanism of action
AGONISTS			
Beta$_2$	↓	↑ Trabecular outflow	Beta-receptors on trabecular cells
		↓ Aqueous formation	Beta-receptor/adenylate cyclase on ciliary epithelial cells
Alpha$_2$	↓	↓ Aqueous formation	Sympathetic presynaptic inhibition/inhibition of adenylate cyclase
Alpha$_1$	↓	—	Arterial vasoconstriction
DA_2	↓	↓ Aqueous formation	(Same as for alpha$_2$-agonists)?
DA_1	↑	?	(Arterial vasodilation)?
ANTAGONISTS			
Beta$_2$	↓	↓ Aqueous formation	Beta-receptor/adenylate cyclase on ciliary epithelial cells?
Alpha$_2$	↓	(↑ Uveoscleral outflow)?	(Venous vasodilation)?
Alpha$_1$	↓	↓ Aqueous formation	
		(↑ Uveoscleral outflow)?	?
DA	↓	(↑ Outflow)?	?
		(↓ Inflow)?	?

of beta-blockers to find an ocular hypotensive agent devoid of beta$_1$ or beta$_2$ side effects with once- or twice-a-day administration is still a worthwhile endeavor. Preliminary findings in animals with some of the alpha-blocker drugs indicates that this may be an important area for long-term investigation.[69] Though not yet proved, there are indications that some of these drugs may work by increasing outflow via the uveoscleral pathway. This mechanism for reducing intraocular pressure is in principle a better therapeutic concept than slowing down the rate of aqueous humor formation, which has the attendant risk of long-term nutritional deficiencies for avascular intraocular tissues.

REFERENCES

1. Ahlquist, RP: A study of the adrenotropic receptors, Am J Physiol 153:586, 1948
2. Araie, M: Acute effects of topical phenylephrine on aqueous humor dynamics and corneal endothelial permeability in man, Jpn J Ophthalmol 27:340, 1983
3. Bartels, SP, and Neufeld, AH: Mechanisms of topical drugs used in the control of open angle glaucoma: clinical pharmacology of the anterior segment. In Holly, F, editor: International ophthalmology clinics, Boston, 1980, Little, Brown
4. Benovic JL, et al: Light-dependent phosphorylation of rhodopsin by β-adrenergic receptor kinase, Nature 321:869, 1986
5. Benovic, JL, Strasser, RH, Caron, MG, and Lefkowitz, RJ: β-adrenergic receptor kinase: identification of a novel protein kinase that phosphorylates the agonist-occupied form of the receptor, Proc Natl Acad Sci USA 83:2797, 1986
6. Bill, A: Autonomic nervous control of uveal blood flow, Acta Physiol Scand 56:70, 1962
7. Bill, A: Effects of norepinephrine, isoproterenol, and sympathetic stimulation on aqueous humor dynamics in vervet monkeys, Exp Eye Res 10:31, 1970
8. Boas, RS, Messenger, M, Mittag, TW, and Podos, SM: The effects of topically applied epinephrine and timolol on intraocular pressure and aqueous humor cyclic-AMP in the rabbit, Exp Eye Res 32:681, 1981
9. Boger, W: The treatment of glaucoma: role of beta-blocking agents, Drugs 18:25, 1979
10. Bond, RA, Charlton, KG, and Clarke, DE: Evidence for a receptor mediated action of norepinephrine distinct from alpha- and beta-adrenoreceptors, Naunyn-Schmiedebergs Arch Pharmacol 334:261, 1986
11. Brubaker, RF, and Gaasterland, D: The effect of isoproterenol on aqueous humor formation in humans, Invest Ophthalmol Vis Sci 25:357, 1984
12. Caprioli, J, et al: Forskolin lowers intraocular pressure by reducing aqueous outflow, Invest Ophthalmol Vis Sci 25:268, 1984
13. Chiou, GCY: Effects of α_1 and α_2 activation on adrenergic receptors on aqueous humor dynamics, Life Sci 32:1699, 1983
14. Chiou, GC-Y: Ocular hypotensive actions of haloperidol, a dopaminergic antagonist, Arch Ophthalmol 102:143, 1984
15. Chu, T-C, and Candia, OA: Effects of adrenergic agonists and cyclic AMP on short circuit current across the isolated rabbit iris-ciliary body, Curr Eye Res 4:523, 1985
16. Coakes, RL, and Brubaker, RS: The mechanism of timolol in lowering intraocular pressure, Arch Ophthalmol 96:2045, 1978
17. Codina, J, Stengel, D, Woo, SLC, and Birnbaumer, L: Beta subunits of the human liver G$_s$, G$_i$ signal-transducing proteins and those of bovine retinal rod cell transducin are identical, FEBS Lett 207:187, 1986
18. Cole, DF: Secretion of aqueous humor, Exp Eye Res Suppl 25:161, 1977
19. De Vries, GW, Mobasser, A, and Wheeler, LA: Stimulation of endogenous cAMP levels in ciliary body by SKF 82526, a novel dopamine receptor agonist, Curr Eye Res 5:449, 1986
20. Dixon, RAF, et al: Cloning of the gene and cDNA for mammalian β-adrenergic receptor and homology with rhodopsin, Nature 321:75, 1986
21. Ehinger, B: Distribution of adrenergic nerves in the eye and some related structures in the cat, Acta Physiol Scand 66:123, 1966
22. Elena, PP, Fredj-Reygrobbelet, D, Moulin, G, and Lapalus, P: Pharmacological characteristic of β-adrenergic sensitive adenylate cyclase in non-pigmented and pigmented cells of bovine ciliary processes, Curr Eye Res 3:1383, 1984
23. Elena, P-P, Kosina-Boix, M, Moulin, G, and Lapalus, P: Autoradiographic localization of beta-adrenergic receptors in rabbit eye, Invest Ophthalmol Vis Sci 28:1436, 1987
24. Furchgott, RF: Role of endothelium in responses of vascular smooth muscle to drugs, Ann Rev Pharmacol Toxicol 24:175, 1984
25. Gaasterland, D, Kupfer, C, Ross, K, and Gabelnick, RL: Studies of aqueous humor in man. III. Measurements in young normal subjects using norepinephrine and isoproterenol, Invest Ophthalmol Vis Sci 12:267, 1973
26. Gregory, DS, Aviado, DG, and Sears, ML: Cervical ganglionectomy alters the circadian rhythm of intraocular pressure in New Zealand white rabbits, Curr Eye Res 4:1273, 1985
27. Gregory, DS, Bausher, LP, Bromberg, BB, and Sears, ML: The beta adrenergic receptors and adenylyl cyclase of rabbit ciliary processes. In Sears, ML, editor: New directions in ophthalmic research, New Haven/London, 1981, Yale University Press
28. Gregory, DS, et al: Intraocular pressure and aqueous flow are decreased by cholera toxin, Invest Ophthalmol Vis Sci 20:371, 1981
29. Hodapp E, et al: The effect of topical clonidine on intraocular pressure, Arch Ophthalmol 99:1208, 1981
30. Innemee, HC, et al: The effect of selective α_1 and α_2-adrenoreceptor stimulation on intraocular pressure

in the conscious rabbit, Naunyn Schmiedebergs Arch Pharmacol 316:294, 1981

31. Jampel, HD, et al: β-adrenergic receptors in human trabecular meshwork. Identification and autoradiographic localization, Invest Ophthalmol Vis Sci (In press)

32. Jumblatt, JE, and North, GT: Potentiation of sympathetic neurosecretion by forskolin and cyclic-AMP in the rabbit iris-ciliary body, Curr Eye Res 5:495, 1986

33. Jumblatt, JE, and Pon, L: Clonidine inhibits adrenergic neurosecretion in the rabbit iris-ciliary body, Invest Ophthalmol Vis Suppl 25:79, 1983

34. Kebabian, JW, and Calne DB: Multiple receptors for dopamine, Nature 277:93, 1979

35. Kobilka, BK, et al: Cloning sequencing, and expression of the gene coding for the human platelet α$_2$-adrenergic receptor, Science 238:650, 1987

36. Kornezis, TA, et al: Effects of a dopamine DA$_1$ receptor agonist, fenoldopam, on human intraocular pressure, Invest Ophthalmol Vis Sci Suppl 28:66, 1987

37. Krupin, T, Feitl, M, and Becker, B: Effect of prazosin on aqueous humor dynamics in rabbits, Arch Ophthalmol 98:1639, 1980

38. Kuhar, MJ: Receptor localization with the microscope. In Yamamura, HI, editor: Neurotransmitter receptor binding, New York, 1985, Raven Press

39. Langham, ME: The intraocular pressure and the pupillary responses of conscious rabbits to racemic erythrol-α-methyl norepinephrine, Exp Eye Res 39:781, 1984

40. Langham, ME: Ocular blood flow and visual loss in glaucomatous eyes. In Krieglstein, GK, editor: Glaucoma update III, Berlin/Heidelberg, 1987, Springer-Verlag

41. Langham, ME, and Diggs, E: Beta-adrenergic responses in the eyes of rabbits, primates and man, Exp Eye Res 19:281, 1974

42. Laties, A, and Jacobowitz, D: A histochemical study of the adrenergic and cholinergic innervation of the anterior segment of the rabbit eye, Invest Ophthalmol Vis Sci 3:592, 1964

43. Lavah, M, Melamed, E, Dofna, Z, and Atlas, D: Localization of β-receptors in the anterior segment of the eye by a fluorescent analog of propranolol, Invest Ophthalmol Vis Sci 17:645, 1978

44. Lee, DA, Brubaker, RF, and Nagataki, S: Acute effect of thymoxamine on aqueous humor formation in the epinephrine-treated normal eye as measured by fluorophotometry, Invest Ophthalmol Vis Sci 24:165, 1983

45. Leopold, IH, and Duzman, E: Observations on the pharmacology of glaucoma, Ann Rev Pharmacol Toxicol 26:401, 1986

46. Lui, HK, and Chiou, GC-Y: Continuous simultaneous and instant display of aqueous humor dynamics with a micro-spectrophotometer and a sensitive drop-counter, Exp Eye Res 32:583, 1981

47. Macri, FJ, and Cevario, SJ: The inhibitory actions of dopamine, hydroxyamphetamine and phenylephrine on aqueous humor formation, Exp Eye Res 26:85, 1976

48. Maurice, D, and Mishima, S: Ocular pharmacokinetics in pharmacology of the eye. In Sears, M, editor: Handbook of experimental pharmacology, Berlin/Heidelberg, 1984, Springer-Verlag

49. McPherson, GA: In vitro selectivity of lisuride and other ergot derivatives for α$_1$ and α$_2$-adrenoreceptors, Eur J Pharmacol 97:151, 1984

50. Mekki, QA, Hassan, SM, and Turner, P: Bromocryptine lowers intraocular pressure without affecting blood pressure, Lancet 2:1250, 1983

51. Minneman, KP, Puttman, RN, and Molinoff, PB: Beta-adrenergic receptor subtypes: properties, distribution and regulation, Annu Rev Neurosci 4:419, 1981

52. Mishima, S: Ocular effects of beta-adrenergic agents, Surv Ophthalmol 27:187, 1982

53. Mittag, TW: Ocular effects of selective alpha-adrenergic agents: a new drug paradox? Am J Ophthalmol 1983:21, 1983

54. Mittag, TW, and Tormay, A: Desensitization of the β-adrenergic receptor-adenylate cyclase complex in rabbit iris-ciliary body induced by topical epinephrine, Exp Eye Res 33:497, 1981

55. Mittag, TW, and Tormay, A: Drug responses of adenylate cyclase in iris-ciliary body determined by adenine labelling, Invest Ophthalmol Vis Sci 26:396, 1985

56. Mittag, TW, Tormay, A, Severin, C, and Podos, SM: Alpha adrenergic antagonists: correlation of the effect on intraocular pressure and on α$_2$-adrenergic receptor binding specificity in the rabbit eye, Exp Eye Res 40:591, 1985

57. Nakaki, T, Nakadate, T, Yamamoto, S, and Kato, R: Alpha-2-adrenergic inhibition of intestinal secretion induced by prostaglandin E, vasoactive intestinal peptide and dibutyryl cyclic AMP in rat jejunum, J Pharmacol Exp Ther 220:637, 1982

58. Nathanson, JA: Adrenergic regulation of intraocular pressure: identification of beta$_2$-adrenergic stimulated adenylate cyclase in ciliary process epithelium, Proc Natl Acad Sci USA 77:7421, 1980

59. Nathanson, JA: Beta-adrenergic regulation of intraocular pressure: ambiguities and insights, Trends Autonomic Pharmacol 3:173, 1984

60. Norton, AL, and Viernstein, LJ: The effect of adrenergic agents on ocular dynamics as a function of administration site, Exp Eye Res 14:154, 1972

61. Page, ED, and Neufeld, AH: Characterization of α- and β-adrenergic receptors in membranes prepared from the rabbit iris before and after the development of supersensitivity, Biochem Pharmacol 27:953, 1978

62. Palkama, A, Uuisitalo, H, and Lehtosalo, L: Innervation of the anterior segment of the eye: functional aspects. In Neurohistochemistry today, New York, 1985, Allan R Liss, Inc

63. Polansky, JR, and Alvarado, JA: Isolation and evaluation of target cells in glaucoma research: hormone receptors and drug responses, Curr Eye Res 4:267, 1985

64. Potter, DE: Adrenergic pharmacology of aqueous humor dynamics, Pharmacol Rev 33:133, 1981

65. Potter, DE, and Burke, JA: Effects of ergoline derivatives on intraocular pressure and iris function in rabbits and monkeys, Curr Eye Res 3:307, 1982

66. Potter, DE, and Burke, JA: In Dopamine Receptor Agonists Symposium sponsored by Smith, Kline and French Laboratories, Philadelphia, 1983, quoted in ref. 1

67. Potter, DE, and Burke, JA: An in vivo model for dissociating α_2- or DA_2-adrenoreceptor activity in an ocular adnexa: utility of the cat nictating membrane preparation, Curr Eye Res 3:1289, 1984

68. Potter, DE, Burke, JA, and Chang, FW: Ocular hypotensive action of ergoline derivatives in rabbits: effects of sympathectomy and domperidone pretreatment, Curr Eye Res 3:307, 1984

69. Reibaldi, A: A new alpha-blocking agent, Glaucoma 6:255, 1984

70. Robin, AL, Pollack, IP, House, B, and Enger, C: Eliminating the acute IOP rise following argon laser glaucoma surgery with topical 1% ALO-2145, Invest Ophthalmol Vis Sci Suppl 28:378, 1987

71. Rowland, JM, and Potter, DE: Adrenergic drugs and intraocular pressure: the hypertensive effect of epinephrine, Ophthalmic Res 12:221, 1980

72. Rowland, JM, and Potter, DE: Steric structure-activity relationships of various adrenergic agonists: ocular and systemic effects, Curr Eye Res 1:25, 1981

73. Ruffolo, RR: Spare α-adrenoreceptors in the peripheral circulation: excitation-contraction coupling, Fed Proc 45:2341, 1986

74. Schmitt, C, Lotti, VJ, Vareilles, P, and LeDouarec, JC: Beta-adrenergic blockers: lack of relationship between antagonism of isoproterenol and lowering of intraocular pressure. In Sears, M, editor: New directions in ophthalmic research, New Haven/London, 1981, Yale University Press

75. Sears, ML: The mechanism of action of adrenergic drugs in glaucoma, Invest Ophthalmol Vis Sci 5:115, 1966

76. Sears, ML, editor: Pharmacology of the eye. Handbook of experimental pharmacology, Berlin/Heidelberg, 1984, Springer-Verlag

77. Sears, M, and Mead, A: A major pathway for the regulation of intraocular pressure, Int Ophthalmol 6:201, 1983

78. Serle, JB, Stein, AJ, Podos, SM, and Severin, CH: Corynanthine and aqueous humor dynamics in rabbits and monkeys, Arch Ophthalmol 102:1385, 1984

79. Shannon, RP, Mead, A, and Sears, A: The effect of dopamine on the intraocular pressure and pupil of the rabbit eye, Invest Ophthalmol Vis Sci 15:371, 1976

80. Siegel, MJ, Lee, P-Y, Podos, SM, and Mittag, TW: Effect of topical pergolide on aqueous dynamics in normal and glaucomatous monkeys, Exp Eye Res 44:277, 1987

81. Smith, BR: Influence of topically applied prazosin on the intraocular pressure of experimental animals, Arch Ophthalmol 97:1133, 1979

82. Steinberg, SF, Jaffe, EA, and Bilezikan, JP: Endothelial cells contain β-adrenoreceptors, Naunyn Schmiedebergs Arch Pharmacol 325:310, 1984

83. Stryer, L, and Bourne, HR: G-proteins: a family of signal transducers, Annu Rev Cell Biol 2:391, 1986

84. Sundler, F, Hakanson, R, Loren, I, and Lundquist, H: Amine storage and function in peptide hormone producing cells, Invest Cell Pathol 3:87, 1980

85. Szalay, J, et al: Effect of β-adrenergic agents on blood vessels of the rat iris. I. Permeability to carbon particles, Exp Eye Res 31:289, 1980

86. Thorig, L, and Bill, A: Effects of BHT-920 in the eye and on regional blood flows in anesthetized and conscious rabbits, Curr Eye Res 5:565, 1986

87. Thorig, L, Hoyng, PF, Timmermans, PBMWM, and van Zwieten, PA: M-7 lowers rabbit intraocular pressure, Ophthalmic Res 17:362, 1985

88. Topper, JE, and Brubaker, RF: Effects of timolol, epinephrine and acetazolamide on the role of aqueous flow during sleep, Invest Ophthalmol Vis Sci Suppl 26:103, 1985

89. van Pinxteren, PCM, and van Alphen, GWHM: Postjunctional adrenergic receptors in the rabbit eye: effects on uveal flow and intraocular pressure in isolated arterially perfused eyes, Curr Eye Res 4:21, 1985

90. Wentworth, WO, and Brubaker, RF: Aqueous humor dynamics in a series of patients with third neuron Horners syndrome, Am J Ophthalmol 92:407, 1981

91. Wettrell, K, Wilke, I, and Pondolfi, M: Effect of β-adrenergic agonists and antagonists on repeated tonometry and episcleral venous pressure, Exp Eye Res 24:613, 1977

Chapter 26

Carbonic Anhydrase Inhibitors

Beth R. Friedland
Thomas H. Maren

Carbonic anhydrase inhibitors have been used in the treatment of glaucoma for nearly 40 years.[45] Friedenwald[15] initially postulated the existence of a ciliary epithelial redox pump responsible for driving an alkaline secretion into the aqueous humor in the posterior chamber. Kinsey[28] measured an abundance of bicarbonate in the posterior chamber aqueous humor of the rabbit. After Wistrand[63] reported the presence of the enzyme carbonic anhydrase in the anterior uveal tract of the rabbit, Becker[8,9] investigated the effect of administration of an inhibitor of the enzyme, acetazolamide, in patients with glaucoma. Acetazolamide decreased intraocular pressure with little or no change in outflow facility.[16]

In 1959 Kinsey and Reddy[29] (Fig. 26-1) showed that carbonic anhydrase inhibition caused a dramatically decreased bicarbonate accumulation rate in rabbit posterior chamber aqueous humor. The magnitude of this change was most apparent in the first 5 to 7 minutes after drug administration. Over the next 20 years, there was considerable discussion as to the mechanism of action of carbonic anhydrase inhibitors because dog, monkey, and human studies revealed no measurable bicarbonate excess in the posterior chamber aqueous humor. Zimmerman et al.[64,65] were able to measure the initial rates of sodium, chloride, and bicarbonate movement in dog and monkey. Under these conditions, just as in the rabbit, measurement of bicarbonate accumulation showed that the ion was formed from CO_2 and moves with sodium from plasma to the posterior chamber (Fig. 26-2). The quantitative analysis of the rates involved has been reviewed elsewhere.[49,50,57]

OCULAR PHYSIOLOGY

The posterior chamber in the eyes of humans, cynomolgus monkeys, and rabbits contains about 50 μL of aqueous humor. Table 26-1 shows rate constants measured by isotopic movement from plasma to posterior chamber aqueous in the monkey.[44,49] The calculated bicarbonate concentration in new fluid is over three times that of plasma. Thirty-seven percent of the sodium ionic movement is accompanied by bicarbonate. After total carbonic anhydrase inhibition, sodium accession into the posterior chamber aqueous humor decreases to 1.3 mmol/min, and bicarbonate accession to 0.7 mmol/min. Chloride movement is only slightly changed, and there is no evidence of exchange mechanisms.[49,64,65] It is, therefore, possible to calculate a catalytic rate for bicarbonate formation of about 3 mmol/min/ml cell volume of bicarbonate. This rate is about 100 times greater than the observed catalytic rate and is consistent with the small amount of enzyme present in the ciliary processes. The concentration of enzyme in the ciliary processes is calculated to be about 3 mmol/L.[48,53] Thus, the dose-response curve for inhibition of carbonic anhydrase begins at 99% inhibition and will be complete at a 99.9% inhibition.[16,40]

Sodium movement is directly linked to bicarbonate synthesis.[23] Because sodium movement is

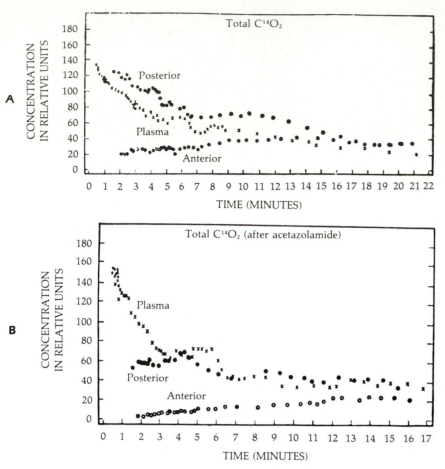

Fig. 26-1 Accumulation of HCO_3^- in aqueous from blood CO_2 and its inhibition by acetazolamide. ^{14}C-labeled bicarbonate and CO_2 were injected at 0 time, and total $^{14}CO_2$ concentration determined in the fluids at times shown. **A,** Normal rabbit. **B,** Acetazolamide (50 mg/kg IV) given 15 minutes before 0 time. In the normal rabbit **A,** total CO_2 is partitioned in its physiologic ratios between posterior chamber aqueous humor and plasma within 1 minute. **B,** shows that with 50 mg/kg acetazolamide, there is a profound delay in accumulation of total CO_2 in posterior chamber aqueous humor. (From Maren, TH. In Drance, SM, and Neufeld, AH: Glaucoma: applied pharmacology in medical treatment, Orlando, FL, 1984, Grune & Stratton)

Fig. 26-2 Accession of ^{14}C to posterior chamber of dog after injection of $H^{14}CO_3^-$ at 0 time. *CPM,* Counts per minute. (From Maren, TH. In Drance, SM, and Neufeld, AH: Glaucoma: applied pharmacology in medical treatment, Orlando, FL, 1984, Grune & Stratton)

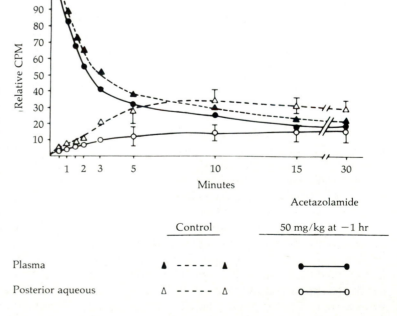

Table 26-1   The accession rates of ions from plasma to posterior aqueous in the cynomolgus monkey: effect of carbonic anhydrase inhibition (CAI)*

		1 Plasma† (mmol)	2 k_{in} (min⁻¹)	3 Accession rate col 1 × col 2 (mmol/min)	4 Calc in new fluid‡ (mmol)	5 Posterior chamber (mmol)
Na⁺	Control	152	0.017	2.7	162	—
	CAI		0.009	1.4	168	—
Cl⁻	Control	103	0.016	1.6	96	115
	CAI		0.012	1.2	144	—
HCO₃⁻	Control	20	0.054	1.1	66	21
	CAI		0.019	0.4	48	—

From Maren, TH: Exp Eye Res (suppl) 25:245, 1977
*50 mg/kg intravenous acetazolamide administration 1 hour before isotope injection.
†Plasma concentration unchanged by CAI.

‡Column 3 × $\dfrac{\text{volume posterior chamber (60 μl)}}{\text{aqueous flow (1 μl/min)}}$ for controls.

Flow 0.5 μl/min during CAI.

isotonic, fluid movement results from the carbonic anhydrase activity (Fig. 26-3). Inhibition of this enzyme reduces aqueous flow and has become the basis for the use of these inhibitors in the treatment of glaucoma.[41]

PHARMACOLOGY

The common feature of the carbonic anhydrase inhibitors is the presence of a free sulfonamide group (-SO₂NH₂) linked to an aromatic ring.[43] The free sulfonamide group competes with the bicarbonate ion in binding to the active site of the enzyme in its acidic form.[62] CO₂ undergoes hydroxylation via an attack of the hydroxyl ion. Organic sulfonamides can effectively block and slow the catalytic conversion of CO₂ to HCO₃⁻.[40,47]

Table 26-2 describes the chemical and pharmacologic properties of clinically used carbonic anhydrase inhibitors.[46] Acetazolamide was mainly introduced into clinical use for its action on renal carbonic anhydrase (Fig. 26-4, Table 26-3). Because it is less diffusible than methazolamide and ethoxzolamide and shows high plasma binding and ionization, acetazolamide is a poor choice for penetration into ocular tissues from the systemic circulation. However, acetazolamide has a high activity against carbonic anhydrase that permits inhibition of ciliary body enzyme when the drug is present in a concentration seven to ten times greater than the enzyme concentration.[17,36] The plasma binding and ionization properties of acetazolamide are an even greater factor when considering this drug for topical administration.

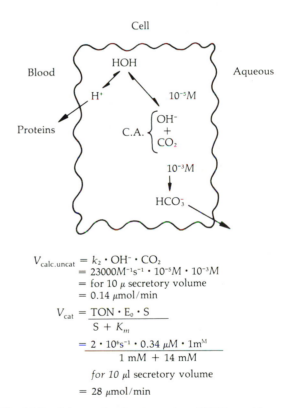

$$V_{\text{calc.uncat}} = k_2 \cdot OH^- \cdot CO_2$$
$$= 23000 M^{-1}s^{-1} \cdot 10^{-5}M \cdot 10^{-3}M$$
$$= \text{for } 10\,\mu \text{ secretory volume}$$
$$= 0.14\ \mu mol/min$$

$$V_{\text{cat}} = \frac{TON \cdot E_0 \cdot S}{S + K_m}$$
$$= \frac{2 \cdot 10^6 s^{-1} \cdot 0.34\ \mu M \cdot 1 m^M}{1\ mM + 14\ mM}$$
$$\textit{for } 10\ \mu l \textit{ secretory volume}$$
$$= 28\ \mu mol/min$$

Fig. 26-3   Schema showing formation of HCO₃⁻ and its quantitative relation to Na⁺ transport. Rate data from experiments of Zimmerman. The velocity of the uncatalyzed reaction is determined from k_2 at 37° C and an assumed pH at the secretory site of 9, PCO₂ of 33 mm Hg, and cell volume of 10 μl. The pH is estimated based on the fact that if it were higher, no enzyme would be needed or revealed by inhibition. (From Friedland, BR, and Maren, TH. In Sears, M, editor: Pharmacology of the eye, Berlin, 1984, Springer-Verlag)

Table 26-2 Properties of carbonic anhydrase inhibitors*

| Name | Structure | $K_i{}^a \times 10^9$ M | pK_{a_1} | Partition coefficient to buffer pH 7.4 | | Solubility in H_2O mM | Human | | k_{in} h^{-1} | |
				Ether	CHCl₃		%† Bound to plasma	f½‡ Plasma hour	rbc§	×10³ Aqueous humor‖
Sulfanilamide		1000	10	0.15	0.02	9	10	6	136	—
Acetazolamide		6	7.4	0.14	10^{-3}	3	95	4	27	2
Methazolamide		8	7.2	0.62	0.06	5	55	15	195	8
Ethoxzolamide		1	8.1	140	25	0.04	96	6	4500	330
Benzolamide		1	3.2	0.001	10^{-4}	0.14	96	2	23	1

From Maren, TH. In Case, RM, Lingard, JM, and Young, JA, editors: Secretion: mechanisms and control, 1984, Manchester University Press[48]
*Against pure carbonic anhydrase C, in hydration.
†At concentrations of 4-40 μM
‡Following oral dose in man.
§From free concentration in plasma to rbc (man).
‖Transcorneal permeability in vivo (rabbit).

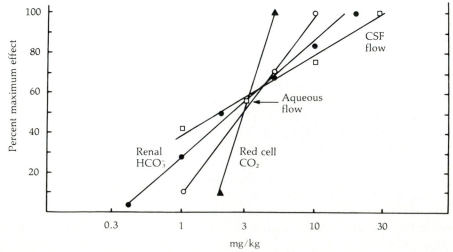

Fig. 26-4 Dose-response studies of acetazolamide in several physiologic systems. (From Friedland, BR, and Maren, TH. In Sears, M, editor: Pharmacology of the eye, Berlin, 1984, Springer-Verlag)

Acetazolamide is actively secreted into the renal tubules and passively reabsorbed by nonionic diffusion.[42] Because a comparable dose of methazolamide does not have as great a renal inhibitory effect, it is associated with much less systemic acidosis.[13,53] In addition, methazolamide, which is not secreted by the kidney, has a wider discrimination of dose-response between the eye and the kidney (Fig. 26-5). Methazolamide is metabolized mainly in the liver, and only 20% to 25% is excreted unchanged.[6,42]

Ethoxzolamide is a weak organic acid, minimally secreted by the renal tubules. About 40% of the drug is secreted unchanged in the dog. Although it has a higher in vitro activity (K_i) against carbonic anhydrase, it is highly bound to plasma proteins. As such it has limited application as a systemic agent but has proved useful as the source of some analogs for topical administration.

Dichlorphenamide is a carbonic anhydrase inhibitor that has a mixed pharmacology with the thiazide diuretics. This agent is also a chloruretic, a potentially hazardous property. Dichlorphenamide can cause loss of chloride and potassium in the urine with a resultant hypokalemia and hypochloremia characteristic of thiazide diuretics. Dichlorphenamide has a high incidence of side effects, particularly headache, and, therefore, is not useful as a carbonic anhydrase inhibitor.[18]

Acetazolamide in the nephrectomized rabbit model[21] lowers intraocular pressure in a dose response fashion. At high doses, 15 to 50 mg/kg acetazolamide causes respiratory acidosis, which appears to add to the pressure lowering effect (see Fig. 26-4). In humans, large doses of acetazolamide do not produce respiratory acidosis unless there is concomitant pulmonary disease.[11] Acetazolamide also produces a mild metabolic acidosis, which may

Table 26-3 Comparison of the effect of graded doses of methazolamide and acetazolamide on intraocular pressure, plasma total CO_2, and citrate excretion

	IOP ↓ mm Hg	Plasma CO_2 mM	Urinary citrate mg/24 h
Normal	—	27.3	554
Methazolamide (every 12 h)			
25 mg	2.6	26.9	386
50 mg	3.2	25.0	324
Acetazolamide (every 6 h)			
62 mg	4	22.0	169
125 mg	4	21.3	120
250 mg	4	21.0	79

From Maren, TH, Haywood, JR, Chapman, SK, and Zimmerman, TJ: Invest Ophthalmol Vis Sci 16:730, 1977[53]

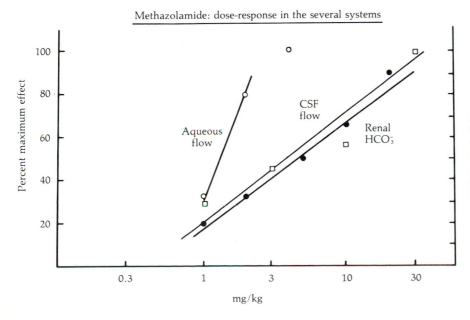

Fig. 26-5 Dose-response study of methazolamide in the eye, cerebrospinal fluid *(CSF)* and kidney. (From Maren, TH. In Drance, SM, and Neufeld, AH: Glaucoma: applied pharmacology in medical treatment, Orlando, FL, 1984, Grune & Stratton)

add to its pressure lowering effect.[32] The effect on the kidney is the major clinical difference between methazolamide and acetazolamide. However, at high doses, greater than 4 mg/kg, methazolamide also inhibits renal carbonic anhydrase[13,53] (see Fig. 26-5).

Some authors have recorded a correlation between the systemic acidosis and the side effects of carbonic anhydrase inhibitors,[13,39] but this association is also disputed.[1] A double-masked study comparing supplemental sodium acetate and placebo showed a minimal effect in reducing side effects in half the patients receiving supplemental sodium acetate.[3] The amount of sodium acetate given (90 mEq/day) did not have a consistent effect on measurable serum CO_2 combining power. There was a trend toward higher concentration of CO_2, but serum chloride levels also increased. Neither serum carbonic anhydrase inhibitor levels nor potassium levels were altered. There is a suggestion that potassium supplementation may be helpful, but sodium chloride supplementation has also been equally effective. No consistent pattern to reduce the side effect of malaise has been found. Notably, patients with comparable metabolic acidosis from renal tubular acidosis, or induced by ammonium chloride ingestion, do not demonstrate such side effects.[18,42] The factors leading to these uncomfortable symptoms appear complex.

CLINICAL APPLICATIONS

Drug Interactions

The reduction in the rate of aqueous humor formation helps to explain some of the additive effects of carbonic anhydrase inhibitors and other types of inflow reducing drugs. Beta-adrenergic antagonists have an additive pressure lowering effect without changes in aqueous outflow.[10,19,24,30]

Resistance to outflow increases at higher intraocular pressures caused by trabecular compression and collapse of Schlemm's canal. Therefore, outflow resistance sometimes improves when intraocular pressure is reduced by carbonic anhydrase inhibitors. This may be the mechanism for the synergistic effects of pilocarpine[19,36] and epinephrine[33] with the carbonic anhydrase inhibitors. This may also explain the role of combined therapy with pilocarpine, an epinephrine preparation, a beta blocker, and a carbonic anhydrase inhibitor.

Clinical Indications

Short-term administration of carbonic anhydrase inhibitors to reduce intraocular pressure can be very effective in the secondary glaucomas because the trabecular outflow channels are often affected by the disease process and unresponsive to medications that increase aqueous outflow. Carbonic anhydrase inhibitors are useful in these conditions, as well as before operations for congenital glaucoma.

In acute angle-closure glaucoma, carbonic anhydrase inhibitors are effective in lowering intraocular pressure. If the patient is nauseated or vomiting, parenteral therapy with intravenous acetazolamide, 250 mg, can be given. The pressure begins to fall within a few minutes, and the effect lasts 2 to 4 hours. As the intraocular pressure decreases, the iridial and ciliary muscles recover from the ischemia of high pressure and the unresponsiveness to topical miotic agents. Topical pilocarpine then becomes effective as a miotic agent, opening a closed anterior chamber angle.

Transient intraocular pressure elevation following cataract surgery may be less common in the era of extracapsular cataract surgery but still is a problem, especially secondary to retained viscoelastic substances or cortical debris. Carbonic anhydrase inhibitors, in conjunction with a topical beta-antagonist, may be useful in preventing or treating the immediate postoperative pressure rise.[12] The elevation in pressure characteristically occurs in the first 6 to 8 hours after surgery and lasts 24 to 48 hours. Pressure control in the immediate postoperative period is essential in patients with glaucomatous damage.

SIDE EFFECTS

The more serious side effects associated with carbonic anhydrase inhibitors include blood dyscrasias, renal stones, and mental changes, such as excitation, confusion, and depression. In the nearly 40 years that carbonic anhydrase inhibitors have been used, only 113 cases of suspected hematopoietic toxicity have been reported. Aplastic anemia with agranulocytosis has been reported as late as 5 or 6 years after initiation of therapy, but in over 50% of the cases this complication occurred in the first 2 months.[31,34,39] A complete blood count including a white blood cell differential has been recommended before, and at frequent intervals after therapy is initiated. However, this recommendation is controversial. Stopping therapy at the first signs of agranulocytosis usually results in a return to a normal hematopoietic status. Other reported side effects include decreased libido,[19,39] hirsutism, and alopecia.[2] A curious side effect of a metallic taste probably relates to inhibition of bicarbonate conversion to CO_2 in the taste buds.[61]

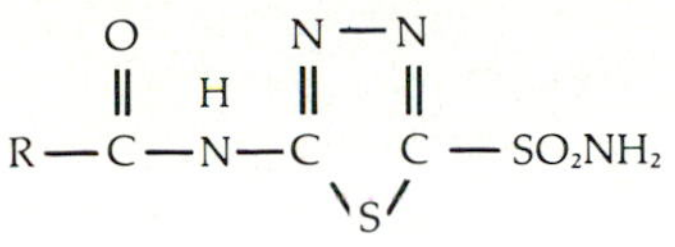

R = CH_3 = Acetazolamide
R = $BrCH_2$ = Bromacetazolamide

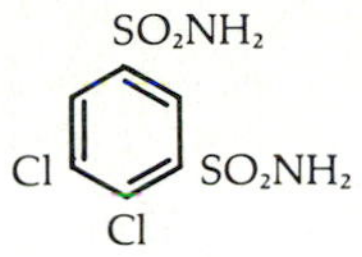

Dichlorphenamide

Benzothiazole-2-sulfonamides

R = 6-ethoxy = Ethoxolamide
R = 6-NH_2
R = 6−O−C_2H_4OH
R = Pivolyl ester of 6-OH

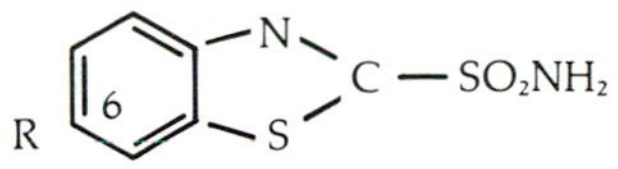

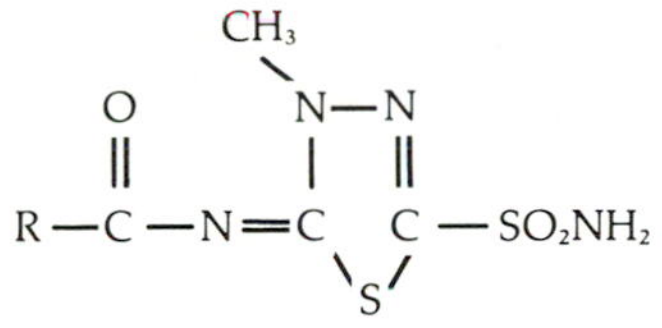

R = CH_3 = Methazolamide
R = CF_3 = Trifluormethazolamide

Fig. 26-6 Structures of four sulfonamides used systemically to treat glaucoma and derivatives now found to be active topically.

The increased incidence of nephrolithiasis is probably related to depression of renal citrate excretion and an increased availability of calcium for insoluble salts. The link between acetazolamide treatment and urinary stones is stronger than the link between methazolamide treatment and urinary stones. Urolithiasis has been reported after the administration of higher dosages of methazolamide, 100 mg three times a day or 200 mg twice a day.[27] Normalization of urinary citrate may reduce the risk of stone formation by reducing the formation of insoluble salts.

Metabolic acidosis alone does not appear to cause a malaise symptom complex. However, because total body sodium is depleted.[19,46] the mild metabolic acidosis may pose a very high risk in patients with (1) diabetes and superimposed ketoacidosis, (2) hepatic insufficiency resulting from decreased ammonia trapping leading to a rise in plasma NH_3,[54] and (3) chronic obstructive pulmonary disease where CO_2 elimination is impaired and a gradient develops between arterial CO_2 and pulmonary alveolar CO_2.[11]

Methazolamide is contraindicated in the presence of hepatic disease because it is metabolized in the liver, increasing the risk of impending hepatic coma.

All carbonic anhydrase inhibitors are contraindicated in the first trimester of pregnancy because of a characteristic limb deformity that has been seen in offspring of rodents that were administered the drug at days 10 and 11 of pregnancy.[25,35] The teratogenicity does not appear to be related to the acidosis. All carbonic anhydrase inhibitors cause this deformity, whereas sulfonamides that do not inhibit carbonic anhydrase do not cause it.

An idiosyncratic transient myopia has been reported with ethoxzolamide and acetazolamide.[7,22] This may be related to ciliary body edema. It is probably unrelated to inhibition of carbonic anhydrase in the lens because acetazolamide penetrates the lens capsule poorly.[18]

The antibacterial and carbonic anhydrase-inhibiting sulfonamides are structurally quite dissimilar,[46] but patients with a history of sensitivity to antibacterial sulfonamides are generally cautioned against using systemic carbonic anhydrase inhibitors.

TOPICAL AGENTS

In dealing with the problem of topical sulfonamides, it has been important to develop compounds with good water and lipid solubility.[26] Acetazolamide, which was initially tested in the 1950s, has a very low lipid solubility and low corneal permeability. Ethoxzolamide is a very lipid soluble but has a relatively low water solubility. The first carbonic anhydrase inhibitor developed with definite activity when applied topically was bromocetazolamide (Fig. 26-6). A 5% solution having a pK of 6, as opposed to a pK of 7.4 for acetazolamide, lowered intraocular pressure when it

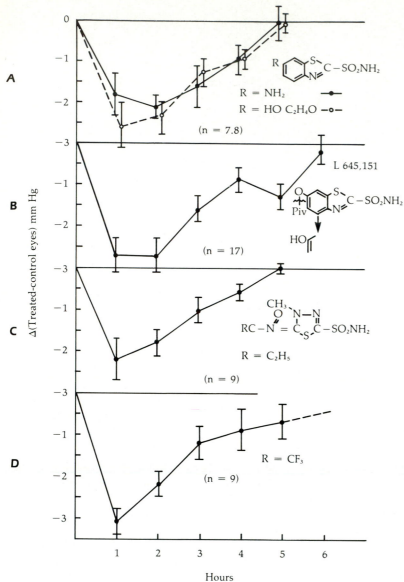

Fig. 26-7 Comparison of intraocular pressure lowering (means ± S.E. mean) in rabbits following 2% suspension (1 drop in 1% hydroxyethylcellulose) of five sulfonamides. **A,** Compounds studied by Lewis et al. (1984, 1986). **B,** Compound of Sugrue et al. (1985). **C** and **D,** Compounds of Maren et al. (1983) and Maren et al. (1987).

Fig. 26-8 Definition and enumeration of rate constants following steady state application of sulfonamides to rabbit cornea: *AC,* Anterior chamber; *PC,* posterior chamber; k_{in}, rate constant from solution laid on cornea; *PC*, the sum of all pathways including k_{in}; k_{out}, rate constant of exit from anterior chamber into blood or tissues; k_h, rate constant of net loss from posterior chamber; *VIT,* vitreous humor. (From Maren, TH. In Drance, SM, and Neufeld, AH: Glaucoma: applied pharmacology in medical treatment, Orlando, FL, 1984, Grune & Stratton)

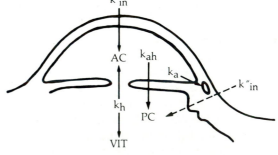

hr^{-1}

	k'_{in} $\rightarrow$ AC	k_{in} $\rightarrow$ PC	k_a out	net k_h out
Bromacetazolamide	4×10^{-4}	1.3×10^{-5}	1.0	0.6
Trifluormethazolamide	0.014	0.0014	0.8	0.8
Trichlormethazolamide	0.08	0.016	0.8	0.3
Ethoxzolamide	0.22	0.17	1.7	1.7

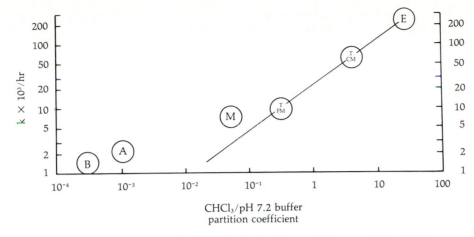

Fig. 26-9 Corneal permeability of sulfanomides in the living rabbit versus lipid solubility accession rate constants to anterior chamber (k_{in}, see Fig. 26-8). *B*, Bromacetazolamide; *A*, acetazolamide; *M*, methazolamide; *TEM*, trifluormethazolamide; *TCM*, trichlormethazolamide; *E*, ethoxzolamide. (Data from Maren, TH, et al: Exp Eye Res 36:457, 1983)

bathed the eye for over 1 hour.[4,51] Unfortunately, the compound was unstable. One group has attempted to focus on amino derivatives of ethoxzolamide, and a 6-hydroxy-C_2H_4OH compound has been tested in rabbits[38,56] and in humans.[37] The pressure lowering effect of the gel formulation, however, is small. Esters of hydroxybenzothiosulfonamides have also been prepared, as well as new ring compounds.[55,58-60]

It is important to achieve drug concentrations in the aqueous humor and ocular tissues on the order of 10 to 30 mmol/L.[50,51] This is identical to the systemic concentrations that cause a pressure lowering effect in the eye. The need to attain high ocular concentrations after administration of carbonic anhydrase inhibitors explains the early negative results occurring after topical delivery of the systemic carbonic anhydrase inhibitors. Drugs of the appropriate class and properties for topical administration are currently being developed. However, all of the drugs available for clinical testing show some degree of corneal toxicity or are only minimally effective. Plasma concentrations are very low.[50] Efforts are underway to find sulfonamide inhibitors that cross the cornea in effective concentrations to inhibit carbonic anhydrase in the ciliary processes (Figs. 26-7 and 26-8). It is necessary to optimize the ratio between water and lipid solubility while maintaining high inhibitory activity (Fig. 26-9). The systemic side effects associated with systemic carbonic anhydrase inhibition are sufficient to warrant continued search for improved topical carbonic anhydrase inhibitors.

REFERENCES

1. Alward, PD, and Wilensky, JT: Determination of acetazolamide compliance in patients with glaucoma, Arch Ophthalmol 99:1973, 1981
2. Aminlari, A: Falling scalp hairs: a side effect of the carbonic anhydrase inhibitor, acetazolamide, Glaucoma 6:41, 1984
3. Arrigg, CA, Epstein, DL, Giovanoni, R, and Grant, WM: The influence of supplemental sodium acetate on carbonic anhydrase inhibitor-induced side effects, Arch Ophthalmol 99:1969, 1981
4. Bar-Ilan, A, Pessah, NI, and Maren, TH: The effects of carbonic anhydrase inhibitors on aqueous humor chemistry and dynamics, Invest Ophthalmol Vis Sci 25:1198, 1984
5. Bar-Ilan, A, Pessah, NI, and Maren, TH: Ocular penetration and hypotensive activity of the topically applied carbonic anhydrase inhibitor L-645,151, J Ocul Pharmacol 2:109, 1986
6. Bayne, WF, et al: Time course and disposition of methazolamide in human plasma and red blood cells, J Pharm Sci 70:75, 1981
7. Beasley, FJ: Transient myopia and retinal edema during ethoxzolamide (Cardrase) therapy, Arch Ophthalmol 68:490, 1962
8. Becker, B: Diamox and the therapy of glaucoma, Am J Ophthalmol 38:16, 1954
9. Becker, B: The effects of the carbonic anhydrase inhibitor, acetazolamide, on the composition of the aqueous humor, Am J Ophthalmol 40:129, 1955
10. Berson, FG, and Epstein, DL: Separate and combined effects of timolol maleate and acetazolamide in open angle glaucoma, Am J Ophthalmol 92:788, 1981
11. Block, ER, and Rostand, RA: Carbonic anhydrase inhibition in glaucoma: hazard or benefit for the chronic lunger? Surv Ophthalmol 23:169, 1978

12. Bryant, WR: Beta blockers and carbonic anhydrase inhibitors for postoperative cataract patients. Proceedings of the American Society of Cataract and Refractive Surgery, 1987

13. Dahlen, K, et al: A repeated dose response study of methazolamide in glaucoma, Arch Ophthalmol 96:2214, 1978

14. Edelhauser, H, and Maren, TH: The permeability of human cornea and sclera to sulfonamides, Invest Ophthal Vis Sci 29(Suppl):3, 1987

15. Friedenwald JS: The formation of the intraocular fluid, Am J Ophthalmol 32:9, 1949

16. Friedenwald, JS: Current studies on acetazolamide (Diamox) and aqueous humor flow, Am J Ophthalmol 39:59, 1955

17. Friedland, BR, Mallonee, J, and Anderson, DR: Short term dose response characteristics of acetazolamide in man, Arch Ophthalmol 95:1809, 1977

18. Friedland, BR, and Maren, TH: The relationship between carbonic anhydrase activity and ion transport in elasmobranch and rabbit lens, Exp Eye Res 33:545, 1981

19. Friedland, BR, and Maren, TH: Carbonic anhydrase: pharmacology of inhibitors and treatment of glaucoma. In Sears, M, editor: Pharmacology of the eye, Berlin, 1984, Springer-Verlag

20. Friedman, Z, Allen, RC, and Ralph, SM: Topical acetazolamide and methazolamide delivered by contact lenses, Arch Ophthalmol 103:963, 1985

21. Friedman, Z, Krupin, T, and Becker, B: Ocular and systemic effects of acetazolamide in nephrectomized rabbits, Invest Ophthalmol Vis Sci 23:209, 1982

22. Galin, MA, Baras, I, and Zweifach, P: Diamox induced myopia, Am J Ophthalmol 54:237, 1962

23. Garg, LC, and Oppelt, WW: The effect of ouabain and acetazolamide on the transport of sodium and chloride from plasma to aqueous humor, J Pharmacol Exp Ther 54:237, 1970

24. Green, K, Bountra, C, Georgiou, P, and House, CR: An electrophysiologic study of rabbit ciliary epithelium, Invest Ophthalmol Vis Sci 26:371, 1985

25. Hallesy, DW, and Layton, WM: Forelimb deformity of rats given dichlorphenamide during pregnancy, Proc Soc Exp Biol Med 126:6, 1969

26. Jankowska, LM, Bar-Ilan, A, and Maren, TH: The relations between ionic and non-ionic diffusion of sulfonamides across the rabbit cornea, Invest Ophthalmol Vis Sci 27:29, 1986

27. Kass, MA, et al: Acetazolamide and urolithiasis, Ophthalmology 88:261, 1981

28. Kinsey, VE: Comparative chemistry of aqueous humor in posterior and anterior chambers of rabbit eye, Arch Ophthalmol 50:401, 1953

29. Kinsey, VE, and Reddy, DVN: Turnover of total carbon dioxide in the aqueous humors and the effect thereon of acetazolamide, Arch Ophthalmol 62:78, 1959

30. Kishida, K, Miwa, Y, and Wata, C: 2-substituted 1, 3, 4-thiadiazole-5-sulfonamides as carbonic anhydrase inhibitors: their effects on the transepithelial potential difference of the isolated rabbit ciliary body and on the intraocular pressure of the living rabbit eye, Exp Eye Res 43:981, 1986

31. Kristinnson, A: Fatal reaction to acetazolamide, Br J Ophthalmol 51:348, 1967

32. Krupin, T, Oestrich, CJ, and Bass, J: Acidosis, alkalosis, and aqueous humor dynamics in rabbits, Invest Ophthalmol Vis Sci 16:997, 1977

33. Kupfer, C, Gaasterland, D, and Ross, K: Studies of aqueous humor dynamics in man. II. Measurements in young normal subjects using acetazolamide and epinephrine, Invest Ophthalmol 10:523, 1971

34. Langlois, IL: Diamox et thrombocytopenie, Arch Ophthalmol (Paris) 26:701, 1966

35. Layton, WM, and Hallesy, DW: Deformity of forelimb in rats: association with high doses of acetazolamide, Science 149:306, 1965

36. Lehmann, B, Linner, G, and Wistrand, PJ: The pharmacokinetics of acetazolamide in relation to its use in the treatment of glaucoma and its effects as an inhibitor of carbonic anhydrase. In Rospe, G, editor: Schering workshop in pharmacokinetics, advances in the biosciences, vol 5, New York, 1969, Pergamon Press

37. Lewis, RA, Schoenwald, RD, Barfknecht, CF, and Phelps CD: Aminozolamide gel: a trial of a topic carbonic anhydrase inhibitor in ocular hypertension, Arch Ophthalmol 104:842, 1986

38. Lewis, RA, et al: Ethoxzolamide analogue gel: a topical carbonic anhydrase inhibitor, Arch Ophthalmol 102:1821, 1984

39. Lichter, PR, Newman, LP, Wheeler, NC, and Beall, OV: Patient tolerance to carbonic anhydrase inhibitors, Am J Ophthalmol 39:885, 1978

40. Lindskog, S, and Wistrand, PJ: Inhibitors of carbonic anhydrase. In Sandler, H, and Smith HJ, editors: Design of enzyme inhibitors as drugs, Oxford, 1987, Oxford University Press

41. Maren, TH: Ionic composition of cerebrospinal fluid and aqueous humor of the dogfish, *Squalus acanthias*. II. Carbonic anhydrase activity and inhibition, Comp Biochem Physiol 5:201, 1962

42. Maren, TH: Carbonic anhydrase: chemistry, physiology, and inhibition, Physiol Rev 47:595, 1967

43. Maren, TH: Relations between structure and biological activity of sulfonamides, Annu Rev Pharmacol Toxicol 16:309, 1976

44. Maren, TH: Ion secretion into the posterior aqueous humor of dogs and monkeys, Exp Eye Res 25(Suppl):245, 1977

45. Maren, TH: An historical account of CO_2 chemistry and the development of carbonic anhydrase inhibitors. The 1979 Theodore Weicker Memorial Award Oration, The Pharmacologist 20:303, 1979

46. Maren, TH: The development of ideas concerning the role of carbonic anhydrase in the secretion of aqueous humor: relation to the treatment of glaucoma. In Drance, SM, and Neufeld, AH, editors:

Glaucoma: applied pharmacology in medical treatment, Orlando, FL, 1984, Grune and Stratton, Inc

47. Maren, TH: The general physiology of reactions catalyzed by carbonic anhydrase and their inhibition by sulfonamides, Ann NY Acad Sci 429:568, 1984

48. Maren, TH: A general view of HCO_3 transport processes in relation to the physiology and biochemistry of carbonic anhydrase. In Case RM, Lingard, JM, and Young, JA, editors: Secretion: mechanisms and control, 1984, Manchester University Press

49. Maren, TH: The kinetics of HCO_3-synthesis related to fluid secretion, pH control and CO_2 elimination. Annu Rev Physiol 50: 1987

50. Maren, TH: Carbonic anhydrase: general perspectives and advances in glaucoma research. Drug Development Research. (Submitted)

51. Maren, TH, and Bar-Ilan, A: The effect of 6-OH benzo[b]thiophene-2-sulfonamide, a new topical carbonic anhydrase inhibitor, on intraocular pressure in rabbits, Invest Ophthalmol Vis Sci 28(Suppl): 1987

52. Maren, TH, Bar-Ilan, A, Caster, KC, and Katritzky, AR: The ocular pharmacology of methazolamide analogs: distribution in the eye and effects on pressure following topical application, J Pharmacol Exp Ther 1986 (Submitted)

53. Maren, TH, Haywood, JR, Chapman, SK, and Zimmerman, TJ: The pharmacology of methazolamide in relation to the treatment of glaucoma, Invest Ophthalmol Vis Sci 16:730, 1977

54. Margo, CE: Acetazolamide and advanced liver disease, Am J Ophthalmol 101:611, 1986

55. Ponticello, GS, Schwam, H, Sugrue, MF, and Baldwin, JJ: Thienothiopyran-2-sulfonamides: topically effective water soluble carbonic anhydrase inhibitors. Presented at 192nd Am Chem Soc National Meeting, Anaheim, (abstract) MEDI 51, 1986.

56. Putnam, ML, et al: Ocular disposition of aminozolamide in the rabbit eye, Invest Ophthalmol Vis Sci 28:1373, 1987

57. Sanyal, G, and Maren, TH: Thermodynamics of carbonic anhydrase catalysis. A comparison between human isoenzymes B and C, J Biol Chem 256:608, 1981

58. Schwam, H, Michelson, SR, Sodney, JM, and Smith, RL: L-645,151, a topically effective ocular hypotensive carbonic anhydrase inhibitor. I. Biochemistry and metabolism. Invest Ophthalmol Vis Sci 25(Suppl):181, 1984

59. Shepard, KL, et al: Benzo[b]thiophene-, benzo[b]furan- and indole-2-sulfonamides: new classes of topically effective carbonic anhydrase inhibitors. Presented at 192nd Am Chem Soc National Meeting, Anaheim, (abstract) MEDI 50, 1986

60. Sugrue, MF, et al: On the pharmacology of L-645,151: a topically effective ocular hypotensive carbonic anhydrase inhibitor, J Pharmacol Exp Ther 232:534, 1985

61. Swenson, ER, and Maren, TH: A quantitative analysis of CO_2 transport at rest and during maximal exercise, Respir Physiol 35:129, 1978

62. Wang, JH: On the catalytic mechanism of carbonic anhydrase. In: Forster, RE, Edsall, JT, Otis, AB, and Roughton, FJM, editors: CO_2: chemical, biochemical and physiological aspects, 1969, Washington, DC, NASA Publication, U. S. Government Printing Office

63. Wistrand, PJ: Carbonic anhydrase in the anterior uvea of the rabbit, Acta Physiol Scand 24:144, 1951

64. Zimmerman, TJ, Garg, LC, Vogh, BP, and Maren, TH: The effect of acetazolamide on the movements of anions into the posterior chamber of the dog eye, J Pharmacol Exp Ther 196:510, 1976

65. Zimmerman, TJ, Garg, LC, Vogh, BP, and Maren, TH: The effect of acetazolamide on the movement of sodium into the posterior chamber of the dog eye, J Pharmacol Exp Ther 199:510, 1976

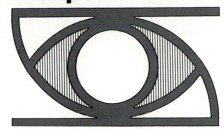

Chapter 27

Hyperosmotic Agents

Marianne E. Feitl
Theodore Krupin

In 1904 Cantonnet[4] first described the use of hypertonic solutions for lowering intraocular pressure. He recommended the oral use of *les substances osmotiques* (sodium chloride and lactose) in the treatment of glaucoma. In 1914 Hertel[12] demonstrated that intravenous administration of concentrated saline was more effective in lowering intraocular pressure. Since saline solutions are rapidly distributed in total body fluids, the osmotic effect was very transitory. Intravenous glucose, sucrose, sorbital, and gum acacia were also investigated as hyperosmotic agents, but toxic side effects limited their use.

The use of intravenous urea to reduce intracranial pressure was reported by Javid[13] in 1956. He later described its effect of lowering both intracranial and intraocular pressure.[14] Galin et al.[8] performed further studies using urea to treat glaucoma. Because of urea's low molecular weight, poor penetration of the blood-aqueous barrier, and fewer side effects, it was widely used as an intravenous hyperosmotic agent.

Mannitol, which was introduced in 1940, was shown by Weiss et al.[29] in 1962 to be an effective, safe agent for lowering intraocular pressure. In 1963 Virno et al.[28] reported that glycerol was an effective oral hyperosmotic for reducing intraocular pressure. Isosorbide, an oral agent that is not metabolized, was introduced in 1967.[2]

Hyperosmotic agents are effective in the short-term treatment of elevated intraocular pressure. They are useful in acute conditions such as angle-closure glaucoma, and in the initial management of some secondary glaucomas presenting with extremely high intraocular pressures. They are most commonly used, however, in the preoperative preparation of the patient for intraocular surgery.

PHARMACOLOGY

Hyperosmotic agents lower intraocular pressure by causing a rapid but transient increase in serum osmolarity of between 20 and 30 mOsm/L. The resulting blood-ocular osmotic gradient draws fluid from the eye via the retinal and uveal vasculature. The decrease in intraocular pressure is primarily caused by a reduction in vitreous volume. Animal studies demonstrate a 3% to 4% reduction in the weight of the vitreous body following administration of various hyperosmotic agents in doses comparable to those used clinically.[25] The decrease in vitreous volume has a greater intraocular pressure–lowering effect in glaucomatous eyes than in eyes with normal intraocular pressure.[1,7]

The effectiveness and duration of action of a hyperosmotic agent is influenced by the following factors:

1. The rate at which the drug is cleared from the systemic circulation by metabolism or excretion
2. The distribution of the drug in either extracellular or intracellular fluid
3. The rate of penetration and the extent to which the drug enters the eye

The magnitude of the blood-ocular osmotic gradient and the duration of that gradient determine the effectiveness of a particular hyperosmotic agent.

Ocular penetration is determined by the permeability of the blood-ocular barrier to the drug and by its molecular size. Agents that penetrate the eye reverse the osmotic gradient so that the osmotic pressure within the eye becomes greater than the osmotic pressure in the blood. This condition results in the movement of fluid into the eye and a rebound increase in intraocular pressure. In addition, with all agents, a transient rebound increase in intraocular pressure may occur if the serum osmolarity falls below that of the dehydrated vitreous body, creating a reversed osmotic gradient that can draw water into the eye.

Hyperosmotic agents may lower intraocular pressure secondary to central effects on the hypothalamus.[17,24] Studies in laboratory animals and humans demonstrated a lowering of intraocular pressure following the administration of small doses of hyperosmotic agents that do not elevate serum osmolarity. This central action may account for the clinical observations of a rapid decrease in intraocular pressure before the establishment of a blood-ocular osmotic gradient, and the decrease in intraocular pressure following low dosage administration of hyperosmotic agents.

ORAL AGENTS (Table 27-1)

Glycerol

Glycerol is the most commonly used oral agent.[7] It is administered as a liquid in dosages of 1 to 1.5 g/kg body weight.[28] Glycerol is denser than water: 1 ml of 100% glycerol = 1.24 g (or 1 g = 0.8 ml glycerol). This should be considered when calculating the total dose by weight of 100% glycerol to be mixed with an equal volume of juice. The percentage dilution of commercial glycerol preparations (grams of glycerol per milliliter) must be considered when determining the total amount to be administered. The onset of action occurs from 10 to 30 minutes after administration, with maximal lowering of intraocular pressure occurring after 45 minutes to 2 hours. The duration of action is approximately 4 to 5 hours. Glycerol is absorbed rapidly and is metabolized by the liver rather than excreted by the kidneys. This produces less diuresis than other hyperosmotic agents. Additionally, the agent is distributed in extracellular water and has poor ocular penetration. These properties enhance its hyperosmotic effect.

Adverse characteristics of glycerol include its sweet taste, which can cause nausea and vomiting. It is somewhat more palatable when given chilled over ice and mixed with orange or lime juice. Of concern is glycerol's caloric content of 4.32 kcal/g. This, combined with the osmotic diuretic effect and resultant dehydration, mandate special caution when used in diabetic patients who may develop hyperglycemia and ketosis.[22]

Isosorbide

Isosorbide is an effective oral hyperosmotic that has fewer side effects than glycerol.[2,16] It is administered in a dosage of 1 to 1.5 g/kg body weight as a 45% (0.45 g/ml) solution.[20,30] Its rate of absorption, time to onset of effect, and duration of action are similar to those of glycerol. Its main advantage over glycerol is that 95% of the drug is excreted unchanged in the urine.[2] Since it is not metabolized, it has no caloric value, and it is therefore recommended over glycerol for use in diabetics.[2] Additionally, isosorbide may produce less nausea and vomiting than other oral agents.[1,21]

Table 27-1 Oral hyperosmotic agents*

Agent	Molecular weight	Dosage (g/kg)	Distribution	Ocular penetration	Advantages	Disadvantages
Glycerol	92	1 to 1.5	Extracellular	Poor	Stable, less diuresis, poor ocular penetration	Nausea, vomiting, calories
Isosorbide	146	1 to 1.5	Total body water	Good	Stable, well tolerated, no caloric value, rapid absorption, nonmetabolized	Penetrates the eye (slowly)
Alcohol	46	0.8 to 1.5 of absolute solution (1 to 2 ml/kg of 40% to 50%)	Total body water	Good	Stable, rapid absorption, palatable, hypotonic diuresis	Nausea, vomiting, calories, diuresis, penetrates the eye (rapidly), CNS effects

*Usually administered in a 50% solution; onset of intraocular pressure reduction slower than intravenous agents.

Ethyl Alcohol

Ethyl alcohol given orally decreases intraocular pressure.[1,23] It may be given straight or as a 40% to 50% solution of ethyl alcohol in juice. In dosages of 1 to 2 ml/kg of the 40% to 50% solution (80 to 100 proof), serum osmolarity increases of 20 to 30 mOsm/L can be achieved. This dosage is adequate to lower intraocular pressure effectively, but it may result in acute alcohol toxicity. The drug is rapidly absorbed from the gastrointestinal tract and distributed in total body water. Alcohol also inhibits the production of ADH (antidiuretic hormone), which induces a hypotonic diuresis. This acts to prolong and increase the osmotic gradient produced, although this is felt to be a minor role. However, alcohol does penetrate the eye rapidly, which limits its pressure-lowering effect and duration. Other adverse effects include nausea, vomiting, and central nervous system effects. Ethyl alcohol is metabolized, and thus it presents a caloric problem similar to that of glycerol. Nonetheless, it may be used in emergency situations when no other agent is available.

INTRAVENOUS AGENTS (Table 27-2)

Intravenous hyperosmotic agents have the advantage of a more rapid onset of action and a greater ocular hypotonic effect than oral agents.[10] They may be effectively administered when a patient has nausea and cannot tolerate oral agents, as may be the situation in acute glaucoma.

Mannitol

Mannitol is one of the most effective hyperosmotic agents for lowering intraocular pressure and is currently the intravenous agent of choice. The recommended intravenous dosage is 1 to 1.5 g/kg body weight of a 10% or 20% solution (i.e., 10 or 20 g/100 ml) at a delivery rate of 3 to 5 ml/minute. However, intravenous mannitol may be an effective ocular hypotensive agent at a lower dosage of 0.5 g/kg body weight. Mannitol has an onset of action of 10 to 30 minutes, a peak effect in about 30 to 60 minutes, and a duration of action of approximately 6 hours. Its distribution is confined to extracellular water with poor penetration into the eye. The drug is rapidly excreted unmetabolized in the urine.[26]

Side effects are infrequent but may be severe. Particular caution is advised in patients with compromised cardiac or renal function. The 20% solution is stable, and in the event of tissue extravasation, is less irritating than intravenous urea.

The major disadvantages of mannitol are the need for intravenous administration and its limited solubility, which necessitates a larger volume of administration than that given with oral agents. It is recommended that the 20% solution be warmed before administration to dissolve crystals, and that a blood filter also be used in the intravenous line. To avoid a potential overdose, excess solution beyond the total desired dose should be removed from the bottle before it is administered.

Urea

Urea may be used intravenously to lower intraocular pressure. It is administered as a 30% solution in a dosage of 2 to 7 ml/kg body weight. It has an onset of action of 15 to 30 minutes, a peak effect in 60 minutes, and a duration of action of 4 to 6 hours. Urea has several disadvantages compared to mannitol. Since it is distributed in all body fluids and penetrates ocular tissue, it may be less effective. Also, these characteristics may lead to a greater rebound effect on intraocular pressure. In the presence of intraocular inflammation, the efficacy of urea is decreased.[9] Urea is unstable, so the solution requires mixing just before use as a 30% urea solution in 10% invert sugar (old solutions decompose to ammonia).[27] If the urea solution extravasates, it may produce thrombophlebitis and skin necrosis.[1]

Table 27-2 Intravenous hyperosmotic agents

Agent	Molecular weight	Dosage (g/kg)	Distribution	Ocular penetration	Advantages	Disadvantages
Mannitol	182	1 to 1.5	Extracellular	Very poor	Stable, rapid action, poor ocular penetration	Large volume, dehydration, diuresis
Urea	60	0.5 to 2	Total body water	Good	Rapid action, nonmetabolized, less cellular dehydration	Unstable, penetrates the eye, slough and phlebitis

CLINICAL USE

Hyperosmotic agents are invaluable in the management of acute angle-closure glaucoma.[10] With greatly elevated intraocular pressure, the iris sphincter may become ischemic and nonreactive to topically administered miotics (e.g., pilocarpine). The effect of hyperosmotic agents, therefore, plays a very important role in lowering the intraocular pressure, which then allows concurrently administered pilocarpine to produce pupillary miosis and to open the iridocorneal angle. In addition, dehydration of the vitreous may result in a deepening of the anterior chamber by allowing the iris and lens to move backward. Glycerol (1 g/kg) or isosorbide (1.5 g/kg) may be given orally in the office, along with topical pilocarpine 1% or 2%. Once the acute attack has been broken, it is safer and easier to proceed with laser or surgical iridectomy.

Secondary glaucomas caused by blunt trauma and hyphema often abate spontaneously in several days as the hyphema resolves. Use of hyperosmotic agents in the interim may lower the intraocular pressure and avoid the need for surgical intervention.[15] In the event that surgery does become necessary, hyperosmotic agents can lower the intraocular pressure preoperatively and prevent optic nerve damage until definitive treatment may be effected.

Hyperosmotic agents play a key role in the therapy of ciliary block glaucoma by dehydrating the vitreous body and reducing the posterior vitreous pressure.[5] The recommended dosage is oral glycerol 1 g/kg body weight or intravenous mannitol 2 g/kg body weight, once or twice daily. In conjunction with this, strong mydriatic agents such as 10% phenylephrine and 2% atropine are given four times daily as well as oral carbonic anhydrase inhibitors. The patient may have to be maintained indefinitely on atropine to prevent recurrences (see Chapter 70).

Oral hyperosmotic agents have been given up to four times daily for periods of weeks for the treatment of transitory secondary glaucomas. For chronic use, isosorbide may be preferable to glycerol to avoid a large caloric load. In neovascular glaucoma and glaucomatous eyes with marked inflammation, intravenous mannitol or oral glycerol penetrate the eye less readily, and are therefore recommended over urea, alcohol, or isosorbide. However, hyperosmotic agents are of limited value when there is disruption of the blood-ocular barrier secondary to a rapid equilibration of the osmotic gradient.

Many clinicians advocate the routine use of preoperative hyperosmotic agents for any type of intraocular surgery. They may be used when hypotony and vitreous dehydration are desired before cataract extraction, corneal transplantation, repair of corneal lacerations, or retinal detachment surgery.[1,10,15]

SIDE EFFECTS

The side effects associated with hyperosmotic agents range from mild to potentially fatal. Severe systemic complications are greater with the intravenous agents.[6] Special caution is advised in the elderly and in all patients with cardiac, renal, or hepatic disease.[6] The most common side effects are headache and back pain. Nausea and vomiting may also be induced with oral agents; these are particularly troublesome when the hyperosmotic agent is given as a preoperative medication.[16] In addition, the diuresis caused by these agents may cause the patient to have to void during the operative procedure. Urinary retention may be seen in patients after intense diuresis. This is most common in older men with prostatic hypertrophy.

Patients with compromised cardiac or renal status may develop circulatory overload with chest pain, pulmonary edema, and congestive heart failure.[3] When decreased renal function precludes the removal of free water, profound hyponatremia can occur and may induce lethargy, obtundation, seizures, and coma.[11] Cellular dehydration may cause agitation, disorientation, and vertigo. Potassium depletion may also be seen.

Hyperosmotic agents must be used with caution in patients with renal failure. Mannitol, which is excreted by the kidneys, can result in a hyperosmotic state caused by lack of mannitol clearance in renal failure.[3] This may lead to cerebrospinal fluid acidosis and neurologic deterioration.[11] Mannitol should not be administered in a total dose of more than 25 to 50 mg in patients with renal failure. Careful observation of renal function, including osmolarity gap (the difference between measured and calculated osmolarity), electrolytes, and urine output, is recommended. Once toxicity is determined in patients with renal insufficiency, extracorporeal hemodialysis is the treatment of choice. This will rapidly remove mannitol from the extracellular space, return plasma osmolality to normal, and correct hyponatremia. Peritoneal dialysis may also be used; however, this method removes mannitol much more slowly.[3]

Other complications include subdural hemorrhage from dehydration, shrinkage of the cerebral cortex, and rupture of the veins between the saggital sinus and the surface of the brain.[18] Hypersensitivity reactions have been attributed to mannitol and include respiratory distress, cyanosis, and hives.[19] Should such a reaction occur, the mannitol infusion should be stopped and supportive treatment such as epinephrine, diphenhydramine, corticosteroids, and aminophylline should be administered.

REFERENCES

1. Becker, B, Kolker, AE, and Krupin, T: Hyperosmotic agents. In Leopold, IM: Symposium on ocular therapy, vol. 3, St. Louis, 1968, The CV Mosby Co
2. Becker, B, Kolker, AE, and Krupin, T: Isosorbide, an oral hyperosmotic agent, Arch Ophthalmol 78:147, 1967
3. Borges, MF, Mochs, J, and Kjellstrand, CM: Mannitol intoxication in patients with renal failure, Arch Intern Med 142:63, 1982
4. Cantonnet, A: Essai de traitement du glaucome par les substances osmotiques, Arch Ophthalmol (Paris) 24:1, 1904
5. Chandler, PA, Simmons, RJ, and Grant, WM: Malignant glaucoma: medical and surgical treatment, Am J Ophthalmol 66:495, 1968
6. D'Alena, P, and Ferguson, W: Adverse effects after glycerol orally and mannitol parenterally, Arch Ophthalmol 75:201, 1966
7. Drance, SM: Effect of oral glycerol on intraocular pressure in normal and glaucomatous eyes, Arch Ophthalmol 72:491, 1964
8. Galin, MA, Aizawa, F, and McLean, JM: Urea as an osmotic ocular hypotensive agent in glaucoma, Arch Ophthalmol 62:347, 1959
9. Galin, MA, and Davidson, R: Hypotensive effect of urea in inflamed and noninflamed eye, Arch Ophthalmol 68:63, 1962
10. Galin, MA, Davidson, R, and Shachter, N: Ophthalmological use of osmotic therapy, Am J Ophthalmol 62:629, 1966
11. Grabie, MT, Gipstein, RM, Adams, DA, and Hepner, GW: Contraindications for mannitol in aphakic glaucoma, Am J Ophthalmol 91:265, 1981
12. Hertel, E: Experimentelle Untersuchungen über die Abhangigkeit des Augendrucks von der Blutbeschaffenheit, v Graefes Arch Ophthalmol 88:197, 1914
13. Javid M, and Settlage, P: Effect of urea on cerebrospinal fluid pressure in human subjects: preliminary report, JAMA 160:943, 1956
14. Javid, M: Urea: new use of an old agent, Surg Clin North Am 38:907, 1958
15. Kolker, AE: Hyperosmotic agents in glaucoma, Invest Ophthalmol 9:418, 1970
16. Krupin, T, Kolker, AE, and Becker, B: A comparison of isosorbide and glycerol for cataract surgery, Am J Ophthalmol 69:737, 1970
17. Krupin, T, Podos, SM, and Becker, B: Effect of optic nerve transection on osmotic alterations of intraocular pressure, Am J Ophthalmol 70:214, 1970
18. Marshall, S, and Hinman, F: Subdural hematoma following administration of urea for diagnosis of hypertension, JAMA 182:813, 1962
19. McNeill, IJ: Hypersensitivity reaction to mannitol, Drug Intell Clin Pharm 19:552, 1985
20. Mehra, K, and Singh, R: Lowering of intraocular pressure by isosorbide: effects of different doses of drug, Arch Ophthalmol 86:623, 1971
21. Mehra, K, Singh, R, Char, JN, and Rajyashree, K: Lowering of intraocular tension: effects of isosorbide and glycerin, Arch Ophthalmol 85:167, 1971
22. Oakley, DE, and Ellis, PP: Glycerol and hyperosmolar nonketotic coma, Am J Ophthalmol 81:469, 1976
23. Peczon, JD: Glaucoma, alcohol, and intraocular pressure, Arch Ophthalmol 73:495, 1965
24. Podos, SM, Krupin, T, and Becker, B: Effect of small-dose hyperosmotic injections on intraocular pressure of small animals and man when optic nerves are transected and intact, Am J Ophthalmol 71:898, 1971
25. Robbins, R, and Galin, MA: Effect of osmotic agents on the vitreous body, Arch Ophthalmol 82:694, 1969
26. Smith, EW, and Drance, SM: Reduction of human intraocular pressure with intravenous mannitol, Arch Ophthalmol 68:734, 1962
27. Tarter, RC, and Linn, JG, Jr: A clinical study of the use of intravenous urea in glaucoma, Am J Ophthalmol 52:323, 1961
28. Virno, M, Cantore, P, Bietti, C, and Bucci, MG: Oral glycerol in ophthalmology: a valuable new method for the reduction of intraocular pressure, Am J Ophthalmol 55:1133, 1963
29. Weiss, DI, Shaffer, RN, and Wise, BL: Mannitol infusion to reduce intraocular pressure, Arch Ophthalmol 68:341, 1962
30. Wisznia, KI, Lazar, M, and Leopold, IM: Oral isosorbide and intraocular pressure, Am J Ophthalmol 70:630, 1970

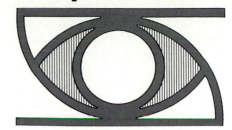

Chapter 28

Alternative and Future Medical Therapy of Glaucoma

Martin B. Wax

The traditional medical treatment of glaucoma is based on the use of several classes of drugs considered efficacious and safe. Long-standing reduction of intraocular pressure in patients with glaucoma is possible with pharmacologic agents such as mixed alpha- and beta-adrenergic agonists (epinephrine and dipivalyl epinephrine), beta-adrenergic antagonists (timolol, betaxolol, and levobunolol), direct (pilocarpine) and indirect (phospholine iodide) cholinergic agonists, and carbonic anhydrase inhibitors (acetazolamide and methazolamide). Despite the promise of additive or more effective reduction of intraocular pressure with laser trabeculoplasty and filtering operations, there remains a constant search to find new classes of pharmacologic drugs that have the ability to lower intraocular pressure. In this chapter, we will discuss three of the most promising of these.

The three classes of drugs—alpha$_2$-selective agonists, cannabinoids, and prostaglandin compounds—all achieve their cellular effects by interacting with receptor-effector mechanisms that share several common components. These are the guanine nucleotide binding proteins. The stimulatory (Gs) and inhibitory (Gi) binding proteins serve to couple the membrane receptors, to which the drug initially binds, to the effector enzyme whose activity is altered (see Chapter 25). As such, these molecular messengers are helpful in providing a unifying framework for the mechanism(s) by which these drugs achieve their cellular effects. However, their physiologic effects on intraocular pressure may be varied and distinct. At this time, few data are available regarding their biochemical and functional interactions with the classes of drugs presently in use.

CLONIDINE AND PARA-AMINOCLONIDINE

Description

Clonidine is an imidazoline derivative used as a potent systemic antihypertensive agent. Clonidine stimulates both central and peripheral alpha$_1$ and alpha$_2$-adrenergic receptors but appears to be a more potent agonist at presynaptic alpha$_2$-adrenergic receptors than at postsynaptic alpha$_1$-adrenergic receptors.[74] Clonidine may not have full agonist activity because it also produces peripheral alpha-adrenergic blockade. Clonidine's ability to reduce systemic blood pressure is attributed to its ability to inhibit central sympathetic outflow by acting on alpha-adrenergic receptors in the lower brainstem region, possibly in the nucleus tractus solitarius.[33] Its agonist activity on alpha$_2$-presynaptic receptors may inhibit neural release of norepinephrine.[71] Activation of alpha$_1$-adrenergic postsynaptic receptors in certain brainstem nuclei may also be associated with inhibition of CNS sympathetic outflow.[32]

557

Para-aminoclonidine hydrochloride is a clonidine derivative and is known generically as apraclonidine or aplonidine hydrochloride. It was granted approval in 1987 by the Food and Drug Administration for acute use following glaucoma laser procedures. It appears similar to the antagonist yohimbine in its selectivity for alpha$_2$-adrenergic receptors; however, the ability of the guanine nucleotide GTP to alter the affinity of para-aminoclonidine for alpha$_2$-adrenergic receptors suggests agonist-specific properties[22].

The density of alpha-adrenergic receptors in the iris/ciliary body of rabbit eyes is approximately 200 to 300 fmol/mg protein (twice that of beta-adrenergic receptors), of which two thirds are alpha$_2$-adrenergic receptors as identified by radioligand studies.[57] Since superior cervical ganglionectomy decreases the total population of alpha-adrenergic receptors in rabbit iris/ciliary body by approximately 10%, it has been suggested that the majority of these are postsynaptic.[60] Mittag has speculated that the large number of alpha$_2$-adrenergic receptors present in the iris/ciliary body may modulate vascular tone, affect aqueous humor formation, or alter uveoscleral outflow. Most of clonidine's effect on the lowering of intraocular pressure appears to be caused by decreased production of aqueous humor rather than increased aqueous humor outflow.[48,50]

Clinical Use

Clonidine lowers both normal and elevated intraocular pressure whether delivered locally or systemically.[36] Directly after topical application, there is a short-term dilation of the conjunctival vessels followed by a persistent and obvious vasoconstriction.[10,64] The effects of topical clonidine on the pupil have been considered negligible,[25,34] but mydriasis has been reported.[48] Initial miosis and prolonged mydriasis occur if toxic levels are reached after systemic administration.[25] The contralateral effect on intraocular pressure after topical clonidine delivery is well noted[39,42,50] and may be caused by a central effect.[43,54]

In patients with primary open-angle glaucoma, both topical 0.125% and 0.25% clonidine hydrochloride were found to effectively lower intraocular pressure, but 2% pilocarpine was slightly more effective than either clonidine concentration.[34] Both concentrations of clonidine, however, reduced systolic and diastolic blood pressures. Significant intraocular pressure lowering (4.4 to 6.1 mm Hg) was noted up to 8 hours after topical application.[39] Although there was no change in resting pulse rate, systolic and diastolic blood pressures were significantly lower after the first day of therapy. Of 21 patients, 10 experienced a decrease in systolic pressure of at least 30 mm Hg. Six patients experienced a decrease in diastolic blood pressure of at least 30 mm Hg. Because systemic clonidine reduced resting cardiac output without changing peripheral vascular resistance, it was feared that this blood pressure change could constitute a dangerous risk for many patients with open-angle glaucoma.

Clonidine, administered to monkeys at a dose that reduced intraocular pressure by 4 to 5 mm Hg, caused a blood flow reduction of 19% in the choroid, 34% in the iris, and 42% in the ciliary body.[10] The authors hypothesized that clonidine-induced vasoconstriction and reduction of systemic blood pressure would have adverse effects on the arterioles supplying the optic nerve head, and thus be undesirable. This concept has severely limited the use of clonidine in this country for the treatment of open-angle glaucoma.

In an effort to achieve satisfactory reduction of intraocular pressure without systemic side effects, minidrops of topical clonidine (both 15 and 70 μl of 0.25% or 0.50% clonidine) all reduced intraocular pressure in patients with primary open-angle glaucoma for at least 5 hours, but only the 70 μl preparations produced systemic hypotension.[62] The authors concluded that, although the 15 μl drop of 0.25% clonidine could, in theory, be used to control glaucoma, a daily application bilaterally would deliver approximately 0.075 mg of clonidine, the oral antihypertensive dose being 0.1 mg/day. Because topical delivery of ophthalmic drops is more akin to an intravenous route of administration, since drops avoid the initial bypass elimination of the liver found with drugs taken orally, the authors questioned whether this dosage would indeed be devoid of systemic effects.

An alternative method of achieving adequate intraocular pressure lowering while minimizing adverse systemic effects is to change the molecular structure of a drug to decrease its systemic absorption. Para-aminoclonidine has sufficiently reduced lipophilicity to allow adequate ocular penetration after topical use with vastly reduced systemic cardiovascular effects, because of a decrease in the ability of the drug to cross the blood-brain barrier. Para-aminoclonidine appears to be a potent ocular hypotensive agent. A 1% solution decreases intraocular pressure almost 40% in normal volunteers.[1] This effect continues with an almost 30% decrease in intraocular pressure at 12 hours. Long-term administration is effective for at least 1 month, and further evaluations in glaucomatous eyes are now in progress.

The new short-term limited-dose uses of aplonidine are promising. Topical 1% aplonidine, given 1 hour before and immediately after anterior segment laser surgery for glaucoma, significantly reduced the incidence of acute postoperative intraocular pressure elevations.[65,66] Aplonidine may have a role in prophylaxis against the potentially devastating complication of elevated intraocular pressure that may occur following argon laser trabeculoplasty or iridectomy.

The use of aplonidine in the treatment of open-angle glaucoma may have high potential. The systemic side effects of aplonidine are similar to those of clonidine and include dry mouth, sedation, dry nasal mucous membranes, orthostatic hypotension, and impotence. Clonidine is contraindicated in patients who are depressed, and may be ineffective in patients concurrently using tricyclic antidepressants.[76]

CANNABINOIDS

Description

The cannabinoids are a family of structurally related compounds naturally synthesized by the hemp plant and include cannabinol, cannabidiol, cannabinolic acid, cannabigerol, cannabicicyclol, and several isomers of tetrahydrocannabinol (THC). The isomer believed to be principally responsible for the characteristic psychoactive effects of marijuana is 1-Δ^9-THC, although the effects of 1-Δ^8-THC are similar. Both exist as viscous, noncrystalline, water-insoluble compounds. Several synthetic analogs appear to be more potent than the naturally occurring compounds.[44]

Ocular Effects

Marijuana, or cannabis, has been used as a herbal medication in many societies for several centuries. It has sedative, analgesic, and anticonvulsant properties. The variability of response to marijuana extracts caused its demise as a treatment modality, and its medical use in this country was terminated by law in 1937. Recently, however, the effectiveness of marijuana, and more specifically its active ingredient, Δ^9-THC, have been shown to have potential efficacious therapeutic applications such as antiemetic effects against the nausea and vomiting induced by cancer chemotherapeutic agents.[67] Limited, legal use of these agents now

exists.[69] The awareness that marijuana had the ability to lower intraocular pressure in humans[37] has spurred a great effort to identify the mechanism by which this effect occurs, and other members of this family of compounds or a delivery system of these drugs to the eye, which can effectively achieve intraocular pressure reduction without the well-known psychotropic side effects that accompany their use.[44] Confirmatory evidence of the intraocular pressure–reducing effect of cannabinoids administered to healthy human subjects has been found by several investigators,[61,63,70] although contradictory evidence has been reported.[23]

In addition to reduction of intraocular pressure, conjunctival injection, decreased tear secretion, and slight miosis were reported in subjects intoxicated with marijuana.[38] The ocular effects of cannabinoids have been reviewed elsewhere.[27,47]

Mechanism of Action

Green et al.[28-31] studied the reduction of intraocular pressure in rabbits given cannabinoids topically and systemically and concluded that both central and peripheral mechanisms were involved. The central component of the ocular hypotensive effect was thought to be mediated at a locus proximal to the superior cervical sympathetic ganglion because it was markedly diminished in ganglionectomized and preganglionectomized eyes of normal rabbits. The peripheral component appeared to involve adrenergic-mediated vasodilation of efferent uveal blood vessels, causing reduced capillary pressure within the ciliary processes, thus decreasing aqueous production. The THC effect is completely abolished by the beta-adrenergic antagonist sotalol and markedly reduced by the alpha-adrenergic antagonist phenoxybenzamine. In addition, the peripheral component appeared to involve alpha-adrenergic-mediated constriction of episcleral vessels that facilitated aqueous outflow, because this effect was blocked by phenoxybenzamine in normal and ganglionectomized eyes. Recent evidence, however, has suggested that the ocular hypotensive effect of at least two THC derivatives in rabbits, namely Δ^9- and Δ^8-THC, is not attributable to a CNS mechanism, but rather to a mechanism involving ocular vascular effects only.[53]

In cultured cells, receptor-mediated inhibition of adenylate cyclase, which required the presence of the guanine nucleotide–binding protein, Gi, was found.[41] The inhibition of adenylate cyclase was abolished by pertussis toxin, which inactivated Gi by ADP-ribosylation of its alpha-subunit. It remains unclear as to whether a specific cellular receptor for cannabinoids exists.

Clinical Usage in Glaucoma

Marijuana inhalation was accompanied by increased heart rate and decreased intraocular and blood pressure in 18 subjects with heterogenous glaucomas. The hypotensive effects appeared in 60 to 90 minutes, and the decrease in intraocular pressure appeared to follow the decrease in blood pressure. In addition to any local effect, the mechanism of lowered intraocular pressure may have involved the decreased perfusion pressure of the ciliary body vasculature as a result of the peripheral vasodilatory properties of marijuana. Postural hypotension, tachycardia, palpitations, and alterations in mental status occurred with such frequency as to suggest that the routine administration of marijuana in the general glaucoma population was not feasible.[55] Further studies confirmed that systemic Δ^9-THC administered either by smoking marijuana or as synthetic THC in soft gelatin capsules, lowered ocular tension in various glaucomas, but at the expense of significant decreases in systolic blood pressure. Topical THC in light mineral oil vehicles, though effective in laboratory animals, was not effective in 0.05% and 0.1% topical solutions when administered to six subjects with primary open-angle glaucoma in a randomized, double-masked protocol.[56]

The potential success of cannabinoid compounds to lower intraocular pressure in the treatment of glaucoma is limited by several obstacles. First, it is not clear which cannabinoids are useful as ocular hypotensive agents. The disagreement in the literature concerning the efficacy of various cannabinoid derivatives to lower intraocular pressure in animals may, in fact, be the result of differences in the animal models used for testing by different laboratories. Topically applied cannabinoids have been disappointing because of their nonaqueous formulations and irritant properties. Although light mineral oil, which has an affinity for corneal epithelium, appears to be an optimum vehicle, topical application of these compounds in mineral oil has shown erratic results in animals. Synthetic water-soluble cannabinoid compounds, such as naboctate, seem effective when given orally in rabbits and humans, but stable topical formulations have not been developed.[40] Most encouraging is the finding that certain topically delivered cannabinoid derivatives, such as the 9,10 epoxide of Δ^9-THC, can lower intraocular pressure more effectively than the parent compound. Furthermore, reduction of intraocular pressure in rabbits is possible with the parenteral administration of the 8,9 epoxide derivative of Δ^8-THC, which has the least CNS activity of the Δ^8-THC metabolites.[21] This suggests that it may be possible to separate the CNS effects from the intraocular pressure–lowering properties of cannabinoid compounds. Further work is necessary to see if this relationship holds true in other animal models, including humans.

PROSTAGLANDINS

Description

Over 30 years ago, Ambache[3,4] reported that a pharmacologically potent substance, "irin," was present in the aqueous extract of rabbit irides and was capable of contracting iris smooth muscle. The iris and subsequently many other ocular structures were found to synthesize the substances now known as prostaglandins (PG), a family of compounds derived from the action of cyclooxygenase on the precursor fatty acid, arachidonate.[5,6,24]

Prostaglandins and Intraocular Pressure

Rarely has there been so large a body of work in any field that appears as dichotomous as that involving the relationship of prostaglandins and intraocular pressure. Early studies that associated prostaglandins with breakdown of the blood-aqueous barrier, iris hyperemia, and the ocular inflammatory response have found that the induced effect on intraocular pressure, mostly in rabbits, was one of ocular hypertension.[7,19,45,72,78] Many investigators thought that the raised intraocular pressure was closely associated with increased aqueous humor protein levels and that local ocular vasodilation and increased permeability of the blood-aqueous barrier were the principle mechanisms by which prostaglandins raised intraocular pressure. Variability of the intraocular pressure response existed between species and routes of administration, and a contralateral response was often observed.[58]

Evidence has accumulated over the last 5 years, however, that contrary to earlier reports, some prostaglandins appear to be highly effective ocular hypotensive agents. Bito[12] has extensively reviewed the ocular effects of prostaglandins with particular emphasis on their role in inflammation and intraocular pressure. The rabbit animal model and the employment of supramaximal concentrations of exogenously administered prostaglandins in experimental protocols are cited as prominent reasons accounting for many earlier findings in which the primary effect of prostaglandins was elevation, rather than lowering, of intraocular pressure in animals.

Topical application of $PGF_{2\alpha}$ reduces intraocular pressure in single- and multiple-dose studies in rabbits, cats, and monkeys.* $PGF_{2\alpha}$ and especially its more lipid soluble isopropyl ester ($PGF_{2\alpha}$-1-isopropyl ester) have strong ocular hypotensive effects on the eyes of normal human volunteers and in patients with the exfoliation syndrome with glaucoma.[26,46,77]

Because the cornea is not readily permeable to organic acids such as $PGF_{2\alpha}$, concentrations of topical drops used for several of the animal experiments previously discussed were relatively high (50 to 200 μg of total drug) and resulted in conjunctival hyperemia, ocular discomfort, and headaches in some human volunteers.[2] Giuffre[26] concluded that the adverse side effects of $PGF_{2\alpha}$ may preclude its use for the management of glaucoma, although it should be noted that flare, cellular response, or miosis were not observed in those patients treated with $PGF_{2\alpha}$-1-isopropyl ester (a total of 0.5 to 5 μg of the drug). The A and B types of prostaglandins are even more potent and lipophilic than the E and F types. A single, 5 μg topical application of PGA_2 resulted in greater and more sustained reduction of intraocular pressure in cats than 100 μg of $PGF_{2\alpha}$, whereas conjunctival hyperemia was considerably shorter in duration than that caused by identical doses of $PGF_{2\alpha}$.[13] These findings suggest that prostaglandin derivatives may possibly be found in an appropriate formulation that provides effective control of intraocular pressure in glaucoma patients with minimal local and systemic side effects.

Mechanisms of Action

Aqueous humor flow rate and episcleral venous pressure were not sufficiently decreased and outflow facility was not sufficiently increased to account for the extent of the intraocular pressure reduction resulting from the use of prostaglandins.[35,46,52,79] These results imply than an increase in uveoscleral outflow may be the mechanism responsible for prostaglandin-induced intraocular pressure reduction.

Studies of prostaglandin interactions with other ocular hypotensive drugs appear to support this concept. It has been suggested that the intraocular pressure–lowering effects of epinephrine in humans may be attributed, at least partially, to in-

creased uveoscleral outflow.[68,75] Topical 2% epinephrine instilled twice daily for 2 weeks to the eyes of patients with glaucoma or ocular hypertension caused an 8.1 ± 1.4 mm Hg reduction of intraocular pressure, but only a 1.9 ± 0.6 mm Hg decrease in patients treated with 25 mg of orally administered indomethacin four times daily.[17]

Systemic treatment with indomethacin for 1 week did not significantly increase intraocular pressure by itself, but when indomethacin treatment was discontinued in those patients receiving topical epinephrine, there was a further reduction in intraocular pressure compared with the placebo-treated group. Because the ocular hypotensive effect of topically applied epinephrine was inhibited by indomethacin, a cyclooxygenase inhibitor, these results suggest that the reduction of intraocular pressure was at least partially mediated by the endogenous production of prostaglandins.

Uveoscleral outflow is affected by the state of contraction of the ciliary muscles[9] and in the cynomolgus monkey is thought to account for approximately 50% of total aqueous drainage.[8] A single application of 1 mg pilocarpine blocked the $PGF_{2\alpha}$-induced ocular hypotensive response in cynomologus monkeys.[20] The authors concluded that $PGF_{2\alpha}$ reduces intraocular pressure by increasing uveoscleral drainage of aqueous humor, because pilocarpine pretreatment contracts the ciliary muscle, closing off the uveoscleral drainage pathway and thus physiologically blocking the $PGF_{2\alpha}$ effect. Topically applied $PGF_{2\alpha}$ in cynomologus monkeys has also been shown to increase uveoscleral outflow significantly.[59] These results are important not only in advocacy of the presumed uveoscleral mechanism of prostaglandin-induced ocular hypotension, but may have profound implications should prostaglandins eventually have widespread clinical use. They suggest that pilocarpine and prostaglandins may not be suitable for combined therapy. We may infer that, should prostaglandins achieve widespread use in the management of glaucoma, they may be of value if conventional outflow facility is damaged to the point whereby pilocarpine can no longer be effective. These considerations are consistent with our current use of drugs that increase uveoscleral outflow, such as atropine, in conditions in which the angle is totally sealed.

REFERENCES

1. Abrams, DA, et al: The safety and efficacy of topical 1% ALO 2145 (p-aminoclonidine hydrochloride) in normal volunteers, Arch Ophthalmol 105:1205, 1987

---

*References 11, 14-16, 18, 51, 52, 59, 73.

2. Alm, A, and Villumsen, J: Intraocular pressure and ocular side effects after prostaglandin F_2 eye drops: a single dose-response study in humans, Proceedings of the International Society of Eye Research 4:14, 1987

3. Ambache, N: Irin, a smooth muscle contracting substance present in rabbit iris, J Physiol (London) 129:65P, 1955

4. Ambache, N: Properties of irin, a physiological constituent of the rabbit iris. J Physiol (London) 135:114, 1957

5. Ambache, N, et al: Thin layer chromatography of spasmogenic unsaturated hydroxy acids from various tissues, J Physiol 185:77P, 1966

6. Anggard, E, and Samuelsson, B: Smooth muscle stimulating lipids in sheep iris: the identification of prostaglandin $F_{2\alpha}$: prostaglandins and related factors 21, Biochem Pharmacol 13:281, 1964

7. Beitch, BR, and Eakins, KE: The effects of prostaglandins on the intraocular pressure of the rabbit, Br J Pharmacol 37:158, 1969

8. Bill, A: Aqueous humor dynamics in monkeys (Macaca irus and Cercopithecus ethiops), Exp Eye Res 11:195, 1971

9. Bill, A: Basic physiology of the drainage of aqueous humor, Exp Eye Res Suppl 25:291, 1977

10. Bill, A, and Heilmann, K: Ocular effects of clonidine in cats and monkeys (macaca irus), Exp Eye Res 21:481, 1975

11. Bito, LZ: Comparison of the ocular hypotensive efficacy of eicosanoids and related compounds, Exp Eye Res 38:181, 1984

12. Bito, LZ: Prostaglandins, other eicosanoids, and their derivatives as potential antiglaucoma agents. In Drance SM, and Neufeld, AH, editors: The medical treatment of glaucomas, New York, 1984 Grune and Stratton

13. Bito, LZ, Baroody, RA, and Miranda, OC: Eicosanoids as a new class of ocular hypotensive agents. 1. The apparent therapeutic advantages of derived prostaglandins of the A and B as compared with primary prostaglandins of the E, F and D type, Exp Eye Res 44:825, 1987

14. Bito, LZ, et al: Long-term maintenance of reduced intraocular pressure by daily or twice daily topical application of prostaglandins to cat or rhesus monkey eyes, Invest Ophthalmol Vis Sci 24:312, 1983

15. Camras, CB, and Bito, LZ: Reduction of intraocular pressure in normal and glaucomatous primate (Aotus trivirgatus) eyes by topically applied prostaglandin $F_{2\alpha}$, Curr Eye Res 1:205, 1981

16. Camras, CB, Bito, LZ, and Eakins, KE: Reduction of intraocular pressure by prostaglandins applied topically to the eyes of conscious rabbits, Invest Ophthalmol Vis Sci 16:1125, 1977

17. Camras, CB, et al: Inhibition of the epinephrine induced reduction of intraocular pressure by systemic indomethacin in humans, Am J Ophthalmol 100:169, 1985

18. Camras, CB, et al: Multiple dosing of prostaglandin $F_{2\alpha}$ or epinephrine on cynomologous monkey eyes. I. Aqueous humor dynamics, Invest Ophthalmol Vis Sci 28:463, 1987

19. Chaing, TS, and Thomas, RP: Ocular hypertension following intravenous infusion by prostaglandin El, Arch Ophthalmol 88:418, 1972

20. Crawford, K, and Kaufman, PL: Pilocarpine antagonizes prostaglandin $F_{2\alpha}$ induced ocular hypotension in monkeys, Arch Ophthalmol 105:1112, 1987

21. ElSohly, MA, et al: Cannabinoids in glaucoma II: the effect of different cannabinoids on intraocular pressure of the rabbit, Curr Eye Res 3:841, 1984

22. Feller, DJ, and Byland, BB: Comparison of alpha$_2$-adrenergic receptors and their regulation in rodents and porcine species, J Pharmacol Exp Ther 228:275, 1984

23. Flom, MC, Adams, AJ, and Jones, RT: Marijuana smoking and reduced pressure in human eyes: drug action or epiphenomenon? Invest Ophthalmol Vis Sci 14:52, 1975

24. Flower, RJ: Prostaglandins and related compounds. In Vane, JR, and Ferreira, SH, editors: Handbook of experimental pharmacology, vol 50, Berlin, 1978, Springer

25. Fraunfelder, FT: Cardiac, vascular, and renal agents. In Fraunfelder, FT, editor: Drug-induced ocular side effects and drug interactions, Philadelphia, 1982, Lea & Febiger

26. Giuffre, G: The effects of prostaglandins $F_{2\alpha}$ in the human eye, v Graefes Arch Klin Exp Ophthalmol, 222:139, 1985

27. Green, K: Current status of basic and clinical marijuana research in ophthalmology. In Leopold, IH, and Burns, RP, editors: Offprints from symposium on ocular therapy, vol 2, New York, 1979, John Wiley

28. Green, K, and Bowman, K: Effect of marijuana and derivatives on intraocular pressure in the rabbit. In Braude, MC, and Szara, S, editors: The pharmacology of marijuana, New York, 1976, Raven Press

29. Green, K, Kim, K, and Bowman, K: Ocular effects of Δ^9-tetrahydrocannabinol. In Cohen, S, and Stillman, RC, editors: The therapeutic potential of marijuana, New York, 1976, Plenum Press

30. Green, K, et al: Cannabinoid action on the eye as mediated through the central nervous system and local adrenergic activity, Exp Eye Res 24:189, 1977

31. Green, W, Wynn, H, and Padgett, D: Effects on Δ^9 tetrahydrocannabinol on ocular blood flow and aqueous humor formation, Exp Eye Res 26:65, 1978

32. Häusler, G: Clonidine-induced inhibition of sympathetic nerve activity: no indication for a central presynaptic or an indirect sympathomeimetic mode of action, Naunyn Schmiedeberg Arch Pharmacol 286:97, 1974

33. Häusler, G: Cardiovascular regulation by central adrenergic mechanisms and its alteration by hypotensive drugs, Circ Res 37:223, 1975

34. Harrison, R, and Kaufmann, CS: Clonidine. Effects of a topically administered solution on intraocular pressure and blood pressure in open-angle glaucoma, Arch Ophthalmol 95:1368, 1977

35. Hayashi, M, Yablonski, ME, and Bito, LZ: Eicosanoids as a new class of ocular hypotensive agents. II. Comparison of the apparent mechanism of the ocular hypostensive effects of A and F type prostaglandins, Invest Ophthalmol Vis Sci 28:1639, 1987

36. Heilmann, K: Special pharmacology. In Heilmann, K and Richardson, KT, editors: Glaucoma, conceptions of a disease, part 5, Philadelphia, 1978, WB Saunders Co

37. Hepler, RS, and Frank, IM: Marijuana smoking and intraocular pressure, JAMA 217:1329, 1971

38. Hepler, RS, Frank, IM, and Ungerleider, JT: Pupillary constriction after marijuana smoking, Am J Ophthalmol 74:1185, 1972

39. Hodapp, E, et al: The effect of topical clonidine on intraocular pressure, Arch Ophthalmol 99:1208, 1981

40. Howes, JF: Antiglaucoma effects of topically and orally administered cannabinoids, In Agurell, S, Dewey, WL, and Willette, RE, editors: The cannabinoids: chemical, pharmacologic, and therapeutic aspects, New York, Academic Press, 1984

41. Howlett, AC, Qualy, JM, and Khachaturian, LL: Involvement of Gi in the inhibition of adenylate cyclase by cannabimimetic drugs, Mol Pharmacol 29:307, 1986

42. Innemee, HC, Hermans, AJM, and van Zweitern, PA: The influence of clonidine on intraocular pressure after topical application to the eyes of anesthetized cats, Graefes Arch Klin Exp Ophthalmol 212:19, 1979

43. Innemee, HC, and van Zweiten, PA: The central ocular hypotensive effect of clonidine, Graefes Arch Clin Exp Ophthalmol 210:93, 1979

44. Jaffe, JH: Drug addiction and drug abuse. In Gilman, AG, Goodman, LS, and Rall, TW, editors: Goodman and Gilman's the pharmacological basis of therapeutics, ed 7, New York, 1985, Macmillan Publishing Co

45. Kelly, RGM, and Starr, M: Effects of prostaglandins and a prostaglandin antagonist on intraocular pressure and protein in the monkey eye, Can J Ophthalmol 6:205, 1971

46. Kerstetter, JR, Brubaker, RF, and Wilson, SE: Prostaglandin $F_{2\alpha}$1-isopropylester effects on aqueous humor dynamics in human subjects, Invest Ophthalmol Vis Sci Suppl 28:266, 1987

47. Korczyn, AD: The ocular effects of cannabinoids, Gen Pharmacol 11:419, 1980

48. Krieglstein, GK, Langham, ME, and Leydhecker, W: The peripheral and central neural actions of clonidine in normal and glaucomatous eyes, Invest Ophthalmol Vis Sci 17:149, 1978

49. Kulkarni, PS, and Srinivasan, BD: Prostaglandins E_3 and D_3 lower intraocular pressure, Invest Ophthalmol Vis Sci 26:1178, 1985

50. Lee, DA, Topper, JE, and Brubaker, RF: Effect on clonidine on aqueous humor flow in normal human eyes, Exp Eye Res 38:239, 1984

51. Lee, P-Y, et al: Pharmacological testing in the laser-induced monkey glaucoma model, Curr Eye Res 4:775, 1985

52. Lee, P-Y, Podos, SM, and Severin, C: Effect of prostaglandin $F_{2\alpha}$ on aqueous humor dynamics of rabbit, cataract, and monkey, Invest Ophthalmol Vis Sci 25:1087, 1984

53. Liu, JHK, and Dacus, AC: Central nervous system and peripheral mechanisms in ocular hypotensive effect of cannabinoids, Arch Ophthalmol 105:245, 1987

54. Liu, JHK, and Neufeld, AH: Study of central regulation of intraocular pressure using ventriculocisternal perfusion, Invest Ophthalmol Vis Sci 26:136, 1985

55. Merritt, JC, et al: Effect on marijuana on intraocular and blood pressure in glaucoma, Ophthalmology 87:222, 1980

56. Merritt, JC, et al: Topical Δ^9-tetrahydrocannabinol and aqueous dynamics in glaucoma, J Clin Pharmacol 21:467S, 1981

57. Mittag, TW, et al: Alpha-adrenergic antagonists: Correlation of the effect on intraocular pressure and on alpha$_2$-adrenergic receptor binding specificity in the rabbit eye, Exp Eye Res 40:591, 1985

58. Neufeld, AH, and Sears, ML: Prostaglandin and eye, Prostaglandins 4:157, 1973

59. Nilsson, FE, Stjernschantz, J, and Bill, A: $PGF_{2\alpha}$ increase uveoscleral outflow, Invest Ophthalmol Vis Sci Suppl 28:284, 1987

60. Page, ED, and Neufeld, AH: Characterization of alpha and beta-adrenergic receptors in membranes prepared from the rabbit iris before and after development of supersensitivity, Biochem Pharmacol 27:953, 1978

61. Perez-Reyes, M, et al: Intravenous administration of cannabinoids and intraocular pressure, In Braude, MC, and Szara, S, editors: The pharmacology of marijuana, New York, 1976, Raven Press

62. Petursson, G, Cole, R, and Hanna, C: Treatment of glaucoma using minidrops of clonidine, Arch Ophthalmol 102:1180, 1984

63. Purnell, WD, and Gregg, JM: Δ^9-tetrahydrocannabinol, euphoria, and intraocular pressure in man, Ann Ophthalmol 7:921, 1975

64. Ralli, R: Clonidine effect on the intraocular pressure and eye circulation, Acta Ophthalmol (Copenh) 125:37, 1975

65. Robin, AL, Pollack, IP, and deFaller, JM: Effects of topical ALO 2145 (p-aminoclonidine hydrochloride) on the acute intraocular pressure rise after argon laser iridotomy, Arch Ophthalmol 105:1208, 1987

66. Robin, AL, et al: Effects of ALO 2145 on intraocular pressure following argon laser trabeculoplasty, Arch Ophthalmol 105:646, 1987

67. Sallan, SE, et al: Antiemetics in patients receiving chemotherapy for cancer, N Engl J Med 302:135, 1980

68. Schenker, HI, et al: Fluorophotometric study of epinephrine and timolol in human subjects, Arch Ophthalmol 99:1212, 1981

69. Scigliano, JA: THC therapeutic research by independent and state-sponsored investigators: a historical review, J Clin Pharmacol 113S, 1981

70. Shapiro, D: The ocular manifestations of the cannabinoids, Ophthalmologica 168:366, 1974

71. Starke, K: Regulation of noradrenaline release by presynaptic receptor systems, Rev Physiol Biochem Pharmacol 77:1, 1977

72. Starr, M: Further studies on the effect of prostaglandin on intraocular pressure of the rabbit, Exp Eye Res 11:170, 1971

73. Stern, FA, and Bito, LZ: Comparison of the hypotensive and other ocular effects of prostaglandins E_2 and $F_{2\alpha}$ on cat and rhesus monkey eyes, Invest Ophthalmol Vis Sci 22:588, 1982

74. Titeler, M, Tedesco, JL, and Seeman, P: Selective labelling of pre-synaptic receptors by ^{3}H-dopamine, ^{3}H-apomorphine and ^{3}H-clonidine; labelling of post-synaptic sites by ^{3}H-neuroleptics, Life Sci 23:587, 1978

75. Townsend, DJ, and Brubaker, RF: Immediate effects of epinephrine on aqueous formation in the normal human eye as measured by fluorophotometry, Invest Ophthalmol Vis Sci 19:256, 1980

76. Van Zweiten, PA: Reduction of the hypotensive effect of clonidine and alpha-methyldopa by various psychtropic drugs, Clin Sci 51:4115, 1976

77. Villumsen, J, and Alm, A: The effect of prostaglandin $F_{2\alpha}$ eye drops in open angle glaucoma, Invest Ophthalmol Vis Sci 28:266, 1987

78. Waitzman, MA, and King, CD: Prostaglandin influences on intraocular pressure and pupil size, Am J Physiol 212:329, 1967

79. Wang, R-F, et al: The ocular hypotensive effects of prostaglandin $F_{2\alpha}$ isopropyl ester (PGF$_{2\alpha}$-IE) and A_2 (PGA$_2$) in glaucomatous monkeys, Invest Ophthalmol Vis Sci 28:266, 1987

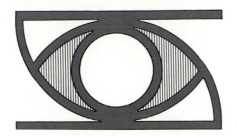

PART IV

LASER SURGERY

29

Clinical Laser Physics

30

Laser Iridectomy and Iridoplasty

31

Laser Treatment in Open-angle Glaucoma

32

Additional Uses of Laser Therapy in Glaucoma

Chapter 29

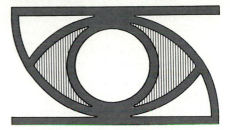

Clinical Laser Physics

Martin A. Mainster

Selection and proper use of ophthalmic laser systems require both familiarity with the various types of clinical instruments and basic knowledge of the biophysical mechanism by which lasers exert their effects on ocular structures. This chapter presents an introduction to light, lasers, and laser-tissue interactions, with particular emphasis on photocoagulation and photodisruption in ophthalmic practice.

BASIC PRINCIPLES

Light

The electromagnetic spectrum is composed of a broad range of radiation frequencies, including ultraviolet radiation, visible light, and infrared radiation. Electromagnetic radiation has wavelike properties that are responsible for large-scale phenomena such as refraction and interference, and particle-like properties that account for such atomic-level phenomena as light absorption and emission by atoms or molecules.

Electromagnetic waves are characterized by their wavelength, λ, the distance between successive peaks of the waves. In free space all electromagnetic radiation travels at the speed of light,* but radiation of different wavelengths interacts with biologic structures in different ways. For example, the cornea is essentially opaque to ultraviolet radiation below 300 nm, but transmits radiation between 300 and 1300 nm quite effectively.[8] In practical terms, if a corneal incision is to be performed with an ultraviolet laser, the wavelength

must be well below 300 nm to avoid damage to the crystalline lens. Similarly, since the crystalline lens protects the retina from potentially hazardous near-ultraviolet light between 300 and 400 nm, the aphakic or pseudophakic eye is at increased risk for photochemical retinal damage, as seen in cases of solar retinitis or welder's maculopathy.[20,22]

The wavelike properties of light are useful in analyzing how light will be affected by optical systems, whereas its particle-like properties are needed to explain how atoms or molecules acquire or release energy. If light is considered to be a stream of discrete particles, or *photons*, it is possible to explain such subatomic phenomena as light absorption or fluorescence.

The energy of a photon is related to its wavelength by Planck's relationship:

$$E = hc/\lambda$$

where h is Planck's constant and c is the speed of light. The electrons of an atom can exist only at a limited number of energy levels, as first proposed by Niels Bohr in 1913.

Generally, when an atom absorbs energy (excitation energy), an outer electron is moved from its normal (ground) energy level to a higher (excited) energy level. If the atom absorbs enough energy, the electron may actually escape from the attraction of the nucleus, producing a free electron and an ion in a process called *ionization*. This occurs during photodisruption with a neodymium:YAG (Nd:YAG) laser, discussed below. Ionization may be regarded as the state of an electron in which there is a continuum of allowed energy levels

---

*Speed of light (c) = 3×10^{10} cm/second.

rather than the discrete number permitted when the electron is bound to the nucleus. This continuum is the basis for the "tunability" of a free-electron laser from the far-ultraviolet to the far-infrared ranges of the spectrum.

If an atom absorbs a photon that has an energy level equal to the difference in energy between two of its adjacent electron energy levels, an electron in the lower level may be excited from the lower to the higher energy level in a process called *stimulated absorption*. Photons causing stimulated absorption can arise from fluorescence or from a flashlamp that produces photons with a continuous range of wavelengths. A flashlamp is used to excite neodymium ions in a Nd:YAG laser. Electrons can also be excited to higher energy levels by processes other than photon absorption. For example, collision with electrons from an electric current is used to excite atoms in an ion (such as argon or krypton) laser or an excimer (such as argon fluoride) laser.

An atom that is excited but not ionized returns quickly to its normal (ground) state when its excited electron falls from an excited energy level to the ground energy level. The excessive energy possessed by the excited atom can be given off in the form of a photon, the energy of which is equal to the energy difference between the electron's excited and ground energy levels ($E_2 - E_1$). This process is termed *spontaneous emission* or *fluorescence*. The wavelength of the emitted photon, from Planck's relationship, is

$$\lambda = hc/(E_2 - E_1)$$

It should be noted that there is no preferred direction for the photons given off in fluorescence, which itself does not produce coherent light.

In general, the return of an electron from an excited, higher energy level to its ground energy level takes place not in a single jump ("transition"), but through alternative, competing pathways, each of which may consist of a sequence of photon-producing transitions and faster nonradiative transitions. Thus photons with several different wavelengths may be produced when a collection of excited atoms of a single type returns to ground state.

In 1917 Albert Einstein postulated that if an atom with an excited electron is struck by a photon, and the photon has an energy equal to the difference between the electron's higher and lower energy levels, then the incoming photon could trigger the atom to return to its ground state by releasing a photon. This process is termed *stimulated emission*. The photon released by the excited atom when the atom returns to its ground state has the same wavelength, direction, and phase as the incoming photon that triggered its release. Thus a single photon can produce two identical photons, and stimulated emission has the potential for producing a chain reaction or "cascade" of photons with identical properties. T.H. Maiman first demonstrated light generated by stimulated emission in 1960, using a ruby crystal in a device that is now known as a laser. The term *laser* is an acronym for *Light Amplification by Stimulated Emission of Radiation*.[33]

The time an atom spends in any one of its many possible excited states is termed the *fluorescent lifetime* of that state. Most lifetimes are very short, typically on the order of 10^{-9} second (nanosecond) or less. Some atoms, however, have an excited energy level with a comparatively longer fluorescent lifetime, referred to as a *metastable* state. Excited atoms must be able to exist in a metastable state to be a useful, active medium for laser operation. Laser photons are generated when electrons make the transition from the metastable energy state to the next lower energy level. In a "four-level" laser system, such as in an argon ion or Nd:YAG laser, the sequence of events is as follows:

1. First the electrons are excited to very high energy levels
2. The electrons then quickly fall through nonradiative transitions to a metastable state: E_3
3. The electrons stay briefly in the metastable state before making the transition to the next lower level: E_2
4. Finally, the electrons fall from E_2 to their ground state (E_1) by very rapid nonradiative transitions

In a four-level system, a collection of excited atoms tends to have more atoms with an electron in its longer-lived metastable state (E_3) than in the next lower state (E_2); this condition is called a *population inversion*.

Lasers

Most atoms or molecules of a crystal or gas exist in the unexcited, ground state. To create a laser beam with a particular type of atom, that atom must have a comparatively long-lived metastable state, and enough energy must be supplied to a collection of those atoms so that more atoms have electrons in the excited metastable state than in the next lower energy level; that is, to produce a population inversion.[38] This population inversion can be induced by transferring energy to the atoms ("pumping" them) in various ways, such as by using a flashlamp or electric current.

A metastable state and population inversion

are necessary but not sufficient conditions for creating a laser beam. In addition, a cylindric or rectangular *resonant cavity* is needed to produce light by stimulated emission, preferentially along a single axis. Resonant cavities are usually constructed by placing atoms or molecules of a particular type in a cavity with a mirror at each end, as shown in Fig. 29-1. The material containing atoms or molecules in an appropriate metastable state is referred to as the laser's *active medium.* A variety of active media are used in gas, liquid, and solid state lasers (Table 29-1). A pumping source, such as a flashlamp or electric current, is then used to produce a population inversion in the resonant cavity.

A certain number of the excited atoms return to their ground state by spontaneous emission (fluorescence). When a photon produced by fluorescence strikes an excited atom, it produces two photons traveling with the same direction, wavelength, and phase. These photons in turn strike other excited atoms, eventually leading to a "cascade" of photons traveling through the cavity. Mirrors at the ends of the cavity redirect these photons back into the cavity along its axis to form the resonance that preferentially produces large numbers of photons traveling along the axis of the cavity. Photons from fluorescence or stimulated emission

that do not travel parallel to the axis of the cavity merely escape from the cavity.

If one of the mirrors at the ends of the cavity is only partially reflecting—known as the *output coupler*—then a fraction of the photons traveling along the axis will escape to produce the laser beam. If more than one wavelength is produced in this manner, as in an argon ion laser, all wavelengths other than the desired one, such as 514.5 nm green, can be suppressed by placing a prism in the cavity to deviate photons other than those with the desired wavelength at an angle to the axis of the cavity.

The design of the resonant cavity affects the energy distribution across the laser beam. This distribution, which is determined by the boundary conditions of the cavity, can have rectangular or cylindric symmetry. For example, the circular beam of a typical argon ion laser tube is produced by a longitudinal discharge between electrodes at both ends of the resonant cavity; that is, the electric discharge is used to pump electrons through the gas parallel to the cavity's axis. The square beam of an excimer laser, however, is produced by a transverse discharge perpendicular to the cavity axis. A much shorter path length is needed to obtain an electric discharge and effective action for

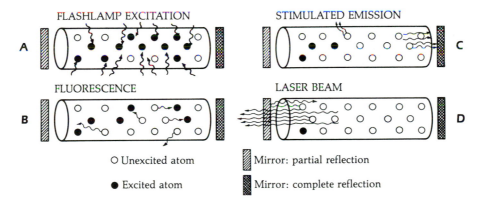

Fig. 29-1 Steps of laser beam production in resonant cavity. **A,** Population inversion in active medium is created by photons from a flashlamp or electrons from an electrical discharge. That is, enough energy is supplied to atoms or molecules in the cavity so that more of them are in an excited metastable state than in their ground state. **B,** Atoms stay briefly in excited state (its fluorescent lifetime) before returning to ground state by spontaneous emission (fluorescence). **C,** If photons from fluorescence travel along axis of cavity and strike an excited atom, stimulated emission will produce two photons traveling along axis of cavity with identical wavelength, direction, and phase. These photons strike other excited atoms, causing further stimulated emission, and producing a cascade of photons with identical properties. Mirrors at end of cavity redirect photons back into cavity along its axis, thereby producing cavity resonance. Photons not traveling along cavity axis (whether from spontaneous or stimulated emission) merely escape from cavity as excess fluorescence. **D,** One of two mirrors at ends of cavity is partly transmitting. This is the output coupler and is designed for the specific cavity and active laser medium. The laser beam is formed when photons traveling along axis of cavity escape through this partly transmitting mirror. (Modified from Worthen, DM: Laser therapies for the glaucomas. In Cairns, JE, editor: Symposium on glaucoma, Trans New Orleans Acad Ophthalmol, St. Louis, 1981, The CV Mosby Co)

Table 29-1 Ophthalmic laser sources

Name	Primary wavelengths (nm)*	Active species	Pumping type†	Use‡	Status§
Argon	488.0 B	Ar ion	ED	PC	C
	514.5 G			PC	C
Carbon dioxide	10,600 IR	CO_2	ED	PV, PC	I,C
Copper vapor	510 G	Cu atom	ED	PC	P
	578 Y			PC	P
Excimer	126-351 UV	Various excimers	ED	PA	E
Erbium:YLF	1228 IR	Er ion	FL	PD	I
Gold vapor	628 R	Au atom	ED	PR, PC	P
Helium-neon	632.8 R	Ne atom	ED	PD aiming, diagnosis‖	C
Krypton	531.0 G	Kr ion	ED	PC	I
	568.2 Y			PC	I
	647.0 R			PC	C
Neodymium:YAG	532 G	Nd ion	FL	PC	E
	650 R			PC	P
	1064 IR			PD, PC	C
	1300 IR			PD	E
Ruby	694.3 R	Cr ion	FL	PD	I
				PC	H

*B, blue; G, green; IR, infrared; Y, yellow; UV, ultraviolet.
†ED, electric discharge; FL, flashlamp.
‡PA, photoablation; PC, photocoagulation; PD, photodisruption; PR, photoradiation; PV, photovaporization.
§C, clinical; E, experimental; H, historical; I, investigational; P, possible clinical use.
‖Laser retinal interferometry, laser Doppler velocimetry, and automated lensometers.

an excimer laser, even with extremely high voltages.

The energy distribution across the beam is characterized by its transverse electromagnetic mode (TEM) structure, which arises from cavity resonances.[33] If an aperture is placed in the beam to limit light output only to the fundamental TEM_∞ mode (a Gaussian or "bell-shaped" distribution of energy across the beam), the cavity produces less total energy, but the laser beam can be focused to a minimum spot size (maximum focal irradiance) for its wavelength. Utilization of the fundamental TEM_∞ mode structure in an Nd:YAG laser permits a maximum focal irradiance for a particular cone angle. Thus for a particular focal irradiance, using the fundamental mode minimizes the exposure of structures anterior and posterior to the focal point.[29]

In addition to its transverse mode structure, a laser beam is characterized by its longitudinal mode structure. Each photon in a laser pulse may be thought of as having traveled back and forth between the ends of the laser cavity for a certain number of transits before leaving the cavity. Separation of the longitudinal modes by *mode locking*

provides a beam with a series or "train" of brief spikes.[29] Each spike in the train consists of a group of photons that have made a particular number of intracavity transits. The peak power of the spikes is considerably higher than the average power output that the cavity would have produced without mode locking.

In general, laser action in a resonant cavity commences almost as soon as pumping begins. If the atoms of the active laser medium have a sufficiently long lifetime in their metastable state, an opaque shutter placed in the resonant cavity can block the formation of a laser beam until an extremely high population inversion is produced. This shutter is known as a *Q-switch*. In Q-switched laser operation, pumping begins (that is, the flashlamp is turned on), but since the Q-switch is closed, a very high population inversion quickly occurs. When the switch is opened (made transparent) for a very brief period shortly after pumping begins, an extremely brief light pulse of very high power escapes from the cavity. Without the Q-switch, (1) only a smaller population inversion is achieved, (2) light production commences almost as soon as pumping begins, and (3) a lengthier light pulse with lower peak power is produced. The comparatively lengthy 0.25 millisecond fluorescent lifetime[29] of the neodymium ion in a Nd:YAG laser is quite useful for Q-switched operation, whereas the much shorter 5 nanosecond (1 nanosecond = 10^{-9} second) lifetime of the argon ion's metastable state is not suitable. Other techniques, such as "cavity dumping," can be used to increase the power output of an ion laser.

Two types of Q-switches are commonly used: a Pockels cell, which is a solid-state device that is switched electronically ("active" Q-switching); and a dye cell that bleaches, or becomes transparent, when exposed to very high irradiances ("passive Q-switching").[29] In addition to Q-switching, the dye cell can also serve to mode lock the laser output, thereby splitting the Q-switched pulse into a train of even briefer spikes (usually 7 to 9), each of which has a higher peak power than that of the Q-switched pulse without mode locking.

Laser Light

Since a laser's resonant cavity amplifies only those photons that travel along its axis, a laser beam is highly directional and has little divergence. Low divergence permits effective focusing of the beam into a small spot of high *irradiance.* (Irradiance = power/unit area and is also termed, less properly, "power density.") Most surgical applications of lasers require very high focal irradiances, as discussed in the next section. The spot size into which a laser beam can be focused is directly proportional to the wavelength of the laser light and to the focal length of the focusing lens. Thus, 193 nm ultraviolet radiation can be focused into a smaller spot than 1064 nm infrared radiation, and Nd:YAG laser radiation can be focused into a smaller spot size by a lens of short focal length rather than by one with a long focal length. The irradiance at a particular wavelength that is obtainable with a laser is millions of times greater than that attainable by filtering the broad spectral output of a conventional incandescent or arc lamp.

Light scattering in the intraocular transit of a laser beam and aberrations in the optical delivery system or in the eye itself can increase the actual spot size, thereby reducing focal irradiance. For example, an increased Nd:YAG laser focal spot size may arise because of light scattering caused by an irregular cornea. This increase can be compensated for by using a contact lens. Light scattering also diminishes contrast in the surgeon's microscopic image. In general, an image is more readily improved by altering the orientation of the slit beam or by reducing the height and width of the beam, rather than by increasing slit-lamp illumination, since increasing illumination only increases veiling back-scattered light.

In addition to having directionality, laser light is also monochromatic and both spatially and temporally coherent. Monochromaticity means that laser light is composed of one or several individual wavelengths (lines), since there are only a limited number of efficient electron transitions from metastable to lower energy levels. Although no line is completely monochromatic (that is, the spectral line width is not zero), laser light is effectively monochromatic for all current ophthalmologic applications. Monochromaticity permits the selection of particular wavelengths for specific applications or target tissues.

Spatial coherence means that there is good phase correlation across the laser beam. That is, if there is a peak in the electromagnetic wave in the center of the laser beam as it crosses an imaginary plane perpendicular to the path of the laser beam, there will also be a peak in the peripheral part of the beam as it crosses the same plane. Spatial coherence is produced primarily by the geometry of the resonant cavity.[33]

Temporal coherence means that the wavelength of the laser beam does not change in time, since differences between electronic energy levels do not change with time. Neither spatial nor temporal coherence is perfect, but they are characterized by a coherence length that is quite long for a highly coherent beam. For example, the coherence length of a helium-neon (He-Ne) laser is 1000 m (for single-mode operation), whereas that of a typical Nd:YAG laser is only 1 cm. Spatial and temporal coherence are essential for diagnostic applications in which laser beams are divided and subsequently recombined, as in retinal interferometry, or compared, as in Doppler velocimetry. Whereas laser beams of high spatial coherence do have low divergence, current surgical applications of the laser do not specifically require spatial and temporal coherence.

LASER EFFECTS

Laser Interactions

Laser light entering biologic tissue is either absorbed or scattered. Scattering affects the resultant distribution of photons in the target tissue,[23] whereas absorption determines the physical effect of the light on the tissue. As noted earlier, the absorption of a photon may alter the energy states of electrons of the atoms in a molecule. In particular, when irradiances lower than those produced by Q-switched lasers are used, photons from ultraviolet or visible radiation generally excite outer shell electrons to higher energy levels. These are the electrons involved in chemical reactions. An excited molecule usually loses this excess electron energy when (1) it participates in a chemical reaction (that is, a photochemical reaction); (2) it collides with another molecule or atom; (3) it releases a photon in spontaneous emission; or (4) the excess electron energy is converted into increased relative motion of the molecule's constituent atoms—a thermal effect. The thermal process results in photon absorption and an increased rate of vibration of atoms relative to their molecule's center of mass, thereby increasing the molecule's vibrational energy level.

Photons produced by infrared radiation differ from those produced by ultraviolet and visible light because, in addition to transferring energy indirectly by exciting electrons to higher energy levels, they can also transfer energy directly to the vibrational energy levels of irradiated molecules. Regardless of whether photons induce molecular vibration indirectly or directly, the net effect of this energy transfer is an increase in the average vibrational motion of the irradiated molecules. The tangible phenomenon of "heat energy" is equivalent at an atomic level to the kinetic energy of the component atoms and molecules of a structure. Light absorption converts photon energy into heat energy, increasing the temperature of the target tissue. Furthermore, since vibrating molecules collide with and transfer energy to neighboring molecules, heat energy quickly diffuses over an area much

larger than that initially irradiated, in a process known as *heat conduction*.

In general, molecules in biologic tissues are opaque to ultraviolet radiation at wavelengths shorter than 300 nm and have strong vibration absorption bands for infrared radiation at wavelengths greater than about 1000 nm.[14] Between 300 and 400 nm only a limited number of biomolecules have moderate absorption. Most biomolecules, however, are effectively transparent between 400 and 1000 nm. Differences in the spectral absorption properties of different molecules permit selective damage to specific components of a target tissue.[23,26]

Laser effects in biologic tissues may be divided into three general categories: (1) photochemical, (2) thermal, and (3) ionizing. Clinical applications of these effects are summarized in Fig. 29-2.

1. For exposures longer than roughly 1 microsecond and low-to-moderate irradiances, laser radiation below 320 nm produces primarily photochemical reactions.[14] In these reactions, photon absorption by outer electrons is needed to provide the excited molecular electronic state from which the chemical reaction can occur.

2. For similar irradiances and exposure durations, laser radiation at longer wavelengths generally produces thermal effects. Thermal effects occur when photon absorption by outer electrons or molecular vibrations produces enough temperature rise to denature biomolecules by breaking the weak van der Waals forces that help to stabilize their complex structures.

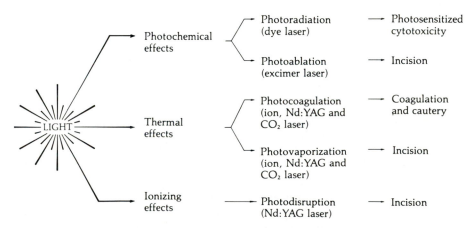

Fig. 29-2 Laser–tissue interactions may be divided into photochemical, thermal, or ionizing effects. (See section in text on laser effects.) (Modified from Worthen, DM: Laser therapies for the glaucomas. In Cairns, JE, editor: Symposium on glaucoma, Transactions of the New Orleans Academy of Ophthalmology, St. Louis, 1981, The CV Mosby Co)

3. At very high irradiances, generally produced by exposure durations shorter than 20 nanoseconds, enough energy is provided to tear electrons from atoms and molecules, thereby ionizing them and inducing secondary mechanical effects.[29]

Although it is useful conceptually to differentiate between photochemical, thermal, and ionizing processes, it is important to recognize that more than one of these processes may be responsible for clinical effects observed at intermediate values of irradiance and exposure time.

Photochemical Effects

Photoradiation

Hematoporphyrin derivative (HpD) is selectively taken up and retained by metabolically active tumor tissue, predisposing this tissue to photochemical damage if the tumor is subsequently irradiated with light between 625 and 635 nm. The exposure of photosensitized tumor tissue is termed *photoradiation therapy* (PRT). Current clinical ophthalmic PRT studies are directed toward the treatment of large choroidal melanomas, which are exposed to 630 nm red light from a rhodamine B dye laser 72 hours after intravenous HpD administration.[17] This irradiation produces an excited state of porphyrin, which interacts with oxygen to produce cytotoxic singlet oxygen. The gold vapor laser producing 628 nm red light is a potentially useful alternative light source for PRT.

Photoablation

Ultraviolet light at wavelengths shorter than 300 nm generally causes photochemical reactions in biologic tissues, because tissues are effectively opaque at these wavelengths. Excimer lasers producing ultraviolet light below 300 nm can provide precise corneal incisions to predetermined depths.[37] This process may be termed photoablation, as photochemical reactions at the target site not only fragment exposed molecules but also volatilize them.

Carbon dioxide lasers produce infrared radiation to which the cornea or any other water-containing tissue is also opaque, but CO_2 lasers incise the cornea by thermal effects, primarily vaporization but with associated coagulation and cautery.[17,21,27] Thus, whereas CO_2 lasers are useful in tractionless incision of vascular tissue, excimer lasers producing ablation but not cautery would have limited value in that application. On the other hand, an excimer laser has the potential to produce much more precise incisions of avascular tissue because photoablation apparently leaves adjacent tissue unaffected, and its short wavelength radiation can be focused into a much smaller spot size.

Thermal Effects

Photocoagulation

Denaturation of biomolecules occurs at an appreciable rate when ambient temperatures are sufficiently high to overcome weak van der Waals forces stabilizing their structure. Whereas some denaturation may occur even at normal body temperature, renewal processes maintain a physiologic equilibrium unless destabilization is favored by a temperature increase or change in the chemical milieu.[14,18,41] In general, (1) nucleic acids are more resistant to thermal injury than collagen, (2) thermal tissue damage requires a 10° to 20° C increase in the tissue temperature,[32,39] and (3) the extent of thermal injury is proportional to the magnitude and duration of the temperature increase. The greater the temperature rise in a target tissue, the less the exposure interval required to produce a burn of given severity.[2,6]

For a particular spot size and duration of exposure, the rise in tissue temperature induced by a laser beam is proportional to the irradiance, which is the ratio of light power delivered to the area exposed. That is,

$$T \propto E$$

where T is temperature rise of the exposed tissue, and

$$E = P/A$$

where E is irradiance, P is the light power delivered to the surface of the tissue, and A is the tissue area exposed.

Temperature rise in an irradiated tissue is also proportional to light absorption by that tissue,[23,26,28] which in turn is determined by how effectively its constituent molecules absorb incident photons of a particular wavelength. For example, the absorption of visible light by melanin in the trabecular meshwork or retinal pigment epithelium make these tissues excellent targets for argon laser photocoagulation. However, the poor absorption of visible light by corneal collagen makes the cornea an effective window for both vision and photocoagulation or photodisruption.[5]

Closure of blood vessels by photocoagulation is caused by light absorption in the blood column, which heats the hemoglobin to a temperature high enough to produce thrombus formation[7] and collagen shrinkage in the wall of a blood vessel and its surrounding connective tissue.[12] Since the blood

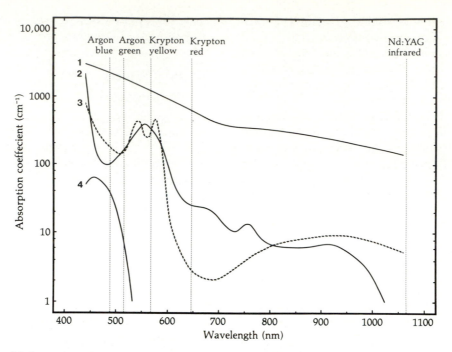

Fig. 29-3 Three primary light absorbers in ocular tissues are melanin *(curve 1),* hemoglobin (reduced, *curve 2;* oxygenated, *curve 3*), and macular xanthophyll *(curve 4).* Absorption coefficients are presented as a function of the wavelength. (Modified from Worthen, DM: Laser therapies for the glaucomas. In Cairns, JE, editor: Symposium on glaucoma, Transactions of the New Orleans Academy of Ophthalmology, St. Louis, 1981, The CV Mosby Co)

column is moving, vessel effects are often located downstream from the actual exposure site or the site of damage to underlying tissues.[40] Light absorption by hemoglobin varies with the wavelength and oxygen saturation, as well as other parameters, as shown in Fig. 29-3. For example, the depth of photon penetration in hemoglobin is 60 μm for argon green light (514.5 nm) but more than 400 μm for Nd:YAG infrared radiation (1064 nm). Thus argon green light is well absorbed in small intraocular blood vessels and is therefore a good instrument for closing them,[3] whereas Nd:YAG infrared radiation deposits only a small fraction of incident radiation in small vessels.[29] On the other hand, continuous-wave or long-pulse (0.2 to 0.5 second) Nd:YAG lasers are useful for treating very large blood vessels, such as in esophageal varices,[10] because infrared light provides uniform bulk heating.

Photovaporization

If very high laser irradiances are used, tissue temperature can quickly reach the boiling point of water, and rapidly expanding water vapor will cause tissue disruption (photovaporization) before

denaturation can cauterize the tissue. In most situations, however, photovaporization (cutting) is accompanied by photocoagulation (cautery). For example, in CO_2 laser surgery, cautery during incision can provide a virtually bloodless operating field.[4,31] Water vaporization tends to stabilize tissue temperature until all the water is boiled off, at which point the temperature increases rapidly and carbonization occurs. Pulsed operation of a CO_2 laser at high repetition rates permits higher peak tissue irradiances than continuous-wave operation and should therefore offer a higher ratio of incision to cautery, with a corresponding decrease in thermal damage to surrounding tissues. The gas bubble seen during laser trabeculoplasty is probably caused by either vaporization of aqueous humor adjacent to the photocoagulation site or "outgassing" (liberation of bound gases) at the site.

The CO_2 laser produces 10,600 nm (10.6 μm) λ infrared radiation, which is absorbed in water-bearing tissue at a rate comparable to the absorption of argon green light in the retinal pigment epithelium.[21] More than 99% of CO_2 laser radiation is absorbed in the first 50 μm of water-containing tissue that is encountered. Thus the cornea is opaque to CO_2 laser radiation, and intraocular applications require an intraocular probe. The limited range (photon penetration depth) of the CO_2 laser can be an advantage in intraocular applications, however, allowing vitreous syneresis and vaporization, or tractionless cautery and incision of fibrovascular bands without damage to adjacent tissues.[9,21,31]

Ionizing Effects

Short-pulse Nd:YAG lasers disrupt transparent tissues by delivering enormous near-infrared (1064 nm) irradiances to tissue targets.[1,11] These irradiances are obtained by using small spot sizes and extremely brief pulses ranging from 30 nanoseconds to 20 picoseconds (1 picosecond = 10^{-12} second). The high irradiance ionizes material in a small volume of space at the focal point of the laser beam, disintegrating it into a collection of ions and electrons called a *plasma*. Plasma may be considered a fourth state of matter that has the mechanical properties of a gas and the electric properties of a metal. Once formed, the plasma first absorbs or scatters radiation arriving later in the pulse, thereby shielding underlying tissues, and then the plasma expands rapidly, producing shock and acoustic (pressure) waves that mechanically disrupt tissues adjacent to the region of disintegration. Additional tissue disruption occurs because of latent stress present in the tissue when the laser incision occurs. Photodisruption is summarized in Fig. 29-4.

Hazards

The eye is vulnerable to photochemical, thermal, or ionizing damage from inadvertent exposure to intense light sources. Safety standards have been developed for ocular exposures to ultraviolet, visible, and infrared radiation.[34] It is clear that standard clinical photocoagulators and photodisruptors are potentially hazardous and that the characteristics of each clinical instrument and procedure must be fully understood to maximize the benefit-to-risk ratio of any laser operation. It is not as widely understood that reflected laser light could pose a hazard to operating room personnel. The surgeon's eyes are effectively protected against "flashback" by a fixed filter in the operating slit-lamp or by a filter with "fail-safe" switching into the field of view during exposures. However, unprotected personnel adjacent to the surgeon are vulnerable to potentially hazardous specular reflections from the surface of a contact lens used in the procedure, even if the lens has an antireflective

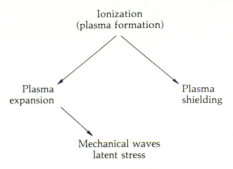

Fig. 29-4 Photodisruption of transparent ocular tissue involves three nonlinear mechanisms.[29] Very high irradiances disintegrate target tissues in focal volume by stripping electrons from atoms and molecules, thereby creating transient plasma of free electrons and ions. (See text.) (Modified from Worthen, DM: Laser therapies for the glaucomas. In Cairns, JE, editor: Symposium on glaucoma, Transactions of the New Orleans Academy of Ophthalmology, St. Louis, 1981, The CV Mosby Co)

coating. For example, in conventional laser photocoagulation, this hazard extends to a distance of 1.6 m from the coated contact lens,[15] and nearby personnel should wear eye protection appropriate for the laser wavelength being used.

For the past two decades, accumulating evidence suggests that photochemical damage from lifelong exposure to ordinary environmental radiation may play a role in the development of certain age-related ocular problems in susceptible individuals. For example, single oxygen formation from photochemical reactions—induced by the ultraviolet light between 300 and 400 nm that passes through the cornea but is absorbed in the crystalline lens—has been implicated in cataractogenesis in experimental animals and in human beings.[16] Similar photochemically generated cytotoxic agents in the retinal pigment epithelium are probably responsible for solar retinitis and welder's maculopathy and may play a significant role in the development of macular degeneration.[13,20,22] Cataract extraction places the aphakic or pseudophakic patient at greater risk to photochemical retinal damage, since potentially hazardous ultraviolet light between 300 and 400 nm previously absorbed by the crystalline lens can now reach the retina.[19,22] This emphasizes the need for properly designing intraocular lenses with an absorption spectrum similar to that of the normal crystalline lens,[22] and for cautioning aphakic or pseudophakic patients to avoid observing the midday sun or welding arcs and to wear appropriate spectacle filters in unusually bright environmental conditions, such as when boating or snow skiing.[20,24]

PHOTOCOAGULATORS

Light absorption in a target tissue determines the efficiency with which laser light energy is converted to heat energy for photocoagulation. The three primary absorbing molecules in ocular tissues are melanin, macular xanthophyll, and hemoglobin (see Fig. 29-3).

Melanin is the best absorber, but since its absorption does not vary substantially between 400 and 700 nm, its absorption spectrum is not a principal factor in selecting a surgical laser system producing visible light. Thus there should be little difference between argon blue-green, argon green, and even krypton red laser trabeculoplasty, in which melanin in the trabecular meshwork is presumably the primary absorber.[35,36] On the other hand, absorption by melanin decreases with increasing wavelength, and so is one of the reasons that a chorioretinal burn becomes deeper as the wavelength increases. In general, the deeper the burn, the more painful and less ophthalmoscopically prominent it is. Argon green is absorbed at the level of the pigment epithelium and choriocapillaris, krypton red produces a deeper lesion, and Nd:YAG causes primary choroidal and even scleral effects.

Macular xanthophyll absorbs well in blue, poorly in green, and minimally in yellow and red light. Thus, if blue light is used for macular photocoagulation, direct inner retinal damage will be produced in addition to the desired pigment epithelial and subretinal lesion.[30] This inner retinal damage not only is a source of needless nerve tissue loss, but also obscures posttreatment fluorescein angiographic detection of persistent or recurrent choroidal neovascularization and obstructs retreatment of neovascularization when present.[23]

Hemoglobin absorbs well in blue, green, and yellow, but poorly in red light. As shown in Fig. 29-3, red light has better absorption in reduced than in oxygenated hemoglobin, which is one reason why retinal veins are more prominent than retinal arteries in monochromatic red ophthalmoscopy. The disadvantages of Nd:YAG infrared radiation for treating small intraocular blood vessels have been discussed earlier. The poor absorption of Nd:YAG radiation by both melanin and reduced hemoglobin may be useful, however, in photocoagulating through heavily pigmented structures or long-standing hemorrhages, provided that very long pulse (0.2 to 0.5 second) or continuous-wave Nd:YAG sources are used so that the potentially hazardous high irradiances of shorter exposures are avoided. In this latter application, it is inter-

esting to note that Nd:YAG infrared radiation actually is better absorbed by oxygenated hemoglobin than krypton red light (see Fig. 29-3) and may therefore be more effective in treating pigmented, vascularized structures. It is important, however, to reemphasize that the safety margin between lesion and iatrogenic hemorrhage becomes progressively smaller as pulse length is shortened.[8] This is a major reason why pulsed ruby laser photocoagulators were superseded by continuous-wave argon laser systems, and why current commercial Nd:YAG photodisruptor systems offering 0.0002 to 0.02 second exposures in a non–Q-switched thermal mode are potentially hazardous for retinal applications.[29]

Clinical laser photocoagulators generally consist of the following:
1. An argon or krypton laser source
2. A fiberoptic or mirror arm apparatus to deliver the laser source output to the slit-lamp delivery system
3. A slit-lamp to view the target tissue and to direct the aiming and treatment beam to a desired location on the target tissue[25]

Fiberoptic delivery systems provide flexible slit-lamp movement and reasonably uniform distribution of power across the focal spot. Mirror arm systems are less flexible, but they preserve the transverse mode structure of the laser beam and thus can provide smaller spot sizes than fiberoptic systems.

Photocoagulator use is facilitated by contact lenses designed for specific clinical applications. These lenses generally have a broad-spectrum antireflective coating that reduces light reflection in the visible spectrum from approximately 4% to less than 1% for normal incidence. The purpose of this coating is to reduce both reflected slit-lamp (white) light and laser light.

1. Slit-lamp light scattered back from the surface of a contact lens reduces the contrast in the surgeon's microscopic image. Since target tissues or localizing structures are often small and have subtle features, it is useful to minimize this scattered white light by using antireflective coatings. As noted, regardless of the contact lens, reducing the slit height and width is usually more effective than increasing slit-lamp illumination for improving microscopic image quality when ocular media are hazy (to minimize veiling back-scattered light).
2. Although clinical photocoagulators have enough power for most applications, a

coated contact lens surface does reduce back-scattering of laser light, thereby reducing the potential hazard to an observer standing behind the contact lens. Reducing back-scattered light also increases contrast in the biomicroscopic image, facilitating target viewing with hazy ocular media.

Wavelengths of current commercial laser photocoagulator systems are shown in Fig. 29-5. Argon laser systems provide bichromatic blue-plus-green (488 nm blue plus 514.5 nm green) or green-only (514.5 nm) light, whereas commercial krypton lasers provide red-only (647 nm) light. Laser systems are now available in argon-only, krypton-only, or argon-plus-krypton configurations. Other potentially useful laser sources not yet available commercially include the following (see Table 29-1): high-power krypton (531 nm green, 568 nm yellow, or 647 nm red); copper vapor (510 nm green or 578 nm yellow); frequency-doubled Nd:YAG (high-frequency, pulsed operation producing 532 nm green); organic dye (tunable, including 631 nm for post-HpD irradiation); gold vapor (628 nm red); and continuous-wave or very-long-pulse Nd:YAG (1064 nm infrared).

Clinical argon and krypton photocoagulators have power, pulse duration, and spot-size settings. Spot-size selector systems are either of the defocus or parfocal type. The cone angle of the beam in a fiberoptic system is generally larger than that in a mirror arm system, and therefore a small axial (anterior or posterior) slit-lamp movement can cause a marked change in the spot-size diameter. For this reason most fiberoptic systems use a parfocal-type spot-size selector, at least for smaller spot sizes, in which the size is varied by changing magnification; the spot size selected is the smallest that can be achieved. Mirror arm systems often use defocus spot-size selectors, in which the spot size is increased merely by posteriorly displacing the focal plane of the treatment beam; since the cone angle is smaller with a mirror arm system, the spot size is less sensitive to small axial slit-lamp movements.

Tissue temperature increase is proportional to irradiance ("power density"). Thus, for a given power setting and exposure time, the spot size determines the temperature increase, and therefore the uniformity and reproducibility of clinical results require accurate spot-size selection. Regardless of the type of spot-size selector that a photocoagulator has, it is important to realize that the spot-size settings are not correct unless the target tissue is properly located at the working distance of the slit-lamp microscope. Since the operator may accommodate and the slit-lamp has a considerable depth of field, it is imperative that the surgeon

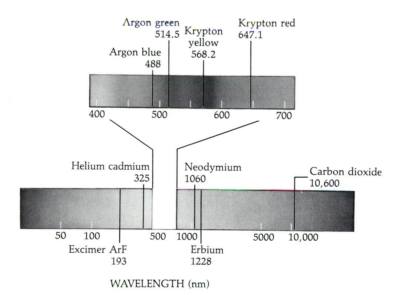

WAVELENGTH (nm)

Fig. 29-5 Current clinical photocoagulators use laser sources that produce visible light, but Nd:YAG lasers in photodisruptor systems generate invisible near-infrared radiation. CO_2 lasers produce much longer wavelength infrared radiation, whereas experimental excimer lasers generate ultraviolet radiation. (Modified from Worthen, DM: Laser therapies for the glaucomas. In Cairns, JE, editor: Symposium on glaucoma, Transactions of the New Orleans Academy of Ophthalmology, St. Louis, 1981, The CV Mosby Co)

determine the proper ocular settings for each instrument and that the instrument itself be properly aligned.

Perhaps the simplest way of ensuring that the ocular settings are correct is to use the aiming bar or reticle supplied by the manufacture, fog (add excess plus power in the ocular), and then slowly decrease ocular power until the aiming bar or reticle first appears sharp. With those ocular settings, the surgeon's unaccommodated retina is conjugate with the working distance of the slit-lamp. If the slit-lamp is then moved forward with the control stick directed back toward the surgeon, until the target tissue is sharply in focus, then the target tissue will be at the slit-lamp working distance, and spot-size settings will be valid. Furthermore, any forward movement of the control stick can only increase the spot size, thereby reducing irradiance and producing a larger spot size of lower peak temperature rise. Nonetheless, if improper ocular settings are used, difficulties may arise—regardless of the type of spot-size selector in the photocoagulator—if slit-lamp movement inadvertently reduces spot size and increases focal irradiance.

PHOTODISRUPTORS

Commercial laser photodisruptors generally consist of the following:

1. A high-power, Q-switched, Nd:YAG laser (with or without mode-locking) that produces invisible, 1064 nm infrared radiation
2. An articulated or directly coupled mirror system that delivers the infrared radiation to the slit-lamp (irradiance is too high for fiberoptic transmission)
3. A low-power, continuous-wave (CW), aiming/focusing, helium-neon (He-Ne) laser that produces 632.8 nm red light
4. A lens system for focusing the Nd:YAG beam into a small spot size at the working distance of the slit-lamp
5. A slit-lamp for aiming and focusing the visible helium-neon (He-Ne) aiming beam and hence the Nd:YAG treatment beam on selected tissue targets[29]

Q-switched, non-mode-locked lasers produce single pulses or bursts of one to nine pulses, each of which is 2 to 14 nanoseconds, depending on the individual photodisruptor. Q-switched, mode-locked lasers produce a train of seven to nine 30 picosecond spikes over roughly a 30 nanosecond pulse interval and can also be used in multiple-pulse, burst operation. Mode-locked photodisruptors are generally more complex instruments, re-

quiring a long resonant cavity and periodic replacement of the dye in the cell used for Q-switching and mode-locking, whereas non-mode-locked systems can be much smaller and use a simple, solid-state Pockels cell for switching.

The treatment beam in an ion laser photocoagulator is merely an intensification of the aiming beam, so there is no possibility of disalignment of the two beams. In a photodisruptor, however, aiming/focusing and treatment beams are produced by two separate sources. The treatment beam is invisible and the clinician must depend on the manufacturer to align the aiming/focusing beam accurately and reliably with the treatment beam. Most manufacturers minimize the number of mechanical linkages connecting the laser sources to the slit-lamp to reduce the possibility of disalignment of the laser beams. Disalignment would be manifested as "beam walk" of the treatment beam around the aiming/focusing beam—differences in their relative positions for different slit-lamp orientations—and the aiming beam would then no longer identify the exact location of the impact site of the treatment beam. Ideally, all components should be connected directly to the location of the treatment beam and directly mounted on the slit-lamp to eliminate disalignment. One simple method of checking alignment is to make test spots on photographic paper that has been exposed and developed. The manufacturer should be consulted promptly any time trouble is suspected.

The photodisruptor aiming/focusing beam must provide not only a visible spot for selecting tissue targets, as in a photocoagulator, but also an accurate and reliable method for placing the beam waist (focal spot) at the axial location of the tissue target. Current photodisruptors use either single-beam or multiple-beam aiming/focusing systems. With a single-beam system, the slit-lamp control stick is moved forward and backward to minimize the size of a red aiming spot on the target tissue. With a multiple-beam system (double or triple beam), the control stick is moved forward or backward until the multiple (two or three) spots fuse into one on the target tissue.

Multiple-beam aiming/focusing systems have an easier and more reproducible end point for axial focusing than single-beam systems. However, even with a single-beam system it is usually possible to open an opacified posterior capsule directly apposed to the posterior surface of a posterior chamber intraocular lens without marking the lens. This can be accomplished by locating the first exposure just posterior to the capsule and using low-energy settings just above breakdown threshold, usually less than 1 mJ. The first exposure not only initiates discission but displaces the capsule posteriorly and provides optically inhomogeneous borders at which the breakdown threshold is reduced. Regardless of the aiming/focusing system used, accurate focusing requires spending enough time before actual therapeutic exposures to determine an orientation of the slit-lamp beam that provides effective direct or retroillumination of the capsule but minimizes the bright specular reflex from the polymethylmethacrylate lens. As with photocoagulators, proper slit-lamp ocular settings should be used at all times.

High irradiances are achieved at the working distance of the slit-lamp, where the aiming/focusing beam is also focused, by using a converging lens to focus the treatment beam into a small spot. Since spot size is proportional to lens focal length, a short focal length lens that provides a large cone angle will produce a small focal spot and high irradiance. Thus, increasing the cone angle increases the focal irradiance and decreases the irradiance at structures anterior and posterior to the focal plane.[29] If the focal length is too short, however, there is little room for a contact lens between the photodisruptor and the patient's cornea, and part of the Nd:YAG beam may be lost at the border of the pupil when midvitreous structures are treated. On the other hand, a long focal length lens provides a small cone angle that facilitates contact lens use and vitreous applications but produces a larger spot size with a lower irradiance in the focal plane and higher irradiance at structures posterior to the focal plane. Clinical Nd:YAG photodisruptor systems represent a balance between the advantages of short and long focal length lenses, with most companies selecting cone angles ranging from 14 to 17 degrees to ensure high focal volume irradiances and low retinal irradiances.[29]

REFERENCES

1. Aron-Rosa, D, Aron, JJ, Griesemann, M, and Thuzel, R: Use of the neodymium-yag laser to open the posterior lens capsule after lens implant surgery: a preliminary report, Am Intraocul Implant Soc J 6:352, 1980
2. Arrhenius, S: Uber die Reaktionsgeschwindigkeit bei der Inversion von Rohrzucker durch Sauren, Z. Physik Chemie 4:226, 1889
3. Bebie, H, Fankhauser, F, Lotmar, W, and Roulier, A: Theoretical estimate of the temperature within irradiated retinal vessels, Acta Ophthalmol 52:13, 1974
4. Beckman, H, and Fuller, TA: Carbon dioxide laser scleral dissection and filtering procedure for glaucoma, Am J Ophthalmol 88:73, 1979
5. Benedek, GB: Theory of transparency of the eye, Appl Opt 10:459, 1971
6. Birngruber, R: Thermal modeling in biological tissues. In Hillenkamp, F, Pratesi, R, and Sacchi, CA, editors: Lasers in biology and medicine, New York, 1980, Plenum Publishing Corp
7. Boergen KP, Birngruber, R, and Hillenkamp, F: Laser-induced endovascular thrombosis as a possibility of selective vessel closure, Ophthalmic Res 13:139, 1981
8. Boettner, EA, and Wolter, JR: Transmission of the ocular media, Ophthalmology 1:776, 1962
9. Bridges, TJ, Patel, CKN, Strand, AR, and Wood, OR, III: Syneresis of vitreous by carbon dioxide laser radiation, Science 219:1217, 1983
10. Dwyer, RM: The technique of gastrointestinal laser endoscopy. In Goldman, L, editor: The biomedical laser: technology and clinical applications, New York, 1981, Springer-Verlag New York, Inc
11. Fankhauser, F, et al: Clinical studies on the efficiency of high power laser radiation upon some structures of the anterior segment of the eye, Int Ophthalmol 3:129, 1981
12. Gorisch, W, and Boergen KP: Heat-induced contraction of blood vessels, Lasers Surg Med 2:1, 1982
13. Ham, WT, Jr, Ruffolo, RJ, Jr, Mueller, HA, and Guerry, D, III: The nature of retinal radiation damage: dependence on wavelength power level and exposure time. Vision Res 20:1105, 1980
14. Hillenkamp, F: Interaction between laser radiation and biological systems. In Hillenkamp, F, Pratesi, R, and Sacchi, CA, editors: Lasers in biology and medicine, New York, 1980, Plenum Publishing Corp
15. Jenkins, DL: Hazard evaluation of the Coherent model 900 photocoagulator laser system, non-ionizing radiation protection special study no. 25-42-0310-79 (NTIS no. ADA 068713) Aberdeen Proving Ground, 1979, U.S. Army Environment Hygiene Agency
16. Lerman, S: Radiant energy and the eye, New York, 1980, Macmillan Publishing Co
17. L'Esperance, FA, Jr: Ophthalmic lasers: photocoagulation, photoradiation, and surgery, ed 2, St Louis, 1983, The CV Mosby Co
18. Mainster, MA: Destructive light adaption, Ann Ophthalmol 2:44, 1970
19. Mainster, MA: Spectral transmittance of intraocular lenses and retinal damage from intense light sources, Am J Ophthalmil 85:167, 1978
20. Mainster, MA: Solar retinitis, photic maculopathy and the pseudophakic eye, Am Intraocular Implant Soc J 4:84, 1978
21. Mainster, MA: Ophthalmic applications of infrared lasers—thermal considerations, Invest Ophthalmol Vis Sci 18:414, 1979
22. Mainster, MA: The spectra, classification, and rationale of ultraviolet protective intraocular lenses, Am J Ophthalmol 102:727, 1986

23. Mainster, MA: Wavelength selection in macular photocoagulation: tissue optics, thermal effects and laser systems, Ophthalmology 93:952, 1986

24. Mainster, MA, Ham, WT, Jr, and Delori, FC: Potential retinal hazards: instrument and environmental light sources, Ophthalmology 90:927, 1983

25. Mainster, MA, Ho, PC, and Mainster, KJ: Argon and krypton laser photocoagulators, Ophthalmology 905:48, 1983

26. Mainster, MA, White, TJ, and Allen, RG: Spectral dependence of retinal damage produced by intense light sources, J Opt Soc Am 60:848, 1970

27. Mainster, MA, White, TJ, and Tips, JH: Corneal thermal response to the CO_2 laser, Appl Opt 9:665, 1970

28. Mainster, MA, et al: Transient thermal behavior in biological systems, Bull Math Biophys 32:303, 1970

29. Mainster, MA, Sliney, DH, Belcher, CD, and Buzney, SM: Laser photodisruptors: damage mechanisms, instrument design and safety, Ophthalmology 90:973, 1983

30. Marshall, J, Hamilton, AM, and Bird, AC: Intraretinal absorption of argon laser irradiation in human monkey retinae, Experientia 30:1355, 1974

31. Miller, JB, Smith, MR, Pincus, F, and Stockert, M: Transvitreal carbon dioxide laser photocautery and vitrectomy, Ophthalmology 85:1195, 1978

32. Priebe, LA, Cain CP, and Welch, AJ: Temperature rise required for the production of minimal lesions in the Macaca mulatta retina, Am J Ophthalmol 79:405, 1975

33. Ready, JF: Industrial applications of lasers, New York, 1978, Academic Press, Inc

34. Sliney, DH, and Wolbarsht, ML: Safety with lasers and other optical sources, New York, 1980, Plenum Publishing Corp

35. Smith, J: Argon laser trabeculoplasty: comparison of biochromatic and monochromatic wavelengths, Ophthalmology 91:355, 1984

36. Spurny, RC, and Lederer, CM: Krypton laser trabeculoplasty: a clinical report, Arch Ophthalmol 102:1626, 1984

37. Trokel, SL, Srinivasan, R, and Braren, B: Excimer laser surgery of the cornea, Am J Ophthalmol 96:710, 1983

38. Weber, JJ: CRC handbook of laser science and technology, vol 1, lasers and masers, Boca Raton, Fla, 1972, CRC Press, Inc

39. White, TJ, et al: Chorioretinal temperature increases from solar observation, Bull Math Biophys 33:1, 1971

40. Wieder, M, Pomerantzeff, O, and Schneider, J: Retinal vessel photocoagulation: a quantitative comparison of argon and krypton laser effects, Invest Ophthalmol Vis Sci 20:418, 1981

41. Young, RW: The Bowman Lecture, 1982, Biological renewal: applications to the eye, Trans Ophthalmol Soc UK 102:42, 1982

Chapter 30

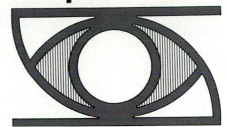

Laser Iridectomy and Iridoplasty

Robert Ritch
Jeffrey Liebmann
Ira S. Solomon

Laser Iridectomy

In the eighteenth century, Boerhave used the thermal effect of light focused through a magnifying glass to burn a hole through paper.[78] In 1916 Verhoef and Bell[122] focused sunlight on the iris and retina. In 1958 McDonald and Light[62] produced patent iridectomies using high-intensity radiant energy from a copper-coated carbon arc, but lenticular opacities were a problem.

In 1956 Meyer-Schwickerath[65] first reported the creation of a patent iridectomy using the xenon arc photocoagulator. In 1960 Hogan and Schwartz[40] and in 1965 Burns[16] also produced patent openings in the iris, but their success was limited by the corneal and lenticular damage caused by the large amounts of applied energy.

The development of laser technology led to the use of monochromatic focused light in anterior segment surgery. The creation of iridectomies with the pulsed ruby laser required less energy than previous methods, with both a shorter duration and lower amplitude of energy emission, and led to further success with this procedure.* In 1973 Beckman and Sugar[8] also attempted to use the neodymium laser, although unsuccessfully, in human irides.

The development of the continuous wave argon laser led to a virtual revolution in the treatment of glaucoma. In 1973 Khuri[49] created patent iridec-

tomies in rabbits. In 1973 Beckman and Sugar[8] reported success in human irides, but the openings were very small and closed with pigment. Others soon reported success in human eyes with angle-closure glaucoma.[2,3,75,110] Difficulties in performing laser iridectomies in dark brown and blue irides were overcome with developments in techniques by Ritch and Podos[82,84] and by Pollack.[74] The ease and convenience of the procedure for both the patient and surgeon and the paucity of severe complications provided the impetus for its rapid acceptance among ophthalmologists. In the early 1980s, argon laser iridectomy became the procedure of choice for performing an iridectomy in angle-closure glaucoma.

More recently, the Neodymium:YAG (Nd:YAG) laser, which causes mechanical disruption of tissue, has been used safely and successfully to create iridectomies in both darkly and lightly pigmented irides.*

INDICATIONS

Laser iridectomy is a safe, effective, and preferred alternative to conventional surgical iridectomy.† It is indicated in the vast majority of situations in which iridectomy is necessary and is the procedure of choice in all forms of angle-closure glaucoma in which pupillary block is presumed

---

*References 9, 24, 69, 70, 135, 136.

*References 51, 56, 67, 106, 120, 129.
†References 3, 4, 25, 30, 33, 52, 59, 66, 71-74, 77, 79, 84, 85, 88, 104, 105, 109, 131, 132, 133.

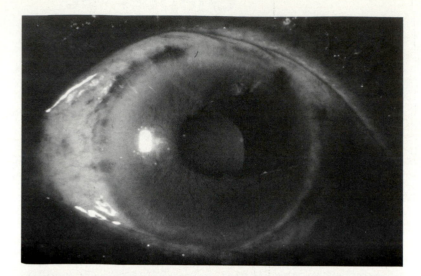

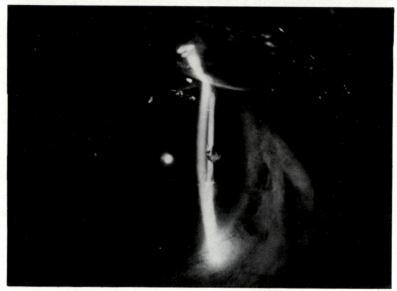

Fig. 30-1   Partial thickness surgical iridectomy.

causative. Full-thickness iris holes can be created in most eyes, relieving pupillary block. The complications associated with intraocular surgery and retrobulbar anesthesia are avoided. In addition, the conjunctiva is left untouched in the event that future filtration surgery is required. Reported success rates have ranged from 60% to 96%.* With present techniques, one should be able to achieve virtually 100% success at penetration of the iris at the initial sitting.[85] Both Nd:YAG and argon lasers appear equally effective.[67,91,106] The various situations that may be encountered follow.

Partial-thickness Surgical Iridectomy

Infrequently, only the iris stroma is removed at the time of surgical iridectomy, leaving the pigment epithelium intact (Fig. 30-1). A full-thickness

iridectomy can be easily made with the argon laser in the immediate postoperative period.[84,115,118]

Malignant (Ciliary Block) Glaucoma after Surgical Iridectomy

Prophylactic laser iridectomy may protect the fellow eye against both an acute attack of angle-closure and the development of malignant glaucoma.

Prophylactic Laser Iridectomy

A prophylactic iridectomy should be performed in the fellow eye of a patient with either primary acute or chronic angle-closure glaucoma. Eyes with spontaneous appositional closure in the presence of a normal intraocular pressure and eyes with narrow angles and positive provocative testing should also have prophylactic laser iridectomy.

---

*References 7, 13, 38, 67, 72, 74, 77, 129, 131.

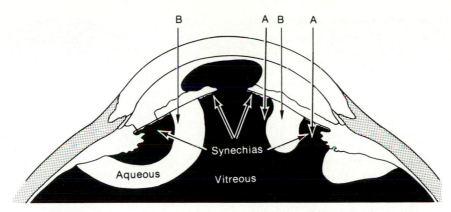

Fig. 30-2 Diagrammatic representation of intermixed pockets of aqueous and vitreous posterior to iris in aphakic pupillary block. (From Anderson, DR, Forster, RK, and Lewis, MK: Arch Ophthalmol 93:434, copyright 1975, American Medical Association)

Acute Angle-closure Glaucoma

Laser iridectomy should be performed after the acute attack has been terminated with medical therapy and the eye is no longer actively inflamed. Medically unresponsive attacks of angle-closure may be successfully treated initially with peripheral iridoplasty, although in some cases the media may be clear enough to perform an iridectomy.[81,82,85,110]

Chronic Angle-closure Glaucoma

Iridectomy can often prevent progressive synechial closure in patients with chronic angle-closure glaucoma. Eyes with appositional angle-closure with or without peripheral anterior synechiae are at risk for progressive trabecular damage as well as an attack of acute angle-closure glaucoma.

Even if the angle appears completely sealed by peripheral anterior synechiae preoperatively, areas of functional meshwork may open after laser iridectomy. Failure of intraocular pressure control by medications before laser iridectomy, particularly if the angle is closed, does not necessarily imply that the intraocular pressure will be uncontrolled by medications after iridectomy. After elimination of pupillary block by the iridectomy, evaluation of the chronic angle-closure is simplified.[28,73,80,86]

Laser iridectomy alone may control the intraocular pressure, or an elevated pressure may persist as a result of prior trabecular damage, warranting continued medical treatment or filtration surgery. It is not possible to predict which eyes will respond favorably; in one series, laser iridectomy reduced the intraocular pressure in 44% of eyes in patients with chronic angle-closure glaucoma.[77]

Combined Mechanism Glaucoma

We use this term to denote continued elevation of intraocular pressure after iridectomy in the ab-

sence of continued appositional closure (i.e., an open-angle component continues after the angle-closure component has been eliminated).

Aphakic or Pseudophakic Pupillary Block

Aphakic and pseudophakic pupillary block may be relieved by laser iridectomy.* In some cases, pockets of aqueous humor and vitreous may both be present posterior to the iris, or broad areas of vitreous may be adherent to the posterior iris (Fig. 30-2). An iridectomy made over an area of vitreous-iris adhesion or apposition will not relieve the pupillary block.[5] Multiple iridectomies may be required before a pocket of aqueous humor is located and the block relieved.[5,84,112] Creating the iridectomy also helps differentiate pupillary block from glaucoma caused by ciliary block (malignant glaucoma, aqueous misdirection), which requires disruption of the anterior hyaloid face or vitrectomy.[23,112] These topics are covered more fully in other chapters.

Before Laser Trabeculoplasty

If a narrow angle makes visualization or treatment of the angle structures difficult, laser iridectomy may be performed if the angle is narrow on the basis of relative pupillary block, often suggested by a peripheral bombé configuration. If the angle is narrow because of a plateau iris configuration or prominent peripheral iris roll, peripheral iridoplasty will be successful at improving visualization of the angle structures.

Nanophthalmos

Eyes with nanophthalmos are at considerable risk for developing angle-closure glaucoma be-

---

*References 5, 18, 26, 68, 98, 125.

cause of anterior chamber crowding. Prophylactic iridectomy may be useful but is not without risk. Peripheral iridoplasty can be useful (see below). Bilateral nonrhegmatogenous retinal detachments have been described following laser iridectomy in these patients[45] and may be attributable to worsening of preexisting retinal or choroidal disease.[113]

CONTRAINDICATIONS

Contraindications to laser iridectomy include moderate corneal edema, corneal opacification, a flat anterior chamber, a completely sealed angle, and angle-closure caused by primary synechial closure of the angle, such as occurs in uveitis, neovascular glaucoma, or the iridocorneal-endothelial (ICE) syndrome. In these cases, pupillary block is not a contributing mechanism.

LASER CONTACT LENSES

Antireflective-coated lenses so facilitate the procedure that their use is almost mandatory.[1,57,73,82] Firm control of the lens reduces saccades and extraneous eye movements that interfere with accurate superimposition of burns. The lens assists in keeping the lids separated, focuses the laser beam, and minimizes loss of laser power caused by reflection. The gonioscopy solution absorbs excess heat delivered to the cornea, decreasing the incidence of corneal burns.

The Abraham lens (Fig. 30-3) consists of a fundus lens with a +66 diopter planoconvex lens button placed on its anterior surface. The button provides magnification without loss of depth of focus. The effective size of a 50 μm spot is reduced to approximately 30 μm, providing higher energy per unit area and permitting the procedure to be performed with a lower total energy. Posterior to the site of focus, the beam is more rapidly defocused, decreasing the potential injury to the posterior segment.[11,100] The Wise lens is similar but has a +103 diopter button, allowing even greater concentration of the laser energy.[128]

PREOPERATIVE TREATMENT

Topical anesthesia virtually always suffices, obviating the trauma and anxiety associated with injections. If the pupil is not already maximally miotic, one or two drops of 4% pilocarpine are given topically. The more dilated the pupil, the thicker the iris stroma at any point, necessitating more burns to achieve penetration or even precluding it.

Preoperative treatment with para-aminoclonidine, aqueous suppressants, or hyperosmotic agents in patients with elevated intraocular pressures or compromised trabecular meshworks is advisable. These patients also require careful monitoring of intraocular pressure postoperatively.

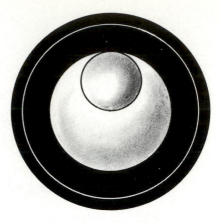

Fig. 30-3 Fundus lens with a high-plus button lens placed eccentrically on a plano surface. Abraham lens has a +66 diopter button, and Wise lens a +103 diopter button.

PERFORMING THE IRIDECTOMY

Irides vary in thickness, color, and number and size of iris crypts and freckles. These characteristics need to be taken into account in order to minimize potential technical difficulties and complications.

Iris color varies from light blue to dark brown. Generally, medium brown irides are the easiest to penetrate with the argon laser. The laser energy is readily absorbed by the iris pigmentation. Light blue and dark brown irides are the most difficult to penetrate.[79,86]

A site about two thirds to three fourths of the distance from the pupil to the iris root should be selected. The iridectomy is best placed between the 10:30 and 1:30 positions. Performing the iridectomy in the base of an iris crypt, where the stroma is thinner, often facilitates penetration. An arcus senilis should be avoided because the density of the arcus causes a drop in laser power across the cornea, and the arcus itself interferes with clear focusing of the beam. Placement under the upper lid is advantageous from an optical point of view to minimize glare and diplopia. Aiming the laser beam away from the fovea is extremely important in limiting the extent of retinal damage. The beam should be perpendicular to the contact lens surface to maximize energy delivery.

TYPES OF BURNS (Table 30-1)
Contraction Burn

This burn contracts the surrounding iris tissue toward, and compacts the stroma at the site of the

Table 30-1 Basic settings for argon laser treatment of angle-closure glaucoma

	Spot size (μm)	Duration (seconds)	Power (mW)
Contraction	500	0.5	200-400
Punch	50	0.01-0.05	800-1500
Penetration	50	0.1-0.2	600-1200
Cleanup	50	0.1-0.2	300

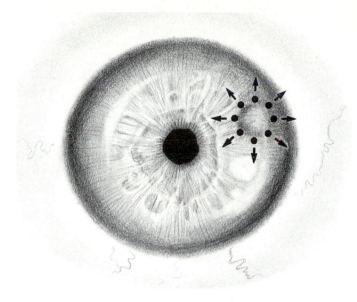

Fig. 30-4 Preliminary stretch burn placement for drumhead technique.

burn. Contraction burns are of low power, large spot size, and long duration and are used to (1) increase the density of iris stroma to facilitate laser energy absorption in blue or light brown irides, (2) create a "hump" on which penetrating burns are placed, and (3) perform peripheral iridoplasty or pupilloplasty.

Settings are 500 μm spot size, 0.5 second duration, and 200 to 400 mW. If bubbles occur or pigment is released into the anterior chamber, the power should be reduced. One should begin with 200 mW in brown irides and 300 mW in light ones, adjusting the power as necessary.

Stretch Burn

This term is now reserved for burns of the order of 200 μm spot size, 0.2 second duration, and 200 mW power, such as those used in the drumhead technique (see following discussion). They function similarly to contraction burns but with much less force and less effectiveness at condensing the iris stroma.

Penetrating Burn

This is a higher-power, small spot size burn designed to destroy iris tissue and create an opening. The settings consist of a 50 μm spot size, 0.1 or 0.2 second duration, and 600 to 1200 mW power. These burns are generally satisfactory for penetrating light and medium brown irides but often cause charring in dark irides.

Punch Burn

This short duration burn is optimal for use in dark irides to avoid charring at the base of the iridectomy site.[83] Although particularly valuable in the thick, dark irides of blacks and Asians,[60,66,131] punch burns produce less thermal effect than penetrating burns and are useful in all types of irides. Posterior synechiae may occur less frequently after the use of punch burns as opposed to penetrating burns.[66]

Cleanup Burn

This is a lower power variation of the penetrating burn and is used after reaching the pigment epithelium.

BASIC TECHNIQUES

A complete discussion of the various techniques for laser iridectomy is beyond the scope of this chapter and is covered fully in reference 85.

Drumhead Technique

In this approach, six to eight stretch burns are placed in a circle around the site selected for penetration to further thin the iris stroma at the selected site and make it more taut (Fig. 30-4). Penetrating burns are then applied in the center of the taut area using a "chipping" technique.

A modified drumhead technique consists of placing a single contraction burn on either side of the selected penetration site (Fig. 30-5). The area between them is tautened and an iridectomy created with penetrating or punch burns using a "chipping" technique (Fig. 30-6). If difficulty in penetration is encountered, the surgeon can easily convert to using punch burns through one of the contraction burns.

Iris Hump Technique

This involves placing a single contraction burn in the stroma to cause a hump to appear on either

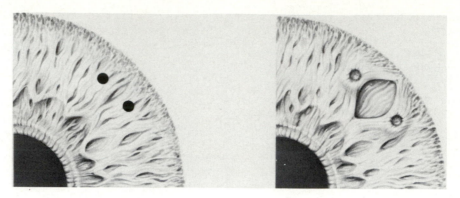

Fig. 30-5 Preliminary contraction burns in region of an oval crypt.

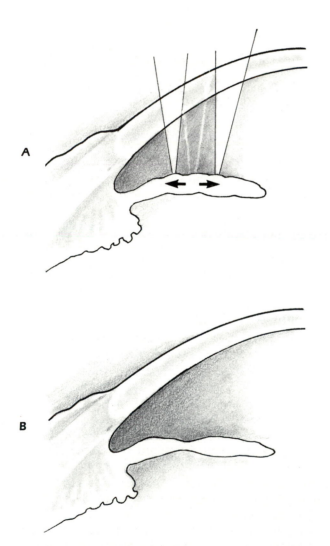

Fig. 30-6 Sagittal section showing effect of contraction burns, **A,** and resultant thinning and tautening of intervening iris stroma, **B.**

side of the burn.[1] A burn of 50 μm spot size, 800 to 1000 mW power, and 0.5 second duration is then placed on the surface of the hump to penetrate it. This burn can be painful to the patient and audible to the surgeon. Abraham recommended the use of retrobulbar anesthesia for this technique, which has not become widely popular.

A similar technique for blue irides was described by Hoskins and Migliazzo, using settings of 0.5 second duration, 1500 mW power, and 50 μm spot size.[42]

Contraction Burn Bed for Penetrating Burns

We have found this technique extremely helpful in lightly pigmented irides without crypts. Two to four contraction burns are placed in a line circumferentially and partially superimposed (Fig. 30-7). Punch burns or penetrating burns are then placed using the contraction burns as a bed for the site of laser iridectomy.[116] In very light irides, this method combined with linear incision usually results in larger iridectomies than attainable with other argon laser techniques.

Linear Incision

This useful technique involves placing a short line of burns circumferentially instead of penetrating at a single spot (Fig. 30-8).[126,127] When the stroma is fully incised in this manner, the iris dilator muscle assists in the separation of the iris pigment epithelium, reducing the necessity of destroying the pigment epithelium with laser energy and creating a larger opening. This is particularly useful in light irides, in which openings made by other techniques are often smaller than those in brown irides and more difficult to enlarge.

Penetration

Our basic approach is to perform linear incision using punch burns for dark brown irides, a mod-

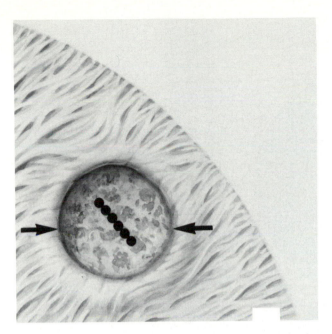

Fig. 30-7 Technique for light irides. Contraction burn *(arrows)* condenses and thins stroma and increases density of pigmentation at site of burn. Second contraction burn may be superimposed on first to enhance this effect. Punch burns are then placed within area of contraction to penetrate stroma.

ified drumhead for medium brown irides, and penetration through contraction burns in combination with linear incision for light irides. Improvisation in technique and choice of laser settings for burns is the key to success. The entire procedure may require anywhere from 1 to 300 burns.

For any iridectomy, the first burn often serves as an indicator for the ease of the procedure. The desired result is the appearance of a small hole with a dark brown base at the site of the burn and dispersion of debris into the anterior chamber. Bubble formation at the site of the burn indicates stromal vaporization. One then simply continues to deliver burns until the stroma has been penetrated (Fig. 30-9).

In the absence of stromal pigmentation, bubble formation and pigment release may be minimal. One clue to the gradual deepening of the iridectomy is a gradual darkening of the base. An orange reflex at the time of beam impact, most commonly seen in irides with little stromal pigmentation, signifies that one is nearing the pigment epithelium.

When the iris pigment epithelium is reached, denser bursts of fine pigment (smoke signals) appear in the anterior chamber. A "mushroom cloud" of pigment mixed with aqueous often slowly balloons into the anterior chamber. Simultaneously, the iris stroma floats backward and the peripheral anterior chamber deepens.

After penetration, the iridectomy may be enlarged and pigment epithelium removed with cleanup burns. Occasionally, an impenetrable cord of stroma is present at the site of the iridectomy. One can create an opening on either side of this cord if it cannot be severed at its base.

At the completion of the iridectomy, the lens capsule should be visible through the opening (Figs. 30-10 to 30-12). If the opening is small and the capsule is not visible, one can often get a sense of depth behind the opening or note a green reflex off the lens capsule when the beam is applied to the opening. Gonioscopy should be performed to assure that the angle is open.

Transillumination is not a reliable indication of success in light irides. If too high a power is used in light irides, it is possible to destroy pigment epithelium without penetrating the stroma. Once this happens, the overlying stroma cannot be penetrated and the surgeon may be fooled into thinking the procedure has been successful. Heijl et al.[34] used transcorneal fluorescein to fill the anterior chamber. Aqueous humor could be seen streaming through the iridectomy site from the posterior to the anterior chamber. The practicality of this technique is limited on a routine basis.

The central anterior chamber depth is unaffected by iridectomy, although deepening of the peripheral chamber may give the subjective impression of central deepening.[43] Any apparent deepening of the anterior chamber may be the result of the postlaser use of cycloplegia and discontinuation of miotics and their respective effects on lens position.

The elevated intraocular pressures associated with laser iridectomy (see following discussion) typically occur in the first 1 to 2 hours postoperatively.[54] It is necessary, therefore, to monitor intraocular pressures during this time. The use of postoperative topical steroids for several days is generally recommended to control inflammation.

Neodymium:YAG Laser Iridectomy

The Nd:YAG laser creates a plasma of free ions and electrons at the site of optical breakdown. This photodisruption releases shock waves that mechanically cause tissue rupture (see Chapter 29). Iris color, which is extremely important in argon laser iridectomy technique, no longer interferes with the creation of the iridectomy.

Suggested settings for Nd:YAG iridectomy have varied from one to four pulses per burst and from 1 to 10 millijoules per burst.* One should

*References 51, 67, 76, 89, 90, 93.

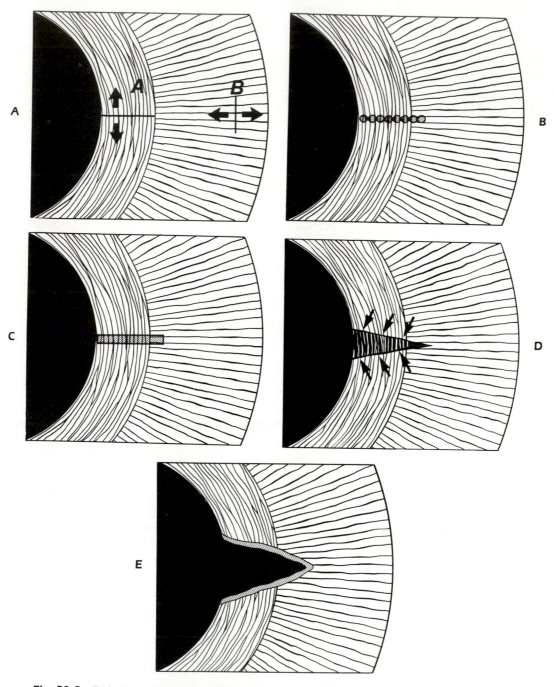

Fig. 30-8 Technique of linear evaporation. **A,** Site for sphincterotomy *(A),* and site for iridectomy *(B).* **B,** Punch burns are placed in a line to mark area through which penetration is desired. **C,** Burns are placed along line, gradually penetrating stroma. **D,** Bridging strands of stroma are incised at base *(arrow).* **E,** Intrinsic tension of muscle pulls wound edges apart, enlarging it. (Courtesy James B. Wise, MD)

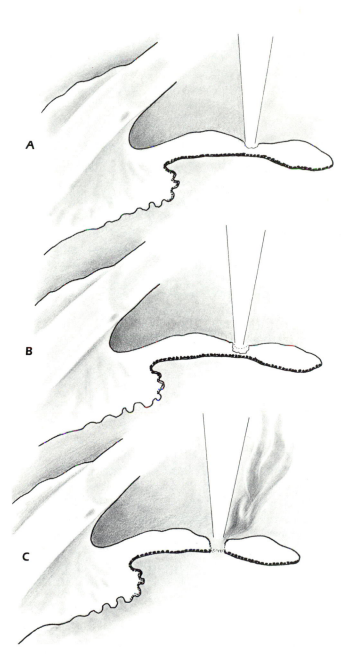

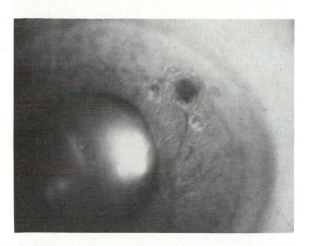

Fig. 30-10 Typical appearance of a moderately sized iridectomy.

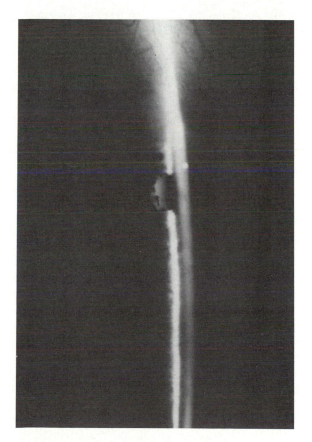

Fig. 30-9 Punch burns or penetrating burns create vaporization and destruction of small portions of iris stroma, **A** and **B,** until pigment epithelium is reached and penetrated, **C.** Pigment ballooning into anterior chamber is enhanced by flow of aqueous humor from posterior chamber through iridectomy.

Fig. 30-11 Slit-lamp view through iridectomy showing slit-beam crossing iris and falling on lens surface.

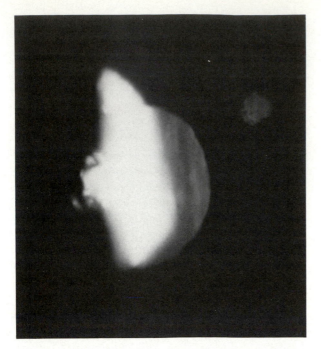

Fig. 30-12 Transillumination with slit-beam through pupil producing a bright reflection through patent iridectomy site.

begin with a single pulse at approximately 1.5 to 3 millijoules. A linear incision technique may also be used with the Nd:YAG laser. The importance of precise focus on the anterior iris stroma cannot be overemphasized; maximal photodisruption is obtained and the possibility of lens injury minimized. The incidence of lens injury is also decreased by choosing a peripheral location.

DIFFICULT SITUATIONS

Landsliding

After initial penetration of the stroma and pigment epithelium, the mechanical effect of the beam hitting the iris may cause additional pigment epithelium to slide into the opening from above. An attempt to remove this results in extensive pigment liberation into the anterior chamber and is frequently followed by refilling of the opening with more pigment. When this occurs, it is best to stop and enlarge the iridectomy at a later date.

Charring

Blackening and coagulation of the stroma at the base of the iridectomy site may occur as a result of thermal effects of argon laser energy on the surface layers of darkly pigmented irides and makes further penetration difficult or impossible. Charring

is minimal or absent when punch burns are used. If extensive charring has taken place, a new site for the iridectomy may need to be chosen.

Marked Corneal Edema

Significant corneal epithelial and stromal edema may preclude the surgeon's ability to achieve a patent iridectomy. Scattering of the laser beam by corneal edema diffuses the laser power, and precise focusing on the iris may be impossible. Higher powers of laser energy are usually necessary, and this may cause corneal endothelial damage.

Extremely Shallow Anterior Chamber

Corneal endothelial burns are generated by heating of the aqueous humor. If the anterior chamber is extremely shallow, corneal endothelial burns may develop rapidly. This situation may be circumvented by using contraction burns to deepen the chamber before the placement of punch burns or penetrating burns. When the anterior chamber is extremely shallow, the power should be reduced and applications not performed too rapidly.

COMPLICATIONS

Blurred Vision

Blurred vision is transitory and occurs in the immediate postlaser period. Possible causes include retinal pigment bleaching, pigment dispersion, anterior segment inflammation, or methylcellulose from the gonioscopy solution.

Pupillary Abnormalities

The pupil may be peaked toward the iridectomy site. The extent of the peaking is greater the closer the iridectomy is to the pupil, the softer the iris, and the greater the energy used in performing the iridectomy. Pupillary distortion is more prominent with the argon laser than with the Nd:YAG laser.[67] It is generally minor, transient, hardly noticeable cosmetically, and not associated with visual difficulties.

Diplopia and Glare

Diplopia and glare are uncommon given the small size of most laser iridectomies, but may develop or worsen if the iridectomy enlarges over time. Diplopia is particularly prone to occur if the iridectomy is placed nasally or temporally. Placement superiorly so that it is covered by the upper lid reduces the frequency of these complaints.[55]

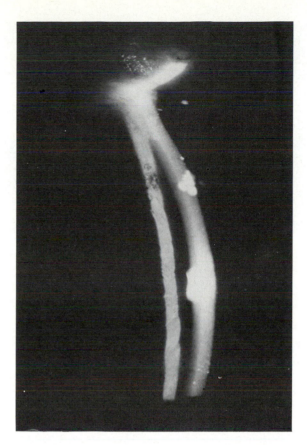

Fig. 30-13 Corneal epithelial burn caused by high laser power density, showing coagulation of epithelium and portions of superficial corneal stroma.

Corneal Damage

Corneal complications include epithelial and endothelial thermal burns, and corneal edema, abrasions, and opacities. Epithelial coagulation and whitening are transient, but may interfere with the delivery of laser energy and make the creation of a patent iridectomy difficult (Fig. 30-13). If epithelial coagulation occurs, an attempt can be made to angle the beam around the burn to complete the iridectomy.[20] If this is not possible, it may become necessary to choose another location for the iridectomy or postpone completion of the iridectomy until the epithelium has healed. Stromal edema and striate keratopathy may also occur.

Endothelial burns are generally dense white with sharp margins and result from the thermal effects of iris photocoagulation (Fig. 30-14). They require more time for resolution and may result in focal endothelial cell loss. However, endothelial cell loss following laser iridectomy has not been found to be statistically significant during follow-up periods of up to 1 year.[37,114,119,130] An increase in mean endothelial cell size and endothelial cell loss associated with the use of greater laser power has been reported.[41]

Although endothelial cell analysis after Nd: YAG iridectomy has also been reported to be unchanged,[101] focal endothelial cell loss has been documented when photodisruption takes place less

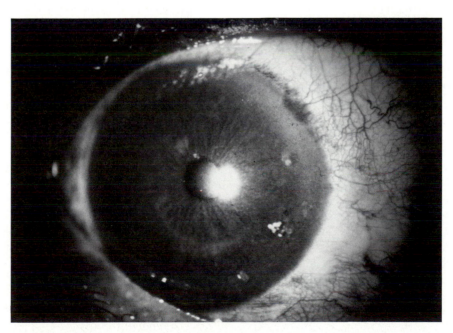

Fig. 30-14 Typical corneal endothelial burn with sharply delineated borders.

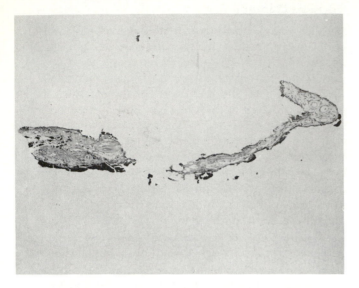

Fig. 30-15 Human iris 6 days after argon laser iridectomy showing pigment filled macrophages in stroma. (×60.) (From Pollack, IP, and Patz, A: Ophthalmic Surg 7:22, 1976)

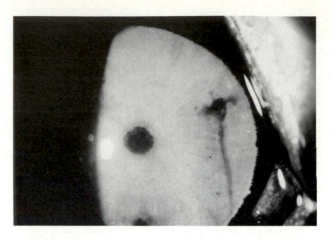

Fig. 30-16 Patent Nd:YAG iridectomy with stream of blood exiting site. (From Pollack, IP, et al: Trans Am Ophthalmol Soc 82:307, 1984)

than 1 mm from the corneal endothelium.[64] Damage to Descemet's membrane occurs when this distance is reduced to 0.1 mm. Damage has also been noted with photodisruption at greater distances from the cornea in rabbit eyes.[48] Kerr Muir and Sherrard found endothelial damage in rabbits to be proportional to the power delivered, mode of delivery, number of bursts, and distance between the cornea and the target tissue.[47]

Anterior Uveitis

Inflammation of the anterior segment is typical in the period following laser surgery and may be mediated to some degree, at least in rabbits, by prostaglandins.[121] The inflammation is usually mild and ceases within several days. Occasionally, it lasts longer than 1 month. Topical corticosteroids are routinely prescribed.

Breakdown in the blood-aqueous barrier has been demonstrated with both the argon and Nd:YAG lasers.[99,103] However, iris angiography in humans 6 months to 3 years after argon laser iridectomy has failed to demonstrate any long-term breakdown.[73]

Initial changes in the iris near the site of the iridectomy include edema, necrosis, loss of melanocytes, the presence of pigment-laden macrophages, and irregular clumps of granules on the pigment epithelial surface[73,75,95] (Fig. 30-15). Histopathologic examination of Nd:YAG laser iridectomies reveals circumscribed holes with limited tissue alteration at the margin, compared with more extensive early edema and tissue destruction after argon laser iridectomy.[94]

Pigment debris accumulates in the trabecular meshwork and decreases with time.[92] The pigment granules initially are located in the extracellular and intracellular spaces and are phagocytosed by the trabecular meshwork cells. The pigment becomes more concentrated in the juxtacanalicular meshwork and is progressively absorbed.

Posterior Synechiae

Posterior synechiae may occur between the pupil and the lens or the iridectomy and the lens. Their formation may be less common after Nd:YAG laser iridectomy.[67] They can be minimized by the use of postoperative topical steroids or broken by postoperative dilation.

Hemorrhage

Bleeding from the iridectomy is rare with the argon laser, because the iris tissue undergoes thermal coagulation. However, hyphema may occur[39] and may occur days after the iridectomy accompanied by a secondary increase in intraocular pressure.[96]

Nd:YAG photodisruption does not coagulate the iris vessels at the site of the iridectomy, and a small hemorrhage at the iridectomy site may occur in as many as 50% of patients[22,61,76] (Fig. 30-16). Bleeding can on occasion be more substantial[29] and may occasionally form small hyphemas, which tend to resolve rapidly. Gentle pressure on the eye with the contact lens may help control the bleeding. The argon laser may be used to coagulate bleeding vessels or may be used before the Nd:YAG laser to coagulate the iris vessels in the location of the anticipated Nd:YAG iridectomy. Iridectomy in eyes with rubeosis should be performed preferentially with the argon laser.

Elevations of Intraocular Pressure

Transient postlaser elevations of intraocular pressure lasting less than 24 hours are common. These are usually mild and easily controlled. However, rapid elevation of the intraocular pressure to high levels may occur immediately after both argon and Nd:YAG iridectomies.* The rise may be sufficiently high and sustained to require filtration surgery.[35]

Although the maximal elevation of intraocular pressure has been reported to occur in the first hour in approximately 70% of patients,[67] others have found that as many as 40% of patients have a maximal pressure elevation during the second hour.[76] A pressure rise greater than 6 mm Hg occurs in up to 40% of patients and to over 30 mm Hg in as many as 30%.[54,76,89,106] No significant difference in postoperative pressure rises has been found between the two types of lasers.[89] The elevation may be related to the amount of energy used, the degree of pigment dispersion, and the preoperative outflow facility. Eyes in which iridectomies are performed prophylactically may have a lower incidence of postoperative pressure elevations.[133]

The pressure elevation may be treated with miotics, topical beta-blocking agents, carbonic anhydrase inhibitors, or oral hyperglycemic agents. Topical indomethacin has not proved efficacious in controlling the postoperative intraocular pressure rise.[132] Topical para-aminoclonidine decreases the duration and magnitude of the rise.[14,91] Treatment with pilocarpine[15,102] or timolol[58] of eyes undergoing Nd:YAG iridectomy has also been reported to reduce the severity of the rise significantly. Inflammatory changes in the trabecular meshwork have been noted histologically after persistent pressure elevation following laser iridectomy.[32] Patients with moderate or severe trabecular compromise are particularly prone to extreme pressure fluctuations and should be monitored closely in the postlaser period. Pretreatment with para-aminoclonidine, aqueous supressants, or hyperosmotic agents should be considered in these patients. Prolonged elevations of intraocular pressure unresponsive to medical therapy are, fortunately, rare.

Tonography performed before and after laser

iridectomy suggests little or no increase in outflow facility.[73,132] Any increase in outflow facility is probably related to relief of pupillary block and reversal of appositional angle-closure.[73]

Lens Opacities

The most common complication of conventional surgical iridectomy is long-term cataract formation or progression, which occurs in over 50% of eyes having had acute angle-closure glaucoma and approximately 30% of fellow eyes undergoing prophylactic surgery.[53] Focal, anterior subcapsular opacities occur after both argon and Nd:YAG iridectomy (Figs. 30-17 to 30-19). Their incidence may be as high as 45%[89,106] and seems to increase with greater amounts of applied energy. Long-term follow-up has shown them to be nonprogressive, and the incidence of visual decrease from cataracts in patients having had laser iridectomy is similar to that in the general population.[88] Histopathologic studies of these opacities are scanty. Electron microscopy of argon laser–induced focal lens changes after panretinal photocoagulation reveals spindle-shaped lesions perpendicular to the lens capsule.[108]

The earlier widespread fear of acute onset of cataract after Nd:YAG iridectomy caused by inadvertent rupture of the lens capsule has not been substantiated. Comparison of argon and Nd:YAG iridectomies in rabbit eyes did not reveal any difference in the rate of cataract formation.[36] Seedor et al[107] reported no lens damage from 71 iridectomies produced in rabbits. Small ruptures of the anterior lens capsule after Nd:YAG iridectomy have been documented histopathologically in patients undergoing intracapsular cataract extraction.[124]

In monkeys the incidence of lens opacities was reduced when Nd:YAG treatment was limited to one or two bursts, each less than 6 millijoules.[27] Limiting the use of the Nd:YAG laser to single burst mode, performing the iridectomy peripherally, and focusing on the anterior iris stroma minimize the chance of lens damage. Animal studies suggest that fibrous proliferation covers the small anterior capsular breaks.[27] Pitting of the anterior lens capsule by the Nd:YAG laser also occurs.[124] These localized lens changes do not affect visual acuity.

Closure of the Iridectomy Site

Closure of a previously patent laser iridectomy may be either delayed or immediate. Immediate closure is caused by occlusion of the opening by circulating debris or landsliding of the pigment epithelium surrounding the iridectomy site.[12]

---

*References 35, 54, 67, 87, 102, 117, 131.

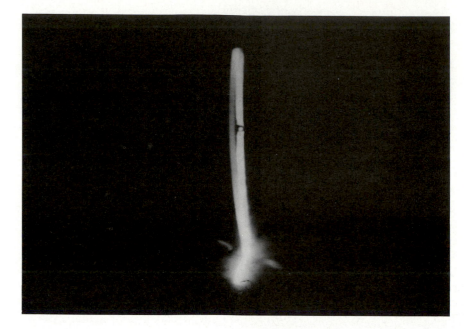

Fig. 30-17 Superficial anterior lens opacity at site of the iridectomy opening.

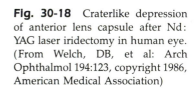

Fig. 30-18 Craterlike depression of anterior lens capsule after Nd: YAG laser iridectomy in human eye. (From Welch, DB, et al: Arch Ophthalmol 194:123, copyright 1986, American Medical Association)

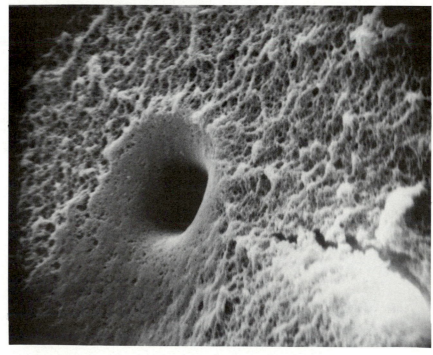

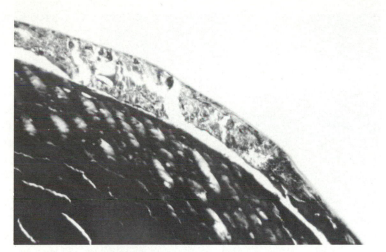

Fig. 30-19 Histologic section through human lens with localized opacity. Lesion is entirely subcapsular and consists of fragmented lens fibers and partial atrophy of lens epithelium. (From Pollack, IP: Ophthalmic Surg 11:506, 1980)

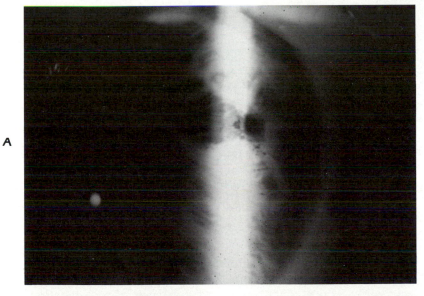

A

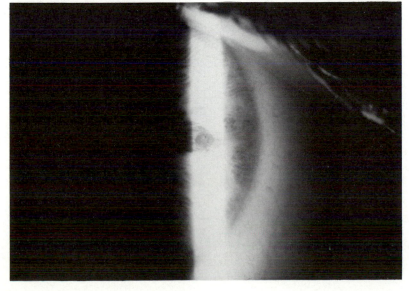

B

Fig. 30-20 Proliferation of pigment at site of laser iridectomy, **A,** easily reopened with cleanup burns, **B.** (From Ritch, R, and Podos, SM: Perspect Ophthalmol 4:129, 1980)

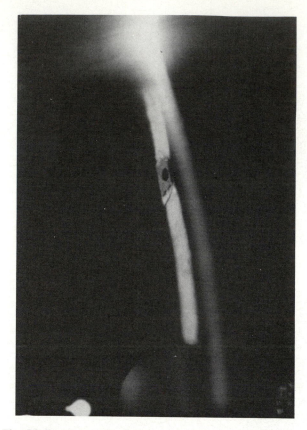

Fig. 30-21 Ingrowth of pigment epithelium from borders of iridectomy and slow closure of opening several months after initial procedure.

Delayed closure is usually caused by localized pigment proliferation occluding the opening (Fig. 30-20). Pigment proliferation is more prominent after argon laser iridectomy and usually occurs within the first 6 to 12 weeks. As many as one third of patients may require retreatment. The iris opening after Nd:YAG laser iridectomy is more irregular, with less pigment dispersion, but late pigment proliferation and closure may occur in as many as 16% of patients.[106] Closure is extremely common in patients with uveitis after either type of laser.

Other causes of late failure include the development of a transparent, thin fibrous membrane occluding the opening and regeneration of iris pigment epithelium from the margins of the iridectomy. This characteristically grows in evenly from the margins of the iridectomy toward the center and does not come forward to occlude the portion of the opening through the stroma (Fig. 30-21). Functional closure may occur with the formation of posterior synechiae.

Retreatment to open the iridectomy is usually easy. Argon laser iridectomies that repeatedly close

over time may remain open after Nd:YAG treatment.[29] Less frequently, laser iridectomies may enlarge over time.[77,97]

Retinal Damage

Photocoagulation of the peripheral retina between the equator and the ora serrata during argon laser iridectomy is significantly reduced by the use of a contact lens.[11] This usually occurs when an opening is being enlarged after iris penetration has been achieved.[77,123] In one study, ophthalmoscopically invisible peripheral retinal damage was detected with static perimetry and fluorescein angiography.[46] However, the authors used much higher energy levels than are ordinarily used and did not use a laser lens.

Inadvertent foveal photocoagulation has been reported,[10] and proper positioning of the laser beam is essential. Choroidal and retinal detachment[21] and nonrhegmatogenous retinal detachment in nanophthalmic eyes[45] have also been reported. Microperforations of the retina may occur with the Nd:YAG laser if the beam is focused to within 2 to 3 mm of the retina.[44]

Other Complications

Sterile hypopyon,[20,111] cystoid macular edema,[17] unexplained loss of central visual acuity[6] and malignant (aqueous misdirection) glaucoma[31] have been reported after laser iridectomy.

Argon Laser Peripheral Iridoplasty

In certain situations, iridectomy either cannot be performed or does not physically eliminate appositional closure. Argon laser peripheral iridoplasty consists of placing a ring of contraction burns circumferentially on the peripheral iris in order to contract the iris stroma between the site of the burn and the angle, thus widening the angle itself (Fig. 30-22). It is a simple and effective means of opening a closed angle in these cases and is extremely useful in reversing an attack of angle-closure glaucoma when medical treatment fails. Complications are minimal.

Early attempts at peripheral iridoplasty were often unsuccessful because of insufficient retraction of the iris away from the trabecular meshwork. Kimbrough et al.[50] described a technique for direct treatment of 360 degrees of the peripheral iris through a gonioscopy lens and termed the procedure *gonioplasty*. Their concept served as the basis for presently used procedures.

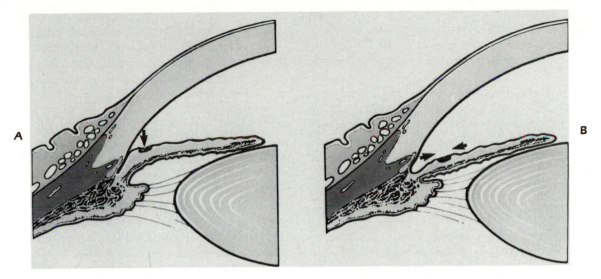

Fig. 30-22 **A,** Contraction burns *(arrows)* placed on peripheral iris lead to **B,** contraction of peripheral iris stroma and opening of angle. These burns break mechanical block caused by apposition of iris to trabecular meshwork.

INDICATIONS

Medically Unbreakable Attacks of Angle-closure Glaucoma

An attack of angle-closure glaucoma that is unresponsive to medical therapy and in which corneal edema, a shallow anterior chamber, or marked inflammation precludes laser iridectomy may be treated effectively with peripheral iridoplasty.

During an attack of angle-closure glaucoma, the iris is directly apposed to the trabecular meshwork. If peripheral anterior synechiae have not formed between the iris and the trabecular meshwork, a contraction burn placed at the periphery of the iris can shrink the iris sufficiently to pull it away from the meshwork. Circumferential treatment of the iris opens the angle in those areas in which there are no peripheral anterior synechiae.

Even when extensive peripheral anterior synechiae are present, the intraocular pressure is usually normalized within an hour or two, perhaps because of associated secretory hypotony. The effect lasts sufficiently long for the cornea and anterior chamber to clear so that, iridectomy can be performed. In cases in which an intumescent lens is responsible for the angle-closure attack, cataract extraction can be postponed until the eye has quieted.

Plateau Iris Syndrome

In this condition, the angle remains appositionally closed or occludable following laser iridectomy (see Chapter 47). The residual angle-closure glaucoma is not caused by pupillary block, but rather by an abnormal iris configuration, which allows the peripheral iris to remain in contact with the angle structures. The presence of a patent iridectomy, which should always be performed first to eliminate any pupillary block component, is necessary before making this diagnosis.

Lens-related Angle-closure Glaucoma

Angle-closure caused by a posterior "push" mechanism (see Chapter 40) is not often responsive to iridectomy, although a component of pupillary block may be present and should be eliminated by iridectomy. These include such types of angle-closure as ciliary block, lens intumescence, anterior subluxation of the lens, or anterior lens displacement secondary to ciliary body edema from panretinal photocoagulation or a scleral buckling procedure. In these situations in which the angle remains appositionally closed after laser iridectomy, the apposition can often be partially or entirely eliminated by iridoplasty. After the angle has been opened and intraocular pressure reduced, cycloplegics may be given cautiously to ascertain the mechanism of the angle-closure.

Adjunct to Laser Trabeculoplasty

When the angle is narrow because of plateau iris configuration or angle-crowding, peripheral iridoplasty can be performed for 360 degrees to retract the iris away from the trabecular meshwork.[82] In eyes in which most of the angle is visible but focal areas of narrowing are present because of iris irregularities or intraepithelial cysts, focal contraction burns are sufficient to widen these areas to permit trabeculoplasty burns to be placed at these sites.[63]

Laser trabeculoplasty can be performed immediately after peripheral iridoplasty when focal coagulation only is necessary. If extensive treatment is necessary, it is better to perform the procedures on separate days because both may be associated with a postlaser rise in intraocular pressure.

Nanophthalmos

Individuals with nanophthalmos are anatomically predisposed to angle-closure glaucoma and may manifest persistent appositional closure following successful laser iridectomy. Peripheral iridoplasty is often sufficient to open the angle and avoid operative surgery, which may have severe complications in these patients.

CONTRAINDICATIONS
Advanced Corneal Edema or Opacification

Moderate degrees of corneal edema are not a contraindication to peripheral iridoplasty when the procedure is performed in order to break a medically unresponsive attack of angle-closure glaucoma. Extensive corneal opacification may present difficulties, because higher powers necessary to cause contraction of the iris may injure the cornea as well. Glycerine may help clear the cornea temporarily.

Flat Anterior Chamber

In this situation, any attempt at photocoagulation of the iris will result in damage to the corneal endothelium. Iridoplasty should not be attempted, since any contraction of the peripheral iris produced would have little or no effect on widening the angle.

TECHNIQUE
Pretreatment Measures

The procedure is performed on an outpatient basis under topical anesthesia. Pilocarpine 4% is applied to stretch the iris maximally. In some cases, because of acute angle-closure or other situation, miosis cannot be fully attained, but usually the iris is sufficiently stretched so that an effective procedure can be performed. Peripheral iridoplasty may be performed for a type of angle-closure that may be worsened by miotics, which cause an increase in lens axial thickness and shallowing of the anterior chamber. Although miotics are contraindicated in maintenance therapy of these types of angle-closure, their administration immediately before the iridoplasty procedure facilitates the procedure. Miotics should not, however, be continued following the procedure.

Laser Parameters

The laser is set to produce contraction burns (500 μm spot size, 0.5 second duration, and 200 to 400 mW power). With the contact lens in place, the surgeon directs the aiming beam to the most peripheral portion of the iris possible. One of the most common errors resulting in failure of the procedure is spot placement in the mid-periphery of the iris rather than the extreme periphery. It is useful to allow a thin crescent of the aiming beam to overlap the sclera at the limbus. The patient may be directed to look in the direction of the beam in order to achieve more peripheral spot placement.

The contraction effect is immediate and usually accompanied by noticeable deepening of the peripheral anterior chamber at the site of the burn. A lack of visible contraction and deepening of the peripheral anterior chamber at any site is suggestive of peripheral anterior synechiae. If bubble formation occurs or if pigment is released into the anterior chamber, the power should be reduced.

Lighter irides generally require more power than darker ones. The surgeon should begin with 200 mW for dark irides and 300 mW for light ones and adjust the power as necessary to obtain visible stromal contraction. Occasionally, in light gray irides, a 200 μm spot size may be more effective in achieving significant stromal contraction. The use of a smaller spot size requires a much larger number of burns to achieve the same result and, particularly with high power settings, may result in stromal destruction and pigment release.

Treatment consists of placing approximately 24 to 36 spots over 360 degrees, leaving approximately 2 spot-diameters between each spot and avoiding large visible radial vessels if possible (Fig. 30-23). Although rare, iris necrosis may occur if too many spots are placed too closely together. If this treatment is insufficient, 20 to 30 more spots may be given at a later sitting.

The presence of an arcus senilis should be ignored. An extremely shallow anterior chamber and corneal edema, which are relative contraindications to laser iridectomy, do not preclude peripheral iridoplasty.

Variations of this procedure have been described using a gonioscopy lens to place burns onto

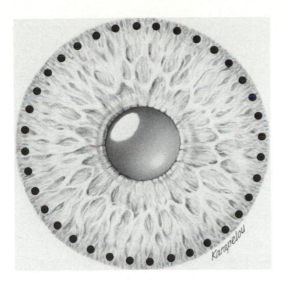

Fig. 30-23 Peripheral iridoplasty using contraction burns. Burns are placed around circumference of iris as peripherally as possible. When each burn is placed, iris stroma contracts toward it from all directions *(arrows)*. Contraction of stroma peripheral to burn site eliminates its contact with trabecular meshwork.

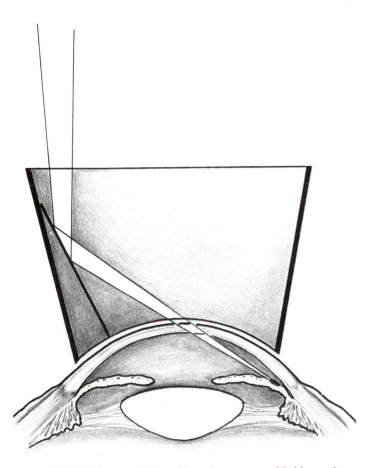

Fig. 30-24 Angulation of beam from mirror of Goldmann lens to treat iris near its root.

the peripheral iris under direct visualization of the angle (Fig. 30-24). Stretch burn settings must be used instead of contraction burns, and the laser beam strikes the peripheral iris tangentially, resulting in a more diffuse burn with less peripheral stromal contraction. These are more likely to result in bubble formation and stromal destruction or inadvertent damage to the trabecular meshwork or scleral spur. Contraction burns placed perpendicular to the peripheral iris through an Abraham lens are sufficient to open the angle in all but a few unusual cases.

Postoperative Treatment

Patients are treated with topical steroids four to six times daily for 3 to 5 days afterward. Intraocular pressure is monitored postoperatively as after any other anterior segment laser procedure and patients treated as necessary if a postlaser rise occurs.

Complications

A mild postoperative iritis is common and responds to topical steroid treatment, seldom lasting more than a few days. The patient may experience transient ocular irritation.

Because iridoplasty is often performed on patients with extremely shallow peripheral anterior chambers, diffuse corneal endothelial burns may occur. As opposed to the dense white, sharply delineated burns seen during laser iridectomy, endothelial burns seen during peripheral iridoplasty are larger and much less opaque. If endothelial burns present a problem early in the procedure, they may be minimized by placing an initial contraction burn more centrally before placing the peripheral burn. This first burn will deepen the anterior chamber peripheral to it, allowing the more peripheral burn to be placed with less adverse consequences. In virtually all cases, the endothelial burns disappear within several days and have not proved to be a major complication. We have seen one case of corneal decompensation following iridoplasty in a patient with preexisting Fuchs' dystrophy.

Hemorrhage has never occurred to our knowledge, presumably because of the lower power density used to produce contraction burns as opposed to destructive ones. A transient rise in intraocular pressure can occur as with other anterior segment laser procedures. Lenticular opacification has not occurred with peripheral iridoplasty, and theoretically this problem would be highly unlikely.

Need for Retreatment

The duration of the effect of the iridoplasty is variable. Long-term effectiveness is possible, but patients need to be followed closely for recurrence of the angle closure, and on occasion, the patients may require retreatment. This is most common in a patient in whom the mechanism of the glaucoma is lens-related because of a posterior "push" mechanism. It is rarely needed in patients with intumescent lenses or plateau iris. Pressure from the lens against the posterior iris may lead to gradual narrowing of the angle, possibly because of further anterior lens movement or to stretching of the iris stroma. Patients should be observed gonioscopically at regular intervals and further treatment given if necessary.

REFERENCES

1. Abraham, RK: Protocol for single-session argon laser iridectomy for angle-closure glaucoma, Int Ophthalmol Clin 21:145, 1981
2. Abraham, RK: Letter to the editor, Ann Ophthalmol 15:673, 1973
3. Abraham, RK, and Miller, GL: Outpatient argon laser iridectomy for angle-closure glaucoma: a two-year study, Trans Am Acad Ophthalmol Otolaryngol 79:OP529, 1975
4. Abraham, RK, and Miller, GL: Outpatient argon iridectomy for angle-closure glaucoma: a 3½ year study, Adv Ophthalmol 34:186, 1977
5. Anderson, DR, Forster, RK, and Lewis, MK: Laser iridotomy for aphakic pupillary block, Arch Ophthalmol 93:434, 1975
6. Balkan, RJ, Zimmerman, TJ, Hesse, RJ, and Steigner, JB: Loss of central visual acuity after laser peripheral iridectomy, Ann Ophthalmol 14:721, 1982
7. Bass, MS, Cleary, CV, Perkins, ES, and Wheeler, CB: Single treatment laser iridotomy, Br J Ophthalmol 63:29, 1979
8. Beckman, H, and Sugar, HS: Laser iridectomy therapy of glaucoma, Arch Ophthalmol 90:453, 1973
9. Beckman, H, et al: Laser iridectomies, Am J Ophthalmol 72:393, 1971
10. Berger, BB: Foveal photocoagulation from laser iridotomy, Ophthalmology 91:1029, 1984
11. Bongard, B, and Pederson, JE: Retinal burns from experimental laser iridotomy, Ophthalmic Surg 16:42, 1985
12. Brainard, JO, Landers, JH, and Shock, JP: Recurrent angle closure glaucoma following a patent 75-micron laser iridotomy: a case report, Ophthalmic Surg 13:1030, 1982
13. Brazier, DJ: Neodymium-YAG laser iridotomy, J Roy Soc Med 79:58, 1986
14. Brown, RH, et al: ALO-2145 reduces the intraocular pressure elevation after anterior segment laser surgery, Ophthalmology 95:378, 1988
15. Brown, SVL, Thomas, JV, Belcher, CD, and Simmons, RJ: Effect of pilocarpine in treatment of intraocular pressure elevation following Neodymium:YAG laser posterior capsulotomy, Ophthalmology 92:354, 1985
16. Burns, RP: Improvement in technique of photocoagulation of the iris, Arch Ophthalmol 74:306, 1965
17. Choplin, NT, and Bene, C: Cystoid macular edema following laser iridotomy, Ann Ophthalmol 15:172, 1983
18. Cinotti, DJ, Reiter, DJ, Maltzman, BA, and Cinotti, AA: Neodymium:YAG laser therapy for pseudophakic pupillary block, J Cat Ref Surg 12:174, 1986
19. Cohen, JS, Bibler, L, and Tucker, D: Hypopyon following laser iridotomy, Ophthalmic Surg 15:604, 1984
20. Cooper, RL, and Constable, IJ: Prevention of corneal burns during high-energy laser iridotomy, Am J Ophthalmol 91:534, 1981
21. Corriveau, LA, Nasr, Y, and Fanous, S: Choroidal and retinal detachment following argon laser iridotomy, Can J Ophthalmol 21:107, 1986
22. Dragon, DM, et al: Neodymium:YAG laser iridotomy in the cynomolgus monkey, Invest Ophthalmol Vis Sci 29:789, 1985
23. Epstein, DL, Steinert, RF, and Puliafito, CA: Neodymium-YAG laser therapy to the anterior hyaloid in aphakic malignant glaucoma, Am J Ophthalmol 98:137, 1984
24. Flocks, M, and Zweng, HC: Laser coagulation of ocular tissues, Arch Ophthalmol 72:604, 1964
25. Floman, N, Berson, D, and Landau, L: Peripheral iridectomy in closed angle glaucoma—late complications, Br J Ophthalmol 61:101, 1977
26. Forman, JS, Ritch, R, Dunn, MW, and Szmyd, L: Pupillary block following posterior chamber lens implantation, Ophthalmic Laser Ther 2:85, 1987
27. Gaasterland, DG, Rodrigues, MM, and Thomas, G: Threshold for lens damage during Q-switched Nd:YAG laser iridectomy: a study of Rhesus monkey eyes, Ophthalmology 92:1616, 1985
28. Gieser, DK, and Wilensky, JT: Laser iridectomy in the management of chronic angle-closure glaucoma, Am J Ophthalmol 98:446, 1984
29. Gilbert, CM, Robin, AL, and Pollack, IP: Letter to the editor, Ophthalmology 91:1123, 1984
30. Go, FJ, Akiba, F, Yamamoto, T, and Kitazawa, Y: Argon laser iridotomy and surgical iridectomy in the treatment of primary angle-closure glaucoma, Jpn J Ophthalmol 28:36, 1984
31. Go, FJ, and Kitazawa, Y: Complications of peripheral iridectomy in primary angle closure glaucoma, Jpn J Ophthalmol 25:222, 1981
32. Greenidge, KC, et al: Acute intraocular pressure elevation after argon laser trabeculoplasty and iridectomy: a clinicopathologic study, Ophthalmic Surg 15:105, 1984
33. Harrad, RA, Stannard, KP, and Shilling, JS: Argon laser iridotomy, Br J Ophthalmol 69:368, 1985

34. Heijl, A, and Holm, O: Technique for testing the patency of laser iridotomies, Acta Ophthalmol 64:251, 1986

35. Henry, JC, Krupin, T, Schultz, J, and Wax, M: Increased intraocular pressure following Neodymium-YAG laser iridectomy (letter), Arch Ophthalmol 104:178, 1986

36. Higginbotham, EJ, and Ogura, Y: Lens clarity after argon and neodymium-YAG laser iridotomy in the rabbit, Arch Ophthalmol 105:540, 1987

37. Hirst, LW, et al: Corneal endothelial changes after argon-laser iridotomy and panretinal photocoagulation, Am J Ophthalmol 93:473, 1982

38. Hitchings, RA: Combined dye and argon laser treatment for narrow angle glaucoma, Trans Ophthalmol Soc UK 104:52, 1985

39. Hodes, BL, Bentivegna, JF, and Weyer, NJ: Hyphema complicating laser iridotomy, Arch Ophthalmol 100:924, 1982

40. Hogan, MF, and Schwartz, A: Experimental photocoagulation of the iris in guinea pigs, Am J Ophthalmol 49:629, 1960

41. Hong, C, Kitazawa, Y, and Tanishima, H: Influence of argon laser treatment of glaucoma on corneal endothelium, Jpn J Ophthalmol 27:567, 1983

42. Hoskins, HD, and Migliazzo, CV: Laser iridectomy—a technique for blue irises, Ophthalmic Surg 15:488, 1984

43. Jacobs, IH, and Krohn, DL: Central anterior chamber depth after laser iridectomy, Am J Ophthalmol 88:865, 1980

44. Jampol, LM, Goldberg, MF, and Jednock, N: Retinal damage from a Q-switched YAG laser, Am J Ophthalmol 96:326, 1983

45. Karjalainen, K, Laatikainen, L, and Raitta, C: Bilateral nonrhegmatogenous retinal detachment following neodymium-YAG laser iridotomies, Arch Ophthalmol 104:1134, 1986

46. Karmon, G, and Savir, H: Retinal damage after argon laser iridotomy, Am J Ophthalmol 101:554, 1986

47. Kerr Muir, MC, and Sherrard, ES: Damage to the corneal endothelium during Nd:YAG photodisruption, Br J Ophthalmol 69:77, 1985

48. Khodadoust, AA, Arkfeld, DF, Caprioli, J, and Sears, ML: Ocular effect of neodymium-YAG laser, Am J Ophthalmol 98:144, 1984

49. Khuri, CH: Argon laser iridectomies, Am J Ophthalmol 76:490, 1973

50. Kimbrough, RL, Trempe, CS, Brockhurst, RJ, and Simmons, RJ: Angle-closure glaucoma in nanophthalmos, Am J Ophthalmol 88:572, 1979

51. Klapper, RM: Q-switched neodymium:YAG laser iridotomy, Ophthalmology 91:1017, 1984

52. Kramer, P, and Ritch, R: The treatment of angle-closure glaucoma revisited, Ann Ophthalmol 16:1101, 1984

53. Krupin, T, Mitchell, KB, Johnson, MF, and Becker, B: The long-term effects of iridectomy for primary acute angle-closure glaucoma, Am J Ophthalmol 86:506, 1978

54. Krupin, T, et al: Acute intraocular pressure response to argon laser iridotomy, Ophthalmology 92:922, 1985

55. Kublin, J, and Simmons, RJ: Use of tinted soft contact lenses to eliminate monocular diplopia secondary to laser iridectomies, Ophthalmic Laser Ther 2:111, 1987

56. Latina, MA, Puliafito, CA, Steinert, RR, and Epstein, DL: Experimental iridotomy with the Q-switched neodymium:YAG laser, Ophthalmology 102:1211, 1984

57. L'Esperance, FA, and James, WA: Argon laser photocoagulation of iris abnormalities, Trans Am Acad Ophthalmol Otolaryngol 79:OP321, 1975

58. Liu, PF, and Hung, PT: Effect of timolol on intraocular pressure elevation following argon laser iridotomy, J Ocul Pharmacol 3:249, 1987

59. Luke, S-K: Complications of peripheral iridectomy, Can J Ophthalmology 4:346, 1969

60. Mandelkorn, RM, Mendelsohn, AD, Olander, KW, and Zimmerman, TJ: Short exposure times in argon laser iridotomy, Ophthalmic Surg 12:805, 1981

61. McAllister, JA, Schwartz, LW, Moster, M, and Spaeth, GL: Laser peripheral iridectomy comparing Q-switched neodymium:YAG with argon, Trans Ophthalmol Soc UK 104:67, 1984

62. McDonald, JE, and Light, A: Photocoagulation of the iris and retina, Arch Ophthalmol 60:384, 1958

63. Metz, D, Ackerman, J, and Kanarek, I: Laser trabeculoplasty enhancement by argon laser iridotomy and/or iridoplasty (letter), Ophthalmic Surg 15:535, 1984

64. Meyer, KT, Pettit, TH, and Straatsma, BR: Corneal endothelial damage with neodymium:YAG laser, Ophthalmology 91:1022, 1984

65. Meyer-Schwickerath, G: Erfahrungen mit der Lichtkoagulation der Metzhaut und der Iris, Doc Ophthalmol 10:91, 1956

66. Mishima, S, Kitazawa, Y, and Shirato, S: Laser therapy for glaucoma, Aust NZ J Ophthalmol 13:225, 1985

67. Moster, MR, et al: Laser iridectomy: a controlled study comparing argon and neodymium:YAG, Ophthalmology 93:20, 1986

68. Patti, JC, and Cinnoti, AA: Iris photocoagulation therapy of aphakic pupillary block, Arch Ophthalmol 93:347, 1975

69. Perkins, ES: Laser iridotomy, Br Med J 2:580, 1970

70. Perkins, ES, and Brown, NA: Iridotomy with a ruby laser, Br J Ophthalmol 57:487, 1973

71. Playfair, TJ, and Watson, PG: Management of chronic or intermittent primary angle-closure glaucoma: a long term follow-up of the results of peripheral iridectomy used as an initial procedure, Br J Ophthalmol 63:23, 1979

72. Podos, SM, et al: Continuous wave argon laser iridectomy in angle-closure glaucoma, Am J Ophthalmol 88:836, 1979

73. Pollack, IP: Use of argon laser energy to produce iridotomies, Ophthalmic Surg 11:506, 1980

74. Pollack, IP: Laser iridotomy: current concepts in techniques and safety, Int Ophthalmol Clin 21:137, 1984

75. Pollack, IP, and Patz, A: Argon laser iridotomy: an experimental and clinical study, Ophthalmic Surg 7:22, 1976

76. Pollack, IP, et al: Use of the neodymium:YAG laser to create iridotomies in monkeys and humans, Trans Am Ophthalmol Soc 82:307, 1984

77. Quigley, HA: Long-term follow-up of laser iridotomy, Ophthalmology 88:218, 1981

78. Raymond, LA: Historical perspective on photocoagulation, Surv Ophthalmol 21:501, 1977

79. Ritch, R: The treatment of angle-closure glaucoma (editorial), Ann Ophthalmol 11:1373, 1979

80. Ritch, R: The treatment of chronic angle-closure glaucoma (editorial), Ann Ophthalmol 13:21, 1981

81. Ritch, R: Argon laser treatment for medically unresponsive attacks of angle-closure glaucoma, Am J Ophthalmol 94:197, 1982

82. Ritch, R: Techniques of argon laser iridectomy and iridoplasty, Palo Alto, 1983, Coherent Medical Press

83. Ritch, R, and Palmberg, P: Argon laser iridectomy in dark irides, Am J Ophthalmol 94:800, 1982

84. Ritch, R, and Podos, SM: Argon laser treatment of angle-closure glaucoma, Perspect Ophthalmol 4:129, 1980

85. Ritch, R, and Solomon, IS: Glaucoma surgery. In L'Esperance, FA, editor: Ophthalmic lasers, ed 3, St. Louis, 1989, The CV Mosby Co

86. Rivera, AH, Brown, RH, and Anderson, DR: Laser iridotomy vs surgical iridectomy: have the indications changed? Arch Ophthalmol 103:1350, 1985

87. Robin, AL: Intraocular pressure rise after iridotomy (letter), Arch Ophthalmol 104:1117, 1986

88. Robin, AL, and Pollack, IP: Argon laser peripheral iridotomies in the treatment of primary angle closure glaucoma: long-term follow-up, Arch Ophthalmol 100:919, 1982

89. Robin, AL, and Pollack, IP: A comparison of neodymium:YAG and argon laser iridotomies, Ophthalmology 91:1011, 1984

90. Robin, AL, and Pollack, IP: Q-switched neodymium-YAG laser iridotomy in patients in whom the argon laser fails, Arch Ophthalmol 104:531, 1986

91. Robin, AL, and Pollack, IP, and DeFaller, JM: Effects of topical ALO 2145 (p-aminoclonidine hydrochloride,) on intraocular pressure rise following argon laser iridotomy, Arch Ophthalmol 105:1208, 1987

92. Robin, AL, et al: Histologic studies of angle structures after laser iridotomy in primates, Arch Ophthalmol 100:1665, 1982

93. Robin, AL, et al: Q-switched neodymium-YAG laser iridotomy: a field trial with a portable laser system, Arch Ophthalmol 102:526, 1986

94. Rodrigues, MM, et al: Histopathology of neodymium:YAG laser iridectomy in humans, Ophthalmology 92:1696, 1985

95. Rodrigues, MM, Streeten, B, Spaeth, GL, and Schwartz, LW: Argon laser iridotomy in primary angle closure or pupillary block glaucoma, Arch Ophthalmol 96:2222, 1978

96. Rubin, L, Arnett, J, and Ritch, R: Delayed hyphema after argon laser iridectomy, Ophthalmic Surg 15:852, 1984

97. Sachs, SW, and Schwartz, B: Enlargement of laser iridotomies over time, Br J Ophthalmol 68:570, 1984

98. Samples, JR, et al: Pupillary block with posterior chamber intraocular lenses, Am Ophthalmol 105:335, 1987

99. Sanders, DR, et al: Studies on the blood-aqueous barrier after argon laser photocoagulation of the iris, Ophthalmology 90:1983

100. Schirmer, KE: Argon laser surgery of the iris, optimized by contact lenses, Arch Ophthalmol 101:1130, 1983

101. Schrems, W, Belcher, CD, and Tomlinson, CP: Changes in the human central corneal endothelium after neodymium:YAG laser surgery, Ophthalmic Laser Ther 1:143, 1986

102. Schrems, W, Eichelbronner, O, and Krieglstein, GK: The immediate IOP response of Nd-YAG-laser iridotomy and its prophylactic treatability, Acta Ophthalmol 92:673, 1984

103. Schrems, W, van Dorp, HP, Wendel, M, and Krieglstein, GK: The effect of YAG laser iridotomy on the blood aqueous barrier in the rabbit, v Graefes Arch Clin Exp Ophthalmol 221:179, 1984

104. Schwartz, LW, and Spaeth, GL: Argon laser iridotomy in primary angle closure or pupillary block glaucoma, Trans Ophthalmol Soc UK 99:257, 1979

105. Schwartz, LW, et al: Argon laser iridotomy in the treatment of patients with primary angle-closure or pupillary block glaucoma: a clinicopathologic study, Ophthalmology 85:294, 1978

106. Schwartz, LW, et al: Neodymium-YAG laser iridectomies in glaucoma associated with closed or occludable angles, Am J Ophthalmol 102:41, 1986

107. Seedor, JA, Greenidge, KC, and Dunn, MW: Neodymium:YAG laser iridectomy and acute cataract formation in the rabbit, Ophthalmic Surg 17:478, 1986

108. Shapiro, A, Tso, MO, and Goldberg, MF: Argon laser-induced cataract, Arch Ophthalmol 102:579, 1984

109. Shields, MB: Laser surgery of the iris. In Textbook of glaucoma, Baltimore, 1987, Williams & Wilkins

110. Shin, DH: Argon laser iris photocoagulation to relieve acute angle-closure glaucoma, Am J Ophthalmol 93:348, 1982

111. Shin, DH: Another hypopyon following laser iridotomy, Ophthalmic Surg 15:968, 1984

112. Shrader, CE, et al: Pupillary and iridovitreal block in pseudophakic eyes, Ophthalmology 91:831, 1984

113. Singh, OS, Belcher, CD, and Simmons, RJ: Nanophthalmic eyes and neodymium-YAG laser iridectomies, Arch Ophthalmol 105:455, 1987

114. Smith, J, and Whitted, P: Corneal endothelial changes after argon laser iridotomy, Am J Ophthalmol 98:153, 1984

115. Snyder, WB, Vaiser, A, and Hutton, WL: Laser iridectomy, Trans Am Acad Ophthalmol Otolaryngol 79:OP381, 1975

116. Stetz, D, Smith, H, Jr, and Ritch, R: A simplified technique for laser iridectomy in blue irides, Am J Ophthalmol 96:249, 1983

117. Taniguchi, T, Rho, SH, Gotoh, Y, and Kitazawa, Y: Intraocular pressure rise following Q-switched Neodymium:YAG laser iridotomy, Ophthalmic Laser Ther 2:99, 1987

118. Tessler, HH, Peyman, GA, Huamonte, F, and Menachof, I: Argon laser iridotomy in incomplete peripheral iridectomy, Am J Ophthalmol 79:1051, 1975

119. Thoming, C, van Buskirk, EM, and Samples, JR: The corneal endothelium after laser therapy for glaucoma, Am J Ophthalmol 103:518, 1987

120. Tomey, KF, Traverso, CE, and Shammas, IV: Neodymium-Yag laser iridotomy in the treatment and prevention of angle closure glaucoma: a review of 373 eyes, Arch Ophthalmol 105:476, 1987

121. Unger, WG, Perkins, ES, and Bass, MS: The response of the rabbit eye to laser irradiation of the iris, Exp Eye Res 25:367, 1974

122. Verhoef, FH, and Bell, L: The pathological effects of radiant energy on the eye, Proc Am Acad Arts Sci 51:630, 1916

123. Watts, GK: Retinal hazards during laser irradiation of the iris, Br J Ophthalmol 55:60, 1971

124. Welch, DB, et al: Lens injury following iridotomy with a Q-switched neodymium-YAG laser, Arch Ophthalmol 194:123, 1986

125. Werner, D, and Kaback, M: Pseudophakic pupillary-block glaucoma, Br J Ophthalmol 61:329, 1977

126. Wise, JB: Iris sphincterotomy, iridotomy, and synechiotomy by linear incision with the argon laser, Ophthalmology 92:641, 1985

127. Wise, JB: Low-energy linear-incision neodymium: YAG laser iridotomy versus linear-incision argon laser iridotomy: a prospective clinical investigation, Ophthalmology 94:1531, 1987

128. Wise, JB, Munnerlyn, CR, and Erickson, PJ: A high-efficiency laser iridotomy-sphincterotomy lens, Am J Ophthalmol 101:546, 1986

129. Wishart, PK, and Hitchings, RA: Neodymium YAG and dye laser iridotomy—a comparative study, Trans Ophthalmol Soc UK 105:521, 1986

130. Wishart, PK, et al: Corneal endothelial changes following short pulsed laser iridotomy and surgical iridectomy, Trans Ophthalmol Soc UK 105:541, 1986

131. Yamamoto, T, Shirato, S, and Kitazawa, Y: Argon laser iridotomy in angle-closure glaucoma: a comparison of two methods, Jpn J Ophthalmol 29:387, 1982

132. Yamamoto, T, Shirato, S, and Kitazawa, Y: Treatment of primary angle-closure glaucoma by argon laser iridotomy: a long-term follow-up, Jpn J Ophthalmol 29:1, 1985

133. Yassur, Y, Melamed, S, Cohen, S, and Ben-Sira, I: Laser iridotomy in closed-angle glaucoma, Arch Ophthalmol 97:1920, 1979

134. Zweng, HC, Little, HL, and Hammond, AH: Complication of argon laser photocoagulation, Tran Am Acad Ophthalmol Otolaryngol 78:OP195, 1974

135. Zweng, HC, et al: Experimental laser photocoagulation, Am J Ophthalmol 58:353, 1964

136. Zweng, HC, et al: Laser photocoagulation of the iris, Arch Ophthalmol 84:193, 1970

Chapter 31

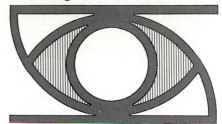
Laser Treatment in Open-angle Glaucoma

Bruce J. Goldstick
Robert N. Weinreb

HISTORICAL PERSPECTIVE

Laser surgery has been used since the early 1970's in an effort to reduce intraocular pressure by treating the trabecular meshwork. Krasnov [35,36] attempted to create holes in the trabecular meshwork with the Q-switched ruby laser, so-called laser puncture, to decrease outflow resistance. He improved outflow facility and lowered intraocular pressure in some patients for as long as 8 months. Worthen and Wickham,[116,126] Ticho,[95] and others[10,25,107,132] used the argon laser to alter the trabecular meshwork. Intraocular pressure was lowered in some patients for more than a year. Although they initially thought this effect was related to increased facility of outflow, the reduced intraocular pressure persisted despite a subsequent reduction in the outflow facility. These early studies did not create widespread enthusiasm because of variable results and complications.

Consistent, long-term effects with argon laser treatment were not realized until Wise and Witter[124] placed evenly spaced, nonpenetrating argon laser burns around the entire circumference of the trabecular meshwork. They theorized that collagen shrinkage and subsequent scarring of the trabecular meshwork tightened the meshwork in the area of each laser burn and reopened the untreated intertrabecular spaces. In over 70% of their patients, intraocular pressure was significantly lowered after 4 years.[123] In black patients and patients older than 70 years, they reported a success rate of 91%.

Subsequently, most clinical investigations of argon laser trabeculoplasty have reported modifications of the original Wise and Witter technique, centering on spot placement, number of applications, laser burn parameters, and prevention of complications.

Recently, attention has been directed to alternative methods of treating open-angle glaucoma with different laser systems. The Nd:YAG laser has proved particularly interesting.

METHODS AND TECHNIQUES OF ARGON LASER TRABECULOPLASTY

Argon laser trabeculoplasty appears to be effective in lowering the intraocular pressure in many eyes with open-angle glaucoma. Optimal treatment parameters have been evaluated by a number of investigators to both maximize benefit and reduce risk to the patient.

Basic Technique

The patient's preoperative glaucoma regimen should be maintained before laser trabeculoplasty. In patients who are not able to tolerate chronic administration of carbonic anhydrase inhibitors, either acetazolamide or methazolamide may be administered approximately 1 to 2 hours before treatment. In eyes with advanced glaucomatous optic nerve damage and visual field loss, a hyperosmotic agent such as oral glycerine or isosorbide may also be helpful in reducing the magnitude of a potential postoperative rise in intraocular pressure (see Chapter 27). Administration of these oral agents may be associated with nausea, vomiting, and headache, and they are often best administered immediately following the procedure.

While the patient sits at a slit-lamp, the eye to be treated is topically anesthetized with 0.5% proparacaine hydrochloride. A mirrored contact lens is placed on the cornea with methylcellulose solution. The three-mirror Goldmann lens with antireflective coating features a dome-shaped mirror angled at 59 degrees for visualizing angle structures. The Ritch trabeculoplasty lens offers two basic mirrors, one inclined at an angle of 59 degrees, which allows a face-on view of the inferior half of the angle, and one inclined at 64 degrees, which allows a similar view of the superior half of the angle.[66] It has two additional mirrors inclined at the same angle with superimposed plano-convex buttons that produce ×1.4 magnification. This effectively reduces spot size from 50 μm to 35 μm and increases the laser energy by a factor of two. Laser energy is delivered through the contact lens to the desired location in the trabecular meshwork.

An attempt is made to space spots equally over the anterior half of the trabecular meshwork. It is important to identify all angle structures at each location to avoid accidental treatment of the cornea or the ciliary body band. Treatment parameters should be set at 50 μm spot size and 0.1 second duration. Treatment should begin at approximately 800 mW. Some surgeons use the same power for all treatments, although most will adjust the treatment according to a reaction endpoint. In the latter case, tissue reactions rather than power settings are used to determine the appropriate energy. The desired response is a blanching of the trabecular meshwork with or without minimal bubble formation. The amount of power necessary is inversely proportional to the degree of pigmentation of the meshwork. If blanching is noted, it is not necessary to further increase the power to obtain bubble formation. The variability of trabecular meshwork pigmentation in different quadrants may require that power settings be changed throughout the treatment session to achieve the desired response. Continuous focusing of the aiming beam on the trabecular meshwork is essential. The beam spot should be circular and the coagulation spot should be the smallest possible size. It is often easiest to start with the goniolens at 12 o'clock (inferior angle) and rotate the lens clockwise, treating the temporal portion of the right eye and the nasal portion of the left eye if only 180

BASIC PROTOCOL FOR ARGON LASER TRABECULOPLASTY

1. Initial treatment session 180 or 360 degrees.
2. Laser burns equally spaced at anterior half of trabecular meshwork.
3. Forty to 50 laser spots (180 degrees); 80 to 100 laser spots (360 degrees).
4. Fifty μm spot size.
5. Spot duration 0.1 seconds.
6. Laser treatment initiated at 800mW. Power either fixed or adjusted to achieve slight blanching or small bubble formation.
7. Intraocular pressure monitored hourly for 3 hours.
8. Intraocular pressure reassessed after 1 week and after 4 to 6 weeks. Second half of trabecular meshwork treated as necessary.

---

degrees is being photocoagulated. The aiming beam should be kept in the central portion of the mirror, and the lens should be rotated after several applications.

After laser treatment, all preoperative glaucoma medications are continued. Mild analgesics are rarely necessary during the immediate postoperative period. Steroids are administered as needed to reduce postoperative inflammation. In the presence of cells and flare, 1% prednisolone may be used four times daily for 4 days beginning at the completion of laser therapy. The intraocular pressure should be monitored for 1 to 3 hours following treatment. The patient is reexamined routinely on the first postoperative day, as well as at 1 week and at 4 to 6 weeks postoperatively. Once the intraocular pressure is stabilized, the physician may attempt to sequentially discontinue some glaucoma medications, particularly carbonic anhydrase inhibitors, based on the clinical status of the patient. The basic technique is summarized in the box above.

Number of Burns and Relationship to Intraocular Pressure

Wise and Witter[102] initially administered 100 to 120 evenly spaced laser burns that were applied on and immediately posterior to the pigmented band of the trabecular meshwork throughout 360 degrees of the circumference. Subsequently, numerous studies have confirmed the reduction of intraocular pressure using this technique.* Intraocular pressure also can increase transiently, rather than decrease, during the immediate postoperative pe-

---

*References 17, 24, 41, 60, 62, 80, 92, 118, and 124.

riod.[28,29,37,114] Significantly, an increase in intraocular pressure during this time has been associated with visual loss in patients with severe glaucomatous damage.[28,114] Since secondary glaucoma has been induced in rhesus monkeys by administering a large number of long-duration laser burns,[20] it appears that delivering excessive energy to the trabecular meshwork can harm rather than benefit the patient. Taking this into account, several studies were undertaken to determine the relationship of the number of laser burns to the amount of intraocular pressure lowering.

By the application of 50 burns to the trabecular meshwork over 180 or 360 degrees of the angle instead of 100 burns over 360 degrees, the maximum rise in intraocular pressure during the immediate postoperative period can be reduced while the beneficial long-term lowering of intraocular pressure is maintained.[28,45,91,92,114] The intraocular pressure rise in eyes treated with fewer laser burns may also be of shorter duration than in eyes treated with 100 burns. Wilensky and Weinreb[119] demonstrated that even 25 burns applied to one quadrant (90 degrees) of the trabecular meshwork may result in a significant decrease in the intraocular pressure in some eyes. An additional 25 burns was additive and the final reduction of intraocular pressure was similar to that obtained in eyes treated with single-treatment sessions of 50 burns. However, one-quadrant therapy has great variability, and long-term studies have not evaluated the efficacy of this treatment modality.

If half-circumference treatment has been performed and additional pressure lowering is needed, evidence suggests that administering laser burns to previously untreated areas of the trabecular meshwork may be beneficial. Horns et al.[28] reported that 67% of their patients were controlled with treatment of just one half of the angle. In eyes that required further lowering of intraocular pressure, they treated an additional 180 degrees. These results were comparable to those obtained in eyes treated throughout 360 degrees in one session. Thomas et al.[91,92] also found a similar success rate in eyes treated in one session with 100 spots throughout 360 degrees and in those treated in two sessions of 50 spots throughout 180 degrees each. Fewer eyes treated in two sessions sustained elevated intraocular pressure during the immediate postoperative period. Similar results have been reported by Klein et al.,[32] who evaluated a two-stage treatment plan in which 180 degrees of trabecular meshwork was treated in each of two sessions spaced 1 month apart (a total of 360 degrees was treated). Several eyes that did not respond adequately to the first treatment had clinically significant decreases in intraocular pressure after the second. Their protocol differed from other researchers in that Klein et al. placed only 35 burns throughout each 180 degrees of the angle.

Placement of Burns

The placement of laser burns has an impact on the extent of postoperative peripheral anterior synechiae. Traverso et al.[97] demonstrated that these synechiae developed in 12% of eyes in which the anterior trabecular meshwork was treated, and 43% of eyes in which the posterior aspect (over Schlemm's canal) of the trabecular meshwork was treated. However, there was no difference in the intraocular pressure–lowering effect in eyes treated by either method. Although the long-term significance of these synechiae is not known, they concluded that laser trabeculoplasty is safer, but no less effective, when performed in the anterior trabecular meshwork rather than in the posterior trabecular meshowrk. Schwartz et al.[81] also reported no difference in treatment effect between eyes treated in the anterior trabecular meshwork and eyes treated similarly in the posterior trabecular meshwork. Anterior placement of burns appears to minimize the early post-laser pressure rise,[45,81] and formation of peripheral anterior synechiae.[97]

Interestingly, there are anecdotal reports of treatment placed directly over the ciliary band. These claim to have excellent results in reducing intraocular pressure with few postoperative complications. However, there has not been a direct controlled comparison of this method with more common methods in which spots are placed over the trabecular meshwork. Such claims are controversial.

Laser Power

Besides the number and location of laser burns administered, the power and wavelength also have been evaluated. Most investigators have used a laser burn with a 50 μm diameter and a duration of 0.1 second during laser trabeculoplasty.* These parameters are similar to those originally used by Wise and Witter.[124] It has been empirically determined that spots should be applied to create a slight blanching with or without the formation of a tiny bubble (Fig. 31-1). Power settings will vary among eyes but generally fall in the 700 to 1200 mW range. Patients with less pigment may require

*References 17, 28, 62, 80, 92, 118, and 124.

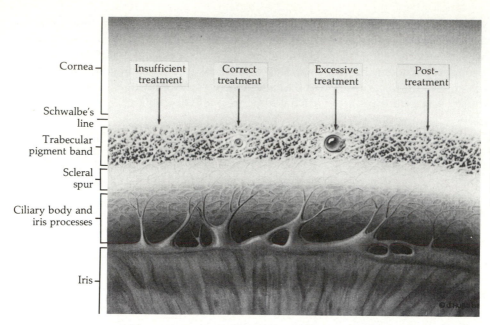

Cornea

Schwalbe's line

Trabecular pigment band

Scleral spur

Ciliary body and iris processes

Iris

Insufficient treatment | Correct treatment | Excessive treatment | Post-treatment

Fig. 31-1 Treatment responses of the trabecular meshwork to light, optimal, and excessive argon laser treatment. (From Schwartz, AL, et al: Ophthalmology 88:203, 1981)

higher power settings to create an effect, whereas those with more heavily pigmented trabecular meshworks may require less power. Another approach uses the same power for all eyes regardless of the trabecular tissue response. Rouhiainen and Terasvirta found the level of power did not affect the lowering of intraocular pressure.[74]

Laser Wavelength

Almost all reports have employed argon blue-green light with a major peak at 488 nm. Smith[85] used the argon green laser and found no difference in postoperative intraocular pressure or complication rate. The krypton laser, however, may possess some theoretic advantages over the argon blue-green laser. Trempe[98] demonstrated less absorption of krypton wavelengths by melanin. Hence, it is theoretically possible that there is greater penetration of heat energy to trabecular tissue adjacent to Schlemm's canal with krypton wavelengths. In addition, there is less scattering and diffraction with these wavelengths as they pass through the cornea. In order to determine their clinical effectiveness, krypton red (647.1 nm) and yellow (568.2 nm) lasers have been used to perform argon laser trabeculoplasty over 180 degrees in a small number of patients.[87] Short-term results have revealed a lowering of intraocular pressure comparable to argon laser trabeculoplasty performed with blue-green wavelengths.[87,129] Further studies are needed to determine the optimum wavelength for perform-

ing laser trabeculoplasty, and perhaps this can be individualized based on certain characteristics of a particular eye.

RESULTS OF ARGON LASER TRABECULOPLASTY

Since Wise and Witter's initial report on the effectiveness of argon laser treatment for open-angle glaucoma, many studies have been published confirming the beneficial effect of this therapeutic modality. Most eyes with uncontrolled open-angle glaucoma and maximal tolerated medical therapy have favorably responded to argon laser trabeculoplasty. Depending on how success is defined in a given study, short-term success has been reported to range from 65% to 97%.* There is no uniform definition for success, however. In some studies, for example, a successful outcome is one in which intraocular pressure is less than a certain value; in others, success is functionally defined as intraocular pressure reduction sufficient to prevent further optic nerve and visual field damage. Clearly, many factors must be considered when evaluating the success of a surgical procedure, including the type of glaucoma (e.g., exfoliation, pigment dispersion, angle recession), whether the eye is phakic or aphakic, the age, sex and race of the patient, the medications administered, and the intraocular pressure before treatment.

---

*References 17, 28, 80, 118, 120, 123.

Pretreatment Intraocular Pressure

The amount of intraocular pressure reduction that one can anticipate after treatment generally correlates with the preoperative intraocular pressure. Eyes with higher intraocular pressure generally have a greater absolute response. This does not imply, however, that eyes with higher pressures will have a greater success rate because these eyes may require an even greater pressure reduction than that attainable by laser treatment. It appears that eyes with intraocular pressures exceeding 30 to 35 mm Hg have a higher failure rate regardless of the definition of success.

Thomas[92] demonstrated an intraocular pressure reduction of 40% to 50% in eyes with intraocular pressures exceeding 30 mm Hg; there was an absolute decrease of as much as 14 to 25 mm Hg, depending on the preoperative pressure. Schwartz[80] reported similar data, showing approximately a 39% intraocular pressure change in eyes with pretreatment values exceeding 30 mm Hg. However, eyes with pretreatment pressures above 35 mm Hg may have a lower absolute change of intraocular pressure than eyes initially between 21 mm Hg and 35 mm Hg.[17] Success rates range only from 45% to 60% if the pretreatment pressure exceeds 30 mm Hg.[17,80,92] Conversely, if pretreatment pressure is below 20 mm Hg, its mean change is much lower (approximately 3 to 4 mm Hg). This should not preclude treatment, however, since even this small change may be sufficient to prevent further deterioration of the optic nerve and visual field.

In most reported series, pretreatment pressures ranged between 20 and 29 mm Hg. In these series, initial success with the procedure ranged between 70% and 90%, and the mean change in intraocular pressure was between 6 and 10 mm Hg (mean of 7 mm Hg).* Thus, argon laser trabeculoplasty appears to be particularly effective in these eyes.

Phakic versus Aphakic Eyes

Aphakic eyes respond less favorably to argon laser trabeculoplasty than phakic ones. Thomas[92] demonstrated only a 59% success rate (mean decrease of 2 mm Hg) in open-angle glaucoma associated with aphakia as compared to an 89% success rate (mean decrease of 7 mm Hg) in phakic eyes with open-angle glaucoma. Horns,[28] however, demonstrated about a 7 mm Hg pressure reduction

in aphakic eyes, which was not significantly different from that found in phakic eyes (7.6 mm Hg). Despite these conflicting reports, both investigators recommended argon laser trabeculoplasty for open-angle glaucoma associated with aphakia. Good results also have been reported with laser trabeculoplasty in aphakic and pseudophakic eyes with open-angle glaucoma after penetrating keratoplasty.[105]

In eyes with both cataracts and uncontrolled glaucoma, it has been suggested that laser trabeculoplasty should be performed before cataract surgery because of the possibility of obtaining a greater response in the phakic eye.[17,124] Controlled data are not available describing the effect of laser trabeculoplasty in pseudophakic eyes (either before or after the lens implant has been placed). Also, there are no data describing differential effects between eyes undergoing extracapsular and intracapsular surgery.

Age of Patient

Patients over 40 years of age appear to respond much more favorably to argon laser trabeculoplasty than younger patients.[17,76,92,131] Thomas[92] and Forbes[17] demonstrated success rates of almost 90% in patients over 40, and Wise found a 91% success rate in patients 70 years or older.

Race and Sex

Most early reports indicated that race or sex did not affect the success rates for laser trabeculoplasty. Krupin et al.[38] reported no apparent difference in the response rate between black and white patients 2 years after treatment. Schwartz[78] followed patients for 2 to 4 years and was unable to find a significant difference. More recently, however, Schwartz[79] found that long-term follow-up success rates were significantly different between blacks and whites. Only 32% of cases involving black patients were successful after 5 years of observation, whereas 65% of cases involving white patients were successful. These data imply that short-term success may be the same for blacks and whites, but with longer observation periods there may be more blacks whose eyes require additional treatment (Fig. 31-2).

Secondary Open-angle Glaucoma

One of the difficulties in analyzing patient response to argon laser trabeculoplasty with secondary forms of open-angle glaucoma is that it is difficult to obtain a large series of patients with these

---

*References 17, 28, 42, 80, 118, 123.

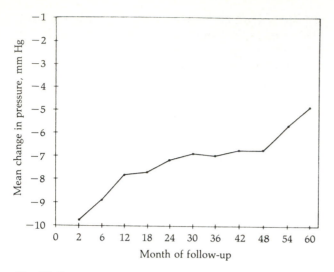

Fig. 31-2 Average intraocular pressure after argon laser trabeculoplasty in black patients over a 5-year period. (From Schwartz, AL, et al: Arch Ophthalmol 103:1482, 1985, copyright 1985, American Medical Association)

conditions, making statistical analysis more difficult. Also, few studies have observed these patients over long periods.

Exfoliation syndrome

Many of the early laser trabeculoplasty studies did not segregate patients with exfoliation from those with primary open-angle glaucoma. Horns et al.[28] reported their results on a large group of glaucomatous eyes[63] with exfoliation and glaucoma. They found a mean reduction of 12.8 mm Hg during a follow-up period of 32 weeks. There was no significant difference in the change of intraocular pressure when compared with phakic eyes with primary open-angle glaucoma. Lieberman[42] successfully treated five of seven exfoliation eyes and lowered intraocular pressure between 5 and 19 mm Hg (mean 10.9 mm Hg). Robin and Pollack[68] reported similar success in four eyes with exfoliation. Other investigators[43,61,98] have confirmed these short-term success rates, and it appears that the early reduction of intraocular pressure is comparable to that obtained with primary open-angle glaucoma. However, Ritch and Podos[67] noted a late sudden elevation of intraocular pressure in 4 of 15 patients with exfoliation, followed for 6 months to 2 years after trabeculoplasty, and suggested that there may be an increased rate of late failures in these patients. Pohjanpelto[61] treated 97 eyes with exfoliation and demonstrated 10 late failures, 2 of which had rubeotic glaucoma from

unrelated causes. The cause of late failure with exfoliation remains unresolved.

Pigmentary glaucoma

Both Horns et al.[28] and Robin and Pollack[68] have demonstrated good responses during the early postoperative period in eyes with pigment dispersion syndrome and glaucoma. Robin and Pollack reported that 11 eyes of 8 patients had a mean intraocular pressure decrease of approximately 11 mm Hg with a follow-up of 7 months.

Lunde[44] studied 13 eyes of 10 patients with pigmentary glaucoma and confirmed this initial decrease of intraocular pressure. However, he observed that five of these eyes had higher levels of pressure an average of 9 months after treatment than before treatment. This tended to occur in older patients and in persons who had glaucoma for longer periods of time. He speculated that the laser may cause further trabecular damage in these eyes because more energy is absorbed by deeply pigmented trabecular meshwork.

Prior filtering surgery

Robin[68] demonstrated a significant reduction of intraocular pressure in six of seven eyes that previously had undergone uncomplicated conventional surgery. Fellman et al.[16] reported that they were able to stabilize visual function in 67% of primary open-angle glaucoma eyes (25 patients, 30 eyes) with failing blebs and progressive posttrabeculectomy field loss. Hence, it appears that even though the structural and functional capabilities of the trabecular meshwork may be altered after filtering surgery, argon laser trabeculoplasty may still have an effect.

Congenital/juvenile glaucoma

Characteristically, patients under 40 years of age have not responded well to argon laser trabeculoplasty. Eyes of young individuals often have significant postoperative inflammation and a paradoxical and prolonged rise in intraocular pressure. Eyes with juvenile open-angle glaucoma have been reported to respond minimally, and 60% to 100% of these individuals have been classified as failures and required subsequent filtering surgery.[17,28,120]

Some eyes with congenital glaucoma (developmental angle anomaly) had lower intraocular pressure after treatment. Spaeth[86] claimed a 63% success rate in eight eyes with congenital glaucoma. Robin and Pollack[68] reported reduced intraocular pressure in two of four treated eyes that had undergone previous goniotomies resulting in initially lower pressure.

Angle recession

The rate of successful treatment for eyes with angle recession may depend on preoperative treatment pressures. Thomas et al.[92] treated four eyes with an average pretreatment pressure of 21.8 mm Hg. There was a subsequent lowering of 5 mm Hg and a 75% success rate in these eyes. Robin and Pollack[68] reported lowering pressure in four eyes with a mean pretreatment pressure of 40 mm Hg; however, treatment was not sufficient to prevent further damage.

Uveitis

Most of the data reporting resultant intraocular pressure in eyes with uveitis after laser trabeculoplasty did not consider the type or severity of the uveitis. In general, these eyes respond poorly.[28,42,68] However, Thomas[92] reported successful outcomes and avoided additional surgery in three of four treated eyes. These observations led Spaeth[86] to speculate that if there is minimal inflammation or structural damage to the trabecular meshwork, an eye may respond favorably to argon laser trabeculoplasty. However, no improvement would be expected in eyes with extensively blocked trabecular meshworks or when the laser trabeculoplasty exacerbates the uveitis.

Miscellaneous

Most observations regarding other secondary glaucomas are based on very few eyes or case reports. Those with iridocorneal endothelial syndrome and trabeculodysgenesis have not responded favorably.[86,92] Eyes with Sturge-Weber syndrome respond variably; Spaeth et al.[86] and Lieberman et al.[42] reported treating three eyes without an adequate response, and Robin and Pollack[68] reported sufficiently reduced pressure in two such eyes. Two eyes with steroid-induced glaucoma did not demonstrate sufficient lowering.[92]

Onset and Duration

Most investigators believe that the optimal effect of argon laser trabeculoplasty occurs within the first 4 to 6 weeks postoperatively. If intraocular pressure is not substantially lower by this time, additional therapy should be initiated to prevent further optic nerve damage.

Several early studies demonstrated a stable intraocular pressure for 6 months to 1 year postoperatively.* Wise[124] reported stable intraocular pressure for up to 4 years in some eyes. Recently, however, the pressure-lowering effect of laser trabeculoplasty has been reported to decrease over time, leading to eventual surgical intervention. Schwartz et al.[79] followed 82 phakic eyes and demonstrated a 46% success rate after 5 years. Interestingly, in this study, eyes of black patients showed only 32% success whereas eyes of white patients were successfully treated in 65% of cases after the 5-year follow-up period. Additional long-term studies are needed to confirm these findings.

Argon laser trabeculoplasty as an initial therapy for glaucoma

The success of argon laser trabeculoplasty in eyes treated with maximal tolerated medical therapy has motivated several studies of laser trabeculoplasty as a primary therapy in glaucoma treatment.[55,73,90,131] If successful, argon laser trabeculoplasty might be more comfortable for the patient and could avoid difficulties with drug treatment compliance. Also, it would eliminate drug-related side effects. Preliminary reports have indicated that 55% to 83% of eyes treated in this manner had successfully lower intraocular pressure without using medication. Mean follow-up periods ranged from 7½ to 12 months. Success rates appeared to correlate with the presence of definable angle landmarks and the level of preoperative intraocular pressure. Complications were similar to those found in medically treated eyes undergoing laser trabeculoplasty. To address the efficacy of this treatment modality, a national multicentered trial (the Glaucoma Laser Trial) is presently being conducted.

Repeat argon laser trabeculoplasty

Several reports have examined the effects of repeating argon laser trabeculoplasty in eyes which have been treated previously throughout 360 degrees.[3,6,54,65,88] Brown et al.[6] and Starita et al.[88] reported a decrease of intraocular pressure in 38% to 53%, respectively, of the eyes in which they repeated treatment. However, there was a risk of sustained intraocular pressure rise of 12% in each study, and this necessitated immediate surgical intervention in some eyes. Therefore, whether to repeat trabeculoplasty remains a controversial issue.

---

*References 17, 28, 42, 80, 92, 118.

COMPLICATIONS OF ARGON LASER TRABECULOPLASTY

A variety of complications may be encountered after laser trabeculoplasty. These include increased intraocular pressure, uveitis, peripheral anterior synechiae, hemorrhage, corneal burns, corneal edema, visual field loss, and pain (see box below).

Elevated Intraocular Pressure

As many as 50% of eyes that undergo laser trabeculoplasty develop elevated intraocular pressure postoperatively. Most often, it is transient and less than 10 mm Hg. However, in a small percentage of eyes the increase can be marked (greater than 20 mm Hg) and may be associated with loss of visual field.[91,114]

The magnitude and frequency of elevated postoperative pressure seems to be related to the amount of treatment administered. Weinreb et al.[113,114] demonstrated that the incidence as well as the magnitude of the postoperative rise in pressure was significantly greater in eyes that had received 100 laser burns (over 360 degrees) compared with 50 laser burns (over 180 degrees). In contrast to the eyes with transient elevations of intraocular pressure in the immediate postoperative period, the pressure in some eyes may increase beginning several days after treatment. Generally, this rise in pressure is not severe (less than 10 mm Hg) and will decrease to pretreatment levels or lower after several weeks. Rarely, the rise in pressure is sustained and requires trabeculectomy. It may be associated with uveitis[42] and formation of peripheral anterior synechiae[120] and is more common in the eyes of patients younger than 40 years old. The incidence of postlaser rises in intraocular pressure is lower when burns are placed along the anterior portion of the trabecular meshwork than when they are placed posteriorly.[45,81]

Whether transient elevated intraocular pressure has an effect on long-term prognosis and treatment is not known. Thomas[92] found a 21% incidence of transient elevated intraocular pressure (ranging between 1 and 19 mm Hg) and commented that these elevations did not reflect failure of laser trabeculoplasty. Forbes,[17] however, found a posttreatment rise greater than 6 mm Hg in 21% of treated eyes and noted that the rate of failure in this group was twice the failure rate of the entire group.

Trabeculectomy specimens have been obtained from several eyes with persistent, medically unresponsive elevation of intraocular pressure following argon laser trabeculoplasty.[22] Histopathologic examination has revealed that there is an inflammatory response that is predominantly confined to the trabecular meshwork; this did not necessarily correlate with the amount of anterior chamber inflammation. Apparently the laser treatment stimulated the release of inflammatory cells and debris into the anterior chamber and the trabecular meshwork. This led to decreased outflow and subsequently increased intraocular pressure.

Many attempts have been made to prevent the immediate rise in postoperative intraocular pressure. Ruderman et al.[75] demonstrated no difference in intraocular pressure response between eyes treated with topically administered prednisolone acetate 1% or placebo before argon laser trabeculoplasty. Pretreatment with topical nonsteroidal agents, the cyclooxygenase inhibitors flurbiprofen and indomethacin, also did not influence the postoperative rise in pressure.[30,58,111,112] The incidence of postlaser elevation of intraocular pressure has been reported to be lower using the Ritch lens compared with the Goldmann lens.[8]

The use of oral hyperosmotic agents may prevent postoperative intraocular pressure increases. Several investigators have used oral isosorbide or glycerol in patients with eyes that have marked visual field loss (i.e., splitting fixation or central island) with good postoperative intraocular pressure control.

The use of 4% pilocarpine immediately after laser trabeculoplasty has been reported to reduce the severity of the postlaser pressure rise.[57] Most recently, the drug para-aminoclonidine, an alpha-agonist, has been shown to reduce the frequency and magnitude of the pressure rise.[3,71] It has been approved by the FDA for this use.

Progressive Visual Field Loss

Visual field loss can progress soon after laser trabeculoplasty. This may be caused by either tran-

---

COMPLICATIONS OF ARGON LASER TRABECULOPLASTY

Elevated intraocular pressure
Progressive visual field loss
Peripheral anterior synechiae
Iritis
Hemorrhage
Corneal abrasion
Corneal edema and endothelial burns
Pain
Syncope/vasovagal response

sient or persistent elevation of intraocular pressure.[114,115] It has been reported to occur also in eyes in which posttreatment intraocular pressure was not elevated above the pretreatment level.[29] Possible mechanisms include (1) inadequate pressure lowering, (2) the occurrence of intraocular pressure spikes not relieved by laser trabeculoplasty or not detected, or (3) visual field loss related to the natural history of the glaucomatous processes or other factors besides intraocular pressure.

Iritis

Iritis may be present in many eyes following laser trabeculoplasty. Generally, it is mild and clears rapidly. Occasionally, it may persist for months. There is evidence that the inflammation correlates with a minimal transient disruption of the blood-aqueous barrier, as measured by fluorophotometry, that occurs following the procedure.[15] Routine topical corticosteroid therapy probably is not indicated unless there is significant postoperative inflammation.

Peripheral Anterior Synechiae

Peripheral anterior synechiae can occur in up to 43% of eyes that have undergone argon laser trabeculoplasty.[97] They appear to occur more frequently when laser burns are placed directly over Schlemm's canal (posterior trabecular meshwork) as compared with similar laser burns placed in the anterior trabecular meshwork. Synechiae are characteristically small and rarely reach beyond the scleral spur. Their presence has not been demonstrated to have any effect on the postoperative intraocular pressure, and their long-term consequence is not known.

Hemorrhage

Hemorrhage is an uncommon problem. It may result from inadvertent photocoagulation of blood

---

CONTRAINDICATIONS FOR ARGON LASER TRABECULOPLASTY

Uncooperative patient
Inadequate visualization
Hazy media
Complete angle-closure
Corneal edema
Uveitic glaucoma*
Juvenile glaucoma*
Less than 35 years old*

---

*Relative contraindications.

vessels in the iris root or from accidentally hitting a circumferential ciliary vessel. Very rarely, blood may be seen emanating from the trabecular meshwork, perhaps the result of reflux from Schlemm's canal. Bleeding usually can be controlled by applying pressure to the eye with the contact lens. If a bleeding site can be identified, it can be photocoagulated with the argon laser (e.g., 200 mW, 200 μm, 0.2 seconds). Thomas[91,92] reported that the hemorrhage did not appear to affect the intraocular pressure response adversely.

Corneal Complications

Corneal abrasions and burns are probably of little significance. Epithelial burns disappear within hours of treatment. Endothelial burns have also been reported and may contribute to focal corneal edema. No change in the postoperative central corneal endothelial cell density has been found 1 to 4 months postoperatively.[96] Corneal edema has been reported in a small number of eyes with an underlying corneal disorder such as Fuchs' endothelial dystrophy[118] or Chandler's syndrome. Also, edema has been reported in association with significant posttreatment elevation of intraocular pressure. The long-term consequence of burns on the corneal endothelium is unknown.

Pain

When the eye is topically anesthetized, pain is uncommon. Inadvertent photocoagulation of the ciliary band may produce pain. There may be postoperative pain and photophobia if significant iritis is present, but this is usually ameliorated with anti-inflammatory treatment.

Contraindications

Argon laser trabeculoplasty should not be performed in uncooperative patients and in patients with inadequate visualization caused by hazy media or corneal edema. The iridocorneal angle must be sufficiently open to perform the treatment. Patients with complete angle-closure will not benefit from laser treatment. Relative contraindications should include those patients with uveitic glaucoma, juvenile glaucoma, and those less than 35 years old. These are summarized in the box at left.

PATHOPHYSIOLOGY OF ARGON LASER TRABECULOPLASTY

Decreased intraocular pressure following laser trabeculoplasty is associated with increased facility of aqueous outflow.[118,128] Initially, it was believed that a direct communication between the anterior chamber and Schlemm's canal was needed to produce this effect. Histopathologic studies have shown this to be incorrect.[50,72]

Although several mechanisms have been proposed, the basis for the improved outflow has not been fully delineated. Wise[123] initially proposed that laser treatment caused shrinkage of the inner "trabecular ring" with resultant separation of the trabecular sheets and opening of the aqueous channels in the trabecular meshwork. Little experimental data exist to support this concept.[50] However, if this hypothesis is correct, it may follow that these shrunken trabecular sheets can pull on the inner wall of Schlemm's canal and open its lumen. This would be important if Moses'[56] theory of glaucoma is correct. He has suggested that the ostia of the collector channels may be occluded by apposition of the inner wall of Schlemm's canal, contributing to trabecular meshwork dysfunction in glaucomatous eyes.

Morphologic changes in the trabecular meshwork immediately following argon laser trabeculoplasty have been studied in nonglaucomatous cynomolgus monkeys. Melamed et al.[53] were able to demonstrate coagulative necrosis of the treated tissue and disruption of trabecular beams with fragmented cells and fibrocellular tissue noted in the juxtacanalicular trabecular meshwork. They speculated that these changes caused the elevated post-treatment intraocular pressure. In this study, trabecular cells were absent from trabecular beams, and some cells were observed in different stages of leaving the beams as well as phagocytizing debris.

Rodrigues et al.[72] have investigated the acute and long-term histopathologic effects of laser trabeculoplasty in specimens obtained at trabeculectomy following laser therapy in human eyes. Early changes were similar to those found in monkeys. There was disruption of trabecular beams and accumulation of cellular and fibrinous debris. The corneal endothelial cells adjacent to the laser burn showed extension of cytoplasmic processes, cytoplasmic edema and nuclear irregularity (Fig. 31-3). One week after treatment, shrinkage of treated uveal and corneoscleral trabecular meshwork was noted in a localized area (50 to 60 μm). Trabecular meshwork away from the area of laser treatment appeared normal. Tissues that were excised at longer intervals after laser treatment (6 months to 1 year) demonstrated confluent areas of fibrosis and abnormally migrating corneal endothelial cells lining the uveal meshwork and occluding the trabecular spaces, possibly obstructing aqueous outflow (Fig. 31-4).

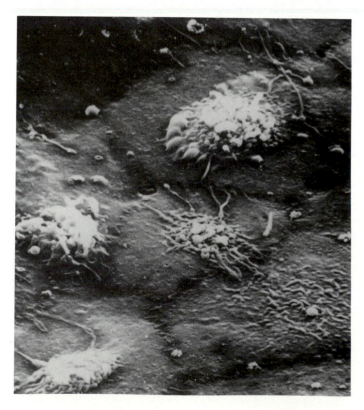

Fig. 31-3 Corneal endothelial cells near Schwalbe's line demonstrating nuclear and cytoplasmic irregularities 24 hours after argon laser treatment. (SEM ×440.) (From Rodrigues, MM, et al: Ophthalmology 89:198, 1982)

In addition to the mechanical and thermal effects of the laser burn, there are biologic effects that are best observed several months following treatment. As previously mentioned, Rodrigues et al.[72] were able to demonstrate areas of fibrosis and migration of corneal endothelial cells (and possibly trabecular cells or fibroblasts) over previously treated areas. Although the fibrosis may cause the meshwork to bow inward and subsequently open Schlemm's canal, it may also result in the formation of a less porous cellular lining.

Some investigators have proposed that the intraocular pressure–lowering effect of laser trabeculoplasty may be a biologic response related to increased or altered production of glycosaminoglycans by trabecular cells lining the aqueous channels. Van Buskirk et al.[101] documented in vitro a change in the synthesis or turnover of the extracellular matrix of the trabeculum following laser trabeculoplasty. The clinical significance of this observation has not been determined.

ALTERNATIVE LASER TREATMENTS

Nd:YAG Laser Angle Treatment/Trabeculopuncture

There are several reports of successful use of Q-switched ruby[35,36] or Nd:YAG[102,104] lasers to penetrate the trabecular meshwork into Schlemm's canal in monkeys. These fistulas, however, close after a short period of time, and the pressures that were initially lowered return to pretreatment levels. Closure appears to be related to scar formation and possible downward migration of corneal endothelial cells.

Limited clinical work has been done with the Q-switched ruby[70] and Nd:YAG[12] lasers. In adult patients with open-angle glaucoma, Epstein et al.[12] were not able to document a substantial long-term pressure-lowering effect using the Nd:YAG laser (2 to 6 mJ) for trabeculopuncture. Gonioscopically, the surgical "holes" appeared to close over several months. In contrast, a dramatic lowering of intraocular pressure was noted in two eyes with juvenile open-angle glaucoma (in one eye, only for a short duration).[51] The authors suggested that this procedure may be helpful in selecting eyes for surgical goniotomy.

Robin and Pollack[70] studied 22 eyes inadequately controlled despite maximal tolerated medical therapy and previous argon laser trabeculoplasty (some had had previous intraocular surgery). Using the Nd:YAG laser to treat the angle with 10 mJ pulses, they reported a significant lowering of intraocular pressure 3 months postoperatively. After 1 year, 46% of eyes were controlled. Long-term follow-up is not yet available, and complications included postoperative intraocular pressure elevation, bleeding from the angle, and posterior displacement of the iris root. These results have not been confirmed. It is not known whether

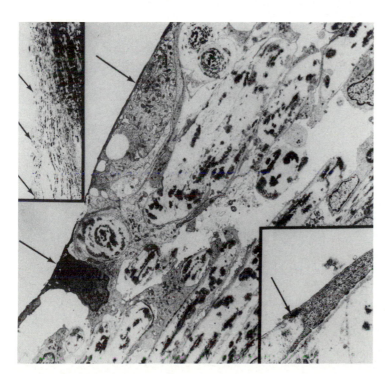

Fig. 31-4 Continuous layer of corneal endothelial cells *(arrows)* lining the inner uveal meshwork 1 year after argon laser treatment. (TEM ×5850.) Upper inset demonstrates junctional complexes *(arrows)* connecting these cells. (Original magnification ×8000.) Lower inset shows corneal endothelial cell extension *(arrows)* across inner uveal meshwork. (Original magnification ×330.) (From Rodrigues, MM, et al: Ophthalmology 89:198, 1982)

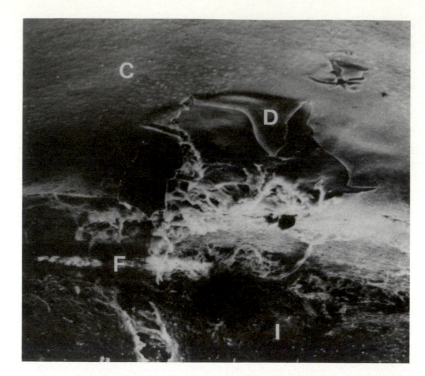

Fig. 31-5 Scanning electron micrograph focusing on changes in Descemet's membrane following Nd:YAG laser sclerostomy. *I*, Iris; *D*, Descemet's membrane; *C*, Cornea; *F*, Fistula. (From March, WF, et al: Arch Ophthalmol 103:860, 1985, copyright 1985, American Medical Association)

Fig. 31-6 Goniophotograph demonstrating high iris insertion in preoperative angle *(right)* with ciliary band becoming visible after treatment with Nd:YAG laser *(left)*. (From Kitazawa, Y, et al: Ophthalmic Surg 16:99, 1985)

the reported intraocular pressure–lowering effect is by the same mechanism proposed for argon laser trabeculoplasty.

Nd:YAG Laser Trabeculotomy/Sclerostomy

The capability of the Nd:YAG laser to produce localized nonthermal damage and to influence nonpigmented tissue provides a theoretic advantage for performing a trabeculotomy or sclerostomy ab interno. Venkatesh[106] has demonstrated in vitro that the Q-switched Nd:YAG laser can create a penetrating opening through trabecular meshwork into Schlemm's canal using 30 mJ of energy (pulse duration of 40 to 50 nsec), while causing minimal damage to adjacent tissue.

The Nd:YAG laser also has been used initially in a two-stage filtering procedure to create a trabeculectomy opening in several eyes.[110] With this procedure, a standard trabeculectomy scleral flap was made, Schlemm's canal was unroofed (or a partial thickness keratectomy made anterior to the trabecular meshwork) without entering the anterior chamber. The conjunctiva was closed, and the patient was treated with the Nd:YAG laser to penetrate the remaining trabecular meshwork and Schlemm's canal the same day or the following morning. Because the eye was never entered, this technique has theoretic advantages over conventional glaucoma surgical procedures including reduced incidence of expulsive hemorrhage, endophthalmitis, and cataract formation.

A one-stage filtering procedure, in which the

Nd:YAG laser is used to create a full-thickness sclerostomy, has been described by March et al. in cynomolgus monkeys,[21,46] rabbits,[46] cadaver eyes,[49] and a human eye before enucleation for malignant melanoma.[47] Using a specially designed contact lens[48] to create an external opening posterior to the conjunctival insertion, the investigators were able to document an immediate reduction in intraocular pressure in human and primate eyes after treatment. In monkey eyes, they reported patent fistulas and increased outflow facility for up to 6 months postoperatively. Pathologic studies[47] have demonstrated splitting along scleral cleavage planes without central corneal endothelial effects (Fig. 31-5). The energy used to create a sclerostomy in this manner is much higher than that characteristically used for posterior capsulotomy, sometimes by eighty-fold. Maximum safe energy levels as well as long-term effects of the Nd:YAG laser have not been determined for the human eye.

Most recently, ab interno fistulization using a contact laser probe has been described.[14,19,26] If such a procedure can prove safe and effective in glaucomatous human eyes, it offers the great advantage of filtration surgery without manipulation of the conjunctiva and reduced potential for postoperative scarring.

Nd:YAG Laser Goniotomy

The Nd:YAG laser has been shown to be effective in lowering intraocular pressure in a limited number of patients with juvenile developmental glaucoma.[31,130] By delivering the laser energy just anterior to the iris insertion, iris tissue can be separated from the trabecular band (Fig. 31-6). Complications include inflammation, hemorrhage, and postoperative intraocular pressure rise; follow-up has been between 1 and 24 weeks.

REFERENCES

1. Beckman, H, Kinoshita, A, Rota, AN, and Sugar, HS: Transcleral ruby laser irradiation of the ciliary body in the treatment of intractable glaucoma, Trans Am Acad Ophthalmol Otolaryngol 76:423, 1972
2. Beckman, H, and Sugar, S: Neodymium laser cyclocoagulation, Arch Ophthalmol 90:27, 1973
3. Bergea, B: Repeated argon laser trabeculoplasty, Acta Ophthalmol 64:246, 1986
4. Bonney, CH, et al: Short-term effects of Q-switched ruby laser on monkey anterior chamber angle, Invest Ophthalmol Vis Sci 22:310, 1982
5. Brown, RH, et al: ALO 2145 reduces the IOP elevation after anterior segment laser surgery, Ophthamology 95:378, 1988
6. Brown, SV, Thomas, JV, and Simmons, RJ: Laser trabeculoplasty retreatment, Am J Ophthalmol 99:8, 1985
7. Brubaker, RF, and Liesgang, TJ: Effect of trabecular photocoagulation on the aqueous humor dynamics of the human eye, Am J Ophthalmol 96:139, 1983
8. Chihara, E: Laser trabeculoplasty using the Ritch goniolens, Jpn J Clin Ophthalmol 40:819, 1986
9. Del Priore, LV, Robin, AL, Pollack, IP: Long-term follow-up of neodymium: YAG laser angle surgery for open-angle glaucoma, Ophthalmology 95:277, 1988
10. Demailly, P, Haut, J, and Bonnet-Boutier, M: Trabeculotomie au laser à l'argon (note preliminaire), Bull Soc Ophthalmol Fr 73:259, 1973
11. Elsas, T, and Harstad, HK: Laser trabeculoplasty in open angle glaucoma, Acta Ophthalmol 61:991, 1983
12. Epstein, DL, Melamed, S, Puliafito, CA, and Steinert, RF: Neodymium:YAG laser trabeculopuncture in open-angle glaucoma, Ophthalmology 92:931, 1985
13. Fankhauser, F, et al: Transscleral cyclophotocoagulation using a Neodymium:YAG laser, Ophthalmic Surg 17:94, 1986
14. Federman, JL, Wilson, RP, Ando, R, Peyman, GA: Contact laser: thermal sclerostomy ab interno, Ophthalmology 18:726, 1987
15. Feller, DB, and Weinreb, RN: Breakdown and reestablishment of blood-aqueous barrier with argon laser trabeculoplasty, Arch Ophthalmol 102:537, 1984
16. Fellman, RL, Starita, RJ, Spaeth, GL, and Poryzees, EM: Argon laser trabeculoplasty following failed trabeculectomy, Ophthalmic Surg 15:195, 1984
17. Forbes, M, and Bansal, RK: Argon laser goniophotocoagulation of the trabecular meshwork in open-angle glaucoma, Trans Am Ophthalmol Soc 79:257, 1981
18. Gaasterland, DE, Bonney, C, Rodrigues, MM, and Kuwabara, T: Long-term effects of Q-switched ruby laser on monkey anterior chamber angle, Invest Ophthalmol Vis Sci 26:129, 1985
19. Gaasterland, DE, Hennings, DR, Boutacoff, TA, and Bilek, C: Ab interno and ab externo filtering operations by laser contact surgery, Ophthalmic Surg 18:254, 1987
20. Gaasterland, D, and Kupfer, C: Experimental glaucoma in rhesus monkey, Invest Ophthalmol Vis Sci 13:455, 1974
21. Gherezghiher, T, March, WF, Koss, MC, and Nordquist, RE: Neodymium-YAG laser sclerostomy in primates, Arch Ophthalmol 103:1543, 1985
22. Greenidge, KC, et al: Acute intraocular pressure elevation after argon laser trabeculoplasty and iridectomy: a clinicopathologic study, Ophthalmic Surg 15:105, 1984
23. Greenidge, KC, Spaeth, GL, and Fiol-Silva, Z: Effect of argon laser trabeculoplasty on the glaucomatous diurnal curve, Ophthalmology 90:800, 1983

24. Gross, BR, and McCole, CE: Argon laser trabecular photocoagulation in the treatment of chronic open-angle glaucoma: a preliminary report, Glaucoma 3:283, 1981

25. Hager, H: Besondere mikrochirurgische Engriffe. II. Erste Erfahrungen mit der Argon-laser-gerat 800, Klin Monatsbl Augenheilkd 163:437, 1973

26. Higginbotham, E, Kao, G, and Peyman, G: Internal sclerostomy with the Nd:YAG contact laser versus thermal sclerostomy in rabbits, Ophthalmol 95:385, 1988

27. Hong, C, Kitazawa, Y, and Tanishima, H: Influence of argon laser treatment of glaucoma on corneal endothelium, Jpn J Ophthalmol 27:567, 1983

28. Horns, DJ, Bellows, AR, Hutchinson, BT, and Allen, RC: Argon laser trabeculoplasty for open angle glaucoma: a retrospective study of 380 eyes, Trans Ophthalmol Soc UK 103:288, 1983

29. Hoskins, HD, et al: Complications of laser trabeculoplasty, Ophthalmology 90:796, 1983

30. Hotchkiss, ML, Robin, AL, Pollack, IP, and Quigley, HA: Non-steroidal anti-inflammatory agents after argon laser trabeculoplasty: a trial with flurbiprofen and indomethacin, Ophthalmology 91:969, 1984

31. Kitazawa, Y, Yumita, A, Shirato, S, and Mishima, S: Q-switched Nd:YAG laser for developmental glaucoma, Ophthalmic Surg 16:99, 1985

32. Klein, HZ, Shields, MB, and Ernest, JT: Two-stage argon laser trabeculoplasty in open angle glaucoma, Am J Ophthalmol 99:392, 1985

33. Koss, MC, March WF, Nordquist, RE, and Gherezghiher, T: Acute intraocular pressure elevation produced by argon laser trabeculoplasty in the cynomolgus monkey, Arch Ophthalmol 102:1699, 1984

34. Krasnov, MM: Laser cyclotrabeculospasis in the system of treatment in glaucoma, Ann Ophthalmol 15:1001, 1983

35. Krasnov, MM: Q-switched laser goniopuncture, Arch Ophthalmol 92:37, 1974

36. Krasnov, MM: Laser puncture of anterior chamber angle in glaucoma, Am J Ophthalmol 75:674, 1973

37. Krupin, T, Kolker, AE, Kass, MA, and Becker, B: Intraocular pressure the day of argon laser trabeculoplasty in primary open-angle glaucoma, Ophthalmology 91:361, 1984

38. Krupin, T, et al: Argon laser trabeculoplasty in black and white patients with primary open angle glaucoma, Ophthalmology 93:811, 1986

39. Lakhanpal, V, Schocket, S, Richards, RD, and Nirankari, VS: Photocoagulation induced lens opacity, Arch Ophthalmol 100:1068, 1982

40. Levene, R: Major early complications of laser trabeculoplasty, Ophthalmic Surg 14:947, 1983

41. Levy, NS, and Bonney, RC: Argon laser therapy in advanced open angle glaucoma, Glaucoma 2:25, 1982

42. Lieberman, MF, Hoskins, HD, and Hetherington, J, Jr: Laser trabeculoplasty and the glaucomas, Ophthalmology 90:790, 1983

43. Logan, P, Burke, E, Joyce, PD, and Eustace, P: Laser trabeculoplasty in the pseudoexfoliation syndrome, Trans Ophthalmol Soc UK 103:586, 1983

44. Lunde, MW: Argon laser trabeculoplasty in pigmentary dispersion syndrome with glaucoma, Am J Ophthalmol 96:721, 1983

45. Lustgarten, J, et al: Laser trabeculoplasty: a prospective study of treatment parameters, Arch Ophthalmol 102:517, 1984

46. March, WF, et al: Creation of filtering blebs with the YAG laser in primates and rabbits, Glaucoma 7:43, 1985

47. March, WF, et al: Histologic study of a Neodymium-YAG laser sclerostomy, Arch Ophthalmol 103:860, 1985

48. March, WF, Gherezghiher, T, Koss, MC, and Nordquist, RD: Experimental YAG laser sclerostomy, Arch Ophthalmol 102:1834, 1985

49. March, WF, Gherezghiher, T, Koss, MC, and Nordquist, RE: Design of new contact lens for YAG laser filtering procedures, Ophthalmic Surg 5:328, 1985

50. Masuyama, Y: Histopathological study of anterior chamber angle after laser trabeculoplasty in cynomolgus monkeys, Acta Soc Ophthalmol Jpn 88:1007, 1984

51. Melamed, S, Latina, MA, and Epstein, DL: Neodymium: YAG laser trabeculopuncture in juvenile open-angle glaucoma, Ophthalmol 94:163, 1987

52. Melamed, S, Pei, J, Puliafito, CA, and Epstein, DL: Q-switched Neodymium-YAG laser trabeculopuncture in monkeys, Arch Ophthalmol 103:129, 1985

53. Melamed, S, Pei, J, and Epstein, DL: Short-term effect of argon laser trabeculoplasty in monkeys, Arch Ophthalmol 103:1546, 1985

54. Messner, D, et al: Repeat argon laser trabeculoplasty, Am J Ophthalmol 103:113, 1986

55. Migdal, C, and Hitchings, R: Primary therapy for chronic simple glaucoma: the role of argon laser trabeculoplasty, Trans Ophthalmol Soc UK 104:62, 1984

56. Moses, RA, and Arnzen, RJ: The trabecular meshwork: a mathematical analysis, Invest Ophthalmol Vis Sci 19:1490, 1980

57. Ofner, S, Samples, JR, and van Buskirk, EM: Pilocarpine and the increase in intraocular pressure after trabeculoplasty, Am J Ophthalmol 97:647, 1984

58. Pappas, HR, et al: Topical indomethacin therapy before argon laser trabeculoplasty, Am J Ophthalmol 99:571, 1985

59. Pederson, JE, and Gaasterland, DE: Laser induced primate glaucoma. I. Progression of cupping, Arch Ophthalmol 102:1689, 1984

60. Pohjanpelto, P: Argon laser treatment of the anterior chamber angle for increased intraocular pressure, Acta Ophthalmol 59:211, 1981

61. Pohjanpelto, P: Late results of laser trabeculoplasty for increased intraocular pressure, Acta Ophthalmol 61:998, 1983

62. Pollack, IP, and Robin, AL: Argon laser trabeculoplasty: its effect on medical control in open angle glaucoma, Ophthalmic Surg 13:637, 1982

63. Pollack, IP, Robin, AL, and Sax, H: The effect of argon laser trabeculoplasty on medical control of primary open angle glaucoma, Ophthalmology 90:785, 1983

64. Quigley, HA, and Hohman, RM: Laser energy levels for trabecular meshwork damage in the primate eye, Invest Ophthalmol Vis Sci 24:1305, 1983

65. Richter, CU, et al: Retreatment with argon laser trabeculoplasty, Ophthalmology 94:1085, 1987

66. Ritch, R: A new lens for argon laser trabeculoplasty, Ophthalmic Surg 16:331, 1985

67. Ritch, R, and Podos, SM: Laser trabeculoplasty in exfoliation syndrome, Bull NY Acad Med 59:339, 1983

68. Robin, AL, and Pollack, IP: Argon laser trabeculoplasty in secondary forms of open angle glaucoma, Arch Ophthalmol 101:382, 1983

69. Robin, AL, and Pollack, IP: The Q-switched ruby laser in glaucoma, Ophthalmology 91:366, 1984

70. Robin, AL, and Pollack, IP: Q-switched Neodymium-YAG laser angle surgery in open-angle glaucoma, Arch Ophthalmol 103:793, 1985

71. Robin, AL, Pollack, IP, House, B, and Enger, C: Effect of ALO 2145 on intraocular pressure following argon laser trabeculoplasty, Arch Ophthalmol 105:656, 1987

72. Rodrigues, MM, Spaeth, GL, and Donohoo, P: Electron microscopy of argon laser therapy in phakic open angle glaucoma, Ophthalmology 89:198, 1982

73. Rosenthal, AR, Chaudhuri, PR, and Chiapella, AP: Laser trabeculoplasty primary therapy in open angle glaucoma: a preliminary report, Arch Ophthalmol 102:699, 1984

74. Rouhiainen, H, and Terasvirta, M: The laser power needed for optimum results in argon laser trabeculoplasty, Acta Ophthalmol 64:254, 1986

75. Ruderman, JM, Zweig, KO, Wilensky, JT, and Weinreb, RN: Effects of corticosteroid pretreatment on argon laser trabeculoplasty, Am J Ophthalmol 96:84, 1983

76. Safran, MJ, Robin, AL, and Pollack, IP: Argon laser trabeculoplasty in younger patients with primary open angle glaucoma, Am J Ophthalmol 97:292, 1984

77. Schrems, W, Glaab-Schrems, E, Krieglstein, GK, and Leydhecker, W: Zur Wirkung der Neodymium-YAG Laserbehandlung beim Offenwinkel-glaukom, Fortschr Ophthalmol 83:382, 1985

78. Schwartz, AL, and Kopelman, J: Four-year experience with argon laser trabecular surgery in uncontrolled open angle glaucoma, Ophthalmology 90:771, 1983

79. Schwartz, AL, Love, DC, and Schwartz, MA: Long-term follow-up of argon laser trabeculoplasty for uncontrolled open angle glaucoma, Arch Ophthalmol 103:1482, 1985

80. Schwartz, AL, Whitter, ME, Bleiman, B, and Martin, D: Argon laser trabecular surgery in uncontrolled phakic open angle glaucoma, Ophthalmology 88:203, 1981

81. Schwartz, LW, Spaeth, GL, Traverso, C, and Greenidge, KD: Variation of techniques on the results of argon laser trabeculoplasty, Ophthalmology 90:781, 1983

82. Sharpe, ED, and Simmons, RJ: Argon laser trabeculoplasty as a means of decreasing intraocular pressure from "normal" levels in glaucomatous eyes, Am J Ophthalmol 99:704, 1985

83. Shirato, S, and Kitazawa, Y: Laser therapy for open-angle glaucoma, Acta Soc Ophthalmol Jpn 84:2101, 1980

84. Shirato, S, Yamamoto, T, and Kitazawa, Y: Argon laser trabeculoplasty in open angle glaucoma, Jpn J Ophthalmol 26:374, 1982

85. Smith, J: Argon laser trabeculoplasty: comparison of bichromatic and monochromatic wavelengths, Ophthalmology 91:355, 1984

86. Spaeth, GL, Fellman, RL, Starita, RJ, and Poryzees, EM: Argon laser trabeculoplasty in the treatment of secondary glaucoma, Trans Am Ophthalmol Soc 81:325, 1983

87. Spurny, RC, and Lederer, CM, Jr: Krypton laser trabeculoplasty, Arch Ophthalmol 102:1626, 1984

88. Starita, RJ, Fellman, RL, Spaeth, GC, and Poryzees, E: The effect of repeating full-circumference argon laser trabeculoplasty, Ophthalmic Surg 15:41, 1984

89. Starita, RJ, Rodrigues, MM, Fellman, RL, and Spaeth, GL: Histopathologic verification of position of laser burns in argon laser trabeculoplasty, Ophthalmic Surg 15:854, 1984

90. Thomas, JV, El-Mofty, A, Hamdy, E, and Simmons, RJ: Argon laser trabeculoplasty as initial therapy for glaucoma, Arch Ophthalmol 102:702, 1984

91. Thomas, JV, Simmons, RJ, and Belcher, CD: Complications of argon laser trabeculoplasty, Glaucoma 4:50, 1982

92. Thomas, JV, Simmons, RJ, and Belcher, CD: Argon laser trabeculoplasty in the pre-surgical glaucoma patient, Ophthalmology 89:187, 1982

93. Ticho, U, et al: Argon laser trabeculotomies in primates: evaluation by histological and perfusion studies, Invest Ophthalmol Vis Sci 17:667, 1978

94. Ticho, U, et al: Low-energy laser trabeculotomies in primates, Exp Eye Res 33:11, 1981

95. Ticho, U, and Zauberman, H: Argon laser application to the angle structures in the glaucomas, Arch Ophthalmol 94:61, 1976

96. Traverso, C, et al: Central corneal endothelial cell density after argon laser trabeculoplasty, Arch Ophthalmol 102:1322, 1984

97. Traverso, CE, Greenidge, KC, and Spaeth, GL: Formation of peripheral anterior synechiae following argon laser trabeculoplasty: a prospective study to determine relationship to position of laser burns, Arch Ophthalmol 102:861, 1984

98. Trempe, CL, Mainster, MA, and Pomerantzeff, O: Macular photocoagulation: optimal wavelength selection, Ophthalmology 89:721, 1982

99. Tuulonen, A: Laser trabeculoplasty as primary therapy in chronic open angle glaucoma, Acta Ophthalmol 62:150, 1984

100. Tuulonen, A, and Airaksinen, PJ: Laser trabeculoplasty in simple and capsular glaucoma, Acta Ophthalmol 61:1009, 1983

101. van Buskirk, EM, Pond, V, Rosenquist, RC, and Acott, T: Argon laser trabeculoplasty: studies of mechanism of action, Ophthalmology 91:1005, 1984

102. van der Zypen, E, Bebie, H, and Fankhauser, F: Morphological studies about the efficiency of laser beams upon the structures of the anterior chamber angle, Int Ophthalmol 2:109, 1979

103. van der Zypen, E, and Fankhauser, F: Lasers in the treatment of chronic simple glaucoma, Trans Ophthalmol Soc UK 102:147, 1972

104. van der Zypen, E, and Fankhauser, F: The ultrastructural features of laser trabeculopuncture and cyclodialysis, Ophthalmol 179:189, 1979

105. van Meter, WS, Allen, RC, Waring, GO, and Stutling, RD: Laser trabeculoplasty for glaucoma in aphakic and pseudophakic eyes after penetrating keratoplasty Arch Ophthalmol 106:185, 1988

106. Venkatesh, S, et al: An in vitro morphological study of Q-switched Neodymium/YAG laser trabeculotomy, Br J Ophthalmol 70:89, 1986

107. Vogel, MH, and Schildberg, P: Histologische Fruhergebnisse nach experimenteller laser Trabekulopunktur, Klin Monatsbl Augenheilkd 163:353, 1973

108. Watson, PG, et al: Argon laser trabeculoplasty or trabeculectomy: a prospective randomized block study, Trans Ophthalmol Soc UK 104:55, 1984

109. Weber, PA, Davidorf, FH, and McDonald, C: Scanning electron microscopy of argon laser trabeculoplasty, Ophthalmic Forum 1:26, 1983

110. Weber, PA, et al: Two-stage Neodymium-YAG laser trabeculotomy, Ophthalmic Surg 14:591, 1983

111. Weinreb, RN, and Drake, MV: Treatment parameters of laser trabeculoplasty, Trans Pacific Coast Oto-Ophthalmol Soc 64:75, 1983

112. Weinreb, RN, et al: Flurbiprofen pretreatment in argon laser trabeculoplasty for primary open angle glaucoma, Arch Ophthalmol 102:1629, 1984

113. Weinreb, RN, Ruderman, J, Juster, R, and Wilensky, JT: Influence of the number of laser burns administered on the early results of argon laser trabeculoplasty, Am J Ophthalmol 95:287, 1983

114. Weinreb, RN, Ruderman, J, Juster, R, and Zweig, K: Immediate intraocular pressure response to argon laser trabeculoplasty, Am J Ophthalmol 95:279, 1983

115. Weinreb, RN, and Wilensky, JT: Clinical aspects of laser trabeculoplasty, Int Ophthalmol Clin 24:79, 1984

116. Wickham, MG, and Worthen, DM: Argon laser trabeculotomy: long-term follow-up, Ophthalmology 86:495, 1979

117. Wickham, MG, Worthen, DM, and Binder, PS: Physiologic effects of laser trabeculotomy in rhesus monkey eyes, Invest Ophthalmol Vis Sci 16:624, 1977

118. Wilensky, JT, and Jampol, L: Laser therapy for open angle glaucoma, Ophthalmology 88:213, 1981

119. Wilensky, JT, and Weinreb, RN: Low-dose trabeculoplasty, Am J Ophthalmol 95:423, 1983

120. Wilensky, JT, and Weinreb, RN: Early and late failures of argon laser trabeculoplasty, Arch Ophthalmol 101:895, 1983

121. Wilensky, JT, Welch, D, and Mirolovich, M: Transcleral cyclocoagulation using a Neodymium:YAG laser, Ophthalmic Surg 16:95, 1985

122. Wise, JB: Long-term control of adult open angle glaucoma by argon laser treatment, Ophthalmology 88:197, 1981

123. Wise, JB: Status of laser treatment of open angle glaucoma, Ann Ophthalmol 13:149, 1981

124. Wise, JB, and Witter, SL: Argon laser therapy for open angle glaucoma: a pilot study, Arch Ophthalmol 97:319, 1979

125. Witschel, B, Danheim, F, and Rassow, B: Experimental studies on laser trabeculo-puncture, Adv Ophthalmol 34:197, 1977

126. Worthen, DM, and Wickham, MG: Argon laser trabeculotomy, Trans Am Acad Ophthalmol Otolaryngol 78:371, 1974

127. Worthen, DM, and Wickham, MG: Laser trabeculotomy in monkeys, Invest Ophthalmol Vis Sci 12:707, 1973

128. Yablonski, ME, Cook, DJ, and Gray, BS: A fluorophotometric study of the effect of argon laser trabeculoplasty on aqueous humor dynamics, Am J Ophthalmol 99:579, 1985

129. Yasuda, N, and Kageyama, M: A comparative study of argon and krypton laser trabeculoplasty in the treatment of open-angle glaucoma, Folia Ophthalmol Jpn 37:764, 1986

130. Yumita, A, Shirato, S, Yamamoto, T, and Kitazawa, Y: Goniotomy with Q-switched Nd:YAG laser in juvenile developmental glaucoma: a preliminary report, Jpn J Ophthalmol 28:349, 1984

131. Zborowski, L, Ritch, R, Podos, SM, and Boas, R: Prognostic features in laser trabeculoplasty, Acta Ophthalmol 62:142, 1984

132. Zweng, HC, and Flocks, M: Experimental photocoagulation of the anterior chamber angle: a preliminary report, Am J Ophthalmol 52:163, 1961

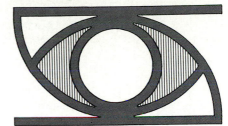

Chapter 32

Additional Uses of Laser Therapy in Glaucoma

Jeffrey Schultz

Ophthalmic lasers have been tremendously advantageous tools in treating patients with glaucoma. Laser iridectomy (see Chapter 30) and argon laser trabeculoplasty (see Chapter 31) have become routine procedures. The ability of the laser to deliver high energy densities of coherent light in a controlled fashion permits the surgeon to create effects ranging from contraction and photocoagulation to photovaporization and photodisruption (see Chapter 29). These separate processes are useful for different techniques in anterior segment laser surgery.

TRANSPUPILLARY ARGON LASER CYCLOPHOTOCOAGULATION

Ciliary body destruction is often considered the procedure of last resort in uncontrolled glaucomas (see Chapter 38). Early attempts at ciliary body destruction involved penetrating cyclodiathermy* and cycloelectrolysis.[54] These procedures were marred by relatively low success rates and high incidences of hypotony. Cyclocryotherapy, although somewhat more successful, is still accompanied by significant incidence of phthisis bulbi and visual loss, especially in neovascular glaucoma.†

Difficulties with cyclodestructive procedures may be related to two factors. First, it is difficult to quantitate the destruction of the ciliary processes via the transscleral route. Second, to achieve the desired effect on the ciliary processes, energy must be delivered through external tissues (conjunctiva, blood vessels, sclera, ciliary body muscles), often damaging their structure.

Direct photocoagulation of ciliary processes offers precision in both knowing the exact number of processes treated and in obtaining a direct effect on the target tissue. Treating via the pupil permits less disruption or destruction of intervening tissue.

This procedure is especially useful for treating glaucoma in aphakia and neovascular, uveitic, and malignant glaucomas when uncontrolled by maximum medical therapy. At least 14 ciliary processes should be visible with maximal dilation to make attempting the procedure worthwhile.[33]

Technique

This procedure is best performed using topical anesthesia. Retrobulbar anesthesia is not necessary and may interfere with the procedure because the patient is often required to alter the position of gaze to better expose the ciliary processes. The pupil is dilated widely before the laser procedure. The treatment can be performed with a Goldmann three-mirror contact lens, a Lee goniolens, or a Ricky cyclo lens. Careful focus is obtained on the tip of the ciliary processes. The laser settings (see box p. 622, top) are adjusted to produce an intense whitening with formation of a central crater at the tips of each process. It is best to avoid treating large

---

*References 2, 20, 42, 62, 70, 71, 72, 76.
†References 8, 9, 11, 21, 26, 48, 49, 55, 75, 78, 81.

```
┌─────────────────────────────────────────┐
│        TRANSPUPILLARY ARGON LASER         │
│         CYCLOPHOTOCOAGULATION             │
│                                           │
│  Spot size          50 to 200 μm          │
│  Duration           0.1 to 0.2 second     │
│  Power              600 to 1000 mW        │
└─────────────────────────────────────────┘
```

```
┌─────────────────────────────────────────┐
│   ARGON LASER TREATMENT OF BLEEDING       │
│           CILIARY PROCESSES               │
│                                           │
│  Spot size          200 μm                │
│  Duration           0.2 second            │
│  Power              150 to 350 mW         │
└─────────────────────────────────────────┘
```

capillaries because they may bleed. If bleeding occurs, the vessel can be coagulated using the appropriate laser settings (see box above). At least 10 to 15 processes, to a maximum of 35 processes (180 degrees) should be treated at one session.

This procedure creates a significant amount of intraocular inflammation, and topical steroids should be applied at least four times a day for at least 3 to 6 days. Cycloplegic drops often help make the eye more comfortable. Retreatment can be performed in 4 to 6 weeks if the intraocular pressure is not lowered adequately.

Results

Lee and Pomerantzeff first attempted this procedure in rabbits with good success.[34] The results of human studies have been mixed.* The success of the procedure may be related to several factors.[33,55] The number of processes treated appears to be critical. In the largest successful series, Lee found that adequate pressure control was not obtained unless at least one fourth of the processes were treated.[33] In many eyes, the procedure is of limited use because an inadequate number of processes are accessible for treatment. Shields,[55] however, has reported success in one case in which only eight processes were treated.

Transvitreal endophotocoagulation using an argon laser probe in conjunction with vitrectomy has been performed in an attempt to increase the number of ciliary processes treated.[45,56,57] Although this allows better access to ciliary processes, it is a

---

*References 4, 10, 31, 33-35, 39, 55, 74.

more invasive procedure and requires lensectomy in phakic patients.

Proper laser settings may also be a significant factor when treating the ciliary processes via the pupil. Subthreshold laser settings can be associated with a whitening of the ciliary processes, which represents only thermal changes at the vitreous base. The angle at which the processes are exposed to the laser beam may also be a significant factor, because this may limit the degree of treatment for each process. Finally, the glaucoma may be important because reports limited to treating only aphakic glaucoma seemed to have higher success rates.

Transpupillary cyclophotocoagulation of the ciliary processes can also be effective in the therapy of malignant glaucoma (see Chapter 70). The mechanism for relieving ciliary block may relate to a laser-induced retraction of the ciliary body.[33]

Complications

Complications are relatively mild.[33] Many patients have transient corneal epithelial changes. This may be related in part to preoperative epithelial edema that is present in many of these patients. Other complications include hemorrhage and mild iritis. Hemorrhage is usually transient and can be stopped with laser photocoagulation. Iritis is usually responsive to topical steroids.

NEODYMIUM: YAG TRANSSCLERAL CYCLOPHOTOCOAGULATION

Transscleral laser cyclodestruction can be performed by delivering light energy through intact sclera to the deeper tissues.[59,60] Beckman reported the use of both pulsed ruby and neodymium lasers for cyclodestruction.[57] The lack of availability of these lasers limited their early use. With the recent availability of Nd:YAG lasers with thermal modes, interest has been revived in this procedure.

The Nd:YAG laser seems ideally suited for transscleral procedures. The 1064 nm light of the Nd:YAG laser penetrates intact sclera better than argon blue (488 nm), argon green (514 nm), or helium-neon (6733 nm).[25,68] Histopathology studies on rabbit eyes show selective destruction of ciliary processes with little damage to overlying structures.[18,77] Clinical studies on human eyes have shown promising results.[19,52]

Technique

This procedure is presently being evaluated, and the optimal technique has yet to be elucidated.[19,52] A Nd:YAG laser with a free running ther-

Nd:YAG TRANSSCLERAL CYCLOPHOTOCOAGULATION	
Spot size	70 μm
Duration	20 msec
Energy	0.5 to 4.2 J
Number	32 to 40

ARGON LASER EXTERNAL TREATMENT OF FAILING BLEB	
Spot size	50 to 100 μm
Duration	0.1 to 0.2 second
Power	300 to 1000 mW

mal mode is required. Treatment is performed with retrobulbar anesthesia. The Nd:YAG beam is retrofocused 3.6 mm posterior to the aiming beam. The aiming beam is then focused at the level of the conjunctiva, 2 mm posterior to the limbus. Treatment is applied using the appropriate laser settings (see box above) using a total of 32 to 40 evenly spaced burns over 360 degrees. Some advocate avoiding the 3 and 9 o'clock positions to avoid possible damage to the long posterior ciliary vessels.[52] There is some suggestion that results may be better at higher energy levels, from 3.5 to 4.2 J.[73]

After the laser procedure, topical steroids and atropine are added to the patient's antiglaucoma regimen. The antiinflammatory drops are tapered according to the clinical course. The treatment can be repeated in 2 weeks if adequate intraocular pressure control is not obtained.

Results

In a 10-year follow-up study using a pulsed ruby laser, Beckman et al. reported success rates of 53% for neovascular glaucoma to 86% for aphakic open-angle glaucoma.[7] Success was defined as an intraocular pressure between 5 and 22 mm Hg. Eyes controlled at 6 months tended to maintain control at 12 months. Of 241 eyes treated, 33 were failures because of elevated pressures and 58 failed because of hypotony. Only 17 of the hypotonous eyes developed phthisis bulbi, however. Although the instances of hypotony were equivalent (12%), a group of eyes treated at a lower energy setting (6 J) had an apparent lower rate of phthisis. In more recent studies by Schwartz[52] and Devenyi[19] using Nd:YAG lasers, success rates of 69% and 62.5% were achieved. In Schwartz's series only 1 of 29 eyes developed hypotony. The lower energy settings by Schwartz (0.5 to 2.75 J) may account for this.

Complications

The most common complications of Nd:YAG transscleral cyclophotocoagulation include con-

junctival edema and intraocular inflammation.[19,52] Hyphema, corneal edema, gas bubbles in the anterior chamber, hypotony, and vitreous hemorrhage are less common complications.

REOPENING FILTRATION FISTULAS

Transconjunctival Treatment with Argon Laser

Failure of glaucoma filtration surgery usually results from external scarring.[1,16,23] Kurata et al.[32] reported success in reestablishing filtration in failing full-thickness filtration procedures with external argon laser treatment. Pigmented tissue was present in the subconjunctival tissue at the site of the previously functioning bleb with this tissue apparently blocking the external sclerostomy site. The internal sclerostomy must be unobstructed for this procedure to be effective.

Technique

The procedure is performed using topical anesthesia. After the patient is positioned at the laser, an Abraham iridectomy lens is positioned over the area of the bleb. Careful focus should be obtained on the subconjunctival pigmented tissue. The laser energy (see box above) is increased until there is subconjunctival pigment dispersion or bubble formation. Successful treatment often results in an immediate elevation of the bleb with lowered intraocular pressure. After treatment it appears prudent to initiate ocular massage to help reestablish flow. Topical steroids are also administered for 4 to 7 days.

Complications

Although there have been no reported complications with this procedure, it is theoretically possible to cause a conjunctival burn or tear that might result in a bleb leak. This can be best avoided by careful focus at the level of the subconjunctival tissue and limiting the laser energy to what is required to produce pigment dispersion or bubble formation.

Internal Treatment of Sclerostomy with the Argon Laser

Although external scarring is the major cause of failure after filtration surgery, failure can also result because of blockage of the internal sclerostomy site.[1] If this blockage is caused by pigmented tissue, it can be treated with the argon laser. This was first reported by Ticho and Ivry in 1977[66] Van Buskirk[67] and Budenz et al.[12] have reported success with the technique.

Technique

After applying topical anesthesia, a goniolens is placed on the eye. Careful focus is obtained on the pigmented tissue inside the sclerostomy. The power settings are adjusted to achieve vaporization of the pigmented tissue (see box below). With adequate treatment, one may often see a widening of the internal sclerostomy if there was a membrane bridging it. When the procedure is successful, there is an immediate lowering of the intraocular pressure associated with elevation of the filtering bleb.

Massage is initiated to encourage flow through the sclerostomy. Topical steroids should be administered for the next 4 to 7 days.

Results and complications

Ticho and Ivry reported success in 5 of 11 eyes treated.[66] Failure was attributed to long-standing external scarring at the drainage site. The previous function of the filter appears to be an important prognostic factor. In addition, eyes in which intraocular pressure lowers with massage seem to be more likely to respond. This may be related to a lack of significant external scarring.

Rarely, an acute pressure rise occurs after the procedure. Mild iritis usually responds to topical steroids.

Internal Treatment of Sclerostomy with the Nd:YAG Laser

Internal blockage is often related to nonpigmented tissue, which may be lens capsule, cortex, vitreous, or fibrous tissue. The ability of the Nd:YAG laser to create photodestruction, independent of tissue pigmentation, makes this an ideal laser for such treatment. Both mode-locked[16] and Q-switched Nd:YAG lasers[12] are suitable for this treatment.

The indications for Nd:YAG laser internal sclerostomy revision are similar to those for argon laser treatment, the one change being that nonpigmented membranes can also be lysed with this laser. A nonfunctioning cycloidialysis cleft can also be revived with a similar technique.[22]

Technique

The procedure is performed with topical anesthesia and either a Goldmann or a specially designed Nd:YAG goniolens. Careful focus is necessary at the level of the membrane blocking the internal sclerostomy to limit damage to adjacent tissue. Energy settings should be adjusted (see box below) to obtain optical breakdown and tissue disruption. Treatment can be applied across the sclerostomy and at the base of the scleral flap if this is accessible through the gonioscopy mirror. This may also open intrascleral channels for aqueous egress.

Postoperative care is the same as for argon laser internal treatment. Massage and topical steroids are started immediately after treatment and continued two to four times daily for at least 4 to 7 days.

Results

Cohn and Aron-Rosa[17] and Prager[47] reported a 100% success in five patients using a mode-locked Nd:YAG laser. Budenz et al.[12] reported success in four of five patients treated with a Q-switched Nd:YAG laser. As with argon laser treatment, success depends on the previous function of the filter.

Complications

Reported complications of this procedure are minor. We have seen patients, however, who have had acute pressure rises after treatment. Mild iritis and occasional hemorrhage can occur, but they are usually self-limited.

ARGON LASER INTERNAL TREATMENT OF FAILING FISTULA	
Spot Size	50 μm
Duration	0.1 second
Power	700 to 1500 mW

Nd:YAG INTERNAL TREATMENT OF FAILING FISTULA	
Mode	Photodisruptive
Energy	3.5 to 5 mJ
Number	100 to 400

ARGON LASER PUPILLOPLASTY

The size, shape, and position of the pupil can be manipulated using light energy to create contraction burns of the iris tissue. Thus, depending on the area of the iris treated, the pupil can either be enlarged (photomydriasis) or pulled toward a better optical position (coreoplasty).

Initial attempts at iris photocoagulation utilized the xenon arc photocoagulator.[13,15,40,46,63] Despite its success, the procedure was complicated by persistent iritis, corneal burns, cataract formation, and progressive iris atrophy. Other attempts at pupilloplasty used the ruby laser[24,43] and the argon laser.[29,36]

Glaucoma patients often have visual dysfunction secondary to miotic therapy. This can be especially pronounced if there is a lens opacity.[82] If pupillary dilation results in an improvement in visual acuity or visual fields or both, or if there is a subjective improvement in vision, the patient can be considered a candidate for argon laser photomydriasis.[65]

In a patient with a subluxed lens, the periphery of the lens may block the pupillary aperture, causing a significant reduction in vision. If the pupil can be moved beyond the periphery of the lens, then vision may dramatically improve with an aphakic correction. Coreoplasty can be successful in these cases.[63,65] In patients with updrawn pupils from any cause, coreoplasty can pull the pupil down toward the visual axis. Finally, laser pupilloplasty can be successful in breaking attacks of acute angle-closure glaucoma associated with pupillary block, especially with anterior chamber intraocular lenses where laser iridotomy has been unsuccessful.[50,58,64,65]

Technique

Argon laser pupilloplasty can (in most cases) be performed with topical anesthesia. A contact lens permits better control of the eye during the procedure. For photomydriasis, the goal is to create contraction burns around the border of the pupil. An attempt is made to cause focal scarring of the iris sphincter without affecting the dilator muscle. The laser settings (see box below left) are adjusted to create a slow contraction of the iris surface without causing vaporization or burning of the iris tissue. One row of 200 μm burns are placed circumferentially near the pupillary border. Care should be taken to avoid light entering the pupil, lest it affect the retina. One row of 500 μm burns is placed just peripheral to the first row. The desired result is a significantly larger pupillary aperture in the face of topical miotic therapy.

Postoperatively, patients are maintained on their previous medical therapy along with a short course of topical steroid therapy. Typically, this includes steroid therapy four times a day for a course of 7 to 10 days.

If there is either a reversal of the initial effect, or a complete lack of initial effect, then the eye can be re-treated. This is usually performed within 1 to 3 weeks after the initial treatment. There may be an advantage in some cases to pretreat the patient with mydriatics before repeating the laser.[29]

Zimmerman et al[82] proposed an alternative treatment by placing contraction burns halfway between the iris root and the pupillary border. They felt that this technique enhanced the pupil's refractoriness to miotics by scarring the dilator muscle fibers only. In addition, there may be some added benefit in eyes with narrow anterior chamber angles in pulling the peripheral iris away from the trabecular meshwork.

This technique involves placing a contiguous row of 500 μm spots halfway between the pupillary border and the iris root. Treatment is performed circumferentially. The power and duration (see box below) are begun at low settings and adjusted to achieve focal contraction of the iris stroma without vaporization or charring. The procedure is repeated in 1 week.

For argon laser coreoplasty,[65] a focal treatment of the iris is performed to either pull the pupillary border back to its original position or to pull it to a better optical position, as in the case of a subluxed lens. One row of contiguous 500 μm spots is placed

---

ARGON LASER PUPILLOPLASTY	
Spot size	200 μm (first row)
	500 μm (additional rows)
Duration	0.2 to 0.5 second
Power	150 to 600 mW

ARGON LASER PHOTOMYDRIASIS (PERIPHERAL TECHNIQUE)	
Spot size	500 μm
Duration	0.05 to 0.2 second
Power	200 mW

just inside the collarette border in the area to be pulled peripherally. Again, the power is adjusted to obtain shrinkage without vaporization or charring. A second row is placed just peripheral to the first row.

Results

L'Esperance treated five eyes with argon laser coreoplasty for updrawn or displaced pupils.[36] In all cases the pupillary border was pulled past the central visual axis. The average visual improvement was three Snellen lines.

James reported on 20 eyes undergoing argon laser photomydriasis.[29] After treatment the average pupil increased from 1.5 mm diameter to about 3 mm. By doubling the radius of the pupil, its area is quadrupled. Despite the fact that only eyes with poor visual prognosis were included in the study, 11 of 20 eyes had visual acuity improve by greater than two Snellen lines. Six of 9 patients showed improvement in their visual fields. Retreatment was required in 6 out of 20 eyes. Although the pupillary effects may be permanent, Sobel et al. feel that laser photomydriasis is often transient and recommend argon laser sphincterotomy for a more permanent effect.[61]

Complications

James et al. found that all treated eyes had a transient plasmoid iritis associated with moderate pigment dispersion.[29] A late iritis (several weeks later) was noted in 15% of eyes undergoing photomydriasis. This responded well to topical steroid therapy. A moderate pressure rise was noted in most patients. One patient who underwent heavy treatment with significant pigment dispersion had an acute pressure rise to 64 mm Hg. This responded to hyperosmotic therapy. Two other patients had persistent pressure elevations of 7 to 10 mm Hg over a few days. One eye developed an iris hemorrhage requiring photocoagulation.

Lens opacity, progressive iris atrophy, and persistent elevated pressure were not noted in at least 8 months of follow-up. No eyes had inadvertent retinal photocoagulation, although this could theoretically happen if light entered the pupil.

ARGON LASER SPHINCTEROTOMY

Wise reported on an alternative method to enlarge the pupil.[79,80] This method involved cutting across the iris sphincter with an argon laser using the linear incision technique with high-power, short-duration spots. The results with this technique tend to be more permanent with fewer complications than photomydriasis.

ARGON LASER SPHINCTEROTOMY	
Spot Size	50 μm
Duration	0.01 to 0.05 second
Power	800 to 1500 mW

Technique

Topical anesthesia and an Abraham or Wise iridectomy lens is placed on the eye. Treatment is begun at low energy settings (see box above) and the power is increased to obtain tissue vaporization. The iris sphincter is treated in a linear fashion, treating the entire length of tissue before retreatment of bridging strands. This permits the strands to be put under tension, facilitating their removal. Care should be taken to limit the energy used to lessen the chance of inducing a lens opacity. Only the iris stromal tissue is treated, leaving the pigment epithelium to pull apart under the tension of the iris sphincter muscle.

Results

Excellent results have been reported by Wise[79,80] and Sobel et al.[61] A large clinical series has not yet been recorded, making both the efficacy and the complications of this procedure difficult to evaluate.

Complications

As with any argon laser therapy to the iris, iritis, acute pressure elevation, lens opacity, and inadvertent retinal burns are possible complications. None were mentioned by Wise in his case reports, although Sobel et al. reported an acute intraocular pressure rise in one eye.[61]

ARGON LASER SUTURE CUTTING

Elevated intraocular pressure in the early postoperative period is a difficult problem after trabeculectomy. In some cases this may be related to excessively tight closure of the scleral flap. If the scleral flap was closed with a black nylon suture, then the argon laser can be used to lyse the suture through intact conjunctiva and release tension on the flap. Lieberman initially reported on the procedure obtaining good success using a four-mirror Zeiss lens.[37] Hoskins and Migliazzo designed a special lens for the procedure.[28]

Because sutures can easily be cut in a controlled fashion, scleral flaps can be closed more tightly, lessening the chance of early postoperative overfiltration. Following the early postoperative period,

```
┌─────────────────────────────────────────┐
│        ARGON LASER SUTURE CUTTING        │
│                                          │
│  Spot size        50 to 100 μm           │
│  Duration         0.02 to 0.1 second     │
│  Power            200 to 600 mW          │
└─────────────────────────────────────────┘
```

```
┌─────────────────────────────────────────────┐
│  ARGON LASER CLOSURE OF CYCLODIALYSIS CLEFT   │
│                                               │
│  Spot size        50 to 200 μm                │
│  Duration         0.1 to 0.2 second           │
│  Power            300 to 800 mW               │
└─────────────────────────────────────────────┘
```

sutures can be sequentially cut, titrating the degree of desired filtration.[51]

The procedure is best utilized in postoperative trabeculectomy patients with an early (1 to 2 weeks) elevated pressure. Other causes of elevated intraocular pressure (internal sclerostomy blockage, choroidal hemorrhage, malignant glaucoma) should be eliminated by examination before laser treatment. Treatment after 2 to 3 weeks may be ineffective, probably because of scarring of the scleral flap.

Suture cutting can also be done as a planned procedure. At the time of surgery, the scleral flap is tightly sutured. After surgery, the sutures are then cut in a controlled fashion to adjust filtration to the desired amount.

Technique

Argon laser suture cutting is performed using topical anesthesia and 2.5% phenylephrine (Neosynephrine) to blanch the superficial conjunctival vessels. A contact lens is helpful to flatten the tissue over the suture and blanch the deeper vessels. The Hoskins lens is specifically designed for this, although a Zeiss four-mirror gonioprism or an Abraham iridotomy lens can be used. After careful focusing, the suture can be cut with a few laser shots resulting in suture retraction (see box above).

After each suture is cut, the patient should be examined at the slit-lamp and the intraocular pressure measured. Ocular massage is often helpful to encourage outflow. Once the desired degree of filtration is obtained, laser treatment is stopped to avoid overfiltration with hypotony and a shallow anterior chamber. Topical steroids are often used in the early postoperative period to lessen external scarring.

Complications

The main complication is excessive filtration with resultant hypotony and a shallow anterior chamber. This usually responds to topical patching over 12 to 24 hours. It is theoretically possible to either tear or burn the conjunctiva, resulting in a wound leak, although this has not yet been reported.

ARGON LASER CLOSURE OF CYCLODIALYSIS CLEFTS

Cyclodialysis clefts can occur as a planned surgical result, an inadvertent complication of intraocular surgery, or as a result of trauma. The resultant hypotony can cause both optic disc and macular edema along with choroidal effusions.[14,38,53] Although cyclodialysis clefts may occasionally close spontaneously, surgical treatment is often necessary.*

Conventional surgical therapy often involves invasive techniques either to close the cyclodialysis cleft directly or to localize the ciliary body detachment. Joondeph first reported using an argon laser to reverse the hypotony associated with an inadvertent cyclodialysis cleft.[30] Since then others have reported success with the procedure.[27,44]

Technique

Topical anesthesia is instilled, and a gonioprism is placed on the eye. For a very shallow chamber, compression gonioscopy can be attempted to deepen the approach to the anterior chamber angle.[44] Laser treatment (see box above) is applied to both the edges and the depths of the cleft, blanching the tissue. After the treatment, topical steroids and cycloplegics are applied for 1 week. If there is no significant improvement, the procedure can be repeated in 1 to 2 weeks.

Results

Of the five reported cases in the literature, all responded well to treatment and over the long-term maintained normal intraocular pressures.[27,30,44] Patients without underlying macular pathologic conditions had dramatic improvements in visual acuity despite the long duration of hypotony before treatment.

Complications

All reported cases developed an acute pressure elevation within the first 2 weeks of treatment associated with closure of the cleft.[27,30,44] This pres-

---

*References 3, 14, 38, 41, 53, 69.

sure rise is usually severe and should be treated with topical beta blockers, systemic carbonic anhydrase inhibitors, and in some cases, a systemic hyperosmotic agent. Fortunately, this complication is usually transient unless there is underlying damage to the outflow pathways.

REFERENCES

1. Addicks, EM, Quigley, HA, Green, WR, and Robin, AL: Histologic characteristics of filtering blebs in glaucomtous eyes, Arch Ophthalmol 101:795, 1983
2. Albaugh, CH, and Dunphy, EB: Cyclodiathermy, Arch Ophthalmol 27:543, 1942
3. Barasch, K, Galin, MA, and Baras, I: Postcyclodialysis hypotony, Am J Ophthalmol 68:644, 1969
4. Bartl, G, Haller, BM, Wocheslander, E, and Hofmann, H: Light and electron microscopic observations after argon laser photocoagulation of ciliary processes, Klin Monatsbl Augenheikd 181;414, 1982
5. Beckman, H, Kinoshita, A, Rota, AN, and Sugar, HS: Transscleral ruby laser irradiation of the ciliary body in the treatment of intractable glaucoma, Trans Am Ophthalmol Otolaryngol 76:423, 1972
6. Beckman, H, and Sugar, HS: Neodymium laser cyclocoagulation, Arch Ophthalmol 90:27, 1973
7. Beckman, H, and Waeltermann: Transscleral ruby laser cyclocoagulation, Am J Ophthalmol 98:788, 1984
8. Bellows, AR: Cyclocryotherapy: Its role in the treatment of glaucoma, Pers Ophthalmol 4:139, 1980
9. Bellows, AR, and Grant, WM: Cyclocryotherapy in advanced inadequately controlled glaucoma, Am J Ophthalmol 75:679, 1973
10. Bernard, JA, et al: Coagulation of the ciliary processes with the argon laser: its use in certain types of hypertonia, Arch Ophthalmol (Paris) 34:577, 1974
11. Bietti, G: Surgical intervention on the ciliary body. New trends for the relief of glaucoma, JAMA 142:889, 1950
12. Budenz, DL, et al.: Laser therapy for internally failing glaucoma filtration surgery, Ophthalmic Laser Ther 1:169, 1986
13. Burns, RP: Improvements in technique of photocoagulation of the iris, Arch Ophthalmol 74:306, 1965
14. Chandler, PA, and Maumenee, AE: A major cause of hypotony, Am J Ophthalmol, 52:609, 1961
15. Cleasby, GW: Photocoagulation coreoplasty, Arch Ophthalmol 83:145, 1970
16. Cohen JS, Shaffer, RN, Hetherington, J, Jr, and Hoskins, D: Revision of filtration surgery, Arch Ophthalmol 95:1612, 1977
17. Cohn, HC, and Aron-Rosa, D: Reopening blocked trabeculectomy sites with the YAG laser, Am J Ophthalmol 95:293, 1983
18. Devenyi, RG, Trope, GE, and Hunter, WH: Neodymium-YAG transscleral cyclocoagulation in rabbit eyes, Br J Ophthalmol 71:441, 1987
19. Deyenyi, RG, Trope, GE, Hunter, WH, and Badeeb, O: Neodymium: YAG transscleral cyclocoagulation in human eyes, Ophthalmology 94:1519, 1987
20. Edmonds, C, de Roeth, A, Jr, and Howard, GM: Histopathologic changes following cyrosurgery and diathermy of the rabbit ciliary body, Am J Opthalmol 69:65, 1970
21. Feibel, RM, and Bigger, JF: Rubeosis iridis and neovascular glaucoma: evaluation of cyclocryotherapy, Am J Ophthalmol 74:862, 1972
22. Fellman, RL, Starita, Rj, and Spaeth, GL: Reopening cyclodialysis cleft with Nd:YAG laser following trabeculectomy, Ophthalmic Surg 15:285, 1984
23. Fitzgerald, JR, and McCarthy, JL: Surgery of the filtering bleb, Arch Ophthalmol 68:453, 1962
24. Flocks, M, and Zweng, HC: Laser coagulation of ocular tissues, Arch Ophthalmol 72:604, 1964
25. Fankhauser, F, et al.: Transscleral cyclophotocoagulation using a neodymium YAG laser, Ophthalmic Surg 17:94, 1986
26. Green, K, Hull, DS, and Bowman, K: Cyclocryotherapy and ocular blood flow, Glaucoma 1:141, 1979
27. Harbin, TS, Jr: Treatment of cycloidialysis clefts with argon laser photocoagulation, Ophthalmology 89:1082, 1982
28. Hoskins, HD, Jr, and Migliazzo, C: Management of failing filtering blebs with the argon laser, Ophthalmic Surg 15:731, 1984
29. James, WA, Jr, DeRoeth, A, Jr, Forbes, M, and L'Esperance, FA, Jr: Argon laser photomydriasis, Am J Ophthalmol 81:62, 1976
30. Joondeph, HC: Management of postoperative and post-traumatic cyclodialysis clefts with argon laser photocoagulation, Ophthalmic Surg 11:186, 1980
31. Klapper, RM, and Dodick, JM: Transpupillary argon laser cyclophotocoagulation, Doc Ophthalmol Proc 36:197, 1984
32. Kurata, F, Krupin, T, and Kolker, AE: Reopening filtration fistulas with transconjunctival argon laser photocoagulation, Am J Ophthalmol 98:340, 1984
33. Lee, P-F: Argon laser photocoagulation of the ciliary processes in cases of aphakic glaucoma, Arch Ophthalmol 97:2135, 1979
34. Lee, P-F, and Pomerantzeff, O: Transpupillary cyclophotocoagulation of rabbit eyes: an experimental approach to glaucoma surgery, Am J Ophthalmol 71:911, 1971
35. Lee, P-F, Shihab, Z, and Eberle, M: Partial ciliary process laser photocoagulation in the management of glaucoma, Lasers Surg Med 1:85, 1980
36. L'Esperance, FA, Jr, and James, WA, Jr: Argon laser photocoagulation of iris abnormalities, Trans Am Acad Ophthalmol Otolaryngol 79:OP321, 1975
37. Lieberman, MF: Suture lysis by laser and goniolens, Am J Ophthalmol, 95:257, 1983
38. Maumenee, AE, and Stark, WJ: Management of persistent hypotony after planned or inadvertent cyclodialysis, Am J Ophthalmol, 71:320, 1971
39. Merritt, JC: Transpupillary photocoagulation of the ciliary processes, Ann Ophthalmol 8:325, 1976
40. Meyer-Schwickerath, G: Light coagulation. M Drance (trans), St Louis, 1960, The CV Mosby Co
41. Miller, SJH: Hypotony following cyclodialysis, Br J Ophthalmol 47:211, 1963

42. Nesterov, AP, and Egorov, EA: Transconjunctival penetrating cyclodiathermy in glaucoma, J Ocul Ther Surg July-Aug:216, 1983

43. Otiti, JM: Photocoagulation of the iris using direct sunlight, Br J Ophthalmol 53:574, 1969

44. Partamian, LG: Treatment of a cyclodialysis cleft with argon laser photocoagulation in a patient with a shallow anterior chamber, Am J Ophthalmol 99:5, 1985

45. Patel, A, Thompson, JT, Michels, RG, and Quigley, HA: Endolaser treatment of the ciliary body for uncontrolled glaucoma, Ophthalmology 93:825, 1986

46. Patti, JC, and Cinotti, AA: Iris photocoagulation therapy of aphakic pupillary block, Arch Ophthalmol 93:347, 1975

47. Praeger, DL: The reopening of closed filtering blebs using the neodymium: YAG laser, Ophthalmology 91:373, 1984

48. Prost, M: Cyclocryotherapy for glaucoma: evaluation of techniques, Surv Ophthalmol 28:93, 1983

49. Quigley, HA: Histologic and physiological studies of cyclocryotherapy in primate and human eyes, Am J Ophthalmol 82:722, 1976

50. Ritch, R: Argon laser treatment for medically unresponsive attacks of angle-closure glaucoma, Am J Ophthalmol 94:197, 1982

51. Savage, JA, and Simmons, RJ: Staged glaucoma filtration surgery with planned early conversion from scleral flap to full-thickness operation using argon laser, Ophthalmic Laser Ther 1:201, 1986

52. Schartz, LW, and Moster, MR: Neodymium: YAG laser transscleral cyclodiathermy, Ophthalmic Laser Ther 1:135, 1986

53. Shaffer, RN, and Weiss, DI: Concerning cyclodialysis and hypotony, Arch Ophthalmol 68:55, 1962

54. Sheppard, LB: Retrociliary cyclodiathermy versus retrociliary cycloelectrolysis: effects on the normal rabbit eye, Am J Ophthalmol, 46:27, 1958

55. Shields, MB: Cyclodestructive surgery for glaucoma: past, present, and future, Trans Am Ophthalmol Soc 83:285, 1985

56. Shields, MB: Discussion of endolaser treatment of the ciliary body for uncontrolled glaucoma, Ophthalmology 93:829, 1986

57. Shields, MB, Chandler, DB, Hickingbotham, D, and Klintworth, GK: Intraocular cyclophotocoagulation; histopathologic evidence in primates, Arch Ophthalmol 103:1731, 1985

58. Shin, DH: Argon laser photocoagulation to relieve acute angle-closure glaucoma, Am J Ophthalmol 93:348, 1982

59. Smith, RS, and Stein, MN: Ocular hazards of transscleral laser radiation. I. Spectral reflection and transmission of the sclera, choroid and retina, Am J Ophthalmol 66:21, 1968

60. Smith, RS, and Stein, MN: Ocular hazards of transscleral laser radiation. II. Intraocular injury produced by ruby and neodymium lasers, Am J Ophthalmol 67:100, 1969

61. Sobel, LI, Ritch, R, and Prince, A: Argon laser sphincterotomy, Ophthalmic Laser Ther 1:87, 1986

62. Stocker, FW: Response of chronic simple glaucoma to treatment with cyclodiathermy puncture, Arch Ophthalmol 34:181, 1945

63. Straatsma, BR, Allen, RA, Pettit, TH, and Hall, MO: Subluxation of the lens treated with iris photocoagulation, Am J Ophthalmol, 61:1312, 1966

64. Theodossiadis, GP: Pupilloplasty in aphakic and pseudophakic pupillary block glaucoma, Trans Ophthalmol Soc UK 104:137, 1984

65. Thomas, JV: Pupilloplasty and photomydriasis. In Belcher, CD, Thomas, JV, and Simmons, RJ, editors: Photocoagulation in glaucoma and anterior segment disease, Baltimore, 1984, Williams & Wilkins

66. Ticho, U, and Ivry, M: Reopening of occluded filtering blebs by argon laser photocoagulation, Am J Ophthalmol 84:413, 1977

67. Van Buskirk, EM: Reopening filtration fistulas with the argon laser, Am J Ophthalmol 94;1, 1982

68. Van Der Zypen, E, and Fankhauser, F: Lasers in the treatment of chronic simple glaucoma, Trans Ophthalmol Soc UK 102:147, 1982

69. Vannas, M, and Vjorkenheim, B: On hypotony following cyclodialysis and its treatment, Acta Ophthalmol 30:63, 1952

70. Vogt, A: Versuche zur intraokularen Druckherabsetzung mittels Diatermieschadigung des Corpus ciliare (Zyklodiatermiestichelung), Klin Monatsbl Augenheilkd 97:672, 1936

71. Vogt, A: Cyclodiathermypuncture in cases of glaucoma, Br J Ophthalmol 24:288, 1940

72. Walton, DS, and Grant, WM: Penetrating cyclodiathermy for filtration, Arch Ophthalmol 83:47, 1970

73. Wandel, T: Personal communication, 1987

74. Weekers, R, et al: Effects of photocoagulation of ciliary body upon ocular tension, Am J Ophthalmol 52:156, 1961

75. Wesley, RE, and Kielar, RA: Cyclocryotherapy in treatment of glaucoma, Glaucoma 3:533, 1980

76. Weve, H: Die Zyklodiathermie das Corpus ciliare bei Glaukom, Zentralbl Ophthalmol 29:562, 1933

77. Wilensky, JT, Welch, D, and Mirolovich, M: Transscleral cyclocoagulation using a neodymium: YAG laser, Ophthalmic Surg, 16:96, 1985

78. Wilkes, TDI, and Fraunfelder, FT: Principles of cryosurgery, Ophthalmic Surg 10:21, 1979

79. Wise, JB: Iris sphincterotomy, iridotomy, and synechiotomy by linear incision with the argon laser, Ophthalmology 92:641, 1985

80. Wise, JB, Munnerlyn, CR, and Erickson, PJ: A high-efficiency laser iridotomy-sphincterotomy lens, Am J Ophthalmol 101:546, 1986

81. Yamishita, H, and Sears, ML: Complications of cyclocryosurgery, Glaucoma 2:273, 1980

82. Zimmerman, TJ, and Wheeler, TM: Miotics: side effects and ways to avoid them, Ophthalmology 89:76, 1982

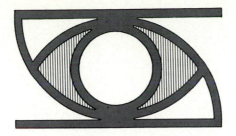

PART FIVE

GLAUCOMA SURGERY

33

Wound Healing in Glaucoma Surgery

34

Conventional Surgical Iridectomy

35

Filtration Surgery

36

Surgical Management of Coexisting Cataract and Glaucoma

37

Surgery for Congenital Glaucoma

38

Cyclodestructive Surgery

39

Setons in Glaucoma Surgery

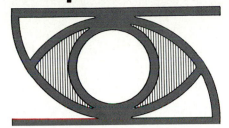

Chapter 33

Wound Healing in Glaucoma Surgery

Richard Kenneth Parrish II
Robert Folberg

The success of surgical procedures designed to treat glaucoma depends on the *prevention* of wound healing. Iridectomy accomplishes its effects because most full-thickness iris wounds do *not* heal. Likewise, the success of glaucoma filtering surgery also depends upon the prevention of limbal wound healing. After performing glaucoma surgery, the ophthalmologist must thwart a healing process that is otherwise an indispensible postoperative ally for almost all other ophthalmic procedures, especially cataract surgery. This chapter focuses on the events that affect wound healing after glaucoma surgery.

IRIDECTOMY

Full-thickness iris wounds tend not to heal regardless of the surgical technique employed to fashion them.[33,38,45,141] Two hypotheses attempt to explain this curious phenomenon. First, the edges of a full-thickness iris wound may be separated by tension generated by the dilator muscle fibers[41] and, in the absence of significant inflammation, this physical separation may contribute to the failure of the iris to heal. When the rabbit iris is incised longitudinally between the major iris arteries and the wound edges are apposed, healing occurs by proliferation of the epithelial layers and stromal fibrocytes.[41] The second hypothesis presumes the presence of an antifibroblastic factor in the aqueous humor.[22] Aqueous humor failed to support the growth of chick and rabbit fibroblasts in tissue culture and rabbit iris in organ culture.[63] The initiation of proliferation of human Tenon's capsule fibro-

blasts in tissue culture was inhibited by aqueous humor obtained from otherwise normal patients who had undergone cataract extraction.[48] The growth of these cells in vitro was stimulated by aqueous humor from eyes with poor prognoses for filtering surgery success, such as neovascular glaucoma.[48] Aqueous humor taken from owl monkey eyes before filtering surgery inhibited the initiation of subconjunctival fibroblast growth in tissue culture, but postoperative aqueous humor supported proliferation.[101] To date, an aqueous humor antifibroblastic substance has not been definitively identified or characterized.

The closure of argon laser iridectomy wounds has been reported.[105,116] The argon laser cuts the iris by generating thermal energy in the stromal melanocytes and, more significantly, in the iris pigment epithelium. The iris pigment epithelium may be stimulated to proliferate in response to the injury and may cover the laser iridectomy site.[105] Regrowth of the iris pigment epithelium over the laser iridectomy site must be distinguished clinically from primary failure to perforate the pigment epithelium. In contrast, the concussive effect of the Nd:YAG laser fashions an iridectomy by disrupting and displacing the pigment epithelium over a larger area than does the argon laser. It is generally accepted that Nd:YAG laser iridectomies, though usually somewhat smaller than argon laser iridectomies, are less likely to close;[61,93,105,116] however, closure of an Nd:YAG laser iridectomy has been reported in association with chronic intraocular inflammation.[115]

Table 33-1   Filtering surgery outcome by age group

Age (years)	Follow-up (months) (mean ± SD)	Outcome				Total successes
		CS	QS	QF	CF	
0-9	32 ± 16	0	0	0	6	0 (0%)
10-19	40 ± 20	3	4	1	11	7 (37%)
20-29	33 ± 21	6	4	2	14	10 (38%)
30-39	30 ± 18	9	8	2	6	17 (68%)
40-49	41 ± 24	17	9	7	8	26 (63%)

From Gressel, MG, Heuer, DK, and Parrish, RK: Trabeculectomy in young patients, Ophthalmology 91:1244, 1984
SD, standard deviation; *CS*, complete success; *QS*, qualified success; *QF*, qualified failure; *CF*, complete failure.

Table 33-2   Series of glaucoma filtering surgery in blacks

Authors	Procedure	Success rate		Success criteria	Follow-up (months)	Age (years)	
						Range	Mean
Bakker and Manku[6]	T	31/39	(80%)	IOP <22 mm Hg	>3	20-75	55.4
	S	29/39	(74%)	IOP <22 mm Hg			
David, Freedman, and Luntz[23]	T	40/47	(85%)	IOP <22 mm Hg	>3	25-73	51.7
Welsh[139]	T	36/49	(73%)	IOP <20 mm Hg	>6	35-75	—
Miller and Barber[84]	T	19/29	(65%)	IOP <20 mm Hg	>3	—	—
Merritt[83]	T(23),S(4),P(9)	70/122	(57%)	IOP <21 mm Hg	>12	0-80	52.3
Ferguson and MacDonald[28]	T	8/36	(22%)	IOP <22 mm Hg	>6	27-76	57.2
Freedman, Shen, and Ahrens[31]	T	42/50	(84%)	IOP <21 mm Hg	>24	40-78	58.5
Thommy and Bhar[134]	T	53/64	(82%)	IOP <20 mm Hg	19	—	56.8
Kietzman[60]	T	106/111	(95%)	IOP <20 mm Hg	>6	36-72	—
	P	164/221	(74%)	IOP <20 mm Hg	>4	—	—
Sandford-Smith[110]	T	165/196	(84%)				
	P	33/51	(65%)	IOP <20 mm Hg	>3	—	—
Ben Sira and Ticho[12]	O	16/27	(60%)				
Ben Ezra and Chirambo[11]	T	25/27	(93%)	IOP <18 mm Hg	>6	—	36
Schimek and Williamson[112]	T	79/100	(79%)	IOP <21 mm Hg	2-12	>50	—
	T	19/23	(83%)	IOP <20 mm Hg	>6	48-83*	66.4*

T, Trabeculectomy; *S*, Scheie Procedure (thermosclerostomy); *P*, Posterior lip sclerectomy; *O*, 9 Lagrange sclerotomies, 6 Scheie procedures, 12 Elliot trephinations; *IOP*, intraocular pressure; —, not specified.
*Age range and mean for overall series, not just blacks.

GLAUCOMA FILTERING OPERATIONS

The following factors interact to influence the outcome of glaucoma filtering procedures:

1. Patient characteristics
   a. Age at the time of surgery
   b. Race
2. The type of glaucoma
3. The type of filtering procedure

Patient Characteristics

Age

Retrospective studies have indicated that filtration surgery is more likely to be successful in older patients rather than in younger ones.[15,39,69,119] In the largest published series of filtering surgery results in young patients, 117 trabeculectomies were performed on 108 eyes of 98 patients aged 50 or younger.[39] Thirty-nine operations (33%) were performed for primary nondevelopmental glaucomas, 50 (43%) for secondary nonneovascular glaucomas, and 17 (15%) for neovascular glaucoma. The results of the surgical outcome by age group are shown in Table 33-1.[39] The 56% overall success of trabeculectomy in nonneovascular eyes in this series is substantially lower than the 75% to 90% success rates reported in primary nonneovascular glaucomas in older patients.[57,104,108,114] The relative success of filtration surgery in the elderly has been attributed to "senescence of wound healing with aging."

Table 33-3 Series of trabeculectomy in aphakic eyes

Authors	Success rate	Success criteria	Follow-up (months)	Age (years) Range	Age (years) Mean
Schwartz and Anderson[114]	4/12 (33%)*†	IOP <20 mm Hg	>4	27-82	60.4
Mehta, Sathe, and Karyekar[81]	16/23 (70%)*	IOP <21 mm Hg	0-16	—	—
Herschler et al.[46]	12/31 (39%)*	IOP <20 mm Hg	12	5-95	47
Singh and Singh[126]	35/40 (88%)*	IOP <20 mm Hg	>9	—	—
Herschler[49]	21/28 (75%)†‡	IOP <21 mm Hg	>6	19-80§	61§
Sharma and Singh[120]	23/25 (92%)*	IOP <22 mm Hg	2	50-80	—
Bellows and Johnstone[8]	12/20 (60%)*†	IOP <21 mm Hg	>5	15-83	61.4
Heuer et al.[51]	32/82 (39%)*	IOP <21 mm Hg with medication IOP <25 mm Hg without medication	>6	6-83	59.1

Modified from Heuer, DK, et al: Trabeculectomy in aphakic eyes, Ophthalmology 91:1045, 1984
IOP, Intraocular pressure; — not specified.
*All cases were trabeculectomies.
†Excluding reoperations and cases of neovascular glaucoma.
‡70% of 47 cases in overall series were trabeculectomies.
§Age range and mean for overall series of 41 patients.

Race

It is widely believed that filtration surgery is less likely to be successful in black patients than in whites. It is not known if the tendency for failure is related to biologic or to socioeconomic factors, such as the accessibility to health care. A tendency toward filtration surgery failure has been reported in black patients from East Africa,* the Caribbean,[53] and from the United States.[31,83,84,112] A sampling of literature on this subject is presented in Table 33-2. In our own experience in treating black patients from the United States and the Caribbean who have excellent access to health care, we still appreciate a pronounced tendency toward filtration surgery failure, suggesting inherent biologic differences in wound healing. It is not known if these differences are related to the predilection for hypertrophic scarring or keloids as seen in some black patients.

To enhance filtration surgery in black and in younger patients, some surgeons advocate excising large portions of Tenon's capsule overlying the filtering site to decrease the reservoir of fibroblasts that can contribute to wound healing.[12,60,139] The theoretical advantages of tenonectomy have not been convincingly confirmed in clinical practice. Maumenee,[77] who initially theorized that bleb failure resulted from the inability of Tenon's capsule to absorb aqueous humor, subsequently concluded that excision did not enhance the filtration success,

but did result in thinner blebs.[78] Kapetansky[58] failed to demonstrate a significant difference in intraocular pressure reduction after trabeculectomy with or without tenonectomy in black and nonblack patients.

Nature of the Glaucoma

Anterior segment neovascularization

The nature of the glaucoma being treated is another factor in the success of filtering surgery. Patients with neovascular glaucoma tend to experience early failure of filtering surgery with closure of the fistula and scarring of the bleb within the first few postoperative weeks.[3,47,50,98] It is possible that the presence of fibrovascular tissue over the surface of the ciliary body, iris, and angle may contribute to wound healing at the filtering site. Panretinal cryoablation or photocoagulation before filtering surgery has been recommended to cause regression of new vessels and to diminish the stimulus for further anterior segment neovascularization.[3] Some have advocated cautery to the iris and ciliary body at the time of filtering surgery to ablate the fibrovascular tissue and enhance surgical success.[47,98]

Inflammation

Patients with active intraocular inflammation either related to an underlying primary uveitis[54,72] or to surgical trauma[32,78] tend to experience early scarring at the filtration site. The postoperative inflammatory response may also enhance wound healing.

---

*References 6, 11, 12, 23, 60, 110, 134, 139.

Table 33-4 Series comparing trabeculectomy to full-thickness procedures

Authors	Procedure	Success rate	Postoperative IOP (mm Hg)	Success criteria	Follow-up (months)	Age (years)	
						Range	Mean
Blondeau and Phelps[13]	T	34/42 (81%)	17.1	<22 mm Hg	12	—	59.3
	S	40/44 (91%)	13.9	<22 mm Hg	12	—	60.1
	T	32/37 (86%)	15.9	<22 mm Hg	24	—	59.3
	S	32/35 (91%)	13.0	<22 mm Hg	24	—	60.1
Lewis and Phelps[71]	T	35/37 (95%)	16.2	<22 mm Hg	60	—	58.6
	S	31/34 (91%)	15.7	<22 mm Hg	60	—	60.0
Shields[121]	T	21/26 (81%)	15	<21 mm Hg	20	6-74	38
	P	20/23 (87%)	14	<21 mm Hg	12	6-81	46
Drance and Vargas[25]	T	33/36 (92%)	—	<20 mm Hg	36	—	—
	S		—	<20 mm Hg	36	—	—
Schwartz, et al.[117]	T	25/27 (93)	—	<20 mm Hg	>6 (20 eyes)	31-82	59.7
	P or Treph	17/22 (77%)	—	<20 mm Hg	>6 (19 eyes)	48-72	61.0
Spaeth and Poryzees[129]	T	10/13 (77%)	22.2*, 17.1†	"Control of glaucoma"	>60	15-80	—
	S	12/13 (92%)	16.5*, 13.5†		>60	15-80	—
Spaeth, Joseph, and Fernandes	T	16/22 (73%)	16.6	"Control of glaucoma"	36	—	59.7
	S	23/27 (85%)	12.3	"Control of glaucoma"	36	—	53.4
Watkins and Brubaker[137]	T	—/49	17	—	>12	15-80	62‡
	Treph	—/27	15	—	>12	38-85	65‡

T, trabeculectomy; S, Scheie procedure (thermosclerostomy); P, posterior lip sclerectomy; Treph, trephination; —, not specified.
*Without medications.
†With medications.
‡Median age.

Aphakia

A high rate of filtering surgery failure has been reported in aphakic eyes. In the largest series of trabeculectomies in aphakic eyes, Heuer et al.[51] reported a success rate of only 39% in 82 aphakic eyes. The results of filtering surgery in several series of aphakic glaucoma patients are summarized in Table 33-3.* It has been suggested that filtering surgery success is greater in eyes rended aphakic by extracapsular cataract surgery than by intracapsular extraction, but this difference has not been demonstrated or reported.

Type of Filtering Procedure

Full-thickness filtering procedures enjoyed great popularity before the introduction of trabeculectomy. The apparent lower incidence of serious complications in the immediate postoperative period after guarded filtration procedures such as trabeculectomy prompted many surgeons to abandon full-thickness procedures.[13] Recently, interest in full-thickness filtering procedures has been revived because, in theory, wound healing after a full-thickness procedure may be less likely to produce scarring at the filtration site than after a trabeculectomy. Table 33-4 summarizes several series in which the results of trabeculectomy are compared to results of various full-thickness procedures. Neither technique has been shown to be clearly superior in achieving intraocular pressure control.*

Regardless of the type of filtering operation selected, surgical and postoperative complications may lead to early closure of the filtering site. Closure of the fistula may also be caused by inadvertent incarceration of the iris, ciliary body processes, vitreous, or lens into the wound at the time of surgery. Although a peripheral iridectomy is usually performed, a nonbasal iridectomy may still permit a narrow flap of iris to rotate anteriorly and to become trapped in the fistula. The poorly supported peripheral iris tissue essentially functions to close off the filtration wound in much the same way that hypoplastic iris in aniridic patients may occlude the filtration angle. Postoperative complications of hyphema, intraocular inflammation, and

*References 8, 46, 49, 51, 81, 114, 120, 126.

*References 13, 25, 71, 117, 121, 128, 129, 137.

flat anterior chamber may further jeopardize patency of the fistula.[77]

The Functional Filtering Bleb

Numerous descriptions have been made of the functional filtration bleb.[2,67,134] Subepithelial clear spaces represent microcystic accumulations of aqueous humor and are the hallmark of the functional filtering bleb. Although the mechanisms of intraocular pressure lowering in filtering blebs have been extensively debated,* it is generally accepted that the aqueous humor in the subconjunctival space either flows transconjunctivally[66] or is absorbed into episcleral and subconjunctival capillaries.[133]

WOUND HEALING IN GLAUCOMA FILTERING PROCEDURES

The surgically fashioned fistula between the anterior chamber and the subconjunctival space may fail to drain aqueous humor successfully because of excessive wound healing of the following three types:

1. The fistula may close with granulation tissue (wound closure) in the immediate postoperative period
2. The fistula may remain patent and the bleb elevated, but aqueous humor may become loculated within the thick-walled cavity during the first few postoperative weeks. This condition, termed exteriorization of the anterior chamber, cyst of Tenon's capsule, "cystic bleb," or encapsulated bleb, does not permit drainage from the bleb into the surrounding subconjunctival space[20,29,79,100,135]
3. The filtration bleb may flatten and scar to the episcleral tissue usually months to years after filtering surgery

Little information is available on the cause and pathogenesis of "cystic bleb" and late bleb scarring. There is, however, an increasingly large volume of information and interest in wound healing in the immediate postoperative period and the remainder of this chapter addresses this subject.

The events of wound healing after filtering surgery are similar to those following injury to other body sites. In most body sites, local injury leads to increased vascular permeability and the subsequent leakage of plasma proteins.[18,70] At the filtration site, plasma proteins may accumulate from damaged conjunctival and episcleral vessels, as well as from the iris, which is evidenced by the usual postoperative flare detected at biomicroscopic examination. The plasma proteins are capable of clotting after they are exposed to tissue factors.[4] Blood from the episclera, iris, or inadvertently traumatized ciliary body may contribute additional quantities of clotting factors as well as platelets, a rich source of clotting promoters,[59] and factors that attract fibroblasts to the site of trauma and induce their replication.[18,59,109]

In the immediate postoperative period, this clot may be detected by gonioscopy as a colorless to gray opacification of the sclerostomy, and it forms a scaffold for the subsequent migration of inflammatory cells. These cells may lyse the clot, but may also secrete factors that recruit fibroblasts.[18,19,26] Fibroblasts and blood vessels may then migrate into the clot. In glaucoma filtering surgery in rabbits,[27,68,85,118] monkeys,[24,40,102,103] dogs,[140] and cats,[106] the fibroblasts and capillaries (granulation tissue) migrate into the fistula primarily from the subconjunctival and episcleral tissues, although fibroblasts may also originate from iris tissue adjacent to or inadvertently incarcerated in the internal sclerostomy opening. The fibroblasts secrete collagen, fibronectin, and glycosaminoglycans to generate an interstitial matrix.[26] With time, the granulation tissue remodels as the vessels decrease in number and caliber.[26] Eventually the fibroblasts and collagen become oriented in a plane parallel to the corneoscleral lamellae.[24]

Strategies to interfere with the process of wound healing after glaucoma filtering surgery may employ one or more of the following techniques:

1. *Minimize trauma to the conjunctiva, episclera, and iris to decrease the leakage of plasma proteins that contribute to clot formation.* The use of serrated rather than toothed tissue forceps to handle the conjunctiva and iris may be preferable to minimize tissue trauma and bleeding. Use of a coaxial bipolar diathermy probe to achieve hemostasis may produce less thermally related necrosis and subsequent inflammation than the standard cautery unit.[50,96]
2. *Pharmacologically increase vascular integrity to diminish the exudation of plasma proteins.* The use of atropine has been advocated after filtering surgery, not only to create cycloplegia, but to normalize the permeability of the blood-aqueous barrier in inflamed eyes.[42] Discontinuation of topical miotic therapy, which may be associated with an increased permeability of the blood-aqueous barrier, has been recommended to

---

*References 9, 10, 16, 66, 122, 130.

diminish postoperative inflammation.[1] Corticosteroids may also reduce the increased permeability of capillaries that is characteristic of inflammation.[43] Inhibition of the early phases of inflammation, including edema, fibrin deposition, capillary dilation, migration of leukocytes, and phagocytic activity, are also beneficial corticosteroid-related effects.[44]

3. *Avoid inadvertent intraocular hemorrhage.* Failure to reflect the conjunctiva sufficiently anteriorly when developing a limbus-based flap may result in poor exposure of the surgical limbus. Subsequently, the incision of the posterior edge of the inner block (trabeculectomy) or the posterior bite (full-thickness procedure) may be made over the ciliary body instead of the anterior chamber. To avoid accidental trauma to the ciliary body, dissection of the conjunctival flap should be carried forward to the anterior limbus, and the trabeculectomy flap should extend into the peripheral cornea.

4. *Prevent iris incarceration into the wound.* Perform as basal an iridectomy as possible without inducing hemorrhage from the iris root or ciliary body.

5. *Splint the wound.* Provide maximal separation of the internal sclerostomy by facilitating aqueous humor flow through the surgical fistula without creating excessive egress of aqueous humor and the sequelae of a flat anterior chamber.

6. *Interfere with the recruitment, migration, and proliferation of fibroblasts.* The most important effect of corticosteroids on wound healing may be their ability to inhibit the recruitment of neutrophils and monocyte-macrophages into the affected area.[97] Additionally, a corticosteroid-induced diminished tendency for neutrophils to adhere to damaged capillary endothelial beds in areas of inflammation has been suggested by in vitro studies that document a decreased adherence of neutrophils to nylon fibers in the presence of glucocorticoids.[73]

7. *Alter synthesis of collagen and other matrix substances by fibroblasts.*

Pharmacologic Modulation of Wound Healing

Recently, attention has focused on pharmacologic techniques to interfere with wound healing and maintain patency of the sclerostomy after trabeculectomy surgery. The following three pharmacologic strategies are presently under investigation:

1. The preoperative[35,36,125] and postoperative[131] administration of glucocorticosteroids to retard scarring
2. The local postoperative administration of antineoplastic agents to reduce fibroblast proliferation[40,74,127]
3. The use of agents to interfere with the synthesis of normal collagen such as beta-aminopropionitrile[92] and penicillamine[14,80]

Corticosteroids

The use of preoperative subconjunctival triamcinolone has been recommended to enhance the likelihood of successful filtering surgery in patients with poor prognoses.[35,36] Intraocular pressure lowering was achieved in 12 of 12 eyes with nonneovascular glaucoma in which subconjunctival triamcinolone, 4 mg, was injected at the intended trabeculectomy site 1 week before surgery. In all cases, discernible filtration blebs, characterized by elevation, relative avascularity, and diffuse subepithelial microcysts, were produced. The authors suggest that a cytocidal effect on fibroblasts and macrophage-induced lysis of connective tissue may explain the apparent beneficial effect of preoperative corticosteroids.[36] Results of a similar nonrandomized pilot study in which a greater amount of preoperative triamcinolone, 12 mg, was injected subconjunctivally in 13 comparable eyes with poor prognoses, five at the time of surgery and eight from 3 to 8 days before surgery, failed to document a substantial beneficial effect.[7] Six of 13 patients achieved intraocular pressure less than 20 mm Hg 3 months after surgery, and three of these six patients required additional antiglaucoma medication.

The beneficial effect of corticosteroids on bleb formation and intraocular pressure lowering was established only recently.[131] In a clinical trial, the effects of no corticosteroids versus topical corticosteroids versus topical and systemic corticosteroids were studied. The mean intraocular pressure 1 year after trabeculectomy was significantly higher in the group that did not receive corticosteroids. The likelihood of producing thin-walled blebs, which was highly associated with lower intraocular pressures, was significantly greater in the corticosteroid-treated groups. No significant difference in intraocular pressure lowering could be demonstrated between the topical and systemic corticosteroid groups.

Antimetabolites

Of the antimetabolites used to decrease fibroblast proliferation after filtering surgery, 5-fluorouracil (5-FU) has received the greatest attention.[40,50,52,138] In a series of aphakic eyes with uncontrolled glaucoma, eyes with neovascular glaucoma, and eyes after prior unsuccessful filtering surgery, Heuer et al.[50] reported an increased success rate after subconjunctival injections of 5-FU were given during the first 14 postoperative days compared to similar patients who had undergone filtering surgery without 5-FU. Sixty-eight per cent of aphakic eyes, 75% of eyes with neovascular glaucoma, and 81% of eyes with previously failed filtering surgery maintained lowered intraocular pressures with a minimum follow-up of 6 months. Life table analysis of the results documented a long-term pressure lowering effect.[107] Despite an apparent beneficial effect, conjunctival epithelial and corneal epithelial defects and conjunctival suture tract leaks complicated the initial postoperative period.[50,52] A controlled clinical study sponsored by the National Eye Institute is presently in progress to determine the long-term efficacy and safety of subconjunctivally injected 5-FU after filtering surgery.[99]

Beta-aminopropionitrile

The initial event in cross-link formation involves oxidative deamination of the epsilon-amino group in certain lysine and hydroxylysine residues to the corresponding aldehyde in a reaction catalysed by lysyl oxidase.[61] Beta-aminopropionitrile (BAPN), a potent inhibitor of the copper-dependent enzyme lysyl oxidase, affects the tensile strength of healing wounds by blocking collagen cross-linking.[37,91,111,124] Topically applied BAPN after glaucoma filtration surgery has been used to decrease the tensile strength of scar tissue obstructing the fistula.[92] In a series of 21 patients, 3 months after surgery the mean intraocular pressure was less than 22 mm Hg in 18 (87%). The long-term effects of BAPN are currently under investigation.

Penicillamine

D-Penicillamine inhibits collagen maturation by interacting with lysine-derived aldehydes, which renders them unavailable for cross-linkage, and by depolymerizing incompletely cross-linked insoluble collagen.[95,123] An inhibitory effect of D-penicillamine on the synthesis of collagen and extracellular secretion has been tested in a tissue culture model of monkey and human conjunctival fibroblasts.[80] Intraperitoneal or topical D-penicillamine

has been used in addition to topical glucocorticoid therapy to promote bleb formation in albino rabbits with limited success.[14] No published clinical trials have been reported to date.

NEW SURGICAL APPROACHES TO FILTERING SURGERY

Beta-irradiation

Renewed interest in the use of beta-radiation has been suggested as a possible means of reducing postoperative proliferation of fibroblasts.* To date, the results have been conflicting and as yet no long-term clinical study has established a clear-cut beneficial effect.

Valves, Tubes, and Shunts

Various valves, tubes, and shunts have been employed to enhance the success of filtering surgery by preventing closure of the limbal filtering site. Krupin et al. popularized the use of a pressure-sensitive undirectional valve implant that was successfully used to control intraocular pressure in 53 of 79 eyes with neovascular glaucoma.[67] Despite maintenance of a patent limbal fistula, external scarring caused bleb failure in 10 eyes. Other authors have reported similar external subconjunctival wound healing,[132] and in one case one internal ostium of the valve was occluded by fibrous connective tissue.[30] To divert aqueous tumor away from anteriorly scarred conjunctiva into the orbital space, Schocket developed an anterior chamber tube shunt that is connected to an encircling band (ACTSEB). This device has been successfully used to control intraocular pressure in 18 of 19 eyes with neovascular glaucoma.[113] Success may be related to the direction of aqueous humor to previously unoperated periorbital tissue.

The most widely used of the devices to divert aqueous humor and promote filtration is the Molteno implant.[86-90] A tube is used to channel aqueous humor from the anterior chamber to a space beneath a circular polymethylmethacrylate plate, which is fixed posterior to the insertion of the rectus muscles. Despite the use of an intensive antifibrotic regimen, including systemic corticosteroids, fluphenamic acid, and colchicine, a considerable fibrovascular response has been shown to encase the implant.[88] The need for supplemental pharmacologic treatment in patients receiving Molteno implants has recently been questioned by others who have reported adequate intraocular

---

*References 17, 21, 32, 55, 56, 94.

pressure lowering without additional antifibrotic agents.[5]

Newer Laser Filtering Operations

To minimize the deleterious effects of tissue handling during *ab externo* surgically fashioned filtering operations, such as trabeculectomy, a full-thickness limbal wound has been fashioned with a Q-switched Nd:YAG laser using an *ab interno* approach in rabbits,[75] monkeys,[34,75] human cadaver eyes,[76] and patients with uncontrolled glaucoma. Whether this approach will result in long-term filtration awaits confirmation. Prior attempts to communicate the anterior chamber with Schlemm's canal have been generally unsuccessful because of subsequent scarring of the internal ostium.[64,65,82,136]

REFERENCES

1. Abraham, SV: Miotic iridocyclitis: its role in the surgical treatment of glaucoma, Am J Ophthalmol 48:634, 1959
2. Addicks, EM, Quigley, HA, Green, WR, and Robin, AL: Histologic characteristics of filtering blebs in glaucomatous eyes, Arch Ophthalmol 101:795, 1983
3. Allen, RC, Bellows, AR, Hutchinson, BT, and Murphy, SD: Filtration surgery in the treatment of neovascular glaucoma, Ophthalmology 89:1181, 1982
4. Bach, R, Nemerson, Y, and Konigsberg, W: Purification and characterization of bovine tissue factor, J Biol Chem 256:8324, 1981
5. Baerveldt, G, and Minckler, D: Molteno implant: clinical experience, pathology and animal studies, Invest Ophthalmol Vis Sci 26(suppl):126, 1985
6. Bakker, NJA, and Manku, SI: Trabeculectomy versus Scheie's operation: a comparative retrospective study in open-angle glaucoma in Kenyans, Br J Ophthalmol 63:643, 1979
7. Ball, SF: Effects of triamcinolone injection, Arch Ophthalmol 104:1749, 1986
8. Bellows, AR, and Johnstone, MA: Surgical management of chronic glaucoma in aphakia, Ophthalmology 90:807, 1983
9. Benedikt, O: Zur Wirkungsweise der Trabekulektomie, Klin Monatsbl Augenheilkd 167:679, 1975
10. Benedikt, O: Die Darstellung des Kammerwasserabflusses normaler und glaukomkranker menschlicher Augendurch Fullung der Vorderkammer mit Fluorescein, v Graefes Arch Klin Exp Ophthalmol 199:45, 1976
11. Ben Ezra, D, and Chirambo, MC: Trabeculectomy, Ann Ophthalmol 10:1101, 1978
12. Ben Sira, I, and Ticho, U: Excision of Tenon's capsule in fistulizing operations on Africans, Am J Ophthalmol 68:336, 1969
13. Blondeau, P, and Phelps, CD: Trabeculectomy vs thermosclerostomy: a randomized prospective clinical trial, Arch Ophthalmol 99:810, 1981
14. Brancato, LJ, and Yablonski, ME: Effect of dexamethasone and D-penicillamine on filtering surgery, Invest Ophthalmol Vis Sci 24(suppl):87, 1983
15. Cadera, W, et al: Filtering surgery in childhood glaucoma, Ophthalmic Surg 15:319, 1984
16. Cairns, JE: Trabeculectomy: preliminary report of a new method, Am J Ophthalmol 66:673, 1968
17. Cameron, ME: Beta irradiation as an adjunct to surgery in refractory glaucoma, Trans Aust Coll Ophthalmol 2:53-60, 1970
18. Clark, RAF, and Colvin, RB: Wound repair. In McDoonagn, J, editor: Plasma fibrinogen structure and function, New York, 1985, Marcel Dekker
19. Clark, RAF: Fibronectin in the skin, J Invest Dermatol 81:475, 1983
20. Cohen, JS, Shaffer, RN, Hetherington, J, Jr., and Hoskins, HD: Revision of filtration surgery, Arch Ophthalmol 95:1612, 1977
21. Cohen, LB, Graham, TF, and Fry, WE: Beta radiation: as an adjunct to glaucoma surgery in the Negro, Am J Ophthalmol 47:54, 1959
22. Daniel, RK: Healing of the iris in rabbits following experimental iridectomy, Arch Ophthalmol 31:292, 1944
23. David, R, Freedman, J, and Luntz, MH: Comparative study of Watson's and Cairns' trabeculectomies in a black population with open angle glaucoma, Br J Ophthalmol 61:117, 1977
24. Desjardins, D, et al: Wound healing after filtering surgery in owl monkeys, Arch Ophthalmol 104:1835, 1986
25. Drance, SM, and Vargas, E: Trabeculectomy and thermosclerectomy: a comparison of two procedures, Can J Ophthalmol 8:413, 1973
26. Dvorak, HF: Tumors: wounds that do not heal: similarities between tumor stroma generation and wound healing, N Eng J Med 315:1650, 1986
27. Ellet, EC: A study of the healing of trephine wounds of the sclera and corneoscleral junction, Trans Sect Ophthalmol, p. 390, 1914
28. Ferguson, JG, Jr., and MacDonald, R, Jr.: Trabeculectomy in blacks: a two-year follow-up, Ophthalmic Surg 8:41, 1977
29. Fitzgerald, JR, and McCarthy, JL: Surgery of the filtering bleb, Arch Ophthalmol 68:453, 1962
30. Folberg, R, Hargett, NA, Weaver, JE, McLean, IW: Filtering valve implant for neovascular glaucoma in proliferative diabetic retinopathy, Ophthalmology 89:286, 1982
31. Freedman, J, Shen, E, and Ahrens, M: Trabeculectomy in a black American glaucoma population, Br J Ophthalmol 60:573, 1976
32. Friedenwald, JS: Some problems in the diagnosis and treatment of glaucoma, Am J Ophthalmol 33:1523, 1950
33. Fuchs, E: Versmml Ophthal Gesell, thesis, Heidelberg, Germany, 1986

34. Gherezghiher, T, March, WF, Koss, MC, and Nordquist RE: Neodymium-YAG laser sclerostomy in primates, Arch Ophthalmol 103:1543, 1985

35. Giangiacomo, J, Adelstein, EH, and Dueker, DK: The effect of preoperative subconjunctival triamcinolone on glaucoma filtration, Invest Ophthalmol Vis Sci 26:126, 1984

36. Giangiacomo, J, Dueker, DK, and Adelstein, EH: The effect of preoperative subconjunctival triamcinolone administration on glaucoma filtration. I. Trabeculectomy following subconjunctival triamcinolone, Arch Ophthalmol 104:838, 1986

37. Gillespie, JA, and Burns, JK: The strength and histology of skin wounds in lathyrism, Br J Surg 46:642, 1959

38. Green, WR: The uveal tract. In Spencer, W, editor: Ophthalmic pathology: an atlas and textbook, vol. 3, Philadelphia, 1986, WB Saunders Co

39. Gressel, MG, Heuer, DK, and Parrish, RK II: Trabeculectomy in young patients, Ophthalmology 91:1242, 1984

40. Gressel, MG, Parrish, RK, II, and Folberg, R: 5-Fluorouracil and glaucoma filtering surgery. I. An animal model, Ophthalmology 91:1242, 1984

41. Hanna, C, and Hampton, RF: Iris wound healing, Arch Ophthalmol 88:296, 1972

42. Havener, WH: Ocular pharmacology, ed 5, Chapter 12, Autonomic drugs, St Louis, 1983, The CV Mosby Co

43. Havener, WH: Ocular pharmacology, ed. 5, Chapter 15, Corticosteroid therapy, St Louis, 1983, The CV Mosby Co

44. Haynes, RC, Jr, and Murad, R: Adrenocorticotropic hormone: adrenocortical steroids and their synthetic analogs; inhibitors of adrenocortical steroid biosynthesis. In Gilman, AG, Goodman, LA, Rall, TW, and Murad, F, editors: Goodman and Gilman's The pharmacological basis of therapeutics, ed 7, New York, 1985, Macmillan Publishing Co

45. Henderson, T: The histology of iridectomy, Ophthalmol Rev 26:191, 1907

46. Herschler, J, et al: Surgical treatment of glaucoma in the aphakic patient. In Emery, JM, editor: Current concepts in cataract surgery: selected proceedings of the Fifth Biennial Cataract Surgical Congress, St Louis, 1978, The CV Mosby Co

47. Herschler, J, and Agness, D: A modified filtering operation for neovascular glaucoma, Arch Ophthalmol 97:2339, 1979

48. Herschler, J, Claflin, AJ, and Fiorentino, G: The effect of aqueous humor on the growth of subconjunctival fibroblasts in tissue culture and its implications for glaucoma surgery, Am J Ophthalmol 89:245, 1980

49. Herschler, J: The effect of total vitrectomy on filtration surgery in the aphakic eye, Ophthalmology 88:229, 1981

50. Heuer, DK, et al: 5-Fluorouracil and glaucoma filtering surgery. II. A pilot study, Ophthalmology 91:384, 1984

51. Heuer, DK, et al: Trabeculectomy in aphakic eyes, Ophthalmology 91:1045, 1984

52. Heuer, DK, et al: 5-Fluorouracil and glaucoma filtering surgery. III. Intermediate follow-up of a pilot study, Ophthalmology 93:1537, 1986

53. Hilgers, JH: Glaucoma surgery in Caribbean negroes on Curacao, Ophthalmic Surg 11:808, 1980

54. Hoskins, HD, Hetherington, J, and Shaffer, RN: Surgical management of the inflammatory glaucomas, Perspect Ophthalmol 1:173, 1977

55. Iliff, CE: Surgical control of glaucoma in the Negro, Am J Ophthalmol 27:731, 1944

56. Iliff, CE, and Haas, JS: Posterior lip sclerectomy, Am J Ophthalmol 54:688, 1962

57. Inaba, A: Long-term results of trabeculectomy in the Japanese: an analysis by life-table method, Jpn J Ophthalmol 26:361, 1982

58. Kapetansky, FM: Trabeculectomy or trabeculectomy plus tenectomy: a comparative study, Glaucoma 2:451, 1980

59. Karpatkin, S, and Holmsen, H: Biochemistry and function of platelets. In Williams, WJ, Beutler, E Erslev, AJ, and Lichtman, MA, editors: Hematology, ed 3, New York, 1983, McGraw-Hill Book Co

60. Kietzman, B: Glaucoma surgery in Nigerian eyes: a five-year study, Ophthalmic Surg 7:52, 1976

61. Kivirkko, K, and Majamaa, K: Synthesis of collagen: chemical regulation of post-translational events. In Ciba Foundation Symposium 114: Fibrosis, London, 1985, Pitman

62. Klapper, RM: Q-switched neodymium:YAG laser iridotomy, Ophthalmology 91:1017, 1984

63. Kornblueth, W, and Tenenbaum, E: The inhibitory effect of aqueous humor on the growth of cells in tissue cultures, Am J Ophthalmol 42:70, 1956

64. Kransov, MM: Laseropuncture of anterior chamber angle in glaucoma, Am J Ophthalmol 75:674, 1973

65. Krasnov, MM: Q-switched laser goniopuncture, Arch Ophthalmol 92:37, 1974

66. Kronfeld, PC: The chemical demonstration of transconjunctival passage of aqueous after antiglaucomatous operations, Am J Ophthalmol 35:38, 1952

67. Krupin, T, et al: Long-term results of valve implants in filtering surgery for eyes with neovascular glaucoma, Am J Ophthalmol 95:775, 1983

68. Kummell, R: Uber das anatomische Verhalten der Narben nach Elliotscher Trepanation bei Kaninchen, Ber Ophthalmol ges 39:205, 1913

69. Kwitko, ML: Glaucoma in infants and children, New York, 1973, Appleton-Century-Crofts

70. Leibovich, SJ, and Ross, R: The role of the macrophage in wound repair: a study with hydrocortisone and antimacrophage serum, Am J Pathol 78:71, 1975

71. Lewis, RA, and Phelps, CD: Trabeculectomy v thermosclerostomy: a five-year follow-up, Arch Ophthalmol 102:533, 1984

72. Liesegang, TJ: Clinical features and prognosis in Fuchs' uveitis syndrome, Arch Ophthalmol 100:1622, 1982

73. MacGregor, RR: Granulocyte adherence changes induced by hemodialysis, endotoxin, epinephrine, and glucocorticosteroids, An Int Med 86:35, 1977

74. Mallick, KS, Hajek, AS, and Parrish, RK, II: Fluorouracil (5-FU) and cytarabine (Ara-C) inhibition of corneal epithelial cell and conjunctival fibroblast proliferation, Arch Ophthalmol 103:1398, 1985

75. March, WF, et al: Creation of filtering blebs with the YAG laser in primates and rabbits, Glaucoma 7:43, 1985

76. March, WF, et al: Histologic study of a neodymium-YAG laser sclerostomy, Arch Ophthalmol 103:860, 1985

77. Maumenee, AE: External filtration operations for glaucoma: the mechanism of function and failure, Trans Am Ophthalmol Soc 58:319, 1960

78. Maumenee, AE: Mechanism of filtration of fistulizing glaucoma procedures. In Transactions of the New Orleans Academy of Ophthalmology: Symposium on glaucoma, St Louis, 1981, The CV Mosby Co

79. McCulloch, C: Surgery of filtering blebs, Int Ophthalmol Clin 7:125, 1967

80. McGuigan, LJB, Quigley, HA, Young, E, and Lutty, GA: Drug effects on proliferation and collagen synthesis of conjunctival fibroblasts, Invest Ophthalmol Vis Sci 26(suppl):125, 1985

81. Mehta, KR, Sathe, SN, and Karyekar, SD: Trabeculectomy ab-externo, Indian J Ophthalmol 22:9, 1974

82. Melamed, S, Pei, J, Puliafito, C, and Epstein, DL: Nd-YAG trabeculopuncture in monkeys, Invest Ophthalmol Vis Sci 25(suppl):92, 1984

83. Merritt, JC: Filtering procedures in American blacks, Ophthalmic Surg 11:91, 1980

84. Miller, RD, and Barber, JC: Trabeculectomy in black patients, Ophthalmic Surg 12:46, 1981

85. Miller, MH, et al: An animal model of filtration surgery, Trans Ophthalmol Soc UK 104:893, 1985

86. Molteno, ACB, Straughan, JL, and Ancker, E: Control of bleb fibrosis after glaucoma surgery by antiinflammatory agents, South African Med J 50:881, 1976

87. Molteno, ACB, Straughan, JL, and Ancker, E: Long tube implants in the management of glaucoma, South African Med J 50:1062, 1976

88. Molteno, ACB, van Rooyen, MMB, and Bartholomew, RS: Implants for draining neovascular glaucoma, Br J Ophthalmol 61:120, 1977

89. Molteno, ACB, Van Biljon, G, and Ancker, E: Two-stage insertion of glaucoma drainage implants, Trans Ophthalmol Soc NZ 31:17, 1979

90. Molteno, ACB: The use of draining implants in resistant cases of glaucoma: late results of 110 operations, Trans Ophthalmol Soc NZ 35:94, 1983

91. Moorhead LC, et al: Effects of topical treatment with β-aminopropionitrile after radial keratotomy in the rabbit, Arch Ophthalmol 102:304, 1984

92. Moorhead, LC, et al: Effects of topically applied beta aminopropionitrile after glaucoma filtration surgery, Invest Ophthalmol Vis Sci 25(suppl):44, 1984

93. Moster, MR, et al: Laser iridectomy: a controlled study comparing argon and neodymium:YAG, Ophthalmology 93:20, 1986

94. Nevarez, J: Personal communication, 1986

95. Nimni, ME: Collagen: structure, function and metabolism in normal and fibrotic tissues, Semin Arthritis Rheum 13:1, 1983

96. Parel, JM, O'Grady, GE, and Machemer, R: A bipolar coaxial microprobe for safe transvitreal diathermy, Arch Ophthalmol 99:494, 1981

97. Parrillo, JE, and Fauci, AS: Mechanisms of glucocorticoid action on immune processes, Ann Rev Pharmacol Toxicol 19:179, 1979

98. Parrish, RK, II, and Herschler, J: Eyes with end-stage neovascular glaucoma; natural history following successful modified filtering operation, Arch Ophthalmol 101:745, 1983

99. Parrish, RK, II: Vital importance of clinical trials, Ophthalmic Surg 17:318, 1986

100. Pederson, JE, and Smith, G: Surgical management of encapsulated filtering blebs, Ophthalmology 92:955, 1985

101. Radius, RL, Herschler, J, Claflin, A, and Fiorentino, G: Aqueous humor after experimental filtering surgery, Am J Ophthalmol 89:250, 1980

102. Regan, EF: Scleral cautery with iridectomy—an experimental study, Trans Am Ophthalmol Soc 61:219, 1963

103. Rich, AM, and McPherson, SD: Trabeculectomy in the owl monkey, Ann Ophthalmol 5:1082, 1973

104. Ridgway, AEA: Trabeculectomy: a follow-up study, Br J Ophthalmol 58:680, 1974

105. Robin, AL, and Pollack, IR: A comparison of neodymium:YAG and argon laser iridotomies, Ophthalmology 91:1011, 1984

106. Rochon-Duvigneaud, MM, and Ducamp, A: Recherches experimentales sur la cicatrisation des trepanations corneo-sclerales, Ann Oculist 150:45, 1913

107. Rockwood, EJ, et al: Life-table analysis of filtering surgery with 5-fluorouracil, Ophthalmology 93(suppl):80, 1986

108. Rollins, DF, and Drance, SM: Five-year follow-up of trabeculectomy in the management of chronic open angle glaucoma. In Transactions of the New Orleans Academy of Ophthalmology, Symposium on glaucoma, St Louis, 1981, The CV Mosby Co

109. Ross, R, Raines, EW, and Bowen-Pope, DF: The biology of platelet-derived growth factor, Cell 46:155, 1986

110. Sandford-Smith, JH: The surgical treatment of open-angle glaucoma in Nigerians, Br J Ophthalmol 62:283, 1978

111. Schilling, ED, and Strong, FM: Isolation, structure, and synthesis of a lathyrus factor from *L odoratus,* J Am Chem Soc 76:2848, 1954

112. Schimek, RA, and Williamson, WR: Trabeculectomy with cautery, Ophthalmic Surg 8:35, 1977

113. Schocket, SS, Lakhanpal, V, and Richards, RD: Anterior chamber tube shunt to an encircling band in the treatment of neovascular glaucoma, Ophthalmology 89:1188, 1982

114. Schwartz, AL, and Anderson, DR: Trabecular surgery, Arch Ophthalmol 92:134, 1974

115. Schwartz, L: Laser iridectomy. In Schwartz, L, Spaeth, GL, and Brown, G, editors: Laser therapy of the anterior segment: a practical approach, Thorofare, NJ, 1984, Slack, Inc

116. Schwartz, LW, et al: Neodymium-YAG laser iridectomies in glaucoma associated with closed or occludable angles, Am J Ophthalmol 102:41, 1986

117. Schwartz, PL, et al: Further experience with trabeculectomy, Ann Ophthalmol 8:207, 1976

118. Seetner, A, and Morin, JD: Healing of trabeculectomies in rabbits, Can J Ophthalmol 14:121, 1979

119. Shaffer, RN, and Weiss, DI: Congenital and pediatric glaucomas, St Louis, 1970, The CV Mosby Co

120. Sharma, SL, and Singh, T: Clinical evaluation of trabeculectomy operation in aphakic glaucoma, Indian J Ophthalmol 29:227, 1981

121. Shields, MB: Trabeculectomy vs full-thickness filtering operation for control of glaucoma, Ophthalmic Surg 11:498, 1980

122. Shields, MB, Bradbury, MJ, Shelburne, JD, and Bell, SW: The permeability of the outer layer of limbus and anterior sclera, Invest Ophthalmol Vis Sci 16:866, 1977

123. Siegel, RC: Lysyl oxidase, Int Connect Tissue Rev 8:73, 1979

124. Siegel, RC, and Martin, RR: Collagen cross-linking: enzymatic synthesis of lysine-derived aldehydes and the production of cross-linked components, J Biol Chem 245:1653, 1970

125. Simmons, RJ: Filtering operations. In Epstein, DL, editor: Chandler and Grant's Glaucoma, Philadelphia, 1986, Lea & Febiger

126. Singh, D, and Singh, M: Pretrabecular filtration in aphakic glaucoma, Indian J Ophthalmol 26:17, 1978

127. Skuta, GL, et al: Invest Ophthalmol Vis Sci 27(suppl):212, 1986

128. Spaeth, GL, Joseph, NH, and Fernandes, E: Trabeculectomy: a reevaluation after three years and a comparison with Scheie's procedure, Trans Am Acad Ophthalmol Otolaryngol 79:349, 1975

129. Spaeth, GL, and Poryzees, E: A comparison between peripheral iridectomy with thermal sclerostomy and trabeculectomy: a controlled study, Br J Ophthalmol 65:783, 1981

130. Spencer, WH: Histologic evaluation of microsurgical glaucoma techniques, Trans Am Acad Ophthalmol Otolaryngol 76:389, 1972

131. Starita, RJ, et al: Short- and long-term effects of postoperative corticosteroids on trabeculectomy, Ophthalmology 92:938, 1985

132. Sutton, GE, Popp, JC, and Records, RE: Krupin-Denver valve and neovascular glaucoma, Trans Ophthalmol Soc UK 102:119, 1982

133. Teng, CC, Chi, HH, and Katzin, HM: Histology and mechanism of filtering operations, Am J Ophthalmol 47:16, 1959

134. Thommy, CP, and Bhar, IS: Trabeculectomy in Nigerian patients with open-angle glaucoma, Br J Ophthalmol 63:636, 1979

135. van Buskirk, EM: Cysts of Tenon's capsule following filtration surgery, Am J Ophthalmol 94:522, 1982

136. van der Zypen, E, and Fankhauser, F: The ultrastructural features of laser trabeculopuncture and cyclodialysis, Ophthalmologica 179:189, 1979

137. Watkins, PH, Jr., and Brubaker, RF: Comparison of partial-thickness and full-thickness filtration procedures in open-angle glaucoma, Am J Ophthalmol 86:756-761, 1978

138. Weinreb, RN: Adjusting the dose of 5-fluorouracil after filtration surgery to minimize the side effects, Ophthalmology 94:564, 1987.

139. Welsh, NH: Trabeculectomy with fistula formation in the African, Br J Ophthalmol 56:32, 1972

140. Wilmer, WH: Discussion on the results of the operative treatment of glaucoma, Trans Ophthalmol Soc UK 47:230, 1927

141. Yanoff, M, and Fine, B: Surgical and nonsurgical trauma. In Duane, TD, and Jaeger, EA, editors: Biomedical foundations of ophthalmology, vol 3 revised ed, Philadelphia, 1985, Harper & Row, Publishers

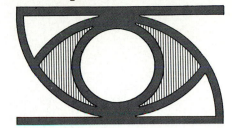

Chapter 34

Conventional Surgical Iridectomy

Jose Morales
Robert Ritch

HISTORICAL DEVELOPMENT

After having noted the hypotensive effect of an iridectomy in cases of corneal staphyloma, von Graefe[41] first reported creating a surgical sector iridectomy for the treatment of acute glaucoma. Subsequently, a large sector iridectomy, in which the iris was torn from its insertion at the root, became the standard approach to the disease.

At the turn of the twentieth century, several surgeons popularized peripheral iridectomy.[19] Curran[7,8] introduced the concept of relative pupillary block. Barkan[3] established the gonioscopic and anatomic basis for the differentiation between open-angle and angle-closure glaucoma and proposed an anatomic classification of the etiology of glaucoma to replace the previous division into inflammatory and noninflammatory types. Peripheral iridectomy rapidly became the treatment of choice for angle-closure glaucoma.[5] Prophylactic iridectomy for a narrow angle in the fellow eyes of patients with acute angle-closure gradually gained acceptance.[18,23] Surgical iridectomy has now largely been replaced by laser iridectomy.* Nevertheless, there are certain instances in which a conventional surgical iridectomy for angle-closure glaucoma is necessary.

INDICATIONS

Peripheral Iridectomy

Conventional surgical iridectomy for angle-closure glaucoma is presently indicated in situa-

*References 1, 14, 21, 27, 29, 30, 39.

tions in which laser iridectomy is not possible because of a lack of technical resources, inability of the patient to sit at the slit-lamp, or inability of the patient to cooperate. Severe corneal edema or leukoma may result in visibility of the iris that is so poor that neither argon nor Nd:YAG laser iridectomy can be successfully performed.

Both argon and Nd:YAG iridectomies may close repeatedly in patients with chronic uveitis, necessitating surgical iridectomy. Consideration should be given to performing a sector iridectomy in such cases. Excision of iris tissue may be necessary for diagnostic or therapeutic purposes, as in the case of suspected malignant iris lesions.[24] Surgical iridectomy is also a routine accompaniment to glaucoma filtering surgery and cataract extraction.

Sector Iridectomy

A sector iridectomy is indicated in a few situations. When the visual axis is occluded by a pupillary membrane or significant distortion or displacement of the pupil, sector iridectomy may be performed alone or in conjunction with sphincterotomy to ensure a large optical opening. A large optical opening is also desirable when the need for repeated disc or retinal examinations and/or treatment is anticipated.

TECHNIQUES

Local anesthesia is appropriate when patient cooperation is adequate and the procedure may be performed on an ambulatory basis.

Either a limbal or clear corneal incision may be used. The limbal approach offers the advantage of

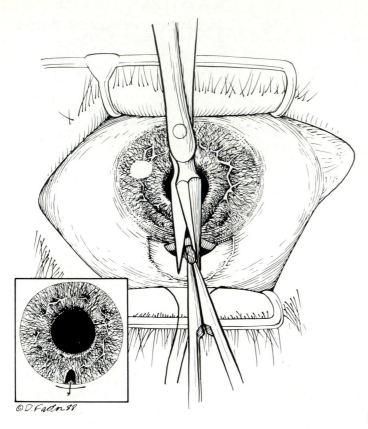

Fig. 34-1 Peripheral iridectomy. After iris tissue has prolapsed, a portion is grasped with forceps and cut with fine scissors. *Inset*, Appearance of the iridectomy after the incision has been closed by a single suture.

Fig. 34-2 Sector iridectomy. Iris is excised after externalization using a hand-over-hand technique. *Inset*, Appearance of iridectomy after closure of incision.

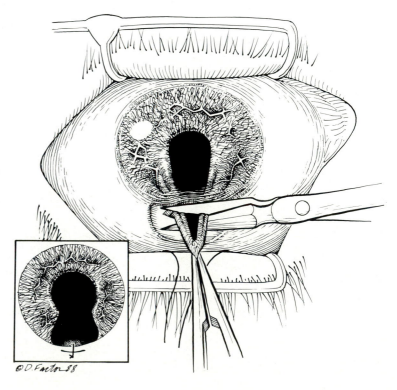

easier prolapse of iris tissue, whereas the corneal approach spares the conjunctiva, which might be important if filtering surgery is needed later.

Beveling of the incision is recommended to facilitate approximation of the wound edges at the end of the procedure. If the incision is made in clear cornea, the angle of the incision should be nearly perpendicular to the globe to facilitate prolapse of the peripheral iris. A 3 mm incision is made in the cornea just anterior to the limbus at the anterior edge of the limbal corneal vessels. In the limbal approach, a small conjunctival peritomy is made in one of the superior quadrants, followed by a beveled, grooved incision approximately 3 mm long at the surgical limbus.

A suture may be preplaced and looped out of the way. This can be grasped by the assistant with tying forceps and used to pull the edges of the incision apart while the surgeon penetrates Descemet's membrane and enters the anterior chamber with a sharp blade.

The assistant can facilitate prolapse of the iris by gentle manipulation of the looped sutures to alternately widen and narrow the incision and by pressure against the back lip of the incision. The iris may not prolapse if the incision is too anterior or posterior, if the eye is hypotonic, if peripheral anterior synechiae are present, or if a hole has been made in the iris inadvertently. If the iris cannot be prolapsed, a fine, smooth forceps is placed within the anterior chamber to grasp the iris for excision. To avoid injury to the lens, the anterior chamber should never be entered with a toothed forceps.

Once prolapsed, the iris is grasped with fine forceps and cut using Vannas or de Wecker scissors (Fig. 34-1). The excised tissue should be inspected to insure that pigmented epithelium has been included by smearing it on the eye drape. Massage over the limbus and cornea in a central direction and/or irrigation of the incision with acetylcholine will facilitate reposition of the iris, resulting in visualization of the iridectomy with a central, regular pupil. A cyclodialysis spatula may be used to liberate iris tissue trapped in the incision without entering the anterior chamber. Reformation of the chamber should be performed by injecting balanced salt solution through a 30-gauge cannula if it is shallow or flat as a result of aqueous loss through the incision. Patency of the iridectomy should be confirmed before closing the wound.

When a sector iridectomy is performed, the iris must be externalized. After the peripheral iris has prolapsed, a gentle hand-over-hand technique may be continued until the sphincter has been exte-

riorized and the pupillary margin exposed. The iris may then be excised (Fig. 34-2).

The corneal incision should be approximated with a 10-0 nylon suture and the knot buried. In the case of a limbal incision, some surgeons pass the suture through the conjunctiva after passing it across the incision to bring the conjunctiva over the incision. Others close conjunctiva separately with an absorbable suture.

Subconjunctival antibiotics and a corticosteroid are injected at the end of the procedure and a topical cycloplegic agent applied. Dilation and cycloplegia are recommended to minimize the chances of posterior synechia formation, ciliary spasm, and malignant glaucoma. Postoperatively, topical antibiotics and corticosteroids are given. Slit-lamp examination and indentation gonioscopy should be performed as soon as possible to evaluate the status and success of the procedure.

COMPLICATIONS

Incomplete Iridectomy

The iris stroma is excised but the pigment epithelium left intact, preventing relief of pupillary block. Residual pigment epithelium can easily be removed with a few low power burns with the argon laser, avoiding the necessity for reoperation.

Photophobia and Glare

Photophobia and glare are not uncommon after both peripheral and sector iridectomy.[2]

Shallow or Flat Anterior Chamber

This is usually secondary to a wound leak,[9,22] which can be detected using the Seidel test. However, the possibilities of malignant glaucoma or choroidal effusion should be considered.

Persistent Subconjunctival Fistula

In cases of a limbal approach, a wound leak may develop underneath the conjunctival flap. This can be avoided by using a beveled incision and by determining that there is adequate wound apposition at the end of the procedure.

Cataract

Cataract formation or progression is a common finding after surgical iridectomy. If the lens is injured during the procedure, cataract formation may be rapid. More common, however, is the development of a cataract over time, which occurs in approximately 50% of eyes having had an acute attack of angle-closure glaucoma and up to 30% of fellow eyes undergoing prophylactic iridectomy.[12,16,20,37] Aqueous flow into the anterior chamber through the iridectomy rather than through the pupil may adversely affect the integrity of the lens.

Bleeding

Small hyphemas frequently occur after surgical iridectomy. Hemorrhage from the iris or ciliary body can usually be controlled by injecting a large air bubble into the anterior chamber. In most cases, they resolve spontaneously. In diabetic patients with rubeosis iridis, the risk of bleeding is significantly higher and the use of bipolar microcautery has been recommended before cutting iris tissue.[17]

Malignant Glaucoma

Malignant glaucoma must be considered when there is a flat anterior chamber and elevated intraocular pressure in the presence of a patent iridectomy. This condition is discussed in detail in Chapter 70.

Other Complications

All the complications of intraocular surgery may occur with surgical iridectomy, albeit rarely. These include iridodialysis, lens dislocation, vitreous loss, endophthalmitis, retrobulbar hemorrhage, stripping of Descemet's membrane, incarceration of iris or ciliary processes in the wound, intralenticular hemorrhage, ptosis, and diplopia.[11,15,22]

FILTRATION SURGERY

Iridectomy is performed in conjunction with filtering procedures primarily to prevent the iris from prolapsing into and occluding the sclerostomy site. It is important that the iridectomy be wider than the trabeculectomy opening. This is discussed in Chapter 35.

CATARACT EXTRACTION

In 1862, Mooren performed an iridectomy in conjunction with extracapsular cataract surgery to decrease such complications as iris prolapse, which probably resulted from pupillary block.[38] In 1879, de Wecker suggested sector iridectomy as a means of clearing the visual axis in cases of thickened capsular remnants after cataract surgery.[38]

A basal iridectomy should always be performed at the time of intracapsular cataract extraction because of the potential for aphakic pupillary block (see Chapter 71). After anterior chamber intraocular lens implantation, the incidence of pupillary block is as high as 4%,[26] whereas in the CORE cases reported in the FDA report on intraocular lenses, the incidence after posterior chamber lens implantation was 0.3%.[36]

At present, controversy has arisen regarding the need to perform a peripheral iridectomy in uneventful cases of extracapsular cataract extraction with a posterior chamber intraocular lens implant.[6,33] Because of the relative rarity of pupillary block after extracapsular cataract extraction and posterior chamber lens implantation, an increasing number of cataract surgeons have advocated omitting peripheral iridectomy as a step in this procedure, arguing that the sum total of complications of surgical iridectomy outweighs that of pupillary block.[32,35] Others are in favor of a peripheral iridectomy in all cases of cataract extraction.[4,6,10]

Complications of surgical iridectomy at the time of cataract extraction include bleeding, increased inflammation, iridodialysis, damage to the intraocular lens, vitreous loss, and postoperative glare and/or diplopia. The complications of pupillary block may be more severe and permanent than those of iridectomy. These complications may involve the integrity of the cataract incision, glaucomatous damage, peripheral anterior synechiae, and continuing need for further treatment of glaucoma due to scarring of and damage to the trabecular meshwork.

Several cases of pupillary block after posterior chamber lens implantation have now been reported.* Pupillary block may result from iris contact with the posterior chamber lens or the anterior capsule, especially if there is significant postoperative inflammation. Vitreous may also prolapse through an inadvertent opening made in the posterior capsule at the time of surgery or after Nd:YAG laser posterior capsulotomy. Weinreb et al.[43] reported six diabetic patients who developed pseudophakic pupillary block after extracapsular cataract extraction without an iridectomy. An increased occurrence of pupillary block in diabetics could be related to increased postoperative inflammation and subsequent formation of posterior synechiae between the iris and the intraocular lens. An angulated lens implant does not prevent pupillary block, which may occur even in the presence of a sector iridectomy.

At the time of cataract extraction, eyes on longstanding miotic therapy frequent dilate poorly or not at all. A sector iridectomy may be created by connecting a peripheral iridectomy with the pupillary sphincter by a radial iridotomy (Fig. 34-3).

---

*References 6, 13, 31, 36, 40, 42, 43.

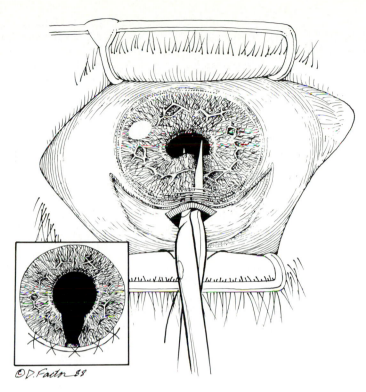

Fig. 34-3 Sector iridotomy. After creation of peripheral iridectomy, scissors are introduced into anterior chamber to connect it to pupil. *Inset*, Postoperative appearance.

A sector iridectomy combined with several spincterotomies may be required to facilitate an adequate anterior capsulotomy, nucleus expression, and posterior intraocular lens insertion. The iridectomy may be sutured at the close of the procedure. However, sector iridectomy in glaucoma patients with intraocular lenses does not produce a significant increase in the amount of glare postoperatively.[25] An iris forceps-scissors has been described for performing an iridotomy during cataract surgery with minimal manipulation of the iris[34] (Fig. 34-4).

Conservative indications for the performance of an iridectomy at the time of extracapsular cataract extraction with posterior chamber intraocular lens implantation include:

1. Preexisting iritis
2. Preexisting glaucoma
3. Miotic pupil
4. Young patient
5. Diabetes mellitus
6. Monocular patients
7. Rupture of the posterior capsule
8. Long or difficult extraction
9. Incomplete removal of cortex
10. Intracapsular or extracapsular cataract extraction without intraocular lens
11. Anterior chamber lens

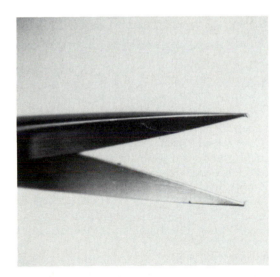

Fig. 34-4 Shields iridotomy scissor-forceps. Note forcep teeth at ends of scissor blades.

REFERENCES

1. Abraham, RK, and Miller, GL: Outpatient argon laser iridectomy for angle closure glaucoma: a two-year study, Trans Am Acad Ophthalmol Otolaryngol 79:259, 1975
2. Allen, JC: Incidence of photophobia in peripheral and sector iridectomy, Am J Ophthalmol 82:316, 1976
3. Barkan, O: Glaucoma: classification, causes, and surgical control, Am J Ophthalmol 21:1099, 1938
4. Champion, R, McDonnell, PJ, and Green, WR: Intraocular lenses. Histopathologic characteristics of a large series of autopsy eyes, Surv Ophthalmol 30:1, 1985
5. Chandler, PA: Narrow-angle glaucoma, Arch Ophthalmol 47:695, 1952
6. Cohen, JS, Osher, RH, Weber, P, and Faulkner, JD: Complications of extracapsular cataract surgery. The indications and risks of peripheral iridectomy, Ophthalmology 91:82, 1984
7. Curran, EJ: A new operation for glaucoma involving a new principle in the etiology and treatment of chronic primary glaucoma, Arch Ophthalmol 49:131, 1920
8. Curran, EJ: Peripheral iridotomy in acute and chronic glaucoma. Some results after ten years duration. Anatomical classification of glaucoma, Trans Ophthalmol Soc UK 51:520, 1931
9. Douglas, WHG, and Strachan, IM: Surgical safety of prophylactic peripheral iridectomy, Br J Ophthalmol 51:459, 1967
10. Emery, JM, and McIntyre, DJ: Extracapsular cataract surgery, St. Louis, 1983, The CV Mosby Co, p 237
11. Feibel, RM, Bigger, JF, and Smith, ME: Intralenticular hemorrhage following iridectomy, Arch Ophthalmol 87:36, 1972
12. Floman, N, Berson, D, and Landau, L: Peripheral iridectomy in closed angle glaucoma, late complications, Br J Ophthalmol 61:101, 1977
13. Forman, JS, Ritch, R, Dunn, MW, and Szmyd, L: Pupillary block following posterior chamber lens implantation, Ophthalmic Laser Therapy 2:85, 1987
14. Gieser DK, and Wilensky JT: Laser iridectomy in the management of chronic angle-closure glaucoma, Am J Ophthalmol 98:446, 1984
15. Go, FJ, and Kitazawa, Y: Complications of peripheral iridectomy in primary angle-closure glaucoma, Jpn J Ophthalmol 25:222, 1981
16. Godel, V, and Regenbogen, L: Cataractogenic factors in patients with primary angle-closure glaucoma after peripheral iridectomy, Am J Ophthalmol 83:180, 1977
17. Hersh SB, and Kass, MA: Iridectomy in rubeosis iridis. Ophthalmic Surg 7:19, 1976
18. Hyams, SW, Friedman, Z, and Keroub, C: Fellow eye in angle-closure glaucoma, Br J Ophthalmol 59:207, 1975
19. Kollner, H: Iridektomie. In Axenfeld, T, and Elschnig, A, editors: Handbuch der Gesamten Augenheilkunde: Augenarztliche Operationslehre. Berlin, 1922, Springer-Verlag, pp 777
20. Krupin, T, Mitchell, KB, Johnson, MF, and Becker, B: The long-term effects of iridectomy for primary angle-closure glaucoma, Am J Ophthalmol 86:506, 1978
21. Latina, MA, Puliafito, CA, Steinert, RR, and Epstein, DL: Experimental iridotomy with the Q-switched neodymium-YAG laser, Arch Ophthalmol 102:1211, 1984
22. Luke, S: Complications of peripheral iridectomy, Can J Ophthalmol 4:346, 1969
23. Mapstone, R: The fellow eye, Br J Ophthalmol 65:410, 1981
24. Margo, CE, and Groden, L: Balloon cell nevus of the iris, Am J Ophthalmol 102:282, 1986
25. McGuigan, LJB, et al: Extracapsular cataract extraction and posterior chamber lens implantation in eyes with preexisting glaucoma, Arch Ophthalmol 104:1301, 1986
26. Moses, L: Complications of rigid anterior chamber implants, Ophthalmology 91:819, 1984
27. Pollack, IP, and Patz, A: Argon laser iridotomy: an experimental and clinical study, Ophthalmic Surg 7:22, 1976
28. Playfair, TJ, and Watson, PG: Management of acute primary angle-closure glaucoma: a long-term follow-up of the results of peripheral iridectomy used as an initial procedure, Br J Ophthalmol 63:17, 1979
29. Podos, SM, et al: Continuous wave argon laser iridectomy in angle-closure glaucoma, Am J Ophthalmol 88:836, 1979
30. Ritch, R, and Podos, SM: Argon laser treatment of angle-closure glaucoma, Perspect Ophthalmol 4:129, 1980
31. Samples, JR, et al: Pupillary block with posterior chamber intraocular lenses, Arch Ophthalmol 105:335, 1987
32. Schulze, RR, and Copeland, JR: Posterior chamber intraocular lens implantation without peripheral iridectomy. A preliminary report, Ophthalmic Surg 13:567, 1982
33. Shepard, DD: Consultation section. Indications for performing an iridectomy, Am Intraocul Implant Soc J 11:301, 1985
34. Shields, MB: Iridotomy scissor-forceps, Am J Ophthalmol 99:609, 1985
35. Simel, PJ: Posterior chamber implants without iridectomy, Am Intraocul Implant Soc J 8:141, 1982
36. Stark, WJ, et al: The FDA report on intraocular lenses, Ophthalmology 90:311, 1983
37. Sugar, HS: Cataract formation and refractive changes after surgery for angle closure glaucoma, Am J Ophthalmol 69:747, 1970
38. The American encyclopedia of ophthalmology, vol 9, Chicago, 1916, Cleveland Press

39. Tomey, KF, Traverso, CE, and Shammas, IV: Neodymium-YAG laser iridotomy in the treatment and
prevention of angle closure glaucoma. A review of
373 eyes, Arch Ophthalmol 105:476, 1987

40. Van Buskirk, EM: Pupillary block after intraocular
lens implantation, Am J Ophthalmol 95:55, 1983

41. Von Graefe, A: Ueber die Iridectomie bei Glaucom
und uber den glaucomatosen Process, v Graefes
Arch Klin Exp Ophthalmol 3:456, 1857

42. Willis, DA, Stewart, RH, and Kimbrough, RL: Pupillary block associated with posterior chamber
lenses, Ophthalmic Surg 16:108, 1985

43. Weinreb, RN, Wasserstrom, JP, Forman, JS, and
Ritch, R: Pseudophakic pupillary block with angle-
closure glaucoma in diabetic patients, Am J Ophthalmol 102:325, 1986

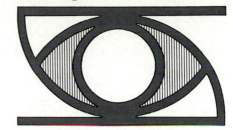

Chapter 35

Filtration Surgery

L. Jay Katz
George L. Spaeth

HISTORICAL PERSPECTIVE (Table 35-1)

The association between glaucoma and elevated intraocular pressure (IOP) was first suggested by Richard Bannister in 1622.[74] Not until the nineteenth century, when this link had become generally accepted, were various surgical attempts made to treat glaucoma by reducing ocular tension. McKenzie (1830) reported a sclerotomy and later a paracentesis, concluding that both were beneficial only temporarily.[74] Critchett[74,165,308] incarcerated iris into a limbal wound to affect a drainage site and termed it "iridodesis." Von Graefe[74,165,308] remarked on the presence of "transparent, vesicle-like prominences" in more than 20% of eyes after peripheral iridectomy, then the standard operation for all types of glaucoma. However, he attributed the reduction of IOP to the peripheral iridectomy alone;

he apparently was unaware of the contribution of the filtration bleb.

The role of a "filtering cicatrix" was probably understood by Louis DeWecker.[165,308] Emphasizing excision of the sclera, rather than of the iris, he wrote in 1869 that he considered an anterior sclerotomy successful only if filtration continued postoperatively. LaGrange[74,108,165,308] performed a "sclerectoiridectomy" to establish a permanent fistula through which aqueous could flow and be absorbed in the subconjunctival space. In 1906 Holth used punch forceps in an anterior lip sclerectomy, and in 1907 he proposed iridencleisis, with iris inclusion into a limbal wound covered by conjunctiva.[108,165,308]

Limbal trephination (Elliot, 1909) became the most popular filtration operation until the 1940s, when it gradually fell out of favor because the very delicate, thin conjunctival bleb which developed frequently ruptured, resulting in late endophthalmitis.[74,105,108,308,310]

Thermal cautery of the scleral wound edges with entry into the anterior chamber (Preziosi, 1924),[74,308,310] and Scheie's modification combined with peripheral iridectomy,[259] a thermal sclerostomy, and posterior lip sclerectomy,[131] were the most widely used glaucoma operations until the guarded filtration procedures were developed.

One such procedure, trabeculectomy, using a partial-thickness scleral flap covering a sclerotomy, was described by Sugar in 1961.[302] Since the intent of the operation was to remove the trabeculum, the suggested site of resistance to outflow, the flap was tightly sutured to prevent any external filtration. All cases were unsuccessful.

Table 35-1 Chronologic history of filtering operations

Date	Surgeon	Procedure
1830	McKenzie	Sclerotomy
1857	Critchett	Iridodesis
1869	Von Graefe	Filtering bleb
1869	DeWecker	Anterior sclerotomy
1906	LaGrange	Sclerecto-iridectomy
1907	Holth	Anterior lip sclerectomy
1907	Holth	Iridencleisis
1909	Elliot	Limbal trephination
1924	Preziosi	Thermal sclerostomy
1958	Scheie	Thermal sclerotomy with iridectomy
1962	Iliff and Haas	Posterior lip sclerectomy
1968	Cairns	Trabeculectomy

Cairns[43] reported successful trabeculectomies using a one-half thickness scleral flap in 17 eyes. The flap was hinged either posteriorly in the sclera or anteriorly at the limbus. After excision of Schlemm's canal and trabecular meshwork, the corneoscleral flap was tightly sutured in place to "secure a watertight union." Subconjunctival blebs, however, developed in six of the eyes. It was unclear at that time whether removing trabecular obstruction or developing subconjunctival or external filtration was the key to relieving the IOP. Watson[331] also reported 44 cases where trabeculectomy with a limbus-based scleral flap yielded filtration blebs in 25 eyes; many of the eyes without apparent blebs were also controlled. Trabeculectomy rapidly became the dominant filtration operation because, although the success rate in lowering IOP was not higher, the incidence of complications was relatively low.

INDICATIONS FOR FILTRATION SURGERY

The decision to perform filtration surgery must be based on a judicious assessment of the following factors:[270,284,288] (1) the magnitude and the duration of IOP elevation, (2) the extent and progression of visual field defects, (3) the extent of damage to the optic nerve head, (4) the patient's own sense of visual function, (5) the course of the contralateral eye with or without treatment, and, (6) the general health and age of the patient.

In general, filtration surgery is indicated when neither medical nor laser therapy is sufficient to control the glaucoma. Medical therapy is deemed insufficient if it cannot maintain the IOP within a range believed low enough to prevent further damage, if it is poorly tolerated, or if compliance is a problem. It has been argued that chronically applied topical medications, especially pilocarpine, may negatively affect future filtration surgery[46] and that earlier surgery rather than long-term medical therapy may be preferable.[35,136]

There are some cases in which laser surgery may be contraindicated[333] or not technically possible. Synechial angle closure, corneal opacification, and poor patient cooperation make argon laser trabeculoplasty technically impossible. Juvenile and secondary glaucomas, such as those associated with angle recession, uveitis, and aniridia, do poorly. Proceeding directly to filtration surgery would be prudent in these cases. If one eye of the patient does not respond to laser trabeculoplasty, it is unwise to perform it in the other eye. Although argon laser trabeculoplasty may lower IOP in many cases, it appears that it does not eliminate, but only delays, the need for surgery.[103] And, although laser trabeculoplasty may lower IOP, it may not lower it enough to prevent further visual loss.

The response of the contralateral eye to filtering surgery is helpful in deciding on the appropriate approach. An uneventful operation and postoperative course in the first eye bodes well for surgery on the fellow eye. But if serious complications, such as suprachoroidal hemorrhage, aqueous misdirection, or rapid cataract progression, occur in the first eye, the fellow eye must be approached cautiously. If vision is significantly impaired by a cataract or keratopathy, filtration surgery may be either performed first or combined with cataract extraction or penetrating keratoplasty.

Unquestionable evidence of optic disc or visual field deterioration makes the decision to intervene surgically less problematic. However, the judgment is primarily based on the surgeon's assessment of the amount of IOP an eye can sustain without further glaucomatous injury. This evaluation is made by considering various factors, most important being the pressure at which damage to the optic disc and visual field has occurred. On occasion, the patient may complain of progressive visual loss or "graying of vision" before any objective determination has been made.

The general and ocular health of a patient are also important factors. Diabetes mellitus, obesity, myopia, or family history of advanced glaucoma argue in favor of intervention. Conversely, it would be difficult to justify surgery for an ill patient with limited expected survival time.

OBJECTIVES

The purposes of surgery are to maintain useful vision and to avoid further glaucomatous damage. The method of achieving these objectives is to lower IOP. Unfortunately, the method is often confused with the purpose. It is essential to recall that the purpose of surgery is not only to lower IOP. Success or failure should be judged in terms of the effect of surgery on the patient's visual function.

"Safe" IOP

The immediate guide for gauging the response to surgery is applanation tonometry. Frequent monitoring helps the surgeon to maintain adequate filtration and to uncover potential problems such as aqueous misdirection. The surgeon defines "safe" IOP individually for each case, taking into account, for example, that a severely damaged optic nerve is probably more susceptible to further damage.[1,111,344] A general rule is that the more advanced the disease, the lower the IOP must be.

Bleb Formation

A filtering bleb is the cornerstone of IOP control in glaucoma.[2,44,67,177,178] Characteristics of the bleb produced depend on the operative technique, postoperative medications, age of the patient, and diagnosis. Full-thickness procedures, such as posterior sclerectomy and thermal sclerostomy, tend to produce very thin, cystic, overhanging blebs. Thicker, more succulent blebs are characteristic of partial-thickness guarded filtration procedures, such as trabeculectomy. Limbus-based conjunctival flaps result in high, easily visible elevations, whereas fornix-based flaps tend to give more diffuse and poorly defined blebs. Antifibrotic agents, such as corticosteroids and antimetabolites (5-fluorouracil), are believed to promote the development of pronounced blebs. Older patients, with thinner Tenon's capsules, tend to develop thinner blebs than younger patients. Some do not develop any apparent bleb. Perhaps in these cases, there is undetected subtle low-lying or posterior blebs, or, perhaps, the aqueous drains by a mechanism other than the subconjunctival route.[86,330]

Retention of Vision

The foremost goal is preservation of sight. One hopes to stabilize a visual field defect, although some have suggested that positive improvement should be the standard.[290] Any encroachment on the central field, the area vital to good visual acuity, is a serious threat. Because cataract progression is a definite risk after filtration surgery, the patient should be forewarned that, although the surgery may be successful in halting glaucomatous progression, there may be a reduction in visual acuity.

Informed Consent—Patient Comprehension of Goals

Informed consent must be obtained before surgery,[162] since decisions regarding care must be made primarily by the patient, not the physician. Since decision making requires knowledge, patient education is vital. The patient must have reasonable expectations and appreciate the intricacies of therapy. Giving "informed consent" implies consenting after being informed of the risks of the procedure. Both the common, minor complications and the rarer, serious complications must be addressed. It should not be taken for granted that a patient who accepts the possibility of enucleation after a potential complication, such as endophthalmitis, somehow automatically will understand that loss of several lines of visual acuity due to cataract is also possible.

Alternative treatments and the prognosis, as well as the natural history of glaucoma with no treatment, must be explained. The patient must be reminded of the basic goal, namely, to preserve, rather than to improve, vision. Communicating this limited goal is surprisingly difficult because patients may assume that this operation, like cataract extraction and corneal transplantation, actually restores sight. The extent of discussion required necessarily varies widely from patient to patient. A few may require nothing more than a recommendation that surgery be performed; others may need many prolonged discussions.

Obtaining a "written operative consent" is not at all the same as obtaining informed consent. Indeed, the former can be used as a way to circumvent the real issue: making sure that the patient has enough information to make a decision that is in his or her best interest. Finally, obtaining informed consent means that the physician is complying with the legal requirement of presenting a patient with various choices.

PATIENT EVALUATION

Diagnosis

Certain generalizations may be made regarding the chances of success with standard filtration surgery according to the type of glaucoma (Table 35-2). The ideal patient would be over 40 years old with a phakic, uninflamed eye, having had no pre-

Table 35-2   *Success of filtering surgery in various glaucomas**

Good (>75%)	Fair (50%)	Poor (<25%)
Primary open-angle glaucoma	Aphakia	Neovascular
Chronic angle-closure glaucoma	Juvenile	Uveitic-active
Exfoliation syndrome	Iridocorneal endothelial syndrome	Congenital
Pigmentary glaucoma	Sturge-Weber syndrome	More than two previous filtration
Fuchs' heterochromia	Repeat filtration	failures
Angle recession	Pseudophakia (anterior chamber IOL)	
Pseudophakia (posterior chamber IOL)	Uveitic-inactive	

*These are rough ranges. Success varies markedly within the diagnostic categories, for example, as in aphakic patients.

vious intraocular surgery. Negative risk factors include youth, intraocular inflammation, previous failure of glaucoma surgery in the same or fellow eye, conjunctival scarring from previous surgery, and aphakia.

The importance of racial differences in response to filtering surgery has been disputed.[51,60,89,189,213] Blacks have often been thought to have a lower success rate than whites. Since scarring of the conjunctiva-Tenon's capsule to the sclera appears to be the major reason for failure, some have suggested routine tenonectomy;[280] others, however, have discounted the value of such a procedure.[141]

Older patients seem to have a higher success rate than younger ones.[112,177,178,213,305] Tenon's capsule, which is mostly connective tissue, thins with age.[305] A decrease in fibroblast concentration may partially explain this phenomenon. Nevertheless, filtering surgery has a role in the younger population, even in those with buphthalmos and congenital glaucoma.[15,262,268,323]

Previous Surgery

Filtering surgery works best in previously unoperated eyes. Eyes with anterior chamber intraocular lenses and no posterior capsule respond as do aphakic eyes. Those with posterior chamber implants and intact posterior capsules, separating aqueous from vitreous, seem to do better.

With each successive filtering operation, the expected surgical success rate falls.[132,139,272] After three or more procedures it may drop to as low as 10%[272] because multiple operations leave fewer unscarred regions of conjunctiva.

Ocular Status

The location of the filtering fistula is partially determined by the configuration of the angle. In the presence of a narrow angle, especially with peripheral anterior synechiae, the excision of the internal corneoscleral block should be more anterior than usual to avoid the iris root and ciliary body.

Conjunctiva that is scarred from previous surgery is difficult to dissect from the underlying sclera; buttonholes in the flap may result. A fornix-based conjunctival flap is often easier to raise; however, we prefer a limbus-based flap even in these cases. Dissection must be meticulous and is usually best accomplished with sharp instruments. Often it is necessary to include the episclera or even a superficial scleral stromal layer in the conjunctival flap to avoid penetrating it. Finding a less adherent area for dissection may sometimes be best.

> **FACTORS SUGGESTING THE NEED FOR URGENT SURGERY***
>
> 1. Rapid deterioration of function or of optic nerve appearance.
> 2. Advanced stage of optic nerve damage (cup/disc ratio greater than 0.8 or area with absent rim).
> 3. Advanced stage of visual field loss (significant deterioration within 10 degrees of fixation).
> 4. Increase in IOP above a level known to cause optic nerve damage.
> 5. Increase in IOP to level considered likely to cause rapid worsening of the disc or field.

*In order of decreasing importance.

Ocular inflammation, such as blepharitis, conjunctivitis, or uveitis, may require postponing the surgery. An external bacterial infection could lead to a bleb infection and endophthalmitis. Inflammation increases vascularity and adhesiveness, lessening the change of developing a lasting functional bleb.

Stage of Glaucoma

The urgency of glaucoma surgery is based on the rapidity with which deterioration is occurring or is expected to occur. For example, a sudden significant worsening of IOP (e.g., from 20 to 40 mm Hg) in a patient with advanced optic nerve damage calls for an urgent lowering of pressure. Factors influencing the urgency are shown in the box above.

The surgeon should not rule out other explanations for apparent progression. For example, further visual field loss may be mimicked by a retinal detachment, paramacular hemorrhage, a branch retinal vein occlusion, focal cataract, change in pupil size, or uncorrected refractive error. Increased optic disc pallor or cupping may be due to ischemic optic neuropathy or a compressive lesion. A thorough preoperative history and examination will often reveal these nonglaucomatous reasons for progression in the visual field or optic nerve head.

PREOPERATIVE PREPARATION

Patient

Certain medications should be discontinued at least 24 hours before the operation, if possible. However, in some advanced glaucoma cases none of the medications is stopped for fear of wiping out central fixation. Short-acting parasympathomimetics, such as pilocarpine, tend to promote inflammation and breakdown of the blood aqueous-barrier and to stimulate contraction of the pupillary sphincter and ciliary body muscle. Paralysis of these muscles is highly important after filtration surgery to help avoid posterior synechiae, pupillary block, flat anterior chambers, and malignant glaucoma. With long-acting parasympathomimetics, such as echothiophate iodide, it is necessary to discontinue use at least 2 weeks before surgery under general anesthesia, not only because they can cause inflammation, but also because they inhibit pseudocholinesterase. This enzyme is responsible for the biodegradation of succinylcholine, a paralyzing agent often used during intubation with general anesthesia. Since the half-life of succinylcholine is significantly increased in the presence of the "irreversible" parasympathomimetics, they can cause prolonged apnea.

Carbonic anhydrase inhibitors and beta-blockers are stopped because they decrease aqueous production, undesirable in the early postoperative period since a good flow of aqueous presumably helps establish a filtration fistula. Oral anticoagulants, such as dicumarol (Coumadin), aspirin, and dipyridamole (Persantine), should be stopped in some cases to minimize a bleeding diathesis. These agents, especially dicumarol, should be stopped only when doing so is in the considered best interest of the patient. If the IOP is above 30 mm Hg, or otherwise thought to be too high, an intravenous hyperosmotic agent, such as mannitol, may be administered at 0.5 to 1 mg/kg over 40 minutes beginning at least 1 hour before surgery (see Chapter 27). This helps prevent sudden, ocular decompression. Theoretically, preventing an acute fall of IOP should reduce the incidence of complications, such as suprachoroidal expulsive hemorrhage, choroidal effusion, and vitreous loss.

Microsurgical Instruments[59]

A working knowledge of the microsurgical instruments is the responsibility of the surgeon and the assistant. The names and purposes of each instrument should be known.

Anesthesia

The choice of local or general anesthesia depends on the medical and psychological status of the patient, the surgeon's reference, and the nature of the operation (Table 35-3).

Local anesthesia[174]

Local injections prevent the generation and conduction of peripheral nerve impulses. Motor, sensory, and autonomic fibers are all blocked, resulting in regional motor paralysis and anesthesia.

Table 35-3 Factors influencing the mode of anesthesia

Factors	Local	General
Patient cooperation	Good	Poor
General health	Poor	Good
Nothing by mouth	Not necessary	Essential
Length of procedure	Short	Long
Anesthesiologist	Inexperienced	Dependable
Previous general anesthesia	Complicated	Uncomplicated
Surgeon's preference	Yes	Yes
Patient's preference	Yes	Yes
Previous retrobulbar hemorrhage	No	Yes
Malignant hyperthermia (personal/family)	Yes	No

Table 35-4 Local anesthetic drugs for retrobulbar anesthesia

Local anesthetics	Concentration (%)	Onset (min)	Duration (hr)
Mepivacaine (Carbocaine)	1, 2*	3-5	2
Lidocaine (Xylocaine)	1, 2*, 4	4-6	1
Etidocaine (Duranest)	½, 1*, 1½	3-5	10
Bupivacaine (Marcaine)	¼, ½, ¾*	5-10	6-12 (8-12 with epinephrine)

*Our preference.

Agents in Table 35-4 are the most commonly used. Sometimes two anesthetics are used to take advantage of the different attributes of both drugs (e.g., duration of action and rapidity of onset). However, this is rarely necessary because the onset of all agents is adequate.

Serious systemic effects involving the central nervous system or cardiovascular system are rarely encountered because the critical dose is usually much higher than the maximum amount routinely employed (a total of 13 to 15 ml). However, respiratory arrest and cardiovascular collapse do occur, especially with retrobulbar injections of bupivacaine.[3,4,9] Anesthetic injection into the optic nerve sheath with posterior spread into the central nervous system can cause brainstem paralysis, obviously a very serious complication.[135,282] Intravascular retrograde injection into the cerebral circulation may also occur, but it is of less concern.[290] Another important factor is the amount (volume and concentration) of anesthetic injected.

Injection technique

FACIAL NERVE BLOCK.   To achieve complete akinesia of the orbicularis oculi and thus prevent any closure of the lids, which could raise IOP, a seventh cranial nerve block is performed. Two common techniques are the modified O'Brien-Spaeth block (Fig. 35-1) and the modified Van Lint approach. The facial nerve has five branches, but only two, the temporal and zygomatic nerve branches, serve the orbicularis oculi muscle. After leaving the stylomastoid foramen, the facial nerve enters the substance of the parotid gland near the angle of the mandible. Injection at this site (the O'Brien technique) causes hemifacial paralysis. In the Spaeth modification of the O'Brien technique, the mandible is palpated posteriorly toward its superior junction. Approximately 10 ml of anesthetic is injected just anterior to this point and then directed toward the lateral canthus. Distal subcutaneous injection at the lateral orbital margin (the modified Van Lint technique) affects only the two branches serving the orbicularis oculi. Five to 7 ml of anesthetic is injected along the lateral orbital wall superiorly and inferiorly. In both these techniques firm pressure allows the anesthetic to diffuse and also provides hemostasis.

RETROBULBAR BLOCK.   Hyaluronidase, an enzyme that breaks down hyaluronic acid, the polysaccharide matrix of tissue interstices, is frequently added to the anesthetic for the retrobulbar injection. This facilitates diffusion of the anesthetic toward the target nerve and thus decreases onset time. Lyophilized, 150 U of the solid material is dissolved in the local anesthetic solution. The completed block immobilizes the muscles supplied by cranial nerves III, IV, and VI and provides a sensory block of the ciliary nerves, anesthetizing the anterior segment. Hyaluronidase should not be used in cases in which greater chemosis is undesirable; in most cases an entirely adequate block can be obtained without it.

A 25-gauge sharp needle (or a blunted Atkinson retrobulbar needle to avoid piercing vessels) is initially directed inferiorly along the inferior orbital rim through the orbital septum and then posteriorly into or adjacent to the retrobulbar muscle cone. After pulling back on the syringe to assure that the needle has not cannulized into a vessel, 3 ml of anesthetic is injected and the needle withdrawn. Firm pressure for several seconds is advisable to limit any potential bleeding.

Many surgeons, especially those in oculoplastics, add epinephrine to the anesthetic solution. A catecholamine vasoconstrictor, epinephrine reduces the perfusion of the anesthetic site, delaying removal of the anesthetic, thereby increasing du-

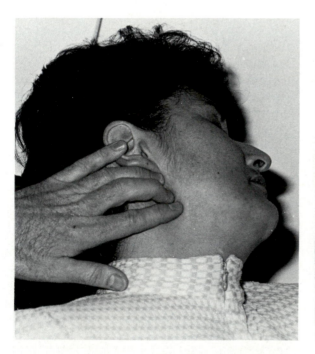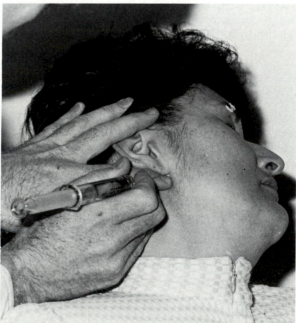

Fig. 35-1   Spaeth modification of O'Brien facial nerve block.

ration of action and decreasing intraoperative bleeding. However, the effect of constricting optic nerve vessels in glaucoma is uncertain and potentially hazardous. Also, bleeding may occur after the effect of the epinephrine has worn off. For these reasons, and because anesthesia of adequate duration can easily be achieved with routinely available anesthetic agents, we believe the use of epinephrine in glaucoma surgery is contraindicated.

Firm pressure on the globe or placement of a Honan balloon or "Superpinky" are common methods of reducing IOP before cataract extraction. However, since even a seemingly insignificant elevation of IOP may be hazardous for certain compromised optic nerves in advanced glaucoma, these methods should be used with caution or not at all in filtration surgery.

GENERAL ANESTHETICS. General anesthesia with endotracheal intubation administered under the supervision of an anesthesiologist involves the careful titration of a mixture of drugs. Neuroleptoanesthesia is the mixture of an inhalation general anesthetic and a neuroleptoanalgesia combination (narcotic plus analgesic). Combination-balanced anesthesia includes a complex array: an ultrashort barbiturate, a narcotic, a neuromuscular blocker, and an inhalational anesthetic. General anesthetics are classified as inhalational or intravenous. (Table 35-5) Deeper anesthesia proceeds through four stages: analgesia, delirium, anesthesia, and respiratory paralysis.

Neuromuscular block facilitates intubation and

makes deep, general anesthesia unnecessary. Nondepolarizing types (e.g., tubocurarine and pancuronium [Pavulon]) directly compete with acetylcholine for muscle receptors. Depolarizing types (e.g., succinylcholine) act indirectly to inhibit muscle stimulation. It should be noted that succinylcholine causes transient ocular hypertension because of sustained extraocular muscle contraction. This ocular hypertension may extrude intraocular tissue through an open wound. Also, as previously noted, echothiophate iodide dramatically prolongs the action of succinylcholine, which is hydrolyzed by pseudocholinesterase. If possible, the echothiophate iodide should be discontinued for at least 2 weeks before surgery. Alternatively, a nonpolarizing blocker could be omitted.

The major difficulties encountered with general anesthesia are adverse intraoperative and postoperative effects (Table 35-6) and prolonged recovery time.

SURGICAL TECHNIQUE

Surgical Anatomy[94]

External layers

Overlying the sclera are two distinct tissue layers, the conjunctiva and Tenon's capsule. There are two potential spaces: sub-Tenon's and subconjunctival. The conjunctiva, a mucous membrane, is lined with nonkeratinized stratified squamous epithelium with a delicate underlying *substantia propria*. The next enveloping coat is the relatively avascular, fibroelastic Tenon's capsule. The sclera is composed of three layers: the episclera, a fine, superficial, vascular connective tissue; the stroma, an avascular, dense array of randomly-oriented collagen lamellae; and the lamina fusca, a thin layer bordering the uvea.

Limbus (Fig. 35-2)

The conjunctiva inserts at the corneoscleral junction, or limbus, marking the anterior limbal border near the end of the corneal Bowman's layer. Tenon's capsule attaches 0.5 to 1 mm farther posteriorly, past a depression, the corneoscleral sulcus. The surgical limbus is up to 1 mm thick and is confined to a 2 mm zone. Extending peripherally, clear cornea becomes a bluish hue for 1 mm before blending into the white sclera. At the junction of the blue and white zones, Descemet's membrane terminates just anterior to Schwalbe's ridge, bordering the anterior trabecular meshwork. The position and dimensions of the limbus, however, vary quite markedly from eye to eye and must always be identified specifically.

Table 35-5 *General anesthetics*

Inhalational	Intravenous
Liquids	Ultrashort-acting barbiturates:
Ether	Thiopental (Pentothal)
Halothane (Flurothane)	Methohexatal (Brevital)
Methoxyflurane (Penthrane)	Thiamylal (Surital)
Enflurane (Ethrane)	Others (Ketamine)
Gases	
Cyclopropane	
Nitrous oxide	

Table 35-6 *Adverse reactions to general anesthetics*

Intraoperative	Postoperative
Systemic hypotension	Nausea, vomiting
Arrhythmia	Hepatitis (halothane)
Respiratory depression	Nephropathy (methoxyflurane)
Malignant hyperthermia	Unpleasant dreams (Ketamine)

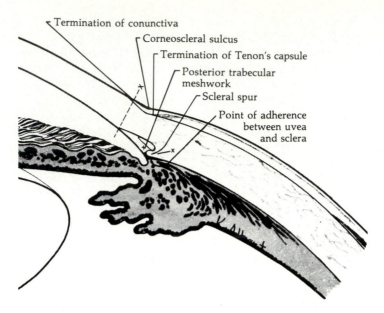

Fig. 35-2 Limbus anatomy.

Uvea

The rich blood supply to the pars plicata makes it prone to hemorrhage. When entry into the vitreous or posterior chamber is necessary, the safe incision site is limited to the pars plana. The standard pars plana approach is initiated 4 mm from the limbus. The only normal areas of adhesion between the uvea and the sclera are at the scleral spur and where the blood vessels penetrate the sclera. The sclera-choroid/ciliary body association is thus a loose one, and the supraciliochoroidal space may easily accumulate fluid as seen in postoperative ciliochoroidal detachments.

Trabeculectomy

The effectiveness of trabeculectomy, as an initial procedure, in lowering IOP to 21 mm Hg or less for primary open-angle glaucoma and for secondary open-angle glaucomas, such as pseudoexfoliation and pigmentary glaucoma is on the order of 80% to 90%.*

Step 1: Exposure of surgical region: A wire speculum is inserted to keep the lids open and adjusted so as not to cause any pressure on the globe. The eyelashes should be out of the surgical field, under the plastic drape.

Step 2: Bridle suture (Fig. 35-3): A traction suture

allows rotation of the globe inferiorly to bring the superior bulbar conjunctiva into view. A closed Lester forceps is slid into the superior fornix where it is opened and directed perpendicularly to the globe, grasping the superior rectus tendon securely. The globe is then rotated inferiorly, and a 4-0 silk suture on a tapered needle is passed under the superior rectus tendon. The suture is then clipped to the drape, keeping the globe in a fixed position.

Step 3: Conjunctival flap: Either a limbal or a fornix-based conjunctival flap is made with Wescott scissors and a nontoothed Pierce-Hoskins forceps. Neither flap is superior to the other in terms of IOP reduction or the ultimate success of the surgery.[186,188,273,319] However, the character of the bleb may be different; with the limbal-based flap, the bleb seems to be more localized and elevated; with the fornix-based flap, it is more diffuse and flatter.

Limbus-based flap (Fig. 35-4)

The conjunctiva is grasped over the superior rectus insertion and elevated, putting the conjunctiva between the forceps and the superior rectus tendon on traction. A buttonhole through conjunctiva is made with sharp dissection, and the incision is extended superiorly 8 mm from, and parallel to, the limbus. Tenon's capsule is next buttonholed and incised 2 mm anterior to the conjunctival incision so as to avoid the anterior ciliary arteries near the superior rectus tendon insertion.

---

*References 29, 31, 43-45, 66, 67, 71, 77, 106, 132, 138, 139, 185, 200, 206, 214, 219, 246, 247, 264, 272, 328, 329, 331, 332, 334, 335, 344, 352.

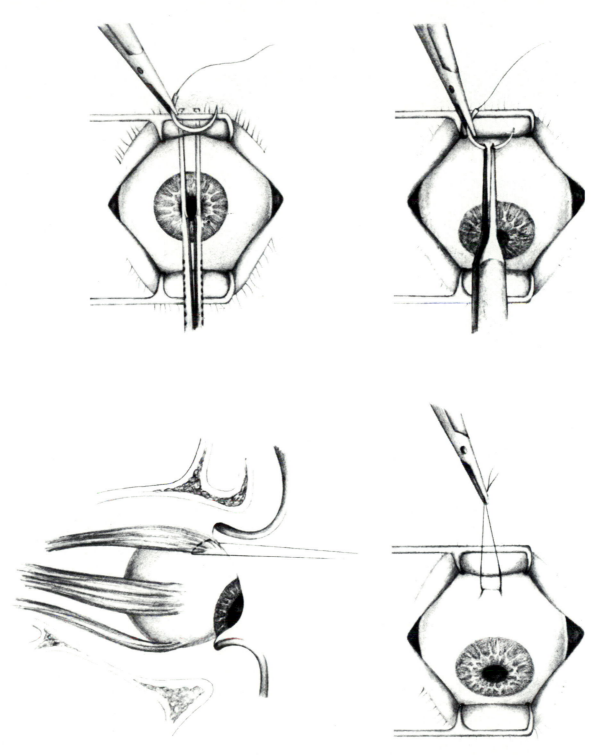

Fig. 35-3 Placement of superior rectus bridle suture.

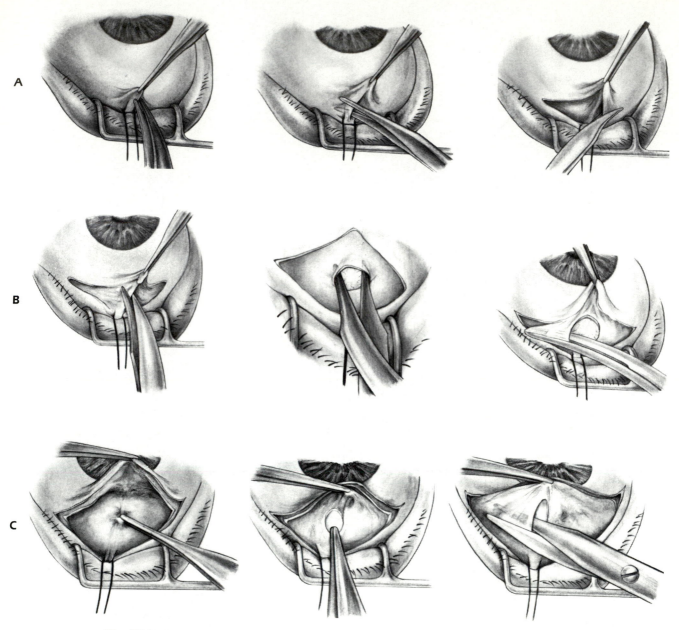

Fig. 35-4 Limbus-based conjunctival flap. **A,** Conjunctival incision; **B,** Tenon's capsule incision; **C,** Episcleral incision.

While the conjunctival flap is elevated, the limbal area is exposed, and the episclera is sharply dissected with Wescott scissors. The conjunctival-Tenon's capsule-episcleral flap is raised in three separate incisions, each deeper layer being incised farther anteriorly (Fig. 35-5). The conjunctival-Tenon's capsule flap is extended anteriorly, either bluntly with a dry cellulose sponge or sharply with a No. 67 Beaver blade. The blade is placed with the flat surface pressed toward the sclera and the sharp tip under the flap. The blade is advanced anteriorly, while cutting, to extend the conjunctival flap anteriorly. If necessary, a superficial lamellar corneal or scleral dissection may be performed. The corneoscleral sulcus should become clearly visible, with no fibers crossing it. The extent of the anterior dissection can be seen by placing the flat part of the surgical blade at the conjunctival flap insertion and draping the flap over the blade (Fig. 35-6). The end point is a clear definition of the surgical limbus

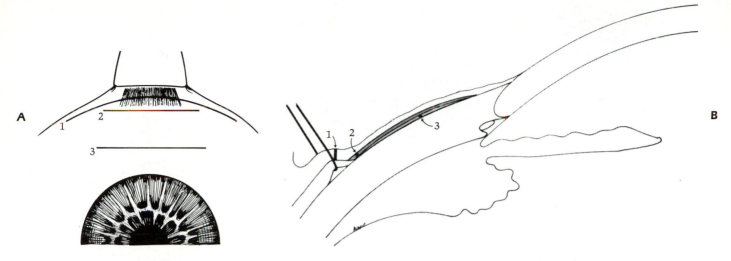

Fig. 35-5 Relative location of incision for conjunctival flap. **A**, Front view. **B**, Side view. *1*, Conjunctival; *2*; Tenon's capsule; *3*, episcleral.

with the three zones of clear, blue and white limbal tissue. In eyes with small anterior segments, or those with preoperatively noted peripheral anterior synechia (as in chronic angle-closure glaucoma), the conjunctival flap must be dissected further anteriorly.

Fornix-based flap (Fig. 35-7)

Disinsertion of the conjunctiva and Tenon's capsule between the 10 and 2 o'clock positions is performed with the Wescott scissors or with a No. 67 Beaver blade. An oblique relaxing incision at one or both of the corners allows the flap to retract superiorly away from the surgical limbus.

Step 4: Scleral flap: After lightly cauterizing every actively bleeding vessel, the scleral flap, measuring 2 to 4 mm circumferentially and 3 to 4 mm radially is demarcated by the wet field cautery (Fig. 35-8). While fixating the globe with a 0.12 mm toothed forceps, the No. 67 Beaver blade, held perpendicularly, incises the sclera to approximately one-half depth. A corneal-based scleral flap is raised by the No. 67 blade, held tangential to the globe (Fig. 35-9). The thickness of the flap is frequently assessed and adjusted according to preference. Guarded blades of predetermined depth may be used to accurately determine scleral flap thickness.[179] The scleral flap is best held with a nontoothed Pierce-Hoskins forceps. This will help avoid a perforation or tear, as might occur with toothed forceps, giving rise to undesired full-thickness drainage. Keeping the area meticulously dry and using relatively high magnification help the

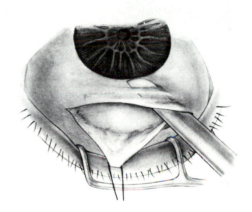

Fig. 35-6 Exposure of limbus.

surgeon raise the flap accurately and safely. A square or triangular flap may be performed; no significant difference in success rate has been reported.[151]

Step 5: Paracentesis track (Fig. 35-10): A corneal paracentesis track is made *before* opening the globe. Grasping the vertical edge of the scleral bed with a 0.12 mm toothed forceps, a 25-gauge sharp disposable 5/8-inch needle on a 3 ml syringe is guided horizontally in clear cornea, starting at the limbus away from the surgical area. The tip of the needle must never be directed toward the iris or lens; it must always be kept *parallel* with the plane of the iris. By pushing down with the shaft of the needle, while holding the syringe and needle parallel to the iris plane, the anterior chamber is entered with the tip not pointed to the lens or iris. Lens injury

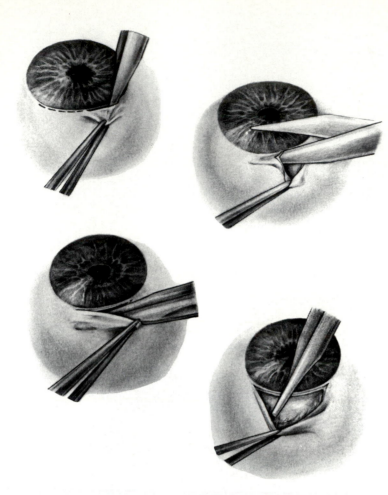

Fig. 35-7   Fornix-based conjunctival flap.

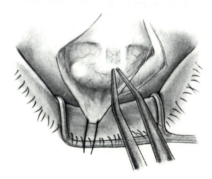

Fig. 35-8   Cauterizing and incising margins of scleral flap site.

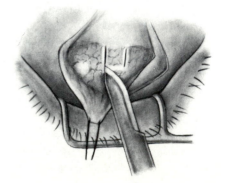

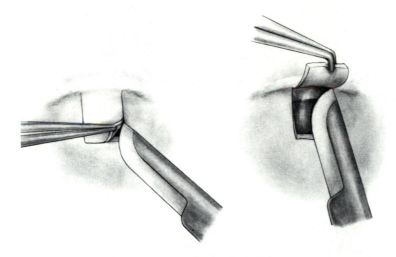

Fig. 35-9 Elevation of scleral flap.

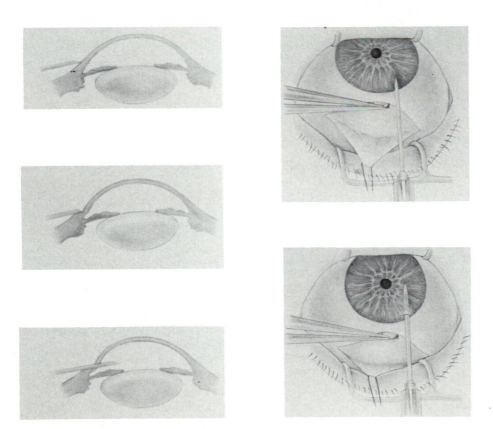

Fig. 35-10 Paracentesis track.

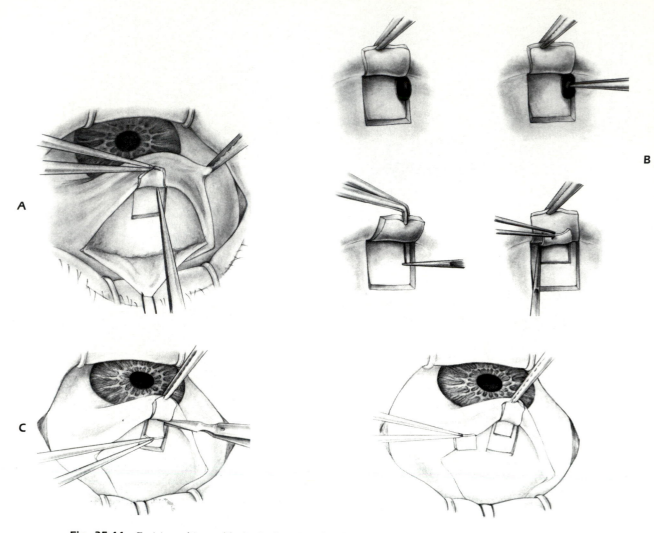

Fig. 35-11 Excision of inner block. **A,** Anterior chamber entry; **B,** Radial and posterior margin incisions; **C,** Anterior margin incision.

is extremely unlikely if the needle point is never directed toward the iris. The track, if properly made 1 to 2 mm through the corneal stroma, is self-sealing.

Step 6: Internal block excision (Fig. 35-11): While the assistant elevates the scleral flap, a radial incision with a No. 67 Beaver or a No. 75 microblade is made from immediately under the flap junction down to the blue-white transition zone, the site of Schwalbe's line. A similar incision can then be made on the other side. One tip of the Vannas scissors is introduced through the radial incision and slid posteriorly.

To minimize bleeding, the posterior incision should be made anterior to the scleral spur and probably even anterior to Schlemm's canal. Moving the incision anteriorly does not decrease the suc-

cess rate. Moving the incision posteriorly increases the incidence of complications (bleeding, cyclodialysis, inflammation), but it does not increase the success rate.[181,294,313]

After the two vertical incisions have been connected posteriorly, the iris may prolapse through the wound. A small iridotomy will allow the iris to fall back out of the way.

While the surgeon firmly pulls the posterior block edge posteriorly (superiorly), the assistant holds the scleral flap, pulling anteriorly (inferiorly). The anterior edge of the block is then cut flush with the flap insertion, as anteriorly as possible. One of the most frequent causes for failure is blockage of the trabeculectomy site by iris or ciliary processes, a result of an incision made too far posteriorly. The scissors should always be held with the

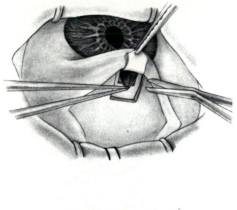

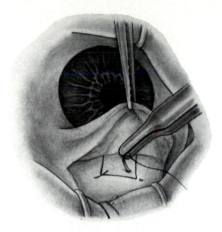

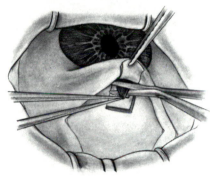

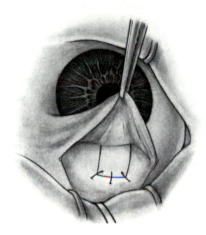

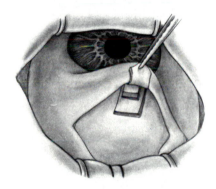

Fig. 35-13 Scleral flap closure.

Fig. 35-12 Peripheral iridectomy.

blades oriented vertically to ensure that the edges will be cut squarely and not shelved.

Step 7: Dilation: The pupillary sphincter and the ciliary body muscle should be completely paralyzed before the conclusion of surgery. This helps assure adequate pupillary dilation, preventing posterior synechiae, which may later interfere with vision or cataract extraction and may predispose to pupillary block. It also facilitates movement of the lens-iris diaphragm posteriorly, decreasing the chance for a flat anterior chamber and malignant (ciliary block) glaucoma. Wide dilation is best done

at the time of surgery because the muscles are already partially paralyzed by the retrobulbar anesthetic, and there is no postoperative inflammation to stimulate muscle spasm.

Atropine 1% topically is the most appropriate agent for achieving cycloplegia in glaucoma surgery. Multiple instillations every 2 to 5 minutes may be used. Phenylephrine may be added to achieve better dilation. The dilating drops may not need to be started until after the iridectomy, but if the patient has used miotics for many years, it is usually appropriate to start topical atropine earlier, in some cases preoperatively.

Step 8: Peripheral iridectomy (Fig. 35-12): A broad, peripheral iridectomy helps avoid iris incarceration into the internal sclerostomy. After the iris is elevated with forceps, it is first pulled away from the DeWecker-Barraquer scissors, and then it is pulled toward them while cutting. In this way a

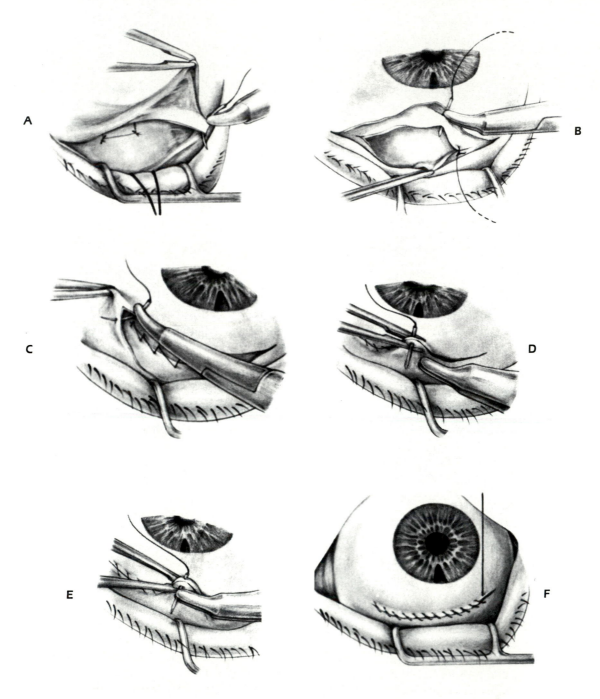

Fig. 35-14 Limbus-based conjunctival flap closure. **A,B,** Tenon's capsule; **C,** externalized suture; **D,E,** conjunctiva; and **F,** completion.

broad iridectomy is created, spanning the full extent of the internal sclerostomy. The iridectomy need not be truly "basal," but it must be large enough to ensure that the edges of the iris do not occlude the trabeculectomy site. Also, it should be noted that a basal iridectomy increases the likelihood of bleeding. The scissor blades should be held circumferentially, cutting along the limbus, not radially toward the pupil. Irrigation into the sclerotomy, and stroking toward the cornea from the limbus with a 21-gauge cannula elbow will free the remaining iris, allowing the return of a round pupil. If bleeding should occur at the iris root or ciliary body, gentle pressure with a cellulose sponge or judicious cautery is usually appropriate. However, the proximity of the zonules and vitreous must be kept in mind.

Step 9: Scleral flap closure and assessment of filtration (Fig. 35-13): The scleral flap is reapproximated to the scleral bed by 10-0 nylon sutures at both corners. The posterior edge usually scars down postoperatively, eventually leaving only the anterior radial edges of the scleral flap leaking. Therefore, the posterior edge is tightly apposed with a third suture. This avoids an increased flow rate that could lead to early postoperative problems, such as a flat anterior chamber, without any long-term benefit. The needle should be passed through the partial thickness flap without the aid of forceps because they may damage the flap. Knots are rotated onto the scleral side. Coating the suture with Healon is helpful when burying the knots. Slipknots may be used to adjust the tightness in the closure to control the rate of outflow.[242]

Using a blunt, 30-gauge cannula, the anterior chamber is reformed through the paracentesis track. Adequacy of filtration at the sides of the scleral flap is judged with cellulose sponges. Attention is directed to the anterior edge of both radial incisions. If the flow is excessive and the anterior chamber shallows, the slipknots are tightened and/or additional sutures are placed. If the leakage seems inadequate, and a firm globe by finger tension is present after reformation, the surgeon may, in decreasing order of preference, (1) loosen the slipknots or remove the permanent tight sutures and replace them with looser sutures; (2) apply cautery to the radial edges of the scleral flap or to the sclera adjacent to the scleral flap anteriorly, causing the wound to gape; (3) make small scleral flap incisions with a Vannas scissor to relax the tension of the flap; or (4) raise the scleral flap again and enlarge the internal block closer to the scleral bed edge.

Step 10: Conjunctival flap closure
LIMBAL-BASED (Fig. 35-14)

Tenon's capsule is closed with five to six running, locking 9-0 polyglactin or 8-0 chromic sutures (Fig. 35-16, *A* and *B*). The suture is then externalized through the conjunctiva at the apex of the conjunctival incision on the left (Fig. 35-16, *C*). A water-tight conjunctival closure is made with multiple nonlocking throws (Fig. 35-16, *D*). Tenon's capsule approximation need not be fastidious because it is intended to provide only structural stability, lessening the likelihood of large overhanging corneal blebs. However, the conjunctival closure must be meticulous in order to prevent a wound leak that could lead to loss of the bleb and a flat anterior chamber.

FORNIX-BASED (Fig. 35-15)

The corneal epithelium is debrided near the limbus with a No. 67 Beaver blade and dry cellulose sponges. This allows better adhesion of the conjunctiva to that region during healing. A 9-0 polyglactin or 10-0 nylon suture is passed through partial thickness sclera at the 9 and 3 o'clock positions, and then through the conjunctival flap margin and tied snugly. The flap is thus brought tightly over the cornea 2 to 3 mm superiorly. Relaxing incisions are also closed tightly. It is essential that the cut edge of the flap be very tightly adherent and taut. If the flap remains loose or if antimetabolite therapy is to be used, interrupted 10-0 nylon sutures are positioned along the limbus, holding the conjunctiva taut with the knots rotated into the cornea.

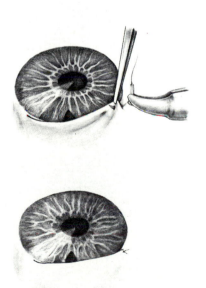

Fig. 35-15 Fornix-based conjunctival flap closure.

Step 11: Reformation of the anterior chamber and bleb elevation (Fig. 35-16): Balanced salt solution is then injected through the paracentesis track with a 30-gauge blunt cannula to deepen the anterior chamber and elevate the filtration bleb. Simultaneously, the IOP is monitored by a finger on the globe. Ideal IOP is approximately 15 to 25 mm Hg. If the bleb does not elevate and the IOP does not rise, there must be a leak, which must be identified and repaired. If the bleb elevates, the IOP does not rise, and the anterior chamber only temporarily deepens, the scleral flap must be sutured more snugly. Conversely, if the bleb does not elevate,

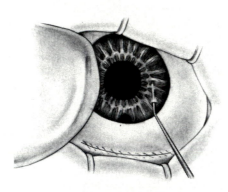

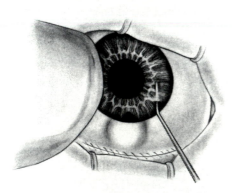

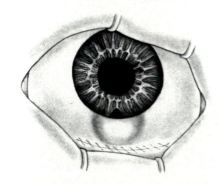

Fig. 35-16 Anterior chamber reformation.

and the IOP rises with deepening of the anterior chamber, the scleral flap must be loosened. Finally, if the bleb does not elevate and the anterior chamber remains shallow with continued elevation of IOP, three possibilities should be considered: aqueous misdirection, suprachoroidal expulsive hemorrhage, or a large choroidal effusion. A posterior sclerotomy 4 to 6 mm from the limbus made inferotemporally may be performed for a choroidal hemorrhage or effusion (Table 35-7).

Step 12: Eye dressing: Atropine ointment and a steroid-antibiotic combination ointment are instilled. If the facial block is still active or filtration is excessive, an eye patch is applied. If a periocular injection of antibiotic or steroid is contemplated, it should be made through the inferior fornix away from the bulbar conjunctiva, since there may be retrograde flow of the injected material into the anterior chamber with potential corneal toxicity. In addition, the surgeon should avoid making any unnecessary holes in the bulbar conjunctiva, because a troublesome wound leak may develop.

Determinants of Flow at the Trabeculectomy Site

The adequacy of filtration may be judged by determining the thickness of the scleral flap, the size of the internal block excised, the scleral flap overlap, and the tightness of the flap closure. The thinner the scleral flap, the more filtration is ob-

Table 35-7 Factors in judging filtration intraoperatively

Bleb	Anterior chamber	IOP*	Problem
High	Deep	Adequate (10-25 mm Hg)	None
Flat	Transiently deep (occasionally deep)	Low (<5 mm Hg)	Wound leak
Elevated	Transiently deep (occasionally remains deep)	Low (<5 mm Hg)	Excessive filtration
Flat	Deep	Elevated (>25 mm Hg)	Inadequate filtration
Flat	Shallow	Elevated (>25 mm Hg)	Aqueous misdirection, Suprachoroidal hemorrhage, Choroidal effusion

*In response to forceful filling of the anterior chamber with balanced salt solution using a 30-gauge cannula through the previously placed paracentesis track.

tained; perhaps some even occurs by transcleral aqueous flow.[60,188,230,244] Neither the size of the scleral flap nor the size of the internal block independently influences the rate of outflow.[213,279,296] However, jointly, in terms of overlap, they are very important. The less the scleral flap overlaps the scleral bed ledge next to the internal sclerotomy, the more freely aqueous will flow, and vice versa. Finally, by adjusting the tension and the number of the scleral flap sutures, the surgeon can titrate the flow. If the sutures are tied too tightly the procedure may fail.[213]

Revisions[304,311]

When reoperations are necessary, the original surgical site usually has significant conjunctival scarring and increased vascularity. It is often easier to reoperate at an adjacent area with less fibrosis. If performed at the same operative site, a fornix-based flap is technically easier. If a limbus-based flap is desired, sharp dissection with a No. 67 Beaver blade is preferable to scissor dissection. It is easy to buttonhole the adherent conjunctiva with scissors. It may also be necessary to create a superficial lamellar episcleral sheet when raising the conjunctival flap. It is often possible to delineate the extent of the conjunctival scarring by gently lifting the conjunctiva with a nontoothed forceps. Another technique is to elevate the conjunctiva by injecting balanced salt solution through a sharp 30-gauge needle away from the surgical region. Since postoperative scarring is even more prevalent with reoperations, an antifibrotic agent is recommended. In addition, large, fibrotic thickened sheets may demand a tenonectomy.

Postoperative Care

Topical medications used in the immediate postoperative period include cycloplegics, corticosteroids, and antibiotics. There are three useful functions of cycloplegics. Paralysis of the ciliary muscle tightens the zonular-iris-lens diaphragm and maximally deepens the anterior chamber. Second, the blood-aqueous barrier is maintained, thereby limiting proteinaceous exudation and cellular infiltration into the anterior chamber. Finally, there is symptomatic relief from the postoperative ciliary spasm. Generally, atropine is used because it is the longest acting. Steroids are used to inhibit inflammation and fibrosis.

A broad-spectrum antibiotic, such as gentamicin, may be used for about 1 week as theoretical prophylaxis against bleb infection and endophthalmitis.

Frequency of evaluation

The first 2 postoperative days are vital for ascertaining the adequacy and extent of filtration.

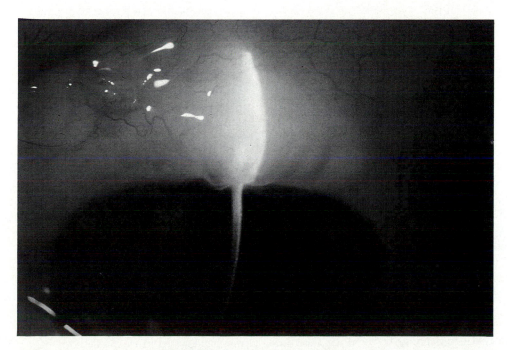

Fig. 35-17   Functioning filtration bleb.

Any critical modifications, such as instilling Healon to reform a flat anterior chamber or performing ocular massage to break early adhesions impeding outflow, are made at this time. These procedures may be more difficult on an outpatient basis, and the complication rate for outpatients may be slightly higher than it is for inpatients.[150] The initial follow-up visits are usually arranged for 1 week, 2 weeks, 1 month, and 2 months.

Assessment

Evaluation should include an assessment of the following parameters:
1. Bleb: (Fig. 35-17) extent and height, ischemia, limbal cysts, microcysts,[4] and possible wound leaks
2. Anterior chamber: hyphema, hypopyon, and depth if shallow. Grade 1—peripheral iris touch; grade 2—iris touch up to the pupillary margin; grade 3—lens-cornea apposition
3. Cornea: clarity, epithelial erosion
4. IOP
5. Presence of choroidal detachment or suprachoroidal hemorrhage
6. Optic disc and macula appearance

SPECIAL MODIFICATIONS
Operative Technique

Aphakia

Filtering procedures are less successful in aphakic eyes, especially in people under 50 years old.[20,121,206,329] A success rate of less than 5% was noted in one study.[121] Some have suggested that the vitreous promotes scarring or mechanically occludes the internal sclerostomy,[117] or that an inhibitor of conjunctival scarring has been lost, perhaps from having removed the lens.[243]

Vitrectomy.[26,117] Initially it seems that combining a total vitrectomy with a trabeculectomy might eliminate any vitreous-induced stimulation toward scarring. However, enthusiasm for total vitrectomies waned after longer follow-up. Frequent complications introduced by total vitrectomy included retinal detachments and vitreous hemorrhages. Long-term success was not increased. Thus, although total vitrectomies are not indicated, an anterior vitrectomy to remove forwardly displaced vitreous, which may mechanically obstruct the sclerostomy site or cause keratopathy with vitreous-cornea touch, is advisable.

Clear cornea trabeculectomy.[47,148] With the aim of avoiding conjunctival manipulation, a clear corneal approach for sclerostomy has been developed and used in a small number of cases. A corneal limbal-based half-thickness corneal flap is raised, and an internal block is excised close to the limbus. Further dissection is carried out posteriorly toward the ciliary body until blood reflux is obvious. Filtration blebs have been observed in some of these cases, indicating that aqueous can flow into the subconjunctival space, even without a direct surgical communication through the sclera. Success, however, has been low, and the procedure cannot be enthusiastically recommended.

Neovascular glaucoma[145]

Rubeotic eyes do not respond well to trabeculectomy because fibrovascularity leads to excessive scarring and hemorrhaging. Panretinal argon laser photocoagulation at an early stage prevents the advancement of anterior neovascularization and often leads to regression of existing iris and angle neovascularization. If the status of the eye permits one to perform panretinal photocoagulation first and wait for regression of iris neovascularization before proceeding with filtration surgery, good results may be obtained.[83] In more advanced situations filtration surgery has a success rate of, at best, 50% to 60%.[8,28,118,194] There have been several modifications aimed at improving the procedure's effectiveness.

Surgical modifications. One modification involves the creation of a very large 8-mm scleral flap and a large internal block excision.[172] A combined pars plana filtration procedure with a lensectomy and vitrectomy has also been proposed.[276] The small series in which these procedures have been used have shown high rates of serious complications.

Carbon dioxide laser. The attractive feature of the carbon dioxide laser is that it provides immediate hemostasis while making incisions. The operative field thus remains bloodless, and instrument manipulation of ocular tissues is unnecessary. At times there may be no need for instruments even to enter the eye. The laser scalpel has decreased the intraoperative complication rate,[16,175,176,316] but unfortunately long-term results appear unchanged.

Sturge-Weber syndrome

In infants or children, in whom the probable mechanism for pressure elevation is an abnormal angle, a goniotomy or trabeculotomy is probably the best procedure. After age 5, the responsible mechanism is more likely elevated episcleral venous pressure, or both an angle anomaly and elevated venous pressure. A combined trabeculotomy and trabeculectomy has been recommended.[32,231] In our experience, trabeculectomy alone works well. The scleral flap must be tightly closed and IOP returned near to normal to prevent excessive bleeding or growth of the choriodal angioma, which predisposes to a flat chamber. This growth is usually only a transient problem; as the IOP rises postoperatively, the enlarged angioma spontaneously shrinks.

Trabeculectomy designed to achieve low IOP

Trabeculectomy, performed in the usual manner, results in a final IOP higher than that achievable by full-thickness procedures. This disadvantage may be partially offset by making the scleral flap very thin (one-fifth the thickness of the sclera), a procedure demanding meticulous surgical technique. More sutures must be placed (usually at least five); these sutures must not penetrate the flap or be tied so tightly that they tear the flap. This is our standard technique.

Primary angle-closure glaucoma and other cases predisposed to flat anterior chamber

Flat anterior chamber and malignant glaucoma occur more often in primary angle-closure glaucoma, in nanophthalmos, in eyes with loose or excessively large lenses, in the exfoliation syndrome, and in patients in whom malignant glaucoma has occurred in the other eye. In these situations we prefer to make the scleral flap thicker than usual and suture it more securely. The flap should be at least one-third the thickness of the sclera. It is essential to assure that the chamber remains formed when filled with balanced salt solution at the end of the procedure. The operation must not be concluded until the chamber remains well formed with saline alone.

Antifibrosis

Tenonectomy

Tenon's capsule, which is especially thick in young patients and in black patients, probably is the major source of fibroblasts in the filtration area. As stated previously, however, a prospective series showed no benefit of performing a tenonectomy during filtration surgery.[141] High-risk patients have not been similarly studied.

Antiinflammatory agents

Corticosteroids seem to decrease the amount of collagen and fibroblast activity,[73,305] to increase outflow facility,[164] and to cause very thin blebs to leak.[303] Topical steroids clearly benefit bleb mor-

phology.[297] A course of 4 weeks of topical steroid therapy is usually sufficient. If used longer, a steroid-induced ocular hypertension may ensue.[287,341] The use of sub-Tenon's or subconjunctival steroid remains disputed. Preoperative injection of triamcinolone into the planned surgical site has been recommended.[102] However, if a subconjunctival hemorrhage should develop in that region, the surgery is jeopardized. The benefit of this technique has not been reproduced by others.[12] Oral steroids are even less attractive,[297] since they may cause profound systemic side effects, even with short-term use. Oral steroids should probably be used only in high risk cases.

We frequently use prostaglandin synthetase inhibitors. Indomethacin topically, however, has proved unexpectedly detrimental to filtration.[210] Given systemically, there is some evidence that these inhibitors help suppress scarring.[216] Currently we prefer sulindac (Clinoril) orally 200 mg twice daily.

Antimetabolites

Antimitotic agents have been tried locally with encouraging results in experimental and pilot clinical studies.[146,147,167,234] 5-Fluorouracil (5-FU) has been injected subconjunctivally immediately after standard filtration surgery[122,336] and has been repeated daily for up to 2 weeks (see Plate III, Fig. 2). Although it does inhibit wound healing in the surgical area, it also inhibits cell replication in undesirable locations, a process that leads to corneal epithelial defects and needle track leaks[157,171] (see Plate III, Fig. 3). Different dosage schedules must be studied. Preliminary experience suggests a good response from the limited use of 5-FU with the administration adjusted for corneal toxicity and wound leak.[337] The routine dosage is 5 mg/day for up to 2 weeks. 5-FU should not be used with a fornix-based conjunctival flap, since persistent wound leak may result unless a watertight closure is made. With limbus-based conjunctival flaps an unusually meticulous closure should also be performed. A nonabsorbable suture, such as nylon, should be used to secure the wound. On a more practical level, it should be kept in mind that receiving routine 5-FU injections is very inconvenient for patients who do not live nearby.

Inhibitors of collagen organization

Agents that interfere with collagen assembly also have been used to retard wound healing.[36,217,218] Beta-amino proprionitrile (BAPN), which inhibits lysine oxidase, an enzyme required for collagen linkage, has been clinically effective.[217,218] Oral colchicine, which blocks the microtubule assembly necessary for cell division and migration, has been used with possible benefit in the antifibrosis regimen of poor risk patients.[216]

Beta radiation

Strontium-90 has been advocated for preventing pterygium recurrence; it has also been applied to the bleb site to curtail fibroblastic activity.[55] Experience has been too limited to determine its effectiveness, but a recent report suggests it is not beneficial.[212]

Maintenance of High Flow Rate

There is a delicate line between ideal flow rate and excessive filtration with a flat anterior chamber. A number of techniques have been devised to approach the ideal flow rate without tipping toward excessive filtration.

Massage

Digital ocular massage raises the IOP, forcing more aqueous through the sclerostomy site.[82,308] With this maneuver, early adhesions may be broken, establishing an increased flow rate via the larger bleb. The surgeon or patient can either press firmly through the upper lid against the cornea for 10 sec, or push with two fingers on either side of the filtration bleb with the eye in down-gaze. However, certain complications may occur, such as iris incarceration in the sclerostomy,[266] hyphema,[222] bleb rupture,[211] or dehiscence of an incisional wound such as a corneal graft.[193] Another technique is to apply focal pressure on the conjunctiva, overlying the radial edge of the scleral flap, using a moistened cotton-tipped application (Figs. 35-18 and 35-19).[318] This deforms the edge of the trabecu-

lectomy flap rather than markedly elevating the IOP. Early scar formation is broken by the misalignment of the flap edge. Theoretically, a thin conjunctival bleb could be lacerated with such focal pressure. We use this maneuver almost routinely and have noted no apparent problems.

Mechanical suction to increase the flow rate in the perioperative period[91,92,93,95] has been found to have no long-term value,[116] and its original proponents no longer recommend it.

Compression shell[276]

Because filtering surgery is designed primarily to increase outflow, once performed, raising the IOP to any significant extent often is difficult, even with copious irrigation through a paracentesis track. A Simmons compression shell, made out of hard polymethylmethacrylate with an internal platform designed to be placed over the fistula track, is intended to slow the flow rate and to maintain the anterior chamber by temporarily increasing the resistance to outflow. The shell may be secured by two sutures inferiorly. The eye is bandaged securely for 3 days with daily changes before the shell is removed. The shell restricts outflow partially by tamponading the filtration area. In this way, a high outflow system can be established while minimizing the risk of immediate flat anterior chamber, profound hypotony, and resulting choroidal effu-

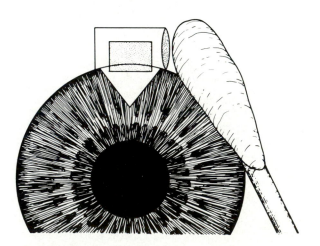

Fig. 35-18 Cotton tip focal massage of filtration site.

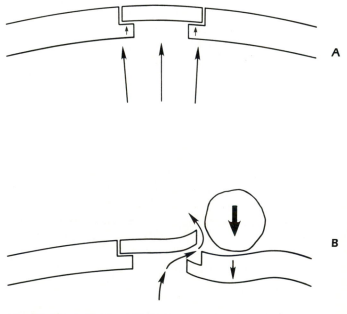

Fig. 35-19 **A,** Raising IOP does not necessarily increase outflow. **B,** Deformation along scleral flap wound edge allows better aqueous outflow.

sion. We currently employ a different type of shell (Fig. 35-20). The shell is designed to compress the bleb but not to traumatize the cornea, which in our experience has been a serious problem with the Simmons shell. Our ring shell appears to predispose to the same low IOPs with extensive diffuse blebs that are characteristic of eyes treated with the Simmons shell.

Releasable sutures

The scleral flap of a trabeculectomy is usually closed securely with several interrupted sutures, allowing only modest outflow. On or after the first postoperative day, the scleral flap sutures may be released by loosening a slipknot or by cutting the sutures with a blade if sutures are externalized or transconjunctivally with the argon laser, using the Hoskins lens.[128,256] The small button on the Hoskins lens is positioned over the flap and flattens the conjunctival bleb, enabling a clear view of the suture. A power setting of 300 to 600 mW at 0.1 sec and a 50 to 100 μm spot size is used. A slipknot with at least one end externalized may be pulled to release the tension and thus allow wound gape at that point of the flap edge.[271,346] The sutures may also be externalized by passing them transcorneally before tying.[346] These sutures may easily be cut with a No. 75 microblade and will then retract into the cornea.

Viscoelastics

Viscoelastic materials, such as sodium hyaluronate, help maintain the anterior chamber for the first day or two, allowing the eye to equilibrate at a low IOP. They also temporarily plug the trabecular outflow system, often a desirable effect in filtering surgery, since it diverts more outflow through the filtration site. Although viscoelastic materials may help in trabeculectomy,[10,24,30,229] some researchers have concluded that they do not.[314,347] We find them useful in difficult cases. For example, in Schocket tube placements they help maintain the anterior chamber in the first 2 days, a period in which there is a relatively high incidence of flat anterior chambers.

Bleb Filtration[37,119,201,243,315]

Mechanisms postulated to account for IOP reduction after filtration surgery include transconjunctival filtration of aqueous, reabsorption through walls of degenerated veins, or movement of aqueous into the superficial conjunctival lymphatics, or into aqueous veins.[22] Outflow may be via Schlemm's canal in a few cases, or perhaps even through uveoscleral drainage. The character and morphology of the bleb is determined by the predominance and combination of these routes.

Guarded filtration procedures have several advantages. If IOP is above episcleral venous pres-

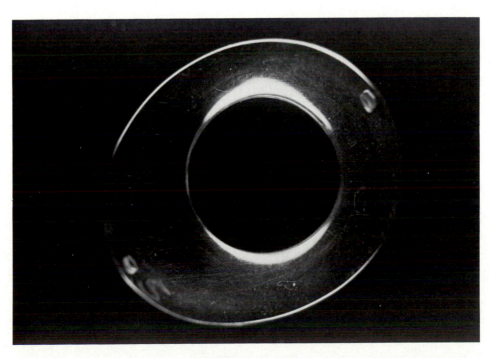

Fig. 35-20   Ring shell.

sure, the physiologic pathways presumably continue to function. Also, the sequence of hypotony, ciliochoroidal separation, aqueous shutdown, persistent hypotony, and scarring is avoided. The continuing production of aqueous and the bathing of the filtration area by the aqueous may assist the possible collagenolytic activity of aqueous to help establish filtration.

Filtration may fail from occlusion of the internal sclerotomy (by iris, Descemet's membrane, vitreous, blood, or ciliary body), or from external scarring of the surface tissue.[123,233] Internal occlusion is largely preventable by proper surgical technique. Fibrosis over the external sclerotomy site, however, is a far more important cause of failure of bleb formation and is harder or impossible to prevent. When a bleb is failing because of internal plugging, eliminating the obstruction may save the operation. This can be accomplished in some cases with the laser or through a transcorneal needle or trans-anterior chamber blade approach.[311]

OTHER FILTRATION PROCEDURES

The preference for trabeculectomy over other filtration procedures is largely a result of the higher complication rate of the unguarded operations. These "full-thickness" procedures were designed to make a direct communication from the anterior chamber to the subconjunctival space. Flat anterior chamber, choroidal detachment, endophthalmitis, and cataract formation are relatively frequent problems, however. The scleral flap of trabeculectomy increases the outflow resistance and decreases the chance of hypotony. However, long-term survival may be poorer with trabeculectomy than it is with full-thickness procedures. Also, and perhaps most important, final IOP is higher with standard types of trabeculectomy than it is with full-thickness procedures. As described, trabeculectomy may be modified to achieve a lower pressure. In almost all cases this is our preferred initial technique. Occasionally, especially when pressure has not been lowered adequately by modified trabeculectomy, a full-thickness procedure appears warranted. Success of glaucoma surgery may be greater in black patients with a Scheie procedure than with a trabeculectomy.

Thermal Sclerostomy*

After fashioning a limbal-based conjunctival flap and cleaning the limbal area so that the corneal

scleral sulcus is clearly defined, a 3 mm line of cautery is placed 1 mm posterior to the corneoscleral sulcus. Alternating blade dissection with cautery, a full-thickness incision is made. The cautery causes wound retraction, ideally resembling a watering trough, creating a 1 mm wound gape. This procedure is a full-thickness operation we usually perform.

In an effort to reduce the likelihood of a flat anterior chamber in the postoperative period, thermal sclerostomies have been performed under a scleral flap.* An internal block is cauterized and incised rather than excised, as it is in trabeculectomy. Cauterization of the scleral edges leads to a more permanent fistulous track.[253] Results are probably comparable to those obtained by trabeculectomy.

Posterior Lip Sclerectomy[107,131,169,198,199]

After the limbal-based conjunctival flap has been reflected, a shelved incision is made through the sclera at the insertion of Tenon's capsule. The incision is extended for a total width of 5 mm with Castroviejo corneoscleral scissors. Using a 1.5-mm Holth punch, two or three bites of complete scleral thickness are taken through the posterior wound margin. The size of the sclerotomy is 1 × 3 mm. A broad-based peripheral iridectomy is made. The conjunctival and Tenon's flap are closed. Reformation of the anterior chamber through a paracentesis track with balanced salt solution deepens the anterior chamber and raises a filtration bleb. The chamber often collapses, however, and depth cannot be maintained. Postoperative care is similar to that with trabeculectomy, except that the patch is left in place until the next day.

Trephination†

Although highly successful in reducing IOP to very low levels, trephination is now rarely recommended because it is difficult to perform, it is associated with a high incidence of cataract progression, and late endophthalmitis has been reported in more than 1% of eyes. The blebs for this procedure are characteristically very thin and likely to tear.

Since this procedure is recommended only in unusual circumstances, suffice it to mention here only that it involves using a trephine to cut a 1 to 1.5 mm button of corneoscleral tissue at the limbus. Care must be taken not to injure the underlying

---

*References 29, 34, 69, 71, 180, 196, 221, 258, 260, 261, 269, 278, 283, 320, 324.

*References 57, 113, 114, 263, 285, 324.
†References 21, 61-63, 78, 134, 168, 240, 295, 300, 326, 330.

iris or lens when entering the anterior chamber. A new approach of internal trephination with an automated instrument passed across the anterior chamber may hold promise for aphakic eyes.[38] No conjunctival manipulation is necessary with this approach.

Iridencleisis*

Iridencleisis is based on the idea that the iris can become a conduit for aqueous flow from the anterior chamber into the subconjunctival space. The iridencleisis was really the first "guarded" filtration procedure, since the outflow of aqueous is retarded by the iris, decreasing the incidence of flat anterior chambers and hypotony.

Iris inclusion into a limbal wound is a highly satisfactory procedure, but it fell into disfavor because it was reported to be associated with a high incidence of sympathetic ophthalmia. However, these reports were generated at a time when iridencleisis was the most popular operation for glaucoma and their validity is questionable. It is an excellent procedure when performed according to Stallard, using iris to plug up the sclerostomy by flapping "the peripheral iridectomy" and avoiding the updrawn pupil that frequently followed the other older methods of iridencleisis. The success rate is high and the complication rate low. Modifications under a scleral flap do not seem to offer any practical advantage over the Stallard iridencleisis.

COMBINED SURGERY†
Filtration Combined with Cataract Extraction

Three approaches are acceptable for removing a visually significant cataract in a glaucomatous eye: cataract extraction alone, filtering surgery followed by cataract extraction, or combined surgery. The latter is often preferable since it requires only one operation, and visual rehabilitation is neither delayed nor threatened by a marked postoperative IOP elevation. Cataract extraction in patients with glaucoma is a very different operation from cataract extraction in healthy eyes. The differences must not be ignored. Spikes of IOP are routine with all types of cataract extraction. In healthy eyes, such rises are relatively small and rarely troublesome. In glaucoma, however, they are larger and almost always dangerous; they may even be catastrophic.

Badly damaged optic nerves cannot tolerate IOPs on the order of 50 mm Hg for more than a few hours without being further permanently damaged. Additionally, glaucomatous eyes, especially those which have been treated for many years, may bleed profusely, have weak zonules, have small pupils that will not dilate, and have flaccid irides that adhere to any adjacent tissue or material.

Extracapsular cataract extraction or phaco-emulsification is usually chosen over intracapsular cataract extraction for three reasons: (1) a smaller incision is required, (2) the intact posterior capsule helps hold the vitreous away from the sclerotomy, and (3) placement of a posterior chamber intraocular lens is possible (the posterior chamber lens is the **only** implant recommended for a glaucoma patient).

Technique

Conjunctival flap

After placing a bridle suture, a fornix or limbus-based conjunctival flap may be fashioned. Surgery with a fornix-based flap is technically easier because it is easier to develop and to close, and the conjunctiva cannot be visualized while the cataract extraction is being performed. On the other hand, a limbus-based flap poses less risk of wound leakage, and postoperative massage may be performed or localized pressure applied without disrupting the adhesion forming between the edge of a fornix-based flap and the underlying sclera or cornea. Also, given the posterior bleb characteristic of a fornix-based flap, it is sometimes difficult to distinguish good filtration from aqueous shutdown in the postoperative period, since both may be associated with low IOP readings and low blebs.

Scleral flap

When a trabeculectomy is performed, a scleral flap is raised and a paracentesis tract made 2 to 3 mm anterior to the limbus temporally.

Limbal groove

A one-half thickness limbal incision is made with a No. 67 or No. 69 blade 1 to 2 mm behind the limbal junction for 10 to 11 mm. A preplaced mattress 8-0 silk suture is placed, dividing the groove into one-third segments. When rapid closure likely will be required (e.g., when there is a predisposition to suprachoroidal expulsive hemorrhage or when there is some danger that the patient may move or cough), it is essential to preplace these sutures before opening the eye. Preplacement is almost mandatory in patients predisposed to expulsive hemorrhage.

---

*References 14, 49, 65, 76, 115, 173, 191, 209, 215, 224, 312.
†References 9, 64, 75, 80, 81, 84, 85, 88, 97, 98, 125, 129, 140, 142, 153, 155, 187, 205, 223, 227, 236, 239, 251, 255, 275, 289, 293, 299, 336, 339, 343.

Anterior chamber entry

The anterior chamber is entered with a No. 75 blade under the scleral flap with a radial incision, as if making the first cut of an internal block excision. A viscoelastic substance is then injected into the anterior chamber to dilate the pupil mechanically, to protect the corneal endothelium, and to keep the anterior chamber formed. Posterior synechiae may be broken with the injection cannula, or if necessary, with a cyclodialysis spatula. If the pupil dilates widely, capsulotomy with an irrigating cystotome may be safely performed.

Pupil enlargement

If the pupil is inadequately dilated for cataract extraction, multiple sphincterotomies, sector keyhole iridotomy, or sector iridectomy may be performed. If only a modest increase in the pupil size is necessary, sphincterotomies with an intraocular scissor (e.g., a Vannas scissor) at three to four locations are adequate. Patients with tiny frozen pupils, usually the result of long-term use of miotics, most often are best managed with a sector iridectomy. After a peripheral iridectomy is performed, the iris is pulled through the wound hand-over-hand using a toothed forceps until the pupillary border is externalized; the iris is then excised with the deWecker-Barraquer scissors. For radial iridotomy, at this point the iris must be incised, not excised.

Anterior capsulotomy

A disposable 25-gauge needle tip bent at a 90-degree angle is used to perform a 360-degree anterior capsulotomy with multiple small cuts. Small strokes are made delicately going from the periphery to the center while rotating the cystotome tip. This maneuver is best performed with two hands. The end result should be about 50 interconnecting capsular tears in a "beer can" opening pattern. To ensure that the anterior capsule is completely free, the cystotome is swept circularly in the regions of the cuts to eliminate any small remaining bridges of capsule. If the pupil cannot be adequately dilated, the bent needle can be attached to a syringe containing sodium hyaluronate (Healon) or another similar agent. This can be injected into the posterior chamber to provide visualization and space for the capsulotomy to be performed with less trauma to the posterior surface of the iris.

Removal of nucleus and cortex

Extracapsular cataract extraction. The wound is enlarged to 10 to 11 mm using corneoscleral scissors held so that a beveled biplane incision is cre-

ated. The 8-0 silk preplaced suture is looped out of the wound. While the cornea is elevated, the anterior lens surface is wiped dry with cellulose sponges. Pressure is placed on the scleral side of the wound with a lens loop at the 12 o'clock position to tilt up the superior pole of the nucleus. If iris remains in the way, it is gently brushed back with cellulose sponges or grasped with a non-toothed forceps and slipped behind the nucleus. Gentle counterpressure at the 6 o'clock limbal position with a strabismus hook or an angled forceps is often necessary in a very soft globe. Since glaucomatous eyes characteristically have weak zonules, the surgeon should employ the minimum pressure necessary to tilt the nucleus into the wound. The assistant then pulls or rotates the nucleus out of the eye with a special lens hook.

We stress the importance of removing the lens nucleus primarily by "pulling it out" rather than by the usual method of "pushing it out." Pulling it out avoids the danger of pushing vitreous out the eye through the ruptured zonules. An excellent lens hook can be made by bending the No. 25 needle used previously as a cystotome. The preplaced mattress suture is then drawn up, cut, and tied, dividing the wound into thirds. The anterior chamber is reformed with balanced salt solution.

Remaining cortical material should be removed by any suitable technique. This may be difficult because of capsular tags or because of poor visualization associated with a small pupil. The surgeon should introduce the irrigation/aspiration tip to aspirate close to the posterior capsule, with the port anterior, irrigating first without aspiration to blow the anterior capsule away so that it will not be sucked into the port.

Phacoemulsification. A small limbal wound can be used with phacoemulsification. Currently, the wound must be enlarged when placing an intraocular lens. However, flexible intraocular lenses are being developed that may make this enlargement unnecessary. A 3 mm wound is made with a No. 55 M Beaver or No. 30 Starpoint blade under the scleral flap. To avoid corneal endothelial injury the nucleus is emulsified in the posterior chamber or pupillary plane. The central nucleus is sculpted to create a ridge inferiorly. The instrument tip should always be kept in view away from the iris and posterior capsule. The nucleus may be manipulated using this ridge to elevate it from the capsule into the pupillary area by a two-handed technique whereby the inferior ridge is depressed, thus elevating the superior pole. This maneuver requires the insertion of an instrument through a separate limbal incision. We prefer a single incision through which we inject sodium hyaluronate under the superior pole of the nucleus; this tilts up the superior edge. Phacoemulsification is then carried out in the pupillary zone. Cortical clean-up is done with the irrigation/aspiration handpiece, using a 0.3 mm aspiration port.

With phacoemulsification (as opposed to extracapsular cataract extraction) only a small incision is required, and thus there will be less postoperative astigmatism and inflammation. Also, with phacoemulsification visual rehabilitation is earlier and more rapid, and zonular stress is minimal. However, phacoemulsification is not recommended for all patients, especially those with very hard nuclei or small pupils. The surgeon must be completely familiar with the instrument and the technique. When improperly used, this technique causes more disastrous complications than any other procedure (e.g., loss of the nucleus in the vitreous cavity, corneal endothelial injury, and iris trauma).

Polishing the posterior capsule. We prefer to polish the posterior capsule despite the risk of rupture because it seems to help prevent subsequent capsule opacifications. Because of weak zonules, however, the capsule is often floppy, making polishing even more hazardous than usual.

Insertion of the posterior chamber intraocular lens

A posteriorly-angulated modified J loop or C loop lens should be used. In sector iridectomies, we prefer using a "no-hole" or two-hole lens rather than a four-hole lens. The latter are difficult to place without one hole showing in the iridectomy. In large eyes in which sulcus fixation is planned, a lens with a large diameter should be used. A lens with flexible haptics is preferable if it is to be placed in the bag. One-piece lenses and the 7 mm lenses with stiffer haptics are less appropriate.

The advantage of the lens with holes is the ease with which it can be dialed into position. The disadvantage is the visual "side effect" of the hole (halos), should it not be covered completely by iris. Thus, in patients needing sector iridectomies, or in those with dilated fixed pupils (e.g., those who have had a severe attack of angle-closure glaucoma), a "no-hole" lens may be preferable.

A 6 to 7 mm opening is adequate for the insertion of most posterior chamber intraocular lenses. Before insertion a viscoelastic material is injected into the posterior chamber. The surgeon must decide whether to place the hyaluronate "in the bag" or anterior to the anterior capsule, collapsing the anterior capsule onto the posterior cap-

sule and thus facilitating placement of the lens into the sulcus. After guiding the inferior haptic behind the iris, the superior haptic is grasped at the tip and inserted with a Kelman forceps and rotated 90 degrees counterclockwise to direct the elbow of the haptic posteriorly behind the iris before releasing it. If there is a sector iridectomy, or if a C loop posterior chamber intraocular lens is used (our preference), one haptic should be carefully placed in the bag. The junction between the haptic and optic is the "leading edge" and is placed into the bag inferiorly, the curled haptic entering the bag to the surgeon's left. The implant should be dialed into position with the haptics resting at the 3 and 9 o'clock positions horizontally.

In patients with the exfoliation syndrome, the zonules are usually weak and the lens partially dislocated; in these cases placement of the lens in the sulcus is probably preferable. In most cases, however, the lens is better placed "in the bag," since this keeps it well centered and may reduce the inflammatory response to the surgery. If the zonules are weak, as in many patients with advanced glaucoma or the exfoliation syndrome, there are advantages to implantation in the sulcus. On the other hand, eyes with 25 mm axial lengths or larger, which are not rare in patients with glaucoma, especially children, sulcus fixation is not advised, since the lens will not be held adequately in position. In these eyes lenses are best placed "in the bag."

Internal block incision and peripheral iridectomy

The corneoscleral wound is closed with interrupted 10-0 nylon sutures. In most cases it is advisable to remove the previously placed viscoelastic material and inject acetylcholine to reduce the pupil size. Air is placed in the anterior chamber to keep the intraocular lens away from the cornea during the removal of the trabeculectomy block. The internal block is then excised with Vannas scissors. After a peripheral iridectomy is made, the scleral flap is reapproximated with three 10-0 nylon sutures, one at each corner and one in the center of the posterior edge.

Testing filtration and wound closure

While irrigating through the paracentesis track, the surgeon checks for a watertight corneoscleral closure with leakage only through the trabeculectomy area. If all is well, the conjunctival flap is closed. If filtration is inadequate, cautery is placed on one or both radial edges of the scleral flap until flow is satisfactory. If filtration is excessive, addi-

---

**STEPS IN COMBINED CATARACT EXTRACTION—
LENS IMPLANTATION—GLAUCOMA
FILTERING SURGERY**

1. Lower IOP with an osmotic agent*
2. Dilate pupil as widely as possible
3. Take necessary steps to assure IOPs below 15 mm Hg
4. Place a superior rectus bridle suture
5. Place inferior rectus bridle suture*
6. Develop conjunctival flap
7. Cauterize bleeders and filtration site
8. Groove sulcus appropriately*
9. Develop scleral flap
10. Make paracentesis track
11. Enter anterior chamber and fill with sodium hyaluronate
12. Perform sector iridectomy*
13. Perform gentle, clean anterior capsulotomy—can opener style
14. Place two 8-0 black silk sutures in groove
15. Open eye with corneoscleral scissors, preserving sutures
16. Remove nucleus with bent needle with no expression
17. Tie 8-0 silk sutures and place one to three 10-0 nylon sutures leaving two entry ports
18. Remove cortical material with irrigation/aspiration and clean capsule
19. Insert hyaluronate ("in the bag")
20. Insert posterior chamber lens
21. Test and adjust position of lens
22. Remove hyaluronate
23. Inject acetylcholine in the anterior chamber
24. Inject air in anterior chamber
25. Perform sclerectomy (and iridectomies if not already done)
26. Close scleral flap
27. Test filtration and adjust as necessary
28. Close corneoscleral incision with 10-0 nylon partially
29. Remove 8-0 black silk sutures
30. Finish closing corneoscleral incision with 10-0 nylon and bury knots
31. Close conjunctiva
32. Fill anterior chamber to restore normal pressure and to develop high bleb, using balanced salt solution
33. Give corticosteroid and antibiotic subconjunctival injections*

*Optional steps depending on circumstances.
NOTE: Only steps 13, and 18 to 23, should be done with coaxial illumination.

---

tional sutures are placed. Irrigation through the paracentesis track should raise a conjunctival bleb and the anterior chamber should remain deep. An IOP of around 10 to 20 mm Hg upon completion is ideal; the eye should soften spontaneously. It is not necessary to flush out the viscoelastic substance completely, since the filtering site is present. A summary of the steps is shown in the box above.

An alternative technique for combined cataract and glaucoma surgery, using the guarded sclerectomy as a modified trabeculectomy, is described in Chapter 36.

Cataract Extraction in Eyes with Filtering Blebs*

The previous comments regarding the likelihood of pressure spikes after cataract extraction in patients with glaucoma must be kept in mind, though such rises are far less likely in these eyes. There are three major techniques of removing the cataract.

Clear corneal approach[228] (Fig. 35-21)

An incision is made through clear cornea immediately anterior to the filtration bleb. One must make this incision quite perpendicularly. If it is beveled, a larger incision is necessary to remove the nucleus. Care must be taken to suture the wound evenly, much in the way a corneal transplant would be sutured. The knots must be rotated into the cornea, but not into the wound itself, since they would be difficult to remove later were they to become caught in the healed incision junction.

The advantage of this technique is that neither the bleb nor any part of the conjunctiva is disturbed; also, it permits the surgeon to work in the familiar superior region. The major disadvantage is that significant corneal astigmatism may result and, because of the slow healing of the cornea, the sutures cannot be released until 6 weeks to 2 months or so postoperatively, delaying the time from surgery to full visual recovery. Also a cornea with marginal endothelial status may be compromised, leading to corneal edema.

Inferior limbal approach[249] (Fig. 35-21)

An inferotemporal conjunctival peritomy is carried out for 10 to 11 mm. A limbal wound is then made as is ordinarily done superiorly for routine cataract extraction. The advantage of this technique is that it avoids a pure corneal incision. However, it is quite awkward for the surgeon who is not used to working in the inferior position. Also, the conjunctiva is manipulated, albeit away from the filtering bleb.

Revision of bleb during cataract extraction (Fig. 35-22)

Another acceptable technique is the performance of the cataract extraction through a standard incision. This requires revising the original filtra-

---

*References 5, 13, 27, 161, 228, 245, 249, 257, 259, 351.

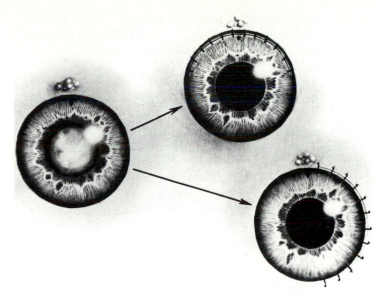

Fig. 35-21 Cataract extraction in eye with filtration bleb.

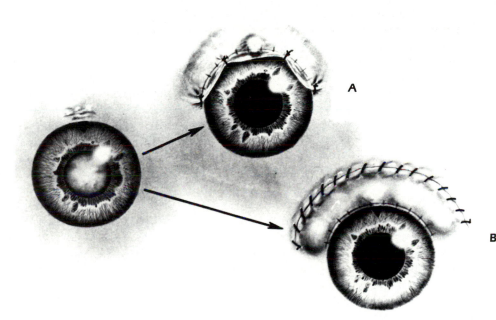

Fig. 35-22 Revision of filtration site and cataract extraction. **A,** Fornix-based conjunctival flap. **B,** Limbus-based conjunctival flap.

tion site and demands meticulous surgical technique to avoid damage to the conjunctiva. This procedure is not recommended for eyes with well-controlled IOP because of a well functioning filtering bleb, since in these eyes it probably more likely leads to loss of adequate filtration. However, in eyes with inadequate filtering blebs this method is preferred, since it allows a better bleb to develop and, more important, helps eliminate the pressure spike that typically follows cataract extraction in patients with glaucoma, and that typically leads to poor visual results in such patients.

Penetrating Keratoplasty with Filtration Surgery

Before a corneal transplant is attempted the IOP must be adequately controlled. If it is not, the chance of a graft surviving is markedly diminished. In addition, many glaucoma medications are toxic to the cornea and promote an inflammatory response postkeratoplasty. The surgeon can either control the IOP before corneal transplantation or combine filtration with the penetrating keratoplasty.[133] We strongly prefer the first approach.

COMPLICATIONS AND THEIR MANAGEMENT

Intraoperative

Conjunctival buttonhole

The location of the conjunctival tear determines the method of repair. If it is located in the center of the conjunctival flap or further posteriorly, a "purse string" with 10-0 or 11-0 nylon is attempted either internally on the undersurface of the conjunctiva or externally if the flap has already been reapproximated. If it is in the limbal area, it may be oversewn with adjacent conjunctiva, sutured directly to the cornea or sclera, closed as a "purse string," or a tissue patch may be applied to it.[130] If not treated it will often lead to a flat anterior chamber and failure of bleb formation.

Scleral flap disinsertion

The scleral flap guarding the sclerostomy may be avulsed during the procedure. If a sclerostomy has not yet been performed, conversion to a posterior lip sclerectomy or thermal sclerostomy may be entertained. However, if a sclerostomy has been performed, these may result in excessive filtration. Meticulous reapproximation of the scleral flap can be attempted with 10-0 or 11-0 nylon suture. If unsuccessful, a Tenon's capsule tissue flap may be sutured over the scleral flap site. It is tied in several locations into partial thickness sclera, spreading it tautly over the scleral flap site.

Vitreous loss

Risk factors for vitreous loss include buphthalmic eyes with thin sclera, high myopia, aphakia, and vitreous loss in the contralateral eye during surgery. The vitreous must be carefully cleaned from the operative site, since it may mechanically plug the sclerostomy. It may also lead to cystoid macular edema if there is traction on the posterior segment. A preventive measure suggested for eyes at high risk is a modified Flieringa's ring.[248] However, we do not use this.

Hyphema[342]

After performing a peripheral iridectomy or traumatizing the ciliary body, blood may fill the anterior chamber from the operative site. Predisposing factors include a blood clotting disorder (perhaps iatrogenic or drug-induced) and elevation of systemic blood pressure. Intraocular cautery should be avoided. However, if a bleeding spot does not stop spontaneously, it must be coagulated. This requires identifying the bleeder carefully. Blind cautery is not helpful. The chance of bleeding is decreased by performing the internal sclerotomy as far anteriorly as possible.

Suprachoroidal expulsive hemorrhage* (Fig. 35-23)

When the patient complains of sudden pain breaking through the local anesthesia, or when a formed anterior chamber collapses suddenly, a suprachoroidal hemorrhage should be suspected. Recognition of a suprachoroidal hemorrhage is essential, since the surgeon must not permit extrusion of ciliary body or retina. The previously placed sutures are closed immediately. At the same time the anesthesiologist is asked to administer acetazolamide 500 mg intravenously and start intravenous mannitol 20%. Closure should be performed as quickly as possible with multiple sutures while intermittently gently repositing the uvea with an iris spatula.

Posterior sclerotomies have been recommended to drain the hemorrhage and allow anterior chamber reformation. They are rarely needed or helpful at the time of surgery. Furthermore, the first order of business is immediate closure of the incision. Even a few seconds delay can transform a good result into a catastrophe. Drainage of the hemorrhage may be necessary later, but it is almost never successful at the time of surgery, since the decompression of the globe predisposes to continued bleeding. Once the eye has been closed, intravenous acetazolamide and mannitol may be used to lower the IOP and restore the eye to satisfactory condition. Prognosis for recovery of vision is good as long as the eye can be closed without loss of uvea.

Descemet's membrane detachment

Small scrolls of Descemet's membrane may be detached at the limbal wound or at the paracentesis track site; these usually require no specific attention, but a large scroll may lead to corneal edema in that region. By injecting air or Healon into the anterior chamber the detached Descemet's scroll is pushed back into place.[68] By reversing needle placement going from the scleral to corneal side, the Descemet's scroll may be secured if needed.

Retrobulbar hemorrhage

After the local anesthetic is given in the retrobulbar space, proptosis with lid ecchymoses and

---

*References 2, 48, 50, 90, 104, 206, 254, 291, 301, 340.

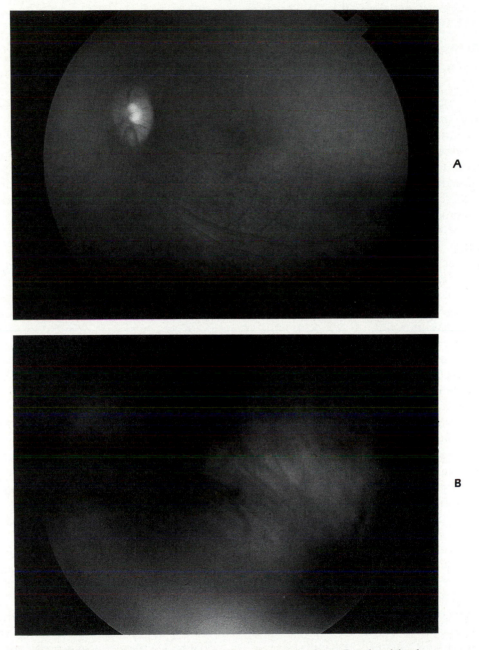

Fig. 35-23   Suprachoroidal hemorrhage. **A,** Posterior pole. **B,** Peripheral fundus.

subconjunctival hemorrhage indicate an orbital hemorrhage. If the IOP rises significantly with a tense orbit, optic nerve compression may ensue. An immediate lateral canthotomy may be necessary; mannitol should be given intravenously. The scheduled surgery should be postponed until the hemorrhage resolves, usually within 2 to 3 weeks. General anesthesia should be considered.

Postoperative

Hypotony and flat anterior chamber*

Low IOP, together with a flat, or shallow, anterior chamber after filtration surgery, may be due to excessive filtration, ciliochoroidal detachment with reduced aqueous production, or wound leak.

If there is excessive filtration, the surgeon may try a light pressure patch or a scleral compression shell to tamponade the scleral flap and reduce the aqueous outflow. Aqueous suppressants may also decrease aqueous production and allow conjunctival scarring, thus limiting the amount of potential filtration. If these methods fail, the persistent flat anterior chamber may lead to corneal decompensation and cataract progression. Usually surgical intervention may be avoided; however, it may be necessary to suture the scleral flap more tightly to limit the amount of filtration.

In case of choroidal detachment with aqueous shutdown, the surgeon should often wait, unless a decrease in bleb size, corneal decompensation, or prolonged shallowing of the anterior chamber become obvious. The grading system commonly used to note anterior chamber depth is grade 1, peripheral iris touch; grade 2, iris touch to the pupillary border; grade 3, corneal-lens or corneal-vitreal touch (Fig. 35-24). Grade 1 flat chambers usually reform spontaneously. Grade 3 chambers always need reformation. Type and timing of treatment of grade 2 chambers is not clear. In these cases the surgeon may simply reform the anterior chamber with air, balanced salt solution, or sodium hyaluronate to keep it formed until the ciliary body and choroid reattach and aqueous production is reestablished. Some surgeons promptly perform choroidal drainage through a sclerotomy 5 to 6 mm from the limbus, combined with an anterior chamber reformation using balanced salt solution.

A wound leak or conjunctival flap perforation may have been undetected at the time of surgery or have resulted postoperatively from the patient

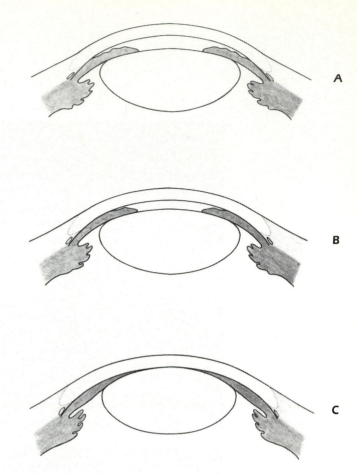

Fig. 35-24 Grading system for flat anterior chamber. **A,** Grade 1—peripheral iris touch. **B,** Grade 2—Pupil touch. **C,** Grade 3—Lens touch.

rubbing a very thin bleb, or from postcautery necrosis, or from wound dehiscence.[54,82,96,235,304] After identifying the site of aqueous leakage by Seidel testing[42,250] (Fig. 35-25 and Plate III, Fig. 3), a mode of correction is chosen on the basis of the location and the character of the filtration bleb. With thin, cystic blebs, a Simmons compression shell is often successful in reforming the anterior chamber and sealing the wound leak (mechanical).[207] Tissue adhesive and a bandage cataract lens may prove helpful with small leaks.[109] Bleb revision and conversion to a fornix-based flap is necessary should a simple closure technique prove unsuccessful. After surgical intervention a pressure patch may be left in place for 2 days.

Aqueous misdirection (malignant glaucoma)[79]

Medical treatment of aqueous misdirection is successful in about 50% of cases. Atrophine 1%,

*References 7, 17, 18, 23, 39, 41, 99, 163, 202, 206, 214, 220, 225, 270, 272, 322, 323.

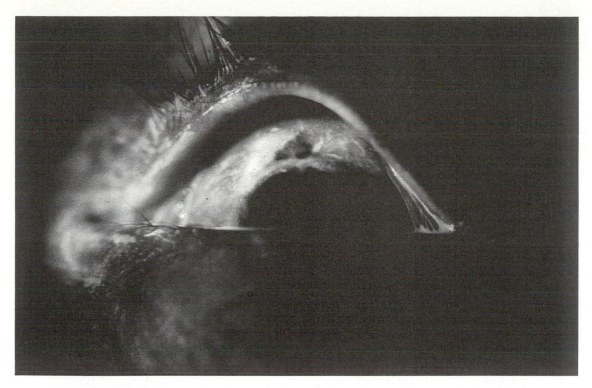

Fig. 35-25   Seidel (+) bleb wound leak.

phenylephrine 2.5%, beta-blockers topically, a hyperosmotic (mannitol IV), and a carbonic anhydrase inhibitor are all given. If conservative means, including argon laser treatment of visible ciliary processes or Nd:YAG laser incision of anterior hyaloid in aphakic eyes are not effective, a pars plana vitrectomy in phakic eyes, and a limbal vitrectomy in aphakic eyes, is one approach. Occasionally a lensectomy must be performed in combination with the vitrectomy. (See further discussion in Chapter 70.)

Bleb infection— endophthalmitis[19,33,144,184,197,309]

A milky white appearing infected bleb is characteristic of postfiltering surgery endophthalmitis. A purulent hypopyon may also be present (Fig. 35-26). In many cases the infection starts in the bleb and spreads into the anterior chamber and finally into the vitreous. Management depends on the type and stage of infection. Infection after surgery may occur early or late. If confined to the anterior segment, topical and periocular injections of antibiotics may suffice. An anterior chamber tap should be performed for Gram stain and culture sensitivity before starting antibiotic therapy. A vitreous tap

should also be performed if there is any indication of vitreal involvement by ophthalmoscopy, slit-lamp biomicroscopy, or ultrasonography. After the antibiotics have been used for a period of 12 to 24 hours, topical steroids should be started promptly and in orally large doses (e.g., 80 mg prednisone orally daily) to preserve the filtration site and prevent scarring. If the vitreous is involved, debulking the organisms, endotoxins, and debris with a vitrectomy and placement of intravitreal antibiotics are recommended.

Tenon's capsule cyst[232,321]

A Tenon's capsule cyst is a fibroblastic overgrowth that results in a tense, opalescent, thick-walled vascular bleb (Fig. 35-27); it is not lined with epithelial cells. It is in direct communication with the anterior chamber. An associated elevation of IOP is usual in the early postoperative period. A Tenon's capsule cyst characteristically resolves spontaneously within 2 to 4 months. Additional medication may be necessary to control IOP during that time. Bleb revision by simple needle incision is only temporarily beneficial. Better but still poor results have been obtained by excising the Tenon's cyst in toto. Where surgery is needed, a second

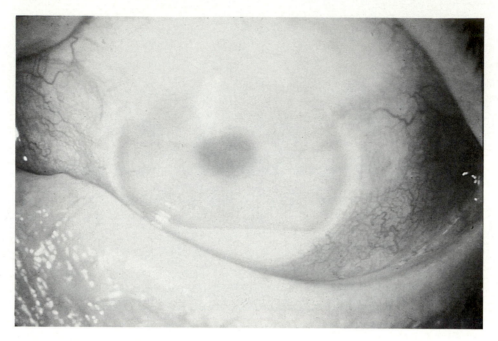

Fig. 35-26 Endophthalmitis in eye with filtering bleb.

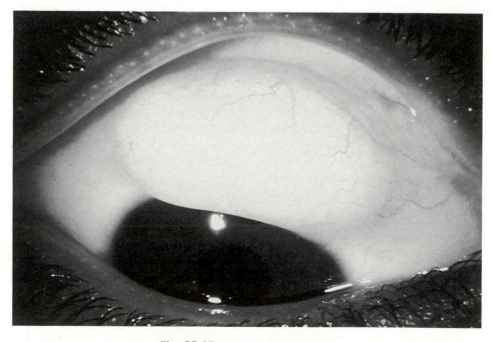

Fig. 35-27 Tenon's capsule cyst.

"new" procedure is usually appropriate, often one that employs an antifibrosis routine.

Cataract*

Substantial progression of cataract occurs in some filtration surgeries. The reported incidence varies from 2% to 53%, reflecting the wide variety of procedures and patient characteristics. It is our impression that uncomplicated surgery in a patient with a clear lens is typically not associated with any increased development of cataract. On the other hand, complicated surgery in a patient with marked nuclear sclerosis is "always" associated with rapid cataract progression. Uncomplicated surgery in a patient with a preexisting cataract usually increases the rate of lens opacification.

Topical steroids play a role in some cases. Topical and systemic steroids given conjointly increase the rate of cataract formation. Direct lens trauma during the operation may be responsible. There is also a strong correlation with flat anterior chamber,[56,67] perhaps through promotion of posterior synechiae.[237]

Visual field loss and loss of central vision[40,124,170,182,338]

Even with reduction of IOP there may be further visual field loss and loss of central acuity in cases with preoperative encroachment on central fixation.[6,158,226] Advanced glaucomatous damage may predispose to fixation loss, especially where field loss already involves fixation. We believe that "wipeout" occurs in around 5% to 10% of cases where field loss involves split fixation preoperatively.

Several recent studies suggest that visual fields may improve in certain eyes after filtration surgery. There are many variables, such as different perimetry techniques, cataract progression, maculopathy, change in pupil size, and use of medications, all of which make postoperative visual field analysis difficult.

Transient IOP elevation†

An IOP rise 3 to 4 weeks postoperatively is common after trabeculectomy. This may be due to the tissue evolution after surgery or to the topical steroids. If there is no Tenon's capsule cyst and filtration is active, the pressure elevation is usually transient and need cause no concern.

---

*References 139, 149, 214, 219, 257, 270, 272, 306, 307, 309, 328.
†References 60, 160, 238, 241, 288, 341.

Corneal dellen[286]

Elevated filtrating blebs, especially if not under the lid, may cause drying of the adjacent cornea, leading to dellen (see Plate III, Fig. 1). Topical lubrication with a bland ointment such as erythromycin is usually effective. When dellen occur in the postoperative period, it is best to use lubricants and wait. Most dellen will gradually clear. Later, when the dellen is the result of a well-established bleb, the problem is much more serious; it can be extremely troublesome to the patient. Cryoapplication,[53,70,309,350] cauterization,[52,152] photocoagulation, and trichloracetic acid[100] have all been applied to the bleb to shrink the tissue, but results have been inconsistent and often disappointing. Revision of the bleb is usually required,[82,262] but it frequently results in less successful filtration. With blebs that extend into the cornea, simple excision may work nicely. Because of the seriousness of this complication, we try to have the filtration site occur under the upper lid whenever possible.

Internal sclerostomy blockage[311]

Iris or a membrane may occlude the opening internally so that filtration is halted. Occasionally vitreous, lens, scleral fragments, or ciliary processes fill the fistula. Carefully inspecting the wound intraoperatively, and keeping the keratosclerectomy as far anterior as possible will avoid most of these problems. However, peripheral anterior synechiae and membrane growth can occur despite careful attention. Argon and Nd:YAG lasers have successfully opened internally sclerostomy sites. In addition, a transcorneal approach with a curved needle and a transanterior chamber approach with a goniotomy-type of blade have also been successful in cases where aqueous outflow is blocked through the internal sclerostomy. The techniques, however, are more easily described than performed; we have had few successes with any of them.

REFERENCES

1. Adebin, S, Simmons, RJ, and Grant, WM: Progressive low-tension glaucoma: treatment to stop glaucomatous cupping and field loss when these progress despite normal intraocular pressure, Ophthalmology 89:1, 1982
2. Abrams, GW, Thomas, MA, Williams, GA, and Burton, TC: Management of postoperative suprachoroidal hemorrhage with continuous-infusion air pump, Arch Ophthalmol 104:1455, 1986
3. Abramov, V, Vakurin, E, Artamonov, V, and Churkin, V: Evolution of surgical operations for open-angle glaucoma, Glaucoma 7:7, 1985

4. Addicks, EM, Quigley, HA, Green, W, and Robin, AL: Histologic characteristics of filtering blebs in glaucomatous eyes, Arch Ophthalmol 101:795, 1983

5. Agarwal, LP: Cataract extraction after postplaced valvular iridencleisis, Ophthalmologica 155:91, 1958

6. Agarwal, SP, and Hendeles, S: Risk of sudden visual loss following trabeculectomy in advanced primary open-angle glaucoma, Br J Ophthalmol 70:97, 1986

7. Allen, JC: Delayed anterior chamber formation after filtering operations, Am J Ophthalmol 62:640, 1966

8. Allen, RC, Bellows, AR, Hutchinson, BT, and Murphy, SD: Filtration surgery in the treatment of neovascular glaucoma, Ophthalmology 89:1181, 1982

9. Alpar, JJ: Cataract extraction in glaucomatous eyes: choice of operative technique, Glaucoma 7:165, 1985

10. Alpar, JJ: Sodium hyaluronate (Healon^R) in glaucoma filtering procedures, Ophthalmic Surg 17:724, 1986

11. Deleted in proofs

12. Ball, SF: Effects of triamcinolone injection, Arch Ophthalmol 104:1749, 1986

13. Baloglou, P, Malta, C, and Asdourian, K: Cataract extraction after filtering operations. Preliminary report on the control of intraocular pressure, Arch Ophthalmol 88:13, 1972

14. Barraquer, JI: Trabeculectomy—intrascleral filtering operation with and without iridencleisis. In Ferrer, OM, editor: Symposium on glaucoma, Springfield IL, Charles C Thomas Publisher 1976

15. Beauchamp, GR, and Parks, MM: Filtering surgery in children: barriers to success, Trans Am Acad Ophthalmol Otolaryngol 86:170, 1979

16. Beckman, H, and Fuller, TA: Carbon dioxide laser scleral dissection and filtering procedure for glaucoma, Am J Ophthalmol 88:73, 1979

17. Bellows, AR, Chylack, LT, Jr, Epstein, DL, and Hutchinson, BT: Choroidal effusion during glaucoma surgery in patients with prominent episcleral vessels, Arch Ophthalmol 97:493, 1979

18. Bellows, AR, Chylack, LT, Jr, and Hutchinson, BT: Choroidal detachment—clinical and manifestation, therapy, and mechanism of formation, Ophthalmology 88:1107, 1981

19. Bellows, AR, and McCulley, JP: Endophthalmitis in aphakic patients with unplanned filtering blebs wearing contact lenses, Ophthalmology 88:839, 1981

20. Bellows, AR, and Johnstone, MA: Surgical management of chronic glaucoma in aphakia, Ophthalmology 90:807, 1983

21. Bencsik, R, Opauzki, A, and Hudomel, I: Effectiveness of trepanotrabeculectomy in glaucoma, Glaucoma 3:42, 1981

22. Benedikt, OP: Drainage mechanism after filtration, Glaucoma 1:71, 1979

23. Berke, SJ, et al: Chronic and recurrent choroidal detachment after glaucoma filtering surgery, Ophthalmology 94:154-162, 1987

24. Berkowitz, P: Surgical wound leaks associated with sodium hyaluronate (Healon^R), Am J Ophthalmol 95:714, 1983

25. Deleted in proofs

26. Billore, OP, Shroff, AP, and Patel, CB: Trabeculectomy combined with pars plana vitrectomy in aphakic glaucoma (a comparative study), Indian J Ophthalmol 31:642, 1983

27. Binkhorst, CF, and Huber, C: Cataract extraction and intraocular lens implantation after fistulizing glaucoma surgery, Am Intraocular Implant Soc J 7:133, 1981

28. Bloch, RK, Hitchings, RA, and Laatikainen, L: Thrombotic glaucoma. Prophylaxis and management, Trans Ophthalmol Soc UK 97:275, 1977

29. Blondeau, P, and Phelps, CD: Trabeculectomy vs thermosclerostomy—a randomized prospective clinical trial, Arch Ophthalmol 99:810, 1981

30. Blondeau, P: Sodium hyaluronate in trabeculectomy: a retrospective study, Can J Ophthalmol 19:306, 1984

31. Blumenthal, M: Surgical approach to the trabeculum, Glaucoma 3:525, 1980

32. Board, RJ, and Shields, MB: Combined trabeculotomy for the management of glaucoma associated with Sturge-Weber syndrome, Ophthalmic surg 12:813, 1981

33. Bohigian, GM, and Olk, RJ: Factors associated with a poor visual result in endophthalmitis, Am J Ophthalmol 101:332, 1986

34. Bounds, GW, Jr, and Minton, LR: Peripheral iridectomy with scleral cautery, Am J Ophthalmol 58:84, 1964

35. Boyd, TAS: A comparison of surgical and conservative treatment in glaucoma simplex, Trans Ophthalmol Soc UK 75:541, 1955

36. Brancato, L, and Yablonski, M: Effect of dexamethasone and D-penicillamine in filtration surgery, Invest Ophthalmol Vis Sci (Suppl) 24:87, 1983

37. Brodeianu, CD: Research on the mechanism of trabeculectomy: the main pathway of the aqueous humor. In Greve, EL, Leydhecker, W, Raitta, C, editors: Second European Glaucoma Symposium, 1984, Helsinki, 1985, Dr. W. Junk Publisher

38. Brown, RM, et al: Internal sclerectomy for glaucoma filtering surgery with automated trephine, Arch Ophthalmol 105:133, 1987

39. Brubaker, RF, and Pederson, JE: Ciliochoroidal detachment, Surv Ophthalmol 27:281, 1985

40. Burke, JW: Field changes after satisfactory filtration operations for glaucoma, Trans Am Ophthalmol Soc 37:149, 1939

41. Burney, EN, Quigley, MA, and Robin, AL: Hypotony and choroidal detachment as late complications of trabeculectomy, Am J Ophthalmol 103:685, 1987

42. Cain, W, Jr, and Sinskey, RM: Detection of anterior chamber leakage with Seidel's test, Arch Ophthalmol 99:2013, 1981

43. Cairns, JE: Trabeculectomy—preliminary report of a new method, Am J Ophthalmol 66:673, 1968

44. Cairns, JE: Surgical treatment of primary open-angle glaucoma, Trans Ophthalmol Soc UK 92:745, 1972

45. Cairns, JE: Trabeculectomy, Trans Am Acad Ophthalmol Otolaryngol 76:384, 1972

46. Cairns, JE: Indications for surgery in glaucoma, Glaucoma 3:307, 1981

47. Cairns, JE: Clear cornea trabeculectomy, Trans Ophthalmol Soc UK 104:142, 1985

48. Cantor, LB, Katz, LJ, and Spaeth, GL: Complications of surgery in glaucoma: suprachoroidal expulsive hemorrhage in glaucoma patients undergoing intraocular surgery, Ophthalmology 92:1265, 1985

49. Cordia, L, Reibaldi, A, and Nacucchi, S: Subscleral iridencleisis in closed-angle glaucoma, Glaucoma 5:114, 1983

50. Carenini, BB, and Musso, M: Intraoperative complications in trabeculectomy, Glaucoma 4:75, 1982

51. Chatterjee, S, and Ansari, MW: Microsurgical trabeculectomy in Ghana, Br J Ophthalmol 56:783, 1972

52. Christensen, RE, and Rundle, HL: Repair of filtering blebs following cataract surgery, Arch Ophthalmol 84:8, 1970

53. Cleasby, GW, Fung, WE, and Webster, RG: Cryosurgical closure of filtering blebs, Arch Ophthalmol 87:319, 1972

54. Cohen, JS, Shaffer, RN, Hetherington, J, and Hoskins, HD: Revision of filtration surgery, Arch Ophthalmol 95:1612, 1977

55. Cohen, LB, Graham, TF, and Fry, WE: Beta radiation as an adjunct to glaucoma surgery in the Negro, Am J Ophthalmol 47:54, 1959

56. Cristiansson, J: Ocular hypotony after fistulizing glaucoma surgery, Acta Ophthalmol (Copenh) 45:837, 1967

57. Dake, CL, and Greve EL: Double flap Scheie (a prospective study of an external filtering operation in glaucoma simplex), Doc Ophthalmol 42:353, 1977

58. Deleted in proofs

59. Daniel, RK: Microsurgery: through the looking glass, N Engl J Med 300:1251, 1979

60. David, R, and Sachs, U: Quantitative trabeculectomy, Br J Ophthalmol 65:457, 1981

61. Dellaporta, A: Experiences with trepanotrabeculectomy, Trans Am Acad Ophthalmol 79:362, 1975

62. Dellaporta, A: Surgical scars after trepanotrabeculectomy, Arch Ophthalmol 99:1063, 1981

63. Dellaporta, A: Scleral trephination for subchoroidal effusion, Arch Ophthalmol 101:1917, 1983

64. Dellaporta, A: Combined trabeculectomy and cataract extraction, Ophthalmic Surg 16:487, 1985

65. Demers, PE: Results of filtering operations for glaucoma, Can J Ophthalmol 2:45, 1967

66. D'Ermo, F, and Bonomi, L: Trabeculectomy: results in the treatment of glaucoma, Ophthalmologica 166:311, 1973

67. D'Ermo, F, Bonomi, L, and Doro, D: A critical analysis of the long-term results of trabeculectomy, Am J Ophthalmol 88:829, 1979

68. Donzis, PB, Karcioglu, ZA, and Insler, MS: Sodium hyaluronate (Healon) in the surgical repair of Descemet's membrane detachment, Ophthalmic Surg 17:735, 1986

69. Douglas, WHG, and Ramsell, TG: Results of preoperative antiglaucomatous treatment and of Scheie's operations, Br J Ophthalmol 53:472, 1969

70. Douvas, NG: Cystoid bleb cryotherapy, Am J Ophthalmol 74:69, 1972

71. Drance, SM, and Vargas, E: Trabeculectomy and thermosclerostomy: a comparison of two procedures, Can J Ophthalmol 8:413, 1973

72. Deleted in proofs

73. Duke-Elder, S, and Ashton, N: Action of cortisone on tissue reactions of inflammation and repair with special reference to the eye, Br J Ophthalmol 35:695, 1954

74. Duke-Elder, S: System of ophthalmology, vol II, Diseases of the lens and vitreous. Glaucoma and hypotony, St. Louis, 1969, The CV Mosby Co

75. Edwards, RS: Trabeculectomy combined with cataract extraction: a follow-up study, Br J Ophthalmol 64:720, 1980

76. El Shewy, TM: Subscleral iridencleisis in open-angle glaucoma, Ophthalmologica 169:285, 1974

77. Eltz, H, and Gloor, B: Trabeculectomy in cases of angle-closure glaucoma—successes and failures, Klin Mbl Angenheilk 177:556, 1980

78. Emmerich, KH, and Busse, H: Long-term results after goniotrephining with scleral flap, Glaucoma 7:252, 1985

79. Epstein, DL: Pseudophakic malignant glaucoma—is it really pseudo-malignant? Am J Ophthalmol 103:231, 1987

80. Eustace, P, Harun, AQSM: Trabeculectomy combined with cataract extraction, Trans Ophthalmol Soc UK 94:1058, 1974

81. Fanous, S, and Brouillette, G: Combined trabeculectomy and cataract extraction: modified technique, Can J Ophthalmol 18:274, 1983

82. Fitzgerald, JR, and McCarthy, JL: Surgery of the filtering bleb, Arch Ophthalmol 68:453, 1962

83. Flanagan, DW, and Blach, RK: Place of panretinal photocoagulation and trabeculectomy in the management of neovascular glaucoma, Br J Ophthalmol 67:526, 1983

84. François, J: A combined operation for glaucoma and cataract, Ophthalmic Surg 1:9, 1970

85. Frankelson, EN, and Shaffer, RN: The management of coexisting cataract and glaucoma, Can J Ophthalmol 9:298, 1974

86. Freedman, J, Shen, E, and Ahrens, M: Trabeculectomy in a black American glaucoma population, Br J Ophthalmol 60:573, 1976

87. Deleted in proofs

88. Freedman, J: Combined cataract and glaucoma surgery, Glaucoma 3:51, 1981

89. Freedman, J, and Kopelowitz, W: Long-term results of trabeculectomy in a black population, Glaucoma 4:123, 1982

90. Frenkel, DEP, and Shin, DH: Prevention and management of delayed suprachoroidal hemorrhage after filtration surgery, Arch Ophthalmol 104:1459, 1986

91. Galin, MA, Baras, I, and McLean, JM: The technique of perilimbal suction cup analysis, Am J Ophthalmol 56:883, 1963

92. Galin, MA, Baras, I, and McLean, JM: The mechanism of external filtration, Am J Ophthalmol 61:63, 1966

93. Galin, MA, Baras, I, and Cavero, R: Stimulation of a filtering bleb, Arch Ophthalmol 74:777, 1965

94. Galin, MA, Boniuk, V, and Robbins, RM: Surgical landmarks in trabeculectomy surgery, Am J Ophthalmol 80:696, 1975

95. Galin, MA, and Hung, PT: Further observations on eccentric perilimbal suction application, Ann Ophthalmol 9:69, 1977

96. Galin, MA, and Hung, PT: Surgical repair of leaking blebs, Am J Ophthalmol 83:328, 1977

97. Galin, MA, and Obstbaum, SA: Combined surgery for cataract and open-angle glaucoma, Int Ophthalmol Clin 21:93, 1981

98. Galin, MA, Obstbaum, SA, Asano, YE, and Maghraby, A: Trabeculectomy, cataract extraction, and intraocular lens implantation, Trans Ophthalmol Soc UK 104:570, 1985

99. Gehring, JR: A new method for re-forming anterior chambers after glaucoma operations, Arch Ophthalmol 68:473, 1962

100. Gehring, JR, and Ciccarelli, EC: Trichloracetic acid treatment of filtering blebs following cataract extraction, Am J Ophthalmol 74:662, 1972

101. Deleted in proofs

102. Giangiacomo, J, Dueker, DK, and Adelstein, E: The effect of preoperative triamcinolone administration on glaucoma filtration. I. Trabeculectomy following subconjuctival triamcinolone, Arch Ophthalmol 104:838, 1986

103. Gilbert, CM, Brown, RH, and Lynch, MG: The effect of argon laser trabeculoplasty on the rate of filtering surgery, Ophthalmology 93:362, 1986

104. Givens, K, and Shields, MB: Suprachoroidal hemorrhage after glaucoma filtering surgery, Am J Ophthalmol 105:689, 1987

105. Deleted in proofs

106. Gloor, B, Niederer, W, and Daicker, B: Trabeculectomy: surgical technique, results, indications, Klin Mbl Augenheilk 170:241, 1977

107. Gorin, G: Use of a thin conjunctival flap in limbosclerectomy, Am J Ophthalmol ??:257, 1971

108. Gradle, HS: A critique of glaucoma operations, Am J Ophthalmol 18:730, 1935

109. Grady, FJ, and Forbes, M: Tissue adhesive for repair of conjunctival buttonhole in glaucoma surgery, Am J Ophthalmol 68:656, 1969

110. Deleted in proofs

111. Grant, WM, and Burke, JF, Jr: Why do some people go blind from glaucoma? Ophthalmology 89:991, 1982

112. Gressel, MG, Heuer, DK, and Parrish, RK, II: Trabeculectomy in young patients, Ophthalmology 91:1242, 1984

113. Greve, EL, and Dake, CL: Four year follow-up of a glaucoma operation. Prospective study of the double flap Scheie, Int Ophthalmol 1:139, 1979

114. Greve, EL, Dake, CL, Klaver, JHJ, and Mutsaerts, EMG: 10 year prospective follow-up of a glaucoma operation. The double flap Scheie in primary open-angle glaucoma. In Greve, EL, Leydhecker, W, Railta, C, editors: Second European Glaucoma Symposium, 1984, Helskini, 1985, Dr. W. Junk Publishers

115. Haisten, MV, and Guyton, J: Iridencleisis, Arch Ophthalmol 61:727, 1959

116. Harris, LS, and Kahanavicz, Y: Unsuccessful eccentric perilimbal suction after filtering surgery, Am J Ophthalmol 79:112, 1975

117. Herschler, J: The effect ot total vitrectomy on filtration surgery in the aphakic eye, Ophthalmology 88:229, 1981

118. Herschler, J, and Agness, D: A modified filtering operation for neovascular glaucoma, Arch Ophthalmol 97:2339, 1979

119. Herschler, J, Claflin, AJ, and Fiorentino, G: The effect of aqueous humor on the growth of subconjunctival fibroblasts in tissue culture and its implications for glaucoma surgery, Am J Ophthalmol 89:245, 1980

120. Deleted in proofs

121. Heuer, DK, et al: Trabeculectomy in aphakic eyes, Ophthalmology 91:1045, 1984

122. Heuer, DK, et al: 5-Fluorouracil and glaucoma filtering surgery. II: A pilot study, Ophthalmology 91:384, 1984

123. Hitchings, RA, and Grierson, I: Clinicopathologic correlation in eyes with failed fistulizing surgery, Trans Ophthalmol Soc UK 103:84, 1983

124. Holmin, C, and Starr-Paulsen, A: The visual field after trabeculectomy—a follow-up study using computerized perimetry, Acta Ophthalmol (Copenh) 622:230, 1984

125. Honrubia, FM, Dominguez, A, Gomez, ML, and Grijalbo, P: Long-term results of combined trabeculectomy and cataract extraction, Glaucoma 6:223, 1984

126. Deleted in proofs

127. Honrubia, FM, Grijalbo, P, Gomez, L, and Tamargo, D: A long-term study of glaucoma, Glaucoma 5:284, 1983

128. Hoskins, HD, and Migliazzo, C: Management of failing filtering blebs with the argon laser, Ophthalmic Surg 15:731, 1984

129. Huber, C, and Reme, CL: Lens implantation combined with trabeculectomy, Trans Ophthalmol Soc UK 104:574, 1985

130. Iliff, CE: Flap perforation in glaucoma surgery sealed by a tissue patch, Arch Glaucoma 71:215, 1964

131. Iliff, CE, and Haas, JS: Posterior lip sclerectomy, Am J Ophthalmol 54:688, 1962

132. Inaba, Z: Long-term results of trabeculectomy in the Japanese: an analysis by life-table method, Jpn J Ophthalmol 26:361, 1982

133. Insler, MS, Cooper, HD, Kastl, PR, and Caldwell, DR: Penetrating keratoplasty with trabeculectomy, Am J Ophthalmol 100:593, 1985

134. Jackson, AH: Lamellar limboscleral trephination in the surgical treatment of glaucoma, Ann Ophthalmol 5:1137, 1973

135. Javitt, JC, et al: Brainstem anesthesia following retrobulbar injection of local anesthetic. Presented 1986 Annual Meeting Am Acad Ophthalmol New Orleans

136. Jay, JL: Earlier trabeculectomy, Trans Ophthalmol Soc UK 103:35, 1983

137. Jay, JL, and Murray, SB: Characteristics of reduction of intraocular pressure after trabeculectomy, Br J Ophthalmol 64:432, 1980

138. Jerndal, T, and Kriisa, V: Results of trabeculectomy for pseudoexfoliation glaucoma, Br J Ophthalmol 58:927, 1974

139. Jerndal, T, and Lundstrom, M: 330 Trabeculectomies—a long time study (3-5½ years), Acta Ophthalmol (Copenh) 58:947, 1980

140. Johns, GE, and Layden, WE: Combined trabeculectomy and cataract extraction, Am J Ophthalmol 88:973, 1979

141. Kapetansky, F: Trabeculectomy or trabeculectomy plus tenectomy: a comparative study, Glaucoma 2:451, 1980

142. Kashyap, BP: Evaluation of combined operation of glaucoma by filtering sinus trabeculectomy and lens extraction for cataract, Aust J Ophthalmol 8:161, 1980

143. Katz, LJ: Ciliochoroidal detachment, Ophthalmic Surg 18:1775, 1987

144. Katz, LJ, Cantor, LB, and Spaeth, GL: Complications of surgery in glaucoma: early and late bacterial endophthalmitis following glaucoma filtering surgery, Ophthalmology 92:959, 1985

145. Katz, LJ, and Spaeth, GL: Surgical management of secondary glaucomas, Ophthalmic Surg 18:826, 1987

146. Kay, J, Litin, B, and Jones, M: Periocular delivery of antimetabolites as adjunctive chemotherapy in filtration surgery, Invest Ophthalmol Vis Sci (Suppl) 25:43, 1984

147. Kay, JS, et al: Delivery of antifibroblast agents as adjuncts to filtration surgery. II. Delivery of 5-Fluorouracil and bleomycin in a collagen implant: pilot study in the rabbit, Ophthalmic Surg 17:796, 1986

148. Keillor, RB, and Molteno, ABC: Twenty-one cases of clear cornea trabeculectomy, Aust NZ J Ophthalmol 14:339, 1986

149. Keroub, C, Hyams, SW, and Rath, E: Study of cataract formation following trabeculectomy, Glaucoma 6:117, 1984

150. Kimbrough, RL, and Stewart, RM: Outpatient trabeculectomy, Ophthalmic Surg 11:379, 1980

151. Kimbrough, RL, Stewart, RM, Decker, WL, and Praeger, TL: Trabeculectomy: square or triangular scleral flap, Ophthalmic Surg 13:753, 1982

152. Kirk, HQ: Cauterization of filtering blebs following cataract extraction, Trans Am Acad Ophthalmol Otolaryngol 77:573, 1973

153. Klemen, UM: Uniphasic glaucoma—cataract surgery: anterior sclerectomy vs trephining, Glaucoma 2:437, 1980

154. Deleted in proofs

155. Klemetti, A, and Kalima, T: Combined trabeculectomy and cataract operation—a follow-up study, Acta Ophthalmol (Copenh) 60:258, 1982

156. Deleted in proofs

157. Knapp, A, Heuer, DK, Stern, GA, and Driebe, WT, Jr: Serious corneal complications of glaucoma filtering surgery with postoperative 5-fluorouracil, Am J Ophthalmol 103:183, 1987

158. Kolker, AE: Visual prognosis in advanced glaucoma: a comparison of medical and surgical therapy for retention of vision in 101 eyes with advanced glaucoma, Trans Am Ophthalmol Soc 75:539, 1977

159. Deleted in proofs

160. Kolker, AE: Discussion of steroid-induced ocular hypertension in patients with filtering blebs, Ophthalmology 87:243, 1980

161. Kondo, T: Cataract extraction after filtering operation, Glaucoma 1:165, 1979

162. Kraushar, MF, and Steinberg, JA: Informed consent—surrender or salvation, Arch Ophthalmol 104:352, 1986

163. Kronfeld, PC: Delayed restoration of the anterior chamber, Am J Ophthalmol 38:453, 1954

164. Kronfeld, P: The effect of topical steroid administration on intraocular pressure and aqueous outflow after fistulizing operations, Trans Am Ophthalmol Soc 62:375, 1964

165. Kronfeld, P: The rise of the filter operations, Surv Ophthalmol 17:168, 1972

166. Deleted in proofs

167. Kwong, E, Litia, B, and Jones, M: Effect of anti-neoplastic drugs on fibroblast proliferation in rabbit aqueous humor, Ophthalmic Surg 15:847, 1984

168. Lambrou, N, and Fronimupoulos, J: Goniotrephination with scleral flap: eight year experience, Glaucoma 3:116, 1981

169. Lamping, KA, Bellows, AR, Hutchinson, BT, and Afran, SI: Long-term evaluation of initial filtration surgery, Ophthalmology 93:91, 1986

170. Lawrence, GA: Surgical treatment of patients with advanced glaucomatous field defects, Arch Ophthalmol 81:804, 1969

171. Lee, PA, Hersh, P, Kersten, D, and Melamed, S: Complications of subconjunctival 5-fluorourcil following glaucoma filtering surgery, Ophthalmol Surg 18(3):187, 1987

172. Lee, P, Shihab, ZM, and Fu, Y: Modified trabeculectomy: a new procedure for neovascular glaucoma, Ophthalmic Surg 11:181, 1980

173. Lennartz, E: Trabeculectomy vs iridencleisis: a two year follow-up, Glaucoma 4:127, 1982

174. Leopold, IH: Advances in anesthesia in ophthalmic surgery, Ophthalmic Surg 5:13, 1974

175. L'Esperance, FA, and Mittl, RN: Carbon dioxide laser trabeculectomy for the treatment of neovascular glaucoma, Trans Am Ophthalmol Soc 80:261, 1982

176. L'Esperance, FA, Mittl, RN, and James, WA: Carbon dioxide laser trabeculostomy for the treatment of neovascular glaucoma, Ophthalmology 90:821, 1983

177. Levene, RZ: Glaucoma filtering surgery: factors that determine pressure control, Ophthalmic Surg 15:475, 1984

178. Levene, RZ: Glaucoma filtering surgery: factors that determine pressure control, Trans Am Ophthalmol Soc 82:282, 1984

179. Levy, NS, Boone, L, and Bonney, RC: Guarded blades and precision in glaucoma filtration surgery, Glaucoma 7:220, 1985

180. Lewis, RA, and Phelps, CD: Trabeculectomy v. thermosclerostomy—a five year follow-up, Arch Ophthalmol 102:533, 1984

181. Leydhecker, W: Surgery and its documentation in glaucoma. In Greve, EL, Leydhecker, W, and Railta, C, editors: Second European Glaucoma Symposium, 1984, Helskini, 1985 Dr. Junk Publisher

182. Lichter, PR, and Ravin, JG: Risks of sudden visual loss after glaucoma surgery, Am J Ophthalmol 78:1009, 1974

183. Deleted in proofs

184. Lobue, TD, Deutsch, TA, and Stein, RM: Moraxella nonliquefaciens endophthalmitis after trabeculectomy, Am J Ophthalmol 99:343, 1985

185. Loewenthal, LM: Trabeculectomy as treatment for glaucoma: a preliminary report, Ann Ophthalmol 9:179, 1977

186. Luntz, MH: Trabeculectomy using a fornix-based conjunctival flap and tightly sutured scleral flap, Ophthalmology 87:985, 1980

187. Luntz, MH, and Berlin, MS: Combined trabeculectomy and cataract extraction—advantages of a modified technique and review of current literature, Trans Ophthalmol Soc UK 100:533, 1980

188. Luntz, MH, and Freedman, J: The fornix-based conjunctival flap in glaucoma filtration surgery, Ophthalmic Surg 11:516, 1980

189. Luntz, MH, and Livingston, DG: Trabeculotomy ab externo and trabeculectomy in congenital and adult onset glaucoma, Am J Ophthalmol 83:177, 1977

190. Deleted in proofs

191. Mackie, EJ, and Rubenstein, K: Iridencleisis in congestive glaucoma, Br J Ophthalmol 38:641, 1954

192. Deleted in proofs

193. MacRae, SM, and Van Buskirk, EM: Late wound dehiscence after penetrating keratoplasty in association with digital massage, Am J Ophthalmol 102:391, 1986

194. Madsen, DH: Experiences in surgical treatment of hemorrhagic glaucoma, Acta Ophthalmol (Copenh) [Suppl] 120:88, 1973

195. Deleted in proofs

196. Malbran, J, and Malbran, E: Surgical management of primary glaucoma—a description of a new technique, Am J Ophthalmol 47:34, 1959

197. Mandelbaum, S, Forster, RK, Gelender, H, and Culbertson, W: Late onset endophthalmitis associated with filtering blebs, Ophthalmology 92:964, 1985

198. Marion, JR, and Shields, MB: Thermal sclerostomy and posterior lip sclerectomy: a comparative study, Ophthalmic Surg 9:67, 1978

199. Marmion, VJ: Anterior sclerectomy, a controlled trial, Trans Ophthalmol Soc UK 89:519, 1969

200. Martenet, AC: Trabeculotomy and trabeculectomy, Klin Mbl Augenheilk 178:292, 1981

201. Maumenee, AE: External filtering operations for glaucoma: the mechanism of function and failure, Trans Am Ophthalmol Soc 58:319, 1960

202. Maumenee, AE, and Schwartz, MF: Acute intraoperative choroidal effusion, Am J Ophthalmol 100:147, 1985

203. Maumenee, AE, and Stark, WJ: Management of persistent hypotony after planned or inadvertent cyclodialysis, Am J Ophthalmol 71:320, 1971

204. Deleted in proofs

205. McMahon, LB, Monica, ML, and Zimmerman, TJ: Posterior chamber pseudophakos in glaucoma patients, Ophthalmic Surg 17:146, 1986

205. McPherson, SD, Cline, JW, and McCurdy, D: Recent advances in glaucoma surgery, trabeculotomy, and trabeculectomy, Ann Ophthalmol 9:91, 1977

207. Melamed, S, et al: The use of glaucoma shell tamponade in leaking filtration blebs, Ophthalmology 93:839, 1986

208. Deleted in proofs

209. Meyer, SJ, and Thorpe, H: Round table conference—complications of ocular surgery, Am J Ophthalmol 47:239, 1959

210. Migdal, C, and Hitchings, R: Effect of antiprostaglandins on glaucoma filtration surgery, Trans Ophthalmol Soc UK 102:129, 1982

211. Miller, GR, and Krustin, J: Ruptured filtering bleb after ocular massage, Arch Ophthalmol 76:363, 1966

212. Miller, MH, Joseph, NH, Wishart, PK, and Hitchings, R: Lack of beneficial effect of intensive topical steroids and beta-irradiation of eyes undergoing repeat trabeculectomy, Ophthalmic Surg 18:508, 1987

213. Miller, RD, Barber, JC: Trabeculectomy in black patients, Ophthalmic Surg 12:46, 1981

214. Mills, KB: Trabeculectomy: a retrospective long-term follow-up of 444 cases, Br J Ophthalmol 65:790, 1981

215. Mishra, RK: A comparative study of sub-episcleral iridencleisis and trabeculectomy, Indian J Ophthalmol 31:680, 1983

216. Molteno, ACB, Ancker, E, and Biljon, GV: Surgical technique for advanced juvenile glaucoma, Arch Ophthalmol 102:51, 1984

217. Moorhead, L, Stewart, R, and Kimbrough, R: Effects of topically applied beta-aminoproprionitrile after glaucoma filtration surgery, Invest Ophthalmol Vis Sci (Suppl) 25:44, 1984

218. Moorhead, LC, Smith, J, Stewart, R, and Kimbrough, R: Effects of beta aminoproprionitrile after glaucoma filtration surgery: pilot human trial, Ann Ophthalmol 19:2235, 1987

219. Murray, SB, and Jay, JL: Trabeculectomy—its role in the management of glaucoma, Trans Ophthalmol Soc UK 99:492, 1979

220. Naccache, R: Delayed re-formation of anterior chamber after trephine operations, Br J Ophthalmol 36:462, 1952

221. Nadel, AJ: Sclerotomy with cautery—a review of 110 operations at the Illinois Eye and Ear Infirmary, Am J Ophthalmol 62:955, 1966

222. Namba, H: Blood reflux into anterior chamber after trabeculectomy, Jpn J Ophthalmol 27:616, 1983

223. Neetens, A: Combined trabeculectomy-cataract surgery, Glaucoma 3:176, 1981

224. Nesterov, AP, Egorov, EA, and Kolesnikova, LN: Valve trabeculectomy and filtering iridocycloretraction in glaucoma. In Greve EL, Leydhecker, W, Railta, CL, editors: Second European Glaucoma Symposium, Helsinki, 1985, Dr. W. Junk Publisher

225. Newhouse, RP, and Beyrer, C: Hypotony as a late complication of trabeculectomy, Ann Ophthalmol 14:685, 1982

226. O'Connell, EJ, and Karseras, AG: Intraocular surgery in advanced glaucoma, Br J Ophthalmol 60:124, 1976

227. Ohanesian, RV, and Kim EW: A prospective study of combined extracapsular cataract extraction, posterior chamber lens implantation, and trabeculectomy, Am Intraocular Implant Soc J 2:142, 1985

228. Oyokawa, RT, and Maumenee, AE: Clear-cornea cataract extraction in eyes with functioning filter blebs, Am J Ophthalmol 93:294, 1962

229. Pape, LG, and Balazs, EA: The use of sodium hyaluronate (Healon®) in human anterior segment surgery, Ophthalmology 87:699, 1980

230. Patel, CB, Billore, OP, and Shroff, AP: Quantitative trabeculectomy, Indian J Ophthalmol 31:793, 1983

231. Patel, CK, Bavishi, AK, and Patel, NC: Further report on trabeculostomy—trabeculectomy with scleral flap, Indian J Ophthalmol 31:749, 1983

232. Pederson, JE, and Smith, SG: Surgical management of encapsulated filtering blebs, Ophthalmology 92:955, 1985

233. Pe'er, J Ticho, V, and Vidaurri, JS: Clinico-histopathological correlation in trabeculectomy. New York, 1984, Excerpta Medica

234. Peiffer, RL, Jr, et al: Myofibroblasts in the healing of filtering wounds in rabbit, dog, and cat, Glaucoma 3:277, 1981

235. Petursson, GJ, and Fraunfelder, FT: Repair of an inadvertent buttonhole or leaking filtering bleb, Arch Ophthalmol 97:926, 1979

236. Peyman, GA, Carney, MD, and Higgenbotham, EJ: Lensectomy and vitrectomy in the presence of filtering blebs, Int Ophthalmol 10:143, 1987

237. Phillips, CI, Clark, CV, and Levy, AM: Posterior synechiae after glaucoma operations: aggravation by shallow anterior chamber and pilocarpine, Br J Ophthalmol 71:428, 1987

238. Portney, GL: Trabeculectomy and postoperative ocular hypertension in secondary angle-closure glaucoma, Am J Ophthalmol 84:145, 1977

239. Praeger, DL: Combined procedure: sub-scleral trabeculectomy with cataract extraction, Ophthalmic Surg 14:134, 1983

240. Prasad, VN, Narian, M, Bist, HK, and Khan, MM: Trepano-trabeculectomy (a combined operation for glaucoma), Indian J Ophthalmol 32:73, 1984

241. Prialnic, M, and Savir, H: Transient ocular hypertension following trabeculectomy, Br J Ophthalmol 63:233, 1979

242. Quigley, HA: Slipknots for trabeculectomy flap closure, Ophthalmic Surg 16:56, 1985

243. Radius, RL, Herschler, J, Claflin, A, and Fiorentino, G: Aqueous humor changes after experimental filtering surgery, Am J Ophthalmol 89:250, 1980

244. Raju, VK: Quantitative trabeculectomy, Br J Ophthalmol 66:474, 1982

245. Regan, EF, and Day, RM: Cataract extraction after filtering procedures, Am J Ophthalmol 71:331, 1971

246. Rehak, S: Microsurgical treatment of primary glaucomas, Glaucoma 4:30, 1982

247. Ridgway, AE: Trabeculectomy—a follow-study, Br J Ophthalmol 58:680, 1974

248. Ritch, R: A modified Flieringa-Legrand ring for use in trabeculectomy, Ann Ophthalmol 13:235, 1981

249. Rizzuti, AB: Cataract following glaucoma surgery—inferior approach—scleral incision, Am J Ophthalmol 47:548, 1959

250. Romanchuk, KG: Seidel's test using 10% fluorescein, Can J Ophthalmol 14:253, 1979

251. Romem, M, Isakow, I, and Dolev, Z: Simultaneous trabeculectomy and cataract extraction, Br J Ophthalmol 66:250, 1982

252. Rosenblatt, RM, May, DR, and Barsoumian, K: Cardiopulmonary arrest after retrobulbar block, Am J Ophthalmol 90:425, 1980

253. Rozsival, P, and Rehak, S: Scleral changes after diathermy and incision (scanning electron microscope study). In Greve, EL, Leydhecker, W, Railta, C, editors: 1985, Second European Glaucoma Symposium, 1984, Helsinki, Dr. W. Junk Publisher

254. Ruderman, JM, Harbin, TS, Jr, and Campbell, DG: Postoperative suprachoroidal hemorrhage following filtration procedures, Arch Ophthalmol 104:201, 1986

255. Sammartino, A: Trabeculectomy according to Cairns' combined with extracapsular lens extraction and intraocular lens implant in the posterior chamber, Ophthalmologica 194:12, 1987

256. Savage, JA, and Simmons, RJ: Staged glaucoma filtration surgery with planned early conversion from scleral flap to full-thickness operation using argon laser, Ophthalmol Laser Ther 1:201, 1986

257. Scheie, HG: A method of cataract extraction following filtering operations for glaucoma, Arch Ophthalmol 55:818, 1956

258. Scheie, HG: Retraction of scleral wound edges—as a fistulizing procedure for glaucoma, Am J Ophthalmol 45:220, 1958

259. Scheie, HG, and Muirhead, JF: Cataract extraction after filtering operations, Arch Ophthalmol 68:67, 1962

260. Scheie, HG: Filtering operations for glaucoma: a comparative study, Am J Ophthalmol 53:571, 1962

261. Scheie, HG: Results of peripheral iridectomy with scleral cautery in congenital and juvenile glaucoma, Arch Ophthalmol 69:13, 1963

262. Scheie, HG, and Guehl, JJ, III: Surgical management of overhanging blebs after filtering procedures, Arch Ophthalmol 97:325, 1979

263. Schimek, RA, and Williamson, WR: Trabeculectomy with cautery, Ophthalmic Surg 8:35, 1977

264. Scuderi, G, Balestrazzi, E, Recupero, SM, and Scorcia, G: Modifications of trabeculectomy, Glaucoma 2:500, 1980

265. Segrest, DR, and Ellis, PP: Iris incarceration associated with digital ocular massage, Ophthalmic Surg 12:349, 1981

266. Shaffer, RN, Hetherington, J, Jr, and Hoskins, HD: Guarded thermal sclerostomy, Am J Ophthalmol 72:769, 1971

267. Shaffer, RN, and Rosenthal, G: Comparison of cataract incidence in normal and glaucomatous population, Am J Ophthalmol 69:740, 1970

268. Shalash, B, El Hoshy, M, and Abd El Azia: Evaluation of trabeculectomy in buphthalmos, Metab Pediatr Syst Ophthalmol 5:167, 1981

269. Shields, MB: Trabeculectomy vs full-thickness filtering operation for glaucoma, Ophthalmic Surg 11:498, 1980

270. Shin, DH: Trabeculectomy, Int Ophthalmol Clin 21:47, 1981

271. Shin, DH: Reversible suture closure of the lamellar scleral flap in trabeculectomy, Ann Ophthalmol 19:51, 1987

272. Shirato, S, Kitazawa, Y, and Mishima, S: A critical analysis of the trabeculectomy results by a prospective follow-up design, Jpn J Ophthalmol 26:468, 1981

273. Shuster, JN, Krupin, T, Kolker, AE, and Becker, B: Limbus v. fornix-based conjunctival flap in trabeculectomy: a long-term randomized study, Arch Ophthalmol 102:361, 1984

274. Simmons, RJ, Thomas, JV, Singh, OS, and Taheri, N: Surgical indications and options in the management of coexisting glaucoma and cataract, Glaucoma 4:92, 1982

275. Simmons, RJ: Filtering surgery. In Chandler, PA, Grant, W, editors: Glaucoma, ed. 2, Philadelphia, 1979, Lea & Febiger

276. Sinclair, SH, Aaberg, TM, and Meredith, TA: A pars plana filtering procedure combined with lensectomy and vitrectomy for neovascular glaucoma, Am J Ophthalmol 93:185, 1982

277. Deleted in proofs

278. Singh, G: Trabeculectomy vs Scheie's operation in chronic simple glaucoma, Glaucoma 3:264, 1981

279. Singh, G: Effect of size of trabeculectomy on intraocular pressure, Glaucoma 5:192, 1983

280. Sira, IB, and Ticho, V: Excision of Tenon's capsule and fistulizing operations on Africans, Am J Ophthalmol 68:336, 1969

281. Deleted in proofs

282. Smith, JL: Retrobulbar marcaine can cause respiratory arrest, J Clin Neuro Ophthalmol 1:171, 1981

283. Smith, R: The comparison between a group of drainage operations and trabeculotomy after a follow-up of five years, Trans Ophthalmol Soc UK 89:511, 1969

284. Smith, RJH: Medical vs surgical therapy in glaucoma simplex, Br J Ophthalmol 56:277, 1972

285. Soll, DB: Intrascleral filtering procedure for glaucoma, Am J Ophthalmol 75:390, 1973

286. Soong, HK, and Quigley, HA: Dellen associated with filtering blebs, Arch Ophthalmol 101:385, 1983

287. Spaeth, GL: A prospective, controlled study to compare the Scheie procedure with Watson's trabeculectomy, Ophthalmic Surg 11:688, 1980

288. Spaeth, GL: Glaucoma Surgery. In Ophthalmic surgery. Principle and practices, Philadelphia, 1983, WB Saunders Co

289. Spaeth, GL: The management of patients with conjoint cataract and glaucoma, Ophthalmic Surg 11:780, 1984

290. Spaeth, GL: The effect of change in intraocular pressure on the natural history of glaucoma: lowering intraocular pressure in glaucoma can result in improvement of visual fields, Trans Ophthalmol Soc UK 104:256, 1985

291. Spaeth, GL: suprachoroidal hemorrhage: no longer a disorder, Ophthalmic Surg 18:329, 1987

292. Spaeth, GL, and Poryzees, E: A comparison between peripheral iridectomy with thermal sclerostomy and trabeculectomy: a controlled study, Br J Ophthalmol 65:783, 1981

293. Spaeth, GL, and Sivalingam, E: The partial-punch: a new combined cataract-glaucoma operation, Ophthalmic Surg 7:53, 1976

294. Spencer, WH: Histologic evaluation of microsurgical glaucoma techniques, Trans Am Acad Ophthalmol Otolaryngol 76:389, 1972

295. Stangos, N, Papathanesiou, A, and Papadoupoulos, N: Goniotrephining in secondary angle-closure glaucoma, Glaucoma 3:67, 1981

296. Starita, RJ, Fellman, RL, Spaeth, GL, and Poryzees, EM: Effect of varying size of scleral flap and corneal block on trabeculectomy, Ophthalmic Surg 15:484, 1984

297. Starita, RJ, et al: Short and long-term effects of postoperative corticosteroids on trabeculectomy, Ophthalmology 92:938, 1985

298. Stewart, RH, and Kimbrough, RL: A method of managing flat anterior chamber following trabeculectomy, Ophthalmic Surg 11:382, 1980.

299. Stewart, RH, and Loftis, MD: Combined cataract extraction and thermal sclerostomy vs combined cataract extraction and trabeculectomy, Ophthalmic Surg 7:93, 1976

300. Stilman, JS: Subscleral trepanation in the treatment of glaucoma, Doc Ophthalmol 44:121, 1977

301. Straatsma, BR, et al: Cataract surgery after expulsive hemorrhage in the fellow eye, Ophthalmic Surg 17:400, 1986

302. Sugar, HS: Experimental trabeculectomy in glaucoma, Am J Ophthalmol 51:623, 1961

303. Sugar, HS: Clinical effect of corticosteroids on conjunctival filtering blebs, Am J Ophthalmol 59:854, 1965

304. Sugar, HS: Complications, repair, and reoperation of antiglaucoma filtering blebs, Am J Ophthalmol 63:825, 1967

305. Sugar, HS: Surgical anatomy of glaucoma, Surv Ophthalmol 13:143, 1968

306. Sugar, HS: Cataract formation and refractive changes after surgery for angle-closure glaucoma, Am J Ophthalmol 69:747, 1970

307. Sugar, HS: Postoperative cataract in successfully filtering glaucomatous eyes, Am J Ophthalmol 69:740, 1970

308. Sugar, HS: Course of successful filtering blebs, Ann Ophthalmol 3:485, 1971

309. Sugar, HS: Postoperative complications of adult glaucoma surgery, Eye Ear Nose Throat Monthly 54:29, 1975

310. Sugar, HS: Filtering operations: an historical review, Glaucoma 3:85, 1981

311. Swan, K: Reopening of non-functioning filters—simplified surgical techniques, Trans Am Acad Ophthalmol Otolaryngol 79:342, 1975

312. Tarkkanen, A, and Eskelin, LE: Iridencleisis—results of 124 consecutive operations for chronic open-angle glaucoma in 1964-1968, Acta Ophthalmol (Copenh) 49:143, 1971

313. Taylor, HR: A histologic survey of trabeculectomy, Am J Ophthalmol 82:733, 1976

314. Teekhasaenee, C, and Ritch, R: The Use of PhEA 34c in trabeculectomy, Ophthalmology 93:487, 1986

315. Teng, CC, Chi, HH, and Katzin, HM: Histology and mechanism of filtering operations, Am J Ophthalmol 47:16, 1959

316. Teng, CC, Chi, HH, and Katzin, HM: Aqueous degenerative effect and protective role of endothelium in eye pathology, Am J Ophthalmol 50:365, 1960

317. Ticho, V, Monselize, M, Levene, S, and Kaye, R: Carbon dioxide laser filtering surgery in hemorrhagic glaucoma, Glaucoma 1:114, 1979

318. Traverso, CE, Greenidge, KC, Spaeth, GL, and Wilson, RP: Focal pressure: a new method to encourage filtration after trabeculectomy, Ophthalmic Surg 15:62, 1984

319. Traverso, CE, Tomey, KF, and Antonios, S: Limbal-vs fornix-based conjunctival trabeculectomy flaps, Am J Ophthalmol 104:28, 1987

320. Tyner, GS, Lahey, DD, Elliff, JE, and Watts, ME: Peripheral iridectomy with scleral cautery—a report on the treatment of forty-two eyes with glaucoma, Arch Ophthalmol 64:268, 1960

321. Van Buskirk, EM: Cysts of Tenon's capsule following filtration surgery, Am J Ophthalmol 94:522, 1982

322. Vela, MA, and Campbell, DG: Hypotony and ciliochoroidal detachment following pharmacologic aqueous suppressant therapy in previously filtered patients, Ophthalmology 92:50, 1985

323. Vengala Rao, K, Madhava Sai, C, and Negendra Babu, BV: Trabeculectomy in congenital glaucoma, Indian J Ophthalmol 32:439, 1984

324. Viswanathan, B, and Brown, IAR: Peripheral iridectomy with scleral cautery for glaucoma, Arch Ophthalmol 93:34, 1975

325. Deleted in proofs

326. Vossen, J, and Neubauer, H: Long-term observations after trephination with scleral flap in glaucoma with threatened point of fixation. In Greve, EL, Leydhecker, W, Railta, C, editors: Second European Glaucoma Symposium, 1984, Helsinki, 1985, Dr. W. Junk Publisher

327. Deleted in proofs

328. Warden, NJ: Long term results of trabeculectomy, Trans Ophthalmol Soc NZ 29:89, 1977

329. Warnock, DC: Trabeculectomy, Trans Ophthalmol Soc NZ 29:85, 1977

330. Watkins, PH, and Brubaker, RF: Comparison of partial-thickness and full-thickness filtration procedures in open-angle glaucoma, Am J Ophthalmol 86:756, 1978

331. Watson, P: Trabeculectomy—a modified ab externo technique, Ann Ophthalmol 2:199, 1970

332. Watson, PG: Trabeculectomy, Dev Ophthalmol 1:61, 1981

333. Watson, PG, et al: Argon laser trabeculoplasty or trabeculectomy—a prospective randomized block study, Trans Ophthalmol Soc UK 104:55, 1984

334. Watson, PG, and Barnett, F: Effectiveness of trabeculectomy in glaucoma, Am J Ophthalmol 79:831, 1975

335. Watson, PG, and Grierson, I: The place of trabeculectomy in the treatment of glaucoma, Ophthalmology 88:175, 1981

336. Wechsler, A, and Robinson, LP: Simultaneous surgical management of cataract and glaucoma, Aust J Ophthalmol 8:151, 1980

337. Weinreb, RN: Adjusting the dose of 5-fluorouracil after filtration surgery to minimize side effects, Ophthalmology 94:564, 1987

338. Werner, EB, Drance, SM, and Schulzer, M: Trabeculectomy and the progression of glaucomatous visual field loss, Arch Ophthalmol 95:1374, 1977

339. West, WM: Combined trabeculectomy and cataract extraction, Aust J Ophthalmol 11:103, 1983

340. Wheeler, TM, and Zimmerman, TJ: Expulsive choroidal hemorrhage in the glaucoma patient, Am J Ophthalmol 19:165, 1987

341. Wilensky, JT, Snyder, D, and Geiser, D: Steroid-induced ocular hypertension in patients with filtering blebs, Ophthalmology 87:240, 1980

342. Wilensky, JT: Late hyphema after filtering surgery for glaucoma, Ophthalmic Surg 14:227, 1983

343. Wiley, RG, Barnebey, HS, and Martin, WG: Combined trabeculectomy, Intracapsular cataract extraction, and lens implantation: a clinical series, Ann Ophthalmol 16:486, 1984

344. Wilson, P: Trabeculectomy: long term follow-up, Br J Ophthalmol 61:535, 1977

345. Wilson, R, Walker, AM, Dueker, DK, and Crick, RP: Risk factors for rate of progression of glaucomatous visual field loss: a computer-based analysis, Arch Ophthalmol 100:737, 1982

346. Wilson, RP, and Spiegel, D: The use of releaseable sutures in glaucoma surgery, personal communication

347. Wilson, RP, and Lloyd, J: The place of sodium hyaluronate in glaucoma surgery, Ophthalmic Surg 17:30, 1986

348. Deleted in proofs

349. Wittpenn, JR, et al: Respiratory arrest following retrobulbar anesthesia, Ophthalmology 93:867, 1986

350. Yannuzzi, LA, and Theodore, FH, Cryotherapy of postcataract blebs, Am J Ophthalmol 76:217, 1973

351. Yasuna, E: Cataract extraction following iridencleisis, Am J Ophthalmol 57:257, 1964

352. Zaidi, AA: Trabeculectomy: a review and 4-year follow-up, Br J Ophthalmol 64:436, 1980

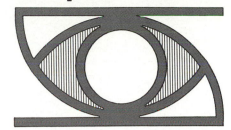

Chapter 36

Surgical Management of Coexisting Cataract and Glaucoma

M. Bruce Shields

The coexistence of a cataract and glaucoma in the same eye is not uncommon. In managing such patients, there are three basic surgical approaches: (1) cataract extraction alone, (2) glaucoma filtering surgery alone (often combined with cataract removal at a later date), and (3) combined cataract and glaucoma surgery as a single procedure. There are advantages and disadvantages to each approach, and the surgeon should consider all of the basic surgical options, selecting the one that seems to be most appropriate for each individual situation.

INDICATIONS

In each case discussed in this chapter, it is assumed that a cataract is present for which extraction is indicated, independent of the glaucoma. This is often difficult to determine in an eye with coexisting glaucoma, because it may be difficult to know how much the glaucoma is contributing to the reduced vision. The potential acuity meter (PAM) has been shown to be helpful in such cases if the glaucomatous damage is mild to moderate and the PAM visual acuity is better than 20/60, whereas the results with advanced visual field loss or a PAM reading worse than 20/60 are not reliable.[1]

When it is decided that cataract surgery is needed, the selection of the specific surgical approach is based primarily on the status of the glaucoma (Fig. 36-1).[33]

Cataract Extraction Alone

When the intraocular pressure is under good control on a well-tolerated, low dose of medication, and glaucomatous damage is mild, most surgeons prefer to perform a cataract extraction alone. This decision, however, should not be made on the assumption that removal of the cataract is likely to improve medical control of the glaucoma. Such a concept developed in the 1960s and early 1970s, when routine cataract techniques were reported to be associated with easier postoperative medical control of the glaucoma.[3,22,27] However, the long-term benefit of cataract extraction on the management of glaucoma has never been proved, and it is generally agreed that any possible benefit is proportionally less with increasing severity of the glaucoma. Furthermore, with the more recent trend toward tighter wound closure with multiple, fine sutures, there is often a transient intraocular pressure rise in the early postoperative period, which may pose a serious threat to the patient with advanced glaucomatous optic atrophy. Intraocular pressure elevation, even for a few days after cataract surgery, may cause additional, irreversible

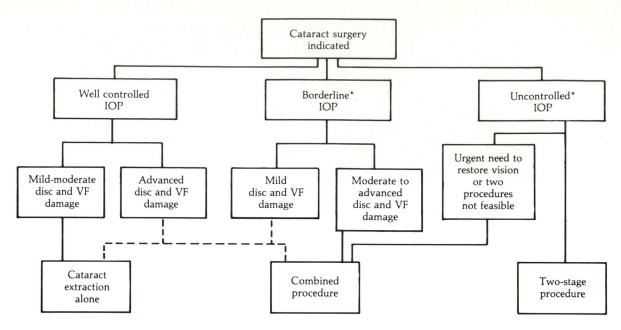

*Despite maximum tolerable medication and laser trabeculoplasty.

Fig. 36-1 Algorithm for one approach to selecting the surgical procedure in patients with coexisting cataract and glaucoma. (*Dotted lines* indicate situations in which decision must be made individually for each patient.) (From Shields, MB: Ophthalmology 93:366, 1986.)

damage to an optic nerve that already has advanced glaucomatous loss. This is also true with extracapsular cataract extraction and posterior chamber intraocular lens implantation and is an important reason for avoiding cataract surgery alone in eyes with advanced glaucomatous damage, even when the preoperative intraocular pressure is well controlled.[18,30]

Modern extracapsular cataract extraction with posterior chamber intraocular lens implantation does not usually have an adverse effect on long-term intraocular pressure control and may actually improve glaucoma control in some cases.[18,36] It should be emphasized, however, that this improvement is unpredictable and usually slight and should not be relied on to improve postoperative glaucoma management in eyes that are poorly controlled preoperatively. Cataract extraction, with or without posterior chamber intraocular lens implantation, does not appear to have an adverse effect on the intraocular pressure reduction obtained by laser trabeculoplasty before cataract surgery.[5] It is important to note, however, that intraocular pressure reduction by laser trabeculoplasty before cataract extraction does not guarantee the prevention of transient pressure elevation that often develops after cataract extraction alone.[10]

Filtering Surgery Alone (Two-stage Approach)

When the glaucoma is uncontrolled despite maximum tolerable medical therapy and poses an immediate threat to the patient's vision, the surgical procedure of choice is the one that has the greatest chance of providing long-term control of the intraocular pressure. In most cases, the next logical step would be laser trabeculoplasty. If this provides good pressure control, with reduction in medical therapy, and if the glaucomatous damage is mild, it might then be reasonable to perform the cataract surgery alone. If pressure control after laser therapy is borderline, or if the glaucomatous damage is advanced, cataract extraction combined with a glaucoma procedure may be in the patient's best interest. If the glaucoma remains uncontrolled, however, the procedure of choice in my experience is filtering surgery alone. This is based on the observation that a filtering procedure, followed by cataract extraction at a later date, has a better chance of long-term pressure control than a filtering procedure performed in combination with cataract surgery.[32] In some cases, the vision may be improved after filtering surgery by eliminating the need for a miotic, thereby postponing the need for cataract surgery. Otherwise, the cataract can be removed 4 to 6 months later as a two-stage approach.

Combined Cataract Extraction and Glaucoma Surgery

Between the two clinically extreme groups of patients (i.e., those patients with good glaucoma control and those with uncontrolled glaucoma despite maximum medical and laser therapy) is a third group of patients with borderline glaucoma status, for whom a combined procedure may be indicated. Often a fine line of judgment is involved in selecting these cases, and surgeons differ on specific criteria. A combined approach might be preferred in the following situations: (1) glaucoma under borderline medical control, with or without prior laser trabeculoplasty, especially when epinephrine is required (due to the postoperative risk of epinephrine maculopathy) or when the patient has significant drug-induced side effects; (2) adequate pressure control, but moderate to advanced glaucomatous damage (due to the risk of further damage with transient postoperative pressure elevation); or (3) uncontrolled glaucoma, despite maximum medical and laser therapy, but an urgent need to restore vision or when two operations are not feasible.

A major benefit of the combined procedure is control of the intraocular pressure during the early postoperative period. As previously noted, the transient rise that may occur after cataract extraction alone can lead to additional loss of vision in eyes that have advanced glaucomatous damage before surgery. On the other hand, it has been my experience that long-term pressure control is not as good with combined surgery as with the two-stage approach. The uncertainty of long-term control after combined surgery has also been noted by others. In one study of 75 patients, 36% had an intraocular pressure above 30 mm Hg during the first 6 months after surgery, and only 12% had a detectable filtering bleb at 12 months.[35] However, by selecting patients who are at least under borderline control before surgery, medical management can be reinstated in the late postoperative period if necessary.

Before deciding on a combined procedure, laser trabeculoplasty, in addition to maximum tolerable medication, should be tried. If the laser therapy results in good intraocular pressure control, with reduction in the need for medical therapy, and if the glaucomatous damage is mild, it may not be necessary to add glaucoma surgery to the cataract extraction. However, as previously noted, intraocular pressure control by laser trabeculoplasty before cataract surgery does not guarantee early or long-term postoperative pressure control,[10] and a combined procedure may still be preferable in cases with borderline intraocular pressure, especially if glaucomatous damage is moderate to advanced.

TECHNIQUES
Cataract Surgery Alone: Special Considerations in Glaucomatous Eyes

Management of chronic miosis and other drug-induced problems

When a cataract extraction is performed in an eye with glaucoma, special considerations must be given to the influence of antiglaucoma medications.[38] The most common drug-induced problem with cataract surgery in the glaucomatous eye is the irreversible miosis from chronic miotic therapy. This has become an even more significant difficulty with the advent of extracapsular surgery, in which adequate pupillary dilation is needed for the anterior capsulotomy. One approach to the problem is to make a sector iridectomy above, often with two inferior sphincterotomies, or multiple sphincterotomies and a peripheral iridectomy.[15] For this step, the corneoscleral incision must be enlarged sufficiently to allow introduction of the iris scissors into the anterior chamber (Fig. 36-2). Temporary ties can then be placed in the corneoscleral sutures to maintain the anterior chamber depth during the anterior capsulotomy. Another technique is a double instrument approach, in which the pupillary portion of the iris is pulled back with an iris retractor while the capsulotomy is being performed. In either case, sodium hyaluronate or another viscoelastic substance is helpful in maintaining the anterior chamber depth, as well as in mechanically dilating the pupil.

Miotics, especially echothiophate iodide, also increase the risk of postoperative iritis; and it may be advisable to change to a different drug 4 to 6 weeks before the surgery. In addition, as previously noted, the risk of epinephrine maculopathy after cataract surgery must be considered in patients who are dependent on this drug preoperatively; combined surgery may be preferred in these cases. Chronic topical drug therapy, especially with adrenergic agents, also increases the risk of intraoperative bleeding, requiring careful hemostasis during the surgery. An intraocular bipolar cautery unit, as used in vitreoretinal surgery, is very useful in these cases for controlling both external and internal bleeding.

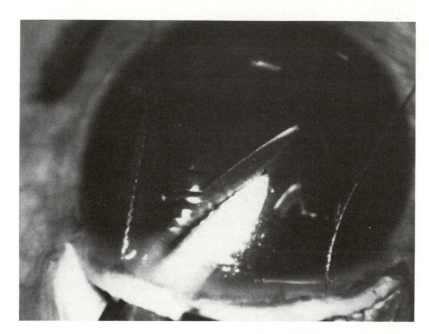

Fig. 36-2 Inferior sphincterotomy being performed with iris scissors through enlarged corneoscleral incision to expand miotic pupil before anterior capsulotomy.

Fig. 36-3 Slit-lamp view of glaucomatous eye after extracapsular cataract extraction in which superior sector iridectomy and inferior sphincterotomies *(arrows)* were created to facilitate anterior capsulotomy. (From Shields, MB: Textbook of glaucoma, ed 2, Baltimore, 1986, Williams & Wilkins.)

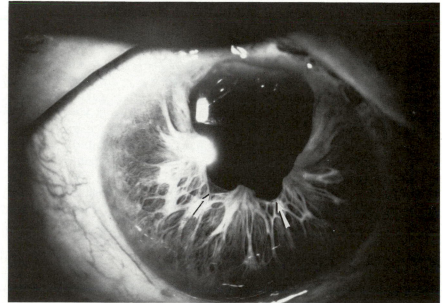

Selection of intraocular lens

Posterior chamber intraocular lenses appear to be well tolerated in glaucomatous eyes, but anterior chamber lenses should be avoided in most cases. If a posterior chamber lens is implanted in an eye with a sector iridectomy, some surgeons will close the iridectomy with one suture. An alternative approach is to rotate the haptics to a horizontal position and leave the iridectomy open. I prefer the latter, since it reduces surgical manipulation and provides a better view of the fundus in the years ahead (Fig. 36-3). Because this technique leaves the patient with a permanently enlarged pupil, an intraocular lens with a 7 mm optic and no holes has the advantage of reducing the distortion and glare that the holes or edge of the optic might create.

Two-stage Procedure

The first stage (i.e., the glaucoma filtering procedure) should be performed according to the surgeon's personal preference. One reasonable technique for the two-stage approach is to place the filtering procedure in the far superior nasal quadrant, so that the subsequent cataract incision can be made in the superior temporal quadrant. As previously noted, a successful filtering operation may eliminate, or at least delay, the need for cataract surgery by allowing discontinuation of miotic therapy, thereby providing improved vision around a central cataract. Otherwise, the cataract surgery can be performed 4 to 6 months after the glaucoma procedure.

When extraction of the cataract becomes necessary in an eye with a functioning filtering bleb, surgeons generally prefer to make the cataract incision away from the bleb, either temporally or inferiorly[2,15] or through a clear corneal incision superiorly.[14,21] These basic approaches appear to be comparable with regard to preservation of the filtering bleb, although the temporal or clear corneal approaches are technically easier for most surgeons, especially when performing extracapsular cataract extraction and posterior chamber intraocular lens implantation. If the cataract wound is placed away from the filtering bleb, a corneoscleral incision beneath a fornix-based flap can be used, thereby reducing the risk of distorting the corneal curvature. If a clear corneal incision is employed, the wound can be closed with either running or interrupted nylon suture (Fig. 36-4). The latter has the advantage of allowing cutting of a suture if postoperative astigmatism is excessive.

Combined Cataract and Glaucoma Surgery

Early combined operations employed full-thickness filtering procedures, and some surgeons still advocate this approach.[24] The main problem with combining full-thickness glaucoma filtering techniques with a cataract extraction, however, is the risk of a transient shallow or flat anterior cham-

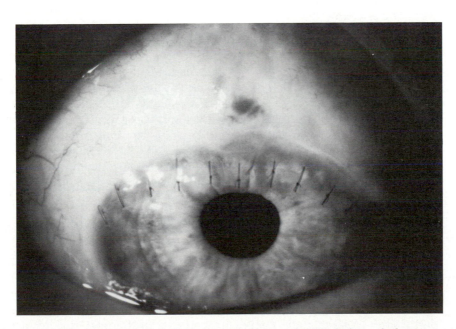

Fig. 36-4   Slit-lamp view of eye with functioning glaucoma filtering bleb in which extracapsular cataract extraction and posterior chamber lens implantation were performed through a clear corneal incision to preserve preexisting bleb.

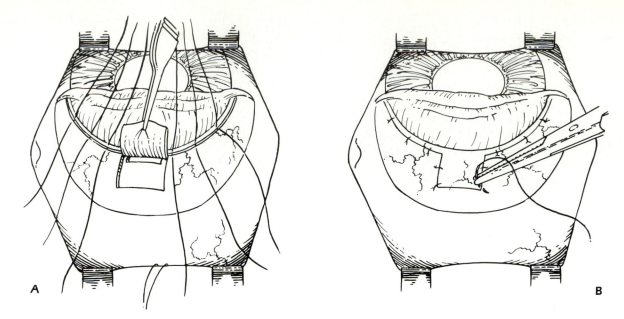

Fig. 36-5 Combined trabeculectomy and cataract extraction. **A,** Partial-thickness scleral flap and deep limbal fistula are prepared and the cataract incision is extended from either side; **B,** Following lens extraction, cataract incision and scleral flap are approximated with multiple sutures. (From Shields, MB: Textbook of glaucoma, ed 2, Baltimore, 1986, Williams & Wilkins.)

ber, which leads to significantly more complications in the inflamed, aphakic, or pseudophakic eye as opposed to glaucoma filtering surgery in a phakic eye. For this reason, the preferred combined operations employ a glaucoma procedure that is less likely to cause loss of the anterior chamber.

Cyclodialysis and cataract extraction

Cyclodialysis combined with cataract extraction has been used for many years, with good results.[8,17,31,34] However, in one large series, an analysis of the postoperative course suggested that the intraocular pressure reduction in many cases was due to the effect of the cataract surgery, rather than the cyclodialysis.[34] Because this effect may be lost with the newer techniques of wound closure, and considering the unpredictable nature of cyclodialysis, most surgeons have turned to a guarded filtering procedure for the glaucoma portion of combined operations.

Combined trabeculectomy and cataract extraction

The protective scleral flap over a limbal fistula, which reduces the chances of an early postoperative flat anterior chamber, makes the guarded filtering operation particularly desirable for combined procedures.* Reported techniques vary con-

siderably, but the basic approach involves preparation of the partial-thickness scleral flap and limbal fistula in the usual manner, followed by extension of the corneoscleral incision from either side of the fistula (Fig. 36-5).

After cataract extraction and intraocular lens implantation, both the scleral flap and corneoscleral incision are closed with multiple sutures. If a limbus-based conjunctival flap is used, it is usually closed with a fine running suture, whereas a fornix-based flap is pulled tightly over the cornea with sutures at either end of the incision. The details of a standard technique for extracapsular cataract extraction and posterior chamber lens implantation combined with a trabeculectomy are provided in Chapter 33. One reported complication with this triple procedure is retraction of the iris behind the lens, especially when surgical enlargement of the pupil is required.[29]

Combined guarded sclerectomy and cataract extraction

In this modification of the standard trabeculectomy and cataract extraction, the anterior lip of a beveled corneoscleral incision serves as the protective scleral flap for the drainage fistula, which is created in the posterior lip of the incision. The concept was introduced by Spaeth and Sivalingam[36] in 1976. I have used it for the past decade, during which time numerous modifica-

---

*References 4, 6, 7, 9, 11-13, 16, 20, 23, 25, 28, 35, 37.

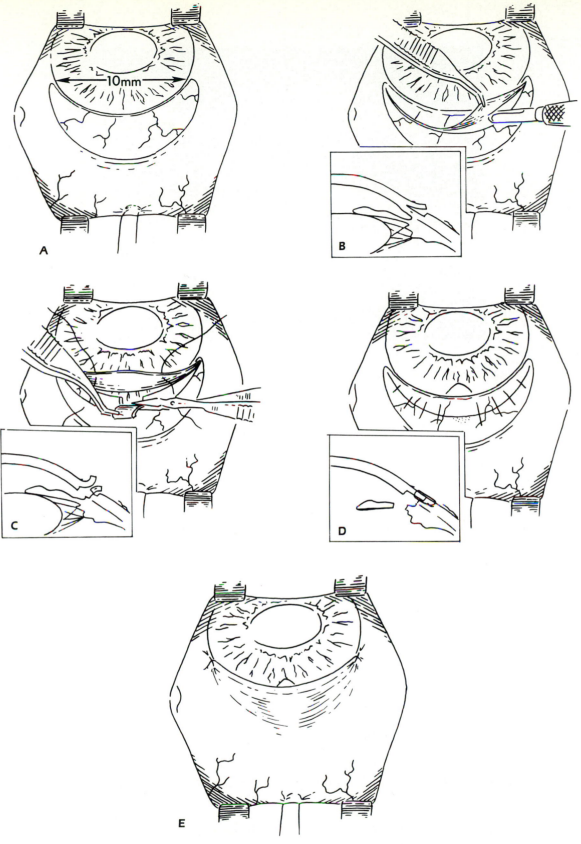

Fig. 36-6 Combined guarded sclerectomy and cataract extraction. **A,** Fornix-based conjunctival flap is created with a chord length at the limbus of 10 mm. **B,** Partial-thickness corneoscleral incision, 10 mm in length, is created with marked bevel. **C,** After extending corneoscleral incision full thickness and extracting the cataract, a fistula is created in posterior lip of corneoscleral incision by making two radial cuts with scissors and then excising the flap of deep limbal tissue at level of scleral spur. **D,** After approximating corneoscleral incision, anterior lip becomes protective scleral flap for underlying fistula. **E,** Free edge of conjunctival flap is pulled tightly over peripheral cornea and secured with two sutures.

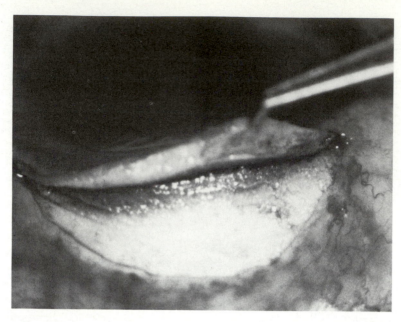

Fig. 36-7 Combined guarded sclerectomy and cataract extraction showing markedly beveled corneoscleral incision.

tions have been made, largely in keeping with the changing trends in cataract surgery.[33,34]

A fornix-based conjunctival flap is preferred, primarily because it facilitates the cataract extraction and intraocular lens implantation without seeming to adversely influence the early or late postoperative course (Fig. 36-6). Other surgeons, however, may prefer a limbus-based flap. With the former technique, a 10 mm chord length is measured at the limbus, and the fornix-based conjunctival flap is kept within these limits. The corneoscleral incision is also 10 mm in length. The initial portion of this incision is perpendicular and approximately one-half scleral thickness, with the two ends of the incision approximately 0.5 mm behind the limbus and the 12 o'clock portion 2 to 3 mm posteriorly. The incision is then beveled forward to the anterior margin of the limbus, creating a broad scleral flap (Fig. 36-7). Two 7-0 sutures of polyglycolic acid are then placed across the incision 3.5 mm to either side of the midline.

If pupillary dilation is sufficient for the anterior capsulotomy, a small stab incision is made in the partial-thickness corneoscleral incision; if the pupil is too small, the corneoscleral incision is extended with scissors to allow creation of inferior sphincterotomies and a superior sector iridotomy as described earlier in this chapter. In either case, after completion of the anterior capsulotomy, the corneoscleral incision is enlarged to the full 10 mm,

the preplaced sutures are looped to either side, and the lens nucleus is expressed. Permanent ties are then placed in the two sutures, and the lens cortex is removed with the standard irrigation-aspiration technique.

The drainage fistula is then created with Vannas scissors. A sclerectomy punch was originally used for this step, but frequently brisk bleeding occurred from inadvertent cutting of the ciliary body. The scissor technique has reduced this complication by allowing better internal visualization of the posterior incision. A fistula approximately 3 mm wide is created at the 12 o'clock position by first making two radial cuts in the posterior lip of the corneoscleral incision, extending back to within about 0.5 mm of the posterior extent of the incision. The flap of deep limbal tissue is then reflected to expose the angle structures and is excised along the scleral spur (Fig. 36-8). The posterior chamber intraocular lens is then implanted. If a sector iridotomy was not previously made, a large peripheral iridectomy is made at this time directly beneath the drainage fistula.

The corneoscleral incision is then approximated with multiple 10-0 nylon sutures, two of which are placed on either side of the fistula. This brings the anterior lip of the corneoscleral incision completely over the fistula, thereby providing the protective scleral flap. The fornix-based conjunctival flap is pulled tightly over the superior cornea

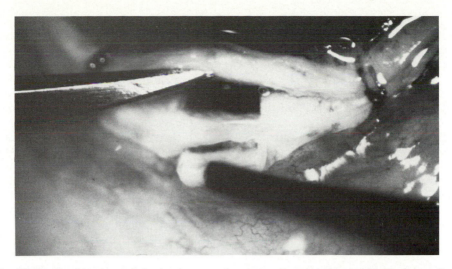

Fig. 36-8 Combined guarded sclerectomy and cataract extraction showing block of deep limbal tissue with pigmented trabecular meshwork excised from posterior lip of corneoscleral incision.

and sutured at either end with 10-0 polyglycolic acid sutures.

The guarded sclerectomy may have some advantages over the standard trabeculectomy in combination with cataract surgery. First, the full extent of the aqueous drainage site is kept several millimeters posterior to the limbus, which may be especially advantageous with the fornix-based conjunctival flap. The posterior corneoscleral incision has also been found to reduce the amount of corneal astigmatism, to the extent that it is now my preferred technique for all cataract extractions. As a result, the guarded sclerectomy adds only one step (creation of the fistula) to the routine cataract procedure, thereby minimizing additional surgical manipulation as compared to a standard trabeculectomy with cataract surgery. The two combined procedures, however, do not appear to differ significantly with regard to early or late intraocular pressure control. It should be emphasized again that a high percentage of patients lose the filtering bleb with time; this possibility must be kept in mind when selecting patients for any form of combined cataract extraction and guarded filtering procedure.

Combined trabeculotomy and cataract extraction

McPherson[19] has reported a technique in which a trabeculotomy is performed through a radial incision at 12 o'clock adjacent to a partial-thickness corneoscleral incision. The cataract wound is then extended full thickness, and the cataract extraction is completed in a standard manner. Good results have been obtained with the preliminary experience.

REFERENCES

1. Asbell, PA, Chiang, B, Amin, A, and Podos, SM: Retinal acuity evaluation with the potential acuity meter in glaucoma patients, Ophthalmology 92:764, 1985
2. Baloglou, P, Matta, C, and Asdourian, K: Cataract extraction after filtering operations, Arch Ophthalmol 88:12, 1972
3. Bigger, JF, and Becker, B: Cataracts and primary open-angle glaucoma: the effect of uncomplicated cataract extraction on glaucoma control, Trans Am Acad Ophthalmol Otolaryngol 75:260, 1971
4. Bregeat, P: Cataract surgery and trabeculectomy at the same time, Klin Monatsbl Augenheilkd 167:505, 1975
5. Brown, SVL, et al: Effect of cataract surgery on intraocular pressure reduction obtained with laser trabeculoplasty, Am J Ophthalmol 100:373, 1985
6. Dellaporta, A: Combined trepano-trabeculectomy and cataract extraction. Trans Am Ophthalmol Soc 69:113, 1971
7. Edwards, RS: Trabeculectomy combined with cataract extraction: a follow-up study, Br J Ophthalmol 64:720, 1980
8. Galin, MA, Baras, I, and Sambursky, J: Glaucoma and cataract. A study of cyclodialysis-lens extraction, Am J Ophthalmol 67:522, 1969
9. Galin, MA, Hung, PT, and Obstbaum, SA: Cataract extraction in glaucoma, Am J Ophthalmol 87:124, 1979

10. Galin, MA, et al: Laser trabeculoplasty and cataract surgery. Trans Ophthalmol Soc UK 104:72, 1984

11. Jay, JL: Extracapsular cataract extraction and posterior chamber intraocular lens insertion combined with trabeculectomy, Br J Ophthalmol 69:487, 1985

12. Jerndal, T, and Lundstrom, M: Trabeculectomy combined with cataract extraction, Am J Ophthalmol 81:227, 1976

13. Johns, GE, and Layden, WE: Combined trabeculectomy and cataract extraction, Am J Ophthalmol 88:973, 1979

14. Kass, MA: Cataract extraction in an eye with a filtering bleb, Ophthalmology 89:871, 1982

15. Kolker, AE, Stewart, RH, and LeBlanc, RP: Cataract extraction in glaucomatous patients, Arch Ophthalmol 84:63, 1970

16. Levene, R: Triple procedure of extracapsular cataract surgery, posterior chamber lens implantation, and glaucoma filter, J Cataract Refract Surg 12:385, 1986

17. McAllister, JA, and Spaeth, GL: Intracapsular cataract extraction with cyclodialysis. A useful procedure, Klin Monatsbl Augenheilkd 184:283, 1984

18. McGuigan, LJB, et al: Extracapsular cataract extraction and posterior chamber lens implantation in eyes with preexisting glaucoma. Arch Ophthalmol 104:1301, 1986

19. McPherson, SD, Jr: Combined trabeculotomy and cataract extraction as a single operation, Trans Am Ophthalmol Soc 74:251, 1976

20. Ohanesian, RV, and Kim, EW: A prospective study of combined extracapsular cataract extraction, posterior chamber lens implantation, and trabeculectomy, Am Intraocular Implant Soc J 11:142, 1985

21. Oyakawa, RT, and Maumenee, AE: Clear-cornea cataract extraction in eyes with functioning filtering blebs, Am J Ophthalmol 93:294, 1982

22. Palimeris, G, Chimonidou, E, Magouritsas, N, and Velissaropoulos, P: Cataract extraction in chronic simple glaucoma. Ophthalmic Surg 5:62, 1974

23. Percival, SPB: Glaucoma triple procedure of extracapsular cataract extraction, posterior chamber lens implantation and trabeculectomy, Br J Ophthalmol 69:99, 1985

24. Pfoff, DS: Simultaneous extracapsular cataract extraction, intraocular lens implantation, and posterior lip sclerectomy filtering procedure in glaucoma patients, CLAO J 10:143, 1984

25. Praeger, DL: Combined procedure: sub-scleral trabeculectomy with cataract extraction. Ophthalmic Surg 14:130, 1983

26. Radius, RL, et al: Pseudophakia and intraocular pressure. Am J Ophthalmol 97:738, 1984

27. Randolph, ME, Maumenee, AE, and Iliff, CE: Cataract extraction in glaucomatous eyes, Am J Ophthalmol 71:328, 1971

28. Rich, W: Cataract extraction with trabeculectomy, Trans Ophthalmol Soc UK 94:458, 1974

29. Rock, RL, and Rylander, HG, III: Spontaneous iris retraction occurring after extracapsular cataract extraction and posterior lens implantation in patients with glaucoma. American Intraocular Implant Society Journal 9:45, 1983

30. Savage, JA, Thomas, JV, Belcher, CD, III, and Simmons, RF: Extracapsular cataract extraction and posterior chamber intraocular lens implantation in glaucomatous eyes, Ophthalmology 92:1506, 1985

31. Shemleva, VV, and Mukhina, EA: Combined cataract extraction and cyclodialysis. Vestn Oftalmol 85:30, 1972

32. Shields, MB: Combined cataract extraction and glaucoma surgery, Ophthalmology 89:231, 1982

33. Shields, MB: Combined cataract extraction and guarded sclerectomy. Reevaluation in the extracapsular era, Ophthalmology 93:366, 1986

34. Shields, MB, and Simmons, RJ: Combined cyclodialysis and cataract extraction, Trans Am Acad Ophthalmol Otolaryngol 81:286, 1976

35. Simmons, ST, et al: Extracapsular cataract extraction and posterior chamber intraocular lens implantation combined with trabeculectomy in patients with glaucoma, Am J Ophthalmol 104:465, 1987

36. Spaeth, GL, and Sivalingam, E: The partial-punch: a new combined cataract-glaucoma operation, Ophthalmic Surg 7:53, 1976

37. Stewart, RH, and Loftis, MD: Combined cataract extraction and thermal sclerostomy versus combined cataract extraction and trabeculectomy, Ophthalmic Surg 7:93, 1976

38. Van Buskirk, EM: Hazards of medical glaucoma therapy in the cataract patient, Ophthalmology 89:238, 1982

Chapter 37

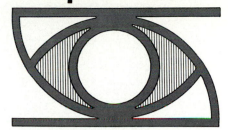

Surgery for Congenital Glaucoma

Maurice H. Luntz
Raymond Harrison

HISTORICAL ASPECTS

The poor prognosis of infantile glaucoma changed dramatically with the introduction of goniotomy by Otto Barkan in 1938.[3] Before this, the outlook had been poor. Anderson[2] quoted Seefelder as saying that "I know of no case of operated hydrophthalmia where undiminished sight has been retained till later life." In reviewing several reported surgical series, he found that one patient in three was blind after surgery.[2,4,7] One patient in three had visual acuity less than 20/200 and one in three had visual acuity better than 20/200. After age 25, no patients had better than 20/100 vision. In the collected series of unoperated patients, only one in four had vision better than 20/200. Two of four were blind by the age of 12. Sixty percent of patients aged 25 to 50 were blind. Barkan[6] reported successful lowering of intraocular pressure in 152 of 196 patients. Other authors have reported similar results with goniotomy.[16]

The introduction of microsurgical techniques in the form of trabeculotomy led to further improvement in the control of intraocular pressure.[24] McPherson[20] reported success in 12 of 15 trabeculotomies and quoted Harms and Dannheim,[14] who had success in 27. Luntz[17] reported a success rate of 96 of 105. Gregersen and Kessing[11] compared results obtained by "macrosurgery" (i.e., goniotomy, trephine, and diathermy) to those obtained with trabeculotomy. Macrosurgery controlled intraocular pressure in 61% of eyes, and microsurgery was successful in 100%. They thought that

trabeculotomy was more successful when performed as a per primum procedure than after goniotomy.

PROGNOSTIC FACTORS

Various factors, such as the age of onset, may affect the prognosis.[8,11,17,19] The earlier in life the disease occurs, the worse the prognosis if untreated. On the other hand, surgery is generally more successful when performed as early as possible. Both of these factors are reflected in many reports on goniotomy.[7,8,11] It is generally accepted that the success of goniotomy is not as good in eyes with significant buphthalmos. Barkan[5] felt that eyes with corneal diameters greater than 15 mm were not suitable for goniotomy. Similarly, Robertson[22] reported 13 of 15 successes in nonbuphthalmic eyes compared with only 3 of 10 successes in buphthalmic eyes.

Although other authors have had the impression that corneal enlargement was a poor prognostic factor in trabeculotomy,[5,11,16] this has not been our experience in a prospective study of 86 eyes so treated.[17,19]

The appearance of the anterior chamber angle is of great prognostic significance.[17] In the same study, eyes with typical angle anomalies did very well, whereas eyes in which the angles appeared cicatrized or had evidence of iridocorneal dysgenesis did poorly.[17,19] The success rate in the first group was 100%, compared with only about 30% in each of the latter two groups.

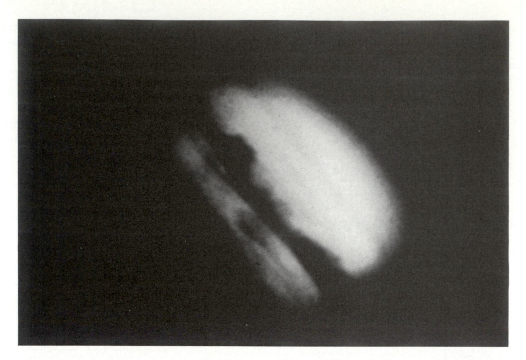

Fig. 37-1 Gonioscopic view of presumed mesodermal (neural crest cell) anomaly of the angle (trabecular dysgenesis). No abnormalities are visible on the posterior corneal surface (uppermost). The trabecular meshwork zone lies approximately in the center of the photograph, characterized by a darkly pigmented, irregular band, presumably mesoderm, lying on the trabecular meshwork. The root of the iris below this band and the posterior corneal surface, which is superior to the band, are normal so that only the trabecular meshwork is affected. A round, brown nodule (iris nevus) is visible on the iris surface at the root of the iris. In this anomaly the prognosis for successful surgery approaches 100%. (From Luntz, MH, Harrison, R, and Schenker, HI: Glaucoma surgery, Baltimore, 1984, Williams & Wilkins)

Classification of Angle Anomalies

Angle anomalies may be divided into three groups.

Group 1

Group 1 anomalies are presumed mesodermal (neural crest cell) anomalies[17] or trabecular dysgenesis.[15] In this group, an angle anomaly involves the trabecular meshwork, leaving the cornea and iris normal. The angle anomaly may be the result of incomplete development of tissue derived from neural crest cells. These patients have the best prognosis for either goniotomy or trabeculotomy, over 90% achieving intraocular pressure control (Fig. 37-1).

Group 2

Group 2 anomalies are cicatricial angle[17,19] or iridotrabecular dysgenesis.[15] In this group, the anomaly and the peripheral iris (Fig. 37-2) involves the trabecular meshwork and is the result of a cicatricial process in the periphery of the anterior chamber angle. These patients have a far poorer prognosis with surgery, particularly goniotomy or trabeculotomy, which have success rates of approximately 30%. Patients undergoing trabeculectomy or combined trabeculotomy-trabeculectomy have a success rate of approximately 50%. When filtration surgery fails, a seton, such as a Molteno implant, is indicated. Some surgeons consider setons as the primary procedure in these patients.[21] Should the seton fail, a cyclodestructive procedure would be indicated.

Group 3

The third group is iridotrabecular-corneal dysgenesis[15,19] in which the anomaly involves cornea, trabeculum, and iris (Fig. 37-3). Examples of this group are Axenfeld-Rieger's and Peters' anomalies. In these eyes, prognosis is also poor with trabeculotomy or goniotomy and better with trabeculectomy, but many of these patients will also finally require a seton or cyclodestructive procedure.

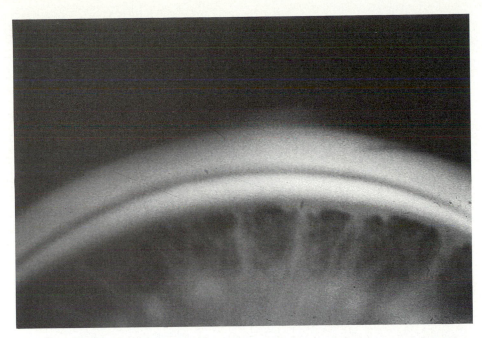

Fig. 37-2   Cicatricial angle (Luntz) or iridotrabecular dysgenesis (Hoskins). Gonioscopic view in a child with congenital glaucoma. At the top, the slit beam illuminates the posterior corneal surface, which apears to be normal. About midway across the posterior corneal surface is a dark band, which is an artifact and should be disregarded. At the lower border of the cornea is a faint brown line, which is Schwalbe's line, and below this is the trabecular meshwork band. In this area, the first prominent structure is a light brown membrane situated at the base of the trabecular meshwork and on the iris root. The upper edge of this membrane is regular and straight, attached to the base of the trabecular meshwork, but the lower edge has a serrated contour and develops a number of small projections, each of which projects downward onto the surface of the iris root. The apex of some of these projections becomes continuous with radial folds of the iris surface. These folds are illuminated by the microscope light, which is focused on the light brown membrane at the trabecular meshwork zone. Therefore, the folds lie on the same horizontal plane as the membrane, which is attached to the base of the trabecular meshwork. Between these folds, the iris surface is dark because it is out of focus and at a level inferior to that of the folds. These dark areas represent troughs of the iris surface. The irregular appearance of the iris is abnormal and denotes that this anomaly involves both the trabecular meshwork and the iris surface (hence iridotrabecular dysgenesis). The appearance of the iris surface is believed to be the result of a cicatricial process that affected the angle during development. The entire limbal area may be involved because Schlemm's canal is closer to the limbus in many of these eyes, being situated 0.5 to 1 mm behind the surgical limbus instead of the usual 2 mm. (From Luntz, MH, Harrison, R, and Schenker, HI: Glaucoma surgery, Baltimore, 1984, Williams & Wilkins)

Even with the use of a seton, the prognosis for successful surgery in groups 2 and 3 probably does not exceed 60%.

Advantages of Trabeculotomy

Patients with angle anomalies of group 1 do well with trabeculotomy or goniotomy and, in these cases, a filtering operation is usually not necessary. Trabeculotomy is our preferred operation for the following reasons[18]:

1. Trabeculotomy has a documented higher success rate than goniotomy. The latter controls intraocular pressure in about 74% of eyes having glaucoma of all degrees of severity, although control may be as high as 85% if eyes with corneal clouding are excluded.[16,23] Trabeculotomy, on the other hand, controls intraocular pressures in over 90%[11,17,20] of eyes with glaucoma of all degrees of severity, although up to three procedures may be necessary.

2. Trabeculotomy is technically easier for a well trained microsurgeon because it does not require the introduction of sharp instruments across the anterior chamber, which increases the risk of damage to other

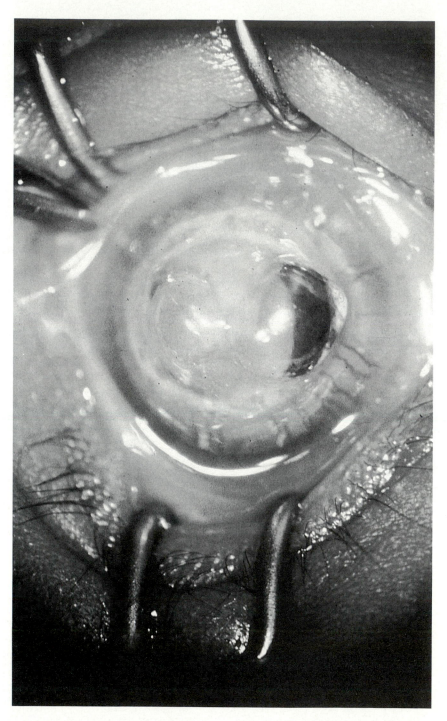

Fig. 37-3   Iridotrabecular-corneal dysgenesis (Luntz, Hoskins) in which the anomaly involves the cornea, trabecular meshwork, and iris. This photograph shows an eye with Peters' anomaly in which the lens and iris are adherent to the posterior corneal surface.

ocular tissue. It can be performed with undiminished accuracy in advanced cases in which the cornea is edematous or scarred and there is poor visibility in the anterior chamber.

3. There is no need for the surgeon to adapt to the visual distortion produced by the operating gonioprism.
4. A trabeculotomy is anatomically more precise in creating an opening between the anterior chamber and Schlemm's canal.
5. The success of trabeculotomy depends only on the type of angle anomaly and is not dependent on the severity of the glaucoma, the size of the cornea, or the presence of corneal edema—all factors that are reported to influence the success of goniotomy.[13,16] It is our operation of choice in those cases known to have a good prognosis, that is, group 1 angle anomalies. Trabeculotomy produces less surgical trauma and the anterior chamber is entered only briefly. There is a lower incidence of postoperative cataract and fewer postoperative complications.[18]

SURGICAL TREATMENT

Preoperative Patient Preparation

Anesthesia

The patient is usually a child and general anesthesia is preferred. Ketamine should be avoided because it may increase intraocular pressure. However, if an examination under anesthesia is performed for diagnostic purposes before surgery, ketamine is an ideal agent and may be followed with intubation and general anesthesia. General anesthesia will lower the intraocular pressure, but an intraocular pressure of over 18 mm Hg with general anesthesia should be regarded as suspiciously high.

Before surgery a careful assessment of intraocular pressure, the corneal diameter, the clinical state of the cornea, the appearance of the iris and lens, and the gonioscopic appearance of the angle must be made. The axial length of the eye may be measured by A-scan ultrasonography. The electrophysiologic activity of the retina and optic nerve may be determined by photopic and scotopic ERG and measurement of the visual evoked potential. The choice of surgical procedure will depend on the type of angle anomaly present. For example, in eyes with a mesodermal anomaly (trabeculodysgenesis) trabeculotomy is the operation of choice.

In eyes with a cicatrized angle (iridotrabeculodysgenesis) or in iridocorneotrabeculodysgenesis a combined trabeculotomy-trabeculectomy will give a better result.

Skin preparation and exposure

After the child is anesthetized, the operative field is prepared using antiseptic solution. The choice of antiseptics is an individual one but there are certain steps we prefer. Both eyes should be cleaned and prepared to ensure that the surgeon or assistant will not touch potentially septic areas while draping the patient and preparing the operative area. Cleansing of the skin should begin with a routine wash using saline, followed by a solution containing a detergent or soap and then by an antiseptic solution. At the end of the skin preparation, all the solutions are removed from the area of the procedure with alcohol followed by saline. After suitably cleansing the operative field, the patient is draped with sterile towels and plastic dressing, exposing the eye. Exposure of the eye can be achieved using a pediatric Barraquer wire speculum. The exposed eye is finally irrigated with an antibiotic solution.

Surgical microscope

A surgical microscope designed for ophthalmic surgery is used for all of the procedures described except ciliodestructive procedures. The magnifications mentioned in the text refer to magnification through the surgical microscope.

SURGICAL TECHNIQUE FOR GONIOTOMY

A gonioscopy lens is fixed to the surface of the cornea.

Goniotomy Lenses

Worst lens (Fig. 37-4)

A popular goniotomy lens is the Worst spherical lens. The lens fits around the limbal area with a flange extending onto the perilimbal conjunctiva. The flange is perforated by four openings, which allow the lens to be sutured to the perilimbal episcleral tissue with 7-0 sutures. The lens has an oval port that permits entry of the goniotomy knife. Once secured to the conjunctiva, the lens straddles the cornea and provides a 2× magnification of the angle.

The operating microscope should be used at relatively low magnification so as not to lose resolution through overmagnification. The Worst lens is connected through a silver cannula and fine polyvinyl chloride (PVC) tube to a syringe or infusion

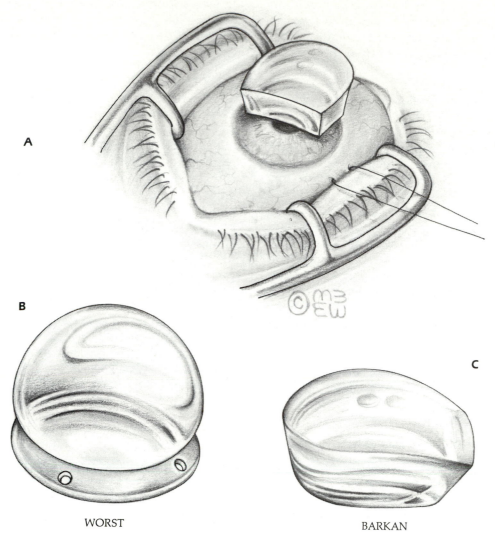

Fig. 37-4 Line drawings illustrating, **B,** the Worst and **C,** the Barkan goniotomy lenses. **A,** shows an eye with a Barkan lens in place on the cornea.

set containing balanced salt solution. The interior of the lens is filled with balanced salt solution to form a fluid bridge between the cornea and the inner surface of the lens. The lens is positioned so that the port through which the knife is introduced is at a convenient spot, if possible facing toward the temporal side.

Barkan and Lister Lenses (Fig. 37-4)

The Barkan lens and the Lister lens are hand-held on the cornea. These are similarly designed prism shaped lenses to allow viewing of the angle with the operating microscope in a vertical position. The inferior surface of the goniotomy lens is spherical with a steeper curvature than the corneal curvature. The space between the corneal surface of the goniotomy lens and the cornea becomes a part of the lens system when filled with balanced salt solution. As these lenses are hand-held and need to be rotated to obtain a view round the angle, it is difficult to maintain the saline meniscus between lens and cornea. For this reason the Lister lens has been modified with a fine silver cannula attached to a PVC tube which is in turn attached to a balanced salt infusion set. Notwithstanding these modifications, it is difficult to visualize the angle adequately and to maintain an air-bubble-free lens-corneal compartment. Breaks in Desce-

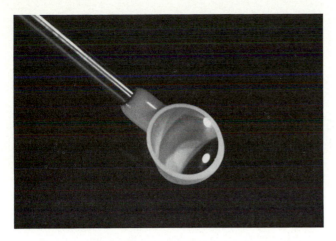

Fig. 37-5 Swan-Jacob Lens.

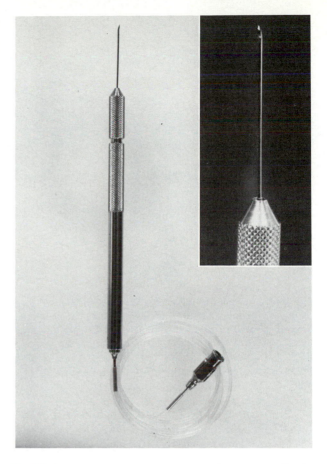

Fig. 37-6 Worst irrigating goniotomy knife. *Inset;* Tip of knife.

met's membrane, scars in the cornea, and thickening of Descemet's membrane may all produce refractile edges that impair the resolving power of the gonioscopic lens system, further reducing visibility.

The need to use a multiple lens system (operating microscope, gonioscopy lens, lens-corneafluid meniscus and cornea) to visualize the angle as well as the above changes in the cornea which reduce visualization all combine to make goniotomy a difficult and hazardous procedure. Use of these prismatic lenses to view the angle also usually requires tilting of the operating microscope, further reducing its resolving power.

Swan-Jacob Lens (Fig. 37-5)

Swan has addressed this problem by designing a gonioscopy lens with a convex anterior surface, allowing observation of the angle with the microscope vertical to the cornea. This reduces distortion when viewing the angle. The lens is small and fits snugly over the center of the cornea without the need for a fluid space between the lens and the cornea, achieved by designing the corneal surface of the lens flatter than the corneal curvature. Unfortunately with large buphthalmic eyes, the direct lens-corneal contact causes distortion of the corneal surface and a distorted view of the angle. The Swan lens has the advantage of being small enough to permit insertion of the gonioscopy knife at the limbus without obstruction by the lens. It also has a metal handle and can be manipulated without obstructing the operative field.

The most widely used gonioscopy lenses are the Worst lens and the Swan-Jacob lens.

Goniotomy Knives

With the lens in position, the next step is to select a suitable goniotomy knife. The goniotomy knife should conform to the following criteria:

1. The blade should not be too wide. The paracentesis incision should not leak after the knife is withdrawn. The average blade width is 1 to 1.5 mm.
2. The blade, which is generally sickle-shaped and resembles a paracentesis blade, is joined to a handle by a tapered shaft with the narrowest portion close to the blade and the widest portion close to the handle. The widest portion should equal but not exceed the width of the blade so that, when the shaft is fully inserted into the eye it will fill the paracentesis opening and prevent loss of fluid and collapse of the anterior chamber. The shaft and blade should be slightly longer than the diameter of the anterior chamber.

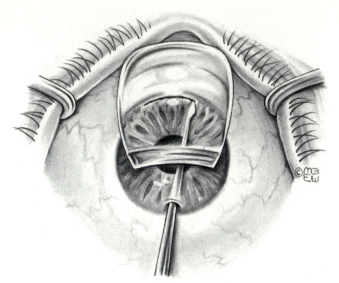

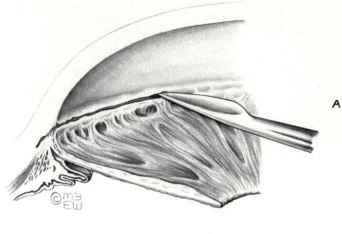 A

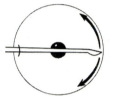 B

Fig. 37-7 Technique for goniotomy. A Barkan lens is in place on the cornea and a Barraquer goniotomy knife has penetrated the cornea just anterior to the limbus at the 12 o'clock position and has been advanced to the anterior trabecular meshwork at the 6 o'clock meridian. The point of the knife penetrates the trabecular meshwork and is then swung to the left and to the right.

Fig. 37-8 **A,** The knife cuts through trabecular meshwork just anterior to the iris root. **B,** The cut extends over approximately one-third of the angle circumference. In this line drawing the cut enters Schlemm's canal, an ideal seldom achieved in clinical practice. The knife cut probably opens an obstructive membrane inside the trabecular meshwork allowing aqueous access to the inner meshwork and Schlemm's canal.

3. A fine metal cannula is attached to the handle and shaft and by a PVC tube to a reservoir filled with balanced salt solution, which is infused during the operation to maintain a deep anterior chamber. Alternatively Healon or a viscoelastic material can be used to fill and maintain the anterior chamber during surgery. In our view, this is not a good alternative as the residual Healon may cause a postoperative rise of intraocular pressure and more severe postoperative iritis.

4. The blade of the knife should have a sharp point for entering the trabecular meshwork and be sharp on both sides to allow it to cut right and left without having to rotate it inside the anterior chamber.

A popular knife is the Barraquer goniotomy knife, which fulfills all these criteria, but another equally popular knife is the Worst knife (Fig. 37-6).

Technique

The goniotomy lens is selected and placed on the cornea (Fig. 37-7) and in the case of the Worst lens, secured with 7-0 silk or vicryl sutures to the perilimbal episcleral tissue. Pretreatment with topical pilocarpine is useful to constrict the pupil, but may shallow the anterior chamber. A gonioscopy knife is selected and the cannula connected via a

PVC tube to balanced salt solution in a 5 cc syringe or an intravenous infusion bottle. All air bubbles are removed from the system. The bottle is hung approximately 100 to 150 cm above the eye and the knife is checked for a suitable rate of infusion, adjusted by the height of the bottle or the force with which the syringe plunger is depressed. The knife is inserted into the anterior chamber through the cornea immediately anterior to the limbus. Under direct visualization, the surgeon ensures a deep anterior chamber and advances the knife across the chamber parallel to the plane of the iris but clear of the iris and lens surface until it reaches the trabecular meshwork in the angle area opposite to the point of insertion (Figs. 37-7 and 37-8). The knife is further advanced until the point enters the trabecular meshwork and is then swung to the left and to the right, incising an area of approximately one-third the circumference of the angle. The incision should be into the trabecular meshwork just anterior to the insertion of the iris. As the knife incises the trabecular meshwork, the iris falls backward and the angle deepens. Great care should be

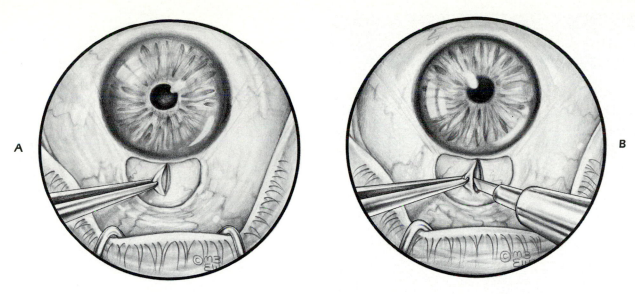

Fig. 37-9 Technique for trabeculotomy. **A,** A line drawing of the trabeculotomy procedure illustrating a fornix-based conjunctival flap 7 mm chord length at the limbus and a radial incision extending 2.5 mm back from the limbus and dissected to half the scleral thickness. **B,** The radial incision is undermined on each side using a diamond knife.

taken to avoid incarcerating the iris on the knife edge or damaging the lens. If iris is incarcerated the knife should be withdrawn and then replaced. If bleeding occurs, the rate of fluid infusion into the chamber should be increased to clear the blood from the area of surgery and tamponade the bleeding vessel. If the saline infusion leaks too rapidly from the anterior chamber and fails to tamponade the bleeder, a large air bubble may be introduced into the chamber to stop the bleeding. After the incision is completed and the chamber is deepened, the knife is carefully withdrawn from the eye, taking care to avoid injury to the iris or the lens. At the end of the procedure, the anterior chamber is filled with balanced salt solution or air to maintain a deep chamber and the goniotomy lens is removed from the eye.

A drop of an antibiotic-corticosteroid preparation is instilled into the conjunctival sac and a patch and shield are applied to the eye.

The day after surgery the anterior chamber should be deep and the pupil reactive. Topical antibiotic-corticosteroid drops are continued until the anterior chamber reaction resolves.

SURGICAL TECHNIQUE FOR TRABECULOTOMY

Conjunctival Flap (5× Magnification)

A fornix-based conjunctival flap of 7 mm is raised at the limbus (Fig. 37-9). The dissection is continued to the sclera, raising conjunctiva, Tenon's capsule and episclera. In this manner, a triangular portion of sclera is exposed, measuring at least 3 mm from its base at the surgical limbus to its apex. The surface of the sclera is cleaned.

Many surgeons prefer a limbus-based conjunctival flap. A fornix-based flap is technically easier, less traumatic to Tenon's capsule, and gives better exposure of the operative field.

To rotate the globe, if necessary, 4-0 Mersilene sutures are passed through lamellar thickness of sclera at each edge of the conjunctival flap at the surgical limbus.

Scleral Dissection (10× Magnification)

Using a sharp knife with a microblade or a diamond knife, an incision is made through half the scleral depth, extending from the surgical limbus at the midpoint of the exposed sclera posteriorly for 2.5 to 3 mm (see Fig. 37-9). Holding one edge of this incision with forceps and rotating it outward to allow greater visibility, the scleral incision is deepened until corneal and trabecular tissue become visible in the depths of the anterior half of the incision. At this point, the incision is undermined on each side to increase the surgical exposure. Once the undermining has been completed, the surgeon has a view of the external surgical landmarks and can proceed to the next step, the dissection of the external wall of the canal of Schlemm. These surgical landmarks are well illustrated in Fig. 37-10.

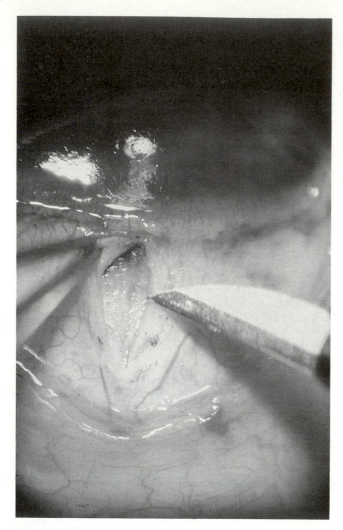

Fig. 37-10 A photograph of a trabeculotomy procedure after gaining adequate exposure by undermining the radial incision on each side. The deeper layers of the sclera are visible and the surgical landmarks can be identified within the deep layers of the incision. Closest to the limbus is a transparent band of deep corneal lamellae. Behind that is a narrow grayish-blue band, which represents the trabecular meshwork. This in turn ceases and is replaced by white, opaque sclera. The junction of the posterior border of the trabecular band and the sclera is the external landmark of the scleral spur and the landmark for finding the canal of Schlemm. The knife points to the landmark for the scleral spur. In most eyes this is situated between 2 and 2.5 mm behind the surgical limbus.

Dissection into Canal (15× Magnification)

Having recognized these landmarks, the next step is to make a radial incision using a diamond knife or microblade (for example, a No. 75 Beaver blade) across the scleral spur at the junction of the lower margin of the trabecular band and the sclera (Fig. 37-11). Transillumination of the globe allows

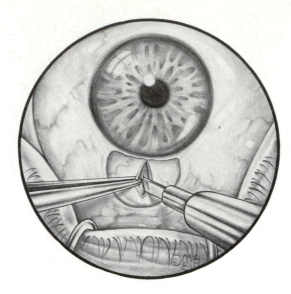

Fig. 37-11 Technique for trabeculotomy. A second radial incision using a diamond knife is made across the scleral spur at the junction of the lower margin of the trabecular band and the sclera. This incision is dissected through the external wall of Schlemm's canal into the limbus.

the surgeon to identify the iris root in most eyes. This is also a useful guide to the canal of Schlemm, which is found just anterior to the root of the iris if the surgical landmarks are not visible or identifiable. The incision is carefully deepened until it is carried through the external wall of Schlemm's canal, at which point there is a gush of aqueous, occasionally mixed with blood. The dissection is carefully continued through the external wall until the inner wall of the canal becomes visible. The inner wall is characteristically slightly pigmented and is composed of crisscrossing fibers. After this point is reached, one blade of a Vannas scissors is passed along the canal and, with the other blade lying superficial to the external wall (Fig. 37-12, *A*), two parallel cuts are made and a strip of the external wall of the canal is excised. The canal is opened for 1.0 to 1.5 mm circumferentially (Fig. 37-12, *B*). The blade of the Vannas scissors should enter the canal with ease and slide along the canal. If not, then further dissection through the external wall is required to avoid producing a false passage. Some surgeons confirm passage into the canal by passing a 6-0 nylon suture into the canal, as described by Smith[24] (Fig. 37-13). The location of the suture should be checked gonioscopically because it can slip into the anterior chamber. We have found this an unnecessary step if the canal is adequately exposed by excising the external wall.

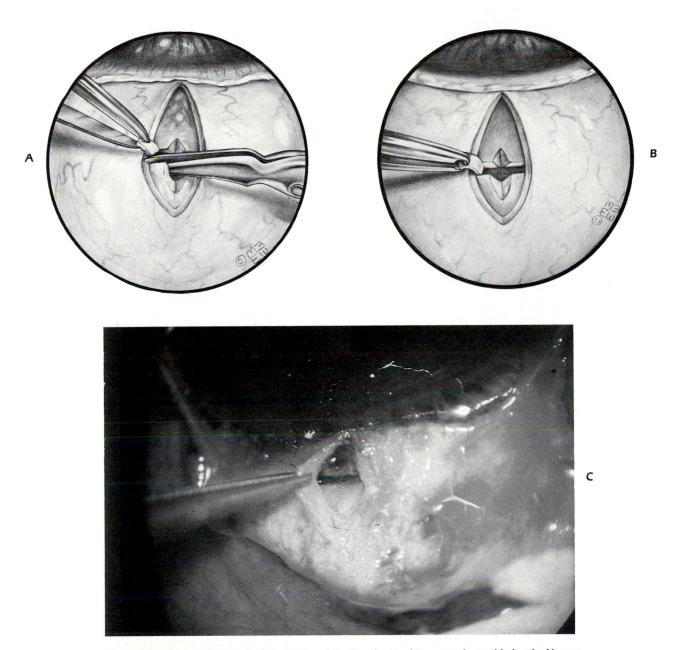

Fig. 37-12 Trabeculotomy technique. **A** and **B,** after the canal is exposed, one blade of a Vannas scissors is passed along the canal, the other blade lying superficial to the external wall, and two parallel cuts are made removing a strip of the external wall of the canal. **C,** Photograph of dissection after removing external wall of Schlemm's canal; the canal is open for 1.0 to 1.5 mm of its circumference.

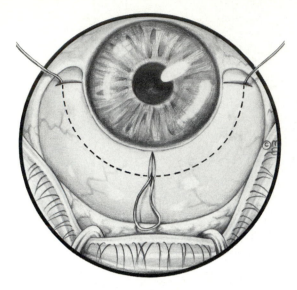

Fig. 37-13 A 6-0 nylon suture is passed along the canal of Schlemm to confirm that the canal has been opened. Adequate enforcement of the canal can usually be confirmed without this step.

Introduction of Trabeculotomy Probe (5× Magnification)

A trabeculotomy probe of the design shown in Fig. 37-14 (Luntz trabeculotomy probe) is introduced. Other designs have been described.[1,9,10,12,13] The lower blade has a diameter of 0.20 mm and fits into the canal; the upper blade lies over the limbus and, if kept resting on the cornea, ensures that the lower blade does not ride downward through the inner wall of the canal or ride upward, creating a false scleral passage. The two blades are separated by 1 mm. The shaft of the probe is divided into three segments so that the central third can be stabilized with the left hand, whereas the right hand rotates the upper and lower thirds around the central third, rotating the probe into the anterior chamber. This will avoid anterior or posterior movement of the probe tip, iris trauma, or disruption of corneal lamellae.

The probe is passed along the canal to the surgeon's left side (Fig. 37-15, *A*) and rotated into the anterior chamber, thus opening this inner wall of the canal (Fig. 37-15, *B*). The same process is repeated on the other side, again rotating the probe into the anterior chamber. The probe is withdrawn; and, if the procedure has been adequately performed, a bridge of the inner wall of the canal of Schlemm remains intact across the area of canal that was unroofed. This bridge prevents the iris prolapsing into the surgical incision so that a peripheral iridectomy is not necessary. If the iris does prolapse into the incision, then a peripheral iridectomy should be performed.

It is important that no force be used when introducing the probe into the canal, as this will create a false passage. If the probe does not slip easily down the canal, it is probably in the sclera because of inadequate dissection of all the fibers of the external wall. The probe should be withdrawn and dissection of the outer wall continued using a microblade or diamond knife until the surgeon is satisfied that all fibers of the outer wall are removed. The probe is then reintroduced into the canal.

During the procedure, the anterior chamber should be formed at all times. As the probe passes into the anterior chamber, disrupting the inner wall of the canal, there should be some slight resistance, and there may be a little intracameral bleeding from the inner wall. The anterior chamber is rarely lost after trabeculotomy. It can be filled with Healon after the first pass of the probe, but, as previously mentioned, we do not favor the use of Healon in the anterior chamber for glaucoma surgery.

As the probe is swung from the canal into the anterior chamber, the surgeon should carefully watch the iris for movement, particularly if the probe passes easily. Movement of the iris or totally unresisted passage of the probe implies that the probe is in the anterior chamber and catching onto the iris root. If not corrected, this may cause an iridodialysis. The probe should be immediately withdrawn without continuing its entry into the anterior chamber and replaced, keeping the tip of the probe slightly anterior so that it does not prematurely rupture the inner wall. The cornea should also be carefully monitored to ensure that the probe is not intrascleral and ripping through sclera, cornea, and Descemet's membrane. This is easy to detect because small air bubbles appear in the cornea as the probe ruptures through corneal lamellae. The probe needs to be repositioned, pushing the tip a little posteriorly.

The important point is that the probe should pass with ease along the canal and from the canal into the anterior chamber without forcing it.

An alternative method[13] is to perform trabeculotomy under a lamellar scleral flap. The radial incisions into Schlemm's canal are made deep to this flap. This technique is useful for combined trabeculotomy and trabeculectomy and is described here. However, for trabeculotomy the radial incision has many advantages.

1. There is no need to dissect a lamellar scleral flap; therefore, there is less surgical trauma.
2. If the canal is not found or if the anterior

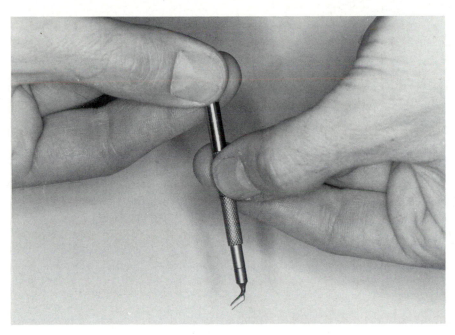

Fig. 37-14   Luntz trabeculotomy probe.

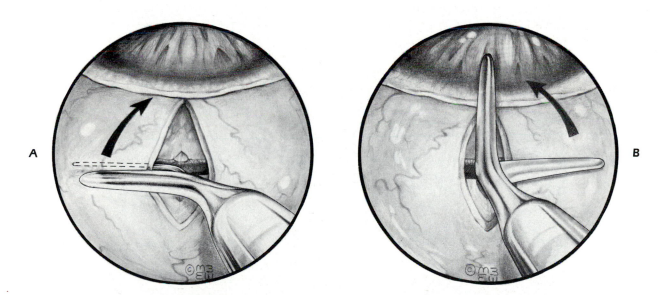

Fig. 37-15   Trabeculotomy technique. **A,** The probe is passed along the canal, the inner probe in the lumen of the canal to the surgeon's left side and then rotated into the anterior chamber *(arrow)*. **B,** A line drawing showing the probe rotated into the anterior chamber from the left side. Then the probe is reinserted into the right side of the lumen of the canal and rotated into the anterior chamber from this side *(arrow)*. No force should be used when introducing the probe into the canal.

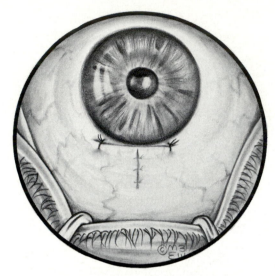

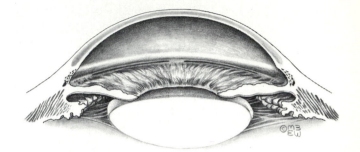

Fig. 37-16 Trabeculotomy technique. The radial scleral incision is closed with three interrupted 9-0 sutures.

Fig. 37-17 Trabeculotomy technique. A line drawing of postoperative gonioscopy showing nasal and temporal ruptures of the inner wall of Schlemm's canal with a bridge of intact inner wall between the nasal and temporal clefts. These clefts are at the scleral spur between the iris root and the anterior trabecular meshwork.

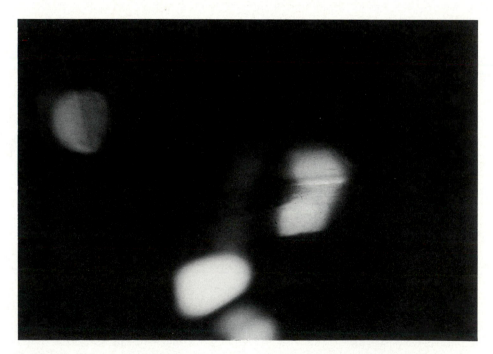

Fig. 37-18 Trabeculotomy technique. A photograph of a gonioscopic evaluation of a cleft of the inner wall of Schlemm's canal after trabeculotomy, as shown in the line drawing in Fig. 37-16. Note that the cleft appears as a white recess as one is looking through the ruptured inner wall directly at the scleral surface of the outer wall.

chamber is accidentally entered, the radial incision can be sutured and another radial incision made at an adjacent site with minimal trauma to the eye. This can be done without raising another conjunctival flap or enlarging the existing conjunctival flap. If the canal cannot be located at one site, it will usually be found at the second incision.

3. In the rare case in which the canal is not found (one case in 110 eyes[19]) the procedure can readily be converted to a guarded trabeculectomy by using the radial incision as one side of the trabeculectomy lamellar scleral flap. The conjunctival flap is not enlarged.

Closure of the Incision

The scleral incision is closed with three interrupted 9-0 virgin silk or nylon sutures (Fig. 37-16). The conjunctival flap is rotated forward to the limbus and secured with a 10-0 nylon suture at each edge of the flap or a running suture for a limbus-based flap. The conjunctival closure is the same as that used for trabeculectomy (Fig. 37-17).

Postoperatively, gonioscopy should be performed to check that the trabeculotomy has been accurately done. The ruptures (nasal and temporal) of the inner wall of Schlemm's canal are visible on gonioscopy as white recesses as one looks through the ruptured inner wall directly to the scleral surface of the outer wall. There is a bridge of intact inner wall between the nasal and temporal dehiscences. The ruptures of the inner wall are placed at the scleral spur between the iris root and the anterior trabecular meshwork (Figs. 37-17 and 37-18).

Postoperative Management

An antibiotic-steroid drop combination is used four times a day for 1 to 2 weeks postoperatively. The day after surgery the eye should be comfortable and the chamber deep. Intraocular pressure is checked in the office or by examination under anesthesia within 6 weeks of the surgical procedure.

SURGICAL TECHNIQUE FOR TRABECULECTOMY

Fornix-based Conjunctival-Tenon's Flap (5× to 7× Magnification)

A fornix-based conjunctival-Tenon's flap 7 mm chord length is raised at the limbus, preferably in the upper nasal quadrant (Fig. 37-19, *A*). A limbus-based flap is an alternative but is significantly more traumatic to Tenon's capsule. The conjunctiva and Tenon's fascia are dissected back in a natural sur-

gical plane between these and the sclera. Some surgeons make a paracentesis incision through the cornea.

Scleral flap (5× to 7× magnification)

The scleral surface is cleaned and a flap 3 mm long and extending 2.5 mm posterior to the limbus is outlined with one or two cautery marks in the exposed sclera. This flap is hinged at the limbus to ensure that the conjunctival and scleral suture lines are separated.

With a diamond knife the scleral flap is incised initially along its posterior border, which is 2.5 mm behind the limbus and this incision is dissected down to the surface of the pars plana (Fig. 37-19, *A*). Next, two one-half thickness radial scleral incisions 3 mm apart are dissected, extending posteriorly for 2.5 mm from the limbus and joining each end of the prepared posterior incision (Fig. 37-19, *B*). The thickness of the sclera can be estimated from the full thickness posterior incision allowing accurate dissection of lamellar scleral flaps of varying thickness. Ideally, the flap should be one-third the scleral thickness, which permits adequate aqueous filtration but avoids the possibility of an excessively thin scleral flap becoming staphylomatous. In patients with a poor prognosis for surgery and in whom better drainage is required, the scleral flap can be dissected thinner than one-third scleral thickness. The dissection of the scleral flap is commenced from the posterior incision at the desired thickness using a Grieshaber No. 68-107 or Beaver No. 75 blade (Fig. 37-19, *C*). Staying in the same surgical plane, the dissection is carried forward to the cornea to just within the surgical limbus. With the lamellar scleral flap retracted, the salient external landmarks are easily recognized in the deeper undissected tissues (Fig. 37-20). A pair of preplaced 10-0 nylon sutures is placed from the two posterior corners of the scleral flap to the posterior corners of the flap bed and subsequently pulled out of the way when the lamellar scleral flap is anteriorly rotated to allow continuation of the trabeculectomy dissection.

Trabeculectomy (10× magnification)

Using a No. 75 Beaver blade or a diamond knife, a square flap of approximately 2 mm containing corneal lamellae and anterior trabecular meshwork is outlined without penetration into the anterior chamber.

Penetration into the anterior chamber is made slowly. The anterior chamber is entered at one corner via a small opening by careful dissection through Descemet's membrane, allowing aqueous

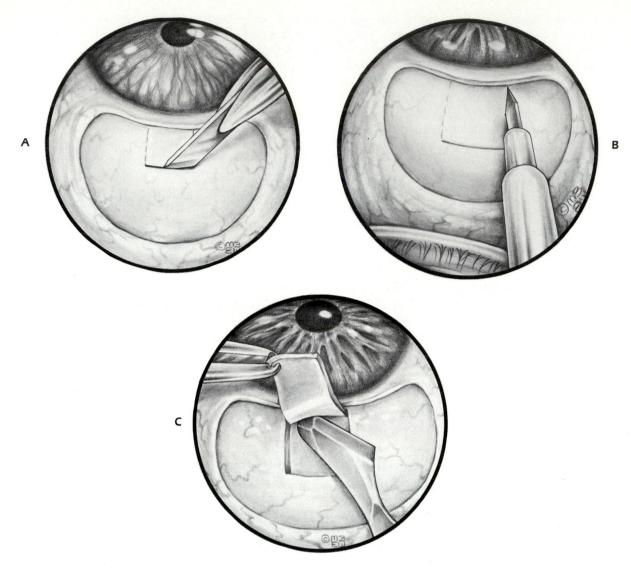

Fig. 37-19 Trabeculectomy technique. **A,** A fornix-based conjunctival flap has been raised. The posterior 3 mm scleral incision, which is parallel to the limbus, is dissected down to the surface of the pars plana. This allows the surgeon to visualize the thickness of the sclera and to accurately dissect the one-third thickness flap. **B,** The two radial incisions are dissected connecting the limbus to the posterior incision. **C,** After estimating the scleral thickness through the posterior incision, a one-third thickness lamellar scleral flap is dissected starting at the posterior incision and carried forward into clear cornea to just within the surgical limbus.

humor to seep slowly out until the eye becomes soft, but without losing the anterior chamber. In buphthalmic eyes, the zonules may be stretched and, with penetration into the anterior chamber, vitreous can prolapse through the zonules into the chamber. The risk of this complication can be reduced by slowly reducing intraocular pressure before completing the trabeculectomy. After the eye has softened, air is injected into the anterior chamber to maintain a moderate depth. The incision into the anterior chamber is enlarged by careful dissection with the microblade until the opening is large enough to introduce a straight or angled Vannas scissor, with which the anterior incision is completed. Then the radial incisions and finally the posterior incision just anterior to the scleral spur and parallel to the limbus are made (Fig. 37-21). Note that iris plugs the trabeculectomy opening, maintaining the anterior chamber, which should remain formed throughout the procedure.

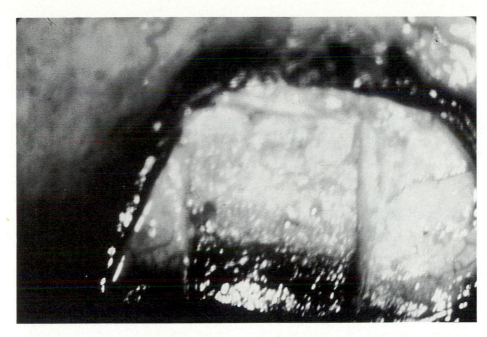

Fig. 37-20 Trabeculectomy technique. Photograph of trabeculectomy through the operating microscope. The cornea is at the upper part of the photograph. The one-third thickness lamellar scleral flap has been dissected and is hinged at the cornea and rotated anteriorly over the cornea exposing deeper structures and the salient anatomic landmarks. Anteriorly the transparent band represents deep corneal lamellae. Posterior to this is a bluish-gray narrower band, which is the landmark for trabecular meshwork. Behind the trabecular meshwork is white sclera with crisscrossing fibers. The most important landmark is the junction of the posterior border of the trabecular band and the sclera representing the external landmark for the scleral spur.

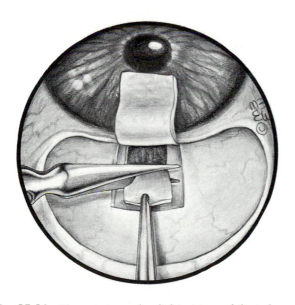

Fig. 37-21 The anterior and radial incisions of the trabeculectomy have been completed, the trabeculectomy flap is hinged posteriorly at the scleral spur, and a posterior incision is completed just anterior to the scleral spur. Note that iris plugs the trabeculectomy opening.

Iridectomy (10× magnification)

An iridectomy is now made. It is imperative that the iridectomy is wider than the trabeculectomy opening to prevent the iris pillars from being pushed into this opening postoperatively. This is achieved by grasping the iris with forceps, moving it to the surgeon's left side and initiating an iridectomy incision with scissors from the right side. As this incision approaches the midway point of the iridectomy, the iris is moved across to the right side, put on stretch, and the iridectomy completed (Fig. 37-22). The anterior chamber is not lost, because it remains filled with air or is refilled with air.

The iridectomy should be made carefully as vitreous may prolapse through a stretched and ruptured zonule and erupt through the iridectomy. If this occurs, a limited vitrectomy must be performed removing all vitreous from the iridectomy and the immediately surrounding iris surface. This is best accomplished using sponges and Vannas scissors.

Closure (5× magnification)

As the iridectomy is completed, the lamellar scleral flap is repositioned by tying the preplaced

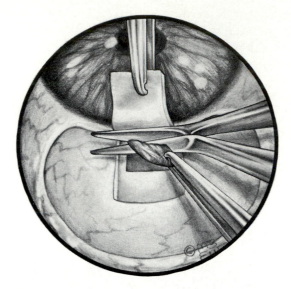

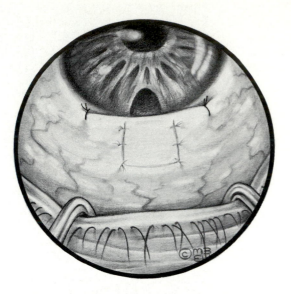

Fig. 37-22 Trabeculectomy technique. Iris is pulled out of the trabeculectomy opening and an iridectomy is made, ensuring that the base of the iridectomy is wider than the trabeculectomy opening. The iris is first pulled to the left, incised halfway across with Vannas scissors and then pulled to the right and the incision completed. The second stage of the iridectomy is demonstrated in this line drawing.

Fig. 37-23 Trabeculectomy technique. Closure of the scleral flap and conjunctival-Tenon's flap. The partial thickness scleral flap is securely sutured with a total of six interrupted 10-0 nylon sutures. The conjunctival-Tenon's flap is rotated anteriorly to the limbus and sutured to the sclera with two 10-0 nylon sutures, one at each end of the flap, ensuring that the cut edge of the flap lies snugly across the limbus.

A
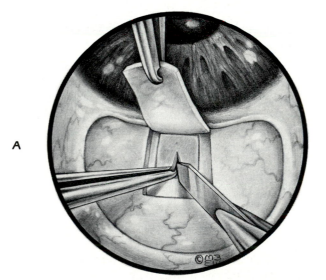

B
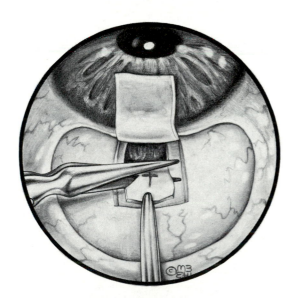

Fig. 37-24 Technique for combined trabeculotomy-trabeculectomy. **A,** A 7 mm wide fornix-based conjunctival-Tenon's flap has been raised, a 2.5 x 3 mm one-third thickness lamellar scleral flap is dissected to within the surgical limbus and anteriorly rotated exposing deeper structures. A 2 x 2 mm trabeculectomy flap is outlined without penetrating the anterior chamber and a central radial incision has been made across the scleral spur and is being dissected into the lumen of Schlemm's canal. **B,** The trabeculotomy has been completed and the anterior and radial incisions for the trabeculectomy flap are completed. The flap is being removed by a posterior incision just anterior to the scleral spur. Note the iris plugging the trabeculectomy opening.

10-0 nylon sutures at the posterior edges of the scleral flap. The anterior chamber is still maintained by the air bubble. Balanced salt solution is injected into the anterior chamber to replace the air bubble. The partial thickness scleral flap is securely sutured using four additional interrupted 10-0 nylon sutures (Fig. 37-23). The conjunctival-Tenon's flap is rotated anteriorly to the limbus and sutured to the episclera and sclera with two 10-0 nylon sutures one at each end of the conjunctival flap, pulling the conjunctival edge taut but not tight across the limbus (Fig. 37-23).

Balanced salt solution is injected under the conjunctival flap to lift it from the sclera. The patient leaves the operating table with an intact anterior chamber and a bleb at the site of the trabeculectomy.

SURGICAL TECHNIQUE FOR TRABECULOTOMY–TRABECULECTOMY

The operation is a combination of the techniques described for trabeculectomy and for trabeculotomy.

Conjunctival and Scleral Flap

A fornix-based 7 mm cord length conjunctival-Tenon's flap is used, identical to that described for trabeculotomy and trabeculectomy. A 2.5 × 3 mm wide one-third thickness lamellar scleral flap is raised in identical manner to that described for trabeculectomy (Fig. 37-24, *A*). The surgical landmarks are identified and a 2 × 2 mm trabeculectomy flap is outlined in the depths of the scleral incision as described for trabeculectomy. The anterior chamber is not penetrated at this point. In the center of the trabeculectomy flap a radial incision is made across the landmark for the scleral spur and this is dissected through the outer wall of the canal of Schlemm into the lumen of the canal as described for a trabeculotomy. The trabeculotomy procedure is then completed into the anterior chamber, following this the trabeculectomy flap is dissected removing the flap just anterior to the scleral spur (Fig. 37-24, *B*). An iridectomy is then performed and the lamellar scleral flap is sutured back into position as described for trabeculectomy. The conjunctival-Tenon's flap is then repositioned as described for trabeculectomy.

Postoperative Management

The postoperative management for trabeculectomy or combined trabeculotomy-trabeculectomy is the same. An antibiotic-steroid drop combination is used four times a day for 2 weeks postoperatively. The day after surgery the eye should be comfortable and the chamber deep. Intraocular pressure is checked in the office or by examination under anesthesia within 6 weeks of the surgical procedure. A cycloplegic (for example Cyclopentolate 1%, bid) is used only if the eye is significantly irritated or if there is significant circumcorneal injection.

SETONS

Setons should be considered in those eyes in which filtering surgery has failed to control intraocular pressure. We prefer the Molteno implant.[21] The inferotemporal area is most suitable for implanting the valve, but it can be placed in any quadrant (Fig. 37-25).

Personal experience with the prosthesis extends over more than 5 years with good results. Molteno et al.[21] use a two-stage technique and postoperatively a regimen of systemic cytotoxins and antiinflammatory agents, but a single-stage technique without the systemic postoperative medications appears to give an equally good surgical result.

CYCLODESTRUCTIVE PROCEDURES

If the Molteno seton fails to control intraocular pressure, a second seton can be inserted. However, if multiple filtration surgery has failed to control intraocular pressure the prognosis for vision in that eye becomes extremely poor. If intraocular pressure is still unduly high, a cyclodestructive procedure should be considered, preferably cyclocryotherapy, therapeutic ultrasound or Nd:YAG laser cyclodestruction. The most widely used is cyclocryotherapy. These procedures are described in detail in Chapter 38.

Indications for a cyclodestructive procedure in congenital, infantile or juvenile glaucoma follow:

1. Failure of repeated filtration surgery.
2. A severely buphthalmic eye with extensive optic nerve pathology and a poor visual prognosis. Filtration surgery in a severely buphthalmic eye has a poor prognosis for success, and when the eye is opened there is a significant risk of vitreous loss from zonular degeneration. The end result may well be vitreous adherence to the incision, contraction of the vitreous, retinal detachment and phthisis. In these eyes cyclodestructive procedures are probably less traumatic.

Cyclodestructive procedures should be applied with caution and in a titrated regimen. Parents should be warned of the high risk of phthisis bulbi

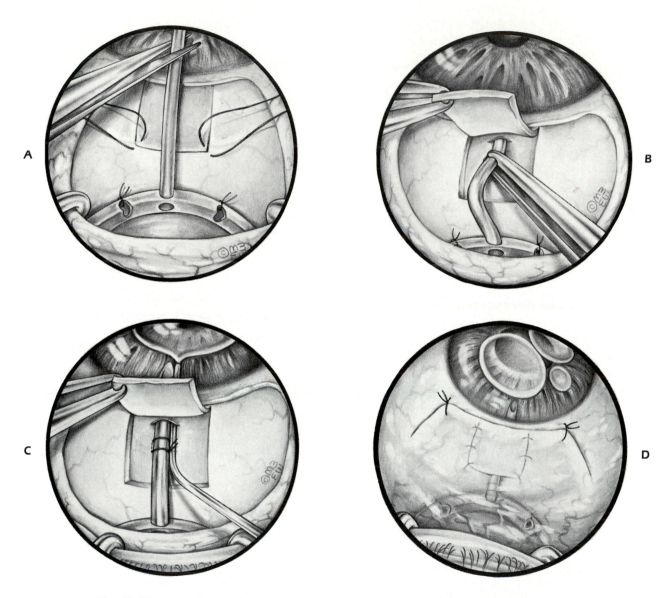

Fig. 37-25 Technique for Molteno implant. **A,** The plate of a Molteno implant has been sutured in place and a lamellar scleral flap dissected. Sutures have been preplaced at the corners of the flap and will be looped out of the way. The tube of the flap is trimmed to size at its anterior end. **B,** The anterior end of the tube is inserted into the anterior chamber through a snug incision. **C,** Sutures are placed through the sclera and looped around the tube of the implant to secure it. **D,** The scleral flap is sutured back in place and the conjunctiva closed. The anterior chamber is reformed.

following these procedures. This is especially true in congenital total aniridia.

Special Considerations

The responsibility of the surgeon does not stop with surgery. Visual rehabilitation is as important in the management of the disease as is intraocular pressure control.[8] Visual rehabilitation involves correction of refractive errors; correction of opacities in the media, such as corneal scarring and cataract; and orthoptic treatment to stimulate the development of binocular vision. These should be undertaken at as early an age as possible.

Children with Sturge-Weber syndrome or nanophthalmos present special problems. In these patients, trabeculotomy is the favored operation, but if this does not control the intraocular pressure then trabeculectomy or combined trabeculotomy-trabeculectomy is done.

Excessive bleeding may occur during surgery from congested episcleral or trabecular meshwork vessels backtracking blood into the canal of Schlemm in Sturge-Weber syndrome. The bleeding is controlled by filling the anterior chamber with air, which tamponades the bleeding.

Nanophthalmic eyes, which are unusually small with microphthalmos and short axial length (less than 18 mm), are particularly prone to develop suprachoroidal hemorrhage or effusion, particularly with trabeculectomy. Posterior sclerotomy incisions in each of the inferior quadrants should be made as a prophylactic measure. If a suprachoroidal effusion does occur, drainage is accomplished through the posterior sclerotomy. The anterior chamber should be kept formed with air (or Healon) during the surgery.

REFERENCES

1. Allen, L, and Burian, HM: Trabeculotomy ab externo. A new glaucoma operation. Technique and results of experimental surgery, Am J Ophthalmol 53:19, 1962
2. Anderson, DR: Trabeculotomy compared to goniotomy for glaucoma in children, Ophthalmology 1:331, 1981
3. Barkan O: Technique of goniotomy, Arch Ophthalmol 19:217, 1938
4. Barkan, O: Operation for congenital glaucoma, Am J Ophthalmol 25:552, 1942
5. Barkan,O: Goniotomy for the relief of congenital glaucoma, Br J Ophthalmol 32:701, 1948
6. Barkan, O: Surgery of congenital glaucoma. Review of 196 eyes operated by goniotomy, Am J Ophthalmol 36:1523, 1953
7. Barkan, O: Goniotomy, Trans Am Acad Ophthalmol Otolaryngol 59:322, 1955
8. Dannheim, R, and Haas, H: Visual acuity and IOP after surgery in congenital glaucome, Klin Manatsbl Augenheilkd 177:296, 1980
9. Della Porta, A: Evaluation of anterior and posterior trabeculodialysis, Am J Ophthalmol 48:294, 1959
10. Dobree, JH: Spatula for trabeculotomy, Br J Ophthalmol 53:861, 1969
11. Gregersen, E, and Kessing, SVV: Congenital glaucoma before and after the introduction of microsurgery. Results of "macrosurgery" 1943-1963 and of microsurgery (trabeculotomy/ectomy) 1970-1974, Arch Ophthalmol 55:422, 1977
12. Hager, H, et al: Experimental principles of trabecular-electro-puncture (TEP), v Graefe's Arch Klin Exp Ophthalmol 185:95, 1972
13. Harms, H, and Dannheim, R: Experience with external trabeculotomy in congenital glaucoma, Dtsch Ophthalmol Ges 69:272, 1969
14. Harms, H, and Dannheim, R: Epicritical consideration of 300 cases of trabeculotomy 'ab externo' Trans Ophthalmol Soc UK 89:491, 1970
15. Hoskins HD, Jr, Shaffer RN, and Hetherington, J: Goniotomy vs trabeculotomy, J Pediatr Ophthalmol Strabismus 21:153, 1984
16. Kwitko, ML: Glaucoma in infants and children, New York, 1973, Appleton-Century-Crofts
17. Luntz, MH: Primary buphthalmos (inflantile glaucoma) treated by trabeculotomy ab extreme, S Afr Arch Ophthalmol 2:219, 1974
18. Luntz, MH: The advantages of trabeculotomy over goniotomy, J Pediatr Ophthalmol Strabismus 2:150, 1984
19. Luntz, MH, and Livingston, DG: Trabeculotomy ab externo and trabeculectomy in congenital and adult-onset glaucoma, Am J Ophthalmol 83:174, 1977
20. McPherson SD, Jr: Results of external trabeculotomy, Am J Ophthalmol 76:918, 1973
21. Molteno, ACB, Van Biljon, G, and Ancker, E: Two-stage insertion of glaucoma drainage implants, TOS NZ 31:17, 1979
22. Robertson, EN, Jr: Therapy of congenital glaucoma, AMA, AO 54:55, 1955
23. Shields, MB: Textbook of glaucoma, ed 2, Baltimore, 1986, Williams & Wilkins
24. Smith, R: A new technique for opening the canal of Schlemm. Preliminary report, Br J Ophthalmol 44:14, 1960

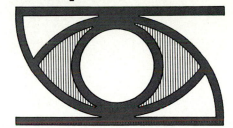

Chapter 38

Cyclodestructive Surgery

A. Robert Bellows
Joseph H. Krug, Jr.

When medical treatment and standard laser and invasive surgical methods fail to control intraocular pressure, cyclodestructive procedures are usually suggested as the only available therapy to preserve vision. These modalities work by decreasing ciliary process secretion of aqueous humor, resulting in a decrease in the intraocular pressure. Accurate determination of the amount of ciliary body destruction necessary to achieve a desired decrease in intraocular pressure (without creating significant ocular complications) remains one of the challenges of cyclodestructive treatment.

Eyes chosen for cyclodestructive procedures often have the poorest prognosis. These include the refractory forms of secondary glaucoma, such as glaucoma in aphakia or pseudophakia, glaucoma associated with uveitis, and neovascular glaucoma, as well as primary and secondary glaucomas after multiple failed filtering procedures.

Intraocular pressure depends on a balance between the adequacy of aqueous secretion and the efficiency of the aqueous outflow channels. When outflow channels are severely compromised, the effect on intraocular pressure of any alteration of aqueous secretion is magnified, and the delicate relationship between the inflow and outflow to regulate intraocular pressure is more critical.

An overly aggressive approach to the destruction of the ciliary body, such as cyclocryotherapy to the entire circumference of the eye, may result in phthisis bulbi[9] and anterior segment necrosis.[40] When energy sources are not accurately directed to the pars plicata, failure to achieve pressure control is frequent.[31] To reduce the frequency and se-

verity of complications after cyclodestructive procedures, accurate applications of various forms of energy sources that can be titrated are being evaluated. Most of the modalities developed to alter ciliary body secretion have been designed to selectively destroy the epithelial layers of the ciliary processes or to interrupt the blood supply of the ciliary body at the base of the ciliary processes. The sources of energy used for cyclodestructive procedures include heat, cold, laser energy, ultrasound, and surgical excision of the ciliary body. Because medical reduction of aqueous secretion with beta-blocking agents and carbonic anhydrase inhibitors remains an important part of glaucoma therapy, it seems quite appropriate that more effort should be expended to identify safer surgical techniques to influence aqueous suppression.

EARLY EXPERIENCE WITH CYCLODESTRUCTIVE SURGERY

The observation that detachment of the ciliary body caused a reduction in intraocular pressure resulting from inhibition of aqueous production was noted by Heine,[35] who proposed cyclodialysis. Shahan and Post[61] applied thermal energy to the perilimbal area to alter the ciliary body and reported a successful decrease of intraocular pressure in normal rabbits and two human eyes with glaucoma. Actual excision of the ciliary body was recommended by Verhoeff[68] as a treatment for glaucoma. He postulated a number of mechanisms for glaucoma control with this technique. However, his surgical excision of the ciliary body did not include the ciliary processes. The use of galvano cau-

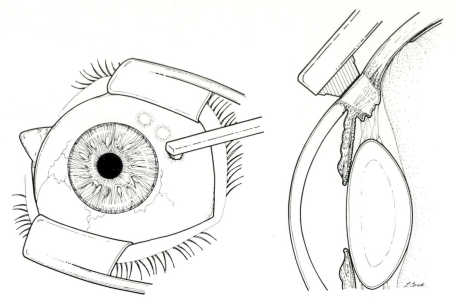

Fig. 38-1 Cyclodiathermy, nonpenetrating.

tery over the ciliary body in an 8 to 10 mm circumferential area was developed by Curran in 1925.[24] His intent with this operation was to (1) establish filtration, (2) interfere with the functioning parts of the ciliary body, and (3) produce a decompression of the "staphyloma." When reporting on a 20-year experience with galvano cautery to treat glaucoma, Fiore[32] was impressed with the pressure-lowering effect but admitted that this form of therapy was often used to treat acute angle-closure glaucoma at a time when peripheral iridectomy was well established as the accepted treatment for this condition.

CYCLODIATHERMY

Weve is credited with developing transscleral surface diathermy (cyclodiathermy) to treat infantile glaucoma, as well as other forms of uncontrolled glaucoma (Fig. 38-1).[76,77] Vogt[69,70] introduced the modification of penetrating cyclodiathermy (Fig. 38-2). He applied a diathermy probe 1.5 to 3.5 mm from the limbus to destroy the ciliary body. Coppez[22,23] showed that the use of diathermy in rabbits destroyed the ciliary body and ciliary body epithelium, resulting in a decrease in aqueous secretion. However, it remained for investigators in the 1950s to demonstrate tonographically that aqueous secretion actually decreased after cyclodiathermy.[58,72,74,76]

The reported results of cyclodiathermy are frequently confusing and contradictory, possibly because of marked differences in technique. The accumulation of information about these procedures often included both surface and penetrating cyclodiathermy for many different types of glaucoma. Although initial enthusiasm was quickly reported[2] and supported,[65,75] careful studies of Troncoso[67] refuted the suspected effect on the ciliary processes and suggested that inflammation and hemorrhage often caused the observed lowering of intraocular pressure. Discouraging results were reported by Marr[45] using partial penetrating diathermy, and surface diathermy. He noted a high incidence of phthisis bulbi and poor pressure control while demonstrating very little histopathologic evidence of ciliary process damage after cyclodiathermy, suggesting that the procedure had little effect on the pars plicata.[45] Berens[12] reported that after cyclodiathermy only 1% of 108 eyes remained controlled during a 7 to 14 year follow-up.[12]

In a detailed review of the available cyclodiathermy procedures, Sugar[66] concluded that long-term success was quite limited. However, despite the accumulated evidence, the procedure remained in popular use until Walton and Grant[71] demonstrated that perforating cyclodiathermy resulted in an equal chance of success or phthisis bulbi (5%), and the remaining eyes had failure of pressure control.[71]

Cyclodiathermy has all but disappeared from the medical literature, except for a recent report by

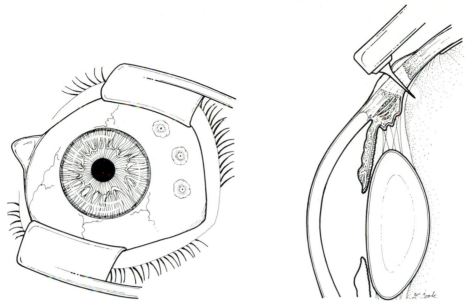

Fig. 38-2 Cyclodiathermy, penetrating.

Nesterov and Egorov.[49] These authors reported 90 eyes with chronic open-angle and angle-closure glaucoma treated with a 3 mm penetrating needle electrode placed 2 to 2.5 mm posterior to the limbus. Eight to ten puncture sites with exposures of 1 to 2 seconds at 8 to 10 W were applied over the lower 180 degrees of the globe. Approximately 65% of these eyes were controlled with or without medication, whereas persistent hypotony occurred in 14 eyes and enucleation was necessary for 9 eyes. When pressure control was considered successful, a small filtration bleb was often observed.

Other techniques using heat or electrical energy have also been developed. Berens[12] designed cycloelectrolysis, a technique to create tissue decompensation using sodium hydroxide with galvanic energy to produce chemical dissolution of the ciliary processes. Angiodiathermy was developed by Acto-Peis,[1] whose procedure required the temporary disinsertion of the horizontal rectus muscles and placement of 8 to 10 puncture sites at the insertion of the muscle in an effort to coagulate the long posterior ciliary arteries. A more direct method designed by Schreck,[59] cilioanalysis, was performed by applying electrical current to a cyclodialysis spatula in the suprachoroidal space to thrombose the ciliary vessels.

All of these techniques have had many variations in methodology and clinical application. The widely disparate results led careful observers to conclude that there is little support for their clinical efficacy at this time.[12,58,71]

CYCLOCRYOTHERAPY

Bietti[13] first recognized that freezing the ciliary body by applying a solid carbon dioxide freezing probe to the conjunctiva in animals and humans resulted in transient lowering of the intraocular pressure (Fig. 38-3). More than 10 years elapsed before animal studies[37,53] demonstrated acute and chronic changes of the ciliary epithelium and ciliary processes after freezing applications. It was also noted that the ciliary epithelium regenerated in some animals, although pigmented eyes were more prone to extensive and permanent tissue destruction. After freezing of the ciliary processes, permanent changes included a marked decrease in stromal vascularity and an extensive disruption of the pigmented and nonpigmented ciliary epithelium.[37]

The first large clinical trial in humans was reported by de Roetth,[26] who established cyclocryotherapy as an effective form of treatment in advanced glaucoma. He also suggested a treatment protocol and provided evidence that retreatment could be helpful, particularly in black patients.[65]

Cyclocryotherapy has become an established form of treatment for advanced glaucoma when all other therapies have failed.[10,14,18,30,41] It is a noninvasive outpatient procedure performed under local

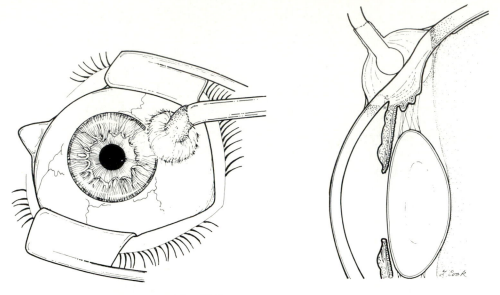

Fig. 38-3 Cyclocryotherapy.

anesthesia. The principal problems with this treatment are the myriad of potential complications and the difficulty in titrating the amount of treatment necessary for a desired pressure lowering effect. The pain that may follow cyclocryotherapy can be severe and often requires potent analgesics. Late complications of vitritis and cystoid macular edema can result in irreversible visual loss and remain the major threat to vision following this procedure.[8]

Many techniques have been suggested for cyclocryotherapy, resulting in a lack of standardization. This is at least partially responsible for the disparity in reported success and in the ability to predict results.* In a review evaluating the various methods of cyclocryotherapy,[54] support for a very specific protocol and adherence to suggested treatment parameters were emphasized.[8]

Technique

A detailed discussion of each important parameter for cyclocryotherapy[8] includes (1) probe placement, (2) size of the probe, (3) temperature of the freeze, (4) duration of the freeze, and (5) number of freeze applications.

Probe placement

Accurate probe placement is essential. Ferry[31] demonstrated that probe placement 4 to 6 mm from the visible limbus results in pars plana cytoarchitectural disruption but ineffective glaucoma con-

---

*References 10, 26, 30, 41, 44, 62.

trol. Burton showed that probe placement over the ciliary processes for 60 seconds at $-75°$ C caused cytoarchitectural disruption in four ciliary processes for each application. When the probe was placed more posteriorly, no ciliary process involvement could be documented.[16] Probe applications 2 mm from the limbus resulted in outflow channel alteration and corneal endothelial changes in experimental animals.[56] A freezing probe placed approximately 2.5 mm from the visible limbus has the optimal chance of being over the pars plicata. On occasion, it is helpful to transilluminate the globe to determine accurately the location of the ciliary body. If an iris coloboma exists, direct visualization of the ice ball during the freeze application is possible.

Probe size

In the physics of freezing, the depth of tissue frozen is equal to the radius of the ice ball minus the radius of the probe tip.[4] It follows that the larger the cryoprobe, the deeper the penetration of the freeze. Cryoprobe tips range from 1.5 to 4 mm, with 2.5 mm being the most common.

Probe temperature

The temperature achieved at the probe tip is not an indication of the actual temperature achieved at the ciliary processes. In a study with monkeys, temperatures at the tips of the ciliary processes did not go below $-17°$ C, when the surface temperature recorded at the probe tip thermocouple was −60° to −80° C. This was true even when freezing applications were applied at −80° C and maintained for 5 minutes.[55] Temperatures lower than −100° C are associated with more frequent and severe complications in humans and experimental animals, although a surface probe temperature of −60° to −80° C is needed to effectively lower the intraocular pressure.

Duration of the freeze

When freezing human eyes for 30 seconds at −70° C with a 2.5 mm probe, crystallization of the valleys between ciliary processes was observed. When the freezing process was applied for 1 minute, using the same sized probe and temperature, a definite ice ball could be visualized involving the entire ciliary processes. Histopathologic disruption of the ciliary epithelium and blood supply was documented after this freezing technique.[16] Experimental evidence has shown that there is approximately a 20 second lag between the onset of freezing at the surface and visualization of some evidence of ice ball penetration of the ciliary process.[56] An appropriate duration of freeze, therefore, should be at least 60 seconds at approximately −80° C when using nitrous oxide as the freezing agent. Additional freeze cycles have been described requiring two different sessions and using two different temperatures,[44] as well as a technique using a freeze, thaw, refreeze cycle.[30,41] No advantage over the single freeze technique has been proven for either of these approaches.

Number of freeze applications

Experimental hypotony has been produced by circumferential cryoapplication in monkeys,[48] and anterior segment necrosis resulted when circumferential cryoapplications were applied in human eyes with neovascular glaucoma.[40] Long-term studies have demonstrated a high incidence of phthisis bulbi and progression to no light perception in patients with neovascular glaucoma who were treated with circumferential cyclocryotherapy.[18,41] In cats treated with 90, 180, or 270 degrees cyclocryotherapy, destruction of the ciliary epithelium was proportionately related to the changes in intraocular pressure and aqueous humor dynamics.[36] It is recommended that six applications of cryotherapy or less be applied to approximately 180 degrees of the globe during each treatment. It has also been urged that not more than 300 degrees of the globe be treated with cyclocryotherapy in an effort to decrease the incidence of phthisis bulbi.[8] The box below outlines a protocol for cyclocryotherapy that

---

CYCLOCRYOTHERAPY PROTOCOL

Retrobulbar anesthesia following sterile preparation
Cryosurgical instrument with nitrous oxide (−80° C)
Glaucoma probe 3.5 to 4 mm applied with the nearest edge 2.5 mm from the limbus
Freeze 180 degrees of the globe with approximately six equidistant points for 1 minute
Soluble dexamethasone injected subconjunctivally in the area of the freeze
Instill atropine 1%, dexamethasone drops, and antibiotic ointment
Warn patient of pain and provide adequate analgesia
Follow-up in 1 day and then weekly with tension check and biomicroscopic evaluation
Continue all antiglaucoma medications until stable
Repeat therapy to treated area and then additional increments of the globe, being mindful not to treat more than 270 degrees

---

we have used for more than 15 years. The modification of adding subconjunctival soluble steroid injection at the completion of the freezing procedures has been important in decreasing the inflammation and postoperative pain.

Indications and Results

The efficacy of cyclocryotherapy has been established in open-angle glaucomas in phakic and aphakic eyes.[10,11,18,62] Approximately 75% of patients with open-angle glaucoma, followed for more than 1 year, demonstrated pressures of 19 mm Hg or less without additional need for surgery.[10] Patients with glaucoma in aphakia, treated with cyclocryotherapy and followed for more than 4 years, maintained intraocular pressures of 19 mm Hg or less in 90% of the eyes studied.[11] More recent studies have demonstrated similar results, although Shields[62] demonstrated a significant loss of vision after cryosurgery.

In the treatment of neovascular glaucoma, cyclocryotherapy was once thought to be the most efficacious way of lowering intraocular pressure and preserving vision.[30] However, the serious complications and the potential for loss of light perception and development of phthisis bulbi prompted Krupin et al.[41] to seek other methods for the therapy of neovascular glaucoma. Cryotherapy for neovascular glaucoma reportedly resulted in adequate pressure control in 64% of 58 eyes, but 17% progressed to phthisis bulbi and 69% had a profound loss of visual acuity.[62] In a larger study, Caprioli et al.[18] reported pressure control in 55% of

96 eyes with neovascular glaucoma while noting that significant loss in vision occurred in more than 70% of these eyes. In addition, many eyes progressed to no light perception and phthisis bulbi. These dismal results with cyclocryotherapy for neovascular glaucoma have prompted us to recommend filtration surgery after panretinal photocoagulation for neovascular glaucoma, which has provided a 60% chance of preserving vision and controlling the intraocular pressure.[3] In patients with neovascular glaucoma, cyclocryotherapy may still be necessary when treating a painful eye with very poor potential for visual function.

Complications

The unpredictability of complications after cyclocryotherapy in eyes with functional vision (better than 20/200 vision) with open-angle glaucoma or glaucoma in aphakia has led to modifications in this form of therapy. Because the development of chronic vitritis or cystoid macular edema can significantly alter vision, we now recommend cyclocryotherapy as a treatment of last resort in patients who have open-angle glaucoma or glaucoma in pseudophakia or aphakia with visual acuity of 20/200 or less.

A transient pressure rise during cyclocryotherapy and in the early postoperative phase is a common complication. Caprioli and Sears[17] suggested maintaining intraocular pressure control with a needle cannula at 25 mm Hg during the procedure and lowering it to 10 mm Hg at the completion of the operation. In the three patients monitored, the intraoperative and early postoperative pressure rise was eliminated by this maneuver. This invasive technique should be considered in eyes with severely compromised optic nerves in an effort to diminish the chance of a high pressure rise during or after cryotherapy.

Additional complications of cyclocryotherapy include transient uveitis, hyphema, and pain, which often result without adverse effect on the therapeutic success of the procedure.[8,9,18,40,41] The most serious complications are vitritis, macular edema, and phthisis bulbi; and efforts should be made to identify and avoid this treatment in highly susceptible eyes.

Cyclocryotherapy remains an important adjunct in the surgical management of advanced glaucoma. Until newer methods of ciliary body destruction using other energy forms can be better evaluated, it will continue to have a place in the management of severe cases of glaucoma.

TRANSSCLERAL, HIGH INTENSITY FOCUSED ULTRASOUND

The pioneering efforts of Coleman et al.[20,21] have expanded the modality of high intensity focused ultrasound to ablate the ciliary body and lower intraocular pressure for the treatment of glaucoma (Fig. 38-4). Purnell et al.[55] developed the first ultrasonic system to destroy the ciliary epithelium for the purpose of controlling glaucoma. With focused ultrasound, retrobulbar anesthesia is required, and a water bath is necessary to suspend a transducer that delivers high intensity ultrasound

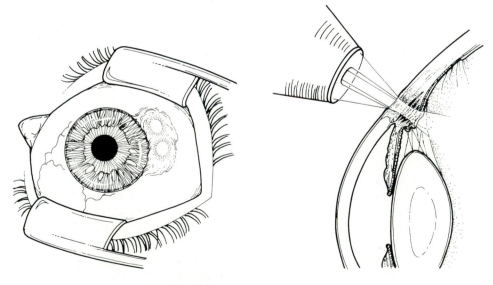

Fig. 38-4 Focused ultrasound.

for a 5-second exposure focused at the level of the ciliary body. In 90% of 170 eyes with advanced glaucoma, intraocular pressure declined to 25 mm Hg or less during the first 3 months after treatment.[21] At 1 year, 56% of these patients had a pressure of 22 mm Hg or less.[15]

The mechanism of high intensity focused ultrasound is not fully understood but theories, in addition to ciliary body ablation, include creation of cyclodialysis cleft and scleral thinning providing a transscleral filtration route. All three of these mechanisms may combine to result in more effective pressure control.[20,21]

Reported complications include phthisis bulbi, scleral thinning, chronic inflammation, corneal changes, and a pressure rise shortly after therapy. Scleral thinning is particularly a problem in children, in whom chronic inflammation and corneal changes have also been observed. Decreased visual acuity in almost 40% of the patients treated, as well as progression to no light perception in five patients, is cause for concern.[15]

Because the costly instrument capable of performing this procedure has had a limited distribution, very few clinical reports on this technique are available. Additional information must be carefully analyzed and evaluated before the efficacy of this technique can be assessed accurately.

LASER THERAPY IN CILIARY BODY DESTRUCTION

Laser energy in the form of heat may be transmitted to the ciliary body in three different routes:

(1) transscleral, with efforts to focus the laser energy at the level of the ciliary body; (2) transpupillary, requiring direct visualization and treatment of the ciliary processes; and (3) endolaser, permitting laser energy to be applied directly to the ciliary processes with an intraocular probe.

Transscleral Laser Cycloablation

The capacity to focus light energy directly on tissues and create heat coagulation of these tissues within the eye was pioneered by Meyer-Schwickerath.[47] Weekers et al.[73] first suggested that photocoagulation to the ciliary body might be effective in controlling intraocular pressure. A pressure-lowering effect was demonstrated in rabbits and in humans using incandescent light. A profound cytoarchitectural alteration of the ciliary body occurred when rabbits were treated with transscleral xenon arc photocoagulation. Clinically, however, the effect of this treatment tended to be transient, and it was concluded that the modality offered no clear advantage over cyclodiathermy.[73] Smith and Stein[64] introduced the application of high intensity monochromatic radiation to the ciliary body. Experimental studies in rabbits using ruby (694.3 nm) and Nd:YAG (1060 nm) lasers demonstrated that transscleral transmission of light energy was most efficacious in the near infrared region. In an extension of this work using the Nd:YAG laser, Beckman produced tissue destruction in the region of the ciliary body in rabbits[5] and humans.[6] In rabbits, a pronounced and prolonged pressure-lowering effect occurred, but there was a high incidence of

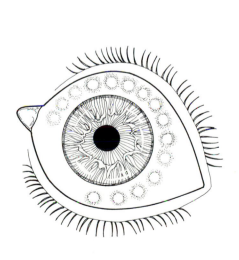

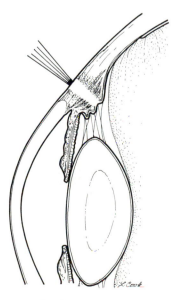

Fig. 38-5 Laser cycloablation, transscleral.

pupillary deformation and cataract formation, particularly in pigmented rabbits.[5] Effective reduction of pain and lowering of the intraocular pressure was also accomplished in 20 human eyes, using the same ruby laser technique.[6] In a 10-year follow-up study of 241 eyes treated with transscleral ruby laser cyclocoagulation, approximately 62% had adequate pressure control (5 to 22 mm Hg).[7] These results seemed to parallel the studies of cyclocryotherapy, with the advantage of less severe pain after the treatment. Aphakic patients responded most successfully, whereas patients with neovascular glaucoma had a poorer pressure response and a higher incidence of serious complications thought to be related to the high energy levels used with ruby laser cyclocoagulation.[7]

The Nd:YAG laser in the thermal mode was used by Beckman and Sugar to perform transscleral cyclocoagulation similar to that with the ruby laser (Fig. 38-5). Initially, 6.5 J of energy, 3.5 mm from the limbus, were applied circumferentially with approximately eight applications per quadrant when treating eyes with advanced glaucoma. This energy source has been extensively studied by Fankhauser et al.[28,29] in animal and human autopsy eyes using 6 to 7 J at maximal defocusing from the conjunctival surface. A beam aimed tangentially 0.5 mm posterior to the visible limbus was found to be most effective by macroscopic examination in altering the ciliary processes. Using much lower energy, Wilensky et al.[78] reduced intraocular pressure in rabbit eyes when 30 burns at 1.5 J were applied transsclerally.

The introduction of commercially available Nd:YAG lasers, with precise focusing and the ability to accurately and reproducibly retroplace peak energy through the slit-lamp has offered a significant advantage over previous laser delivery systems. Standard energy delivery, beam diameter, core angle, and pulse length have improved the control for this procedure. Enhanced scleral transmission results at a wave length of 1016 nm and offers greater heat penetration to the ciliary body. The depth of penetration can be controlled by defocusing the laser light and altering the cone angle of the energy delivered. It is hoped that the careful control of these parameters will result in improved capacity to titrate the energy delivered.

Clinical trials designed to evaluate this procedure are limited.[25,27,60] Most authors place the beam 1 to 3 mm posterior to the visible limbus, using a setting that will maximally defocus the therapeutic laser from the aiming laser. In the studies reported, 360-degree laser applications have been common, and authors attempt to create approximately eight burns per quadrant. Schwartz and Moster[60] used a lower energy, of 0.5 to 2.75 J and achieved a 69% success rate in controlling the intraocular pressure at 22 mm Hg or less, with a lower incidence of hypotony and phthisis bulbi than was reported with treatments at higher energy levels. Half of the eyes required only one treatment session, and severe pain was not reported as a major complication; iritis was common but easily treated.

In a study of 24 patients with 20/400 vision or less, Devenyi et al.[27] used a protocol of 360-degree treatment with 40 burns, placed 2 to 3 mm posterior to the limbus, with a pulse duration of 20 msec and an energy of 1.8 to 3.0 J. This was effective in lowering the intraocular pressure to 25 mm Hg or less in 62.5% of the treated eyes. Conjunctival edema, corneal edema, and iritis were present in all cases; whereas hyphema and hypopyon occurred in 12 eyes and cleared spontaneously. Vitreous hemorrhage occurred in three eyes and represented a serious complication. Postoperative

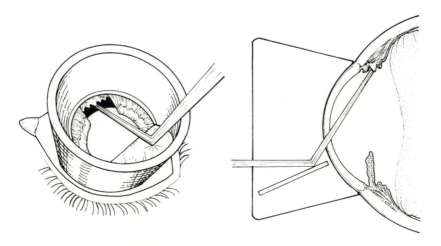

Fig. 38-6 Laser cycloablation, transpupillary.

pain was prominent but phthisis bulbi had not been observed in this small sample with a mean follow-up of 8.8 months.

Cyrlin et al.[25] used 6.4 to 7.5 J and found that the higher energy levels resulted in greater potential for success. Earlier studies in animals had demonstrated a dose dependency and correlated with ciliary body architectural change. In this study, a significant number of patients had a decrease in visual acuity, and six eyes progressed to no light perception. Hypotony of less than 5 mm Hg occurred in 26% of the eyes 1 year after the treatment. These serious complications make selection of eyes for this procedure a critical variable, and the amount of energy delivered appears to be one of the major variables that should be standardized.

Transpupillary Laser Cycloablation

The focus of laser energy through the anterior chamber to the ciliary processes can be accomplished in some eyes with transpupillary photocoagulation (Fig. 38-6). This technique has been evaluated in rabbits and humans but is limited by the requirement that the ciliary processes must be visible by gonioscopy.[39,42,43,46] Argon laser energy can be applied through a gonioprism to the visible ciliary processes, using blanching and pigment disruption as the desired visible tissue response. Limitations of this technique include the need to visualize and treat a sufficient number of ciliary processes and a sufficient amount of each ciliary ridge. The angle of visualization provided by gonioscopy usually only exposes the anterior tip of the ridge, leaving a functional portion of untreated posterior ciliary process.[62] As a result, even when this procedure has been used to treat a majority of the ciliary processes, the resultant lowering of intraocular pressure has been unpredictable. Even when scleral indentation permits adequate visualization of the ciliary processes through a widely dilated pupil, favorable results have not been uniformly achieved. The direct visualization of laser application was expected to allow improved accuracy of laser delivery with better quantitation and fewer complications. Indeed, with this technique there is no obvious damage to sclera or conjunctiva, but heat coagulation of the overlying vitreous base may result in retinal detachment.

Laser Endophotocoagulation Cycloablation

The most sophisticated and involved method of applying energy to the ciliary body is accomplished with an endolaser probe after cataract and vitreous surgery[52,62] (Fig. 38-7). The development of the intraocular laser to create chorioretinal burns has led to the use of the endolaser energy to coagulate the ciliary body.[19,33] Reports by Parel et al.[52] demonstrated that during a pars plana vitrectomy, blue-green argon laser energy can be directly applied to the ciliary processes with a fiberoptic probe for more than 180 degrees. This was sufficient to lower the intraocular pressure to below 21 mm Hg in 14 of 18 eyes. Transient vitreous hemorrhage, choroidal detachment, and hypotony were reported complications. The need for aphakia and an extensive vitrectomy represent significant limitations of this technique. Transparency of the cornea and dilation of the pupil are needed for visualization of the processes and may also be lim-

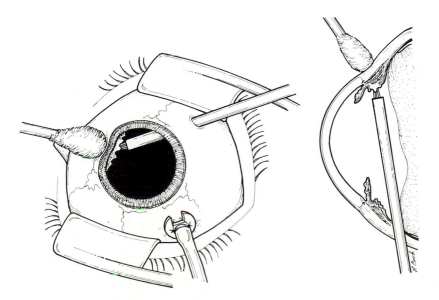

Fig. 38-7   Laser cycloablation, transvitreal.

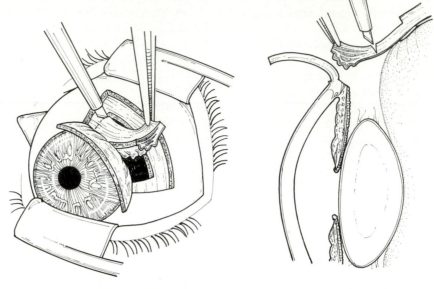

Fig. 38-8 Cyclectomy.

itations with this form of therapy. Because of the problems associated with visualization, Shields[62,63] has used an endoscopic instrument[50,51] to permit direct visualization of the ciliary processes. In the aphakic eye with an anterior vitrectomy, ciliary processes can be viewed 180 degrees away from the entry site of the needle scope, which provides a 1.7 mm diameter view with focusing on the ciliary processes. Monkey eyes studied immediately after treatment with this technique demonstrated epithelial layer destruction and stromal hemorrhage. After 1 to 8 months, partial ciliary epithelial destruction and intrastromal pigment alteration with fibrosis was observed. The efficacy of this technique was demonstrated in a small clinical trial,[62] although larger trials are pending results of transscleral cyclophotocoagulation, which may obviate a need for the invasive approach (Personal communication, M. Bruce Shields, M.D.).

EXCISION OF THE CILIARY BODY

Excision of the ciliary body, the most definitive ciliary body ablative procedure, involves surgical removal of the ciliary processes and ciliary muscle (Fig. 38-8). Until recently, this form of ciliary body excision has been reserved for iridocyclectomy to treat iris or ciliary body tumors.[38] An early report of Verhoeff[68] is somewhat misleading in that the author reported on seven eyes with advanced glaucoma that had surgical removal of the pars plana portion of the ciliary body and a resultant lowering of the intraocular pressure. The author pointed out

that the ciliary processes were not present in the specimens removed during surgery. He postulated a number of reasons for the pressure-lowering effect after this operation, but it is unlikely that alteration of aqueous secretion occurred with this technique.

One of the major deterrents to this procedure has been the observation that removal of more than one quadrant of the ciliary body will frequently result in phthisis bulbi and even loss of the eye.[38] Recently, Sautter and Demeler[57] described removal of the ciliary body in 90 eyes. All of these eyes had had multiple previous antiglaucoma procedures before surgical cyclectomy. During the follow-up, 60 eyes had intraocular pressures of 19 mm Hg or lower, whereas seven had a pressure below 22 mm Hg. Ciliary body excision was not successful in 13 eyes, although only nine were considered frank failures, with intraocular pressures of greater than 40 mm Hg. Vitreous hemorrhage and expulsive hemorrhage complicated the intraoperative period, and wound dehiscence and vitreous hemorrhage were responsible for problems during the postoperative stage. In a smaller series, 12 of 22 eyes with secondary and angle-closure glaucoma had a permanent lowering of the intraocular pressure, and two eyes became atrophic and blind.[34]

The excision of the pars plicata is a major surgical undertaking, and evaluation of more clinical data would be helpful before recommending this procedure.

REFERENCES

1. Arato, S: Angiodiathermy and its application in glaucoma, Ophthalmologica 120:325, 1950
2. Albaugh CH, and Dunphy EB: Cyclodiathermy, an operation for the treatment of glaucoma, Arch Ophthalmol 27:543, 1942
3. Allen, RC, Bellows, AR, Hutchinson, BT, and Murphy, SD: Filtration surgery in the treatment of neovascular glaucoma, Ophthalmology 89:1181, 1982
4. Amoils, SP: Cryosurgery in ophthalmology. In Hughes, WF, editor: The year book of ophthalmology, Chicago, 1975, Year Book Medical Publishers
5. Beckman, H, et al: Trans-scleral ruby laser irradiation of the ciliary body in the treatment of intractable glaucoma, Trans Am Acad Ophthalmol Otolaryngol 46:423, 1972
6. Beckman, H, and Sugar, HS: Neodymium laser cyclocoagulation, Arch Ophthalmol 90:27, 1973
7. Beckman, H, and Waeltermann, J: Trans-scleral ruby laser cyclocoagulation, Am J Ophthalmol 98:788, 1984
8. Bellows, AR: Cyclocryotherapy for glaucoma, Int Ophthalmol Clin 21:99, 1981
9. Bellows, AR: In Epstein, Dl, editor: Glaucoma, Philadelphia, 1986, Lea & Febiger
10. Bellows, AR, and Grant, WM: Cyclocryotherapy in advanced inadequately controlled glaucoma, Am J Ophthalmol 75:679, 1973
11. Bellows, AR, and Grant, WM: Cyclocryotherapy of chronic open angle glaucoma in aphakic eyes, Am J Ophthalmol 85:615, 1978
12. Berens, C: Glaucoma surgery: an evaluation of cycloelectrolysis and cyclodiathermy, Arch Ophthalmol 54:548, 1955
13. Bietti, G: Surgical intervention on the ciliary body: new trends for the relief of glaucoma, JAMA 142:889, 1950
14. Binder, PS, Abel, R Jr, and Kaufman, HE: Cyclocryotherapy for glaucoma after penetrating keratoplasty, Am J Ophthalmol 79:4890, 1975
15. Burgess, SEP, Silverman, RH, and Coleman, DJ: Treatment of glaucoma with high intensity focused ultrasound, Ophthalmology 93:831, 1986
16. Burton, TC: Cyclocryotherapy. In Blodi, FC, editor: Current concepts of ophthalmology, vol 4, St. Louis, 1974, The CV Mosby Co
17. Caprioli, J, and Sears, ML: Regulation of intraocular pressure during cyclocryotherapy for advanced glaucoma, Am J Ophthalmol 101:542, 1986
18. Caprioli, J, Strang, SL, Spaeth, GL, and Poryzees, EF: Cyclocryotherapy in the treatment of advanced glaucoma, Ophthalmology 92:947, 1985
19. Charles, S: Endophotocoagulation, Retina 1:117, 1981
20. Coleman, DJ, et al: Therapeutic ultrasound in the treatment of glaucoma. I. Experimental model, Ophthalmology 92:339, 1985
21. Coleman, DJ, et al: Therapeutic ultrasound in the treatment of glaucoma. II. Clinical applications, Ophthalmology 92:347, 1985
22. Coppez, H: La technique de la diathermie en ophthalmologie, Bull Soc Belge Ophthalmol 55:91, 1927
23. Coppez, H: Au sujet des applications chirurgicales de la diathermie en ophthalmologie, Bull Soc Belge Ophthalmol 58:56, 1929
24. Curran, EJ: Subconjunctival cauterization of the sclera over the ciliary body with the galvano cautery to reduce intraocular pressure in advanced glaucoma, Arch Ophthalmol 54:321, 1925
25. Cyrlin, MN, Beckman, H, and Czedik, C: Nd:YAG laser trans-scleral cyclocoagulation treatment for severe glaucoma, Arch Ophthalmol (In press)
26. deRoetth, A Jr: Cryosurgery for treatment of advanced chronic simple glaucoma, Am J Ophthalmol 66:1041, 1968
27. Devenyi, RG, Trope, GE, Hunter, WH, and Badeeb, O: Neodymium:YAG transcleral cycloablation in human eyes, Ophthalmology 94:1519, 1987
28. Fankhauser, F, Van der Zypen, E, Kwasniewska, S, and Loertscher, H: The effect of thermal mode Nd:YAG laser irradiation on vessels and ocular tissues, Ophthalmology 92:419, 1985
29. Fankhauser, F, et al: Transcleral cyclophotocoagulation using a Neodymium YAG laser, Ophthalmic Surg 17:94, 1986
30. Feibel, RM, and Bigger, JF: Rubeosis iridis in neovascular glaucoma: evaluation of cyclocryotherapy, Am J Ophthalmol 74:862, 1972
31. Ferry, AP: Histopathologic observations on human eyes following cyclocryotherapy for glaucoma, Trans Am Acad Ophthalmol Otolaryngol 83:OP113, 1977
32. Fiore, T: Igni-Skler-Ciliarotomie, Zentralbl. f.d. ges. Ophthal, 22:780, 1930
33. Fleishman, JA, Schwartz, M, and Dixon, JA: Argon laser endophotocoagulation, an intraoperative trans-pars plana technique, Arch Ophthalmol 99:1610, 1981
34. Freyler, H, and Scheimbauer, I: Excision of the ciliary body (Sautter Procedure) as a last resort in secondary glaucoma, Klin Monsatsbl Augenheilkd 179:473, 1981
35. Heine, L: Die Cyklodialyse, eine neue Glaukomoperation, Deutsche Med Wochenschr 31:824, 1905
36. Higginbotham, EJ, et al: The effects of cyclocryotherapy on aqueous humor dynamics in cats (In press)
37. Howard, GM, and deRoeth, AJ: Histopathologic changes following cryotherapy of the rabbit ciliary body, Am J Ophthalmol 64:700, 1967
38. Surgery of the iris and the ciliary body, Basel, 1975, S Karger
39. Klapper, RM, and Dodick, JM: Transpupillary argon laser cyclophotocoagulation, Doc Ophthalmol 36:197, 1984
40. Krupin, T, Johnson, MF, and Bowman, K: Anterior segment ischemia after cyclocryotherapy, Am J Ophthalmol 84:426, 1977

41. Krupin, T, Mitchell, KB, and Becker, B: Cyclocryotherapy in neovascular glaucoma, Am J Ophthalmol 86:24, 1978

42. Lee, PF: Argon laser photocoagulation of ciliary processes in cases of aphakic glaucoma, Arch Ophthalmol 97:2135, 1979

43. Lee, PF, and Pomerantzeff, O: Transpupillary cyclophotocoagulation of rabbit eyes: an experimental approach to glaucoma surgery, Am J Ophthalmol 71:911, 1971

44. Lynn, JR: Trabeculectomy ab externo versus cyclocryosurgery in glaucoma. In Transactions of the New Orleans Academy of Ophthalmology: Symposium on glaucoma, St. Louis, 1975, The CV Mosby Co

45. Marr, WG: The treatment of glaucoma with cyclodiathermy, Am J Ophthalmol 32:241, 1949

46. Merritt, JC: Transpupillary photocoagulation of the ciliary processes, Ann Ophthalmol 8:325, 1976

47. Meyer-Schwickerath, G: Lichtcoagulation, Buech Augenorst 33:1, 1959

48. Minckler, DS, and Tso, MOM: Experimental papilledema produced by cyclocryotherapy, Am J Ophthalmol 82:577, 1976

49. Nesterov, AP, and Egorov, EA: Transconjunctival penetrating cyclodiathermy in glaucoma, J Ocul Therapy-Surg, p. 216, 1983

50. Norris, J, and Cleasby, GW: An endoscope for ophthalmology, Am J Ophthalmol 85:420, 1978

51. Norris, J, et al: Intraocular endoscopic surgery, Am J Ophthalmol 91:603, 1981

52. Patel, A, Thompson, JT, Michaels, RG, and Quigley, HA: Endolaser treatment of the ciliary body for uncontrolled glaucoma, Ophthalmology 93:825, 1986

53. Polack, FM, and de Roetth, A Jr: Effect of freezing on the ciliary body (cyclocryotherapy), Invest Ophthalmol Vis Sci 3:164, 1964

54. Prost, M: Cyclocryotherapy for glaucoma. Evaluations of techniques, Surv Ophthalmol 28:93, 1983

55. Purnell, EW, et al: Focal chorioretinitis produced by ultrasound, Invest Ophthalmol Vis Sci 3:657, 1964

56. Quigley, HA: Histologic and physiologic studies of cyclocryotherapy in primate and human eyes, Am J Ophthalmol 82:722, 1976

57. Sautter, H, and Demeler, U: Antiglaucomatous ciliary body excision, Am J Ophthalmol 98:344, 1984

58. Scheie, HG, Frayer, WC, and Spencer, KW: Cyclodiathermy, Arch *Ophthalmol* 53:839, 1955

59. Schreck, E: Cilio-anolyse und Cilio-cycloanalyse: Eine neue Glaukomoperation, Arch f Ophth 149:95, 1949

60. Schwartz, LW, and Moster, MR: Neodymium YAG laser: transscleral cyclodiathermy, Ophthalmic Laser Therapy 1:135, 1986

61. Shahan, WE, and Post, L: Thermophore studies in glaucoma, Am J Ophthalmol 4:109, 1921

62. Shields, MB: Cyclodestructive surgery for glaucoma: past, present and future, Trans Am Ophthalmol Soc 83:283, 1985

63. Shields, MB, Chandler, DB, Hickingbotham, D, and Klintworth, GK: Histopathologic evaluation of endoscopic cyclophotocoagulation in primates, Arch Ophthalmol 103:1731, 1985

64. Smith, RS, and Stein, MN: Ocular hazards of transscleral laser radiation. II. Intraocular injury produced by ruby and neodymium lasers, Am J Ophthalmol 67:100, 1969

65. Stocker, FW: Response of chronic simple glaucoma and treatment with cyclodiathermy puncture, Arch Ophthalmol 34:181, 1945

66. Sugar, HS: The glaucomas, New York, 1957, Harper & Brathus

67. Troncoso, M: Diathermic surgery of the ciliary body in glaucoma: experimental and clinical observations, Am J Ophthalmol 29:269, 1946

68. Verhoeff, FH: Cyclectomy: a new operation for glaucoma, Arch Ophthalmol 53:228, 1924

69. Vogt, A: Versuche zur intraokularen Drucknerabsetzung mittels Diatermieschadigung des Corpus ciliare (Zyklodiathermiestichelung) Klin Mbl Augenheilkd 97:672, 1936

70. Vogt, A: Zyklodiathermiestichelung, Schweiz med Wochneschr 66:593, 1936

71. Walton, DS, and Grant, WM: Penetrating cyclodiathermy for filtration, Arch Ophthalmol 83:47, 1970

72. Weekers, R, and Delmarcelle, Y: Ocular hypotony due to reduced aqueous flow, Ophthalmologica 125:425, 1953

73. Weekers, R, et al: Effects of photocoagulation of ciliary body upon ocular tension, Am J Ophthalmol 52:156, 1961

74. Weekers, R, and Prijot, E: Investigation of the mode of action of retrociliary diathermy by means of the electronic tonometric pressure test, Bull Soc Belge Ophthalmol 99:924, 1951

75. Weekers, L, Weekers, R, and Heintz, A: Les effects tensionnels eloigne' de la cyclodiathermie non perforante dans de traitement du glaucome chronicum, Bull Soc Belge Ophthalmol 92:210, 1949

76. Weve, HJM: Clinische Lessen, Ned Tidjschr Geneesk 76:5335, 1932

77. Weve, HJM: Zyklodiathermie das corpus ciliare bei Glaukom, Zentralbl Ophthalmol 29:562, 1933

78. Wilensky, JT, Welch, D, and Mirolovich, M: Transscleral cyclocoagulation using a neodymium YAG laser, Ophthalmic Surg 16:95, 1985

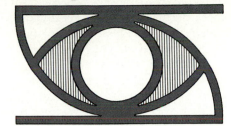

Chapter 39

Setons in Glaucoma Surgery

Theodore Krupin
Scott M. Spector

The aim of glaucoma filtration surgery is to produce an opening at the limbus (a sclerostomy or sclerectomy) to allow aqueous humor to flow from the anterior chamber to the subconjunctival-Tenon's tissue space. The opening bypasses the site of increased resistance to aqueous flow within the conventional outflow system. The surgical opening provides a low resistance pathway for the flow of aqueous humor and the establishment of an external filtration bleb. Filtration surgery reduces intraocular pressure below 21 mm Hg in 73% to 95% of patients with uncomplicated open-angle or chronic angle-closure glaucoma.* However, filtration surgery is less successful in eyes with certain types of secondary glaucoma (e.g., neovascular glaucoma,[1,7] uveitic glaucoma,[8] and glaucoma in aphakia[4]) and in eyes with previously failed filtration surgery.[9]

Failure of filtration surgery can occur internally or externally. The fistula may close by incarceration of the iris, ciliary body processes, vitreous, lens, or by the formation of scar tissue. External scarring of the conjunctival, Tenon's, or scleral tissues results in an encapsulated or a flattened nonfunctioning bleb. Pharmacologic modulation of wound healing after filtration surgery has been studied to prevent or reduce scarring and bleb failure (see Chapter 33).

Various types of foreign materials and devices have been implanted to facilitate drainage after filtration surgery in eyes with a poor surgical prognosis. These have been used in an attempt to (1) prevent closure of the fistula; (2) prevent fibrosis of the subconjunctival-Tenon's tissue bleb site; and (3) provide a shunt for aqueous humor from the anterior chamber to the suprachoroidal space, the subconjunctival space, and even to a venous channel or the lacrimal sac. In general, most of these procedures have been associated with poor long-term results, either secondary to excessive postoperative inflammation or foreign body reaction, leading to bleb scarring. These procedures are presented in this chapter for historical interest. The currently used plastic implants, which place an open tube into the anterior chamber as a conduit for aqueous humor flow to the subconjunctival space, are reported in greater detail.

ANTERIOR CHAMBER SETONS

Many attempts have been made to implant foreign materials across the anterior chamber or into a cyclodialysis cleft. In 1907, Rollett and Moreau[28] performed a double paracentesis and used horse hair through the corneal punctures to treat two patients with painful absolute glaucoma. Zorab[46] reported placing a double silk loop covered with a conjunctival flap through a superior keratome incision 2 mm behind the limbus. He called the procedure "aqueoplasty." Modifications were reported by Mayou[19] and Wood,[44] both of whom reported good results in patients with absolute glaucoma. Other materials that have been placed within sclerostomy openings and the subconjunctival space include gold, tantalum, platinum, and various plastics.

Vail reported placing a silk suture from the vit-

*References 2-4, 16, 34, 35, 42.

reous cavity to Tenon's space to treat absolute glaucoma.[45] This suture was removed at 3 months. He stated that the glaucoma did not return for the 2 years before the patient's death.

Implants that have been placed within a cyclodialysis cleft include platinum wire, horse hair, Supramid, polyethylene, gelatin film, and Teflon.[25,29,36,40,43] Strips of magnesium or a tantalum foil were used by Troncosco.[40,41] The cyclodialysis implants were associated with poor results and extensive intraocular reaction. These implants did not improve the relatively low rate of intraocular pressure lowering after a cyclodialysis procedure.

ANTERIOR CHAMBER SHUNT TO A DISTANT SITE

Plastic tube shunts have been used to connect the anterior chamber to distant sites for the drainage of aqueous humor. Mascati[18] connected the anterior chamber tube to the lacrimal sac, and Rajah-Sivayoham[26] connected a silicone tube into the superficial temporal vein. Lee and Wong[14] described an aqueous-venous shunt using a collagen tube inserted into an intrascleral portion of a vortex vein. Obvious difficulties with these procedures include erosion of the extraocular tube and reflux of contents into the anterior chamber. Although initial results with these shunts have been excellent, there have been no long-term follow-up studies and, to our knowledge, they are no longer in use.

TRANSLIMBAL SETONS

A silk thread was the first device to be placed translimbally from the anterior chamber to the subconjunctival space. As previously stated, this procedure was reported by Zorab[46] in 1912 and was called aqueoplasty. This pioneering work was followed by a larger number of translimbally placed materials: various plastic rods and plates, studs and plates of gold, tantalum, glass, platinum, gold leaf, and silk.[2,15,27,37,38] These devices were used in an attempt to prevent closure of the sclerostomy and to act as a "wick" to promote flow of aqueous humor through the anterior chamber opening. However, most of these devices were associated with postoperative inflammation and uniformly poor results.

TRANSLIMBAL TUBE SHUNTS

Open plastic tubes implanted through a sclerostomy incision connecting the anterior chamber with the subconjunctival space at the limbus provide several functions. The open end of the tube,

and not the entry incision, becomes the effective "sclerostomy," which can be situated in the anterior chamber away from the iridocorneal angle. In eyes with peripheral anterior synechiae and a sealed angle, the tube permits access to the anterior chamber and a pathway for aqueous humor to be shunted from the eye. Although scarring occurs around the tube at the site of entry into the anterior chamber, the lumen of the tube remains open, thereby maintaining a patent communication to the external bleb. Difficulties encountered with this type of implant include obstruction of the anterior chamber end of the tube by the iris, lens, or inflammatory debris; obstruction of the lumen by inflammatory or blood products; and scarring around the external part of the tube. In addition, an open tube provides minimal resistance to aqueous flow, which is usually excessive immediately after surgery, often leading to a flat anterior chamber, hypotony, and choroidal detachment or hemorrhage.

Before the introduction of microsurgery and subscleral procedures, open tubes were inserted at the limbus into the anterior chamber. Their external end was fixated to the sclera and covered with conjunctiva.[17,27] These procedures were associated with scarring of the bleb, which is reduced if the external part of the tube is covered with a partial thickness scleral flap. Two such implants currently used are the open tube reported by Honrubia et al.[16] and the pressure-sensitive glaucoma valve implant described by Krupin et al.[10-12]

In the procedure reported by Honrubia et al.[7] an open silicone tube is placed through the sclerostomy of a trabeculectomy.[6] This procedure is reported to have an 85% success rate in eyes with neovascular glaucoma. Complications associated with excessive aqueous humor flow in an open tube occur with this procedure.

Krupin et al.[12] described a valve implant for use in filtration surgery. The original design of the short glaucoma valve implant consisted of an open anterior chamber Supramid tube. This was attached to a Silastic tube with a sealed end containing horizontal and vertical slits which functioned as a pressure-sensitive and unidirectional valve (Fig. 39-1). This design has been modified so that the implant now consists of a one-piece Silastic tube. The open end of the tube (outer diameter 0.6 mm, inner diameter 0.3 mm) is placed within the anterior chamber. The external valve end, which has an opening pressure of approximately 12 mm Hg and a closing pressure 1 to 2 mm Hg lower, remains outside the eye under a scleral lamellar flap. This implant was successful in lowering in-

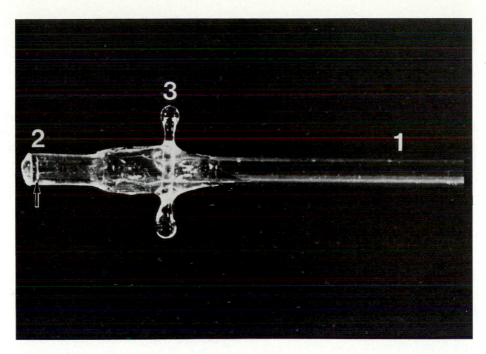

Fig. 39-1 Short glaucoma valve implant consisting of *(1)* an open tube that is placed into anterior chamber, *(2)* a sealed valve end with horizontal and vertical slits *(arrow)* that remains outside eye under a scleral lamellar flap, and *(3)* horizontal side arms for fixation of device. (From Krupin, T: Surgical treatment of glaucoma with the Krupin-Denver valve. In Cairns, CE, editor: Glaucoma, vol 1, London, 1986, Grune & Stratton)

traocular pressure in 67% to 89% of eyes with neovascular glaucoma or prior failure after filtration surgery.[3,11,12] Approximately 50% of the eyes were controlled without postoperative glaucoma medications (see Plate III, Fig. 4).

The devices described by Honrubia and Krupin are designed to produce an anterior limbal bleb. The procedures do not address external bleb scarring, the major cause for their failure. Recent developments in the use of setons in filtration surgery use an anterior chamber tube but attempt to modify external scarring by creating a large area for filtration posterior to the limbus.

POSTERIOR TUBE SHUNTS

Molteno[21] was the first to relate successful filtration surgery more to maintaining a functioning bleb than to maintaining a functioning fistula. His pioneering work on the control of bleb inflammation and fibrosis included the use of postoperative topical and systemic corticosteroids, a systemic prostaglandin synthetase inhibitor (fluphenamic acid), and a systemic antimitotic agent (colchicine).[22] These agents were used in conjunction with his implant, which consists of a large posterior episcleral plate that functions as a bleb-promoting de-

vice. While Molteno's drug regimen is not commonly used by other surgeons, his concepts of bleb scarring were important to current investigations on pharmacologic modulation of wound healing (see Chapter 33).

Molteno's concept of an external bleb-promoting device is incorporated into three other currently used surgical implants as discussed by Schocket et., Krupin et al., Hitchings et al.[5,13,31] These employ a plastic anterior chamber tube as a shunt to a posterior episcleral device. The external portion of these implants normally becomes encapsulated with scar tissue. Aqueous humor flows into this enclosed cavity, which essentially is a large Tenon's cyst. However, there is adequate exchange of aqueous humor across the large surface area of the cyst.[33]

Results with the four types of posterior tube filtration implants (in eyes with a poor surgical prognosis) have been encouraging, particularly in neovascular glaucoma and after failure of prior filtration surgery. In all of these implants, the open end of the tube is sufficiently within the anterior chamber, placing the effective sclerostomy away from the iridocorneal angle. The tube permits access to the anterior chamber in eyes with peripheral

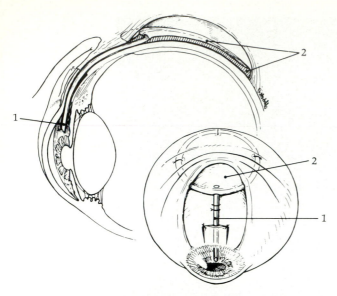

Fig. 39-2 Molteno drainage implant consisting of (1) an open tube that extends 2 to 4 mm into anterior chamber, and (2) a thin plastic episcleral plate 13 mm in diameter. (From Krupin, T: Setons in glaucoma surgery. In Waltman, SR, et al, editors: Surgery of the eye, vol 1, New York, 1988, Churchill Livingstone. Reprinted by permission)

anterior synechiae and a sealed chamber angle. The tube also prevents scarring and closure of the sclerostomy. These procedures also create a large, external, encapsulated bleb, which usually provides a sufficient drainage area for aqueous humor and subsequent reduction in intraocular pressure. The posterior filtration site also avoids the limbal area, which may be important in eyes with prior surgery and conjunctival scarring.

Molteno Implant[21,22] (Fig. 39-2)

The Molteno implant consists of an open silicone rubber tube (outer diameter 0.6 mm, inner diameter 0.3 mm) that is attached to and opens onto the upper surface of a thin, acrylic episcleral plate, 13 mm in diameter. The edge of the plate has a thickened rim 0.7 mm high that is perforated to permit attachment to the sclera. Two-plate implants, which are connected by a silicone tube, are available.

Implantation is performed via a fornix-based conjunctival flap, which is dissected to expose the equator of the globe. A rectangular half-thickness limbus-based 8 mm scleral flap is prepared. The episcleral plate is placed into Tenon's space and sutured to the sclera. The silicone tube is laid radially across the scleral flap, and excess tube is cut off so that the tube overlaps the limbus by 2 mm. The anterior chamber is entered parallel to the iris

plane with a 2 mm keratome, and the tube is inserted into the anterior chamber. The scleral flap is sutured. Tenon's tissue and conjunctiva are drawn forward and sutured to the limbus. Many surgeons have modified Molteno's technique by omitting the scleral flap, using a 23-gauge needle to enter the anterior chamber and covering the tube at the limbus with a scleral patch graft.[20,39]

Molteno et al.[24] recommend a two-stage operation to avoid a flat anterior chamber, which may be associated with placing the open tube into the chamber before the development of fibrosis around the episcleral plate. In the first stage, the plate is inserted beneath Tenon's capsule and the end of the anterior chamber tube tucked underneath a horizontal rectus muscle. Later, the conjunctiva is reopened, the tube is identified, and it is then inserted into the chamber. Other surgeons perform a one-stage implantation and attempt to reduce early flow through the tube by placing suture ties around either the internal or external portions of the tube.[20,39] Later, the suture is cut with a surgical knife or laser. Although Molteno still recommends postoperative therapy with systemic prednisone (10 mg three times a day); fluphenamic acid (200 mg three times a day); and colchicine (0.5 mg three times a day), as well as topical epinephrine 2%, atropine 1%, and dexamethasone 0.1% four times a day for 6 weeks, most surgeons omit the systemic regimen and the topical epinephrine.

The success rate ranges from 50% to 94% in eyes with neovascular glaucoma, other types of secondary glaucoma, and in eyes with prior filtration failure.[20,23,24,39] The major complication is a persistent flat anterior chamber associated with the one-stage implantation. Attempts at reducing this complication with suture ligatures around the tube have not been very successful. Delayed suprachoroidal hemorrhage has been associated with prolonged hypotony. The two-stage implantation avoids these complications; however, intraocular pressure remains uncontrolled until the second stage is performed approximately 4 to 6 weeks later. Therefore, as previously stated, most surgeons using this device perform a primary and not a two-stage implantation. Conjunctival erosion with exposure of the implant can occur, requiring removal of the device.

Schocket Procedure (Fig. 39-3)

Schocket et al.[30-32] described a procedure whereby an anterior chamber tube shunt is attached to an encircling band. The 30 mm long Silastic tube (outer diameter 0.64 mm, inner diameter 0.3 mm)

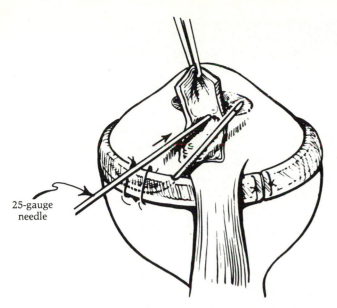

Fig. 39-3 Schocket anterior chamber tube shunt to an encircling band. Anterior chamber tube is placed into chamber through a tract incision made with a 25-gauge needle. (From Schocket, SS, et al: Ophthalmol 92:553, 1985)

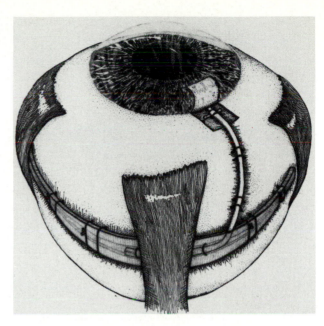

Fig. 39-4 Long Krupin-Denver valve implant. Valve end is sutured within groove of a No. 220 Silastic exoplant, which is sutured with groove side against sclera. Open tube is placed under scleral flap into anterior chamber. (From Krupin, T: Surgical treatment of glaucoma with the Krupin-Denver valve. In Cairns, CE, editor: Glaucoma, vol 1, London, 1986, Grune & Stratton)

is sutured into the grooved portion of a No. 20 silicone band with the tube extending 15 mm from the wall of the band.

A 360-degree peritomy is made 4 to 5 mm posterior to the limbus, except for the superior nasal quadrant, where the conjunctival incision is extended posteriorly 8 to 10 mm. A vitreous tap is performed 4 to 5 mm from the limbus using a 25-gauge needle, to prevent excessive intraocular pressure increase after securing the band. The 360 degree band is placed grooved side toward the sclera, beneath the rectus muscles. Several 5-0 Supramid mattress sutures are placed in each quadrant so that the anterior band edge is 10 to 12 mm from the limbus. The tube emerges nasal to the superior rectus muscle. The ends of the band are united with a mattress suture. A 4×4 mm scleral flap is prepared. The tube is cut obliquely to a length to extend 3 mm into the anterior chamber, which is entered with a 23-gauge needle. The chamber is filled with a viscoelastic substance and the tube inserted anterior to the iris surface. The scleral flap and conjunctiva are closed.

Surgical success reported by Schocket et al.[32] was 96% in eyes with neovascular glaucoma and with previous failed glaucoma surgery. Most of the cases were controlled without glaucoma medications. However, 75% of the patients had a prolonged (5 to 16 days) postoperative flat anterior chamber. Attempts to reduce aqueous humor flow

by suture ligatures has met with limited success.[30] Blockage of the tube with blood or protein debris has been reported. Laser or surgical intervention is indicated to bring about return of function of the implant. Improper position of the tube can result in corneal contact and decompensation and necessitates surgical modification or removal.

Long Glaucoma Valve Implant[13]

The original design of the glaucoma valve implant has been modified to provide a filtration area posterior to the limbus. The implant consists of an open Silastic tube (outer diameter 0.6 mm, inner diameter 0.3 mm), which is placed into the anterior chamber. The tube is approximately 20 mm long with the external end sealed closed. This end contains vertical and horizontal slits that function as a unidirectional and pressure-sensitive valve with an opening pressure of approximately 11 mm Hg and a closing pressure of approximately 9 mm Hg. The valve end is sutured within the grooved portion of a No. 220 Silastic exoplant (Fig. 39-4), which is attached to the globe, grooved side down, for 160 degrees to 180 degrees in length.

A superior or inferior 180-degree conjunctival peritomy is performed with the conjunctiva dissected posteriorly. The superior (or inferior) and

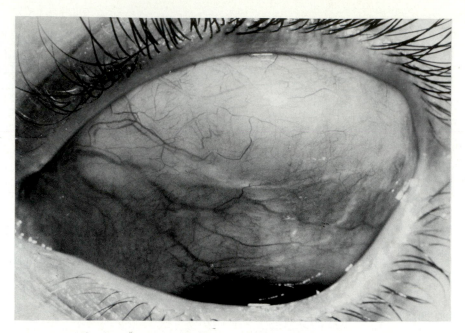

Fig. 39-5 Posterior bleb extending over area of scleral exoplant 2 years following surgery with a long Krupin-Denver glaucoma valve implant.

both horizontal rectus muscles are isolated. The band is placed beneath the vertical rectus muscle with the grooved side against the sclera and positioned so that the tube exists from the band to one side of the vertical muscle (Fig. 39-4). The anterior edge of the band is placed 10 to 12 mm from the limbus and is fixated to the sclera with 5-0 Dacron mattress sutures, at least two on either side of the vertical muscle. The band is cut so that each end extends up to or just below the horizontal rectus muscle. A 4 to 5 mm square lamellar scleral flap is dissected at the limbus into clear cornea and a paracentesis performed away from this site. The scleral flap is retracted and entry made into the anterior chamber with a microvitreoretinal blade. The open end of the tube is cut to a length that will extend into the anterior chamber. After placement within the chamber, the tube is fixated within the scleral bed with 10-0 nylon sutures, and the scleral flap and conjunctiva are closed.

Surgical success (intraocular pressure <21 mm Hg) in eyes followed for over 1 year was 77% for neovascular glaucoma and 82% for eyes with secondary nonneovascular glaucoma or primary glaucoma in which prior filtration surgery had failed. These eyes had a large posterior bleb extending over the area of the Silastic band (Fig. 39-5). Failures (intraocular pressure greater than 21 mm Hg) were secondary to internal occlusion of the anterior chamber tube by iris or inflammatory debris or to scarring over the external Silastic band.

The external valve end of the implant is constructed to provide resistance to flow of aqueous humor. However, postoperative choroidal detachment with associated reduction in intraocular pressure still occurs in eyes with severe glaucoma. This complication is less frequent than in eyes undergoing a Molteno or Schocket implant. In addition, the incidence of a flat anterior chamber with tube contact to either the cornea or lens is only 5% with the long valve implant. This latter complication requires drainage of the choroidal detachment and reformation of the anterior chamber.

One-piece Valved Silicone Exoplant

Hitchings et al.[5] have described the use of a valved tube attached to a silicone exoplant. The silicone anterior chamber tube has an outer diameter of 0.64 mm and an inner diameter of 0.3 mm. A slit in the side of the tube functions as the valve, with an opening pressure between 4 and 20 mm Hg. The tube is attached with silicone rubber adhesive to a rubber strap which is 9 mm wide, 1 mm thick, and 85 mm long.

Placement of the silicone exoplant and the anterior chamber tube are similar to that previously described for the long glaucoma valve implant. The authors report similiar intraocular pressures after the use of either a 180 degree or 360 degree plate. Although incorporation of the valve would appear to decrease bulk flow of aqueous humor, the device is still associated with postoperative hypotony and choroidal detachment. However, as previously described for the long glaucoma valve implant, use of a valved implant reduces the frequency and magnitude of these complications when compared to the open tubes used in the Molteno or Schocket implants.

SUMMARY

It is difficult to compare the success rates of the current long tube implants. These devices have been used in various subgroups of glaucoma patients whose disease is difficult to manage. Intraocular pressure results with the long posterior tube filtration implants are encouraging. However, these devices should be reserved for eyes with poor surgical prognosis or prior filtration failure. It should be noted that controlled studies have not been performed for any of the implant procedures. Neovascular glaucoma in an only eye or in an eye with visual potential is the only condition for which we recommend any of these implants as the primary procedure. In all other types of glaucoma, conventional filtration surgery and procedures that do not require setons should be performed initially. However, these implants do provide a useful alternative surgical procedure for controlling intraocular pressure in eyes with recalcitrant glaucoma.

REFERENCES

1. Allen, RC, Bellows, AR, Hutchinson, BT, and Murphy, SD: Filtration surgery in the treatment of neovascular glaucoma, Ophthalmology 89:1181, 1982
2. Epstein, E: Fibrosing response to aqueous, Br J Ophthalmol 43:641, 1959
3. Forestier, F: Technique chirurgicale récente du traitement du glaucome néo-vasculaire: "Valve de Krupin-Denver," Clinique Ophthalmogique 2:2, 1983
4. Heuer, DK, et al: Trabeculectomy in aphakic eyes, Ophthalmology 91:1045, 1984
5. Hitchings, RA, et al: Use of a one-piece valved tube and variable surface area explant for glaucoma drainage surgery, Ophthalmology 94:1079, 1987
6. Honrubia, FM, et al: Surgical treatment of neovascular glaucoma, Trans Ophthalmol Soc UK 99:89, 1979
7. Hoskins, HD: Neovascular glaucoma. Current concepts, Trans Am Acad Ophthalmol Otolaryngol 78:330, 1974
8. Hoskins, HD, Hetherington, J, and Shaffer, RN: Surgical management of the inflammatory glaucomas, Perspectives in Ophthalmology 1:173, 1977
9. Kolker, AE, and Hetherington, J, Jr: Becker-Shaffer's diagnosis and therapy of the glaucomas, ed 5, St. Louis, 1983, CV Mosby Co
10. Krupin, T, et al: Filtering valve implant for eyes with neovascular glaucoma, Am J Ophthalmol 89:338, 1980
11. Krupin, T, et al: Long-term results of valve implants in filtering surgery for eyes with neovascular glaucoma, Am J Ophthalmol 95:775, 1983
12. Krupin, T, et al: Valve implants in filtering surgery. A preliminary report, Am J Ophthalmol 81:232, 1976
13. Krupin, T, et al: A long Krupin-Denver valve implant attached to a 180° scleral explant for glaucoma surgery, Ophthalmology (In press)
14. Lee, P-F, and Wong, W-T: Aqueous-venous shunt for glaucoma: report of 15 cases, Ann Ophthalmol 6:1083, 1974
15. Lehman, RN, and McCaslin, MF: Gelatin film used as a seton in glaucoma, Am J Ophthalmol 47:609, 1959
16. Lewis, RA, and Phelps, CD: Trabeculectomy vs thermosclerostomy: a five-year follow-up, Arch Ophthalmol 102:533, 1984
17. MacDonald, RK, and Pierce, HF: Silicone setons, Am J Ophthalmol 59:635, 1965
18. Mascati, NT: A new surgical approach for the control of a class of glaucomas, Int Surg 47:10, 1967
19. Mayou, MS: A note of Zorab's operation of aqueoplasty, Ophthalmoscope 10:254, 1912
20. Minckler, DS, Baerveldt, G, and Heuer, DK: Clinical experience with the Molteno implant in complicated glaucoma cases, Invest Ophthalmol Vis Sci (Suppl) 28:270, 1987
21. Molteno, ACB: New implant for glaucoma clinical trial, Br J Ophthalmol 53:606, 1971
22. Molteno, ACB: Mechanisms of intraocular inflammation, Trans Ophthalmol Soc NZ 32:69, 1980
23. Molteno, ACB, Ancker, E, and Bartholomew, RS: Drainage operations for neovascular glaucoma, Trans Ophthalmol Soc NZ 32:101, 1980
24. Molteno, ACB, Van Biljon, G, and Ancker, E: Two stage insertion of glaucoma drainage implants, Trans Ophthalmol Soc NZ 31:17, 1979
25. Pinnan, G, and Boniuk, M: Cyclodialysis with Teflon tube implants, Am J Ophthalmol 68:879, 1969
26. Rajah-Sivayoham, S-S: Camero-venous shunt for secondary glaucoma following orbital venous obstruction, Br J Ophthalmol 52:843, 1968
27. Richards, RD, and Van Bijsterveld, OP: Artificial drainage tubes for glaucoma, Am J Ophthalmol 60:405, 1965
28. Rollett, M, and Moreau, M: Traitement de hypopyon par le drainage capillaire de la cambre antérieure, Rev Gen Ophthalmol 25:481, 1906
29. Row, H: Operation to control glaucoma: preliminary report, Arch Ophthalmol 12:325, 1934
30. Schocket, SS: Investigations of the reasons for success and failure in the anterior shunt-to-the-encircling-band procedure in the treatment of refractory glaucoma, Trans Am Ophthalmol Soc 84:743, 1986
31. Schocket, SS, Lakhanpal, V, and Richards, RD: Anterior chamber tube shunt to an encircling band in the treatment of neovascular glaucoma, Ophthalmology 89:1188, 1982

32. Schocket, SS, et al: Anterior chamber tube shunt to an encircling band in the treatment of neovascular glaucoma and other refractory glaucomas: a long-term study, Ophthalmology 92:553, 1985

33. Shammas, A, et al: The Molteno implant—a model for study of artificial aqueous drainage, Invest Ophthalmol Vis Sci (Suppl) 28:378, 1987

34. Shields, MB: Trabeculectomy vs full-thickness filtering operation for control of glaucoma, Ophthalmic Surg 11:498, 1980

35. Spaeth, GL, and Poryzees, E: A comparison between peripheral iridectomy with thermal sclerostomy and trabeculectomy: a controlled study, Br J Ophthalmol 65:783, 1981

36. Stefansson, J: An operation for glaucoma, Am J Ophthalmol 8:681, 1925

37. Stone, W: Alloplasty in surgery of the eye, I, New Engl J Med 258:486, 1958

38. Stone, W: Alloplasty in surgery of the eye, II, New Engl J Med 258:533, 1958

39. Traverso, CE, et al: The Molteno draining implant for the management of complicated glaucoma cases, Ophthalmology Suppl 94:80, 1987

40. Troncosco, MU: Cyclodialysis with insertion of a metal implant in the treatment of glaucoma, Arch Ophthalmol 23:270, 1940

41. Troncosco, MU: Use of tantalum implants for inducing a permanent hypotony in rabbits eyes, Am J Ophthalmol 32:499, 1949

42. Watkins, PH, and Brubaker, RF: Comparison of partial-thickness and full-thickness filtration procedures in open-angle glaucoma, Am J Ophthalmol 86:756, 1978

43. Wolfe, OR, and Blaess, MJ: Seton operation in glaucoma, Am J Ophthalmol 19:400, 1936

44. Wood, CA: The sclerocorneal seton in the treatment of glaucoma, Ophthal Rec Chicago 24:235, 1915

45. Vail, DT: Retained silk thread or 'seton' drainage from vitreous chamber to tenon's lymph channel for the relief of glaucoma, Ophthal Rec Chicago 24:184, 1915

46. Zorab, A: The reduction of tension in chronic glaucoma, Ophthalmoscope 10:258, 1912

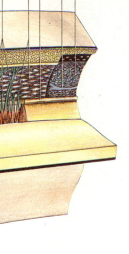

Fig. 1 Architecture of trabecular meshwork. Ciliary muscle *(1)*; sclera *(2)*; collector channel *(3)*; Schlemm's canal *(4)*; cornea *(5)*; iris root *(6)*; iris processes *(7)*; uveal meshwork *(8)*; corneal endothelium *(9)*; Schwalbe's line *(10)*; anterior ciliary muscle tendons *(11)*; corneoscleral meshwork *(12)*; scleral spur *(13)*; Sondermann's channel *(14)*; cribriform layer *(15)*. (From Rohen, JW, and Unger, HM: Mainz, Nr., 3 Wiesbaden, 1959, Steiner Verlag.) (Chapter 2)

A

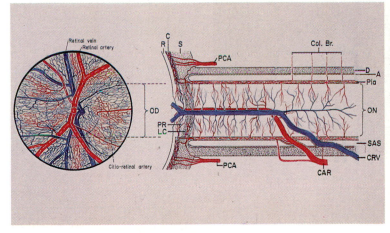

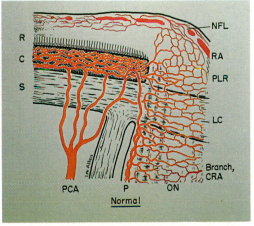

B

Fig. 2 Blood supply of anterior part of optic nerve. **A** also shows, on left side, ophthalmoscopic view of optic disc, adjacent retina. Choroid *(C)*; central retinal artery *(CRA)*; lamina cribrosa *(LC)*; surface nerve fiber layer of disc *(NFL)*; optic disc *(OD)*; optic nerve *(ON)*; pia *(P)*; posterior ciliary artery *(PCA)*; prelaminar region *(PLR/PR)*; retina *(R)*; retinal arteriole *(RA)*; sclera *(S)*. (**A** from Hayreh, SS: Arch Ophthalmol 95:1565, 1977; **B** from Hayrah, SS. In Heilmann, M, and Richardson, KT: Glaucoma: conceptions of a disease, Stuttgart, 1978, Georg Thieme Publishers.) (Chapter 5)

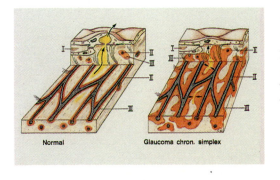

Fig. 3 Development of SD-plaques *(III)* from sheaths of subendothelial elastic-like fiber network *(II)* in normal and glaucomatous eyes. Type I plaques *(I)* are probably remnants of basement membrane material. Endothelium of Schlemm's canal *(E)*. (From Rohen, JW: Ophthalmology 90:758, 1983. With permission of the American Academy of Ophthalmology.) (Chapter 2)

PLATE I

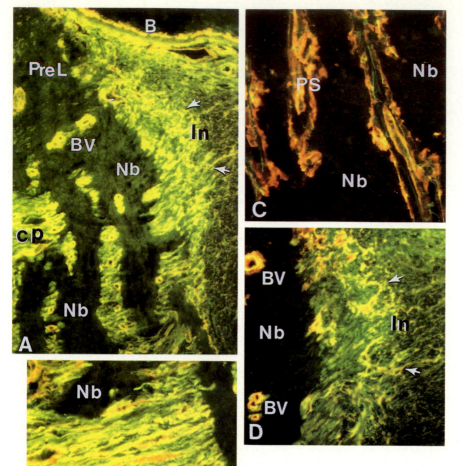

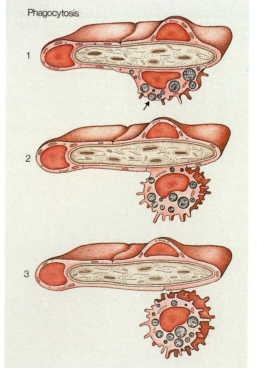

Fig. 4 Double immunofluorescent staining for human collagen type IV (rhodamine label, orange-yellow) and elastin (fluorescein label, green). **A,** Sagittal section of optic nerve head. Prelaminar region *(PreL)*; blood vessel *(BV)*; nerve bundle *(NB)*; cribriform plates *(cp)*; insertion region *(In)*. **B,** Detail of cribriform plates in sagittal section. Note linear staining for elastin and collagen type IV. (×100.) **C,** Pial septa in postlaminar region in sagittal section. Pial setpa *(PS)*. **D,** Detail of insertion region in sagittal section; note that collagen type IV stained material extends into sclera. Arrows point to elastin fibers in cross section. (×100.) (From Hernandez, MR, Luo, XX, Igoe, F, and Neufeld, AH: Am J Ophthalmol 4:564, 1987.) (Chapter 6)

Fig. 5 Trabecular lamellae showing different stages of phagocytosis after repeated injections of foreign material. **A,** Activated trabecular cell *(arrow)* with increased amount of endoplasmic reticulum. **B,** Phagocytosing trabecular cell separating from trabecular lamellae. (Chapter 2)

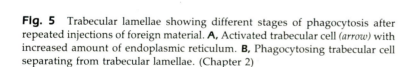

PLATE I, cont'd.

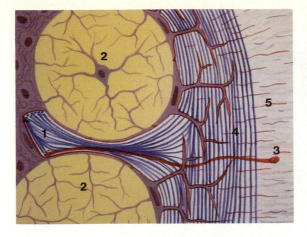

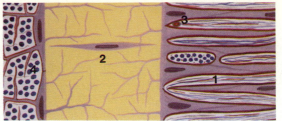

Fig. 1 Lamina cribrosa showing the different extracellular matrix components and their relationships with nerve bundles, astrocytes, and surrounding tissues. **A,** Cross section of lamina cribrosa. Cribriform plates *(1)*; nerve bundles *(2)*; blood vessels *(3)*; insertion region *(4)*; sclera *(5).* Color code: *red,* basement membranes; *lavender,* astrocytes; *blue,* elastic fibers; *gray,* interstitial collagen. **B,** Sagittal section of lamina cribrosa. (From Hernandez, MR, Luo, XX, Igoe, F, and Neufeld, AH: Am J Ophthalmol 4:564, 1987.) (Chapter 6)

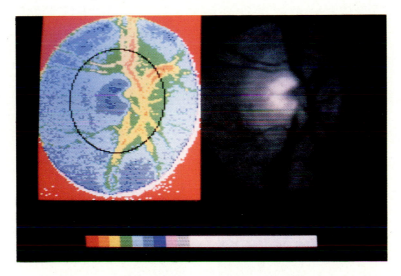

Fig. 2 Color-coded "pallor map" of optic nerve head derived from video images in red and green light. Colors toward right of scale indicate increasing values for pallor. (Chapters 22 and 23)

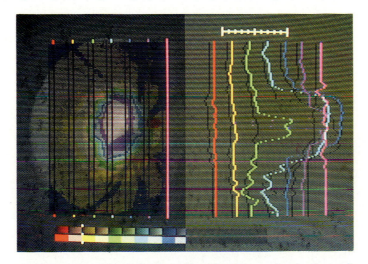

Fig. 3 Corresponding cross-sectional depth profiles of optic nerve head redrawn from computer display derived from digital image analysis of simultaneously recorded striped video images. Scale at right indicates 1.0 mm in depth. (Chapter 23)

PLATE II

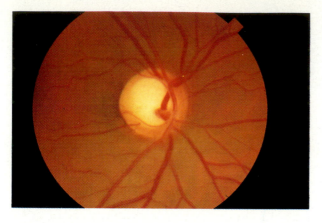

Fig. 4 Large physiologic cup in a 16-year-old white male patient with normal intraocular pressure and no eye disease. Note irregularity in neural rim width. (Chapter 22)

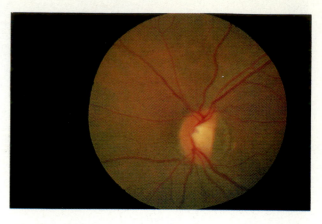

Fig. 5 "Gray crescent." Retinal pigment epithelium extends onto disc, giving appearance of a tilted disc. In patient with elevated intraocular pressure, this could be misinterpreted as glaucomatous cupping. Disc is actually circular, and temporal rim is of normal width. (Chapter 22)

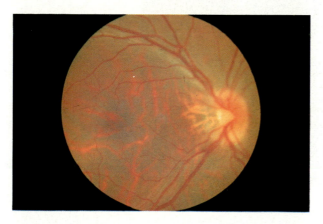

Fig. 6 True tilted disc. Note temporal chorioretinal atrophy. (Chapter 22)

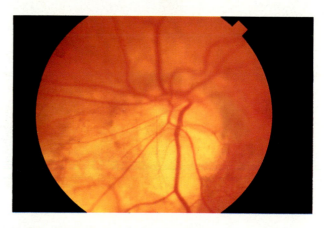

Fig. 7 Markedly tilted disc in patient with high myopia. (Chapter 22)

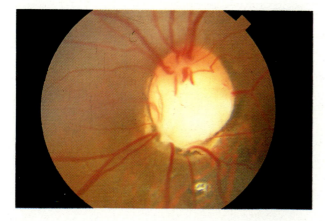

Fig. 8 Coloboma of optic nerve head, which could be misinterpreted as glaucomatous cupping in patient with elevated intraocular pressure. (Chapter 22)

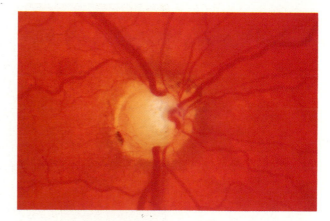

Fig. 9 Total glaucomatous cupping. (Chapter 22)

PLATE II, cont'd.

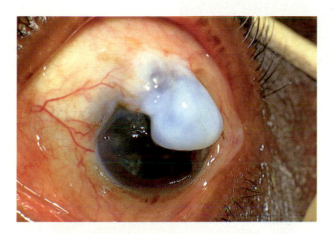

Fig. 1 Hypertrophic, overhanging filtering bleb after trabeculectomy. (Chapter 35)

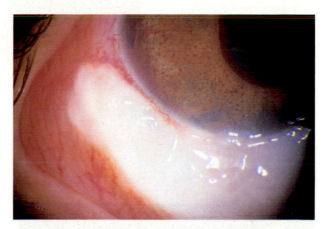

Fig. 2 Diffuse, inferior, cystic ischemic filtering bleb after trabeculectomy with 5-fluorouracil in patient with iris nevus syndrome, angle-recession, and uveitis. Note marked conjunctival erythema surrounding bleb. (Chapter 35)

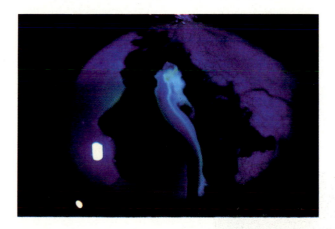

Fig. 3 Positive Seidel test in patient with leaking filtration bleb after trabeculectomy with 5-fluorouracil. (Chapter 35)

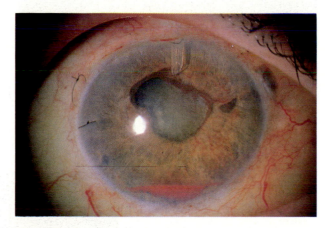

Fig. 4 Krupin-Denver valve in eye with iris rubeosis and neovascular glaucoma. Preoperative intraocular pressure was 62 mm Hg. Intraocular pressure was 16 mm Hg 4 months later at time of photograph. Small hyphema is caused by recurrent bleeding from iris vessels. (Chapter 39)

PLATE III

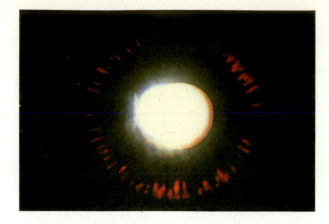

Fig. 5   Midperipheral, slitlike, radial iris transillumination in pigmentary glaucoma. (Chapter 55)

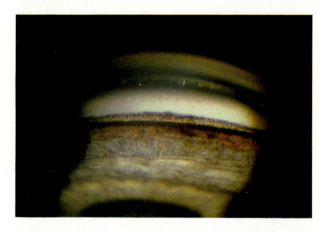

Fig. 6   Dense pigmentation of trabecular meshwork and Schwalbe's line in 14-year-old girl with pigmentary glaucoma. Note markedly posterior iris insertion and peripherally concave configuration to iris. (Chapter 55)

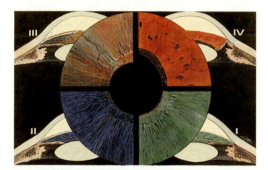

Fig. 7   The phases and mechanisms of neovascular glaucoma. **I,** Early rubeosis iridis. **II,** Moderate rubeosis iridis. **III,** Advanced rubeosis iridis with angle neovascularization. **IV,** More advanced neovascular glaucoma. (From Wand, M, Dueker, DK, Aiello, LM, and Grant, WM: Am J Ophthalmol 86:332, 1978. Published with permission from the American Journal of Ophthalmology. Copyright by the Ophthalmic Publishing Co.) (Chapter 60)

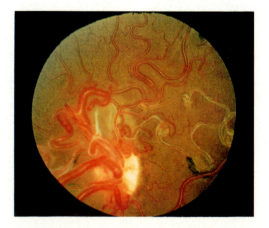

Fig. 8   Optic disc in Wyburn-Mason syndrome. (Chapter 52)

PLATE III, cont'd.

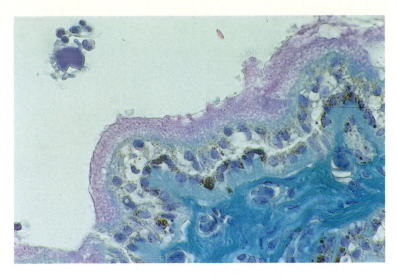

Fig. 1 Exfoliation material on ciliary body. (Chapter 56)

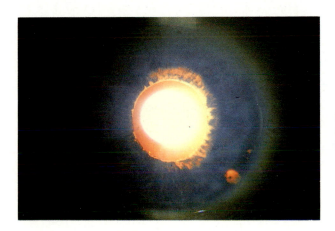

Fig. 2 Moth-eaten sphincter transillumination defects in exfoliation syndrome. To lower right is laser iridectomy seen by transillumination. (Chapter 56)

Fig. 3 Pars plicata of ciliary body and zonules in exfoliation syndrome. Exfoliation material covers these structures. Zonules are weakened, frayed, and broken. (Chapter 56)

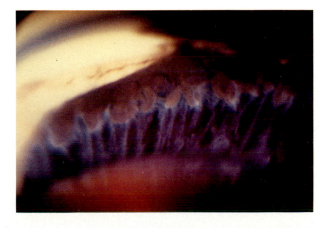

PLATE IV

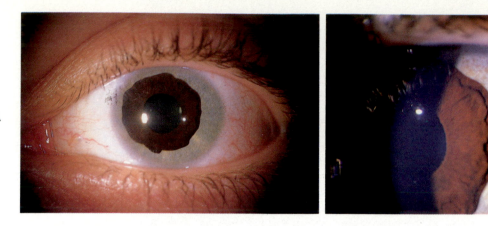

A   B

Fig. 4 **A,** Congenital ectropion uveae and juvenile glaucoma in 16-year-old male patient with Prader-Willi syndrome. **B,** Magnified view of **A** showing marked iris stromal hypoplasia and congenital ectropion uveae extending over collarette onto iris stromal surface. (From Futterweit, W, et al: JAMA 255:3280, 1986.) (Chapters 52 and 53)

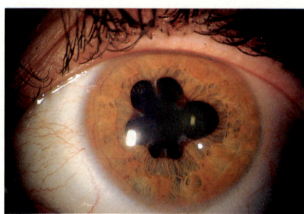

Fig. 5 Posterior synechiae to lens in patient with chronic uveitis. (Chapter 67)

Fig. 6 Inferiorly subluxated lens. (Chapter 58)

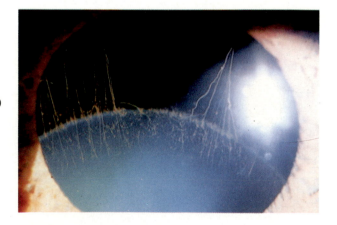

Index

A

Abrasion, corneal, 781
  argon laser trabeculoplasty and,
    613
Absolute calibration, 369
Absolute glaucoma, 844-845
Absolute threshold, 186
Accommodation, pilocarpine-induced,
    224
Accommodative spasm, 518
ACE; *see* Angiotensin-converting en-
    zyme
Acetazolamide, 1173
  acute angle-closure glaucoma and,
    855-856, 856
  argon laser peripheral iridoplasty and,
    605-606
  ciliochoroidal detachment and, 286
  congenital glaucoma and, 782-783
  hypotony and, 287
  intraocular pressure and, 302
  malignant glaucoma and, 1256
  pharmacology and, 541, 543-544
  pilocarpine and, 518
  sickle cell hemoglobinopathy and,
    1153
  trabecular meshwork and, 222
  zonular glaucoma and, 1268
Acetophenazine, 1170
Acetylcholine
  carbachol and, 518
  open-angle glaucoma after cataract ex-
    traction and, 1268
  zonular glaucoma and, 1268
Acetylcholine esterase
  anticholinesterase agents and, 520
  cholinergic nerve and, 258
Acetylsalicylic acid, 657, 1173-1174, 1179
Achromatic function, ganglion cell, 181
Acid burn, 1233
Acidosis, 544, 545

Acquired immune deficiency syndrome
  angle-closure glaucoma and, 1051,
    1156
  tonometer and, 307
Acromegaly, 1141-1142
ACTH; *see* Adrenocorticotropic hormone
Acuity; *see* Visual acuity
Acuity perimetry, 188-189
Acute angle-closure glaucoma, 841; *see*
    also Angle-closure glaucoma
  anticholinesterase agents and, 520
  episcleritis and, 1190
  hyperosmotic agent and, 554
  influenza and, 1156
  laser iridectomy and, 583
  treatment of, 855-859
Acute open-angle glaucoma; *see also*
    Open-angle glaucoma
  episcleritis and, 1189-1190
  mumps and, 1156
Acyclovir, 1219
Adaptation, local retinal, 374
Adaptation level, 187
Adenocarcinoma, 1122-1123
Adenoma, adrenal, 1142
  nonpigmented ciliary epithelium and,
    1122-1123
Adenosine monophosphate, cyclic
  adrenergic receptors and, 524-525
  beta-adrenergic agents and, 530, 532
  trabecular meshwork and, 225
Adhesion
  iridocorneal
    iridocorneal epithelial syndrome
      and, 977
    Peters' anomaly and, 897
  iris to lens and, 1206
Adrenal adenoma, 1142
Adrenergic agonist, 523-537
  alpha
    angle-closure glaucoma and, 862

Adrenergic agonist—cont'd
  alpha—cont'd
    episcleral venous pressure and,
      1131
    norepinephrine and, 526
    pigmentary glaucoma and, 993
  angle-closure glaucoma and, 856
  aqueous flow and, 342, 862
  beta, 530
  catecholamine receptors and, 523-528
  future directions and, 534-535
  ghost cell glaucoma and, 1246
  intraocular pressure and, 528-534
  open-angle glaucoma and, 815-816,
    817
Adrenergic antagonist
  alpha
    intraocular pressure and, 533
    pigmentary glaucoma and, 993
  beta; *see* Beta-adrenergic blocking
    agent
Adrenergic innervation, 258
  aqueous humor and, 224-225, 270
  ciliary body and, 84-85, 261
  limbus and, 265
  trabecular meshwork and, 263-264
  uveal blood vessel and, 262
Adrenocortical steroid, 302
Adrenocorticotropic hormone, 1142
Afferent input, 267-268
Age
  angle-closure glaucoma and, 834
  argon laser trabeculoplasty and, 609
  circadian variation in intraocular pres-
    sure and, 328-329
  collagen and, 164
  exfoliation syndrome and, 997
  intraocular pressure and, 301
  juxtacanalicular tissue and, 171
  lamina cribrosa and, 176-177
  low-tension glaucoma and, 804

Age—cont'd
  outflow system and, 52-54
  pigmentary glaucoma and, 983
  visual thresholds and, 384
  wound healing and, 634
Agonist, adrenergic; see Adrenergic agonist
Air chamber technique, 1129
Air jet method, 253
Air-tear interface, 339-340
Albumin
  anterior chamber and, 337
  binding of fluorescein to, 340-341
Alcohol
  ethyl, 553
  injection and, 1100
Algorithm
  kinetic perimetry and, 378-379
  static automated perimetry and, 376-378
Alkali burn, 1233-1235
Alkylamine, 1171
Alpha-adrenergic agonist
  angle-closure glaucoma and, 862
  episcleral venous pressure and, 1131
  norepinephrine and, 526
  pigmentary glaucoma and, 993
Alpha-adrenergic antagonist
  intraocular pressure and, 533
  pigmentary glaucoma and, 993
Alpha-adrenergic receptor, 558
Alpha-chymotrypsin, 1179
  cataract extraction and, 1268
  phacolytic glaucoma and, 1019
Alpha-methylnorepinephrine, 529
Amblyopia
  aniridia and, 881
  congenital glaucoma and, 784
  Peters' anomaly and, 901
Amine precursor uptake and decarboxylation cell, 266
Amino acid metabolism, 934
Amitriptyline, 1171
Amorphous corneal dystrophy, 976
AMP; see Adenosine monophosphate, cyclic
Amphetamine, 1172
Amyl nitrate, 1175
Amyloidosis
  exfoliation syndrome and, 1008
  familial, 1154-1155
Analog stereophotogrammetry, 498
Anastomosis
  optic nerve and, 158-159
  posterior ciliary artery and, 137, 141-156
Anemia, aplastic, 544
Anesthesia, 1177-1178
  argon laser peripheral iridoplasty and, 598
  congenital glaucoma and, 711, 775
  filtration surgery and, 657
  intraocular pressure and, 302
  laser iridectomy and, 584
  retrobulbar, 1020

Anesthesia—cont'd
  transpupillary argon laser cyclophotocoagulation and, 621-622
Angiodiathermy, 731
Angioedema, hereditary, 935-936
Angiogenesis
  neovascular glaucoma and, 1077
  retinal pigment epithelial cells, 1078
Angiography
  fluorescein, 133-161, 507; See also Blood flow, optic nerve and
  neovascular glaucoma and, 1070-1071
Angioma, retinal, 921-922
Angiomatosis, encephalotrigeminal, 913-920
Angiomatosis retinae, 921-922
Angiotensin-converting enzyme, 1216
Angle; see also Angle-closure glaucoma; Open-angle glaucoma
  aqueous humor and, 41
  Axenfeld-Rieger syndrome and, 888
  classification of, 708-709
  congenital glaucoma and, 769
  development of, 9-12
  endothelization and, 1328-1329
  exfoliation syndrome and, 1001-1003
  gonioscopy and, 345-360; see also Gonioscopy
  grading depth of, 355-356
  intraocular lens implantation and, 1289-1291
  iridocorneal epithelial syndrome and, 967
  nerves and, 262-265
  normal development of, 767-769
  phacolytic glaucoma and, 1018
  visual, of test object, 363
Angle-closure glaucoma, 825-864
  absolute, 844-845
  acquired immune deficiency syndrome and, 1051, 1156
  anatomy and, 825-827
  aphakia and, 1271-1278
  carbonic anhydrase inhibitors and, 544
  central retinal vein occlusion and, 1050-1051
  chronic, 843-844
  epidemiology and, 834-835
  episcleritis and, 1190
  examination of, 830-831, 832
  Fuchs' endothelial dystrophy and, 978
  history of, 825
  hyperosmotic agent, 554
  influenza and, 1156
  laser iridectomy and, 583
  laser iridecoplasty and, 597
  malignant glaucoma and, 1251
  microspherophakia and, 1035-1036
  nanophthalmos and, 1049-1050
  neovascular glaucoma and, 1070
    treatment of, 1095
  pathology and, 847-852
  penetrating keratoplasty and, 1342
  physiology and, 827, 829, 830

Angle-closure glaucoma—cont'd
  posterior polymorphous dystrophy and, 975-976
  posterior scleritis and, 1201-1202
  primary, 825-864
    classification of, 751-752
    clinical types of, 839-853
    filtration surgery and, 673
    lens intumescence and, 1027-1028
    mechanism and epidemiology and, 825-837
    scleritis and, 1199
    treatment of, 855-864
  retina and
    cystic macular degeneration and, 946
    photocoagulation and, 1051-1052
    retinopathy of prematurity and, 947
    scleral buckling procedure and, 1052-1052
  secondary, 846-847
    classification of, 753, 755
    syphilis and, 1214
    traumatic lens dislocation and, 1041
    treatment of, 855-864
Angular aqueous plexus, 15
Angular neurocristopathy, 23-37
Anhidrosis, 270
Aniridia, 869-883
  aqueous humor outflow and, 223
  Axenfeld-Rieger syndrome versus, 894
  classification of, 869-873
  clinical findings and, 873-877, 879
  histopathology and, 879-881
  management of, 881-882
Ankylosing spondylitis, 1216-1217
Anomaloscope, 189
Anomaly
  angle and, 708-709
  encephalotrigeminal angiomatosis and, 916, 919
  iris and corneal, 776
  iris vessel and, 765-766
  mesodermal angle, 984
  skeletal, 1040
Anoxia, 899
Antagonist
  alpha-adrenergic
    intraocular pressure and, 533
    pigmentary glaucoma and, 993
  beta; see Beta-adrenergic blocking agent
Antazoline, 1171, 1172
Anterior capsulotomy, 678
Anterior chamber; see also Angle
  anatomy and, 3, 241
  aspiration and, 1246
  cataract extraction and filtration and, 678
  central retinal vein occlusion and, 1050
  chronic angle-closure glaucoma and, 844
  cleavage and
    Axenfeld-Rieger syndrome; see Axenfeld-Rieger syndrome

Anterior chamber—cont'd
  cleavage and—cont'd
    Peters' anomaly and, 899
  curettage and, 1313, 1316
  ectopia lentis and, 1030-1031
  epithelial cyst and, 1300-1301
  exfoliation syndrome and, 1001-1003
  extremely shallow, 590
  flat
    argon laser peripheral iridoplasty
      and, 598
    conventional iridectomy and, 647
    filtration surgery and, 673
  fluorophotometry and, 337-344
  ghost cell glaucoma and, 1245
  hyphema and, 1244
  hypotony and, 684
  intraocular lens implantation and,
    1289-1291
  iridectomy and; see Iridectomy
  lens dislocation and, 1036-1037
  pigmentary glaucoma and, 982, 983
  posterior polymorphous dystrophy
    and, 976
  reformation of, 670
  scleral buckling procedure and, 1053
  seton and, 741-742
  shunt and, 639, 742
  vitreous and, 1269
Anterior hyaloid
  angle-closure glaucoma and, 1277
  diabetic retinopathy and, 1086
  posterior capsule and, 1086, 1087
  rupture of, 1269
  vitreous hemorrhage and, 1242
Anterior lens; see Lens
Anterior limbus, 22-23
Anterior scleritis, 1191
  posterior scleritis and, 1193-1194
Anterior segment
  developmental anatomy of, 6-8
  embryology of, 3-40; see also Embryol-
    ogy of anterior segment
  exfoliation syndrome and, 1005
  inflammation and
    laser iridectomy and, 594
    uveitis and, 1209
  sarcoid uveitis, 1215
  wound healing and, 635
Anterior synechia
  peripheral; see Peripheral anterior syn-
    echia
  Peters' anomaly and, 899
Anterior uveal tract, 85-90
  arthritis and, 1216-1218
  laser iridectomy and, 594
Antiarrhythmic agent, 1174
Antibiotic, 1173-1174
  filtration surgery and, 671
Antibody
  anti—neuron-specific enolase, 23-24
  extracellular matrix and, 166
Anticholinergic activity, 519-520, 1170,
  1171
  aniridia and, 881

Anticholinergic activity—cont'd
  parasympathomimetic agent and, 1176
  trabecular meshwork and, 222
Anticoagulant, 657
Antidepressant, 1171
  acute angle-closure glaucoma and, 841
Antidiuretic hormone, 553
Antifibrosis, 673-674
Antigen, HLA-B27, 1216
Antihistamine, 1171-1172
Antihypertensive agent, 1178
Antiinflammatory agent, 673
Antimetabolite
  fibroblast and, 673
  filtering surgery and, 639
Anti—neuron-specific enolase antibody,
  23-24
Antiparkinsonian drug, 1172
Antiprostaglandin, 1178-1179
Antireflective contact lens
  laser iridectomy and, 584
  photocoagulator and, 576
Antispasmolytic agent, 1173
Aphakia, 1265-1283; see also Extracapsu-
    lar lens extraction; Intracapsular
    lens extraction
  angle-closure glaucoma and, 1271-1278
  argon laser trabeculoplasty and, 609
  diabetic retinopathy and, 1086
  epinephrine maculopathy and, 815-816
  filtration surgery and, 672, 677-681
  ghost cell glaucoma and, 1244
  glaucoma surgery and, 699
  keratoplasty and, 1339
  management of, 1278-1280
  open-angle glaucoma and, 1266-1271
  phacolytic glaucoma and, 1020
  pupillary block and, 583
  single-procedure extraction and, 697-
    698, 699, 701
  vitreous surgery and, 1260-1261
  wound healing and, 636
Aplastic anemia, 544
Aplonidine, 559
Apostilb, 381
Applanation tonometry, 304-311
  retinal detachment and, 1056
APUD; see Amine precursor uptake and
    decarboxylation
Aqueous flare
  cyclodialysis and, 284
  iridocyclitis and, 282
Aqueous humor
  angle-closure glaucoma and, 827
    acute, 843, 855-856
  calcitonin gene-related peptide and,
    262
  cataract surgery and, 1290
  catecholamine and, 529
  encephalotrigeminal angiomatosis
    and, 916, 919
  epinephrine and, 270
  episcleral venous pressure and, 249-
    256
  epithelial ingrowth and, 1316

Aqueous humor—cont'd
  fluorophotometry and, 337-344
  formation of, 199-218
  Fuchs' dystrophy and, 977
  glaucomatocyclitic crisis and, 1211
  hypotony and, 281-290
  low-tension glaucoma and, 803-804
  misdirection of, 684-685
  outflow and, 41-74, 219-239; see also
    Outflow
  oxytalanosis of, 997
  Peters' anomaly and, 900
  phacolytic glaucoma and, 1019
  posterior diversion of, 1251-1252
  trabecular meshwork and, 166
  ultrafiltration and secretion and, 261
  uveitis and, 1205
  uveoscleral outflow and, 241-247
  vasoactive intestinal peptide and, 262
Aqueous plexus, angular, 15
Aqueous vessel, 1128
  episcleral venous pressure and, 250
  vein of Archer and, 1127
Aqueousplasty, 741
Arachnoid, 113, 115
Arc perimetry, 361
Archer's aqueous vein, 1127
Arcuate scotoma, 394, 396
Arcus senilis, 598
Argemona mexicana, 1179
  neovascular glaucoma and, 1099-1100
Argon endophotocoagulator, 1093-1094
Argon laser; see also Laser
  cyclodialysis cleft and, 627-628
  cyclophotocoagulation, 1099-1100
    open-angle glaucoma and, 819
    transpupillary, 621-622
  iridectomy and, 633
  peripheral iridoplasty and, 596-600
    scleral buckling procedure and,
      1053
  photocoagulation and, 577
    angle-closure glaucoma and, 1051
    epithelial ingrowth and, 1313, 1315
  pupilloplasty and, 625-626
  sclerostomy with, 624
  sphincterotomy, 626
  suture cutting and, 626-627
  trabecular meshwork and, 232
  trabeculoplasty and, 605-615; see also
    Trabeculoplasty
    aphakia and, 1279
    exfoliation syndrome and, 1011
    peripheral iridoplasty and, 597-598
  transconjunctival treatment with, 623-
    624
Arteriole
  capillary anastomosis and, 159
  ciliary body and, 81, 83
  ciliopapillary, 135
Arteriovenous anastomosis, 918
Arteriovenous fistula, 920
Artery; see specific artery
Arthritis
  anterior uveitis and, 1216-1218

Arthritis—cont'd
    familial histiocytic dermatoarthritis and, 935
Arthroophthalmopathy, progressive hereditary, 939
Artifact, lens rim, 440
Ash leaf sign, 922
Asian patient, 834, 840
Aspiration
    epithelial ingrowth and, 1316
    ghost cell glaucoma and, 1246
    hyphema and, 1227
Aspirin, 1173-1174, 1179
    filtration surgery and, 657
Astrocyte
    cribriform plates and, 172-173, 176
    intraorbital optic nerve and, 115
    lamina choroidalis and, 109
    lamina cribrosa and, 173
    lamina scleralis and, 111
    optic nerve head neuroglia and, 105, 108
    peripapillary hamartoma and, 922
Astroglia, 113, 115
Asymmetry of cupping, 472
Ataxia, 873
Atherosclerosis, 1087-1088
Atopic dermatitis, 934
Atrophy
    encephalotrigeminal angiomatosis and, 914
    iridocorneal epithelial syndrome and, 963-973
    peripapillary, 478-479
Atropine, 1176
    ciliary block glaucoma and, 554
    malignant glaucoma and, 1256
    misdirection of, 684-685
    neovascular glaucoma and, 1095
    trabecular meshwork and, 224
        trabeculectomy and, 667
    uveitis and, 1207, 1208
    uveoscleral outflow and, 245-246
    vitreous surgery and, 1261
Attachment factor, 165
Aulhorn's curve of light sense, 364-365
Autofluorescence of cornea, 340
Automated infusion-suction instrumentation, 1262
Automated perimetry, 403-466
    algorithm and, 376-378
    data presentation and, 414-418
    examination for glaucoma and, 418-431
    glaucomatous field defects and, 432
    goals of, 403-404
    history and, 403, 403
    interpretation of, 432-466
    methods of, 404-405
    test strategies and, 405-413
Autonomic drug, 1175-1177
Autoregulation of optic nerve blood flow, 124-125, 136
Autosomal dominant aniridia, 869-873
Axenfeld-Rieger syndrome, 25-27, 885-896
    iridocorneal epithelial syndrome and, 972-973

Axenfeld's syndrome, 767
Axial centrifugal vascular system, 135
Axial length
    angle-closure glaucoma and, 826
    congenital glaucoma and, 777
Axial myopia
    congenital glaucoma and, 779
    tilted disc and, 781
Axon
    diameter of, 125
    lamina choroidalis and, 110
    lamina scleralis and, 111-113
    number of, 495
    optic disc and, 103
    optic nerve and, 107, 109, 116, 118, 120, 123
    retina and, 95-100, 102
    trabecular, 263
Axoplasmic flow, 102

B

Bacitracin, 1174
Background, calibration of, 369
Background illumination, 387, 404-405
Background noise, 186
Band keratopathy, 1304-1305
Banding, 52-53
BAPN; see Beta-aminoproprionitrile
Barbiturate, 1172
Barkan lens, 712-713
Barkan membrane, 31, 34
Barrier
    blood-aqueous; see Blood-aqueous barrier
    posterior capsule-anterior hyaloid, 1086, 1087
Basal cell nevus syndrome, 924
    multiple, 938
Basement membrane
    characteristics of, 163-164
    exfoliation syndrome and, 997, 1008
    intraorbital optic nerve and, 114, 115
    lamina scleralis and, 111
    neovascular glaucoma and, 1073
    primary open-angle glaucoma and, 60
    subendothelial region and, 167, 171
    trabecular beams and, 171
Beam, 570
    photodisruptor aiming/focusing, 578-579
    trabecular meshwork, 166-167, 171
Benign reactive lymphoid hyperplasia, 1123
Benzalkonium chloride, 518
Beta radiation
    fibroblast and, 674
    filtering surgery and, 639
Beta-adrenergic agonist, 530
Beta-adrenergic blocking agent
    acute angle-closure glaucoma and, 856
    aphakia and, 1278
    aqueous flow and, 342
        misdirection and, 685
    central retinal vein occlusion, 1148
    chemical burn and, 1234, 1235

Beta-adrenergic blocking agent—cont'd
    episcleral venous pressure and, 1135
    exfoliation syndrome and, 1011
    filtration surgery and, 657
    ghost cell glaucoma and, 1246
    hyphema and, 1227
        open-angle glaucoma after cataract extraction and, 1270
    intraocular pressure and, 532-533
    iridocorneal epithelial syndrome and, 977
    lens-induced glaucoma and, 1023
    low-tension glaucoma and, 809
    malignant glaucoma and, 1256
    open-angle glaucoma and, 815, 817
        cataract extraction and, 1268
        initial therapy and, 81
    pigmentary glaucoma and, 993-994
    pilocarpine and, 518
    pseudophakic glaucoma and, 1294
Beta-adrenergic receptor
    aqueous humor and, 270
    trabecular meshwork and, 221
Beta-aminoproprionitrile
    fibroblast and, 673-674
    filtering surgery and, 639
Beta-Hypophamine; see Vasopressin
Betaine, 1040
Betaxolol, 782-783, 784
BHT-920, 531
Bicarbonate
    aqueous humor and, 203
    rate of formation of, 539
Biochemistry
    extracellular matrix and, 165-166
    trabecular meshwork, 222
Biomechanics, outflow, 231-232
Biopsy, iris, 1313
Biorhythm; see Circadian variation in intraocular pressure
Bjerrum scotoma, 436, 438
    nerve fiber bundle defect and, 394
Black patient, wound healing in, 635
Blackening, laser iridectomy and, 590
Bleb
    cataract extraction and, 680-681, 701
    corticosteroid and, 638
    cystic, 637
    elevation and, 670
    formation of, 655
    functional filtering, 637
    infection and, 685, 686
    intraocular pressure and, 675-676
    neovascular glaucoma and, 1095, 1096
Bleeding; see Hemorrhage
Blepharospasm, 773
Blind spot
    history and, 361, 393
    monitoring and, 404
    nerve fiber bundle defect and, 394
Block
    facial nerve, 658
    iridovitreal, 1254
    pupillary; see Pupillary block

Block excision, 666-667
Blockage, sclerotomy, 687
Blood cell
  erythrocyte and
    ghost cell glaucoma and; *see* Ghost
      cell glaucoma
    sickle cell disease and, 1153
    trabecular meshwork and, 229
  white, 1246
    iridocorneal epithelial syndrome
      and, 972
    neovascular glaucoma and, 1077
Blood disorder, 1152-1154
Blood flow
  lamina choroidalis and, 109-110
  optic nerve and, 133-161
    glaucoma and, 123-125
    lamina cribrosa and, 133
    misconceptions about, 158-159
    optic nerve head and, 135-136
    posterior ciliary artery and, 136-
      158
    prelaminar region and, 133, 135
    retrolaminar region and, 135
    surface layer of nerve fibers and,
      135
    retinal nerve fiber layer and, 92,
      95
Blood glucose
  diabetic retinopathy and, 1085
  neovascular glaucoma and, 1091
Blood pressure
  diabetic retinopathy and, 1085
  ciliary body and, 84
  intraocular pressure and, 1151
    correlation between, 200
  low-tension glaucoma and, 804
  posterior ciliary artery and, 152
  retinal blood flow and, 95
  optic nerve and, 136
Blood test, 808
Blood vessel; *see also* specific vessel
  adrenergic receptors and, 527
  intraorbital optic nerve and, 114, 115
  iris and
    aqueous humor and, 41-42
    congenital glaucoma and, 765-766
    exfoliation syndrome and, 1001
  lamina scleralis and, 111
  limbal, 265
  nerve distribution and, 261
  optic nerve head and, 107
  photocoagulation and, 573-574
Blood-aqueous barrier
  ciliary body and, 88, 89, 90
  epithelial ingrowth and, 1313
  hypotony and, 287
  laser and, 594
Blood-induced glaucoma, 1239-1247
Blood-retinal barrier, 1070-1071
Blood-to-aqueous transfer rate, 201-
  202
Blue
  color pairing and, 183-185
  glaucoma and, 190

Blunt trauma, 1225-1232
  ghost cell glaucoma and, 1244
  gonioscopy and, 358
Blurred vision
  laser iridectomy and, 590
  threshold and, 387
Body
  ciliary; *see* Ciliary body
  geniculate, 119, 120
Bombé, iris; *see* Iris bombé
Bone
  Klippel-Trenaunay-Weber syndrome
    and, 920
  osteogenesis imperfecta and, 938-939
Border tissue, 111
Bourneville's disease, 922
Bowman's zone, 8
Bradycardia, 520
Branch retinal vein occlusion, 1147
Bridle suture, 660, 661
Brightness in perimetry, 370-372
Brittle bone disease, 938-939
Bromide, 201
Brompheniramine, 1171, 1172
Bruch's membrane, 158
Bruit, cervical, 1088
Bud, endothelial, 1073
Bundle, nerve fiber, 394, 396
Buphthalmos
  definition of, 763
  encephalotrigeminal angiomatosis
    and, 915-916
  neurofibromatosis and, 911, 912
Bupivacaine, 657
Burinamide, 1172
Burn
  chemical, 1202-1203, 1233-1235
  laser
    corneal, 591, 592, 585, 586, 613
    iridectomy and, 586-587, 589
    pupilloplasty and, 625
    trabecular meshwork and, 232, 606-
      607
Burned-out glaucoma, 807
Button, donor, 1340
Buttonhole, conjunctival, 682
Butyrophenone, 1170
Bypass, carotid, 1088

C

Café-au-lait spot, 906
Caffeine, 1172
  intraocular pressure and, 303,
    815
Calcification, cerebral, 914
Calcitonin gene-related peptide, 260
  aqueous humor and, 262
Calcium
  adrenergic receptors and, 524-525
  aqueous humor and, 229
  ATPase and, 207, 210
  ciliary epithelial cells and, 88
Calcium channel blocker, 1174
Calibration, 369-370
Camera, 496

cAMP; *see* Cyclic adenosine monophosphate
Campimetry
  benefits and inaccuracies of, 373-
    374
  perimetry versus, 368
Canal
  optic
    anatomy and, 102-103
    optic nerve and, 118
  Schlemm's; *see* Schlemm's canal
Cannabinoid, 559-560
Capillary
  anastomosis and, 158-159
  ciliary body and, 80-85
  endothelial cell and, 92
  lamina choroidalis and, 109-110
  lamina scleralis and, 111
  neovascular glaucoma and, 1077
  retinal nerve fiber layer and, 95
Capsule, lens; *see also* Capsulotomy
  development of, 6-8
  diabetic retinopathy and, 1086
  exfoliation and, 1009
  laser iridectomy and, 587
  persistent hyperplastic primary vitre-
    ous and, 944
  phacoanaphylaxis and, 1024
Capsulotomy
  anterior, 678
  Nd:YAG laser
    angle-closure glaucoma after cata-
      ract extraction and, 1278
    diabetic retinopathy and, 1086
    lens-induced glaucoma and, 1021-
      1022
Caput-medusa, 1131
Carbachol, 518-519, 1176
  open-angle glaucoma after cataract ex-
    traction and, 1268
Carbon dioxide laser, 573
  filtration surgery and, 672
  neovascular glaucoma and, 1095
Carbonic anhydrase inhibitor, 539-
  549; *see also* Acetazolamide
  acute angle-closure glaucoma and,
    855-856
  aphakia and, 1278
  aqueous flow and, 342
    misdirection and, 685
  argon laser peripheral iridoplasty and,
    605-606
  Axenfeld-Rieger syndrome and, 895
  central retinal vein occlusion and,
    1050, 1148
  chemical burn and, 1234
  episcleral venous pressure and, 1135
  filtration surgery and, 657
  ghost cell glaucoma and, 1246
  hyphema and, 1227, 1270
  iridocorneal epithelial syndrome and,
    977
  lens-induced glaucoma and, 1023
  low-tension glaucoma and, 809
  malignant glaucoma and, 1256

Carbonic anhydrase inhibitor—cont'd
  open-angle glaucoma and, 816
    cataract extraction and, 1268, 1270
    initial therapy and, 816-817
  pigmentary glaucoma and, 994
  pseudophakic glaucoma and, 1294
  sickle cell hemoglobinopathy and,
    1153
Cardiac agent, 1174
Cardiac function
  hyperosmotic agents and, 554
  Marfan syndrome and, 1038
Cardiac glycoside, 213
Carotid artery
  fistula and, 1132-1133
  low-tension glaucoma and, 808
  occlusion and, 155
    hypotony and, 287
    neovascular glaucoma and, 1087-
      1088
    prophylaxis and, 1091
Cataract, 444-445
  anticholinesterase agents and, 520
  arthritis and, 1218
  atopic dermatitis and, 934
  automated perimetry and, 432
  chemical burn and, 1235
  exfoliation syndrome and, 998
  Fuchs' heterochromic cyclitis and,
    1210
  Hallermann-Streiff syndrome and, 935
  hypermature, 230
  iridectomy and, 648
    conventional, 647
    Nd:YAG laser, 595
  iris retraction syndrome and, 1051
  Lowe's syndrome and, 936
  open-angle glaucoma and, 819, 1017-
    1026
  phacoanaphylaxis and, 1024
  progression of, 687
  retrocorneal membrane and, 1324
  surgical management of, 697-706
  telangiectasia-cataracta syndrome and,
    938
  unequal, 1028
Cataract extraction; see Aphakia; Extra-
    capsular lens extraction; Intracap-
    sular lens extraction
Catecholamine, 523-537
  future directions and, 534-535
  intraocular pressure and, 528-534
  receptors and, 523-528
Cation ionophore, 287
Cautery, 1096
Cavernous sinus, 1132-1133
Cavity, resonant, 568-570
CCK; see Cholecystokinin-gastrin
Cell
  blood; see Blood cell
  endothelial; see Endothelium
  epithelial; see Epithelium
  ganglion; see Ganglion cell
  iridocorneal epithelial syndrome and,
    967

Cell—cont'd
  neural crest, 5, 8
  opercular, 42-43
  paracrine, 266
    catecholamines and, 525-526
  photoreceptor, 363-364
  trabecular; see Trabecular meshwork
Cell-extracellular matrix interaction, 1313
Cell-induced facility decrease, 229-230
Cellular membrane, 972
Central 10-degree field, 429
Central 30-degree program, 418, 423
Central corneal leukoma, 897
Central field test pattern, 406
Central nervous system, 257-279; see also
    Nervous system
Central pallor, 475-476
Central retinal artery; see Retinal artery
Central retinal vein occlusion; see Retinal
    vein, occlusion and
Central vision loss, 687
Central-only test, 422
Centrifugal vascular system, 135
Cerebellar ataxia, 873
Cerebral calcification, 914
Cerebrohepatorenal syndrome of Zell-
    weger, 940
Cerebrovascular disease, 450, 1148
Cervical bruit, 1088
Cervical ganglion, 258
Cervical sympathetic nerve, 269, 270
CGRP; see Calcitonin gene-related pep-
    tide
Chamber, anterior; see Anterior chamber
Chandler's syndrome, 963, 964, 967, 972
Chandler's technique, 1258-1262
Change analysis printout, 463, 465
Channel
  emissarial, 241-242
  transcellular, 221
Charring, 590
Chelator, 229
Chemical burn to cornea, 1202-1203
Chemical injury, 1233-1235
Chemical sympathectomy, 529
Chemoattractant, 1078
Chiasm
  compressive lesion of, 807
  intraorbital optic nerve and, 118-119
Chloprothixene, 1170
Chloral hydrate, 1177-1178
Chloride
  aqueous humor and, 200, 203
  bicarbonate and, 539
Chloroprocaine, 520
Chlorothen, 1172
Chlorpheniramine, 1171
Chlorpromazine, 1170
Chlorthalidone, 1173, 1178
Chlorthiazide, 1178
Cholecystokinin-gastrin, 260
Cholinergic agent, 515-521
  aniridia and, 881
  aphakia and, 1279
  aqueous humor outflow and, 222-223

Cholinergic agent—cont'd
  pseudophakic glaucoma and, 1294
Cholinergic nerve, 258
  chamber angle and, 263
  ciliary body and, 84-85
Cholinesterase, 1278-1279
Cholinomimetic effect, 224
Choriocapillaris, 1092
Chorioretinal scar, 449
Chorioretinitis, 1215
Choroid
  blood pressure and, 152
  detachment and
    cataract extraction and, 1276
    filtration surgery and, 684
    scleral buckling procedure and, 1053
  encephalotrigeminal angiomatosis and
    effusion and, 920
    hemangioma and, 915, 916
  effusion and
    encephalotrigeminal angiomatosis
      and, 920
    posterior scleritis and, 1201-1202
  innervation and, 261
  melanoma and, 1115-1116
  metastasis and, 1118-1119
  separation and
    malignant glaucoma and, 1253-1254,
      1255
    sclerotomy and, 1258
  watershed zone and, 147-149, 152
Choroidal artery, peripapillary
  prelaminar region and, 133, 135
  retrolaminar region and, 135
Choroidal lamina cribrosa, 172
Choroidal vein, 261
Chromatic-achromatic classification of
    ganglion cell, 181, 183
Chromophobe pituitary adenoma, 1142
Chromophore, 183
Chromosome
  aniridia and, 870
  disorder, 931-932
  neurofibromatosis and, 906-907
  ring, 933-934
Chronic angle-closure glaucoma, 843-844
  laser iridectomy and, 583
  treatment of, 860
Chronic ocular ischemia, 1088
Chronic open-angle glaucoma
  diurnal variation and, 806
  ghost cell glaucoma and, 1246
  scotoma and, 398, 400
Chronobiology of intraocular pressure,
    319-320
Chymotrypsin, 1179
Cicatricial angle, 708
Cigarette smoking, 302-303
Cilia, 43
Ciliary artery
  anatomy and, 80-85
  lamina cribrosa and, 133
  posterior
    retrolaminar region and, 135
    variations of, 136-158

Ciliary block glaucoma, 847; *see also* Malignant glaucoma
  hyperosmotic agent and, 554
  surgical iridectomy and, 582
Ciliary body
  alpha-adrenergic receptor and, 558
  anatomy of, 77-80
  angle-closure glaucoma and, 827, 850
  aniridia and, 882
  aqueous humor and, 41, 201
  carotid artery occlusive disease and, 1088
  central retinal vein occlusion and, 1050
  destruction of, 729-740; *see also* Cyclodestructive surgery
  detachment and, 282, 284
  development of, 10
  epithelium, 85-90
    ingrowth and, 1305
  exfoliation syndrome and, 1003
  freezing of, 731-734
  malignant glaucoma and, 847
  melanocytoma and, 1116
  melanoma and, 1113-1115
  metastasis and, 1117-1118
  microvasculature, 80-85
  mucopolysaccharidosis and, 67
  nerve distribution and, 261
  pigmentary glaucoma and, 64, 67
  radiation and, 1155
  scleral buckling procedure and, 1053
  traumatic lens dislocation and, 1042
  uveitis and, 1205
  venous drainage and, 1128
Ciliary epithelium
  aqueous humor and, 41
  ATPase and, 206-210
  tumors of, 1121-1123
  ultrastructure and, 85-90
Ciliary ganglion, 257
Ciliary muscle
  adrenergic mechanism and, 84, 224
  capillaries and, 85
  cholinergic mechanism and, 84, 222-223
  cribriform meshwork and, 231
  trabecular meshwork and, 16, 46-50, 224
Ciliary process
  adrenergic and cholinergic nerve endings and, 84
  arterioles and, 83
  capillaries and, 85
  microvasculature and, 80
  malignant glaucoma and, 1252
  Marfan syndrome and, 1039
  nerve distribution and, 261
  persistent hyperplastic primary vitreous and, 944
  photocoagulation and, 1279
Ciliary-iris region, 16, 18
Cilioanalysis, 731

Ciliochoroidal detachment
  hypotony and, 285-286
  uveoscleral outflow and, 246
Ciliodestructive procedure
  congenital glaucoma and, 725, 727
  open-angle glaucoma and, 819
Ciliopapillary arteriole, 135
Cilioretinal artery, 133, 135
Cimetidine, 1172
Circadian variation in intraocular pressure, 319-336
  aqueous flow and, 341-342
  characteristics of, 324-332
  chronobiology of, 319-320
  clinical application of, 332-333
  methods of measurement of, 320-324
Circle
  intramuscular, 81
  of Zinn and Haller
    lamina cribrosa and, 133
    retrolaminar region and, 135
Circulation; *see* Blood flow
Classification of angle anomaly, 708-709
Cleanup burn, 585
Cleavage, anterior chamber
  Axenfeld-Rieger syndrome and, 885
  Peters' anomaly and, 899
Cleft
  cyclodialysis, 627-628
  Schlemm's canal and, 50
Clinoril; *see* Sulindac
Clonidine, 1178
  episcleral venous pressure and, 1131
  intraocular pressure and, 531
  pharmacology and, 557
Closed system lensectomy, 1042
Clot
  filtering operation and, 637
  hyphema and, 1225
CLV; *see* Corrected loss variance
Coagulation; *see* Photocoagulation
Coating, antireflective
  iridectomy and, 584
  photocoagulator and, 576
Cocaine, 1177-1178
Cogan-Reese syndrome, 963, 964, 970, 971, 972
Colistin, 1174
Collagen
  age and, 52
  angle-closure glaucoma and, 1049-1050
  extracellular matrix and, 164
  fibroblast and, 673-674
  iridocorneal epithelial syndrome and, 967
  lamina cribrosa and, 173, 176
  lamina scleralis and, 111
  lattice, 60
  sclera and, 22
  trabecular beams and, 167, 171
    age and, 54
Collagen vascular disorder, 1151
Collector channel, 50-52
Color of optic nerve, 503-505
Color testing, 189-191

Color testing—cont'd
  basis of, 183-185
  intraocular lens implantation and, 1293-1294
Coma, 855
Combined mechanism glaucoma, 846
  treatment of, 861
Compact zone, 241
Complex pigmentary glaucoma, 997
Compression shell, 674-675
Compressive lesion, 807
Computed tomography
  low-tension glaucoma and, 808
  orbital varices, 1132
Computerized image analysis, 499-503
  automated perimetry and, 404
Computerized static perimetry, 186-187
Conduction, heat, 572
Cone
  color vision and, 183
  ganglion cell and, 89, 91
  glassy, 1325
  number of, 363-364
  visual process and, 180
Congenital disorder; *see also* Congenital glaucoma
  chromosomal abnormality and, 931-934
  color perception and, 189-190
  ectropion uveae and, 940
    Axenfeld-Rieger syndrome versus, 895
    Prader-Willi syndrome and, 934
  embryologic basis for, 23-37
  encephaloophthalmic dysplasia, 936
  hemangiomatosis and, 924
  hereditary endothelial dystrophy and, 779
  iris hypoplasia and, 894
  low-tension glaucoma and, 807
  mucopolysaccharidosis and, 67-69
  ocular, 940-951
  posterior polymorphous dystrophy and, 974
  rubella and, 1156
  syphilis and, 1213-1214
  of unknown etiology and, 934-940
Congenital glaucoma, 25, 759-785
  aniridia and, 874
  argon laser trabeculoplasty and, 610-611
  classification of, 752, 763-767
  clinical presentation and, 773
  differential diagnosis and, 779-781
  epidemiology and, 767
  examination and, 773-777
  hemangiomatosis and, 924
  histopathology and, 767-771
  history of, 761-762
  iridocorneal epithelial syndrome and, 976
  management and, 781-784
  neurofibromatosis and, 909, 911-913
  Peters' anomaly and, 900
  surgery for, 707-727

Congenital glaucoma—cont'd
  surgery for—cont'd
    ciliodestructive procedure and, 725,
      727
    conjunctival and scleral flap and,
      725
    goniotomy and, 711-715
    history and, 707
    postoperative management and, 725
    prognosis and, 707-711
    setons and, 725
    trabeculectomy and, 721-725
    trabeculotomy and, 715-721
  terminology and, 7762-763
  trabecular meshwork and, 31, 35
Congestive glaucoma; see Neovascular
  glaucoma
Coniophotocoagulation, 1094
Conjunctiva
  encephalotrigeminal angiomatosis
    and, 919
  epithelium and, 22-23
  exfoliation syndrome and, 998-999,
    1008, 1009
  filtration surgery and, 656, 659
  ghost cell glaucoma and, 1245
  telangiectasis and, 1155
Conjunctival buttonhole, 682
Conjunctival flap
  cataract extraction and filtration and,
    677
  congenital glaucoma and, 725
  fornix-based
    closure and, 669
    sclerotomy and cataract extraction
      and, 704
  perforation and, 684
  sclerotomy and, 1258
  trabeculectomy and, 660, 662-663, 669
  trabeculotomy and, 715
Conjunctivitis
  infant and, 781
  Reiter's syndrome and, 1218
Connective tissue
  extraocular optic nerve and, 113, 115
  lamina scleralis and, 111
Connexon, 88
Consanguinity, 1035
Consent, informed, 655
Constant force applanation tonometry,
  311-312
Contact lens
  laser iridectomy and, 584
  photocoagulator and, 576
Continuous measuring device, 312
Contraction
  argon laser peripheral iridoplasty and,
    598
  ciliary muscle, 224
  neovascular glaucoma and, 1073
Contraction burn, laser
  iridectomy and, 585, 586
  pupilloplasty and, 625
Contrast sensitivity, temporal, 189
Contusion, 1041

Cornea
  abrasion and, 781
  amorphous dystrophy and, 976
  angle-closure glaucoma, 848
  aniridia and, 874, 878
  applanation tonometry and, 304-311
  argon laser trabeculoplasty and, 613
  autofluorescence of, 340
  Axenfeld-Rieger syndrome and, 886-
    888
  chemical burn and, 1202-1203, 1235
  congenital glaucoma and, 773, 776
  cystinosis and, 934
  dellen and, 687
  development of, 8-10
  ectoderm and, 3
  edema and; see Corneal edema
  enlargement of, 770-771, 779
  endothelium and
    exfoliation syndrome and, 999
    nonfiltering trabecular meshwork
      and, 43
    pigment and, 982
    posterior polymorphous dystrophy
      and, 28
    proliferation and, 1324-1325
    staining of, 23-24
  epithelium and
    exfoliation syndrome and, 999
    Fuchs' endothelial dystrophy and,
      977-978
    ingrowth and, 1305
    iridocorneal epithelial syndrome
      and, 963-973
    pigment and, 982
    posterior polymorphous dystrophy
      and, 974-977
  exfoliation syndrome and, 998-999
  fibrous ingrowth and, 1322, 1323-1324
  ghost cell glaucoma and, 1245
  intraocular lens implantation and, 1289
  iridocorneal epithelial syndrome and,
    964, 965, 967, 973
  laser iridectomy and, 591, 594
  leukoma and, 897
  Meesman's dystrophy and, 781
  megalocornea and, 766-767
  mesodermal dysgenesis of; see Axen-
    feld-Rieger syndrome
  microcornea and, 941, 943
  penetrating keratoplasty and, 1344
  Peters' anomaly and, 25, 28, 897, 899,
    900
  posterior polymorphous dystrophy
    and, 974
  reflectivity and, 339-340
  sclerocornea and, 949-951
  staphyloma and, 940
  stromal development and, 22
Cornea guttata, 977
Cornea plana, 940-941
Corneal edema
  acute angle-closure glaucoma and, 841
  argon laser peripheral iridoplasty and,
    598

Corneal edema—cont'd
  congenital glaucoma and, 784
  laser iridectomy and, 590
Corneoplasty, 625-626
Corneoscleral incision, 704
Corneoscleral limbus, 21; see Limbus
Corneoscleral meshwork, 16, 18, 45
Corneoscleral suture, 1267
Corneotrabeculodysgenesis, 766-767
Corpuscle, sensory, 267
Corrected loss variance, 383
Corrected pattern standard deviation,
  451
Cortex, lens
  extracapsular extraction and, 678-679
  retained, 1021-1023
Corticosteroid-induced glaucoma, 1161-
  1168; see also Steroid
  arthritis and, 1218
  episcleritis and, 1189
  open-angle glaucoma and, 1270
  outflow pathway and, 67
  scleritis and, 1197, 1199
  uveitis-induced glaucoma and, 1294
Corticotropin, 1173-1174
Cortisol, 231
Coumadin; see Dicumarol
Counseling, genetic, 881
Coupler, output, 569
Cranial nerve, 268-269
Creeping angle-closure, 844
Crest, neural; see Neural crest
Cribiform cell, 46
Cribiform layer
  age and, 53
  ciliary muscle and, 231
  morphology and, 43-45
  outflow resistance and, 49-50
  pigmentary glaucoma and, 64, 67
  pseudoexfoliative glaucoma and, 64
Cribiform plate, 172-173, 176
Cryoablation, 635
Cryotherapy; see also Cyclocryotherapy
  ciliary body and, 731-734
  epithelial ingrowth and, 1317
  panretinal, 1094
Cryothermy, 1301
Crystal
  corneal, 934
  cytinosis and, 1151
Cup, optic
  angle-closure glaucoma and, 851-
    852
  congenital glaucoma and, 781
  Cushing's syndrome and, 1142
  development of, 7, 8
  disc rim and, 496-497
  enlargement of, 470, 472
  infant eye and, 771, 778
  low-tension glaucoma and, 800, 803
  mechanism of, 172
  retinal detachment and, 1056
Cup-disc ratio, 495
  topography and, 505-506
Cupola distance, 405

Curettage, anterior chamber, 1313, 1316
Curve
 angle-closure glaucoma and, 827
 fluctuation and, 382-383
 learning, 426, 442
Cushing's syndrome, 1142-1143
Cuticular membrane, 1232
Cyclic adenosine monophosphate
 adrenergic receptors and, 524-525
 beta-adrenergic agents, 530, 532
 trabecular meshwork and, 225
Cyclitis
 Fuchs' heterochromic, 1209-1211
 neovascular glaucoma and, 1090
 rubeosis iridis and, 1069
 recurrent mild, 1211
Cyclizine, 1171, 1172
Cycloablation
 endophotocoagulation, 737-738
 transpupillary laser, 737
 transscleral laser, 735-737
Cyclocryotherapy, 731-734
 aniridia and, 882
 aphakia and, 1280
 chemical burn and, 1235
 neovascular glaucoma and, 1098-1099
 open-angle glaucoma and, 819
 pseudophakic glaucoma and, 1295
Cyclodestructive surgery, 729-740
 congenital glaucoma and, 784
 cyclocryotherapy and; see Cyclocryotherapy
 cyclodiathermy and, 730-731
 history and, 729-730
 laser and, 735-738
 surgical excision and, 738
 ultrasound and, 734-735
Cyclodialysis
 aphakia and, 1280
 argon laser closure of cleft and, 627-
  628
 cataract extraction and, 702
 hypotony and, 284-285
 open-angle glaucoma and, 819
 pseudophakic glaucoma and, 1295
 uveoscleral outflow and, 246
Cyclodiathermy, 730-731
Cyclopentolate, 1176
 intraocular pressure and, 303
 uveitis and, 1208
Cyclophotocoagulation
 Nd:YAG transscleral, 622-623
 neovascular glaucoma and, 1099-
  1100
 transpupillary argon laser, 621-622
 open-angle glaucoma and, 819
Cycloplegia
 angle-closure glaucoma and, 857, 859
 bucking procedure and, 1053
 central retinal vein occlusion and,
  1050, 1148
 ciliochoroidal detachment and, 286
 filtration surgery and, 671
 lens dislocation and, 1036
 lens-induced glaucoma and, 1023

Cycloplegia—cont'd
 malignant glaucoma and, 1256, 1261
 pseudophakic glaucoma and, 1294
 uveitis and, 1207, 1208
 vitreous surgery and, 1261
Cyst
 epithelial, 1300-1303
 iris, 520; see also Epithelium, proliferation of
 Tenon's capsule, 685-687
Cystathionine beta-synthase deficiency,
  1040
Cystic bleb, 637
Cystic macular degeneration, 946
Cystinosis, 934, 1151
Cytochalasin
 aqueous humor and, 231
 outflow resistance and, 226, 228
Cytoplasm, 109

D

D-15 test, 189
Dark adaptation, 186, 187
Dark room test, 861-862
Daylight vision, 365
Decibel versus apostilb, 381
Decompression, vortex vein, 1050
Defect; see Anomaly
Degeneration, retinal, 946
deGrouchy's syndrome, 932
Deletion, chromosome 18 and, 932
Dellen, corneal, 687
Demecarium bromide, 519
Dendritic field of ganglion cell synapse,
  89
Dental-ocular-cutaneous syndrome, 935
Depolarization, membrane, 213
Dermatitis, atopic, 934
Dermatoarthritis, 935
Dermatologic disorder, 1156
Descemetization, 1324-1329
Descemet's membrane
 anterior trabecular meshwork and,
  43
 congenital glaucoma and, 773
 detachment and, 682
 development of, 9
 epithelial ingrowth and, 1316-1317
 fibrous ingrowth and, 1324
 Fuchs' dystrophy and, 977
 gonioscopy and, 351, 713
 obstetrical trauma and, 779
 Peters' anomaly and, 897, 898, 899
 posterior polymorphous dystrophy
  and, 975
 Schwalbe's line and, 20
 tears of, 784
Descemet's tubes, 1325
Desmosome, 87-88
Detachment
 choroidal
  angle-closure glaucoma after cataract extraction and, 1276
  filtration surgery and, 684
 ciliary body, 282, 284

Detachment—cont'd
 ciliochoroidal, 285-286
 Descemet's membrane, 682
 posterior vitreous, 1275
 retinal; see Retinal detachment
 scleral, 1053
Developmental disorder, 867-960
 angle anomaly and, 610-611
 aniridia and, 869-883; see also Aniridia
 Axenfeld-Rieger syndrome and, 885-896
 congenital disorders and, 931-960; see
  also Congenital disorder
 embryologic basis for, 23-37
 Peter's anomaly and, 897-903
 phakomatosis and, 905-929; see also
  Phakomatosis
Developmental glaucoma, 752; see also
  Congenital glaucoma
Dexamethasone
 angle-closure glaucoma and, 858
 aqueous humor and, 231
 trabecular meshwork and, 172
Dextran, 243, 244
Diabetes mellitus, 1143; see also Diabetic
  retinopathy
 neovascular glaucoma and; see Neo-
  vascular glaucoma
 pupillary block and, 648
Diabetic retinopathy
 photocoagulation and, 1051
 pituitary ablation and, 1100
 prophylaxis and, 1091
Dialysate of plasma, 200
Diamox; see Acetazolamide
Diarrhea, 520
Diathermy, 730-731
Diazepam, 302
Dibenamine; see Dibenzylchlorethamine
Dibenzoxepin, 1170
Dibenzylchlorethamine, 1175
Dibucaine, 520
Dichlorphenamide, 543
Dicon perimeter, 404
Dicumarol, 657
Diencephalon, 270-271
Diet in homocystinuria, 1040
Diffuse congenital hemangiomatosis, 924
Diffuse scleritis, 1191
Diffusion, 244
Digilab perimeter, 404
Digital ocular massage, 674
Digitalis, 1174
5β-Dihydrocortisol, 1164
Diisopropyl fluorophosphate, 519
Dilation
 exfoliation syndrome and, 1011
 pupillary, 1207
 trabeculectomy and, 667
Dilator muscle, 829-830
Diltiazem, 1174
Dimenhydrinate, 1171
Diphenhydramine, 1171, 1172
Dipivefrin
 miotic-induced angle-closure glau-
  coma and, 860

Dipivefrin—cont'd
  open-angle glaucoma and, 816
Diplopia, 590
Dipyridamole, 657
Direct gonioscopy, 346, 347
Disc; see Optic disc
Discrimination testing, 188-189
Dislocation, lens, 1028, 1030-1042
  blunt trauma and, 1228
Disopyramide phosphate, 1174
Disseminated hamartomatosis; see
    Phakomatosis
Dissolution of iris, 972-973
Diurnal pressure variation; see Circadian
    variation in intraocular pressure
Dominant aniridia, 869-873
Domperidone, 534
Donor button, 1340
Dopamine, 258, 1172, 1175
Dopamine receptor antagonist, 534
Dopaminergic drug
  adrenergic receptors and, 523-525
  intraocular pressure and, 531-532
Down's syndrome, 932-933
Doxepin, 1171
Doxylamine, 1172
Draeger applanation tonometer, 308
Drainage device
  congenital glaucoma and, 784
  neovascular glaucoma and, 1096-
    1098
Dressing, 670
Dropsy, epidemic, 1179-1180
Drug
  adrenergic, 523-537; see also Adrener-
    gic agonist; Beta-adrenergic block-
    ing agent
  aqueous flow and, 231-232, 342
  carbonic anhydrase inhibitors and; see
    Carbonic anhydrase inhibitor
  cataract extraction and, 699
  cholinergic agents and, 515-521
    aniridia and, 881
    aphakia and, 1279
    pseudophakic glaucoma and, 1294
  episcleral venous pressure and, 1130-
    1131
  hyperosmotic agent and; see Hyperos-
    motic agent
  intraocular pressure and, 302-303
  nonsteroidal, 1169-1184; see also Non-
    steroidal drug
  open-angle glaucoma and, 815
  steroid and; see Steroid
  uveoscleral outflow and, 245-246
  wound healing and, 637-638
Drumhead technique, 585
D-tubocurarine, 302
Dynamic Seidel test, 1313, 1314
Dyscephalic mandibulooculofacial syn-
    drome, 935
Dysgenesis
  iridotrabecular, 708, 710
  mesodermal; see Axenfeld-Rieger syn-
    drome

Dysplasia
  encephaloophthalmic, 936
  oculodentodigital, 938
    Axenfeld-Rieger syndrome versus,
      894
Dysrhythmic agent, 1174
Dystrophy
  endothelial
    congenital glaucoma and, 779
    Peters' anomaly and, 900
  familial renal-retinal, 939
  Fuchs', 977
  Meesman's corneal, 781
  myotonic, 286-287
  posterior amorphous corneal, 976
  posterior polymorphous, 28-31, 974-
    977
    Axenfeld-Rieger syndrome versus,
      894
    congenital glaucoma and, 779

E
Echothiophate, 519, 1176
  cataract extraction and, 699
  filtration surgery and, 657
Ectoderm, 3
  upper lid and, 23
Ectopia lentis, 1028, 1030-1042
Ectopia lentis et pupillae, 1033
  Axenfeld-Rieger syndrome versus,
    895
Ectropion uveae
  Axenfeld-Rieger syndrome versus, 895
  congenital, 940
  epithelial ingrowth and, 1310
  neovascular glaucoma and, 1063
  Prader-Willi syndrome and, 934
Eczema, 934
Edema
  cataract extraction and, 1267
  corneal; see Corneal edema
  optic disc and, 287
EDTA, 229
Edward's syndrome, 932
Effusion
  choroidal
    encephalotrigeminal angiomatosis
      and, 920
    posterior scleritis and, 1201-1202
  uveal, 1049-1050
Ehlers-Danlos syndrome, 1041
Eight-ball hyphema, 1244
Elasticity, 829
Elastic-like fiber, 53
Elastin
  characteristics of, 164-165
  lamina cribrosa and, 173, 176
  trabecular beams and, 171
Elastosis, 1008
Electrical injury, 1236
Electrical response, 193
Electrocautery, 920
Electromagnetic radiation, 567, 570
Electron, 568
Electrophysiology, 191-193

Electrophysiology—cont'd
  ganglion cell and, 89, 91-92
Electroretinogram, 191-193
Electroshock therapy, 302
Elschnig's membrane, 105
Embolism, 1040
Embryology of anterior segment, 3-40
Embryonic tissue in neurofibromatosis,
    911-912
Embryotoxon, 351
Emissarial channel, 241-242
Emission, stimulated, 568
Encephalofacial hemangiomatosis, 1123
Encephaloophthalmic dysplasia, 936
Encephalotrigeminal angiomatosis, 913-
    920
Endarterectomy, carotid, 1088
Endocrine disorder, 1141-1147
Endocrine cells, 266
Endoderm, 3
Endophotocoagulation
  cycloablation and, 737-738
  neovascular glaucoma and, 1093-1094
  vitrectomy and, 622
Endophthalmitis
  external wound leaks and, 282
  filtration surgery and, 685, 686
  Horner's syndrome and, 270
Endothelial bud, 1073
Endothelium
  Axenfeld-Rieger syndrome and, 25,
    893
  basement membrane and, 1008
  capillary, 92
  corneal; see Cornea, endothelium and
  descemetization and, 1324-1329
  development of, 12
  dystrophy and
    hereditary congenital, 779
    Peters' anomaly and, 900
  extracellular matrix of cribriform
    plates and, 176
  intraorbital optic nerve and, 114, 115
  iridocorneal endothelial syndrome
    and; see Iridocorneal endothelial
    syndrome
  laser burn and, 591
  mucopolysaccharidosis and, 67, 69
  neovascular glaucoma and, 1070
  pigmentary glaucoma and, 987
  Schlemm's canal and, 14, 46, 50-51
  Sturge-Weber syndrome and, 31
  trabecular meshwork and, 16, 225-226
    beta-adrenergic agonists and, 530
    morphology and, 43-45
    origin of, 23
  vascular, 527, 530
Enolase
  neuron-specific, 23
  trabecular meshwork and, 221-222
Ephedrine, 1175
Epidemic dropsy, 1179-1180
Epinephrine, 1175
  adrenergic mechanism and, 224
  aphakia and, 1278-1279

Epinephrine—cont'd
  aqueous humor and, 270, 342
  cataract extraction and, 699
  chemical burn and, 1234
  denervation and, 529
  episcleral venous pressure and, 1131
  indomethacin and, 560
  low-tension glaucoma and, 809
  maculopathy and, 815-816
  miotic-induced angle-closure glau-
    coma and, 860
  open-angle glaucoma and, 529-530
  pigmentary glaucoma and, 993
  pseudophakic glaucoma and, 1294
  retrobulbar block and, 658-659
  sickle cell hemoglobinopathy and,
    1153
  trabecular meshwork and, 225
  uveoscleral outflow and, 245-246
Epiphora, 779, 781
Episclera, 919
  vasculitis and, 1197
Episcleral venous pressure, 249-256,
    1127-1140
  anatomy and, 1127-1128
  hypotony and, 281
  increased, 1131-1137
  measurement of, 1128-1130
  pathophysiology and, 1130
  pharmacologic agents, 1130-1131
  postural change, 1130
  tonography and, 293
Episcleritis, 1188-1190
Epithelial cell
  cornea and, 8
  retinal pigment, 1092
Epithelial cyst, 1300-1303
Epithelial downgrowth, 1291
Epithelial ingrowth, 1303-1320
  clinical findings and, 1303-1305
  diagnosis and, 1313, 1316
  histopathology and, 1305-1310
  incidence of, 1303
  management and, 1317-1320
  mechanism of glaucoma and, 1313
  open-angle glaucoma and, 1271
  pathogenesis and, 1310-1313
    trauma and, 1232
Epithelium
  aqueous humor transport and, 213
  ciliary
    aqueous humor and, 41
    ATPase and, 206-210
    tumors of, 1121-1123
    ultrastructure of, 85-90
  conjunctival, 22-23
  ingrowth and; see Epithelial ingrowth
  iris pigment, 1236
  laser iridectomy and, 587, 591
  Peters' anomaly and, 898
  pigmentary
    ciliary body and, 86
    NA/K-ATPase and, 206-207
    tumors of, 1123
  proliferation of, 1299-1320

Epithelium—cont'd
  proliferation of—cont'd
    anticholinesterase and, 520
    epithelial cysts, 1300-1303
    historical review and, 1299-1300
    ingrowth and, 1303-1320; see also
      Epithelial ingrowth
    pearl tumors and, 1300
  tumors of, 1123
Epsilon aminocaproic acid, 1225
Equation, Goldmann's, 1130
ERG; see Electroretinogram
Erythrocyte
  ghost cell glaucoma and; see also
    Ghost cell glaucoma
  sickle cell hemoglobinopathy and,
    1153
  trabecular meshwork and, 229
Eserine, 1176
Eskimos, 834
Estrogen, 1178
Ethanol, 815
Ethanolamine, 1171
Ethoxzolamide
  pharmacology and, 543
  topical, 545, 547
Ethyl alcohol, 553
Ethylenediamine, 1171
Evoked potential, 193
Evoked response, 1293
Excavation, disc, 505-506
Exercise, intraocular pressure and, 302
Exfoliation syndrome
  argon laser trabeculoplasty and, 610
  clinical picture and, 998-1005
  epidemiology and, 997-998
  glaucoma mechanism and, 1008-1011
  history of, 997
  management and, 1011
  pathophysiology and, 1005-1008
  posterior chamber intraocular lens
    and, 679
Exophthalmos, 909
Explant, 746-747
Expulsive hemorrhage
  encephalotrigeminal angiomatosis
    and, 920
  filtration surgery and, 682, 683
Extracapsular lens extraction
  diabetic retinopathy and, 1086
  filtration and, 677, 678
  intraocular lens implantation and,
    1289
  intraocular pressure and, 698
  nanophthalmos and, 1050
  peripheral iridectomy and, 648
  phacolytic glaucoma and, 1021
Extracellular matrix, 163-178
  characteristics of, 163-164
  crest cells and, 5-6
  macromolecules of, 164-166
  optic nerve head and, 172-177
  trabecular meshwork and, 166-172
Extraction of lens
  dislocated, 1042

Extraction of lens—cont'd
  extracapsular; see Extracapsular lens
    extraction
  intracapsular; see Intracapsular lens
    extraction
Extraocular anomaly, 889-890
Extraocular optic nerve, 113-119
Extravascular water, 201
Eyelid
  development of, 22-23
  hemangioma and, 1133-1134
  intraocular pressure and, 302

F
Facial anhidrosis, 270
Facial nerve
  filtration surgery and, 658
  intraocular pressure and, 268-269
Facial vein, 1127
Factor VIII-related antigen, 23-24
False negative response in automated
    perimetry, 403-404
Familial disease; see Hereditary disorder
Family history, 803
Far-field pattern ERG response, 193
Farnsworth-Munsell 100-hue test, 189
Fazadinium, 302
Fetal alcohol syndrome, 935
Fever, hemorrhagic, 1155
Fiber
  adrenergic nerve, 258
  collagen; see Collagen
  elastin and, 164-165
  nerve; see Nerve fiber
  zonular
    ectopia lentis and, 1031
    pigmentary glaucoma and, 982
Fiber plexus, cribriform, 49-50
Fiberoptic delivery system, 576
Fibril
  primary open-angle glaucoma and, 55
  pseudoexfoliative glaucoma and, 64, 65
Fibrillopathica epitheliocapsularis, 997
Fibrinolysin inhibitor, 1225
Fibroblast
  ciliary muscle and, 47
  exfoliation syndrome and, 1008
  extracellular matrix of cribriform
    plates and, 176
  lamina scleralis and, 111
  scleral, 22
  wound healing and, 638
Fibroblastoid cell, 176
Fibroelastic ligament, 176
Fibronectin
  characteristics of, 165
  crest cells and, 5-6
  Schlemm's canal and, 46
Fibrosis
  argon laser trabeculoplasty and, 615
  failure of bleb formation and, 676
Fibrous ingrowth, 1321-1324
Fibrous membrane, 596
Fibrous proliferation, 1271
Fibrovascular membrane, 1067, 1073

Field; *see* Visual field
Fifth cranial nerve, 268
Filament, 87
Filamentous collagen, 164
Filtering bleb; *see* Bleb
Filtering trabecular meshwork; *see* Trabecular meshwork
Filtration surgery, 653-696
  angle-closure glaucoma and nanophthalmos and, 1050
  aniridia and, 882
  aphakia and, 1279
  argon laser trabeculoplasty and, 610
  cataract and, 698-699, 701-702
  chemical burn and, 1235
  choroidal separation and, 1253-1254
  complications and, 682-687
  congenital glaucoma and, 783
  corticosteroid-induced glaucoma and, 1165
  episcleral venous pressure and, 1137
  history of, 653-654
  hypotony and, 282
  indications for, 654
  intraocular lens implantation and, 1286
  iridectomy and; *see* Iridectomy
    acute angle-closure glaucoma and, 859
  iridocorneal epithelial syndrome and, 973, 977
  low-tension glaucoma and, 809
  modifications to, 672-676
  neovascular glaucoma and, 1095-1096, 1096-1098
  objectives of, 654-655
  open-angle glaucoma and, 819
  other surgery combined with, 677-681
  patient evaluation and, 655-656
  preoperative preparation for, 656-659
  pseudophakic glaucoma and, 1295
  reopening of fistula and, 623-624
  seton and, 741-748
  syphilis and, 1214
  trabeculectomy and; *see* Trabeculectomy
  uveitis and, 1209
  wound healing and, 634-639
Fistula
  arteriovenous, 1132-1133
    Klippel-Trenaunay-Weber syndrome and, 920
  reopening of, 623-624
  sclerotomy and cataract extraction and, 704
  subconjunctival, 647
  wound and, 282, 637
Fixation
  automated perimetry and, 403-404
  visual field testing and, 368
Flake, glaucoma, 850-851
Flap
  conjunctival, 715
  lamellar scleral, 718, 721

Flap—cont'd
  scleral, 682
Flare, aqueous
  cyclodialysis and, 284
  iridocyclitis and, 282
Flat anterior chamber
  argon laser peripheral iridoplasty and, 598
  conventional iridectomy and, 647
  filtration surgery and, 673
  hypotony and, 684
Floater, 1056
Fluctuation
  automated perimetry and, 404
  scatter versus, 382-384
Fluid
  aqueous humor and; *see* Aqueous humor
  sclerotomy and, 1258-1259
  suprachoroidal, 285-286
Fluorescein
  angle-closure glaucoma and, 1276
  aqueous flow by, 337-344
  blood supply studies and, 133-161; *see also* Blood flow, optic nerve and
  epithelial ingrowth and, 1304
  fluorophotometry and, 337-344
  neovascular glaucoma and, 1070-1071
  optic nerve head and, 505
  quantitative studies and, 507
  uveoscleral outflow and, 243, 244
Fluorescent lifetime, 568
Fluoromethalone, 1207
Fluorophotometry; *see* Fluorescein
5-Fluorouracil
  fibroblast and, 673
  filtering surgery and, 639
  neovascular glaucoma and, 1098
Fluphenazine, 1170
Foreign body
  exfoliation syndrome and, 1009, 1011
  penetrating injury and, 1232-1233
Fornix-based conjunctival flap
  congenital glaucoma and, 721-725
  sclerotomy and cataract extraction and, 704
  trabeculectomy and, 663-667, 669
Four-mirror gonioscopy, 348, 831, 833, 834
Fovea, 89
Framingham Eye Study
  blood pressure and, 1151
  exfoliation syndrome and, 997
  low-tension glaucoma and, 805
Francois dyscephalic syndrome, 935
Freezing; *see* Cryotherapy; Cyclocryotherapy
5-FU; *see* 5-Fluorouracil
Fuchs' endothelial dystrophy, 977
Fuchs' heterochromic iridocyclitis
  neovascular glaucoma and, 1090
  rubeosis iridis and, 1069
Full-field test, 422
Full-thickness procedure, 819

Full-thresholding examination, 405, 412, 413
Functional testing
  basic elements of visual process and, 180-185
  electrophysiology and, 191-193
  psychophysics and, 185-191
Fundus photography, 495-496

G
Galanin, 260
Galanin-LI nerve fiber, 265
  ciliary body blood vessel and, 262
Gallamine, 302
Ganglion cell
  anatomy and pathophysiology of, 89-92
  axonal transport in retina and, 97-98
  ciliary, 257
  classification of, 181-183
  retina and, 364
    topographic anatomy and, 95
  superior cervical, 258
  trigeminal, 257
Gap junction
  ciliary epithelium and, 87-88
  optic nerve head neuroglia and, 105, 107
  Schlemm's canal and, 50
Gas, intravitreal, 1055
Gastrointestinal drug effect, 520
Gaze in thyrotropic ophthalmopathy, 1143
Gel, pilocarpine, 816; *see also* Pilocarpine
General anesthetic, 1177-1178
  congenital glaucoma and, 775
  filtration surgery and, 659
Genetic counseling, 881
Geniculate body, 119, 120
Genitourinary anomaly, 871
Germ-layer theory of development, 3
Ghost cell glaucoma, 1239-1247
  neovascular glaucoma and, 1070
  open-angle glaucoma and, 1270
  trauma and, 1228
Giant vacuole, 221
Gland
  lacrimal, 1215
  parotid, 1220
  pituitary, 889-890
  thyroid, 1135, 1137, 1143-1144
Glare
  conventional iridectomy and, 647
  laser iridectomy and, 590
Glassy cone, 1325
Glaucoma capsulare, 997
Glaucoma test, 408
Glaucomatocyclitic crisis, 1210, 1212-1213
Glaukomflecken, 850-851
Glial cell
  glaucoma and, 120
  intraorbital optic nerve and, 115
Glial neoplasm, 907, 909
Glial process, 107

Glioma, 1090
Global index, 383
Globe in Marfan syndrome, 1038
Glucocorticoid; *see also* Steroid
    aqueous humor and, 230-231
    Cushing's syndrome and, 1142-1143
    trabecular meshwork and, 172
Glucose
    diabetic retinopathy and, 1085
    neovascular glaucoma and, 1091
Glutamyl transpeptidase, 524-525
Glycemia
    diabetic retinopathy and, 1085
    neovascular glaucoma and, 1091
Glycerine
    argon laser peripheral iridoplasty and,
        605-606
    pseudophakic glaucoma and, 1294
Glycerol
    ciliary block glaucoma and, 554
    malignant glaucoma and, 1256
    oral, 552
Glycoprotein, 6
Glycosaminoglycan
    angle-closure glaucoma and, 1049-1050
    characteristics of, 165
    glucocorticoid and, 1164
    lamina scleralis and, 111
    mucopolysaccharidosis and, 67
    trabecular meshwork and, 46, 171
Glycoside, cardiac, 213
Goldmann equation, 220, 1130
Goldmann lens
    indirect gonioscopy and, 347-348
    three-mirror, 606
Goldmann perimeter, 370-372
Goldmann tonometer, 304-307
Goniodysgenesis, 941
Gonioplasty, 596
Gonioscopy, 345-360
    anatomy and interpretation of, 351-354
    angle-closure glaucoma and, 831, 833,
        834
        acute, 857-858
        cataract extraction and, 1278
    Axenfeld-Rieger syndrome and, 888
    congenital glaucoma and, 776
    epithelial ingrowth and, 1305
    findings of, 356-358
    ghost cell glaucoma and, 1245
    grading angle depth of, 355-356
    indentation, 857-858, 859
    intraocular lens implantation and,
        1287, 1293
    lens-induced glaucoma and, 1028
    Marfan syndrome and, 1038
    methods of, 345-351
Goniosynechialysis, 859
Goniotomy
    aniridia and, 881-882
    congenital glaucoma and, 711-715,
        771, 781, 783
    encephalotrigeminal angiomatosis
        and, 920
    Nd:YAG laser, 617

Goniotomy—cont'd
    neurofibromatosis and, 913
    results of, 707
    Sturge-Weber syndrome and, 672-673
    uveitis and, 1209
G-protein, 523-525
Granule, pigment, 64
Granulomatous inflammation, 1023-
    1024
Graves' disease, 1143
Gray scale, 419, 420, 421, 424
Green
    color pairing and, 183-185
    glaucoma and, 190
Groove
    limbal, 677
    retinal nerve fiber layer and, 482
Ground substance, 111
Growth factor, 1313
Growth hormone, 1143-1144
GTP; *see* Glutamyl transpeptidase

H

Haab's striae, 976
Haag-Streit slit-lamp, 830-831
Haldol; *see* Haloperidol
Hallermann-Streiff syndrome, 935
Halo around light, 840
Haloperidol, 1170, 1171
    intraocular pressure and, 534
Halothane, 1177-1178
Hamartoma, 922
Hamartomatosis, 1123; *see also* Phakoma-
    tosis
Haptic, 1255, 1293
Harmartia, 919
Healing, 633-644
    inhibitor of, 783-784
Healon; *see* Hyaluronic acid
Heat conduction, 572
Heinz bodies, 1246
Hemangioma
    angiomatosis retinae and, 921, 922
    encephalotrigeminal angiomatosis
        and, 914, 915, 916
    Klippel-Trenaunay-Weber syndrome
        and, 920
    episcleral venous pressure and, 1133-
        1134
Hemangiomatosis
    diffuse congenital, 924
    encephalofacial, 1123
Hematologic disorder, 1152-1154
Hematoporphyrin derivative, 573
Hemodialysis, 1151
Hemodynamic crisis, 804
Hemoglobin
    ghost cell glaucoma and, 1241
    light absorption by, 574
    photocoagulation and, 576
    sickle cell, 1152-1154
Hemolytic glaucoma, 1246
Hemorrhage
    argon laser peripheral iridoplasty and,
        599

Hemorrhage—cont'd
    argon laser trabeculoplasty and,
        613
    choroid and
        encephalotrigeminal angiomatosis
            and, 920
        hemangioma and, 916
    chronic drug therapy and, 699
    episcleral venous pressure and, 1137
    fibrous ingrowth and, 1324
    goniotomy and, 715
    hyphema and; *see* Hyphema
    iridectomy and, 648
        laser, 594-595
    optic disc and, 476-478
        low-tension glaucoma and, 802
    retrobulbar, 682, 684
    suprachoroidal
        filtration surgery and, 682, 683
        sclerotomy and, 1258-1259
    vitreous, 1152
    wound healing and, 638
Hemorrhagic fever, 1155
Hemorrhagic glaucoma; *see* Neovascular
    glaucoma
Hemorrhagic retinopathy, 1078-1079
Hemosiderin, 1239, 1246
Hepatic dysfunction, 940
Hereditary disorder
    angioedema and, 935-936
    angle-closure glaucoma and, 834
    congenital glaucoma and, 767
    deep dystrophy of cornea and, 974
    ectopia lentis and, 1033-1036, 1038-
        1039
    endothelial dystrophy and, 779
    exfoliation syndrome and, 998
    intraocular pressure and, 302
    Klippel-Trenaunay-Weber syndrome
        and, 920
    ocular hypertension and, 792-793
    Peters' anomaly and, 897-898, 900
    pigmentary glaucoma and, 982
    progressive arthroophthalmopathy
        and, 939
    tuberous sclerosis and, 922
    Von-Hippel-Landau syndrome and,
        922
Herpes zoster, 1155-1156, 1219
Herpesvirus, 1218-1219
    keratitis and, 1203
    posterior cornea and, 974
Heterochromia, 1111
Heterochromic cyclitis, Fuchs', 1069,
    1090
Hexamethonium, 1173-1174, 1178
    trabecular meshwork and, 225
High intensity focused ultrasound, 734-
    735
Histamine, 1171-1172
Histidine isoleucine, 259
Histiocytic dermatoarthritis, 935
HLA-B27 antigen, 1216
Homatropine, 1176
    pigmentary glaucoma and, 992

Homatropine—cont'd
  uveitis and, 1207
Home tonometry, 312
  circadian variation and, 322
Homocystinuria, 1039-1041
Hormone, 1178
  antidiuretic, 553
  intraocular pressure and, 302
Horner's syndrome
  catecholamine and, 529
  cervical sympathetic denervation and, 270
HpD; see Hematoporphyrin derivative
Humphrey perimeter, 408
Humphrey visual field indices, 454, 462-466
Hyaloid, anterior, 1086, 1087
Hyaloidectomy, anterior, 1277
Hyaluronic acid, 1179
  extracellular matrix and, 165
  open-angle glaucoma and, 1268-1269
  pseudophakic glaucoma and, 1295
  trabecular meshwork and, 46, 171-172
Hyaluronidase
  filtration surgery and, 658
  outflow resistance and, 229
Hydralazine, 1173-1174, 1178
Hydraulic model of aqueous humor, 220
Hydrochlorothiazide, 1173, 1178
Hydrophthalmia, 763
Hydroxyamphetamine, 1175, 1176
Hyperchromic heterochromic, 1111
Hyperemia
  acute angle-closure glaucoma and, 841-842
  alpha-adrenergic antagonists and, 533
Hyperlysinemia, 1041
Hypermature cataract
  phacolytic glaucoma and, 1018
  trabecular meshwork and, 230
Hyperosmotic agent, 551-555; see also Osmotic agent
  angle-closure glaucoma and
    acute, 855
      cataract extraction and, 1276
  aqueous misdirection and, 685
  lens dislocation and, 1036
  pilocarpine and, 518
  sickle cell hemoglobinopathy and, 1153
  traumatic lens dislocation and, 1041
Hyperosmotic sodium gradient, 206-207
Hyperpigmentation
  dental-ocular-cutaneous syndrome and, 935
  oculodermal melanocystosis and, 922-924
Hyperplasia
  benign reactive lymphoid, 1123
  iris stroma and, 765
  primary vitreous and, 944-946
  vascular, 920
Hypertension
  ocular; see Intraocular pressure
  systemic

Hypertension—cont'd
  systemic—cont'd
    diabetic retinopathy and, 1085
    intraocular pressure and, 1151
    low-tension glaucoma and, 804
Hyperthyroidism, 1143
Hypertonic solution, 551
Hypertrophy, 920
Hyperviscosity syndrome, 1152
Hyphema
  blunt trauma and, 1225-1228
  conventional iridectomy and, 648
  filtration surgery and, 682
  ghost cell glaucoma and, 1244
  hyperosmotic agent and, 554
  open-angle glaucoma after cataract extraction and, 1269-1270
  retrocorneal membrane and, 1324
  sickle cell hemoglobinopathy and, 1153, 1154
Hypoperfusion, vascular, 984
Hypoplasia
  aniridia and, 879
  iris and, 894
Hypopyon, 685
Hypospadias, 890
Hypotensive response
  alpha-adrenergic antagonists and, 533
  pilocarpine and, 518
Hypothalamus, 271
Hypothyroidism, 1147
Hypotony, 281-290
  epithelial ingrowth and, 1313
  filtration surgery and, 684
  iris retraction syndrome and, 1051
  malignant glaucoma and, 1254
  myotonic dystrophy and, 1156
  neovascular glaucoma and, 1097, 1098-1099
Hypoxia, 1077

I
ICE; see Iridocorneal epithelial syndrome
I-Diodrast, 202-203
Idoxuridine, 1219
Illumination
  automated perimetry and, 404-405
  color testing and, 190
  retinal, 89, 91
Image analysis, computerized, 499-503
Image intensification, 496
Imidazoline derivative, 557-559
Imipramine, 1171
Immunocytochemical technique, 166
Immunohistochemistry
  chamber angle and, 263
  neuropeptides and, 258-259
Immunoreactive nerve fiber, 264-265
Immunosuppressive therapy, 1208
Implant, valve
  long glaucoma, 745-746
  Molteno, 744
    congenital glaucoma and, 784
    filtering surgery and, 639-640
    seton and, 725, 726

Implant, valve—cont'd
  pressure-sensitive unidirectional, 639
  neovascular glaucoma and, 1096-1098
  translimbal tube shunt and, 742-743
Implantation, lens, 1285-1297
  intraocular pressure and, 698
  pupillary block and, 648
Incarcerated iris
  goniotomy and, 715
  Peters' anomaly and, 900
  wound healing and, 638
Incision
  closure of, 721
  corneoscleral, 704
  laser iridectomy and, 586, 588
Indentation gonioscopy, 353-354
  angle-closure glaucoma and, 831, 833, 834
    acute, 857-858, 859
Indentation tonometry, Schiøtz, 303-304
Indirect gonioscopy, 346, 347-348
Indomethacin
  glaucomatocyclitic crisis and, 1212-1213
  laser iridectomy and, 595
  prostaglandin and, 560
Infant diagnostic lens, 774-775
Infantile glaucoma; see also Congenital glaucoma
  definition of, 762
  trabecular meshwork and, 34
Infection
  bleb and, 685, 686
  corneal, 1203
  intrauterine, 899
  viral, 1155-1156
Inferior ophthalmic vein, 1127
Inflammation; see also Uveitis
  angle-closure glaucoma and, 858
  aphakia and, 1279
  epithelial cyst and, 1301
  epithelial ingrowth and, 1312
  fibrous ingrowth and, 1322
  gonioscopy and, 356
  granulomatous, 1023-1024
  laser iridectomy and, 594
  lens implantation and, 1291
  neovascular glaucoma and, 1077
  open-angle glaucoma and, 1270
  pseudophakic glaucoma versus, 1294
  retrobulbar, 1143
  rubeosis iridis and, 1069-1070
  trauma and, 1228
  wound healing and, 635-636
Influenza, 1156
Informed consent, 655
Infrared radiation, 572, 573
Ingrowth
  epithelial; see Epithelial ingrowth
  fibrous, 1321-1324
Inhaler, 1175
Injection
  alcohol, 1100
  steroid, 1163, 1165, 1207

Insertion, iris
  congenital glaucoma and, 776
  trabeculodysgenesis and, 763-764
Insulin-dependent diabetes, 1083, 1085
Intensity
  color testing and, 190
  perimetry and, 370-372
  stimulus, 405
  test object, 379
Intercellular communication, 525
Intercellular epithelial junction, 87-88, 89
Interconnecting cell, 364
Interface, optical, 339-340
Intermittent angle-closure glaucoma,
    839-840
  treatment of, 860
Internal block excision, 666-667
Internal block incision, 679
Internal carotid artery; see Carotid artery
Interstimulus time, 405
Interstitial keratitis
  congenital syphilis and, 1214
  syphilis and, 1213
Interstitial matrix, 163-164
Intestinal polypeptide, vasoactive, 259
Intracapsular lens extraction
  diabetic retinopathy and, 1086
  phacolytic glaucoma and, 1021
  pupillary block and, 1271
Intractable glaucoma, 1313
Intramuscular circle, 81
Intraocular bleeding; see Hemorrhage
Intraocular inflammation; see Inflamma-
    tion; Uveitis
Intraocular lens; see Lens
Intraocular pressure, 301-318
  angle-closure glaucoma after cataract
    extraction and, 1276
  aphakia and, 1266-1268
  blood pressure and, 200, 1151
  carotid artery occlusive disease and,
    1088
  carotid sinus-cavernous sinus fistula
    and, 1132
  central retinal vein occlusion and,
    1081-1082, 1147
  chemical burn and, 1234
  chronic angle-closure glaucoma and,
    844
  ciliary body and, 84
  circadian variation in, 319-336; see also
    Circadian variation in intraocular
    pressure
  color testing and, 190-191
  congenital glaucoma and, 769-770
    diagnosis of, 775
  corticosteroid-induced glaucoma and,
    1161-1165
  cyclocryotherapy and, 734
    neovascular glaucoma and, 1098-
    1099
  deformation of optic nerve head and,
    506
  diurnal curve of; see Circadian varia-
    tion in intraocular pressure

Intraocular pressure—cont'd
  drug therapy and, 515-566; see also
    Drug
  encephalotrigeminal angiomatosis
    and, 916, 919
  endocrine disorder and, 1141-1147
  epidemiology of, 789-795
  episcleral venous pressure and, 250,
    1130
  exfoliation syndrome and, 1003, 1005
  factors influencing, 301-303
  filtration surgery and, 687
  foreign body and, 1232-1233
  Fuchs' dystrophy and, 977
  ghost cell glaucoma and, 1239, 1244-
    1245
  glaukomflecken and, 850
  hemodialysis and, 1151
  hypotony and, 281-290
  increased pallor and, 507
  infant eye and, 770-771
  intraocular lens implantation and,
    1287
  iridectomy and, 859
    laser, 587, 595, 612
  low-tension glaucoma and, 803-804
  malignant glaucoma and, 1253
  Nd:YAG laser posterior capsulotomy
    and, 1021-1022
  neovascular glaucoma and, 1069
  nervous system and, 257-279
  open-angle glaucoma and, 813, 814-
    815
    aphakia and, 1266-1268
  penetrating keratoplasty and, 1345-
    1346
  phacolytic glaucoma and, 1018, 1019,
    1020
  pigmentary glaucoma and, 983, 985
  pilocarpine and, 518
  retinal blood flow and, 95
  retinal detachment and, 1048-1049
  sickle cell trait and, 1152-1153, 1154
  tonography and, 291
  trabecular block and, 1205-1206
  trabeculectomy and, 673
  trabeculoplasty and, 609
  trauma and, 1225-1237, 1230
  uveoscleral outflow and, 245
Intraocular tumor, 1111-1124; see Tumor
Intrascleral vessel, 1128
Intrauterine infection, 899
Intravenous hyperosmotic agent, 553
Intraventricular perfusion study, 271-272
Inulin, 202
Invaginated gap junction, 88
Invagination, 221
Ion laser photocoagulator, 578
Ion transport, 213
Ionizing effect of laser, 575
Ionophore, 287
I-Rayopake, 202-203
Iridectomy
  acute angle-closure glaucoma and,
    858-859, 860

Iridectomy—cont'd
  central retinal vein occlusion, 1148
  conventional, 645-651
  haptics of intraocular lens and, 1255
  laser; see Laser iridectomy
  malignant glaucoma and, 1258, 1262
  neovascular glaucoma and, 1096
  new vessels around, 1064
  peripheral
    internal block and, 679
    lens implantation and, 1290-1291
  prophylactic, 860
  pseudophakic glaucoma and, 1295
  pupillary block and, 1254
  retinopathy of prematurity and, 947,
    949
  scleral buckling procedure and, 1053
  trabeculectomy and, 723
  uveitis and, 1209
  vitreous in, 1279
  wound healing and, 633
Iridencleisis, 677
Iridociliary exfoliation, 997
Iridocorneal adhesion
  epithelial syndrome and, 977
  Peters' anomaly and, 897
Iridocorneal angle, 349, 351
Iridocorneal endothelial syndrome, 28,
    29, 963-973
  argon laser trabeculoplasty and, 611
  Axenfeld-Rieger syndrome versus, 894
Iridocyclitis
  exfoliation syndrome and, 1009
  hypotony and, 282-284
  uveoscleral outflow and, 246
Iridolenticular apposition, 1027
Iridoplasty
  acute angle-closure glaucoma and,
    858, 859
  argon laser peripheral, 596-600
Iridoschisis, 941
  angle-closure glaucoma and, 849-850
  Axenfeld-Rieger syndrome versus, 895
  iridocorneal epithelial syndrome and,
    972-973
Iridotrabecular dysgenesis, 708
  congenital glaucoma and, 764-766
Iridotrabecular meshwork, 18
Iridotrabecular-corneal dysgenesis, 708,
    710
Iridovitreal block, 1254
Iris
  adhesion and, 1206
  adrenergic mechanism and, 224
  alpha-adrenergic receptor and, 558
  angle-closure glaucoma and, 828-829,
    848-850
    chronic, 844
  aniridia and, 869-884; see also Aniridia
  aqueous humor and, 41-42
  Axenfeld-Rieger syndrome and, 888-
    889, 890
  biopsy and, 1313
  congenital glaucoma and, 776
  congenital hypoplasia and, 894

Iris—cont'd
  development of, 10
  epithelial ingrowth and, 1305, 1308-
      1309, 1313
  exfoliation syndrome and, 1000-1001
  fibrous ingrowth and, 1322
  heterochromia and, 1209-1210
  incarceration and
      goniotomy and, 715
      Peters' anomaly and, 900
      wound and, 638, 1323
  intraocular lens implantation and,
      1289
  Marfan syndrome and, 1038
  melanocytoma and, 1116, 1117
  melanoma and, 1111-1113
  mesodermal dysgenesis of; see Axen-
      feld-Rieger syndrome
  metastasis and, 1117-1118
  neovascular glaucoma and, 1063-1110;
      see also Neovascular glaucoma
  pigment epithelium and, 1236
  pigmentary glaucoma and, 64, 981-995
  plateau, 845-846
      treatment of, 861
  primary open-angle glaucoma and, 58
  retraction syndrome and, 1051
  stroma hyperplasia and, 765
  structural defect of, 766
  Sturge-Weber syndrome and, 31
  thrombosis and, 1155
  trabecular meshwork and, 18-20
  trabeculodysgenesis and, 764
Iris bombé
  chronic angle-closure glaucoma and,
      843
  ectopia lentis and, 1031
  lens-induced glaucoma and, 1027,
      1028
  pseudophakia and, 1254
  cyst and, 1299-1320; see also Epithe-
      lium, proliferation of
Iris nevus syndrome, 963, 971, 972
Iris plane implant, 1294-1295
Iris retraction syndrome, 286
Iritis
  argon laser peripheral iridoplasty and,
      599
  argon laser pupilloplasty and, 626
  argon laser trabeculoplasty and, 613
  exfoliation syndrome and, 1009
Irradiance, 571
Irradiation, 1155, 1235-1236
Irrigation of anterior chamber, 1245
Ischemia, 1147-1151
  autoregulation of blood supply and,
      136
      cerebrovascular disease and, 1148
      chronic ocular, 1088
  optic neuropathy and, 807
      posterior ciliary artery and, 137-156
  retinal, 1078-1079
Island of vision, 439
  Traquair's, 368
Isoflurophate, 1176

Isoleucine, 259
Isoproterenol
  aqueous flow and, 342
  intraocular pressure and, 530
Isopter, 366, 367
  contraction of, 394
  intermediate, 372
  scatter and, 382
Isosorbide
  acute angle-closure glaucoma and, 855
  argon laser peripheral iridoplasty and,
      605-606
  malignant glaucoma and, 1256
  oral, 552
  transitory secondary glaucoma and,
      554

J
Jacoby's border tissue, 111
Juvenile glaucoma; see also Congenital
      glaucoma
  argon laser trabeculoplasty and, 610-
      611
  definition of, 762
Juvenile rheumatoid arthritis, 1217
Juxtacanalicular tissue
  development of, 12
  trabecular meshwork and, 166-167,
      171
      morphology and, 43-45

K
Kanamycin, 1174
Keratitis, 1202-1203
  congenital syphilis and, 1214
Keratitis bullosa interna, 974
Keratocyte
  Peters' anomaly and, 898
  sclera and, 22
  staining of, 23-24
Keratolenticular adherence, 897
Keratopathy, band, 1304-1305
Keratoplasty, penetrating, 1337-1347
  filtration surgery and, 681
  iridocorneal epithelial syndrome and,
      973
Keratouveitis, 1203
  herpes simplex, 1218-1219
Ketamine, 1177-1178
  congenital glaucoma and, 711, 775
Khaki colored cells, 1243-1244, 1246
Kidney
  familial renal-retinal dystrophy and,
      939
  polycystic, 940
Kinetic perimetry, 186
  algorithm for, 378-379
  benefits and inaccuracies of, 373-
      374
  history and, 361
  static perimetry versus, 368
Klippel-Trenaunay-Weber syndrome,
      920-921
Knife, goniotomy, 713-714
Koeppe gonioscopy, 1009

Krause's syndrome, 936
Krupin-Denver implant, 1097-1098
Krypton photocoagulator, 577
Kuhnt's border tissue of, 111

L
Lacrimal gland, 1215
Lactose, 551
Lamella, 173
Lamellar scleral flap, 718, 721
Lamina, 120, 123
Lamina choroidalis, 103, 109
Lamina cribrosa
  baring of, 472, 474
  blood supply and, 133
  extracellular matrix and, 172, 172-177
  intraocular pressure and, 506
Lamina scleralis, 111-112
  anatomy and pathophysiology of, 103
Laminin, 165
Landsliding, 590
Laser, 565-629
  aniridia and, 882
  argon; see Argon laser
  aphakia and, 1279
  Axenfeld-Rieger syndrome and, 895
  carbon dioxide
      filtration surgery and, 672
      neovascular glaucoma and, 1095
  ciliary body destruction and, 735-738
  encephalotrigeminal angiomatosis
      and, 920
  epithelial cyst and, 1303
  exfoliation syndrome and, 1011
  filtration surgery and, 654
      fistula and, 623-624
  iridectomy and, 581-596; see also Laser
      iridectomy
  malignant glaucoma and, 1256-1257
  Nd:YAG; see Nd:YAG laser
  open-angle glaucoma and, 605-620
  peripheral iridoplasty and, 596-600
      scleral buckling procedure and,
          1053
  photocoagulation and; see Photocoagu-
      lation
  physics and, 567-580
  pupilloplasty, 625-626
      cataract extraction and, 1276-1277
  trabeculectomy and
      iridocorneal epithelial syndrome
          and, 973
      pigmentary glaucoma and, 994
  trabeculoplasty and; see Trabeculo-
      plasty, laser
  transscleral cyclophotocoagulation
      and, 622-623
  transpupillary cyclophotocoagulation
      and, 621-622
Laser iridectomy
  angle-closure glaucoma and
      cataract extraction and, 1277
      chronic, 860
      nanophthalmos and, 1050
  lens dislocation and, 1036, 1042

Laser iridectomy—cont'd
  malignant glaucoma in fellow eye
    and, 1262
  narrow angle and, 861
  pseudophakic glaucoma and, 1295
  uveitis and, 1209
Lattice collagen, 60
Leak, wound, 281-282
Learning curve, 426, 442
Lectin, 1008
LED; see Light emitting diode instru-
    ment
Lens; see also Cataract
  adhesion and, 1206
  angle-closure glaucoma and, 826-827,
    828, 850-851
  aniridia and, 874, 879
  development of, 6-8
  dislocation of, 1028, 1030-1042
  epithelial ingrowth and, 1312
  exfoliation syndrome and, 1003, 1006-
    1008
  goniotomy, 711-712
  homocystinuria and, 1040
  implantation and, 1285-1297
    epithelial ingrowth and, 1306,
      1312
    pupillary block and, 648
  indirect gonioscopy and, 347-348
  infant diagnostic, 774-775
  intumescence and, 1027-1028
  iridectomy and, 701
  Lowe's syndrome and, 936
  opacities and; see also Cataract
    automated perimetry and, 432
    laser iridectomy and, 592, 595
  rim artifact and, 440
Lens capsule
  exfoliation and, 1009
  laser iridectomy and, 587
  persistent hyperplastic primary vitre-
    ous and, 944
  phacoanaphylaxis and, 1024
  pseudoexfoliation and, 997
  rupture of, 1232
  subluxation and, 1228
Lens extraction
  extracapsular; see Extracapsular lens
    extraction
  intracapsular
    diabetic retinopathy and, 1086
    phacolytic glaucoma and, 1021
    pupillary block and, 1271
Lens-induced glaucoma, 1270
  angle-closure, 846-847
  open-angle glaucoma, 1017-1026
Lens-iris diaphragm, 1228
Lenticular abnormality, 899, 900
Leukemia, 1123
Leukocyte, 1077
Levodopa, 1172
Lid
  development of, 22-23
  hemangioma and, 1133-1134
  intraocular pressure and, 302

Ligament
  fibroelastic, 176
  pectinate, 42
Light
  ganglion cell and, 89, 91
  halo around, 840
  laser and, 567-568, 571
  perimetry and, 187, 372
  sense of, 394
  threshold versus sensitivity and, 381
Light emitting diode instrument, 404-
    405
Limbal blood vessel, 265
Limbal groove, 677
Limbus
  congenital glaucoma and, 770-771
  development of, 12-23
  filtration surgery and, 659
  scleritis and, 1195, 1197
  trephination and, 653
Limbus-based flap
  sclerotomy and cataract extraction
    and, 704
  trabeculectomy and, 660, 662-663
Line, Schwalbe's, 20
Lister lens, 712-713
Lithium, 201
Liver, 940
Local anesthesia; see Anesthesia
Long glaucoma valve implant, 745-746
Lowe's syndrome, 936, 937
Low-tension glaucoma, 797-812
  clinical picture of, 800-805
  corticosteroid-induced glaucoma and,
    1163
  definition of, 797-798
  diagnosis and evaluation of, 806-808
  epidemiology and, 805-806
  history and, 797
  outflow pathway and, 60, 62-64
  posterior ciliary artery and, 152
  treatment and, 808-809
LSD; see Lysergic acid diethylamide
Luminance, 365
  perimetry and, 387
Lymphatics, 241-242
Lymphocyte
  iridocorneal epithelial syndrome and,
    972
  neovascular glaucoma and, 1077
Lymphoid tumor, 1123
Lysergic acid diethylamide, 303, 1173
Lysozyme, 1008

M
Mackay-Marg tonometer, 309-310
Macrocornea, 766
Macromolecule-induced facility de-
    crease, 230
Macrophage
  ghost cell glaucoma and, 1239
  lens-induced glaucoma and, 1017,
    1017
  phacolytic glaucoma and, 1019
  trabecular meshwork and, 46, 229

Macula
  edema of optic disc and, 287
  epinephrine and, 699, 815-816
  hypoplasia and, 879
  lesion of, 450
  retinal degeneration and, 946
  xanthophyll and, 576
Magnesium, 229
Maklakov applanation tonometer, 311
Malformation of anterior segment, 763
Malignancy; see Tumor
Malignant glaucoma, 648, 847, 1251-1262
  angle-closure glaucoma after cataract
    extraction and, 1277
  filtration surgery and, 684-685
  hyaloid membrane and, 1086
  surgical iridectomy and, 582
Mandibulooculofacial syndrome, dys-
    cephalic, 935
Mannitol
  acute angle-closure glaucoma and, 855
  aqueous misdirection and, 685
  filtration surgery and, 657
  hyperosmotic agent and, 551
  intravenous, 553
  malignant glaucoma and, 1256
  renal failure and, 554
  zonular glaucoma and, 1268
Manual perimetric calibration, 369-370
Marfan syndrome, 1038-1039
  cystathionine beta-synthase deficiency
    and, 1040
Marijuana, 559
Marker, neuronal transmitter, 525
Massage, 674
Matrix, extracellular; see Extracellular
    matrix
Matrix vesicle, 58-59
Mature cataract, 1018
MD; see Mean defect
Mean defect
  calculations of, 383
  visual field indices and, 451
Mean sensitivity, 451
Medulloepithelioma, 1122
Meesman's corneal dystrophy, 781
Megalocornea, 766-767, 941
  congenital glaucoma and, 779
Megaloglobus, 1038
Megalophthalmos, 941
Melanin, 576
Melanocytoma, 1116
Melanocytosis, 922-924
Melanoma
  neovascular glaucoma and, 1089-1090
  uveal tract and, 1111-1116
Melanosis of iris, 973
Membrane
  Axenfeld-Rieger syndrome and, 890
  Barkan's, 31, 34
  basement; see Basement membrane
  Bruch's, 158
  ciliary body and, 213
  of Elschnig, 105
  fibrous, 596

Membrane—cont'd
  fibrovascular, 1067
  iridocorneal epithelial syndrome and,
      967, 969, 972
  pupillary, 8
  retrocorneal, 1322, 1323-1324
  subendothelial, 43
Meningoblastoma, 907, 909
Menstrual period, 1178
Mental retardation
  aniridia and, 871
  encephalotrigeminal angiomatosis
      and, 914
Mephenisin, 1172
Mesenchymal cell, neural crest-derived
  anterior segment anomaly and, 23
  cornea development and, 8
  outer limbus and, 22-23
Mesenchymal tissue
  embryology and, 5
  sclera and, 22
  Schlemm's canal and, 12-15, 16
  trabecular meshwork and, 15, 16, 18
Meshwork, trabecular; see Trabecular
      meshwork
Mesoderm, 3
  lids and, 23
  Schlemm's canal and, 24
  sclera and, 22
Mesodermal anomaly
  classification of, 708
  cornea and iris and; see Axenfeld-Rie-
      ger syndrome
  hereditary dystrophy and, 974
  pigmentary glaucoma and, 984
Mesodermal mesenchyme, 5-6
  Schlemm's canal and, 12-15, 16
Messenger RNA, 1164
Metabolic disease
  carbonic anhydrase inhibitors and, 545
  congenital glaucoma and, 779
Metaraminol, 1175
Metastable state of atom, 568-569
Metastasis, 1116-1119
Methapyrilene, 1171
Methazolamide
  argon laser peripheral iridoplasty and,
      605-606
  carbonic anhydrase inhibitors and, 545
  dose-response and, 543
  sickle cell hemoglobinopathy and, 1153
Methionine, 1040
Methoxamine, 1175
  intraocular pressure and, 530-531
Methoxyflurane, 1177-1178
Methylnorepinephrine, 529
Methylphenidate, 1172
Methylxanthine, 1173
Metiamide, 1172
Mexican poppy, 1179
Meyer-Schwickerath syndrome, 938
Microcirculation
  ciliary body, 84-85
  optic nerve head and, 125
  retinal nerve fiber layer and, 92

Microcornea, 941, 943
  aniridia and, 874
  congenital glaucoma and, 766
Microdensitometric measurement, 503-
      505
Microelectrode study, 213
Microfibril, 1008
Micrognathia-glossoptosis syndrome, 939
Microphthalmos, 942, 943, 944
Micropinocytosis, 221
Microscopy
  epithelial ingrowth and, 1313, 1314
  surgical, 711
Microspherophakia, 1033-1035
Microsurgical instrument, 657
Microvasculature, 80-83, 85
Midget cell, 89
Migraine, 805
Millilambert, 381
Minor tranquilizer, 1172
Miosis
  alpha-adrenergic antagonists and, 533
  automated perimetry and, 432
  carbachol and, 518
  Horner's syndrome and, 270
  irreversible, 699
  lens subluxation and, 1228
  pilocarpine and, 517
  pseudophakic glaucoma and, 1294
Miotic agent
  angle-closure glaucoma, 849
    acute, 856
    cataract extraction and, 1276
    nanophthalmos and, 1050
    treatment of, 860
  aniridia and, 881
  aphakia and, 1279
  congenital glaucoma and, 784
  exfoliation syndrome and, 1011
  hypotony and, 287
  intraocular lens implantation and,
      1287
  iridocorneal epithelial syndrome and,
      977
  lens dislocation and, 1036
  lens-induced glaucoma and, 1023
  open-angle glaucoma and, 816, 817
    initial therapy and, 816-817
    retinal detachment and, 1056
  penetrating keratoplasty and, 1344-
      1345
  pigmentary glaucoma and, 993
  trabecular meshwork and, 48
  traumatic lens dislocation and, 1041
  uveitis and, 1208
  vitreous and
    in anterior chamber and, 1269
    malignant glaucoma and, 1261
Modulation transfer, 189
Molteno implant, 744, 1096-1098
  congenital glaucoma and, 784
  filtering surgery and, 639-640
  seton and, 725, 726
Monoamine oxidase inhibitor, 1170, 1171
  amphetamine and, 1172-1173

Monoarticular-onset juvenile rheumatoid
      arthritis, 1217
Monochromaticity, 571
Monoclonal antibody, 166
Mood-altering agents, 1172-1173
Morning glory syndrome, 943-944
Morphine, 1172
Mucocutaneous lesion, 1218
Mucopolysaccharidosis, 165
  outflow pathway and, 67-69
  Peters' anomaly and, 900
Mulberry lesion, 922
Multiple level test, 405
  automated perimetry and, 410
Mumps, 1156, 1220
Muscarinic agent, 268
Muscarinic receptor, 516
Muscle
  ciliary; see Ciliary muscle
  dilator, 829-830
  neurofibromatosis and, 909
  sphincter
    angle-closure glaucoma, 849
    neovascular glaucoma and, 1073
Muscle relaxant, 302
Multiple basal cell nevus syndrome, 938
Mydriatic agent, 1176-1177
  acute angle-closure glaucoma and,
      857, 862
    cataract extraction and, 1276
  ciliary block glaucoma and, 554
  cocaine and, 1177-1178
  malignant glaucoma and, 1256
  pigmentary glaucoma and, 985-986
  traumatic lens dislocation and, 1041
  uveitis and, 1208
  vitreous in anterior chamber and, 1269
Myelin, 123
Myopia
  axial, 781
  carbonic anhydrase inhibitors and,
      545
  congenital glaucoma and, 773, 779
  intraocular pressure and, 302
  low-tension glaucoma and, 803-804
  open-angle glaucoma and retinal de-
      tachment and, 1056
  optic disc damage and, 819
  pigmentary glaucoma and, 983, 991
  Stickler's syndrome and, 1058
  sulfa drugs and, 1173
Myotonic dystrophy, 286-287, 1156

N

NA/K-ATPase; see Sodium pump, so-
      dium/potassium-adenosine tri-
      phosphatase and
Nanophthalmos, 942, 943, 944
  argon laser peripheral iridoplasty and,
      598
  laser iridectomy and, 583-584
  retinal degeneration and, 946
    angle-closure glaucoma and, 1049-
      1050
  surgery and, 727

Naphazoline, 1175
Narrow angle, 1176
Nasal angle, 349-350
Nasal step, 434, 436, 437
    nerve fiber bundle defect and, 394
Nd:YAG laser, 568; see also Laser
    angle-closure glaucoma after cataract
        extraction and, 1278
    capsulotomy
        angle-closure glaucoma and, 1277
        diabetic retinopathy and, 1086
        open-angle glaucoma after cataract
            extraction and, 1271
    ciliary body destruction and, 735-736
    goniotomy and, 617
    ionizing effect of, 575
    iridectomy and
        cataract after, 587, 590, 595
        wound closure and, 633
    iridovitreal block and, 1254
    lens-induced glaucoma and, 1021-
        1023
    malignant glaucoma and, 1257
    Q-switched, 640
    sclerostomy with, 624
    trabeculopuncture and, 615-616
    trabeculotomy/sclerostomy, 616-617
    transscleral cyclophotocoagulation
        and, 622-623
Necrosis, iris stroma, 848-849
Necrotizing anterior scleritis, 1191-1192
Neomycin sulfate, 1174
Neosynephrine, 859
Neovascular glaucoma, 1063-1110
    cataract extraction and, 1278
    causes of, 1078-1090
    clinical picture and, 1063-1069
    differential diagnosis and, 1069-1070
    episcleral venous pressure and, 1137
    fluorescein studies and, 1070-1071
    ghost cell glaucoma and, 1246
    history and terminology and, 1063
    hyperosmotic agent and, 554
    management of, 1090-1101
    pathogenesis and, 1077-1078
    pathology and, 1071-1076
    posterior scleritis and, 1202
    scleritis and, 1201
    trabeculectomy and, 672
Neovascularization
    anterior segment, 635
    intraocular lens implantation and,
        1293
Nephrolithiasis, 545
Nephronophthisis, 939
Nephropathia epidemica, 1155
Nerve; see Nerve fiber; Nervous system;
    Optic nerve
Nerve block, facial, 658
Nerve ending, 84-85
Nerve fiber
    bundle defect and, 394, 396
    galanin-LI, 265
    number of, 495
    retina and, 92-102, 481-487

Nerve fiber—cont'd
    substance P immunoreactive, 264-265
    surface layer of, 135
Nerve growth factor, 906-907
Nerve head, retinal, 481-482
Nervous system, 257-279
    central, 270-272
    ciliary body and, 261-262
    limbal blood vessels and, 265
    neurotransmitters and neuromodula-
        tors in ocular nerves and, 257-260
    paracrine cells and, 266
    peripheral, 266-270
    trabecular meshwork and, 262-265
Neural crest
    aniridia and, 881
    anomaly and, 708
    Axenfeld-Rieger syndrome and, 25,
        894
    embryology and, 5
Neural crest-derived mesenchymal cell,
    5-6, 22-23
    cornea development and, 8
Neurocristopathy, 23-37
Neuroectoderm
    aniridia and, 881
    dysplasia and, 906-913
    keratocytes and, 24
Neurofibroma, 906-913, 1123
    Sturge-Weber syndrome and, 31
Neurofilament, 97-98
Neuroglia
    ganglion cell and, 92
    lamina choroidalis and, 109
    lamina scleralis and, 111
    optic nerve head and, 105-107
    retina and, 92
Neurologic disorder, 1156
Neuromodulator in ocular nerve, 257-
    260
Neuromuscular block, 659
Neuronal transmitter marker, 525
Neuron-specific enolase, 23
Neuropathy, optic
    ischemia and, 807
    posterior ciliary artery and, 137-156
Neuropeptide
    peripheral nervous system and, 258-
        259
    Y, 259
        intraocular pressure and, 267
Neuropeptide Y–like immunoreactive
    neuron
    ciliary process and, 262
    trabecular meshwork and, 264
Neurotransmitter, 257-260
Nevus
    basal cell nevus syndrome and, 924,
        938
    iris, 963, 971, 972
    uveal, 1116
Nevus flammeus, 914
Nieden's syndrome, 938
Nifedipine, 1174
Night vision, 365

Nitrate, 1174-1175
Nitroglycerin, 1175
Nitroprusside, 287
Nitrous oxide, 1177-1178
Nodular anterior scleritis, 1191
Nodular episcleritis, 1189
Nodule
    Cogan-Reese syndrome and, 963,
        972
    iridocorneal epithelial syndrome and,
        973
Noncontact tonometer, 311-312
Nonfibrous collagen, 164
Nonfiltering meshwork, 42-43
Nonglaucomatous optic nerve disease,
    807
Nonglaucomatous visual field loss, 443
Noninsulin-dependent diabetes, 1083,
    1085
Nonmalignant neoplasm, 1154
Nonpigmented ciliary epithelium
    beta-adrenergic agonists and, 530
    NA/K-ATPase and, 206-207
    tumors of, 1121-1123
Nonproliferative retinopathy, 1152
Nonrhegmatogenous retinal detach-
    ment, 1115
Nonsteroidal drug, 1169-1184
    acetylsalicylic acid and, 1179
    adjuvant to surgery and, 1179
    anesthetic, 1177-1178
    antibiotics, 1173-1174
    antidepressant, 1171
    antihistamine, 1171-1172
    antihypertensive agent, 1178
    antiparkinsonian, 1172
    antiprostaglandin and, 1178-1179
    antispasmolytic, 1173
    autonomic, 1175-1177
    cardiac agents and, 1174
    epidemic dropsy and, 1179-1180
    hormonal agent, 1178
    mood-altering, 1172-1173
    psychotropic, 1170-1171
    tobacco and, 1179
    uveitis and, 1208
    vasoactive, 1174-1175
Norepinephrine, 1175
    alpha-adrenergic agonists and, 526
    aqueous humor and, 224
    denervation and, 529
    trabecular meshwork and, 225
Norgesic; see Orphenadrine citrate
Norpace; see Disopyramide phosphate
NPY; see Neuropeptide, Y
NPY-LI; see Neuropeptide Y–like immu-
    noreactive neuron
NSE; see Neuron-specific enolase
Nuclear sclerosis, 851
Nucleus, 678-679
Nystagmus, 881

O

Obstetrical trauma, 779
Occlusion; see also Ischemia

Occlusion—cont'd
capillary, 1077
hypotony and, 287
retinal artery, 98, 100, 102
retinal vein; see Retinal vein
Octopus perimeter, 372
G1 program on, 408
multiple-level test and, 410
test strategies and, 405
visual field indices and, 451-453, 455-461
Ocular disease, 963-1124
corneal endothelial disorder and, 963-980
exfoliation syndrome and, 997-1015
intraocular tumors and, 1111-1124
len-induced glaucoma and, 1017-1026
lens intumescence and dislocation and, 1027-1045
neovascular glaucoma and, 1063-1110
pigmentary glaucoma and, 981-995; see also Pigmentary glaucoma
Ocular hypertension; see Intraocular pressure
Ocular nerves, peripheral, 257-260
Ocular surgery; see Surgery
Oculodentodigital dysplasia, 938
Axenfeld-Rieger syndrome versus, 894
Oculodermal melanocytosis, 922-924
Oculomotor nerve, 268-269
Ocusert
open-angle glaucoma and, 816
plateau iris and, 861
O'Brien-Spaeth block, 658
Oil, silicone, 1055
Oligodendroglia, 115
One-piece valved silicone explant, 746-747
Opacity
automated perimetry and, 432
congenital glaucoma and, 766
corneal, 598
lens, 592, 595
posterior polymorphous dystrophy and, 974
Open-angle glaucoma, 787-822
aphakia and, 1266-1271
central retinal vein occlusion and, 1081
circadian variation in intraocular pressure and, 325
clonidine and, 558
color testing and, 190
corticosteroid-induced glaucoma and, 1163-1164
dermatologic disorder and, 1156
epidemiology and, 789-795
epinephrine and, 529-530
episcleritis and, 1189-1190
estrogen-progesterone and, 1178
exercise and, 302
exfoliation syndrome and, 1008-1009
features of, 751
Fuchs' endothelial dystrophy and, 977-978

Open-angle glaucoma—cont'd
ghost cell glaucoma and, 1246
glaucomatocyclitic crisis and, 1211
growth hormone and, 1142
laser treatment in, 605-620
lens-induced, 1017-1026
low-tension, 797-812; see also Low-tension glaucoma
mumps and, 1156
myopia and, 302
outflow pathways in, 54-60, 225
posterior polymorphous dystrophy and, 976
radiation therapy and, 1235-1236
retinal detachment and, 1048-1049
rhegmatogenous retinal detachment and, 1055-1057
sanguinarine and, 1179-1180
scleritis and, 1194-1199
secondary
argon laser trabeculoplasty and, 609-611
classification of, 753, 755
Stickler's syndrome and, 1057-1058
sympathomimetic agent and, 1175
syphilis and, 1214
thyroid and, 1147
trabecular meshwork and, 172
trauma and, 1230, 1232
treatment of, 813-821
drugs and, 815-818
escalation of therapy and, 815
laser trabeculoplasty and, 818
lifestyle issues and, 815
monitoring and, 819-820
pressure control guidelines and, 814-815
surgery and, 818-819
Opercular cell, 42-43
Ophthalmic artery, 80
Ophthalmic vein, 1127
Ophthalmodynamometry, 1133
Ophthalmopathy, thyroid, 1135, 1136, 1143-1147
Ophthalmoscopy, 777
Opioid peptide, 259-260
Opponent color perception, 183-185
Optic canal
anatomy and pathophysiology of, 102-103
intraorbital optic nerve and, 118
Optic cup; see Cup, optic
Optic disc
anatomy and, 468-470
baring of lamina cribrosa and, 472, 474
enlargement of optic cup and, 470-472
evaluation of, 467-468
examination techniques and, 480-481
filtration surgery and, 654
hypotony and, 287
low-tension, 800-803
measurement of changes in, 495-511
myopic patient and, 819-820
neovascular glaucoma and, 1090

Optic disc—cont'd
open-angle glaucoma and, 814-815
pallor and, 474-476
angle-closure glaucoma and, 851-852
measurement of, 503-505, 507
peripapillary atrophy and, 478-479
retinal detachment and, 1056
staphylomatous, 944
vascular changes and, 476-478
Optic nerve
abnormalities, 781
angle-closure glaucoma and, 851-852
scleral buckling procedure and, 1053
aniridia and, 879
blood supply of, 133-161
extraocular
anatomy and pathophysiology of, 113-119
glaucoma and, 119-125
intraocular lens implantation and, 1293, 1294
intraocular pressure and, 270
low-tension glaucoma and, 807
neurofibromatosis and, 909
open-angle glaucoma and, 814-815
Optic nerve head
acute angle-closure glaucoma and, 841-842
anatomy and pathophysiology of, 105-113
color and, 503-505
Cushing's syndrome and, 1142
extracellular matrix and, 163-166, 172-176, 172-177
fluorescein angiography and, 505
future research and, 508
glaucoma and, 120
peripapillary choroid artery and, 158
quantitative measurements of, 495-511
topography and, 496-503
Optic primordium, 6
Optic tract, and, 118-119
Optic vesicle, 6-8
Optical interface, 339-340
Orbit
disorders of, 1155
neurofibromatosis and, 909
sarcoidosis and, 1215
venous drainage of, 1127-1128
varices and, 1132
Orphenadrine citrate, 1171, 1171-1172
Osmolality of serum, 302
Osmotic agent, 1294; see also Hyperosmotic agent
lens-induced glaucoma and, 1023
malignant glaucoma and, 1253
Osmotic pressure, 200
Osteogenesis imperfecta, 938-939
Osterberg's plot of rod and cone, 365-366
Ouabain
ATPase and, 207, 210
ciliary body and, 213
Na/K-ATPase and, 210-211, 213-216
short-circuit current and, 213, 215, 216

Ouabain—cont'd
  vanadate and, 213
Outer wall endothelium, 50-51
Outflow
  carbonic anhydrase inhibitors and, 544
  corticosteroid and, 67, 1164
  Fuchs' dystrophy and, 977
  low-tension glaucoma and, 60, 62-64
  mucopolysaccharidosis and, 67-69
  normal pathways of, 41-54
  open-angle glaucoma and, 54-60
  Peters' anomaly and, 900
  pigmentary glaucoma and, 64, 66, 67
  pressure-dependent, 219-239
    adrenergic mechanisms and, 224-225
    biomechanics and pharmacologic responses and, 231-232
    cholinergic mechanisms and, 222-223
    corticosteroid and, 230-231
    fluid mechanics and, 219-221
    innervation of, 221-222
    resistance and, 225-230
    Schlemm's canal and, 221
    underperfusion and, 222
  pseudoexfoliative glaucoma and, 64
  thyrotropic ophthalmopathy and, 1143
  trabecular meshwork and, 166
  uveoscleral, 241-247
    prostaglandin and, 560
Output coupler, 569
Oxygen
  episcleral venous pressure and, 1131
  retina and, 1092
Oxytalan, 1008
Oxytalanosis of aqueous, 997

P
Pachymeter, 831
Pain
  argon laser trabeculoplasty and, 613
  iridocorneal epithelial syndrome and, 964
  open-angle glaucoma after cataract extraction and, 1267
  scleritis and, 1190-1191
Pallor of optic disc, 474-476
  angle-closure glaucoma and, 851-852
  measurement of, 503-505, 507
Palsy, 909
Pancuronium, 659
Panretinal cryotherapy, 635
  neovascular glaucoma and, 1091-1093, 1094, 1095
Para-aminoclonidine
  laser iridectomy and, 595
  pharmacology and, 557
Para-aminohippuric acid, 202-203
Paracellular pathway, 221
Paracentesis
  ghost cell glaucoma and, 1245
  hyphema and, 1227
  sickle cell hemoglobinopathy and, 1154
  trabeculectomy and, 663, 665, 666
Paracentral scotoma, 394, 439

Paracrine cell, 266
  catecholamines and, 525-526
Paragyline, 1171
Paraldehyde, 1172
Parasitic disease, 1156
Parasympathetic effect
  ciliary body and, 84-85, 261
  intraocular pressure and, 268
Parasympatholytic agent, 1176-1177
Parasympathomimetic agent, 515-518, 1176
  filtration surgery and, 656-657
  ghost cell glaucoma and, 1246
  hypotony and, 287
Parkes-Weber syndrome, 920
Parotid gland, 1220
Pars plana lensectomy, 1042
Pars plana vitrectomy, 1262
Pars plicata, 77, 78
Partial deletion syndrome, chromosome 18, 932
Partial-thickness surgical iridectomy, 582
Particulate sieving, 221
Particulate-induced facility decrease, 229-230
PAS; see Peripheral anterior synechia
Patau's syndrome, 931-932
Patching, pressure, 1276
Pattern electroretinogram, 192-193
Pattern on Humphrey perimeter, 408
Pattern standard deviation, 451
Pavulon; see Pancuronium
PCA; see Posterior ciliary artery
Peak intraocular pressure, 326-329
Pearl tumor, 1300
Pectinate ligament, 42
Pedunculated nodule, 972
Penetrating injury, 1232-1233
  ghost cell glaucoma and, 1244
Penetrating keratoplasty, 1337-1347
  filtration surgery and, 681
  iridocorneal epithelial syndrome and, 973
  Peters' anomaly and, 901
Penicillamine, 639
Penicillin, 1174
Penlight beam, 830
Peptidase, 258
Peptide, 258, 259; see also Neuropeptide
Peptide histidine isoleucine, 259
Perception, color, 189-191
Perfluorocarbon gas, 1055
Perforation, conjunctival flap, 684
Perfusion study, intraventricular, 271-272
Pericyte, 176
Perimetry, 361-466; see also Visual field
  automated, 403-466; see also Automated perimetry
  chemical burn and, 1235
  history and, 361, 393
  interpretation of results and, 380-382
  normal gradient of, 362-368
  optic nerve fiber loss and, 179
  physiologic basis for, 384-389
  scatter versus fluctuation and, 382-384

Perimetry—cont'd
  static, 374-378
    computerized, 186-187
    duration of test in, 373
    kinetic perimetry versus, 368
    Octopus and, 372
  test parameters in, 369-380
  threshold technique and, 186-187
Periocular corticosteroid injection, 1163, 1165
Peripapillary astrocytic hamartoma, 922
Peripapillary atrophy, 478-479
Peripapillary choroid
  optic nerve head and, 158
  watershed zone and, 152
Peripapillary choroid artery, 133, 135
Peripheral angle, 354
Peripheral anterior chamber, 831
Peripheral anterior synechia, 1206
  angle-closure glaucoma and
    acute, 841
    cataract extraction and, 1277-1278
    chronic, 843
    examination of, 833
    intermittent, 840, 841
  argon laser trabeculoplasty and, 613
  iridocorneal epithelial syndrome and, 967
  gonioscopy and, 356
  penetrating injury and, 1232
Peripheral centripetal vascular system, 135
Peripheral corneal thickness, 1344
Peripheral iridectomy, 645
  internal block incision and, 679
  lens implantation and, 1290-1291
  trabeculectomy and, 667, 669
Peripheral iridoplasty
  angle-closure glaucoma and, 858, 859
  argon laser, 596-600
Peripheral nervous system
  eye and, 257
  intraocular pressure and, 266-270
  neuropeptide and co-transmission in, 258-259
Peripupillary neovascularization, 1064; see also Neovascular glaucoma
Periumbilical skin, 890
Perkins applanation tonometer, 308
Permeability to water, 200-201
Perphenazine, 1170
Persantine; see Dipyridamole
Persistent hyperplastic primary vitreous, 944-946
Peters' anomaly, 25, 28, 897-903
  Axenfeld-Rieger syndrome versus, 894
Pfaundler-Hurler disease, 67
Pfeifer-Weber-Christian syndrome, 939-940
Phacoanaphylaxis, 1023-1024
Phacoemulsification, 677, 678-679
Phacolytic glaucoma, 1017-1021
  trabecular meshwork and, 230
Phakic eye
  argon laser trabeculoplasty and, 609

Phakic eye—cont'd
  ghost cell glaucoma and, 1244
Phakomatosis, 25, 905-929, 1123
  angiomatosis retinae and, 921-922
  basal cell nevus syndrome and, 924
  diffuse congenital hemangiomatosis
    and, 924
  encephalotrigeminal angiomatosis
    and, 913-920
  Klippel-Trenaunay-Weber syndrome
    and, 920-921
  neurofibromatosis and, 906-913
  oculodermal melanocytosis and, 922-
    924
  tuberous sclerosis and, 922
Pharmacokinetics, 528
Pharmacology; see Drug
Phasic ganglion cell, 181
Phenelzine, 1171
Phenformin, 1173-1174
Pheniramine, 1172, 1175
Phenothiazine tranquilizer, 1170, 1171
Phenylephrine, 1175
  angle-closure glaucoma and, 862
    scleral buckling procedure and, 1053
  aqueous misdirection and, 685
  ciliary block glaucoma and, 554
  intraocular pressure and, 530-531
  malignant glaucoma and, 1256
  pigmentary glaucoma and, 985
  uveitis and, 1208
Phenylephrine-pilocarpine test, 862
Phenytoin, 1172
Phlebolith, 1132
Phosphate, 203
Phospholine iodide; see Echothiophate
Photoablation, 573
Photochemical effect, 573
Photocoagulation, 573-578
  ciliary process and, 1279
  diabetes and, 1086
  encephalotrigeminal angiomatosis
    and, 920
  epithelial cyst and, 1303
  epithelial ingrowth and, 1313, 1315
  filtering surgery and, 635
  open-angle glaucoma and, 819
  retinal
    angle-closure glaucoma and, 1051-
      1052
    neovascular glaucoma and, 1091,
      1091-1093, 1095
Photodisruptor, 578-579
Photogrammetry
  accuracy of, 503
  optic cup and, 506
  optic nerve and, 497-499
Photographic techniques, 495-511
  optic disc changes and, 480-481
  retinal nerve fiber layer and, 487
Photometry, 365
Photomydriasis, argon laser, 625
Photon, 567-568
  capture of, 183
Photopapillometry, 504-505

Photophobia
  aniridia and, 873-874
  causes of, 779, 781
  congenital glaucoma and, 773
  conventional iridectomy and, 647
Photopic threshold, 187
Photopic vision, 365
Photopigment, 180
Photopigment chromophore, 183
Photoradiation, 573
Photoreceptor
  number of, 363-364
  visual process and, 180
Photostimulation, 89, 91
Photovaporization, 574-575
Photophobia, 881
Physics, laser, 567-580
  hazards and, 575
  ionizing effects and, 575
  laser interactions and, 571-572
  light and, 567-568, 571
  photochemical effects and, 573
  photocoagulators and, 576-578
  photodistributors and, 578-579
  thermal effects and, 573-575
Pia, 113, 115
Pial septum, 173, 176
Pial vessel, 135
Pierre Robin syndrome, 939
  Stickler's syndrome and, 1058
Pigment; see also Pigmentary glaucoma
  angle-closure glaucoma and, 833
    chronic, 844
  Cogan-Reese syndrome and, 972
  electrical injury and, 1236
  epithelium and
    ciliary body and, 86
    NA/K-ATPase and, 206-207
    tumors of, 1123
  exfoliation syndrome and, 1000-1001,
    1003, 1009
  familial amyloidosis and, 1154
  irradiation and, 1155
  laser iridectomy and, 593, 594
  retinal
    chemoattractant and, 1078
    photochemical reaction and, 575
    photocoagulation and, 1092
  oculodermal melanocystosis and, 922-
    924
  trabecular meshwork and, 229
    gonioscopy and, 358
  vitreous and, 1048
Pigmentary glaucoma, 981-995
  argon laser trabeculoplasty and,
    610
  clinical features of, 981-982
  complex, 997; see also Exfoliation syn-
    drome
  differential diagnosis and, 992-993
  history of, 981
  intraocular lens implantation and,
    1291
  management and, 993-994
  natural history and, 982-984

Pigmentary glaucoma—cont'd
  outflow pathway and, 64, 66, 67, 225
  pathophysiology and, 984-992
  retinal detachment and, 1057
Pilocarpine, 515-518, 1176
  accommodation and, 224
  angle-closure glaucoma and, 862
    acute, 856
  aqueous humor and, 222, 224, 342
  argon laser peripheral iridoplasty and,
    598
  Axenfeld-Rieger syndrome and, 895
  congenital glaucoma and, 784
  episcleral venous pressure and, 1135
  filtration surgery and, 656-657
  hyperosmotic agent and, 554
  lens dislocation and, 1036
  lens-induced glaucoma and, 1023
  low-tension glaucoma and, 809
  open-angle glaucoma and, 816
  plateau iris and, 861
  prostaglandin and, 560
  trabecular meshwork and, 225
  zonular glaucoma and, 1268
Piperazine, 1171, 1172
Pituitary gland, 1141-1142
  Axenfeld-Rieger syndrome and, 889-
    890
  neovascular glaucoma and, 1100
Planimetric measurement, 496-497
Plaque
  cribriform layer and, 53-54
  juxtacanalicular tissue and, 171
  sheath-derived, 55-58
Plasma, 200, 201
Plasmoid aqueous, 1267
Plastic tube shunt, 742
Plate, cribriform, 172-173, 176
Plateau iris syndrome, 845-846
  argon laser peripheral iridoplasty and,
    597
  treatment of, 861
Platelet dysfunction, 1152
Plexiform neuroma, 906, 907, 908, 909-
    911
Plexus
  angular aqueous, 15
  fiber, 49-50
Pneumatonometer, 311
  chemical burn and, 1235
POAG; see Open-angle glaucoma
Poisoning, salicylic, 1179
Polishing of posterior capsule, 679
Polyarticular-onset juvenile rheumatoid
    arthritis, 1217
Polyclonal antibody, 166
Polycystic kidney, 940
Polycythemia, 1152
Polymixin B, 1174
Polymorphous dystrophy, posterior; see
    Posterior polymorphous dystro-
    phy
Polypeptide, vasoactive intestinal, 259
Polythiazide, 1178
Polyvinyl chloride tube, 711-712

Pore
  inner wall endothelium, 54
  trabecular meshwork and, 43-45
  transcellular channels and, 221
Posner-Schlossman syndrome, 1211-1213
Posterior amorphous corneal dystrophy, 976
Posterior capsule
  diabetic retinopathy and, 1086
  lens-induced glaucoma and, 1021-1022
  polishing of, 679
Posterior capsule-anterior hyaloid barrier, 1086, 1087
Posterior chamber
  aqueous humor and, 41
  lens dislocation and, 1037
  physiology and, 539-541
  intraocular lens implant and, 1289
    insertion of, 679
    intraocular pressure and, 698
    iridectomy and, 701
    pseudophakic glaucoma and, 1294-1295
    pupillary block and, 648
Posterior ciliary artery
  retrolaminar region and, 135
  variations of, 136-158
Posterior embryotoxon, 351; see also Axenfeld-Rieger syndrome
Posterior lip sclerectomy, 676
Posterior polymorphous dystrophy, 24-25, 28-31, 974-977
  Axenfeld-Rieger syndrome versus, 894
  congenital glaucoma and, 779
  iridocorneal epithelial syndrome and, 972
Posterior push mechanism, 597
Posterior scleritis, 1193-1202
Posterior sclerotomy
  hemorrhage and, 682
  malignant glaucoma and, 1257
Posterior segment
  aniridia and, 879
  sarcoid uveitis, 1215
Posterior stroma, 897
Posterior synechia, 1206
  angle-closure glaucoma and, 850
  laser iridectomy and, 594
Posterior tube shunt, 743-747
Posterior vitreous detachment, 1275
Postganglionic nerve of ciliary ganglion, 257
Postreceptor organization, 180-183
Postural change
  episcleral venous pressure and, 1130
  intraocular pressure and, 302
Potassium, 544
PPMD; see Posterior polymorphous dystrophy
Prader-Willi syndrome, 934
Prazosin, 533
Preceptor factor, 190
Prednisolone
  angle-closure glaucoma and, 858

Prednisolone—cont'd
  injection and, 1207-1208
Pregnancy, 545
Prelaminar area
  anatomy and, 172
  blood supply and, 133, 135
Premature infant, 947-949
Preoperative preparation, 656-659
Presentation time, 405
Pressure
  blood; see Blood pressure
  episcleral venous; see Episcleral venous pressure
  intraocular; see Intraocular pressure
  osmotic, 200
Pressure chamber method, 252, 1129
Pressure patching, 1276
Pressure-dependent outflow; see Outflow
Pressure-induced axon damage, 120-125
Pressure-sensitive unidirectional valve implant, 639
Pretrabecular secondary glaucoma, 755
Primary glaucoma, 757-866
  angle-closure; see Angle-closure glaucoma
  classification of, 751-752
  congenital, 759-785; see also Congenital glaucoma
  filtration surgery and, 673
  open-angle; see Open-angle glaucoma
Primordial endothelial tissue, 25
Primordium, optic, 6
Probe
  cyclocryotherapy and, 732-733
  trabeculotomy, 718, 721
Procaine, 520
Procaine penicillin, 1174
Process
  ciliary; see Ciliary process
  glial, 107
Prochlorperazine, 1170, 1173-1174
Progesterone, 1178
Progression of glaucomatous damage, 396-401
Progressive arthroophthalmopathy, hereditary, 939
Progressive iris atrophy, 963-973
Projection perimeter, 404
Proliferative retinopathy, 1152
Promethazine, 1170, 1171, 1172, 1173-1174
Prone provocative test, 862
Prophylactic laser iridectomy, 582
Propicamide, 1176
Prophylactic iridectomy, 860
Prostaglandin
  antiprostaglandin and, 1178-1179
  aqueous humor and, 231
  corticosteroid-induced glaucoma and, 1164
  neovascular glaucoma and, 1077
  pharmacology and, 560-561
  trigeminal nerve and, 268
  uveitis and, 1205-1206

Protease, 229
Protein
  extracellular matrix and; see Extracellular matrix
  G, 523-525
  trabecular meshwork and, 230
Proteinemia, 1152
Proteoglycan
  basement membrane and, 1008
  characteristics of, 165
  neovascular glaucoma and, 1077
  open-angle glaucoma and, 58
  trabecular meshwork and, 171
Proteoglycosaminoglycan, 1008
Protriptyline, 1171
Provocative test
  angle-closure glaucoma and, 861-862
  tolazoline and, 1175
Pseudoexfoliation
  familial amyloidosis and, 1154
  lens capsule and, 997
  outflow and, 64, 65, 225
  pigmentary glaucoma and, 993
  rubeosis iridis and, 1069
Pseudofacility
  aqueous humor and, 220
  tonography and, 293
Pseudohypopyon, 1245
Pseudophakia
  epinephrine maculopathy and, 815-816
  iris bombé and, 1254
  open-angle glaucoma and, 1271
  pupillary block and, 583
Pseudophakic correction, 1285-1297
Psychological effect, 387, 389
Psychophysics, 179, 185-191
Psychotropic agent, 1170-1171
Pterygopalatine ganglion, 268-269
Ptosis, 443
  aniridia and, 874
  Horner's syndrome and, 270
Pulmonary embolism, 1040
Pulsating exophthalmos, 909
Pump, sodium, 199-218; see also Sodium pump
Punch burn, 585, 586-587, 589
Punctum adherens, 87
Puncture hole, 232
Pupil
  contraction of; see Miosis; Miotic agent
  dilation and; see Mydriatic agent
  ectopia lentis et pupillae and, 1033
  enlargement of, 678
  epithelial ingrowth and, 1305
  exfoliation syndrome and, 1000-1001
  intraocular lens implantation and, 1289
  laser iridectomy and, 590
  microcoria and, 941
  miotic, 432
  size of
    automated perimetry and, 446-447
    static perimetry and, 386, 387

Pupillary block
  angle-closure glaucoma and, 827, 829, 830
    aphakia and, 1271-1276
  chemical burn and, 1234-1235
  cystinosis and, 934
  epithelial ingrowth and, 1313
  lens dislocation and, 1037
  lens implantation and, 1290
  lens subluxation and, 1228
  malignant glaucoma and, 1254, 1255
  Peters' anomaly and, 899
  plateau iris and, 845
  posterior chamber lens implantation and, 648
  pseudophakic
    glaucoma and, 1294, 1295
    laser iridectomy and, 583
  relative to absolute, 841
  scleral buckling procedure and, 1053
  scleritis and, 1200-1201
  traumatic lens dislocation and, 1041
  uveitis and, 1209
  vitreous and, 1274-1275
Pupillary border, exfoliation syndrome and, 1009
Pupillary membrane, 8
Pupillary tuft, 1073
Pupilloplasty, laser, 625-626
  angle-closure glaucoma and, 1276-1277
Purulent hypopyon, 685
Push mechanism, posterior, 597
PVC; see Polyvinyl chloride tube
Pyridoxine, 1040

Q
Q-switch, 570-571
Q-switched Nd:YAG laser
  filtering operation and, 640
  trabeculotomy/sclerostomy and, 616
Q-switched non-mode-locked laser, 578
Q-switched ruby laser, 615
Quantify defect screening test, 412
Quinidine, 1174

R
Racial differences
  angle-closure glaucoma and, 834
  argon laser trabeculoplasty and, 609
  intraocular pressure and, 301-302
  low-tension glaucoma and, 804
  pigmentary glaucoma and, 983, 991-992
  wound healing and, 635
Radiation, 1155
  electromagnetic, 567; see also Laser
  epithelial ingrowth and, 1317
  fibroblast and, 674
Ranitidine, 1172
Reaction time, visual, 373-374
Reactive lymphoid hyperplasia, 1123
Rebleeding, 1225, 1227
Receptor
  catecholamine, 523-528

Receptor—cont'd
  color perception and, 190
  ganglion cell and, 89, 91
  retina and, 364
  visual process and, 180
Recession, angle, 611
Red
  color pairing and, 183-185
  glaucoma and, 190
Red blood cell
  ghost cell glaucoma and; see Ghost cell glaucoma
  sickle cell disease and, 1153
  trabecular meshwork and, 229
Red dextran, 243
Redox, 201
Reflectometry, 504-505
Refractive error
  angle-closure glaucoma and, 825-826, 835
  aniridia and, 881
  low-tension glaucoma and, 803-804
  perimetry and, 384-387
Reis-Bückler's dystrophy, 781
Reiter's syndrome, 1218
Releasable suture, 675
Reliability of patient
  automated perimetry and, 403-404, 440-441
  interpretation of, 432
Reliability factor in automated perimetry, 414
Renal disorder, 1151, 1155
  familial renal-retinal dystrophy and, 939
  hyperosmotic agent and, 554
Renal-retinal dystrophy, 939
Reoperation, 671
  argon laser trabeculoplasty and, 611
Reserpine, 1172
Resistance, outflow
  carbonic anhydrase inhibitors and, 544
  trabecular meshwork and, 225-230
Resonant cavity, 568-570
Respiratory disorder, 815
Restrictive airway disease, 520
Retained lens cortex, 1021-1023
Retardation
  aniridia and, 871
  encephalotrigeminal angiomatosis and, 914
Retina, 1047-1061
  anatomy and pathophysiology of, 89-102
  angiomatosis and, 921-922
  angle-closure glaucoma and, 851-852
  capillary anastomosis and, 159
  central retinal vein occlusion and; see Retinal vein occlusion
  degeneration and, 946
  detachment and; see Retinal detachment
  ectoderm and, 3
  electroretinogram and, 191-193

Retina—cont'd
  familial renal-retinal dystrophy and, 939
  laser iridectomy and, 596
  optic nerve head and, 172
  pigment epithelium and
    chemoattractant and, 1078
    photochemical reaction and, 575
    photocoagulation and, 1092
  static perimetry and, 374
  traumatic dialysis and, 1228
  tumor of, 1119-1121
  visual field and, 363-366
Retinal artery
  axonal transport and, 98, 100, 102
  lamina choroidalis and, 109-110
  optic nerve head and, 107
  watershed zone and, 154
Retinal detachment
  angle-closure glaucoma and, 1049-1050
  choroidal melanoma and, 1115
  homocystinuria and, 1040
  hypotony and, 286
  iris retraction syndrome and, 1051
  Marfan syndrome and, 1039
  neovascular glaucoma and, 1090
  open-angle glaucoma and, 1048-1049
    Stickler's syndrome and, 1057-1058
  pigmentary glaucoma and, 1057
  postvitrectomy rubeosis iridis and, 1087
  scleral buckling procedure and, 1052
Retinal nerve fiber, 481-487
  glaucoma and, 120
Retinal vein
  anatomy and, 1128
  occlusion and, 1147
    carotid artery occlusion and, 1068
    neovascular glaucoma and, 1063, 1069, 1073, 1078-1082
    photocoagulation before cataract surgery and, 1087
    transient angle-closure glaucoma and, 1050-1051
Retinitis pigmentosa, 449, 1057
Retinoblastoma, 1120-1121
  neovascular glaucoma and, 1090
  Wilms' tumor versus, 871
Retinopathy
  diabetic, 1082-1083, 1085
    pituitary ablation and, 1100
  of prematurity, 947-949
  sickle cell, 1152-1154
Retraction syndrome, iris, 286
Retrobulbar anesthetic
  complications of, 657
  filtration surgery and, 658-659
  phacolytic glaucoma and, 1020
Retrobulbar hemorrhage, 682, 684
Retrobulbar inflammation, 1143
Retrocorneal membrane, 1322, 1323-1324
Retrolaminar region
  blood supply and, 135
  optic nerve head and, 172
Rhegmatogenous retinal detachment; see Retinal detachment

Rheumatoid arthritis, 1217

Rhodopsin, 180

Rhythm, circadian; see Circadian variation of intraocular pressure

Rieger's anomaly, 885

Rigidity, ocular, 293

Rim, disc, 496-497

Ring
  gonioscopy and, 351
  trabecular, 614

Ring chromosome 6 syndrome, 933-934

Ritalin; see Methylphenidate

Ritch trabeculoplasty lens, 606

RMS; see Root mean square

RNA, 1164

Rod
  ganglion cell and, 89, 91
  visual process and, 180

Rodenstock Optic Disk Analyzer, 476, 506

Root mean square, 383
  automated perimetry and, 404

Rubella, 1219-1220
  congenital, 1156

Rubeosis iridis, 1064, 1065, 1074; see also Neovascular glaucoma
  cataract extraction and, 1086
  cerebrovascular disease and, 1148
  diabetes and, 1083
  Fuchs' heterochromic cyclitis and, 1069, 1210
  melanoma and, 1089
  postvitrectomy, 1087
  radiation and, 1155
  retinal vein occlusion and, 1147
  retinoblastoma and, 1090
  sickle cell hemoglobinopathy and, 1152
  trabeculectomy and, 672

Rubinstein-Taybi syndrome, 939

Ruby laser, 1051

Rudimentary stump of iris, 874

Rupture
  anterior hyaloid face and, 1269
  lens capsule and, 1232

S

Salbutamol, 342

Salicylic poisoning, 1179

Saline solution, 551

Salivary gland, 1220

Sampaolesi line, 351

Sanguinarine, 1179-1180

Sarcoid uveitis, 1215

Scar
  inhibitors of, 783-784
  scotoma and, 449
  reopening of filtration fistula and, 623

Scatter
  fluctuation versus, 382-384
  laser and, 571-572

Scheie system, 355

Schiøtz tonometry
  home, 322

Schiøtz tonometry—cont'd
  indention, 303-304

Schlemm's canal
  aqueous humor and, 41
    pressure-dependent outflow and, 221
  Axenfeld-Rieger syndrome and, 25
  congenital glaucoma and, 31, 35-36
  corticosteroid-induced glaucoma and, 67
  cribriform layer and, 50
  development of, 12-20
  dissection in, 716
  encephalotrigeminal angiomatosis and, 919
  endothelial lining of, 46
  fibronectin and, 46
  fluid movement across, 221
  mesoderm and, 24
  morphology and, 50-52
  neurofibromatosis and, 912
  open-angle glaucoma and, 55
  outflow resistance and, 225
  Peters' anomaly and, 28
  pilocarpine-induced alterations and, 224
  plaques and, 54
  pseudoexfoliative glaucoma and, 64, 65
  sickle cell hemoglobinopathy and, 1153
  Sturge-Weber syndrome and, 31
  trabecular meshwork and
    low-tension glaucoma and, 60, 62, 64

Schocket procedure, 744-745

Schocket tube, 675

Schwalbe's line, 20
  Axenfeld-Rieger syndrome and, 886, 888, 890, 892
  gonioscopy and, 351
  Peters' anomaly and, 899-900

Schwalbe's line cell, 43

Schwartz's syndrome, 1048-1049

Scissors, Vannas, 704

Sclera
  angle-closure glaucoma and, 1049-1050
  development of, 21, 22
  lamina cribrosa and, 173
  optic nerve and, 120, 123
  thermal cautery of, 653
  trabeculotomy and, 715
  wound leaks and, 282

Scleral buckling procedure, 1052-1053

Scleral canal, 103

Scleral flap
  cataract extraction and filtration and, 677
    closure and, 669
    trabeculectomy and, 669
  congenital glaucoma and, 725
  disinsertion and, 682
  trabeculectomy and, 663, 665
    congenital glaucoma and, 721
    lamellar, 718, 721

Scleral lamina cribrosa, 172

Scleral spur, 18-20
  cholinergic mechanism and, 222-223
  gonioscopy and, 351

Sclerectomy, 653
  bleb and, 655
  cataract extraction and, 702-705
  posterior lip, 676
  trabeculectomy versus, 705

Scleritis, 1190-1202

Sclerocornea, 949-951
  congenital glaucoma and, 778, 779

Scleromalacia performans, 1193

Sclerosis
  nuclear, 851
  tuberous, 922

Sclerostomy
  argon laser, 624
  Nd:YAG laser, 616-617, 624
  thermal, 676
    open-angle glaucoma and, 819

Sclerotomy
  filtration surgery and, 687
  malignant glaucoma and, 1257, 1258

Scopolamine, 1176
  uveitis and, 1207, 1208

Scotoma
  Bjerrum, 436, 438
  chorioretinal scar and, 449
  history and, 361
  paracentral, 394, 439
  Seidel, 435

Scotopic threshold, 187

Scotopic vision, 365

Screening
  advanced glaucoma and, 427, 428
  advantage of, 405
  automated perimetry and, 415, 418
  ocular hypertension and, 791
  quantifying defect and, 412
  suprathreshold, 381-382
  thresholding and, 425

SD-plaque material, 60, 62, 64

Secondary glaucoma, 865-1348
  angle-closure, 846-847
    peripheral anterior synechia and, 1202
    scleritis and, 1199-1200
  arthritis and, 1217-1218
  classification of, 752-755
  corticosteroid-induced, 1161-1168
  developmental disorders and, 867-960; see also Developmental disorder
  drugs and,
  exfoliation syndrome and, 1009
  Fuchs' heterochromic cyclitis and, 1210
  hyperosmotic agent and, 554
  inflammation and, 1185-1247
  low-tension glaucoma and, 806-807
  nonsteroidal drugs and, 1169-1184
  ocular disease and, 961-1124; see also Ocular disease
  ocular surgery and, 1249-1347; see also Surgery

Secondary glaucoma—cont'd
  open-angle
    argon laser trabeculoplasty and, 609-611
      scleritis and, 1194-1199
    sarcoiditis and, 1215
    syphilis and, 1214
    systemic disease and, 1147-1160
    viral uveitis and, 1218
Secretion, 199-205
Sector iridectomy, 645
  angle-closure glaucoma after cataract extraction and, 1277
  cataract extraction and, 648-649
Seidel scotoma, 435
Seidel test
  epithelial ingrowth and, 1313, 1314
  wound fistula and, 282, 283
Self-tonometry, 322-324
Senile exfoliation, 997
Senior-Loken syndrome, 939
Sensitivity
  mean, 451
  spatial contrast, 187
  temporal contrast, 189
  visual
    perimetry and, 380-381
    refractive error and, 387
Sensory input, 267-268
Sensory nerve
  chamber angle and, 264-265
  ciliary body blood vessel and, 262
  neuropeptide in, 260
Septum
  pial, 173, 176
  fiber bundle, 105
Serotonin, 258
Serum osmolality, 302
Seton, 741-748
  congenital glaucoma and, 725, 726
Sex
  angle-closure glaucoma and, 834
  argon laser trabeculoplasty and, 609
  circadian variation in intraocular pressure and, 329
  intraocular pressure and, 301-302
  low-tension glaucoma and, 804
  pigmentary glaucoma and, 983, 991
Shaffer system, 355
  angle-closure glaucoma and, 833
Sheath of elastic-like fiber, 53
Sheath-derived plaque, 55-58
Short-circuit current, 213, 215, 216
Short-term fluctuation, 383
  automated perimetry and, 404
Shunt
  anterior chamber, 742
  filtering surgery and, 639
  posterior tube, 743-747
  translimbal tube, 742-743
Sickle cell hemoglobinopathy, 1152-1154
  hyphema and, 1227
Sieving, particulate, 221
Signal coupling efficiency, 527-528

Signal transduction system, 523
Silicone explant, 746-747
Silicone oil, 1055
Silicone tube
  neovascular glaucoma and, 1097
  translimbal tube shunt and, 742
Sinequan; see Doxepin
Sinus, cavernous, 1132-1133
Skeletal anomaly, 1040
Skin
  basal cell nevus syndrome and, 924
  dental-ocular-cutaneous syndrome and, 935
  periumbilical, 890
  upper lid and, 23
Sleep, 840
Slit-lamp
  Haag-Streit, 830-831
  intraocular lens implantation and, 1291, 1293
  photocoagulator and, 576-578
Smith-Leber-Niesnamoff method, 200
Smoking, 1179
  intraocular pressure and, 302-303
Sodium azide, 287
Sodium bicarbonate and, 539, 541
Sodium chloride, 551
Sodium hyaluronate
  cataract extraction and, 699
  filtration surgery and, 675
  open-angle glaucoma after cataract extraction and, 1268-1269
Sodium nitroprusside
  hypotony and, 287
  homocystinuria and, 1040-1041
Sodium pump, 199-218
  historical perspective and, 199-205
  sodium/potassium-adenosine triphosphatase and, 205-216
    localization of, 206-210
    studies of, 210-216
    vanadate and, 213
Soft tissue hypertrophy, 920
Somitomere, 6
SP; see Substance P
Spaeth system, 355-356
Spasm, accommodative, 518
Spatial coherence, 571
Spatial vision, 187-189
Specular microscopy, 1313, 1314
Spherical lens, Worst, 711-712
Sphincter muscle
  angle-closure glaucoma, 830, 849
  neovascular glaucoma and, 1073
Sphincterotomy
  argon laser, 626
  cataract extraction and, 699, 700
Sphygmomanometer, 1129
Spironolactone, 1173-1174, 1178
Splint, 638
Spondylitis, ankylosing, 1216-1217
Spur, scleral, 18-20
  cholinergic mechanism and, 222-223
  gonioscopy and, 351

Squamous epithelium, 1310
Squeezing of lid, 302
Standard deviation, pattern, 451
Standardization of test condition, 403-404
Staphyloma, 940
Staphylomatous optic disc, 944
Static perimetry, 374-378
  computerized, 186-187
  duration of test in, 373
  history and, 361, 393
  kinetic perimetry versus, 368
  Octopus and, 372
Status dysraphicus, 1211
Stent, 1096-1098
Step, nasal, 434, 436, 437
  nerve fiber bundle defect and, 394
Stepped Suprathreshold test, 411
Stereochronoscopy, 496
Stereophotogrammetry, 497-499
Stereoscopic fundus photography, 495-496
Stereoscopic video image, 499
Sterilization, 307
Steroid; see also Corticosteroid-induced glaucoma
  angle-closure glaucoma and, 1053
  aqueous humor and, 230-231
  argon laser and
    peripheral iridoplasty and, 599
    pupilloplasty and, 625
  arthritis and, 1217
  atopic dermatitis and, 934
  central retinal vein occlusion and, 1148, 1150
  chemical burn and, 1234
  ciliochoroidal detachment and, 286
  fibroblast and, 673
  fibrous ingrowth and, 1324
  filtering surgery and, 638, 671
  ghost cell glaucoma and, 1245
  herpes zoster and, 1219
  inflammation and, 1228
  intraocular pressure and, 302
  lens-induced glaucoma and, 1023
  neovascular glaucoma and, 1095
  phacolytic glaucoma and, 1020
  pigmentary glaucoma and, 984
  retinal detachment and, 1055, 1056-1057
  sarcoidosis and, 1216
  uveitis and, 1207-1208
  vitreous surgery and, 1261
Stickler's syndrome, 939
Still's disease, 1217
Stimulated emission, 568
Stimulus, 370-372
  size of, 430
    automated perimetry and, 405
    visual field and, 387, 388
  threshold versus sensitivity and, 380-381
Stocker-Holt dystrophy, 781
Strabismus, 881

Straining, 302
Streptomycin sulfate, 1174
Stress
    acute angle-closure glaucoma and,
        841
    open-angle glaucoma and, 815
Stretch burn
    iridectomy and, 585, 586
    iridoplasty and, 599
Stretching, corneal, 773
    megalocornea, 766-767
Stroma
    ciliary, 85
    conjunctival epithelium and, 22
    cornea development and, 8-9, 22
    fluorescence in, 340
    iris
        aqueous humor and, 41-42
        congenital glaucoma and, 765
    laser iridectomy and, 590
    mid limbal, 20, 22
    Peters' anomaly and, 897, 898
    scleral, 22
    uveal, 1119
Strontium 90, 674
Strophanthidin, 213
Stump of iris, 874
Sturge-Weber syndrome, 25, 30, 31, 32-
        33, 913-920
    episcleral venous pressure and, 1133-
        1134
    filtration surgery and, 672-673
    surgery and, 727
    tumors and, 1123
Subacute angle-closure glaucoma, 860
Subconjunctival fistula, 647
Subconjunctival injection, 1207
Subendothelial membrane, 43
Subendothelium, 167, 171
Subluxation, lens, 1028
    blunt trauma and, 1228
Substance P, 260
Substance P immunoreactive nerve fiber,
        264-265
Sub-Tenon injection, 1207
Succinylcholine, 1177-1178
    anticholinesterase agents and, 520
    filtration surgery and, 659
    intraocular pressure and, 302
Suction effect, 347
Sulcus, ciliary, 77
Sulfa drug, 1173-1174
Sulfite oxidase deficiency, 1041
Sulfonamide
    carbonic anhydrase inhibitors and, 541
    structures of, 545
Sulfur hexafluoride, 1054-1055
Sulindac, 673
Summation
    kinetic perimetry and, 374
    perimeter and, 373
Superior cervical ganglion, 258
Superior ophthalmic vein, 1127
Superior vena cava syndrome, 1134-1135
Suprachoroidal fluid, 285-286

Suprachoroidal hemorrhage, 1255
    aphakic eye undergoing filtration and,
        1279
    expulsive, 682, 683
Suprachoroidal space
    anatomy and, 241
    sclerotomy and, 1258
Supraciliary fluid, 285
Supraciliary space, 241
Suprathreshold screening, 381-382
    stepped, 411
Surface layer of nerve fiber, 135
Surgery
    angle-closure glaucoma and na-
        nophthalmos and, 1050
    aniridia and, 881-882
    aphakia and, 1279
    Axenfeld-Rieger syndrome and, 895
    ciliary body and, 738
    congenital glaucoma and, 707-727,
        781-782; see also Congenital glau-
        coma
    cyclodialysis and, 284-285
    episcleral venous pressure and, 1135,
        1137
    epithelial cyst and, 1301-1303
    epithelial ingrowth and, 1317
    exfoliation syndrome and, 1011
    fibrous ingrowth and, 1324
    filtering; see Filtration surgery
    ghost cell glaucoma and, 1244-1245
    glaucoma associated with, 1249-
        1347
        aphakia and, 1265-1283; see also
            Aphakia
        intraocular lens implantation and,
            1285-1297
        malignant glaucoma and, 1251-
            1262
        penetrating keratoplasty and, 1337-
            1347
        proliferation and, 1299-1335
    glaucoma treatment and, 631-749
        cataract and, 697-706
        congenital glaucoma and, 707-727
        conventional iridectomy and, 645-
            651
        cyclodestructive, 729-740
        filtration and, 653-696
        setons in, 741-748
        wound healing and, 633-643
    hypotony and, 287
    iridectomy; see Iridectomy
    laser, 565-629; see Laser
    neovascular glaucoma and, 1095
    neurofibromatosis and, 913
    open-angle glaucoma and, 818-819
    phacoanaphylaxis and, 1024
    phacolytic glaucoma and, 1020-1021
    pigmentary glaucoma and, 994
    pseudophakic glaucoma and, 1294-
        1295
    retinal detachment and, 1054-1055
        neovascular glaucoma and, 1090
    uveitis and, 1209

Suture
    bridle, 660, 661
    corneoscleral, 1267
    releasable, 675
    tension of, 1343-1344
    through-and-through, 1339
Suture-cutting, laser 626-627
Suxamethonium, 302
Swan-Jacob lens, 713
Sympathectomy, chemical, 529
Sympathetic nerve
    ciliary body and, 84-85
    intraocular pressure and, 269-270
Sympathomimetic agent, 1175-1176
    uveitis and, 1207
Synapse, 89
Synechia, 1206
    angle-closure glaucoma and, 1053
    neovascular glaucoma and, 1067, 1073
        treatment of, 1095
    peripheral anterior; see Peripheral an-
        terior synechia
    Peters' anomaly and, 899
    posterior, 594
Synthetic drainage device, 784
Syphilis, 1213-1214
    interstitial keratitis and, 1203
Syringomyelia, 1211

T
Tapetoretinal degeneration, 939
Tear
    ciliary body and, 1230
    congenital glaucoma and, 773
    Descemet's membrane and, 784
Telangiectasia-cataracta syndrome, 938
Telangiectasis, 1155
TEM; see Transverse electromagnetic
        mode
Temperature
    cyclocryotherapy probe and, 732-733
    irradiated tissue and, 573
Temporal angle, 349-350
Temporal coherence, 571
Temporal contrast sensitivity, 189
Temporal vision, 187-189
Tendon, ciliary muscle, 47
Tenon's capsule
    cyst and, 685-687
    filtration surgery and, 659
    posterior lip sclerectomy and, 676
    sclerotomy and, 1258
Tenonectomy, 673
Tenon's flap, 721-725
Tension
    intraocular; see Intraocular pressure
    suture, 1343-1344
Terbutaline, 342
Testing
    color vision, 183-185
    functional, 179-197
    visual field, 369-380; see also Perimetry;
        Visual field
Tetracaine, 520
Tetracycline, 1173-1174

Tetrahydrocannabinol, 559-560
Tetrahydrozoline, 1175
THC; see Tetrahydrocannabinol
Theobromine methylxanthine, 1173
Theophylline, 1173
Thermal cautery of scleral wound edge, 653
Thermal effect, 573-574
Thermal sclerostomy, 676
    open-angle glaucoma and, 819
Thiocholine, 258
    chamber angle and, 263
Thiocyanate, 201
Thioridazine, 1170
Thiothixene, 1170
Thioxanthene, 1170
Third cranial nerve, 268
Three-dimensional model, 368
Three-mirror Goldmann lens, 606
Threshold testing, 185-187, 425
    scatter versus fluctuation and, 382
    static perimetry and, 376-377
Thromboembolism, 1040
Thrombosis, iris, 1155
Thrombotic glaucoma; see Neovascular glaucoma
Through-and-through suture, 1339
Thymoxamine
    acute angle-closure glaucoma and, 856
    intraocular pressure and, 533
    pigmentary glaucoma and, 993
Thyroid disease, 1143-1144
Thyroid ophthalmopathy, 1135, 1136
Tilting of lens, 1041
Timolol
    aqueous flow and, 342
    ciliochoroidal detachment and, 286
    congenital glaucoma and, 782, 784
    lens-induced glaucoma and, 1023
    malignant glaucoma and, 1256
Tobacco, 1179
    intraocular pressure and, 302-303
Tolazoline, 1175
Tomography, 808
Tonic ganglion cell, 181
Tonography, 291-297
    cyclodialysis and, 284
Tonometry, 303-312
    congenital glaucoma and, 775
    retinal detachment and, 1056
Tono-Pen, 310-311
Tooth, 889, 890
Topical agent, 545, 547
    anesthesia and, 1177-1178
        cyclophotocoagulation and, 621-622
        iridectomy and, 584
        iridoplasty and, 598
    bleeding after cataract extraction and, 699
    cannabinoid and, 560
    intraocular responses and, 528
    laser iridectomy and, 595
    prostaglandin and, 560

Topical agent—cont'd
    steroid and
        central retinal vein occlusion and, 1050
        ciliochoroidal detachment and, 286
        fibroblast and, 673
        peripheral iridoplasty and, 599
        pigmentary glaucoma and, 984
        pupilloplasty and, 625
Topography of optic nerve, 496-503, 505-507
Trabecular meshwork
    adrenergic mechanism and, 224-225
    age and, 53
    anterior chamber angle and, 12
    aqueous humor and, 219, 220-221
    Axenfeld-Rieger syndrome and, 25, 890
    beta-adrenergic agonists and, 530
    biochemistry and, 222
    blunt trauma and, 358
    chemical burn and, 1234
    congenital glaucoma and, 31, 35-36
    corticosteroid-induced glaucoma and, 67
    development of, 15-18
    dysgenesis and; see Trabeculodysgenesis
    encephalotrigeminal angiomatosis and, 919
    episcleral venous pressure and, 249
    epithelial ingrowth and, 1313
    exfoliation and, 64, 1001, 1003, 1005
    extracellular matrix and, 163-172
    familial amyloidosis and, 1154
    Fuchs' heterochromic cyclitis and, 1210
    gonioscopy and, 349
    infantile glaucoma and, 34
    innervation and, 221-222
    Intraocular pressure and;, 1205-1206
    iridocorneal endothelial syndrome and, 28
    iris melanoma and, 1111, 1113
    low-tension glaucoma and, 60, 62, 64
    mucopolysaccharidosis and, 67
    neovascular glaucoma and, 1067
    nerve fibers in, 267
    nerves and, 262-265
    normal development of, 767, 769
    normal eyes and, 42-50
    open-angle glaucoma and, 55, 59
    origin of, 23
    penetrating keratoplasty and, 1338-1340, 1342
    peripheral anterior synechia and, 1206
    Peters' anomaly and, 28
    pigmentary glaucoma and, 64, 67, 984, 986, 987, 988, 989, 993
    secondary glaucoma and, 753, 755
    Sturge-Weber syndrome and, 31
    trauma and, 1228-1230
Trabeculectomy, 660-676
    aniridia and, 882
    aphakia and, 1279
    cataract extraction and, 702, 705
    congenital glaucoma and, 771, 781

Trabeculectomy—cont'd
    encephalotrigeminal angiomatosis and, 920
    exfoliation syndrome and, 1011
    history of, 653-655
    hyphema and, 1227-1228
    laser
        iridocorneal epithelial syndrome and, 973
        pigmentary glaucoma and, 994
    neurofibromatosis and, 913
    open-angle glaucoma and, 819
    sclerectomy versus, 705
Trabeculodialysis, 1209
Trabeculodysgenesis
    argon laser trabeculoplasty and, 611
    classification of, 708
    congenital glaucoma and, 763-764
Trabeculoplasty, laser, 605-615
    aphakia and, 1279
    cataract extraction and, 698
    complications of, 612-613
    exfoliation syndrome and, 1011
    iridocorneal epithelial syndrome and, 977
    laser iridectomy and, 583
    low-tension glaucoma and, 809
    methods and techniques of, 605-608
    open-angle glaucoma and, 818
    pathophysiology of, 613-615
    peripheral iridoplasty and, 597-598
    pseudophakic glaucoma and, 1295
    results of, 608-611
Trabeculopuncture, 615-616
Trabeculotomy
    congenital glaucoma and, 709, 711
        technique for, 715-721
    encephalotrigeminal angiomatosis and, 920
    results of, 707
    Sturge-Weber syndrome and, 672-673
    sclerotomy and, 616-617
    trabeculectomy and, 724, 725
Tracer, 244
Tranquilizer, 1170
Transcapillary pressure, 1137
Transcellular channel, 221
    aqueous humor and, 221
    ATPase and, 207
Transconjunctival treatment with argon laser, 623-624
Transduction system, signal, 523
Transient angle-closure glaucoma, 1050-1051
Transillumination, 587
Translimbal seton, 742
Translimbal tube shunt, 742-743
Transmitter marker, neuronal, 525
Transport
    axonal, 96-100, 102
    transcellular, 207
Transpupillary laser cyclophotocoagulation, 621-622
    neovascular glaucoma and, 1099-1100
    open-angle glaucoma and, 819

Transpupillary laser cycloablation, 737
Transscleral cyclophotocoagulation
  Nd:YAG, 622-623
  open-angle glaucoma and, 819
Transscleral high intensity focused ultrasound, 734-735
Transscleral laser cycloablation, 735-737
Transverse electromagnetic mode, 570
Transvitreal endophotocoagulation, 622
Tranylcypromide sulfate, 1171
Traquair's island of vision, 368
Trauma
  blunt, 1225-1232
  chemical injury and, 1233-1235
  ghost cell glaucoma and, 1244
  gonioscopy and, 358
  hyperosmotic agent and, 554
  intraocular pressure and, 1225-1237
  lens location and, 1041
  neovascular glaucoma and, 1064, 1066
  obstetrical, 779
  penetrating injury and, 1232-1233
  phacolytic glaucoma and, 1020
  radiation therapy and, 1235-1236
Trephination
  filtration and, 676-677
  limbal, 653
  open-angle glaucoma and, 819
  penetrating keratoplasty and, 1343
Triamcinolone, 638
Trichlormethiazide, 1173, 1178
Tricyclic antidepressant, 1171
Trifluoperazine, 1170
Triflupromazine, 1170
Trifluridine, 1219
Trigeminal ganglion, 257
  neuropeptide and, 260
Trigeminal nerve, 268
Trigonometric angle, 351
Trihexyphenidyl, 1172
Tripelennamine, 1171, 1172
Trisomy 13 syndrome, 931-932
Trisomy 18 syndrome, 932
Trisomy 21, 932-933
Trisomy G syndrome, 932-933
Tropicamide
  angle-closure glaucoma and, 862
  uveitis and, 1208
Tube
  anterior chamber and, 742
  Descemet's, 1325
  filtering surgery and, 639
  polyvinyl chloride, 711-712
  posterior, 743-747
  Schocket, 675
  silicone, 1097
  translimbal, 742-743
Tuberous sclerosis, 922
Tubocurarine, 659
Tuft, pupillary, 1073
Tumor, 1154
  basal cell nevus syndrome and, 924
  hamartomatosis and, 1123

Tumor—cont'd
  lymphoid, 1123
  neovascular glaucoma and, 1077, 1089-1090
  neurofibromatosis and, 906-913
  nonpigmentary ciliary epithelium and, 1121-1123
  pearl, 1300
  pigmented epithelium and, 1123
  pituitary, 1143-1144
  retina and, 1119-1121
  superior vena cava syndrome and, 1135
  uveal tract and, 1111-1119
  Wilms', 871
Turner's syndrome, 933

U
Ullrich's syndrome, 932
Ultrafiltration, 261
  aqueous humor and, 199-200, 202, 220
Ultrasonography
  open-angle glaucoma and, 819
  orbital varices, 1132
  transscleral high intensity focused, 734-735
Ultraviolet light; see Laser
Urea
  aqueous humor and, 200, 201
  hyperosmotic agent and, 551
  intravenous, 553
Urethritis, 1218
Urolithiasis, 545
User-defined program, 431
User-defined test, 409, 410
Uvea
  adrenergic innervation to, 262
  anatomy of, 85-90
  congenital ectropion uveae and, 940
    Axenfeld-Rieger syndrome versus, 895
  development of, 16, 18
  ectoderm and, 3
  exfoliation and, 997
  filtration surgery and, 660
  melanoma and, 1089
  morphology of, 45-46
  open-angle glaucoma and, 60
  Prader-Willi syndrome and, 934
  retinal detachment and, 1049-1050
  tumors of, 1111-1119
Uveitis, 1205-1223
  arthritis and, 1216-1218
  Fuchs' heterochromic cyclitis and, 1209-1211
  ghost cell glaucoma and, 1246
  intraocular pressure and, 1205-1206
  laser iridectomy and, 594
  laser trabeculoplasty and, 611
  management of, 1206-1209
  open-angle glaucoma and, 1270
  phacoanaphylaxis and, 1023-1024
  Posner-Schlossman syndrome and, 1211-1213
  sarcoid, 1215-1216

Uveitis—cont'd
  scleritis and, 1199
  syphilis and, 1213-1214
  trabecular meshwork and, 230
  viral, 1218-1220
Uveoscleral outflow, 41, 219, 220-221, 241-247, 281
  episcleral venous pressure and, 249
  prostaglandin and, 560

V
Vacuole
  giant, 221
  inner wall endothelium, 54
  Schlemm's canal and, 12, 14, 15, 50
Valsalva maneuver, 302
Valve implant; see Implant, valve
Valved silicone explant, 746-747
Van Herick technique, 356
Van Lint technique, 658
Vanadate, 213
Vannas scissors, 704
Vaporization, 574; see also Laser
Variable force applanation tonometry, 304-307
Varices, 1132
  Klippel-Trenaunay-Weber syndrome and, 920
Vascular disease, 1147-1151
  collagen and, 1151
  congenital glaucoma and, 765-766
  encephalotrigeminal angiomatosis and, 916, 919
  hypotony and, 287
  Klippel-Trenaunay-Weber syndrome and, 920
  low-tension glaucoma and, 804
  optic disc and, 476
Vascular endothelial cell, 530
Vascular system
  adrenergic receptors and, 224, 527
  ciliary body and, 80-85
  episcleral vessels and, 1197
  epithelial ingrowth and, 1305
  intraocular lens implantation and, 1293
  pigmentary glaucoma and, 984
  uveitis and, 1206
Vasoactive agent, 1174-1175
Vasoactive intestinal polypeptide, 259
  ciliary body and, 262
Vasoconstrictor, 1175
Vasodilator, 1174-1175
Vasopressin, 1175
Vein
  aqueous, 250
  choroidal, 261
  facial, 1127
  optic nerve head and, 107
  retinal; see Retinal vein
Venomanometer, 1129
  episcleral, 252-253
Venous pressure, episcleral; see Episcleral venous pressure
Venous stasis retinopathy, 1078-1079

Verapamil, 1174
Vesicle
  axonal transport in retina and, 97-98
  optic, 6-8
Vessel, blood; see Blood vessel; *specific vessel*
Vidarabine, 1219
Video camera, 496
Video image
  computerized image analysis of, 499
  disc pallor measurement and, 505
VIP; see Vasoactive intestinal polypeptide
VIP-LI nerve fiber, 261-262, 263
Viral infection, 1155-1156
  uveitis and, 1218
Viscoelastic agent, 1179
  filtration surgery and, 675
  open-angle glaucoma after cataract extraction and, 1268-1269
Vision
  basic elements of, 180-185
  blurred, 590
Visual acuity
  aniridia and, 874
  intraocular lens implantation and, 1288-1289
  neovascular glaucoma and, 1069
  thyrotropic ophthalmopathy and, 1143, 1146, 1147
Visual evoked response, 193
  intraocular lens implantation and, 1293
Visual field
  absence of, 448
  angle-closure glaucoma and, 842
  argon laser trabeculoplasty and, 612-613
  circadian variation in intraocular pressure and, 325
  Cushing's syndrome and, 1142
  examination of, 1143, 1147
    change and, 451-466
    color deficit and, 190-191
    congenital glaucoma and, 774
    test pattern and, 407
    threshold technique and, 186-187
  filtration surgery and, 654, 687
  glaucomatous, 393-402
  intraocular lens implantation and, 1293
  low-tension glaucoma and, 803
  normal, 361-391
    history and, 361
    interpretation of results and, 380-382
    normal gradient of, 362-368
    physiologic basis for, 384-389
    scatter versus fluctuation and, 382-384

Visual field—cont'd
  normal—cont'd
    test parameters in, 369-380
    open-angle glaucoma and, 814-815, 820
Visual reaction time, 373-374
Visual sensitivity
  perimetry and, 380-381
  refractive error and, 387
Visual threshold, 382
Vitrectomy
  diabetic retinopathy and, 1087
  epithelial ingrowth and, 1316
  filtration surgery and, 672
  ghost cell glaucoma and, 1243
  malignant glaucoma and, 1262
  transvitreal endophotocoagulation and, 622
Vitrectomy-lensectomy, 1024
Vitreociliary block, 1277
Vitreoretinal degeneration, 1058
Vitreous
  cataract extraction and, 1269
  epithelial ingrowth and, 1307
  fibrous ingrowth and, 1322
  filtration surgery and, 682
  fluorescein leakage and, 1070
  ghost cell glaucoma and, 1239-1242, 1246
  iridectomy and, 1279
  lens dislocation and, 1038
  malignant glaucoma and, 1252, 1259-1261
  neovascular glaucoma and, 1071
  persistent hyperplastic primary, 944-946
  phacolytic glaucoma and, 1018
  Schwartz's syndrome and, 1048
  sickle cell hemoglobinopathy and, 1152
Von Recklinghausen's disease, 906-913
Von-Hippel-Landau syndrome, 921-922
Vortex vein
  anatomy and, 1128
  angle-closure glaucoma and nanophthalmos and, 1050

W

Wagner's disease, 1058
Water
  aqueous humor and, 200-201
  laser and, 574
Watershed zone, 137, 141-156
Wave, electromagnetic, 567
Wavelength
  argon laser trabeculoplasty and, 608
  laser photocoagulator and, 577
  photon catches and, 183-184
Weber-Christian syndrome, 939-940
Weber's law, 365

Wedge-shaped defects, 482
Weill-Marchesani syndrome, 1033-1035
Weyer's syndrome, 938
White blood cell, 1246
  iridocorneal epithelial syndrome and, 972
  neovascular glaucoma and, 1077
Wilms' tumor, 871
Wolf's syndrome, 932
Worst goniotomy lens, 711-712
Wound
  cataract extraction and, 1276
    angle-closure glaucoma , 1276
    open-angle glaucoma and, 1267
  healing and, 633-644
  hypotony and, 281-282
  leak and, 684, 685
  testing and, 679-680
Wound-incarcerated tissue
  epithelial ingrowth and, 1305
  fibrous ingrowth and, 1323
W-type ganglion cell, 91-92

X

X chromosome, 933
Xanthophyll, 576
Xenon arc laser, 1303
Xenon endophotocoagulator, 1093
X-type ganglion cell, 91

Y

Yellow
  color pairing and, 183-185
  glaucoma and, 190
Y-type ganglion cell, 91

Z

Zeiss goniolens, 347-348, 350-351
  acute angle-closure glaucoma and, 857-858
  indentation gonioscopy and, 353-354
Zeiss-Nordenson camera, 496
Zellweger syndrome, 940
Zonulae occludens, 88
Zonular fiber
  ectopia lentis and, 1031
  pigmentary glaucoma and, 982
Zonular fragment, 229-230
Zonule
  angle-closure glaucoma and, 828, 851
  ciliary, 77
  exfoliation syndrome and, 1003, 1006-1008
  microspherophakia and, 1035
  traumatic lens dislocation and, 1041
Zonulytic glaucoma, 1268